PHYSICAL ACTIVITY AND FITNESS

President's Council on Physical Fitness and Sports

NUTRITION

National Institutes of Health; Food and Drug Administration

TOBACCO

Centers for Disease Control and Prevention

ALCOHOL AND OTHER DRUGS

Alcohol, Drug Abuse, and Mental Health Administration

FAMILY PLANNING

Office of Population Affairs

MENTAL HEALTH AND MENTAL DISORDERS

Alcohol, Drug Abuse, and Mental Health Administration

VIOLENT AND ABUSIVE BEHAVIOR

Centers for Disease Control and Prevention

EDUCATIONAL AND COMMUNITY-BASED PROGRAMS

Centers for Disease Control and Prevention; Health Resources and Services Administration

UNINTENTIONAL INJURIES

Centers for Disease Control and Prevention

OCCUPATIONAL SAFETY AND HEALTH

Centers for Disease Control and Prevention

ENVIRONMENTAL HEALTH

National Institutes of Health; Centers for Disease Control and Prevention

FOOD AND DRUG SAFETY

Food and Drug Administraion

ORAL HEALTH

National Institutes of Health; Centers for Disease Control and Prevention

MATERNAL AND INFANT HEALTH

Health Resources and Services Administration

HEART DISEASE AND STROKE

National Institutes of Health

CANCER

National Institutes of Health

DIABETES AND CHRONIC DISABLING CONDITIONS

National Institutes of Health; Centers for Disease Control and Prevention

HIV INFECTION

National AIDS Program Office

SEXUALLY TRANSMITTED DISEASES

Centers for Disease Control and Prevention

IMMUNIZATION AND INFECTIOUS DISEASES

Centers for Disease Control and Prevention

CLINICAL PREVENTIVE SERVICES

Health Resources and Services Administration; Centers for Disease Control and Prevention

SURVEILLANCE AND DATA SYSTEMS

Centers for Disease Control and Prevention

Community Health Nursing

Promoting Health of Aggregates, Families, and Individuals

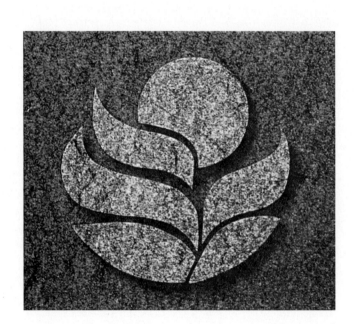

Community Health Nursing

Promoting Health of Aggregates, Families, and Individuals

Marcia Stanhope, RN, DSN, FAAN

Professor and Director
Division of Community Health Nursing and Administration
College of Nursing
University of Kentucky
Lexington, Kentucky

Jeanette Lancaster, RN, PhD, FAAN

Dean and Sadie Heath Cabaniss Professor
School of Nursing
University of Virginia
Charlottesville, Virginia

FOURTH EDITION

Illustrated

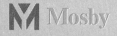 Mosby

St. Louis Baltimore Boston Carlsbad Chicago Naples New York Philadelphia Portland
London Madrid Mexico City Singapore Sydney Tokyo Toronto Wiesbaden

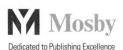

Dedicated to Publishing Excellence

A Times Mirror
Company

Publisher: Nancy L. Coon
Editor: Loren S. Wilson
Associate Developmental Editor: Brian Dennison
Project Manager: Patricia Tannian
Production: Graphic World Publishing Services
Book Design Manager: Gail Morey Hudson
Manufacturing Manager: David Graybill
Cover Designer: Carol Haddonberry

FOURTH EDITION

Printed in the United States of America
Composition by Graphic World, Inc.
Printing/binding by Von Hoffmann Press, Inc.

Mosby–Year Book, Inc.
11830 Westline Industrial Drive
St. Louis, Missouri 63146

Library of Congress Cataloging in Publication Data

Community health nursing : promoting health of aggregates, families,
  and individuals / [edited by] Marcia Stanhope, Jeanette Lancaster.
  —4th ed.
      p.   cm.
  Includes bibliographical references and index.
  ISBN 0-8151-8142-6
  1. Community health nursing.   I. Stanhope, Marcia.
II. Lancaster, Jeanette.
  [DNLM: 1. Community Health Nursing—United States.   WY 106 C7356
1995]
RT95.C6562   1995
610.73′43—dc20
DNLM/DLC
for Library of Congress   95-39516
                                                                CIP

95 96 97 98 99 / 9 8 7 6 5 4 3 2 1

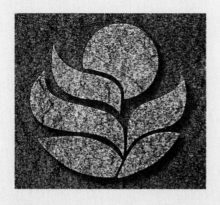

Contributors

TERESA ACQUAVIVA, RN, MSN

Family Nurse Practitioner
Community Medical Center
Washington, D.C.

DYAN A. ARETAKIS, RN, MSN, FNP

Project Director, Teen Health Center
University of Virginia
Charlottesville, Virginia

SARA BARGER, DPA, RN, FAAN

Dean, Capstone College of Nursing
University of Alabama
Tuscaloosa, Alabama

PATRICIA C. BIRCHFIELD, RN, DSN, CANP, CGNP

Associate Professor, College of Nursing
University of Kentucky
Lexington, Kentucky

JEANNE A. BUCSELA, MS, MLib

Technical Writer/Editor
Agency for Toxic Substances and Disease Registry
United States Public Health Service
Atlanta, Georgia

ANGELINE BUSHY, RN, PhD, CS

Associate Professor, Division of Community Health
College of Nursing, University of Utah
Salt Lake City, Utah

JACQUELYN C. CAMPBELL, RN, PhD, FAAN

Anna D. Wolf Endowed Professor
School of Nursing, Johns Hopkins University
Baltimore, Maryland

ANN H. CARY, RN, MPH, PhD, A-CCC

Doctor of Philosophy in Nursing Program Coordinator
George Mason University
College of Nursing and Health
Fairfax, Virginia

MARCIA K. COWAN, RN, MSN, CPNP

Pediatric Nurse Practitioner
The Pediatric Center
Tullahoma, Tennessee

CYNTHIA E. DEGAZON, RN, PhD

Associate Professor, Hunter-Bellevue School of Nursing
Hunter College of the City University
New York, New York

LOUISE IVANOR DENNIS, BS, MSN

Associate Professor, School of Nursing
Purdue University
West Lafayette, Indiana

BEVERLY COLLORA FLYNN, RN, PhD, FAAN

Professor, Community Health Nursing, School of Nursing
Director, Institute of Action Research for Community Health
Head, World Health Organization Collaborating
Center in Healthy Cities
Indiana University
Indianapolis, Indiana

DOUGLAS CHARLES FORNESS, BA, MA

Mental Health Counselor
University of Virginia
Charlottesville, Virginia

SARA T. FRY, RN, PhD, FAAN

Henry R. Luce Professor of Nursing Ethics
School of Nursing, Boston College
Boston, Massachusetts

CAROL Z. GARRISON, PhD

Professor of Epidemiology, Associate Provost and Dean of
the Graduate School
University of South Carolina
Columbia, South Carolina

JEAN GOEPPINGER, RN, PhD, FAAN

Professor and Chairperson
Department of Community and Mental Health
School of Nursing, University of North Carolina
Chapel Hill, North Carolina

PATTY J. HALE, RN, PhD

Assistant Professor, School of Nursing
University of Virginia
Charlottesville, Virginia

SHIRLEY M.H. HANSON, RN, PMHNP, PhD, FAAN, CFLE, MFT

Professor, School of Nursing
Oregon Health Sciences University
Portland, Oregon

SUSAN B. HASSMILLER, RN, PhD

Executive Director, United States Public Health Service
Primary Care Policy Fellowship and Society
Bureau of Health Professions
Rockville, Maryland

BETH F. HIBBS, RN, MPH

Environmental Health Scientist
Agency for Toxic Substances and Disease Registry
United States Public Health Service
Atlanta, Georgia

PATRICIA B. HOWARD, RN, PhD, CNAA

Assistant Professor, College of Nursing
University of Kentucky
Lexington, Kentucky

KATHLEEN HUTTLINGER, RN, PhD

Director, Transcultural Program
Wayne State University
Detroit, Michigan

JUDITH B. IGOE, RN, MS, FAAN

Associate Professor, Director, School Health Programs
University of Colorado, School of Nursing
Denver, Colorado

KIM DUPREE JONES, RNc, MN, FNP

Family Nurse Practitioner/Assistant Professor, School of Nursing
Georgia State University
Atlanta, Georgia

LINDA CORSON JONES, RN, PhD, FAAN

Professor and Coordinator Research
Graduate Nursing Program
Louisiana State University Medical Center
New Orleans, Louisiana

JOANNA R. KAAKINEN, RN, PhD

Associate Professor, School of Nursing
University of Portland
Portland, Oregon

THOMAS KIPPENBROCK, RN, EdD

Associate Professor, Assistant Dean
School of Nursing, University of Nebraska
Medical Center-Kearney Division
Kearney, Nebraska

JOYCE SPLANN KROTHE, RN, DNS

Assistant Professor, Indiana University
School of Nursing
Indianapolis, Indiana

PAMELA A. KULBOK, RN, DNSc

Associate Professor, School of Nursing
University of Virginia
Charlottesville, Virginia

SHIRLEY CLOUTIER LAFFREY, RN, MPH, PhD

Associate Professor, School of Nursing
The University of Texas at Austin
Austin, Texas

JEANETTE LANCASTER, RN, PhD, FAAN

Sadie Heath Cabaniss Professor of Nursing
Dean, School of Nursing, University of Virginia
Charlottesville, Virginia

KÄREN M. LANDENBURGER, RN, PhD

Assistant Professor, Tacoma Campus–Nursing Program
University of Washington
Tacoma, Washington

PEGGYE GUESS LASSITER, RN, BSN, MSN

Assistant Professor, College of Nursing
Howard University
Washington, D.C.

SUSAN C. LONG-MARIN, DVM, MPH

Epidemiologist
Mechlenburg County Health Department
Charlotte, North Carolina

CAROL J. LOVELAND-CHERRY, RN, PhD, FAAN

Associate Professor, Director, Division II
School of Nursing, University of Michigan
Ann Arbor, Michigan

LOIS W. LOWRY, RN, DNSc

Associate Professor, Interim Associate Dean for
Undergraduate Studies, College of Nursing
University of South Florida
Health Sciences Center
Tampa, Florida

MAX R. LUM, MPA, EdD

Director of Communications
National Institute for Occupational Safety and Health
Washington, D.C.

KAREN S. MARTIN, RN, MSN, FAAN

Health Care Consultant
Omaha, Nebraska

MARY LYNN MATHRE, RN, MSN, CARN

Nurse Consultant, Addictions Consult Services
University of Virginia Health Sciences Center
Charlottesville, Virginia

MARY ANN McCLELLAN, RN, MN, CFLE

Assistant Professor, College of Nursing
University of Oklahoma
Oklahoma City, Oklahoma

ROBERT E. McKEOWN, PhD

Assistant Professor, Department of Epidemiology
  and Biostatistics
School of Public Health
University of South Carolina
Columbia, South Carolina

DIANE M. NARKUNAS, MPH

Health Education Specialist
Division of Health Education
Agency for Toxic Substances and Disease Registry
United States Public Health Service
Atlanta, Georgia

LISA ONEGA, RN, PhD, CS, FNP

Post-doctoral Fellow, College of Nursing
University of Iowa
Iowa City, Iowa

CHARLENE C. OSSLER, RN, PhD

Director, Managed Care Services
ROSS Stores, Inc./ICS
Newark, California

LYNELLE PHILLIPS, RN, MPH

Environmental Health Scientist
Agency for Toxic Substances and Disease Registry
United States Public Health Service
Atlanta, Georgia

MOLLY ROSE, RN, PhD, FNP

Associate Professor
Medical College of Pennsylvania/Hahnemann University
School of Nursing
Philadelphia, Pennsylvania

CHERYL PANDOLF SCHENK, RN, MN, CS

Adult Nurse Practitioner/Assistant Professor, School of
Nursing
Georgia State University
Atlanta, Georgia

JULIANN G. SEBASTIAN, RN, PhD, CS

Associate Professor, College of Nursing
University of Kentucky
Lexington, Kentucky

GEORGE F. SHUSTER III, RN, DNSc

Associate Professor, College of Nursing
University of New Mexico
Albuquerque, New Mexico

SUDIE E. SPEER, RN, BS, MS

Level III Staff Nurse, Home Care
The Children's Hospital
Denver, Colorado

MARCIA K. STANHOPE, RN, DSN, FAAN, c

Professor and Director
Community Health Nursing and Administration Division
College of Nursing, University of Kentucky
Lexington, Kentucky

FRANCISCO S. SY, MD, DrPH

Associate Professor, Graduate Director
Department of Epidemiology and Biostatistics
School of Public Health
University of South Carolina
Columbia, South Carolina

SHIRLEEN TRABEAUX, RN, MN

Instructor, School of Nursing
Undergraduate Program
Louisiana State University Medical Center
New Orleans, Louisiana

CAROLYN A. WILLIAMS, RN, PhD, FAAN

Dean and Professor, College of Nursing
University of Kentucky
Lexington, Kentucky

JUDITH LUPO WOLD, RN, PhD

Associate Professor
Director of Undergraduate Programs
School of Nursing, Georgia State University
Atlanta, Georgia

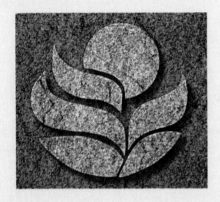

Reviewers

PATRICIA L. ACKERMAN, RN, PhD

Associate Professor, California State University
Sacramento, California

ARNETTE ANDERSON, RN, PhD

Faculty of Nursing, University of Alberta
Edmonton, Alberta, Canada

JoELLEN BRANNAN, RN, MSN, CS

Assistant Professor of Nursing
MacMurray College
Jacksonville, Illinois

DIANE BUCHANAN, RN, DNS

Assistant Professor, Faculty of Nursing
University of Alberta
Edmonton, Alberta, Canada

SHARON DAVIS BURT, PHN, MSN

Lecturer, School of Nursing
San Diego State University
San Diego, California

BARBARA CROSSMAN, MSN, RN

Assistant Professor, College of Nursing
Valdosta State University
Valdosta, Georgia

MARGARET R. EDWARDS, RN, DSN

Professor and Level Coordinator, School of Nursing
Northeast Louisiana University
Monroe, Louisiana

GRACE ERRINGTON, RN, MSPH

Nursing Faculty, Texas Woman's University
Dallas, Texas

MARILYN S. FETTER, RN, PhD, CS

Assistant Professor, College of Nursing
Villanova University
Villanova, Pennsylvania

NANCEY E. M. FRANCE, RN, PhD

Associate Professor, Graduate Nursing
Department of Nursing, Murray State University
Murray, Kentucky

BARBARA GRAHAM, RN, EdD

Associate Professor Emeritus
School of Nursing, University of Virginia
Charlottesville, Virginia

ELLA BEHLING GROSS, RN, MSN

Assistant Professor Nursing, Neumann College
Aston, Pennsylvania

GLORIA A. HARMAN, RN, PhD, c

Assistant Professor
Frances Payne Bolton School of Nursing
Case Western Reserve University
Cleveland, Ohio

KATHRYN THOMAS JORDAN, RN, MPH

Assistant Professor, Community Health Nursing
School of Nursing, Belmont University
Nashville, Tennessee

KATHERINE LAUX KAISER, RN, PhD

Assistant Professor, College of Nursing
University of Nebraska Medical Center
Omaha, Nebraska

ELIZABETH K. KEECH, RN, PhD

Assistant Professor, College of Nursing
Villanova University
Villanova, Pennsylvania

RITA J. LOURIE, RN, MSN

Assistant Professor, Department of Nursing
Temple University
Philadelphia, Pennsylvania

KELLY MAYO, RN, PhD

Assistant Professor
Medical University of South Carolina
Charleston, South Carolina

TERRY R. MISENER, RNCS, FNP, PhD, FAAN

Professor, College of Nursing
University of South Carolina
Columbia, South Carolina

BARBARA JOYCE-NAGATA, RN, PhD

Associate Professor of Nursing
Beth-El College of Nursing
Colorado Springs, Colorado

JEAN NAGELKERK, RN, PhD

Associate Professor, Grand Valley State University
Allendale, Michigan

LINDA L. NELSON, RN, MS

Practitioner–Teacher, College of Nursing
Rush University
Chicago, Illinois

DIANE L. OKESON, RN, BSN, MM, ARNP, CNS, Doctoral Student

Assistant Professor of Nursing
Southwestern College
Winfield, Kansas

CAROL ORMOND, RN, MSN, CNAA, CS, FNP

Assistant Professor, School of Nursing
Georgia College
Milledgeville, Georgia

C. VIRGINIA PALMER, RN, DNSc

Assistant Professor, Millersville University
Millersville, Pennsylvania

CAROLE A. PEPA, RN, PhD

Assistant Professor, Valparaiso University
Valparaiso, Indiana

MARGARET S. POPPE, RN, MS

Instructor of Community Health Nursing
Ursuline College
Pepper Pike, Ohio

ROSANNE H. PRUITT, PhD, RNCS

Associate Professor, Clemson University
Clemson, South Carolina

LINDA REUTTER, RN, PhD

Associate Professor, Faculty of Nursing
University of Alberta
Edmonton, Alberta, Canada

JULIE FISHER ROBERTSON, RN, EdD

Assistant Professor, School of Nursing
Northern Illinois University
Dekalb, Illinois

MARY W. RODE, RN, MSN

Associate Professor of Nursing
University of Evansville
Evansville, Indiana

JOANNE F. RUTH, MS, RNC

Associate Professor
Beth-El College of Nursing
Colorado Springs, Colorado

ANN E. SCANNEL, MSN, RNC

Instructor, Community Health Nursing
Saint Anselm College
Manchester, New Hampshire

KATHRYN W. SULLIVAN, RN, MA, MSN, PhD, CNAA

Professor, Research College of Nursing
Kansas City, Missouri

ELSA MEYER TANSEY, RN, DrPH

Associate Professor, Community Health Nursing
College of Nursing, Prairie View A & M University
Houston, Texas

ANITA NARCISO THROWE, RN, MS, CS

Associate Professor
Medical University of South Carolina Satellite Program
Francis Marion University
Florence, South Carolina

WILLIAM R. WHETSTONE, RN, PhD

Professor and Assistant Chair, Division of Nursing
California State University-Dominguez Hills
Carson, California

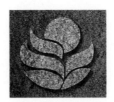

This edition of the text is dedicated to all the faculty, students, and public health and community health nurses who have used the text to benefit student learning and to promote the health of client aggregates. Your comments and suggestions through three editions of the text have been helpful to us in trying to make the content appropriate and applicable to education and practice. Through the years we have heard what you have said to us, and we hope you find your suggestions reflected in subsequent editions. My family and friends continue to be an invaluable support, especially the Smokie Mountain Boy, Patti, Sam, and Glenn. Thanks for understanding my limited availability for social events. A special thanks to Kerrie Schnapf and Peg Teachey for trying to assist me in getting projects completed. They have a monumental task. Jeanette, I am happy to be able to say that you are my friend.

Marcia Stanhope

No one of us succeeds in the goals for our lives and careers without the support, encouragement, and friendship of many caring people. As I reflect back over my many years in nursing, I realize there have been many family and friends who have inspired, urged, and prodded me to achieve as much as was humanly possible. Special thanks to my parents, Howard and Glada Miller, who simply thought nothing was impossible and who were always so pleased by my accomplishments no matter how large or small. Over the years, my husband, Wade, and my daughters, Melinda and Jennifer, have been tremendous sources of inspiration and colleagueship. While I am indebted to many, three people stand out as caring, giving, and supporting over time: Virginia Jarratt, my first dean; Marcia Stanhope, friend and colleague through four editions of this text; and Brenda Belcher, my assistant and "right-hand woman." Thanks to each of you for being such a wonderful friend and supporter.

Jeanette Lancaster

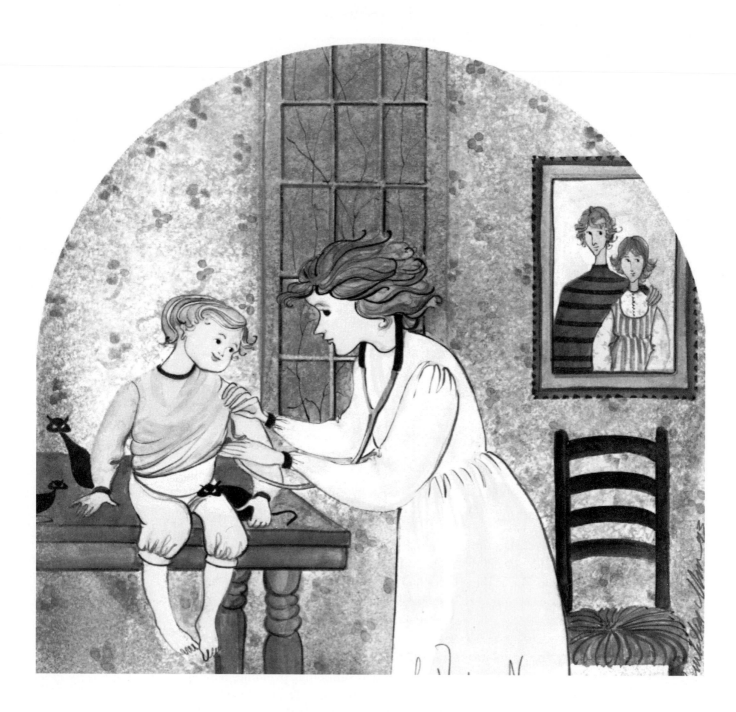

Visiting Nurse, by P. Buckley Moss
Copyright 1993, P. Buckley Moss
From the archives of the P. Buckley Moss Museum
Waynesboro, Virginia

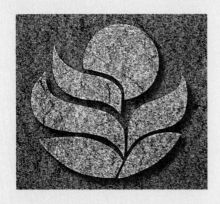

Foreword

The challenge of today's nursing educator is the preparation of the practitioners and leaders of the future. Rather than focus on giving lectures and providing "content," the model of the effective educator is increasingly being conceptualized as that of a "coach" whose expertise is directed to assessing the needs of students and identifying resources and opportunities that they can use in addressing their learning needs. Although a wide range of materials and experiences may be useful in assisting students to meet their goals, the need for a progressive, authoritative, and readable textbook persists. Stanhope and Lancaster's fourth edition of *Community Health Nursing: Promoting Health of Aggregates, Families, and Individuals* remains a compelling choice.

This latest edition of what has become a classic resource in the field of community health nursing maintains the strengths of the three previous editions and incorporates new material to deal with current health problems and management strategies. In one single volume the user has access to guidance from acknowledged experts and leaders in community health nursing, who consider a wide range of topics from the history of the field and conceptual foundations to models for program planning and evaluation. In addition, contemporary epidemics and concerns such as AIDS, adolescent pregnancy, substance abuse, and homelessness are addressed as are the latest approaches to advocacy, nursing diagnosis, and case management in community-based services.

The provision of high quality, direct care nursing service to individuals is the heart of nursing, but for a profession that aspires to make a difference, a focus that is limited to direct care clinical concerns at the individual level is not a sufficient response to the present and future health care needs of the nation. If nursing is to have a positive and significant impact, its practitioners must become seriously involved in structuring the political agenda and adopting strategies to deal with promoting health and providing health care services at the community level. With the aging of the population, the growing recognition that the ever increasing cost of medical care must be slowed, and the introduction of capitated managed care, it has never been more important to focus attention on community-based, population-focused approaches to health promotion and disease prevention. For those who seek to understand the elements and strategies inherent in such practice, which is the essence of community health nursing, and for those who seek to prepare for the challenges and rewards that go with it, Stanhope and Lancaster's text continues to be the resource of choice.

Carolyn A. Williams, RN, PhD, FAAN

Dean and Professor
College of Nursing
University of Kentucky
Lexington, Kentucky

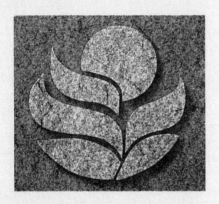

Preface

For a long time, the health care system in the United States, especially the public health system, has been in trouble. It has been widely accepted that a good health care system should address cost, quality of care, and access to health care. In recent years, considerable time and attention have been devoted to what is called "health care reform." In truth, what is actually being reformed is the way in which medical care is organized, financed, and delivered. Still lacking is a commitment to the actual reformation of the entire health care system.

Despite the fact that more money is spent per capita in the United States for health care than in any other country, Americans are not the healthiest of all people. Life-style continues to play an enormous role in morbidity and mortality. For example, half of all deaths in the United States are attributed to tobacco, alcohol, illicit drug use, diet and activity patterns, microbial agents, toxic agents, firearms, sexual behavior, and motor vehicle accidents. Over the years, the most significant improvements in the health of the population have come from advances in public health such as improved sanitation, food pasteurization, refrigeration, immunizations, and the emphasis on personal life-style and environmental factors that affect health.

The need to focus our attention on health promotion, life-style factors, and disease prevention led to the development of a healthy public policy for the nation. This policy was designed by a large number of people representing a wide range of groups interested in health. The policy is reflected in the document *Healthy People 2000,* which identifies a comprehensive set of national health promotion and disease prevention objectives.

The most effective disease prevention and health promotion strategies designed to change personal life-styles are developed by the establishment of partnerships between government, business, voluntary organizations, consumers, and healthcare providers. These partnerships aim to reduce health disparities among Americans by targeting care to children, minorities, elderly, and the uninsured; to increase the healthy life-span of Americans; and to achieve access to preventive services. The overall goal is to develop healthy communities. The development of healthy communities requires commitment from individuals, families, the communities themselves, and society through the development of health policy that supports better health care, the design of improved health education, and the financing of strategies to alter health status.

What does this mean for community health nursing? Because people do not always know how to maximize their health status, the challenge of nursing is to be a catalyst for change. Community health nursing is a practice that is continuous and comprehensive. Directed toward all age groups, community health nursing takes place in a wide variety of settings and includes health education, maintenance, restoration, coordination, management, and evaluation of care of individuals, families, and aggregates, including communities.

To meet the demands of a constantly changing health care system, nurses must be visionary in designing their roles and identifying their practice areas. To do this effectively, the nurse must understand concepts and theories of public health, the changing health care system, the actual and potential roles and responsibilities of nurses and other health care providers, the importance of health promotion and disease prevention orientation, and the necessity to involve consumers in the planning, implementation, and evaluation of health care efforts.

◆ ◆ ◆

Since its initial publication 12 years ago, *Community Health Nursing* has achieved wide acceptance and popularity among community health nursing students and nursing faculty in baccalaureate, BSN-completion, and graduate programs. The text was written to provide nursing students and practicing nurses with a comprehensive source book that provides a foundation for designing community health nursing strategies for individuals, families, and aggregates, including communities. The unifying theme for the book is the integration of health promotion and disease prevention concepts into the multifaceted role of the community health nurse. The prevention focus emphasizes traditional public health practice with increased attention to the effects of the internal and external environment and life-style on health.

ORGANIZATION

The text is divided into seven sections. *Part One*, Perspectives in Health Care Delivery and Community Health Nursing, describes the historical and current status of the health care delivery system both domestically and internationally.

Part Two, Influences on Health Care Delivery and Community Health Nursing, addresses specific issues and societal concerns that affect community health nursing practice.

Part Three, Conceptual Frameworks Applied to Community Health Nursing Practice, provides conceptual models for community health nursing practice, and selected models from nursing and related sciences are also discussed.

Part Four, Issues and Approaches in Aggregate Health Care, examines managing the health care of groups in the community.

Part Five, Issues and Approaches in Family and Individual Health Care, presents risk factors and health problems for families and individuals throughout the lifespan.

Part Six, Vulnerability: Predisposing Factors, covers specific health care needs and issues for populations at risk, such as the homeless and the poor.

Part Seven, Community Health Nursing: Roles and Functions, examines diversity in the role of community health nurses and describes the rapidly changing roles, functions, and practice settings.

NEW TO THIS EDITION

Numerous new chapters have been included in the fourth edition of *Community Health Nursing* to ensure that the text remains a complete and comprehensive resource:

- Chapter 4, International Health Care, compares and contrasts health care systems in the United Kingdom, Canada, Sweden, and Cuba and discusses major world health problems.
- Chapter 16, Community Health Nursing in Rural Environments, discusses current health status and specific health needs of rural populations.
- Chapter 17, Health Promotion Through Healthy Cities, describes the history and future of the international healthy cities movement and provides insight on how to better care for people in urban settings.
- Chapter 18, Nursing Centers, describes the services provided by this emerging community setting and discusses the populations they serve.
- Chapter 20, Disaster Management, discusses the role of the community health nurse in disaster response and preparedness.

- Women's Health and Men's Health are discussed in two separate chapters (Chapters 28 and 29) to focus on the unique health concerns of each group.
- Chapter 25, Family Health Risks, and Chapter 26, Family Health Assessment, provide strategies for identifying risks and assessing health status of families.
- The new Part Six, Vulnerability: Predisposing Factors, includes new chapters on Poverty (Chapter 33), Teen Pregnancy (Chapter 34), and Migrant Health Issues (Chapter 35) to provide a better understanding of these at-risk aggregates.

Additional new features include the following:

- Focused information on providing "culturally competent care" to aggregates, families, and individuals in Chapter 7, Cultural Diversity and Community Health Nursing Practice.
- *Healthy People 2000* objectives, and community health nursing interventions designed to obtain them, incorporated in appropriate chapters throughout the text.
- Eye-catching color illustrations and an open, colorful design to make the book more inviting and "user-friendly" for both students and instructors.

PEDAGOGY

Each chapter is organized for easy use by students and faculty. Chapters begin with an **outline** to alert students to the structure and content of the chapter. Also at the beginning of the chapter are **objectives,** which guide student learning and assist faculty in knowing what students should gain from the content. **Key terms** are identified at the beginning of the chapter and defined either in the chapter or in the glossary to assist the student in understanding unfamiliar terminology. Each chapter includes a **"Did You Know?"** box to provide students with a fact of interest and lend insight into the topic of the chapter. **"What Do You Think?"** boxes present a controversial issue about the chapter topic and are designed to stimulate debate and discussion. **Research Briefs** in each chapter illustrate the use and application of the latest research findings in community health and nursing. **Clinical Applications** at the end of each chapter provide the reader with an understanding of how to apply chapter content in the clinical setting through the presentation of a case situation. **Key Concepts** provide a summary in list form of the most important points made in the chapter. The **Critical Thinking Activities** stimulate student learning by suggesting a variety of activities that encourage both independent and collaborative effort. The **Bibliography** offers both references used to develop chapter materials and additional readings to expand the student's knowledge of the chapter topics.

TEACHING AND LEARNING PACKAGE

A number of ancillaries have been developed to assist instructors and students in the teaching and learning process. These include an instructor's resource manual (which includes 75 transparency masters) and test bank, a computerized test bank, an eight-part community health nursing video series, and a quick reference to community health nursing.

ACKNOWLEDGMENTS

We would like to thank our families, friends, and colleagues who supported us in the completion of this edition. Special thanks go to our co-workers at the University of Kentucky College of Nursing and the University of Virginia School of Nursing who provided generous support and assistance. We also thank Loren Stevenson Wilson and Brian Dennison at Mosby–Year Book, Inc. and the peer reviewers for their time and thoughtfulness in completing the revisions.

We would like to extend special thanks to the contributors of edition three of the book. Their expertise and commitment to community health nursing continue to be reflected in this edition: Wade Lancaster (health care system); Beverly McElmurry, Susan M. Swider, and Prapin Watanakij (primary health care); Eleanor Bauwens and Sandra Anderson (social and cultural influences); Gwendolen Lee (conceptual models and program management); Linda Shortridge and Barbara Valanis (epidemiology); Nancy J. Scheet (nursing diagnosis); Joan Turner and Myra Lovvorn (communicable disease); Diane Boyer and Irma Heppner (mental health); Rosemary Johnson (family); Julia Balzer (family health promotion); Nancy Dickenson-Hazard (child health); Patricia Starck and Geneva W. Morris (adults); Delois Skipwith (older adults); Karen Labuhn (self-health care); Kathleen Beckman Blomquist (health promotion); Phyllis Graves (stress management); Cynthia S. Selleck, Ann T. Sirles, and Rebecca H. Sloan (family nurse practitioner); Roberta K. Lee (manager); Rena Alford (consultant); and Mary N. Albrecht (home health).

Marcia Stanhope
Jeanette Lancaster

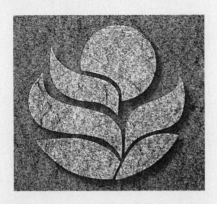

Student Preface

Despite the fact that more money is spent per capita on health care in the United States than in any other country, Americans are not the healthiest of all people. One-half of all deaths in the United States can be attributed to tobacco, alcohol, illicit drug use, diet and activity patterns, toxic agents, sexual behavior, microbial agents, firearms, and motor vehicle accidents. Over the years, health promotion and disease prevention efforts, such as those outlined in the government document *Healthy People 2000*, have yielded the most significant improvements to this trend. With a goal of improving the nation's health while keeping costs down, government, business, voluntary organizations, consumers, and health providers are viewing health promotion and disease prevention strategies as critically important to the future of health care.

What Does This Mean For You, the Student Nurse?

To face the challenges of a changing health care system, you will need to take a close look at practice areas you may not have considered when you enrolled in nursing school. You will need to understand public health and the changing dynamics of the health care system. You will need to know your role as a nurse and the role of other health care providers. But most important, you will need to know the importance of health promotion and disease prevention strategies and the importance of involving your client, the consumer, in the planning, implementation, and evaluation of these efforts.

Community Health Nursing: Promoting Health of Aggregates, Families, and Individuals, fourth edition is the resource you will need to guide you through the future of nursing with confidence.

KEY FEATURES
What You Need to Know

You will not find another community health nursing text with both the depth and breadth of information of *Community Health Nursing*. The text covers traditional community health nursing topics such as community assessment and epidemiology, as well as contemporary issues such as substance abuse and AIDS.

Vulnerable Populations Coverage

This edition of *Community Health Nursing* includes a new Part Six on vulnerable populations—that is, aggregates at risk. The homeless, migrant workers, pregnant teens, and other vulnerable groups are approached with an eye on health promotion and disease prevention to help you better understand their unique problems and health care needs.

Readable and Student-Friendly

Each chapter has been carefully written and edited with you, the student, in mind. An eye-catching, colorful design and several learning aids have been added to make your learning experience enjoyable and worthwhile.

The learning aids in *Community Health Nursing* are designed to help you get the most out of each chapter and help you tackle concepts and issues central to community health nursing. The following pages graphically display the features you will find most helpful.

Begin your study of each chapter by looking over the **Objectives.** As you read each objective, challenge yourself to write down what you do know already. If you have a tentative written response to each (just a word or two or perhaps a big question mark in some cases!), you will have a focus to help you concentrate. Study of the chapter becomes a quest to fill in this new or partial knowledge. After reading the chapter, test yourself against these objectives.

Each chapter begins with a list of **Key Terms** to be encountered in the chapter. Reviewing these before reading the chapter will let you know the kinds of topics coming under discussion and the kinds of terms that will loom as most important in your understanding of the chapter content.

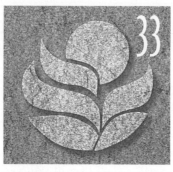

33 Poverty and Homelessness

Teresa Acquaviva • Jeanette Lancaster

Objectives

After reading this chapter, the student should be able to do the following:

- Analyze the concept of poverty.
- Discuss patients' perceptions about poverty and health.
- Describe the social, political, cultural, and environmental factors that influence poverty.
- Discuss the effects of poverty on the health and well being of individuals, families, and communities.
- Analyze the concept of homelessness.
- Discuss patients' perceptions about homelessness and health.
- Describe the social, political, cultural, and environmental factors that influence homelessness.
- Discuss the effects of homelessness on the health and well being of individuals, families, and communities.
- Discuss community health nursing interventions for poor and homeless individuals.

Key Terms

Aid to Families with Dependent Children (AFDC)
deinstitutionalization
feminization of poverty
homelessness
Interagency Council on the Homeless
near poor
neighborhood poverty
persistent poverty
poverty
poverty guidelines
poverty thresholds
Stewart B. McKinney Assistance Act
subjective poverty
Women, Infants and Children (WIC)

Outline

641

By reviewing the **Outline** before reading, you will have a preview of what is ahead and what is to be emphasized in the chapter. The outlines also offer helpful bridges in understanding how topics are interrelated. Looking over the outline after you have read the chapter provides a mini-review that helps you see the chapter content and the connections more globally.

Throughout each chapter, **Key Terms** will appear in bold-faced type the first time each is used for quick and easy reference.

---

cooperation is needed to ensure that the goal of health for all by the year 2000 is reached.

Health promotion had become a key strategy for the goal of health by the time the *Ottawa Charter for Health Promotion* was adopted in 1986. This charter provided a clear definition of health promotion and the framework for the Healthy Cities movement (*Twenty Steps for Developing a Healthy Cities Project*, 1992; Ashton, 1992). *Health Promotion* was officially defined as the "process of enabling people to take control over and to improve their health" (*Ottawa Charter for Health Promotion*, 1986, p.1). This is accomplished through enabling community members to increase control over and assume more responsibility for health; mediating between public, private, voluntary, and community sectors; and advocating on behalf of people powerless to make the necessary changes to promote health.

Five elements make up the strategic framework provided by the Charter and are listed in order of priority for health promotion action. The elements include building healthy public policy, creating supportive environments, strengthening community action, developing personal skills, and reorienting health services. Healthy public policy refers to public policy for health that is based on an ecological perspective and multisectoral and participatory strategies (Pederson, Edwards, Kelner, Marshall, & Allison, 1988). Healthy public policy is future oriented and deals with local health problems as well as global health issues. In contrast, medical policy is mainly concerned with the existing medical care system and use of technology and biomedical science to treat disease. Creating supportive environments refers to physical, political, economic, and social systems that will support the community's health. Strengthening community action refers to promoting the community's capacity, ability, and opportunity to take appropriate action to protect and improve the health of the community. Developing personal skills is helping people develop the lifestyle skills they need to be healthy. Reorienting health services refers to changing the focus of health services toward primary health care, health promotion, disease prevention, and community-based care.

The CITYNET-Healthy Cities process is an adaptation of the European and Canadian models of Healthy Cities in the United States. The nine step **CITYNET**

process includes the following: building the partnership for health, obtaining community commitment, developing the Healthy City Committee, developing leadership in Healthy Cities, assessing the community, community-wide planning for health, community action for health, providing data-based information to policy makers, and monitoring and evaluating Healthy City initiatives (Rider, Flynn, Yuska, Ray, & Rains, 1993).

MODELS OF COMMUNITY PRACTICE

The assumptions that professionals have about communities shape the implementation of the Healthy Cities process. Rothman and Tropman (1987) propose three distinct models of community practice: locality development, social planning, and social action. Locality development is a process-oriented model that emphasizes consensus, cooperation, and building group identity and a sense of community. Social planning stresses rational-empirical problem solving, usually by outside professional experts. The authors note that social planning does not focus on building community capacity or fostering fundamental social change. Social action, on the other hand, aims to increase the problem-solving ability of the community along with concrete actions to correct the imbalance of power and privilege of an oppressed or disadvantaged group in the community (Minkler, 1990). Although it is argued that these models of community practice are not mutually exclusive, efforts generally can be categorized within one.

Arnstein (1969) depicted a ladder of citizen participation with the lower levels of participation as manipulation, therapy, and informing. The higher levels of participation include partnership, delegated power, and citizen control.

> **What Do You Think?**
>
> Community participation in health decisions is more effective in promoting healthy public policy than decision-making by outside professional experts.

These models of community practice can be summarized as top-down and bottom-up approaches. In a top-down approach, experts and health professionals take the lead in identifying community health problems and implementing programs with little input from individuals for whom these programs are being planned. A bottom-up approach utilizes broad-based community problem solving that includes health professionals, local officials, service providers, and other community members including those at risk for health problems.

> **Did You Know?**
>
> Implementing the steps of the CITYNET-Healthy Cities process will enable nurses to gain an understanding of the linkages between health, community, and the policy process. Benefits to the community include increased access to services and improved health status, thus promoting equity in health.

The **Did You Know?** boxes are brief facts of interest that provide food for thought and discussion. Research has proven that we learn more by interacting in a community of learners than we learn by studying in isolation. So, we encourage you to respond to these boxes in a discussion with at least one other student.

The **What Do You Think?** box in each chapter will challenge you to examine a controversial issue about the chapter content. Use these boxes to generate discussions with other students. As you encourage the opinions of others and express opinions of your own on these relevant topics, the chapter material truly becomes your own in terms of knowledge.

Located at the end of each chapter, the **Clinical Application** presents a fascinating, detailed case study that personalizes the usual client scenario, lending it a face, a name, and a personality to help the content of each chapter come alive. Challenge yourself to raise questions about each "case" that force you to relate specific strategies from the chapter to a seemingly real client or situation.

720   *Vulnerability Predisposing Factors*

 ## Clinical Application

Luis, age 53, is a migrant farmworker harvesting vegetables during late July on a large farm in southeastern US. One evening, Luis asks if he can talk with Terry, a community health nurse, who is in the medical van parked outside the trailer camp where he lives. He states he has had continuous upper abdominal pain for the last 3 weeks and is losing weight. He tells Terry that he had this problem in Mexico and the doctor has given him pills so he can work. He must work as he supports his wife, who recently fell from some farm machinery and has not been able to work because of the pain in her hip as a result. He claims he is also responsible for 10 year old twins, his grandchildren, since their parents were killed in a car accident six months ago. His grandchildren attend school when there is no work in the fields. He does not know the last time the children were examined or if they have had their immunizations. He believes his grandchildren are healthy but does notice that they cough frequently, especially when he smokes or it is dusty outside. He just wants medicine that will take away the pain. Terry refers Luis inside the van to be evaluated by the nurse practitioner. Concerned about his wife and grandchildren, Terry asks if she can visit their home. Luis reluctantly gives his permission for the visit and wants to be present. They agree that midday the next day would be an agreeable time.

After being evaluated by the nurse practitioner, Luis leaves. The nurse practitioner and Terry discuss Luis and his family. The NP is concerned about Luis in that he had significant abdominal tenderness and a positive test for occult blood in his stool. He needs further evaluation and diagnostic tests. She discussed the need for further evaluation but Luis is very resistant. The community health nurse is concerned about Luis' wife and the health of the grandchildren. She is also concerned that the environment at the camp might be affecting the health of the children. The nurses know

Luis and his family are not eligible for support programs such as Medicaid or Worker's Compensation. Both are familiar with the Migrant Health Program in their community and will use this as a resource for Luis and his family. Together, they agree that during the home visit, Terry can discuss their concerns and see what Luis and his family might agree to.

The next day, Terry visits the trailer where Luis and his family live. With Luis there, his wife, Eugelia, greets the nurse warmly. Eugelia states she fell about 10 days ago and had some pain in her right hip and difficulty moving her leg. She has gradually resumed moving about in the trailer and is feeling better. The nurse notes there is no bruising or compromise to neurological functioning and there is full ROM of lower extremities without pain. With Luis' permission they discuss the results of the exam yesterday. Luis comments he has no transportation, no money, and he does not want the farmers to know he is sick. He fears that the farmers will not allow him to work if they know he is ill. Terry asks if he would consider it if she could arrange a doctor to evaluate him after work hours. She also assures him of confidentiality. Terry asks Luis and Eugelia if she can visit again to bring more information. Luis tells Terry she can visit Eugelia only if he knows when she is coming. When leaving the trailer, Eugelia tells the nurse she is very concerned about her husband. She is also concerned about her grandchildren—they often cough and have used "nose and breathing medicine" in the past. The children have been working through most of the year and have fallen behind in school. She states she wants a better life for her children. In looking at the trailer and trailer park, Terry has environmental concerns for this family as well. It is dusty and there is trash surrounding the camp. Terry notes that there is a broken window in the trailer and the window air conditioning unit is not functioning.

Key Concepts

- A migrant farm worker is a laborer whose principal employment involves moving from farm to farm planting or harvesting agriculture and attaining temporary housing.
- Estimates of number of migrant farm workers are between three and five million in the United States. These numbers are controversial due to inconsistency in defining farm workers and limitations in obtaining data.
- The life expectancy of the migrant farm worker is 49 as opposed to 75 years of age for U.S. residents.

- When harvesting is completed the farm worker becomes simultaneously homeless and unemployed. Forced migration to find employment leaves little time or energy to seek out and improve living standards.
- Hispanic women are subject to oppression through both political action and expectations of their own families and communities.
- Children of migrant farm workers may need to work for the family's economic survival.

When you have finished reading the chapter, **Key Concepts** offer you a summary of the chapter's most important content in a list format. If one concept is less familiar to you than the rest, review that section of the chapter. Make sure that you understand each concept *and* the related details from the chapter.

Hands-on application of what you have encountered in a textbook still provides the most meaningful reinforcement of new material. **Critical Thinking Activities** send you out of the classroom and into the library or community setting. Use these to practice and develop your analytical skills.

The **Bibliography** can give you additional reading opportunities and can be used as automatic "working bibliographies" for your own original research. When choosing a subject covered in one of the chapters, start with the materials listed in the bibliography and expand your source list from there.

Critical Thinking Activities

1. Interview health care workers and determine their definition of migrant farm worker. Health care workers could include: social workers, nurses, physicians and registered dieticians. Compare and contrast their definitions.
2. Interview community leaders to determine the presence of migrant farm workers in your area. Compare and contrast information about migrant farm workers by interviewing teachers, clergy and politicians versus migrant outreach workers, Wage and Hour personnel, Department of Labor personnel and Migrant Head Start program employees.
3. Consult your library to review vital statistics and census tract data to confirm the presence of migrant workers documented in your area. Are there any contradictions between documented statistics and your interview in activity number two? Why is it difficult to account for (no less track) migrant farm workers?
4. Determine eligibility for Medicaid and Aid to Families with Dependent Children services. You may consult the county health department and the state office. Do migrant workers in your state qualify?
5. Design a clinic to provide health care to migrant workers in your area. What services would you provide? What hours would you operate?

Bibliography

Bishop M, Harrison M: *Farm labor camp outreach project: a step toward meeting the healthcare needs of the Hispanic farm worker in Oregon,* 1987, Unpublished report.

Cassetta R: Needs of migrant health workers challenge RNs, *Amer Nurs* 6(6), 34, 1994.

Caudle, P. (1993). Providing Culturally Sensitive Health Care to Hispanic Clients. *The Nurse Practitioner.* 18(12), 40-51.

Crawford, L. H. (1994). *Linkages Between the Health Care System and Mexican-American Migrant Farm Workers.* Unpublished doctoral dissertation, Georgia State University, Atlanta, Georgia.

Decker, S., Knight, L. (1990). Functional Health Assessment: A Seasonal Migrant Farm Worker Community. *Journal of Community Health Nursing.* 7(3), 141-151.

de la Rosa, M. (1989). Health care needs of Hispanic Americans and the responsiveness of the health care system. *Health and Social Work.* 14.105-113.

Duggar, B. (1990). Access of Migrant and Seasonal Farm workers to Medicaid Covered Health Care Services. *Unpublished paper.*

Galarneau, C. ed. (1993). Under the Weather: Farm Worker Health, National Advisory Council on Migrant health, Bureau of Primary Health Care. U.S. Department of Health and Human Services.

Larson, K. & Watkins, E. (1990). *Migrant and Lay Health Programs: Their Role and Impact.* North Carolina: University of North Carolina at Chapel Hill Press.

Littlefield, C. & Stout, C. (1989). A Survey of Colorado's Migrant Farm workers: Access to Healthcare. *International Migration Review.* 21(3), 688-707.

Marin, B. (1990). AIDS Prevention for Non Puerto Rican Hispanics. In C. Leukefeld, R. Batjes, and Z. Amsel (Eds.), *AIDS and Intervenous Drug Use: Community Interventions and Prevention* (pp. 35-52). New York: Hemisphere.

Medicaid and Migrant Farm Worker Families: Analysis of Barriers and Recommendations for Change. (1991). Washington, D.C.: National Association of Community Health Centers.

National Migrant Resource Program, Inc. *Migrant and Seasonal Farm Worker Health Objectives for the Year 2000, April 1990.*

Smith, K. (1986). The Hazards of Migrant Farm Work: An Overview for the Rural Public Health Nurse. *Public Health Nursing,* 3, 48-56.

Smith, L. S. (1988). Ethnic Differences in Knowledge of Sexually Transmitted Diseases in North American Blacks and Mexican American Migrant Farm Workers. *Research in Nursing and Health,* 11, 51-58.

Staff, Division of Community and Migrant Health, Bureau of Primary Care, Department of Health and Human Services, 1994.

The Helsinki Commission. (1993). *Migrant Farm Workers in the United States, Briefings of the Commission on Security and Cooperation in Europe,* (ISBN Publication No. 0-16-040822-9). Washington, DC.: U.S. Government Printing Office.

U.S. Department of Health and Human Services. (1993) *1993 Recommendations of the National Advisory Council on Migrant Health.* National Advisory Council in Migrant Health. National Migrant Resource Program, Austin, Texas.

U.S. Department of Health and Human Services. (1994) *1994 Update to the Recommendations of the National Advisory Council on Migrant Health.* National Advisory Council in Migrant Health. National Migrant Resource Program, Austin, Texas.

Watkins, E. & Larson, K. (1991). *Migrant Lay Health Advisors: A Strategy for Health Promotion, A Final Report.* North Carolina: University of North Carolina at Chapel Hill.

QUICK REFERENCE TO
COMMUNITY HEALTH NURSING

This handy little book is our gift to you and comes with every copy of *Community Health Nursing.* This portable and accessible reference tool focuses on "need to know" information and is ideal for the clinical component of your community health nursing course. The quick reference includes tools for community, family, and individual assessment, tips for the home visit, and so much more.

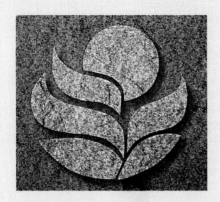

Contents

Part One Perspectives in Health Care Delivery and Community Health Nursing

Since the late 1800s, community health nurses have been leaders in improving the quality of health care for individuals, families, and communities. It has become clear that community health nursing throughout the world, from one country to another, has more similarities than differences.

In September 1990 Secretary of Health and Human Services Louis Sullivan called together in Washington, D.C. over 1500 leaders of 300 national organizations and governmental agencies to announce the Health Objectives for the Nation for the Year 2000. Based upon the success in achieving the first set of objectives for the nation (the 1990 objectives), there is every reason to believe that these latest objectives will improve the overall health of the nation and that community health nurses can play an important role in helping to achieve these objectives.

If community health nurses are to be an effective force in promoting the health of Americans, it is necessary to understand the history of community health nursing and the current status of the public health system. In 1994 the public health nursing specialty celebrated its one hundredth birthday. It was recognized that the challenges currently facing community health nurses are similar to those facing nurses in earlier times. The approaches that have proved successful in the past often can be modified and implemented to deal with contemporary challenges. We can learn not only from the past but also from others.

Part One presents information about significant factors affecting health in the United States. Some contrasts and comparisons in health care are made. To influence the national health care agenda and play an instrumental role in changing the level and quality of services and the priorities for funding requires informed, courageous, and committed nurses. The chapters in Part One are designed to provide crucial information so that community health nurses can make a difference in health care by understanding the roles of public health nurses, community health nurses, and nurses in community-based practice, as well as the roles of the public health system in contrast to the primary health care system.

Chapter 2 explains exactly what makes community health nursing unique. Often people confuse community health nursing with community-based practice. There is a core of knowledge known as public health that forms the foundation for community health nursing. Working with people in the community may not necessarily be community health nursing simply because care of an individual client or the acute care focus is moved from the hospital to the community. ▼

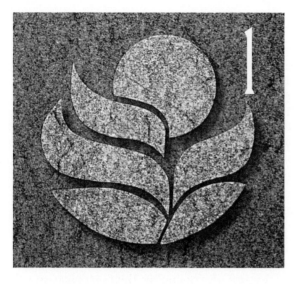

1

The History of Community Health and Community Health Nursing

Jeanette Lancaster

Objectives ▼

After reading this chapter, the student should be able to do the following:

◆ Trace health ideas and practices from the pre-Hellenistic era through the colonial period.
◆ Discuss the pivotal role that Florence Nightingale played in the development of nursing and the subsequent development of community health nursing.
◆ Identify two key nursing leaders who led in the development of community health nursing in the United States.
◆ Outline the role of two major nursing organizations in the development of community health nursing in the United States.
◆ Describe community health nursing practice in the nineteenth century.
◆ Discuss the status of community health nursing practice in the twentieth century.

Outline ▼

The roles of the community health nurse are varied and challenging. Many of the current roles can be traced to the early nineteenth century when public health efforts focused on environmental conditions such as sanitation, control of communicable diseases, education in personal hygiene, disease prevention, and care of sick persons in their homes. Although health threats from communicable diseases, the environment, chronic illnesses, and the aging process have changed over time, the foundational principles and goals of community health nursing have not changed. Many diseases, such as diphtheria, cholera, and typhoid fever, have been controlled in developed countries; however, they have been replaced by hepatitis, acquired immunodeficiency syndrome (AIDS), and a resurgence of diseases such as measles and tuberculosis. Similarly, the environment in industrialized countries is no longer polluted with garbage in the streets but now is threatened by overcrowded garbage dumps; seepage of garbage into the waters that feed crops; and toxins in the air, water, and soil. In addition, instead of experiencing illnesses related to the physical toll of manual labor on their bodies, individuals now experience debilitating diseases that are often stress related. Finally, as the population of the United States ages and desires to remain at home in spite of decreased family and community resources, different community health care needs emerge (New York Visiting Nurse Service, 1994).

Throughout history the roles of the community health nurse have changed to respond effectively to the prevailing public health problems. The roles have been dynamic and multifaceted and have relied heavily on the science of public health. Part of the appeal of community health nursing is the result of the autonomy of the practice and the use of problem-solving and decision-making skills in the role.

To understand the current scope of community health nursing in the United States, it is necessary to briefly trace the history of Western health care from pre-Hellenistic times to the present. The early role of the community health nurse in the United States was patterned after the European model of nursing; therefore the origins of the discipline of nursing and its foundational development in Europe are described. The need for community health nurses, practice of community health nursing, and organizations influencing community health nursing in the United States during the nineteenth century are outlined. Finally, the evolution of community health nursing in the United States in the twentieth century is described.

HISTORICAL REVIEW OF HEALTH CARE PRACTICES

A brief review of the dominant cultural ideas and practices of each era helps to explain the antecedents of the current community health care system. The patterns of health care in previous eras are reflected in the current patterns of modern Western medical and nursing practice. Although the health beliefs and practices of numerous civilizations and cultures could be described, this chapter focuses on the following:
1. Pre-Hellenistic
2. Hellenistic
3. Roman
4. Middle Ages
5. Renaissance
6. Industrial Revolution
7. Colonial

Pre-Hellenistic Era

People have always been concerned with the events surrounding birth, death, and illness. With few exceptions, primitive tribes had a certain amount of group spirit and a sense of hygiene. In their struggles to exist, early people tried to understand disease so that they could cope with disease-producing agents. However, their success was limited, since their health practices were largely based on magic and superstition rather than on facts about the cause and effect of actions and the subsequent health consequences. Priests cared for both health and religious needs and were highly esteemed (Kalisch and Kalisch, 1986).

Rudiments of community health can be traced to the earliest recorded civilizations. The ancient Babylonians believed that illness was caused by sin and failure to please the gods and that disease was a punishment for sinning (Dolan, 1978). Sick persons were seen as unclean and in need of purification; therefore temples became the seat of medical care. In spite of their primitive practices, the Babylonians emphasized hygiene and possessed some medical skills such as the use of medications to treat sick persons. Later, the Egyptians of about 1000 BC used principles based on observation and empirical knowledge rather than on magic. They also developed and systematized a variety of pharmaceutic preparations, constructed earth closets and public drainage systems, and embalmed dead persons. In addition, the Mosaic health code of the Hebrews is clearly reflected in the Old Testament. This code discussed many aspects of individual, family, and community hygiene and provided a basis for practices to maintain health and prolong life. Also, Hebrew women participated in carefully planned programs of visiting sick individuals in their homes and caring for them by bringing physical and spiritual refreshment to the sick person and the family (Rosen, 1958).

Hellenistic Period

The early Greeks viewed people as part of nature and believed health resulted from a harmonious relationship with nature. They saw health care delivery as a responsibility of a civilized society. As a guide to their medical practice, the Greeks established a code of medical ethics. Hippocrates has been described as the "father of medicine" because he empirically attempted to systematize and demystify the treatment of illness. He also linked health with the balance of individuals and their environment (Kalisch and Kalisch, 1986). In addition, the Greeks paid attention to personal cleanliness, exercise, diet, and sanitation.

The first notation of women being associated with healing is found in connection with the Greek mythological character of Aesculapius, who eventually became deified as the god of healing. One of his five children, Hygeia, became the goddess of health and another, Panacea, the restorer of health. In later Greek civilizations, healing occurred largely in shrines where patients congregated and were looked after by attendants called "basket healers" (Deloughery, 1977).

The first clear-cut evidence of acute communicable disease is recorded in classical Greek literature. There are numerous references to severe sore throats that often ended in death. The Greek work *Kynanche* mentioned acute inflammatory processes of the throat and larynx and referred to what is probably now known as diphtheria. In ancient Greece, medicine was an itinerant vocation, with practitioners going from town to town, knocking on doors and offering their services. Larger cities appointed physicians and paid for their services from public funds (Rosen, 1958).

Roman Empire

The Roman view of health shared many concepts with the Greeks yet focused much more on pragmatic application of ideas rather than astute observation and a continual search for new knowledge. The Roman Empire is remembered for its administrative and engineering efforts. According to Pellegrino (1963), Romans viewed medicine from a community health and social medicine perspective. They emphasized regulation of medical practice, punishment for negligence, drainage of swamps, provision of pure water, establishment of sewage systems, and supervision of street cleaning and public food preparation.

Appius Claudius Crassus Caecus, who built the first great Roman road, the Appian Way, was responsible for bringing a supply of water to Rome by means of an aqueduct (Rosen, 1958). To monitor the purity of water, settling basins were established at points along the aqueduct to allow sediment to deposit. When the water reached Rome, it was received in large reservoirs from which smaller reservoirs emerged so that water could be segregated according to its purpose. The Romans not only valued pure water but also had sewage systems in major cities. The Romans developed community health services with an effective and systematic organization, which continued to function as the empire disintegrated. In addition, at the peak of the Roman Empire women visited and cared for sick persons. Special hospitals were established when it became impractical to shelter patients in the bishops' houses, which had previously been their practice (Pellegrino, 1963).

Middle Ages

The decline of the Greco-Roman era led to both a decay of urban culture and a disintegration of community health organization and practice (Rosen, 1958). The period between 500 and 1500 AD was a heterogeneous phase in history during which superstitions dominated thinking yet advances such as the development of health care facilities originated. As cities grew, people built great walls to protect themselves against invasions by hostile groups. These encircling walls, while necessary for safety and protection, also led to considerable crowding and poor sanitary and hygienic conditions. Clean water supplies and elimination of refuse in the streets were difficult to ensure. Thus communicable diseases such as measles, smallpox, diphtheria, and bubonic plague were prevalent.

With the dawn of the Christian era, a new conceptualization of human beings influenced health practices. The early Christian church believed that the Roman and Greek ways pampered the body at the expense of the soul. Disease was seen as punishment for sin (Kalisch and Kalisch, 1986).

During this era thinking reverted to mysticism and superstition. Religious persecution of those who tried to introduce new ideas occurred. Progress in medicine came to a halt. People considered it immoral to look at their bodies. People seldom bathed and often wore dirty clothes. Sanitation was not viewed as important. Refuse and body wastes were allowed to accumulate near dwellings. However, despite this reversal in thinking about health, hospitals for poor and neglected individuals were developed (Rosen, 1958).

The rise of monasteries and convents as places for caring for sick persons led to the early development of nursing activities. Between 1091 and 1291, the first male and female nurses joined military orders during the Crusades. As the early Christian church developed, those individuals who had devoted their lives to Christian service cared for poor, fatherless, and sick persons. Initially they cared for all three groups under the same roof. However, the knowledge that the Crusaders gained from the Arabs led to the establishment of hospitals. Early hospitals were known as Hotels Dieu, with the best known being in Paris. During this era several orders of nuns provided simple nursing care directed primarily toward meeting the patient's physiologic needs (Griffin and Griffin, 1973). Health education and personal hygiene knowledge also increased during the later portion of the Middle Ages. Books were written about healthful living that encouraged moderate eating to promote health.

Renaissance

The great epidemics of the Middle Ages led to attitudes of fatalism and a general depressed attitude toward health. However, during the Renaissance people started opening their minds to new ideas. Thus between 1500 and 1700 medicine began to advance. In general, the Renaissance was characterized

Table 1-1 Milestones in History of Community Health and Community Health Nursing: 1600-1865

Year	Milestone
1601	Elizabethan Poor Law written
1617	Sisterhood of the Dames de Charite organized in France by St. Vincent de Paul
1789	Baltimore Health Department established
1812	Sisters of Mercy established in Dublin where nuns visited the poor
1813	Ladies Benevolent Society of Charleston, South Carolina founded
1850	Shattuck Report prepared on the status of medical education
1851	Florence Nightingale went to Kaiserwerth
1855	Quarantine Board established in New Orleans; beginning of tuberculosis campaign in the United States
1859	District nursing established in Liverpool by William Rathbone
1860	Florence Nightingale Training School for Nurses established at St. Thomas Hospital in London; nursing program started at New England Hospital
1864	Beginning of Red Cross

by achievements in the arts and scholarly efforts, as well as by a rise in commerce and industry. Belief in humanism developed. Human dignity and worth began to influence health practices (Kalisch and Kalisch, 1986).

The Renaissance ushered in a new period of history during which community health as it is currently known was begun (Rosen, 1958) (Table 1-1). The many technological advances designed to treat the epidemics of the Middle Ages provided the impetus and resources necessary for the changes that took place in the Renaissance. These changes, although not directly influencing community health, supplemented the foundation of modern community health.

A matter of serious debate during the Renaissance was whether diseases prominent at the time—including scarlet fever, rickets, scurvy, syphilis, smallpox, and malaria—were caused by contagion or constitution. The invention of the microscope by Anton van Leeuwenhoek in the late seventeenth century supported the contagion view by permitting the observation of microorganisms in soil and water (Rosen, 1958).

Although establishment of a systematic national health policy in Europe failed, health problems began to be analyzed and proposals for national action were set forth (Rosen, 1958). William Perry contributed significantly with his belief that communicable disease

control would save infant lives and improve the lives of the people. Although this idea made sense, there was no way of enforcing it, since local authorities had no jurisdiction outside their boundaries and ships frequently brought contagious diseases into the ports (Rosen, 1958).

During the Renaissance, town and city residents attempted to keep streets clean. Communities had no systems of sewage disposal. Private enterprises supplied water. Towns provided assistance for sick and lame persons. During this period, hospitals became places not only to care for sick patients but also to study and teach medicine. These advances were the forerunners to later scientific discoveries (Kalisch and Kalisch, 1986).

Industrial Revolution

The Industrial Revolution, with its emphasis on power and profits, reversed many of the gains of the Renaissance. Also, as urban populations grew because of the emphasis on industry and production, the number of people needing health care outpaced the voluntary and often piecemeal efforts to provide services. The 80 years between 1750 and 1830 influenced the future design of community health because of the upheaval and change prevalent at that time (Rosen, 1958).

The population increased dramatically. Major problems included a high infant mortality, neglect and often murder of illegitimate infants, poor working conditions, diseases of certain occupations, and the growing incidence of mental illness.

Early hospitals in the United States include the 1731 establishment of Blockley Hospital, later known as Philadelphia General, was established to receive sick, poor, insane, imprisoned and orphaned individuals. In 1737 Charity Hospital was established in New Orleans. In 1751 Pennsylvania Hospital was founded in Philadelphia to admit acutely ill or injured people (Dolan, 1978). Most early hospitals in the United States were begun on the Northeast coast, following the pattern of settlement in the United States. Community-minded citizens established New York Hospital in 1771, and the Philadelphia Dispensary opened in 1786 because of the efforts of the Quakers (Dolan, 1978).

During the eighteenth century, people with mental illness were locked in jails, workhouses, or madhouses. An early defender of mentally ill persons, Vincenzo Chiarugi, brought about major reforms at St. Bonifacio in Florence, Italy, where in 1788 he established a system in which properly trained nurses cared for mentally ill persons under the direct supervision of a physician (Rosen, 1958). Other such asylums followed suit, providing patients with kindness, physical exercise, good food, and fresh air (Kalisch and Kalisch, 1986). In 1770 Eastern State Hospital, known as the "Lunnatick Hospital," was established in Williamsburg, Virginia. This was one of the first American state hospitals for mentally ill persons.

The Industrial Revolution witnessed tremendous advances in transportation, communication, and other forms of technology. Modern public health efforts began in England. The prevailing social problem of that time was caring for poor persons. The Elizabethan Poor Law of 1601 guaranteed medical and nursing care for poor, blind, and lame individuals. A Commission of Inquiry on the Poor Laws was established and administered by Edwin Chadwick, who subsequently devoted his entire career to helping poor persons. Chadwick campaigned vigorously to get bills passed in Parliament that would not only help poor people but also eliminate some of the unsanitary environmental conditions of that time.

Early forerunners of community health nursing are found in the work of the first two nursing orders in the British Isles. Mary Aikenhead (Sister Mary Augustine) started the Irish Sisters of Charity in Dublin in 1812, where the nuns visited among the poor population. The Sisters of Mercy founded a home for destitute girls and visited sick persons in their homes (Kalisch and Kalisch, 1986).

Toward the end of the Industrial Revolution, women performing nursing functions changed from a caring group of women largely supported by a religious order to a group often referred to as the "dregs of the community: dirty, drunken, and dishonest" (Swinson, 1965). Charles Dickens in *Martin Chuzzlewit* provided a lasting impression of nursing in the eighteenth century with his description of Sairy Gamp, a drunk, untrained servant who reportedly provided a semblance of nursing care.

Colonial Period

During the Industrial Revolution in Europe, events occurred that influenced the course of community health in what would later be the United States of America. Epidemics, especially smallpox, occurred in the early years of North American settlement. Possibly the colonists were able to settle in North America because the diseases they brought with them were fatal to natives, who lacked immunity to them. Early colonial community health efforts included the collection of vital statistics, improved sanitation, and the avoidance of exotic diseases brought in from trade routes. However, the colonists lacked a continuing and organized mechanism for ensuring that community health efforts would be supported and enforced (Rosen, 1958).

Because of the pressure to establish a federation of states, community health received little attention before the American Revolution. After the American Revolution, the threat of a variety of diseases, especially yellow fever, influenced the establishment of official boards of health. By the end of the eighteenth century New York City, with a population of 75,000, had established a public health committee for monitoring water quality, sewer construction, drainage of marshes, planting of trees and vegetables,

construction of a masonry wall along the waterfront, and burial of the dead (Rosen, 1958).

NURSING DEVELOPED BY NIGHTINGALE

Although concern about health and the care of individuals in the community has existed throughout the centuries, the organized discipline of nursing was not developed until the mid-1800s in England by **Florence Nightingale.** Nightingale's vision and model of nursing guided the development of nursing, and ultimately community health nursing, in the United States. This section outlines the need for nurses, the origins of organized nursing, and principles of nursing.

Need for Nurses

The Crimean War, which started in March of 1854 and ended in February of 1856, began over Russia's displacement of the Turkish sultan. The mission of the Turkish sultan was to protect Christian shrines in the Middle East. The nations of Great Britain, Turkey, France, and Austria entered the war against Russia. Many Irish Catholic men joined the British to fight against the Russians because they believed that the war was primarily a religious war. Although approximately one-third of all British soldiers were Irish Catholics, in general the British disliked and oppressed the Irish and feared the spread of Catholicism. Therefore in part, although British hospitals to care for sick and wounded soldiers were established in Scutari during the Crimean War, the care of soldiers was appalling (Palmer, 1983). Cramped quarters, filth, lice, rats, vermin, insufficient food, stale air, and inadequate medical supplies were the norm (Kalisch and Kalisch, 1986).

Word of the conditions of the sick and injured soldiers at Scutari reached England by way of letters from soldiers and an expose written by William Howard Russell, a reporter for *The Times.* As a result of learning about these conditions, the public demanded that the government do something to improve the care of sick and wounded soldiers. Because of her wealth, social and political power, and knowledge of hospitals, Florence Nightingale was asked by the Roman Catholic church and the British government to go to Scutari to improve conditions for the sick and injured soldiers. She agreed to go to Scutari and took 40 ladies, 117 hired nurses, and 15 paid servants with her. Nightingale attributed the drop in mortality from 415 per 1000 at the beginning of the war to 11.5 per 1000 at the end of the war to the nursing care that soldiers received (Cohen, 1984; Palmer, 1983).

Origins of Organized Nursing

As described, Florence Nightingale organized nursing care for the soldiers in the Crimean War, many of whom were Irish Catholics. Thus the roots of organized nursing were grounded in the provision of health care to poor, discriminated against, and powerless individuals. Often, as community health nursing has developed, community health nurses have been the only advocates for disadvantaged individuals. Like Nightingale, community health nurses typically identify health care needs that affect the entire population, mobilize resources, and organize themselves and the community to meet these needs.

After the Crimean War, Nightingale organized hospital nursing and nursing education in hospitals. Nightingale not only focused on the role of hospital nursing but also emphasized community health nursing. She coined the phrase "health nursing" to emphasize that nursing should strive to promote health and prevent illness. In addition, she worked with **William Rathbone,** the British philanthropist, who founded the first district nursing association in Liverpool between 1859 and 1862. Because of the outstanding nursing care provided to his dying wife, Rathbone promoted the establishment of a district nursing service. Based on his experience, Rathbone concluded that many people with long-term illnesses could be better cared for in their own homes than in a hospital. Subsequently at Rathbone's urging, the Liverpool Relief Society divided the city into nursing districts and assigned a committee of "Friendly Visitors" to each district to provide health care to needy people (Kalisch and Kalisch, 1977). Based on the Liverpool experience, Rathbone wrote a book entitled *Social Organization of Effort in Works of Benevolence and Public Charity by a Man of Business,* in which he outlined a philosophy for home health care. Rathbone's work spurred Florence Nightingale to publish a pamphlet on nursing entitled *Suggestions for Improving Nursing Service,* which recommended steps to take to provide nursing care in the home (Bullough and Bullough, 1964). Eventually, as a result of Nightingale and Rathbone's efforts, district nursing was organized nationally and spread throughout England. In addition, Nightingale wrote community health nursing articles entitled "Village Sanitation" and "District Nursing" (Dock, 1922, reprinted).

Principles of Nursing

In her famous book *Notes on Nursing: What it is, and What it is not,* Nightingale (1946, reprinted) stated that the task of nursing was to "put the constitution in such a state as that it will have no disease, or that it can recover from disease." She identified principles that continue to guide not only the practice of nursing in general but especially the practice of community health nursing. Nightingale outlined the following five essential points in securing the health of households and in ultimately promoting health: (1) pure air, (2) pure water, (3) efficient drainage, (4) cleanliness, and (5) light. She also identified that proper nutrition, rest, sanitation, and hygiene are necessary for health. Community health nurses continue to focus on the role of health promotion, disease prevention, and environment as they deliver care to their patients.

COMMUNITY HEALTH NURSING IN THE UNITED STATES IN THE NINETEENTH CENTURY

Community health nursing developed in the United States in the nineteenth century. This section describes the societal need that influenced nurses to establish community-based practices. It also highlights the two types of community-based nursing practices that were common at the time: (1) visiting nurses and (2) settlement houses. In addition, organizations dedicated to improving health care in the United States during the nineteenth century are outlined.

Need for Community Health Nursing

Although the United States grew tremendously between 1800 and 1850, community health efforts did not keep pace. During this period, threats to health escalated as epidemics of smallpox, yellow fever, cholera, typhoid, and typhus entered the country along with the influx of migrants from many parts of the world. To illustrate the seriousness of conditions, in New York City in 1880, on average, 16 individuals lived in one small tenement house and the death rate was more than 25 per 1000. At the same time, hospitals were generally unsanitary and staffed by poorly trained workers. Hospitals were places where people, especially poor people, went to die. In fact, many people developed infections and died after surgery in the early hospitals (Kalisch and Kalisch, 1986). Because of these poor health care conditions, community health care reform efforts began in the late 1800s.

Just as cities in the United States began to establish community health efforts, an influx of immigrants poured in from Europe. These immigrants taxed the stability of cities, especially those on the east coast. Housing and sanitation became major problems. As urban communities grew and their sanitary conditions worsened, conflict arose between those wanting health reform and those wishing to maintain the status quo. A number of voluntary health associations, such as the National Tuberculosis Association, developed to mobilize forces to promote health within the community (Kalisch and Kalisch, 1986).

Community Health Nursing Practice

Meanwhile, community health nursing in the United States was beginning to organize to meet urban health care needs. Nurses became active as visiting nurses and in establishing community-based **settlement houses. Visiting nurses** went to individuals' homes and delivered nursing and health care services. Other nurses ran settlement houses. These nurses typically lived in the settlement houses, which were located in the areas that they served. Settlement houses were

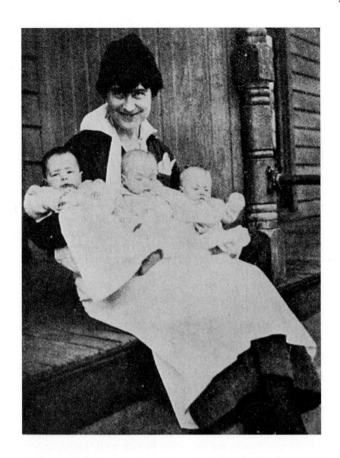

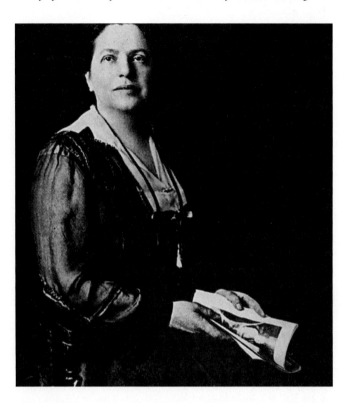

FIGURE 1-2

Lillian Wald. (Photo courtesy the Visiting Nurse Service of New York.)

FIGURE 1-1

Teaching well-child care was a significant public health nursing role. (Photo courtesy Instructional Visiting Nurse Association of Richmond, Va.)

developed based on the philosophy that the most effective way to help poor people improve their health was for educated people to live among them and teach by example, as well as by instruction in better health care. These houses were the hub of health care programs, education, and individual and family care in a community (Kalisch and Kalisch, 1986).

The first nurses to visit in homes were in New York. In 1877 the Women's Board of the New York Mission hired Frances Root, a graduate of Bellevue Hospital's first nursing class, to visit sick poor persons and to provide nursing care and religious instruction to them (Bullough and Bullough, 1964). In 1878 the Ethical Culture Society of New York hired four nurses to work in dispensaries. Thus began ambulatory care nursing. In the next few years visiting nurse associations were established in Buffalo (1885), Philadelphia (1886), and Boston (1886). These visiting nurses strictly followed physicians' orders, gave selected treatments, and kept temperature and pulse records. Because their visits were brief, the nurses soon recognized the need to teach family members basic elements of care (Bullough and Bullough, 1964). Thus from the beginning, community health nursing included teaching and prevention. As seen in Figure 1-1, visiting nurses provided home health services to mothers and their babies.

Meanwhile in 1886, two women in Boston approached the Women's Education Association to seek support for **district nursing.** They used the term *instructive district nursing* to emphasize the relationship of nursing to health education and to increase their likelihood of receiving support from this group. They then met with representatives of the Boston Dispensary, which was providing free medical care to poor persons according to the dispensary district in which they lived. Through these efforts, in February of 1886 the first district nurse was hired in Boston. As the number of district nurses increased, they worked closely with physicians to carry out medical orders. Patients paid no fees. In 1888 the Instructive District Nursing Association became incorporated as an independent voluntary agency to provide care to sick poor persons under the direction of a trained physician. These nurses also taught families to take better care of themselves and their neighbors by living a wholesome life (Brainard, 1922).

During this era, wealthy people became interested in charitable activities and began to fund settlement houses in the poorer sections of many larger cities. These settlement houses offered a variety of services for members of the community. For example, in 1893 **Lillian Wald** and her friend Mary Brewster, both trained nurses and wealthy women, organized a visiting nursing service for the poor population of New York (see box on p. 10 and Figure 1-2). Eventually, this settlement house became known as the

Lillian Wald: First Public Health Nurse in the United States

Community health nursing evolved in the United States in the late nineteenth and early twentieth centuries largely because of the pioneering work of Lillian Wald. Born on March 10, 1867, Lillian Wald decided to become a nurse after Vassar College refused to admit her at 16 years of age. She graduated in 1891 from the New York Hospital Training School for Nurses and spent the next year working at the New York Juvenile Asylum. To supplement what she thought had been inadequate training in the sciences, she enrolled in the Woman's Medical College in New York (Frachel, 1988).

Having grown up in a warm, nurturing family in Rochester, New York, her work in New York City introduced her to an entirely different side of life. In 1883, while conducting a class in home nursing for immigrant families on the Lower East Side of New York, Wald was asked by a small child to visit her sick mother. Wald found the mother in bed, having hemorrhaged for 2 days. This home visit confirmed for Wald all of the injustices in society and the differences in health care for poor persons versus those persons able to pay (Frachel, 1988).

She simply could not tolerate seeing poor people with no access to health care. With her friend Mary Brewster and the financial support of two wealthy laypeople, Mrs. Solomon Loeb and Joseph H. Schiff, she moved to the East Side and occupied the top floor of a tenement house on Jefferson Street. This move eventually led to the establishment of Henry Street Settlement. In the beginning, Wald and Brewster helped individual families. Wald believed that the nurse's visit "should be like that of a very interested friend rather than that of an impersonal, paid visitor" (Dolan, 1978).

Ever discontent to deal only with the present and convinced that environmental conditions as well as social conditions were the causes of ill health and poverty, Wald became actively involved in using epidemiological methods to campaign for health-promoting social policies. Not only did she write *The House on Henry Street* to describe her own public health nursing work but also she led in the development of payment by insurance companies for nursing services (Frachel, 1988).

In 1909, along with Lee Fraskel, Lillian Wald established the first community health nursing program for workers at the Metropolitan Life Insurance Company. Believing that keeping workers healthier would increase their productivity, she urged that nurses at agencies such as Henry Street Settlement provide skilled nursing care. Wald convinced the company that it would be more economical to use the services of community health nurses than to employ their own nurses. She also convinced them that services could be available to anyone desiring them, with fees graduated according to the ability to pay. This nursing service designed by Wald continued for 44 years and contributed several significant accomplishments to community health nursing, including the following (Frachel, 1988):
1. Providing home nursing care on a fee-for-service basis
2. Establishing an effective cost-accounting system for visiting nurses
3. Using advertisements in both newspapers and the radio to recruit nurses
4. Reducing mortality from infectious diseases

Lillian Wald also believed that the nursing efforts at Henry Street Settlement should be aligned with an official health agency. Therefore she arranged for nurses to wear an insignia that signified that they served under the auspices of the board of health. Also, she established rural health nursing services through the Red Cross. Her other accomplishments included helping to establish the Children's Bureau and fighting in New York City for better tenement living conditions, city recreation centers, parks, pure food laws, graded classes for mentally handicapped children, and assistance to immigrants (Backer, 1993; Dock, 1922; Frachel, 1988; Zerwekh, 1992).

Henry Street Settlement (Zerwekh, 1992). Meanwhile, other settlement houses were being established in many other cities throughout the United States.

Community Health Organizations

During the middle of the nineteenth century, the nation's attention focused on attacking community health problems and improving urban living conditions. Founded in 1847, the American Medical Association (AMA) responded to pressure to form a hygiene committee in 1848 to carry out sanitary surveys and to develop a system for collecting vital statistics. The American Public Health Association began in 1872 and focused on interdisciplinary efforts, published a variety of health promotion and illness prevention materials, and lobbied for improved public health (Pickett and Hanlon, 1990) (Table 1-2). Local health departments were established at this time in cities and targeted the elimination of environmental hazards associated with poor living conditions, crowding, and the close proximity of slaughterhouses to homes. Local health departments subsequently developed in rural areas (Kalisch and Kalisch, 1986).

Concurrently, efforts in Massachusetts produced the famous **Shattuck Report.** This report was published in 1850 by the Massachusetts Sanitary Commission. Major recommendations called for the following (Kalisch and Kalisch, 1986):
1. The establishment of a state health department and local health boards in every town
2. Sanitary surveys
3. Varying kinds of vital statistics
4. Environmental sanitation
5. Food, drug, and communicable disease control
6. Well-child care including immunizations and health education (Figure 1-3)
7. Proposals on smoke and alcohol control, town planning, and the teaching of preventive medicine in medical schools.

Although the Shattuck Report now receives credit as a noteworthy and farsighted document, it was virtually ignored in its own time. Implementation of the actions recommended by the report came 19 years after its publication.

Simultaneously, nurses were organizing into national groups. In 1893 Isabel Hampton Robb led the effort to establish the **Society of Superintendents of**

Table 1-2 Milestones in History of Community Health and Community Health Nursing: 1866-1945

Year	Milestone
1866	New York Metropolitan Board of Health established
1872	American Public Health Association established
1877	Women's Board of the New York Mission hires Frances Root to visit the sick poor
1879	New York Ethical Society places trained nurses in dispensaries
1885	District Nursing Association established in Buffalo
1886	District nursing begun in Philadelphia and Boston
1893	Lillian Wald and her friend, Mary Brewster, organized a visiting nursing service for the poor of New York, which later became the famous Henry Street Settlement; Society of Superintendents of Training Schools of Nurses in the United States and Canada was established (in 1912 became known as the National League for Nursing)
1895	Associated Alumnae of Training Schools for Nurses established (in 1911 became the American Nurses' Association)
1902	School nursing started in New York (Lina Rogers)
1903	First nurse practice acts
1910	Public health nursing program instituted at Teachers College, Columbia University, in New York
1912	National Organization for Public Health Nursing formed with Lillian Wald as first president
1914	First undergraduate nursing education course in public offered by Adelaide Nutting at Teacher's College
1918	Vassar Camp School for Nurses organized; U.S. Public Health Service (USPHS) establishes division of public health nursing to work in the war effort
1919	Textbook, *Public Health Nursing*, written by Mary S. Gardner
1925	Frontier Nursing Service using nurse-midwives established
1934	Pearl McIver becomes first nurse employed by USPHS
1935	Passage of Social Security Act
1941	Beginning of World War II
1943	Passage of Bolton-Bailey Act for nursing education and Cadet Nurse Program established; Division of Nursing begun at USPHS; Lucille Petry appointed chief of Cadet Nurse Corps
1944	First basic program in nursing accredited as including sufficient public health content

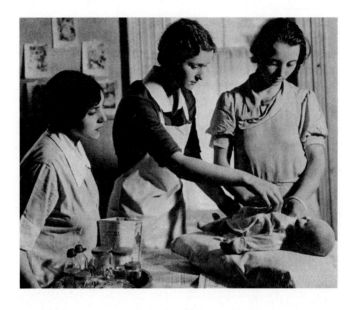

FIGURE 1-3
Public health nurse demonstrating well-child care during a home visit. (Photo courtesy the Visiting Nurse Service of New York.)

Training Schools of Nurses in the United States and Canada. The society, which later became the **National League for Nursing** (NLN), established training standards and promoted collegial relationships among nurses. Two years later the **Associated Alumnae of Training Schools for Nurses,** which later became the **American Nurses Association** (ANA), was organized to strengthen the union of nursing organizations, improve nursing education, and promote ethical standards in nursing (Dock, 1922; Dock and Steward, 1983).

COMMUNITY HEALTH NURSING IN THE UNITED STATES IN THE TWENTIETH CENTURY

In the twentieth century, community health nursing in the United States has continued to evolve and adapt to meet the health care needs of the nation. This section is organized into four time periods: (1) 1900 to World War I, (2) World War I to World War II, (3) World War II to 1960, and (4) 1960 to the present.

1900 to World War I

In 1911 a joint committee was appointed, composed of representatives of the ANA (at that time called the Associated Alumnae of Training Schools for Nurses) and the NLN (known as the Society of Superintendents of Training Schools for Nurses) to standardize nursing services outside the hospital. Lillian Wald chaired and Mary Gardner served as secretary of this committee. The committee recommended that a new organization be formed to meet the needs of community health nurses. They subsequently invited 800 agencies known to be involved in community health nursing activities to send delegates to an organizational meeting in Chicago in June of 1912. A heated debate commenced as to the name and purpose of this organization; however, at noon on June 7, 1912, the delegates unanimously voted the **National Organization for Public Health Nursing** (NOPHN) into existence with Lillian Wald as its first president (Dock, 1922).

Did You Know?

Public health agencies were among the earliest major enterprises run by women in the United States. Early public health nurses were effective managers, clinicians, and fund-raisers as they began services to provide care for the country's neediest segment of the population.

The new organization sought, "to standardize public health nursing activities on a high level and coordinate all efforts in the field" (Deloughery, 1977). Specifically, one task of this organization was to standardize community health nursing education. Because diploma schools of nursing emphasized hospital care of patients, community health nursing at this time required special education. Debate ensued as to whether community health nurses needed a basic nursing education or just specialized training in home care. Nursing leaders decided that all nurses needed some community health content. Thus basic undergraduate courses were required to include the topic of community health nursing (Dock, 1922).

As community health nursing grew into a specialized and respected area of nursing, it became apparent that the inclusion of this content in basic curricula was insufficient. In 1914 Mary Adelaide Nutting offered the first postgraduate nursing course in community health at Teachers College in affiliation with the Henry Street Settlement (Deloughery, 1977). When this turned out to be successful, other nursing schools developed specialized postgraduate training programs for community health nurses.

Meanwhile, advances in the practice of community health nursing occurred. Community health nurses were the primary staff members of local health departments. Likewise, they (community health nurses) assumed a leadership role in collaborating on health care issues with citizens, nurses, and other health care providers. During the early portion of the twentieth century the scope of community health nursing included disease prevention, health promotion, and family-oriented services (Kalisch and Kalisch, 1986). This type of nursing care serves as a prototype of contemporary community health nursing (see Figure 1-4).

 ### Research Brief

Hamilton D: Research and reform: Community nursing and the Framingham tuberculosis project, 1914-1923, *Nurs Res* 41(1):8-13, 1992.

The relationship between nursing and Metropolitan Life Insurance Company is both interesting and reflective of a range of historical events in nursing. Metropolitan Life led the insurance industry in the provision of nursing care in the home for its policyholders. A friend of Lillian Wald's, Lee Frankel, headed the welfare department at Metropolitan. She proposed that nurses could assess illness, teach health practices, and effectively collect data from policyholders. On June 9, 1909, the first Henry Street nurse made a home visit to a policyholder. By 1914 Metropolitan provided home nursing care to policyholders in 1804 cities. The original idea was for the company to contract for services with existing nursing agencies. However, in 1910 the Metropolitan Visiting Nurse service was established in St. Paul, Minnesota, and these nurses became "Met nurses." They not only provided care to policy-holders that may have lengthened their lives, but also collected immense amounts of data that were invaluable to the insurance industry.

The author describes the relationship among the insurance company, nurses, and policyholders in the study of tuberculosis that began in Framingham, Massachusetts, in 1916. The article is not about tuberculosis but rather is about nursing and how since the early 1900s other groups have tried to be in control.

World War I to World War II

The onset of World War I in 1914 threatened the role of community health nurses. The large numbers of nurses involved in the war left very few nurses to practice in the community setting. However, the American Red Cross helped to sustain community health nursing by establishing a roster of nurses who could be enlisted to supply health care. During the war the NOPHN loaned a nurse to the U.S. Public Health Service to establish a community health nursing program for military outposts, which led to the first community health nursing program sponsored by the federal government (Shyrock, 1959; Wilner et al., 1978).

In 1918 during World War I, the Vassar Camp School for Nurses started as a unique and patriotic aspect of nursing education. The American Red Cross and the Council of National Defense jointly supported this novel program, which proposed that nursing education could be shortened from three years to two years for college graduates. The Vassar Camp School, modeled after the Plattsburg Military Camp in New York, gave intensive training to college graduates so that they could become army reserve officers and meet urgent wartime needs. A total of 435 graduates

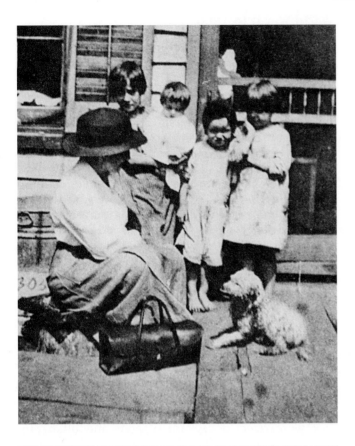

FIGURE 1-4

Early public health nurses provided a range of services for families. (Photo courtesy Instructional Visiting Nurse Association of Richmond, Va.)

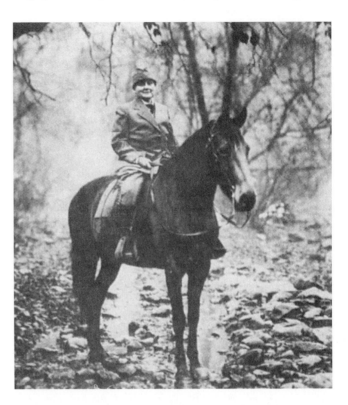

FIGURE 1-5

Mary Breckinridge, founder of the Frontier Nursing Service. (Photo courtesy the Frontier Nursing Service of Wendover, Ky.)

of this program represented many colleges across the United States. The program ended when peace was declared (Buhler-Wilkerson, 1989; Dock, 1922; Kalisch and Kalisch, 1986; Shyrock, 1959; Wilner et al., 1978).

After World War I, many changes occurred that subsequently affected community health nursing. Despite the economic constraints of the depression, this era witnessed many advancements in community health nursing. Because of limited local and national resources, many people volunteered to assist others. These volunteers rapidly learned the value of community health nursing. Also, many federally funded relief projects utilized nurses, which led to the need for these federally employed nurses to provide consultation to the states. In 1934 Pearl McIver became the first nurse employed by the U.S. Public Health Service to provide consultation services to state health departments (Buhler-Wilkerson, 1985; Buhler-Wilkerson, 1989; Kalisch and Kalisch, 1986).

In addition, in the early post–World War I years, the **Frontier Nursing Service** (FNS) was developed by **Mary Breckinridge** (see box on p. 14 and Figure 1-5). The FNS was characterized by a unique pioneering spirit and was influential in the development of community health programs geared toward improv-

ing the health care of a rural and often inaccessible population in the Appalachian sections of Kentucky (Browne, 1966; Tirpak, 1975).

Meanwhile, substantial changes took place at the federal level, affecting the structure of community health resources. The federal **Social Security Act of 1935** was the first of these changes. Title VI of the act affected the scope of community health through its original mission to assist states and their subdivisions in the establishment and maintenance of adequate community health services. These services included the training of personnel for both state and local health activities (Buhler-Wilkerson, 1985; Kalisch and Kalisch, 1986).

As the Social Security Act of 1935 attempted to overcome the national setbacks of the depression, it expanded community health nursing. Title VI stipulated protection and health promotion for all people, creating two particularly valuable provisions. First, it appropriated $8 million to assist states, counties, and medical districts to establish and maintain adequate health services, as well as to train public health workers. A second major provision was the allocation of $2 million for the research and the investigation of disease and sanitation. This act also provided funds for the education and employment of community health nurses (Kalisch and Kalisch, 1986).

Mary Breckinridge and the Frontier Nursing Service

Born in 1881 into the fifth generation of a Kentucky family, Mary Breckinridge devoted her life to the establishment of the Frontier Nursing Service (FNS). Learning from her grandmother, who used a large part of her fortune to improve the education of southern children, Breckinridge later used money left to her by her grandmother to start the FNS (Browne, 1966).

Tutored in childhood and later attending private schools, Mary Breckinridge did not consider becoming a nurse until her husband died. In 1907 she began studying nursing at St. Luke's Hospital School of Nursing in New York. She later married for a second time and had two children. Her son died at the age of 4 years, and her daughter died at birth. From the time of her son's death in 1918, she devoted her energy to promoting the health care of disadvantaged women and children (Browne, 1966).

After World War I and her work in postwar France, she returned to the United States passionate about helping the neglected children of rural America. To prepare herself for what would become her life's work, she studied for 1 year at Teacher's College, Columbia University, to learn more about community health nursing (Browne, 1966).

Early in 1925 she returned to Kentucky. She decided that the mountains of Kentucky were an excellent place to demonstrate the value of community health nursing to remote, disadvantaged families. She thought that if she could establish a nursing center in rural Kentucky, this effort could then be duplicated anywhere. The first health center was established in a five-room cabin in Hyden, Kentucky. Establishing the center took not only nursing skills but also the construction of the center and later the hospital and other buildings; it required extensive knowledge about securing a water supply, disposing of sewage, getting electric power, and securing a mountain area in which landslides occurred (Browne, 1966). Despite many obstacles inherent in building in the mountains, six outpost nursing centers were built between 1927 and 1930. The FNS hospital in Hyden, Kentucky, was completed in 1928, and physicians began entering service. Payment of fees ranged from labor and supplies to funds raised through annual family dues, philanthropy, and fund-raising efforts of Mary Breckinridge (Frontier Nursing Service, 1978; Holloway, 1975).

The FNS established medical, surgical, and dental clinics; provided nursing and midwifery services 24 hours a day; and served nearly 10,000 people spread out over 700 square miles. At the suggestion of a supportive physician, baseline data were obtained on infant and maternal mortality before beginning services. The reduced mortality following the inception of the FNS is especially remarkable considering the environmental conditions in which these rural Kentuckians lived. Many homes had no heat, electricity, or running water. Often physicians were located over 40 miles from their patients (Frontier Nursing Service, 1978; Tirpak, 1975).

During the 1930s, nurses lived and saw patients from one of the six outposts and often had to make their visits on horseback. Like her nurses, Mary Breckinridge traveled many miles through the mountains of Kentucky on her horse, Babette, providing food, supplies, and health care to mountain families (Browne, 1966).

Over the years several hundred nurses have worked at the FNS. Despite the fact that Mary Breckinridge died in 1965, the FNS has continued to grow and provide needed services to people in the mountains of Kentucky. This service continues today as a vital and creative way to deliver community health services to rural families.

World War II to 1960

The onset of World War II in 1941 accelerated the need for nurses. Many nurses joined the Army and Navy Nurse Corps. Substantial funding was provided by the Bolton Act of 1943 to establish the Cadet Nurses Corps. The National Nursing Council, which comprised six national nursing organizations and was assisted by the U.S. Department of Education, received $1 million to expand facilities for nursing education. The U.S. Public Health Service managed these nursing education funds. During this time, community health nursing expanded its scope of practice. Community health nurses moved into rural areas, and many official agencies began to provide bedside nursing care (Buhler-Wilkerson, 1985; Kalisch and Kalisch, 1986).

Many changes after World War II subsequently affected community health nursing (Table 1-3). These changes included a more prosperous economy, prohibition, and increasing use of the automobile. Where community health nurses had previously made visits on foot, in horse-drawn buggies, or on bicycles, automobiles made it possible to see far more people. Also, wartime service had called national attention to the poor health of young and middle-aged males. Approximately 29% of all men called up for military service were rejected because of poor and often preventable health conditions (Kalisch and Kalisch, 1986; Roberts and Heinrich, 1985).

As veterans returned home from the war, because of the level of military health care that they had received, they expected a higher quality of health care. Local health departments were soon faced with a group of patients who expected services and with a sudden increase in emotional problems, accidents, alcoholism, and other health problems not previously considered to be in their treatment domain (Roberts and Heinrich, 1985). Funds were increased and targeted to specific health problems such as venereal disease, cancer, tuberculosis, and mental illness. Likewise, funding through the GI bill was available to send veterans to school, and many veterans chose community health (Kalisch and Kalisch, 1986).

One considerable setback in this decade was the dilution of community health content in nursing curricula. Students received limited information on groups and the community as a unit of service. Instead, nursing education focused heavily on the care of individuals, which meant that new graduates were not adequately prepared to work in community health without considerable agency orientation and teaching (National Organization for Public Health Nursing, 1944). Training for Nurses for National Defense, the GI Bill, the Nurse Training Act of 1943, and Public Health and Professional Nurse Traineeships provided additional educational funds (McNeil, 1967).

After World War II, local health departments increased dramatically. By 1955, 72% of all counties in the continental United States had full-time local health services. Community health nurses constituted

Table 1-3 Milestones in History of Community Health and Community Health Nursing: 1946-1995

Year	Milestone
1946	Nurses classified as professionals by U.S. Civil Service Commission; Hill-Burton Act approved providing funds for hospital construction in underserved areas and requiring these hospitals to provide care to poor people for a designated number of years; passage of National Mental Health Act
1948	NLN established accrediting service for nursing education programs
1950	25,091 nurses employed in public health
1951	NLN recommended that college-based nursing education programs include public health content
1960	NLN established criteria for evaluation of educational programs in nursing that lead to BSN and MS degrees
1964	Passage of Economic Opportunity Act; public health nurse defined by the ANA as a graduate of a BSN program; Congress amended Social Security Act to include Medicare and Medicaid
1965	ANA position paper recommended that nursing education take place in institutions of higher learning
1977	Passage of Rural Health Clinic Services Act, which provided indirect reimbursement for nurse practitioners in rural health clinics
1978	Establishment of Association of Graduate Faculty in Community Health Nursing/Public Health Nursing (later renamed as Association of Community Health Nursing Educators)
1980	Medicaid amendment to the Social Security Act to provide direct reimbursement for nurse practitioners in rural health clinics; both ANA and APHA developed statements on the role and conceptual foundations of community health nursing
1983	Beginning of Medicare prospective payments
1985	National Center for Nursing Research established in National Institutes of Health (NIH)
1988	Institute of Medicine published *The Future of Public Health*
1990	Association of Community Health Nursing Educators published *Essentials of Baccalaureate Nursing Education*
1991	Over 60 nursing organizations joined forces to support health care reform and published a document entitled *Nursing's Agenda for Health Care Reform*
1993	*American Health Security Act of 1993* published as a blueprint for national health care reform; the national effort, however, failed, leaving states and the private sector to design their own programs
1994	NCNR began the National Institute for Nursing within the National Institutes of Health

a large proportion of the staff in these health departments. During the 1950s there was considerable interest in nurse-midwifery, equality and advancement of black nurses in community health nursing, cost analysis methods and studies, inclusion of nursing services in health insurance programs, and better coordination of organized nursing (Roberts and Henrich, 1985).

In 1946 a committee of representatives from agencies interested in community health met to establish guidelines for this area of nursing ("Desirable organization," 1946). These guidelines became necessary because community health nursing evolved in an unplanned fashion with sponsorship by many voluntary agencies, thereby leading to a great deal of overlap of services. The guidelines took into account this history of community health nursing and proposed that a population of 50,000 be required to support a community health program and that there should be one nurse for each 2200 people. Other principles addressed were that the function of community health nursing should include health teaching, disease control, and care of the sick and that the community should adopt one of the following organizational patterns ("Desirable organization," 1946):

1. All community health nurse services administered by the local health department
2. Preventive health care provided by health departments and home health care provided by a cooperating voluntary agency
3. A combination service jointly administered and financed by official and voluntary agencies with all services provided by one group of community health nurses

1960 to the Present

The 1960s witnessed a revolution in health care that affected community health and community health nursing. In 1964 the passage of the Economic Opportunity Act provided funds for neighborhood health centers, Head Start, and many other community action programs. Funding was also increased for maternal and child health, mental health and mental retardation, and community health training. In 1965 Congress amended the Social Security Act to include health insurance benefits for the elderly (Medicare) and increased care for the poor (Medicaid). Unfortunately, the revised Social Security Act did not include coverage for preventive services, and home health care was compensated for only when ordered by the physician. However, this latter coverage prompted the rapid proliferation of home health care agencies. Many local and state health departments rapidly changed their policies to allow them to provide reimbursable home care. This often led to the decline of their health promotion and disease prevention activities. From 1960 to 1968 the number of official agencies that provided home care services grew from 250 to 1328, and the number of for-profit agencies also increased (Kalisch and Kalisch, 1986).

Two additional major factors influenced community health nursing during the 1960s: (1) the development of the nurse practitioner movement and (2) the call for the evaluation of the effectiveness of community health programs. The nurse practitioner movement began in 1965 at the University of Colorado and opened a new era for nursing's involvement in primary health care. Initially, the nurse practitioner was a community health nurse with additional skills in the diagnosis and treatment of common illnesses. Although many nurse practitioners remained in community health, others migrated to a variety of clinical areas. Those who remained in community health have made sustained contributions in providing primary health care to people in rural areas, inner cities, and other medically underserved areas (Roberts and Heinrich, 1985).

The enthusiasm of the 1960s continued into the 1970s. Prevention regained prominence at the federal level. The individual orientation of health care in the 1960s gave way in the 1970s to a review of what broader views needed to be considered to provide comprehensive health care services. Evaluation of the effectiveness of care was emphasized. Nursing was viewed as a powerful force in improving the health care of communities. Nurse practitioners became increasingly accepted as cost-effective providers of primary health care services. Educational programs to prepare nurse practitioners grew. In general, community health nursing and nursing in general were on the move. Nurses made significant contributions to the hospice movement, the development of birthing centers, day care for elderly and disabled persons, drug abuse programs, and rehabilitation services in long-term care (Roberts and Heinrich, 1985).

During the 1980s concern grew about the high costs of health care in the United States. Health promotion and disease prevention programs received less priority as funding was shifted to meet the escalating costs of hospital care and medical procedures. The use of ambulatory services including health maintenance organizations was encouraged. Home health care and the services of nurse practitioners grew. People were encouraged to assume more responsibility for their own health status. Health education, always a part of community health nursing, became increasingly popular. Consumer groups urged laws to prohibit unhealthy practices in public such as smoking and driving under the influence of alcohol.

As federal and state funds grew scarce, the presence of nurses in official public health agencies diminished. However, community health nurses, steadfast in their determination to improve the health care of Americans, have pressed for greater involvement in official and private agencies (Kalisch and Kalisch, 1986; Roberts and Heinrich, 1985).

The establishment in 1985 of the National Center for Nursing Research (NCNR) within the National Institutes of Health in Washington, D.C., has been a major tool in promoting the work of nurses. Through research, nurses can document the quality of care they provide by looking at the cost-effectiveness of their actions and also at the outcomes of nursing intervention. Because of the concerted efforts of many nurses, the NCNR was approved for official institute status within the National Institutes of Health in 1993 and became the National Institute of Nursing (NIN).

By the latter part of the 1980s public health had reached an all-time low in terms of its effectiveness in carrying out its mission and affecting health. The seriousness of what had happened was most vividly described in the report of the Institute of Medicine (IOM) entitled *The Future of Public Health* (1988). Essentially, the study group assigned by the IOM to thoughtfully determine the state of public health in the United States found public health to be "in disarray" (IOM, 1988, p. 10). The study group concluded that although there was widespread agreement about what the mission of public health should be, there was little consensus on how to translate that mission into action. In fact, they found that the mix and level of public health services varied from place to place in the United States (Williams, 1995).

The IOM report stated that the core public health functions were assessment, policy development, and assurance. Assessment means that public health agencies should "collect, assemble, analyze and make available information on the health of the community, including statistics on health status, community health needs, and epidemiological and other studies of health problems" (IOM, 1988, p. 7). The report also recommended that public health agencies become actively involved in helping to develop comprehensive public health policies. Assurance meant that public health agencies should assure their constituents that they would either provide agreed on services or encourage actions to see that some other entity provides the services.

In addition to the landmark document by the IOM on the future of public health, two additional documents by the Public Health Service, *Healthy People 2000: National Health Promotion and Disease Prevention Objectives* (1991) and *Healthy Communities 2000: Model Standards* (1991), were published to influence goal setting in public health. The first document, *Healthy People 2000* (1991), set forth a national strategy for significantly improving health in the years to come by describing strategies for preventing major chronic illness, injuries, and infectious diseases. Specific goals and objectives were established, and time frames for accomplishing them were set forth. The strategies recommended by this document are summarized in Appendix A. Implementation of the strategies called for in these documents has had considerable influence on community health nursing, and many of the objectives and strategies for their accomplishment are described in chapters throughout this text.

The 1990s have been a decade of debate about health care. The central issues have involved cost, quality, and access. Although there has been considerable interest in universal coverage, neither individuals nor employers are willing to pay for this level of service. Public health was a minor point of discussion during the health care reform debate of the early 1990s. The core content of the debate centered around economics, with most suggested strategies dealing with reform of medical care, not health care reform.

In 1991 the American Nurses Association, the American Association of Colleges of Nursing, the National League for Nursing, and more than 60 other

specialty nursing organizations joined to support health care reform. The document resulting from this historic joint effort of more than 60 nursing organizations set forth a range of efforts designed to build a healthy nation through improved primary care and public health efforts. In addition, key health care issues such as access, quality, and cost were also addressed. Similarly, in 1993 a blue-ribbon group assembled by President Bill Clinton and with Mrs. Clinton serving as chair published *The American Health Security Act*. This act, although not supported in Congress, did address a range of issues and concerns in health care, especially the organization and delivery of medical care. The act also stimulated considerable activity both at the state level and within the private sector to reform health care. However, the aims of public health were never clearly considered in the act, leaving a visible void in the design of a comprehensive program for health care.

Public health nursing celebrated "A Century of Caring" in 1993. This significant anniversary provided an opportunity for many organizations and professional groups to reflect on the many and varied contributions made over the years by nurses in this specialty area. Two excellent photograph books were published in 1993 to celebrate the centennial. They are *A Century of Caring: a Celebration of Public Health Nursing in the United States, 1883-1993* (U.S. Public Health Service, Division of Nursing, Bureau of Health Professions, 1993) and *Healing at Home: Visiting Nurse Service of New York, 1893-1993* (Denker, 1994). Both of these photo essays pointed out how courageous, caring, and committed public health nurses have been for the past 100 years. They traced many of the specific contributions that these nurses have made as they have, often with minimal support and few resources, sought to serve people who frequently have nearly overwhelming health problems. A major common theme of public health nursing has been and continues to be: reaching out to care for the health of people in need (U.S. Public Health Service, 1993).

What Do You Think?

What is needed in health care reform is attention to health, especially attention to public health. The focus has typically been on medical care reform with particular attention to the financing of care.

Key Concepts

- ◆ An understanding of the dominant cultural ideas of each era since early recorded history is useful in understanding the antecedents of the current community health care system.
- ◆ Rudiments of community health can be traced to the earliest civilizations.
- ◆ With the dawn of the Christian era, a new conceptualization of human beings influenced health practices. The early church believed that the Roman and Greek ways pampered the body at the expense of the soul. Disease was viewed as a punishment for sin.
- ◆ The Renaissance ushered in a new period of

history during which community health as currently known began.
- ◆ The Industrial Revolution witnessed tremendous advances in transportation, communication, and other forms of technology. Modern public health efforts began in England, the first modern industrial nation.
- ◆ The first salaried visiting nurse in the United States was Frances Root, who was hired in 1887 by the Women's Branch of the New York City Mission to provide home health care to sick persons.

Continued.

Key Concepts—cont'd

◆ Lillian Wald organized visiting nursing in New York in the nineteenth century, established the unique program at the Henry Street Settlement, and was responsible for many improvements in living conditions in New York City.

◆ The early twentieth century witnessed multiple improvements that both directly and indirectly affected health status.

◆ Several significant events influenced the further development of community health efforts in the first half of the twentieth century, including two major wars and an economic depression.

◆ The Frontier Nursing Service (FNS) was influential in the development of community health programs and was characterized by a unique pioneering spirit.

◆ As the Social Security Act of 1935 attempted to overcome the national setbacks of the depression, it expanded community health nursing.

◆ Over the years, community health nursing has evolved from a home care service characterized as being delivered by caring women who ministered to both the health and spiritual needs of individuals and families to a broadly based, population-focused discipline that considers individuals, families, groups, and communities as it scope of practice.

Critical Thinking Activities

1. Write a summary of what you believe were Lillian Wald's greatest contributions to community health nursing.

2. If you were Lillian Wald and chose to devote your energy to critical forces affecting the health of Americans, what would be your three highest priority efforts?

3. Of the three efforts, take one and develop a realistic plan for implementation and evaluation.

4. Telephone or visit one voluntary agency in your community and describe its purpose, source of funding, major programs or services, and eligibility of recipients of services.

5. Interview three nurses employed in community health nursing to determine how they currently define their role.

Bibliography

Backer BA: Lillian Wald: connecting caring with action, *Nurs Health Care* 14:122-128, 1993.

Brainard AM: *Evolution of public health nursing*, Philadelphia, 1922, Saunders.

Browne H: A tribute to Mary Breckenridge, *Nurs Outlook* 14:54-55, May 1966.

Buhler-Wilkerson J: Public health nursing: then and now, *Am J Pub Health* 75:1155-1161, 1985.

Buhler-Wilkerson J: *False dawn: the rise and decline of public health nursing, 1900-1930*, New York, 1989, Garland Publishing.

Bullough V, Bullough B: *The emergence of modern nursing*, New York, 1964, Macmillan.

Cohen IB: Florence Nightingale, *Sci Am* 250(3):128-137, 1984.

Deloughery GL: *History and trend of professional nursing*, ed 8, St Louis, 1977, Mosby–Year Book.

Denker EP (editor): *Healing at home: visiting Nurse Service of New York, 1893-1993*, New York, 1994, The Carl and Lily Pforzheimer Foundation.

Desirable organization for public health nursing for family service, *Pub Health Nurs* 38:387-389, Aug 1946.

Dickens C: In Furbank PN (editor): *Martin Chuzzlewit*, New York, 1975, Penguin Books.

Dock LL: The history of public health nursing (reprinted by The American Public Health Association from *The public health nurse*, 1922).

Dock L, Steward I: *A short history of nursing*, ed 4, New York, 1983, GP Putnam's Sons.

Dolan J: *History of nursing*, ed 14, Philadelphia, 1978, Saunders.

Frachel RR: A new profession: the evolution of public health nursing, *Pub Health Nurs* 5(2):86-90, 1988.

Griffin GJ, Griffin JK: *History and trends of professional nursing*, ed 7, St Louis, 1973, Mosby–Year Book.

Healthy People 2000: national health promotion and disease prevention objectives, Washington, DC, 1991, USDHHS, Public Health Service.

Holloway JB: Frontier Nursing Service 1925-1975, *J Ky Med Assoc* 13:491-492, Sept 1975.

Institute of Medicine: *The future of public health*, Washington, DC 1988, National Academy of Science.

Kalisch P, Kalisch BJ: *Nursing involvement in the health planning process*, DHEW pub no HRA 78-25, Hyattsville, Md, 1977, US Department of Health, Education and Welfare.

Kalisch P, Kalisch BJ: *The advance of American nursing*, ed 2, Boston, 1986, Little, Brown & Co.

McNeil EE: *Transition in public health nursing*, John Sundwall Lecture, University of Michigan, Feb 27, 1967.

National Organization for Public Health Nursing: Approval of Skidmore College of Nursing as preparing students for public health nursing, *Pub Health Nurs* 36:371, July 1944.

New York Visiting Nurse Service: Healing at home, *Nurs Health Care* 15:66-73, 1994.

Nightingale F: *Notes on nursing: what it is, and what it is not*, Philadelphia, 1946, Lippincott (reprinted).

Palmer IS: *Florence Nightingale and the first organized delivery of nursing services*, Washington, DC, 1983, American Association of Colleges of Nursing.

Pellegrino ED: Medicine, history, and the idea of man, *Ann Am Acad Pol Soc Sci* 346:9-20, March 1963.

Pickett G, Hanlon JJ: *Public health administration and practice*, ed 9 St Louis, 1990, Times Mirror/Mosby College Publishing.

Roberts DE, Heinrich J: Public health nursing comes of age, *Am J Pub Health* 75(10):1162-1172, 1985.

Rosen G: *A history of public health,* New York, 1958, MD Publications.

Shyrock H: *The history of nursing,* Philadelphia, 1959, Saunders.

Swinson A: *The history of public health,* Exeter, England, 1965, A Wheaton & Co.

Tirpak H: The Frontier Nursing Service—fifty years in the mountains, *Nurs Outlook* 33:308-310, May 1975.

US Public Health Service, Division of Nursing, Bureau of Health Professions: *A century of caring: a celebration of public health nursing in the United States, 1883-1993,* Washington, DC, 1993, US Government Printing Office.

US Public Health Service, US Department of Health and Human Services: *Healthy communities 2000: model standards,* Washington, DC, 1991, US Government Printing Office.

Williams CA: Beyond the Institute of Medicine report: a critical analysis and public health forecast, *Fam Comm Health* 18(1):12-21, 1995.

Wilner DM, Walkey RP, O'Neill EJ: *Introduction to public health,* ed 7, New York, 1978, Macmillan.

Zerwekh JV: Public health nursing legacy: historical practical wisdom, *Nurs Health Care* 13:84-91, 1992.

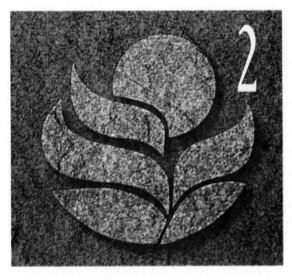

Community-Based Population-Focused Practice: The Foundation of Specialization in Public Health Nursing

Carolyn A. Williams

Key Terms

aggregate
community health nurse
Core Functions Project
Health Services Pyramid
noninstitutional populations
nursing roles
population
population-focused practice
public health
public health nurse
public health nursing specialist
subpopulations

Objectives ▼

After reading this chapter, the student should be able to do the following:

◆ State the mission and core functions of public health and the essential public health services.
◆ Describe specialization in public health nursing and community health nursing and the practice goals of each.
◆ Contrast clinical community health nursing practice with population-focused practice.
◆ Describe what is meant by population-focused practice.
◆ Name barriers to acceptance of population-focused practice.
◆ State key opportunities for population-focused practice.

Outline ▼

As America looks toward the twenty-first century, its citizens and health professionals are experiencing major changes in health care delivery. Despite the failure of the Clinton administration's efforts to reform health care, other federal, state, and private market forces are transforming the health care system. Questions about access to care, the ability to maintain insurance coverage, quality, and health care costs represent key forces for reform at the federal and state levels as well as in the private sector. In this context a community-based, population-focused approach to planning, delivering, and evaluating nursing care has never been more important. This is a crucial time for public health nursing and community health nursing, a time of opportunity and challenge. The issue of cost compounded with the changing demography of the United States population, specifically the aging of the population, is expected to put ever-escalating pressures on resources available for health care. Finally, and of paramount importance to the public health community, is the emergence of modern-day epidemics and causes of mortality, many of which affect the young, infants and teenagers and most of which are preventable.

PUBLIC HEALTH PRACTICE: THE FOUNDATION FOR HEALTHY POPULATIONS AND COMMUNITIES

During the last two years much attention has been directed to various proposals designed to reform what has generally been referred to as the health care system in America. A more accurate description of these proposals reveals that they have focused on cost containment in medical care financing and strategies for providing health insurance coverage to a higher proportion of the population. Since medical treatment is estimated to account for approximately 99% of the nation's aggregate health expenditures (U.S. Public Health Service, 1993) it is understandable that such an emphasis would prevail. But what if one is looking in the wrong place for maximum benefits for minimal expenditures? The truth is, that's exactly what is happening! As stated in the U.S. Public Health Services Report on the Core Functions of Public Health, reform of the medical insurance system is necessary, but it is not sufficient for improving the health of Americans. "Historically, gains in the health of populations have derived largely from changes in the safety and adequacy of food supplies, in the provision of safe water, in sewage disposal, and in personal behavior, including reproductive behavior. . . . The dramatic gain in life expectancy for Americans over the course of this century, from less than 50 years in 1900 to more than 75 years in 1990, is attributed primarily to improvements in sanitation, the control of infectious diseases through immunizations, and other public health activities" (U.S. Public Health Service, 1993). The report further states that "population-based preventive programs launched in the 1970s are also largely responsi-

ble for the more recent changes in tobacco use, blood pressure control, dietary patterns (except obesity), automobile safety restraint, and injury control measures that have fostered declines of more than 50% in stroke deaths, 40% in coronary heart disease deaths, and 25% in overall death rates for children" (U.S. Public Health Service, 1993).

Did You Know?

The concept of using a population/aggregate approach in the practice of community health nursing began to be seriously discussed in the 1970s.

Another way of comparing the impact of medical treatment with the benefits of public health practice is to look at the extent to which early deaths can be prevented. The U.S. Public Health Service estimates that medical treatment can prevent only about 10% of all early deaths in the United States. Yet, "population-wide public health approaches have the potential to help prevent some 70 percent of early deaths in America through measures targeted to the factors that contribute to those deaths. Many of these contributing factors are behavioral such as tobacco use and diet and sedentary lifestyles; others are environmental in nature" (U.S. Public Health Service, 1995).

Public health practice is a great buy! The U.S. Public Health Service estimated in 1993 that only 0.9% of all national health expenditures support population-based public health functions, yet as we have just seen, the impact is enormous. Unfortunately, the public is largely unaware of the contributions of public health practice. Also, the proportion of expenditures for public health activities has actually declined by approximately 25% over the last ten years! Some of this decline has been attributed to the fact that over the last two decades public health agencies have had to provide personal care services to shore up shortfalls in the delivery system. The result is a shift of resources and energy away from public health's traditional and unique population-wide perspective (U.S. Public Health Service, 1995). Because of its importance in influencing the health of the population and in providing a strong foundation for the health care system, the U.S. Public Health Service and other groups are vigorously advocating a renewed emphasis on the population-wide essential functions and services of public health that have made the greatest impact on improving the health of the entire population. As part of this effort, the statement presented in Figure 2-1 was developed by a work group made up of representatives of various federal agencies and organizations concerned about public health. The list of essential services presented in Figure 2-1 represents a specification and illustration of the fundamental obligations of public health for the core functions of assessment, assur-

PUBLIC HEALTH IN AMERICA

Vision:
Healthy people in healthy communities

Mission:
Promote physical and mental health and prevent disease, injury, and disability

Public health

- ❖ Prevents epidemics and the spread of disease
- ❖ Protects against environmental hazards
- ❖ Prevents injuries
- ❖ Promotes and encourages healthy behaviors
- ❖ Responds to disasters and assists communities in recovery
- ❖ Assures the quality and accessibility of health services

Essential public health services

- ❖ Monitors health status to identify community health problems
- ❖ Diagnoses and investigates health problems and health hazards in the community
- ❖ Informs, educates, and empowers people about health issues
- ❖ Mobilizes community partnerships to identify and solve health problems
- ❖ Develops policies and plans that support individual and community health efforts
- ❖ Enforces laws and regulations that protect health and ensure safety
- ❖ Links people to needed personal health services and assures the provision of health care when otherwise unavailable
- ❖ Assures a competent public health and personal health care workforce
- ❖ Evaluates effectiveness, accessibility, and quality of personal and population-based health services
- ❖ Researches for new insights and innovative solutions to health problems

Source: Essential Public Health Services Work Group of the Core
              Public Health Functions Steering Committee

Membership: American Public Health Association
              Association of State and Territorial Health Officials
              National Association of County and City Health Officials
              Institute of Medicine, National Academy of Sciences
              Association of Schools of Public Health
              Public Health Foundation
              National Association of State Alcohol and Drug Abuse Directors
              National Association of State Mental Health Program Directors
              U.S. Public Health Service
                Centers for Disease Control and Prevention
                Health Resources and Services Administration
                Office of the Assistant Secretary for Health
                Substance Abuse and Mental Health Services Administration
                Agency for Health Care Policy and Research
                Indian Health Service
                Food and Drug Administration

FIGURE 2-1
Public health in America.

ance, and policy development discussed above. More complete discussions can be found in the bibliography (U.S. Public Health Service, 1993, 1995).

In 1988 the Institute of Medicine published a report on the future of public health. In that report **public health** was defined as "what we, as a society, do collectively to assure the conditions in which people can be healthy" (Institute of Medicine, 1995). The committee stated that the aim of public health was "to generate organized community effort to address the public interest in health by applying scientific and technical knowledge to prevent disease and promote health" (Institute of Medicine, 1995). It was clearly acknowledged that the mission could be accomplished by many groups, public and private, and by individuals, but the idea was put forth that government has a special function and that is "to see to it that vital elements are in place and that the mission is adequately addressed" (Institute of Medicine, 1995). To clarify the governmental role in fulfilling the mission, the report stated that assessment, policy development, and assurance are the core functions at all levels of government. Assessment refers to systematic data collection on the population, monitoring of the population's health status, and making information available on the health of the community. Policy development refers to the need to provide leadership in developing policies which support the health of the population, including the use of the scientific knowledge base in decision-making about policy. Assurance refers to the role of public health in making sure that essential community-wide health services are available, which may include providing essential personal health services for those who would otherwise not receive them. Assurance also refers to making sure that a competent public health and personal health care workforce is available. Those involved in the **Core Functions Project,** a subgroup of the U.S. Public Health Service, also developed a useful illustration, the **Health Services Pyramid** (See Figure 2-2) which shows that population-based public health programs focusing on disease prevention, health protection, and health promotion provide a foundation upon which primary, secondary, and tertiary health care services rest. All levels of services shown in the pyramid are important to the health of the population and thus must be part of a health care system with health as a goal, "but the greater the effectiveness of services in the lower tiers, the greater is the capability of higher tiers to contribute efficiently to health improvement" (U.S. Public Health Service, Prevention Report, 1995). Because of the importance of the foundational public health programs, members of the Core Functions Project argued that "financing any tier of the overall health care system at the expense of those below it undermines the system's integrity" (U.S. Public Health Service, 1995).

New initiatives designed to enable public health practitioners to be more effective in actualizing the core functions of assessment and assurance are now

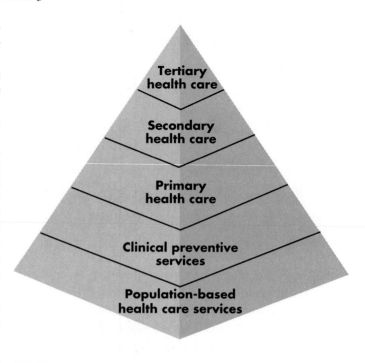

FIGURE 2-2
Health services pyramid.

underway at the national level. The Institute of Medicine has initiated a project on public health performance monitoring. They plan to organize two workshops and produce a report. The first workshop will focus on a review of "indicators that are currently being used to assess population health status and risk factors and to measure the performance of state and local public health agencies PHS programs, and health plans in providing population-based core public health functions, and in promoting individual health education and access to preventive health care services" (IOM, Board on Health Promotion, 1995). The second workshop will focus on public health indicators that can be measured in national information systems and "identify data sources for other important public health indicators. . . that can not be measured through such a system. It is anticipated that the report of the project will include policy recommendations and integrated sets of indicators.

The second initiative is the Guideline Development Project for public health practice which has been undertaken by the Council on Linkages Between Academia and Public health practice, based at Johns Hopkins University and funded by the Kellogg Foundation (Council on Linkages Between Academia and Public Health Practice, 1995). This effort is directed at developing a methodology for generating public health practice guidelines which are usable and practical. Both of these efforts are important because they hold promise for putting tools and methods into the hands of public health practitioners, many of whom are public health nursing specialists, to enable them to be more effective in dealing with their core responsibilities.

THE RELATIONSHIP BETWEEN PUBLIC HEALTH NURSING AND COMMUNITY HEALTH NURSING

Is it important to distinguish between public health nursing and community health nursing? Diverse opinions abound as to what public health nursing and community health nursing are and how they relate to each other. Many individuals use the terms as though they were completely interchangeable. Some wish to minimize the differences because they feel that focusing on distinctions is trivial. However, some clarification is useful to grasp the importance of a population-focused approach, to understand its relationship to the success of nursing strategies directed toward community-based clients, and to be clear about the choices available in nursing roles. It may be helpful to define what is meant by the term "population" and to comment on what is meant by population-focused practice. A basic definition of a **population** or **aggregate** is a collection of individuals who have in common one or more personal or environmental characteristics. Thus those who are members of a community defined either in terms of geography (e.g., county) or a special interest (e.g., children attending a particular school) can be seen as constituting a population. Frequently it is useful to identify **subpopulations** within the larger population. Examples include high-risk infants under the age of 1, unmarried pregnant adolescents, or individuals exposed to a particular event such as a chemical spill. The basic notion in **population-focused practice** is that problems are defined (diagnoses) and solutions (interventions) are proposed for defined populations or subpopulations as opposed to diagnoses and intervention/treatment carried out at the patient or client level.

By contrast, much of the material in current community health textbooks presents the view that the focus of community health nursing is on providing services to individual persons and individual families in community settings. This emphasis is also the predominant focus of the American Nurses Association's statement, *A Conceptual Model of Community Health Nursing*, which was developed by the Division of Community Health Nursing (ANA, 1980).

Several distinctions relevant to this discussion are set forth in the ANA conceptual model. First, the statement identifies two categories of nurses in community health: generalists prepared at the baccalaureate level who practice in community health settings and specialists in community health nursing who have master's level preparation or beyond. The practice of the generalists is described as follows (ANA, 1980):

The nursing process is applied to the client, who may be an individual, family, group, or community. While working with individual clients, the nurse keeps the community perspective in mind.

In describing the scope of practice for community health nursing, the major objectives of the community health nurse are stated as "the preservation and improvement of the health of a community" (ANA, 1980). One way to look at the relationship between public health nursing and community health nursing is to view public health nursing as a specialized field of practice with certain attributes within the broad arena of community health nursing. This view is consistent with recommendations developed at a Consensus Conference on the Essentials of Public Health Nursing Practice and Education, sponsored by the Division of Nursing and held in Washington, D.C., in September 1984 (1985).

One of the most interesting outcomes of the conference was consensus on the use of the terms *community health nurse* and *public health nurse*. It was agreed that the term **community health nurse** could apply to all nurses who practice in the community, whether or not they have had preparation in public health nursing. Thus, nurses providing tertiary care in a home setting, school nurses, nurses in clinic settings, in fact, any nurse who does not practice in an institutional setting falls into the category of "community health nurse." Nurses with a master's degree or a doctorate degree who are practicing in community settings can be referred to as "community health nurse specialists" regardless of the area of nursing in which the degree was earned. According to the conference statement, "the degree may be in any area of nursing, such as maternal-child health, psychiatric-mental health, or medical-surgical nursing or some subspecialty of any clinical area" (Consensus Conference, 1985, p. 4).

What Do You Think?

Are public health nursing, community health nursing, and community based nursing practice all the same?

In contrast to the focus on the setting as the key variable in defining the community health nurse, **public health nurse** was defined in terms of educational preparation. The participants of the consensus conference agreed "that the term 'public health nurse' should be used to describe a person who has received specific educational preparation and supervised clinical practice in public health nursing" (Consensus Conference, 1985, p. 4). At the basic or entry level, a public health nurse is one who "holds a baccalaureate degree in nursing that includes this educational preparation; this nurse may or may not practice in an official health agency but has the initial qualifications to do so" (Consensus Conference, 1985, p. 4). Specialists in public health nursing are defined as those who are prepared at the graduate level, either master's or doctoral, "with a focus in the public health sciences" (Consensus Conference, 1985, p. 4).

If one takes seriously the definitions of the community health nurse and the public health nurse agreed to in the 1984 consensus conference, it is clear that the setting in which one practices is viewed as the feature distinguishing community health nurses from other nurses. However, setting is not used to set apart public health nurses; here type of preparation is the distinguishing feature. Using setting as a distinguishing feature for community health nursing is problematic for several reasons.

First, the way community is equated with "noninstitutionalization" leads to further confusion. According to the statement, an individual who has received preparation in any clinical or subclinical area and who practices in a noninstitutional setting can be seen as a community health nursing specialist. Such a broad view may indeed be consistent with the way things have been perceived, but it is not clear that the distinction of setting is very meaningful. For example, two nurses could have completed a master's program in medical-surgical nursing with a subspecialization in nephrology. They both could be providing the same clinical services to similar populations, including home visits. But the nurse who is employed in a dialysis center would be viewed as a community health nursing specialist and the nurse working in the hospital-based dialysis center would not be seen as such a specialist.

Another problem with the use of setting as a distinguishing feature is that so much shifting and reorganization is occurring in the health care system that the institutional/noninstitutional distinction made in the consensus statement is outdated. Is a hospital-linked health maintenance organization an institutional setting? How does one define a hospital-based home care agency? For these reasons the use of setting to distinguish areas of specialization for nurses with graduate preparation has serious problems.

Public Health Nursing as a Field of Practice, an Area of Specialization

For the most part, the discussion to this point has focused on general definitions of the roles of community health nurses and public health nurses as opposed to the "field" of community health nursing and the "field" of public health nursing or the arenas encompassed by specialization in either "field." It is reasonable to ask, is community health nursing really a specialty area? It was suggested by those participating in the consensus conference mentioned above that "the term" 'community health nursing' came into broad use when the American Nurses Association sought to create a unit within the organization to which nurses working in scattered community settings could belong. These settings included "doctors' offices, work sites, schools, street clinics, and other similar community locations where nursing functions are carried out" (ANA, 1980, p. 3). The consensus conference report went on to elaborate that the term 'community health nurse' is simply an umbrella term used for all nurses who work in the community, including those who have formal preparation in public health nursing.

In essence, public health nursing requires specific educational preparation and community health nursing denotes a setting for the practice of nursing" (Consensus Conference, 1985, p. 4). If one accepts this view it may be difficult to see community health nursing as a discrete specialty. Thus, rather than calling graduate-prepared nurses who simply work in community settings "community health nurse specialists," it might be more clear and more appropriate to refer to these nurses in a manner that is more in keeping with their area of practice specialization (e.g., ambulatory pediatrics, nurse midwifery, or school nursing). In contrast, a case can be made that public health nursing clearly is an area of specialization. What makes it so? The focus of practice, detailed below, and special knowledge supporting the practice set public health nursing apart from other areas of nursing practice.

With regard to the nature of practice, four characteristics are particularly salient: (1) the focus on populations that are free-living in the community as opposed to those that are institutionalized; (2) the predominant emphasis on strategies for health promotion, health maintenance, and disease prevention; (3) the concern for the connection between health status of the population and the living environment (physical, biological, sociocultural); and (4) The use of political processes to affect public policy as a major intervention strategy for achieving goals.

In 1981 the public health nursing section of the American Public Health Association put forth a statement on the Definition and Role of Public Health Nursing in the Delivery of Health Care, which clearly describes the field of specialization. Central elements of their definition were as follows:

Public health nursing synthesizes the body of knowledge from the public health sciences and professional nursing theories. The implicit over-riding goal is to improve the health of the community. . . . Public Health Nursing practice is a systematic process by which:

1. The health and health care needs of a population are assessed in collaboration with other disciplines in order to identify subpopulations (aggregates), families, and individuals at increased risk of illness, disability, or premature death.
2. A plan for intervention is developed to meet these needs, which includes resources available and those activities that contribute to health and its recovery, the prevention of illness, disability, and premature death.
3. A health care plan is implemented effectively, efficiently, and equitably.
4. An evaluation is made to determine the extent to which these activities have an impact on the health status of the population (APHA, pp. 3-4).

With regard to preparation as mentioned earlier, the **public health nursing specialist** was defined by the 1984 consensus conference as one "prepared at the graduate level with a focus in the public health sciences; such a person holds a master's or doctoral degree, and may or may not practice in an official public health agency, but is qualified to do so, (Consensus

Conference, 1985, p. 4)." In the consensus statement it was specifically pointed out that the public health nursing specialist "should be able to work with population groups and to assess and intervene successfully at the aggregate level," (Consensus Conference, 1985, p. 11). Areas deemed essential for the preparation of such specialists were "Epidemiology, Biostatistics, Nursing theory, Management theory, Change theory, Economics, Politics, Public health administration, Community assessment, Program planning and evaluation, Interventions at the aggregate level, Research, History of public health, and Issues in public health" (Consensus Conference, 1985, p. 11).

Population-Focused Practice Versus Practice Focused on Individuals

It is proposed that the fundamental factors that distinguish specialization in public health nursing from other areas of nursing specialization are as follows: A focus on **populations** which are free living in the community as opposed to those institutionalized for episodes of care; a focus on strategies for health promotion, health maintenance, and disease prevention; and the use of strategies which take into account the broad social/po-

litical context in which community problems occur and are resolved. A population focus is historically consistent with public health philosophy and is reflected in the definition of public health nursing developed by the Public Health Nursing Section and officially adopted by the American Public Health Association (APHA, 1981). That statement defines the goal of public health nursing as "improving the health of the entire community" (APHA, 1981, p 4). Of particular significance is the APHA statement "Identifying subgroups (aggregates) within the population which are at high risk of illness, disability, or premature death and directing resources toward these groups is the most effective approach for accomplishing the goal of public health nursing" (AHPA, 1981, p 4). Such practice is built on but is different from basic clinical nursing practice.

Basic professional education in nursing, medicine, and other clinical disciplines focuses primarily on developing competence in decision-making at the level of the *individual* client—assessing health status, making management decision (ideally with the client), and evaluating the effects of care. In Figure 2-3, this basic educational focus on the individual is depicted by the individuals in any sub-population (see the *a* arrows). However, three levels of problem definition are

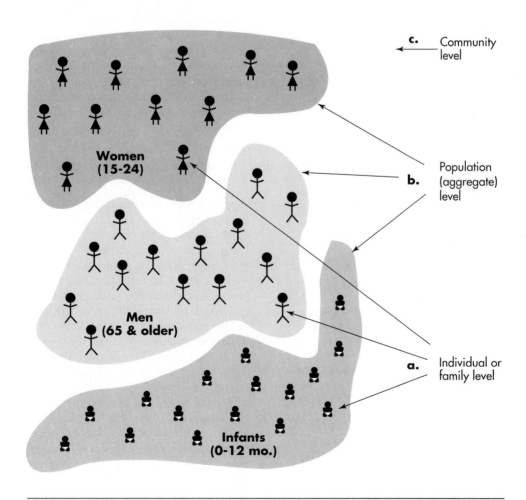

FIGURE 2-3
Levels of practice.

illustrated in Figure 2-3. For example, individual nurse clinicians, nurse practitioners, and sometimes public health nurses focus attention on individuals they see either in a home or clinic setting. Thus, their emphasis is on problem definition and resolution for individuals, each individual seen one at a time. However, it can be seen in Figure 2-3 that the individuals are grouped into three separate sub-populations, each of which has a characteristic in common (see the *b* arrows). Sub-populations such as these are frequently the focus of attention of public health nursing specialists who define problems at the sub-population or aggregate level as opposed to an individual level.

Research Brief

Olds D, Kitzman H: Can Home Visitation Improve the Health of Women and Children at Environmental Risk? *Pediatrics* 86(1):1990.

The purpose of this study was to review seven research studies related to randomized trials of prenatal and infancy home visitation programs for socially disadvantaged women and children. Three factors were examined to determine the success of the programs: 1) the underlying causal model of influences on maternal and child outcomes; 2) the corresponding content and structure of the services, and 3) the degree to which the population served is at environmental, behavioral, or psychosocial risk for the particular problem under consideration. This analysis focused only on review of research related to a primary prevention focus of improving the outcomes of pregnancy or the health or development of socially disadvantaged young children and their mothers.

The study fundings indicated that some home visitation programs were effective in improving women's health related behaviors during pregnancy, the birth weight and length of gestation of babies born to smokers and young adolescents, parents' interaction with their children, and children's developmental status; reducing the incidence of child abuse and neglect, childhood behavioral problems, emergency department visits and hospitalizations for injury, and unintended subsequent pregnancies; and increasing mothers' participation in the work force. The more effective programs employed nurses who began visiting during pregnancy, who visited frequently and long enough to establish a therapeutic alliance with families and who addressed the systems of behavioral and psychosocial factors that influence maternal and child outcomes. They also targeted families at greater risk for health problems by virtue of the parents' poverty and lack of personal and social resources.

This study clearly shows the importance of looking at the interaction between the social and psychological environment (ecological model) and health status. Another important feature is that it illustrates the desirability of targeting services to high-risk sub-populations.

Population-level decision-making is different from decision-making in clinical care and demands the specialized preparation described above. For example, in a clinical direct-care situation the nurse may determine that a client is hypertensive and explore options for intervention. At the population level the questions would include the following:
- What is the prevalence of hypertension among various age, race, and sex groups?
- Which subpopulations have the highest rates of untreated hypertension?
- What programs could reduce the problem of untreated hypertension and thereby lower the risk of further cardiovascular morbidity and mortality?

Usually, those who specialize in public health nursing are concerned with more than one subpopulation. Frequently, they are concerned with the health of the entire community, which is depicted in Figure 2-3 as all of the subgroups within a given community (see arrow *c*). Naturally, in the real world there are many more subgroups than those reflected in Figure 2-3. Those concerned with the health of a given community must ultimately consider the total population which is made up of multiple and sometimes overlapping subpopulations. Such an example could be adolescents at risk for unplanned pregnancies which would overlap with the female population age 15 to 24. A subpopulation which would overlap with infants under one year of age would be children from 0 to 6 years of age. In addition, a population focus requires consideration of those who may need particular services but have not entered the health care system (e.g., children without immunizations or patients with untreated hypertension).

The Arenas for Specialization in Public Health Nursing and Community Health Nursing

A very broad understanding of public health should include some concern for all populations within the community, both free-living and institutionalized. Further, it should consider the match between the health needs of the population and the health care resources in the community, including those services offered in institutional settings. Although all direct care providers may contribute to the community's health in the broadest sense, not all are primarily concerned with the population focus, or the "big picture." Thus all nurses in a given community, including those working in hospitals, physicians' offices, and health clinics, theoretically would be contributing positively to the health of the community. However, the special contributions of public health specialists are to look at the community as a whole, raise questions about its overall health status and factors associated with that status, and work to improve the population's health status.

The prevalent view of public health nurses historically and at present is that they provide direct care services, including health education, to persons or family units outside of institutional settings, either in the client's home or in a clinic environment. Such practice falls into the upper right quadrant *(section B)* in Figure 2-4. However, if one accepts the argument made earlier for specialization in public health nursing, such community-based population focused practice places specialization in public health nursing in the upper left quadrant *(section A)* in Figure 2-4. In addition to the population focus, there are three more reasons that the most important practice arena for public heath nursing is represented in the upper left quadrant of Figure 2-4. First, preventive strategies can have the greatest impact on **noninstitutionalized populations**, which represent the majority of a community most of the time. Second, the major interface between health status and the environment (physical, biological, sociocultural) occurs in the noninstitutional population. Third, for philosophical, historical, and economic reasons population-focused practice is most likely to flourish in organizational structures that serve noninstitutionalized populations (health departments, health maintenance organizations, health centers, etc.).

What roles in the care system would public health nursing specialists have? Options include Director of Nursing for a health department, Director of the Health Department, State Commissioner for Health, or Director of Maternal and Child Health services for a state or local health department. Although nurses have in the past occupied and currently do occupy all of these roles, they are in the minority. Frequently, nurses who do occupy these roles are not seen as public health nursing specialists. Where does the staff public health nurse fit into the scheme? It is suggested that the staff public health nurse is not a public health nurse specialist. Although she or he works in the context of a public health program, the focus of the practice is in dealing with individual patients and individual families, thus the arena for practice is in *section B* of the diagram.

Figure 2-4 also shows that specialization in public health nursing as it has been defined in this chapter is a part of the broader field of community health nursing. In the middle of the diagram is a box labeled specialization in community health nursing. It is partly in *section A* and partly in *section B*. This suggests that there is a need and a place for specialization in community health nursing that is more focused than the definition put forth in the consensus conference discussed earlier in the chapter. Such specialization would include some responsibilities for providing direct care services and some responsibilities for dealing with subpopulations in the community. Preparation for such specialization would include master's preparation in a direct-care clinical area (e.g., family nurse practitioner) and some work in the public health sciences. Examples of roles such specialists might have include case manager, supervisor in a home health agency, school nurse, occupational health nurse, parish nurse, and a nurse practitioner who also manages a nursing clinic.

Section C and *section D* represent nurses who focus on institutionalized populations. Nurses who provide direct care in hospital settings fall into *section D,* and those who are responsible for the administration of nursing services in institutional settings fall into *section C.*

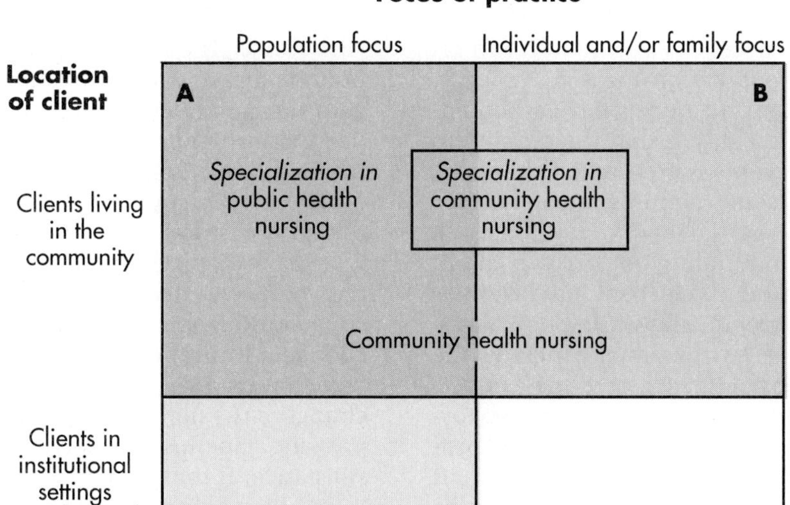

Focus of practice

FIGURE 2-4
Arenas of practice.

The Need to Think Broadly About Roles in Public Health Nursing

Within public health and community nursing circles there has been a tendency to talk about public health nursing and community health nursing from the point of view of a role, such as the public health nursing role or the community health nursing specialist. This is limiting. In discussing such **nursing roles** there is an enormous preoccupation with a direct care provider orientation. Even in discussions about how a practice can become more population-focused, it is interesting that the focus frequently is on how an individual practitioner, such as a staff nurse in an agency, can adopt such a practice focus. Rarely is attention given to how nurse administrators in public health (one role for public health nursing specialists) might reorient their practice toward a population focus, which is more critical and possible for an administrator than for the staff nurse. This is because in many agencies nursing administrators, supervisors, or others (sometimes program directors who are not nurses) make the key decisions about how staff nurses will spend their time—what types of clients will be seen and under what circumstances.

With regard to public health nursing administrators, those who are prepared to practice in a population-focused manner should be more effective than those who are not prepared to do so. In addition, staff public health nurses would benefit from having a clear understanding of population-focused practice for three reasons. First, it would give them professional satisfaction in being able to put their own clinical activities into perspective, to see how what they do clinically contributes at the population level. Second, it would help them understand and appreciate the practice of their associates who are population-focused specialists. Third, it would give them a firmer basis for providing clinical input to decision making at the program or agency level, a necessary contribution to effective and efficient population-focused practice. Clearly it is desirable that staff nurses have a population perspective, but the reality is that their ability to make decision at that level is more limited than that of the nurse who has some administrative responsibility.

Another problem with thinking too narrowly about nursing roles is that present role conceptualizations are frequently too limited to allow for population-focused practice. Also, roles that might include the type of decision making being suggested may not be defined as nursing roles. Examples include directorships of health departments, state or regional programs, and units of health planning and evaluation. If population-focused public health nursing is to be taken seriously and strategies for its implementation (assessment, intervention, and evaluation) are to be applied at the population level, more consideration must be given to organized systems for assessing population needs and managing care. Such a view of public health nursing clearly places those who specialize in this area in the position of dealing with health care policy. In other words, public health nurse specialists must move into situations in which policy formation is a recognized component; however, to do this, some nurses may have to assume positions outside of what are usually considered nursing positions or nursing roles. This is true because, at present, much of the policy-making that directly affects provision of nursing services to certain populations occurs outside the range of what are normally referred to as nursing roles.

Defining nursing roles so that they fit into the present way of structuring nursing services may have unfortunate limitations. For the immediate future it may be more useful to concentrate on identifying the skills and knowledge needed to make decisions in population-focused practice. It is also more important to define where in the broader community and health care system such decisions are made and to develop nurses with the substantive knowledge, skills, and political finesse necessary for success in such positions. Some of these positions are within nursing settings, particularly roles such as administrator of the nursing service and top level staff nurse administrators, but as suggested earlier, other such positions may be outside of what are traditionally viewed as nursing roles.

CHALLENGES FOR THE FUTURE

There are several barriers to the full development of specialization in public health nursing, and our challenge is to address them. One of the most serious is the "mind-set" of many nurses that the only role for a nurse is at the bedside or at the client's side, the direct care role. Clearly, the heart of nursing is the direct care provided in personal contacts with clients. On the other hand, two things should be clear to the observant nurse. The first is that whether a nurse is able to provide direct care services to a given client is contingent on a number of decisions on the part of individuals within and without of the care system. Second, nursing needs to be involved in those fundamental decisions. Perhaps the one-to-one focus of nursing and past cultural expectations of the "proper role" of women influenced nurses to view less positively indirect modes of contributing, such as administration, consultation, and research. However, two things have changed: In all fields, in and out of nursing, women have taken on every role imaginable. The second change is the population of male nurses is consistently growing. So this old barrier no longer has cultural substance. It must fall.

Another barrier to the type of practice implied in population-focused public health nursing is the structure within which nurses work and the process of role socialization that occurs within those structures. The fact that a particular role might not exist within the nursing unit may suggest that it is undesirable or impossible for nurses. For example, nurses interested in using political strategies to effect changes in health-related policy, an activity clearly within the practice domain of public health nursing, may run into a number of barriers if the goals disrupt the agenda of other groups within the health care arena. Such groups may use subtle but effective maneuvers to lead nurses to conclude that involvement takes them from the client and is not in their own or the client's best interests.

Another barrier is that relatively few nurses receive graduate level preparation in the concepts and strategies of disciplines basic to public health (e.g., epidemiology, biostatistics, community development, service administration, and policy formation). One of the problems mentioned earlier, which continues to be a problem in master's level preparation for public health nursing, is that in many programs the skills necessary for population assessment and management are not given the in-depth treatment accorded other components of the curriculum, particularly the direct care aspects. In short, with few exceptions, within the graduate programs in public health nursing and community health nursing, there is no aggressive effort to develop population-focused skills that are commensurate with the need (Josten et al, 1995). The bias of many nurses seems to be that these skills are less important than clinical skills. However, these skills are as essential as direct care skills; they are just as difficult to develop and they should be given more attention in graduate programs that prepare nurses for specialization in public health nursing.

The massive organizational changes occurring in the delivery system present a unique opportunity to establish new roles for nurse leaders who are prepared to think in population terms. In the 1980s Starr described the developing trend toward the use of private capital in financing health care, particularly institutional-based care and other health-related businesses. The movement can be thought of as the "industrialization" of health care, which until recently has operated very much like a "cottage industry." The implications and consequences of this movement, which has as a goal providing investors a return on their equity, are enormous. Major developments include more attention on primary care and community-based care delivery in a variety of settings, less emphasis on speciality care, the development of partnerships, alliances, and other linkages across settings in an effort to build integrated systems which would provide a broad range of services for the population which it serves; and a growing adoption of capitation (insurers agree to pay providers a fixed sum for each person per month or per year, independent of the costs actually incurred), as a reimbursement strategy. With the spread of capitation there is a growing interest throughout the health care system in the concept of populations, sometimes referred to by financial officers and others as "covered lives," (e.g. individuals with insurance which pays on a capitated basis). For public health specialists it is a new experience to see

individuals involved in the "business" aspects of health care and frequently employed by hospitals thinking in population terms and taking a population approach to decision-making.

This new focus on populations coupled with the integration that is occurring in some health care systems will likely create new roles for individuals, hopefully nurses, who will span in-patient and community-based settings and will focus on providing a wide range of services to the population served by the system. Such a role might be Director of Patient Care Services for a health care system. In addition to those who will have the administrative responsibility for a large programmatic area, there will be a demand for individuals who can design programs of preventive and clinical services to be offered to targeted subpopulations within the system. Who will decide what services will be given to which subpopulation by which providers? Large systems and consultant firms are currently offering courses designed to prepare physicians for such roles (Advisory Board Company 1994). What about nurses? How will they be prepared for what is ahead?

It is interesting that just as physician leaders are recognizing that some physicians need to be prepared to use population-oriented methods (epidemiology and biostatistics) to make evidence-based decisions in the development of programs and protocols, the attention being given to preparing nurses for administrative decision-making seems to be declining. This may be due to the lack of federal support for preparing nurse administrators and to the growing popularity of nurse practitioner programs. However, it is time that nurse leaders gave more attention to preparing nurses for leadership in this area. Perhaps it is time to forge the creative synthesis between specialization in public health nursing and nursing administration suggested sometime ago (Williams, 1985). One basis for suggesting this is that regardless of how the population is defined, there will be a growing need for nurses with population level assessment, management, and evaluation skills. Another basis is to accept the prediction that the primary focus of the health care system of the future will be on community-based strategies for health promotion and disease prevention, primary care, and much of secondary care. Our response should be to direct more attention to developing the specialty of public health nursing as a way of providing nursing leadership. To prepare for such population-focused decision-making will entail more attention to master's and doctoral level programs with a strong basis in the public health sciences.

Some observers of the public health scene anticipated that if universal coverage became a reality, public health practitioners could turn over the delivery of personal primary care services to others (HMO's, health plans, etc.) and go back to the core public health functions. However, as described earlier, assurance, making sure that basic services are available to all is a core function of public health. Thus, even under the condition of universal coverage there would still be a need to monitor subpopulations in the community to ensure that necessary care is available and when it is not, to see that it is provided. Universal coverage did not become a reality. Due to pressures in the health care system to cut costs and not shift costs, there is now a growing concern that the problem of access to basic primary care will get worse before it gets better, particularly for special, vulnerable populations (the homeless, the frail, the elderly, and persons with HIV).

The history of public health nursing shows that a common feature of those considered as leaders are individuals who moved forward to deal with unresolved problems in a positive, proactive way. This is the legacy of Lillian Wald at the Henry Street Settlement

and many others who have met need with innovation. Within the context of the core public health function of assurance, there clearly is an opportunity for public health nursing to develop population-based outreach programs directed to "the matching of the needs of vulnerable groups in the community with the services that hold promise for helping them" (Aiken and Salmon, p. 328). As a specialty, public health nursing can have a positive impact on the health status of populations, but to do so "it will be necessary to have broad vision; to prepare nurses for leadership roles in policy making and in the design, development, management, monitoring, and evaluation of population-focused health care systems and to develop strategies to support nurses in these roles" (Williams, 1992).

Clinical Application

The basic thesis of this chapter is that population-focused nursing practice is different from clinical nursing care delivered in the community. If one accepts the thesis of this chapter that specialization in public health nursing is population-focused and encompasses a unique body of knowledge, then it is useful to debate where and how public health nursing specialists practice and how their practice compares with what has been defined as specialization in community health nursing.

In your community health class, debate with classmates whether there are nurses in the following categories who are practicing population-focused nursing:
1. School nursing
2. Staff nurses in home care

3. Director of nursing for a home care agency
4. Nurse practitioners in a health maintenance organization
5. Vice-President of nursing in a hospital
6. Staff nurses in a public health clinic or community health center
7. Director of nursing in a health department

Which are (are not) public health or community health specialists? Why are they considered (not considered) specialists?

Choose three categories on the list and interview at least one nurse in each category. Determine what their scope of practice is. Are they carrying out population-focused practice? Could they? How?

Key Concepts

- Public Health is "what we, as a society, do collectively to assure the conditions in which people can be healthy."
- Assessment, policy development, and assurance are the core public health functions at all levels of government.
- Assessment refers to systematic data collection on the population, monitoring of the population's health status, and making information available on the health of the community.
- Policy development refers to the need to provide leadership in developing policies which support the health of the population, including the use of the scientific knowledge base in decision-making about policy.

- Assurance refers to the role of public health in making sure that essential community-wide health services are available, which may include providing essential personal health services for those who would otherwise not receive them. Assurance also refers to making sure that a competent public health and personal health care work force is available.
- Setting is frequently viewed as the feature that distinguishes public health nursing from other nursing specialties. A more useful approach is to use characteristics such as the following: a focus on populations that are free-living in the community; the emphasis on prevention; the concern for the interface between health

Key Concepts—cont'd

status of the population and the living environment (physical, biological, sociocultural); and the use of political processes to affect public policy as a major intervention strategy for achieving goals.

◆ According to the 1984 Consensus Conference sponsored by the Nursing Division for the Department of Health and Human Services, specialists in public health nursing are defined as those who are prepared at the graduate level, either master's or doctoral, "with a focus in the public health sciences" (Consensus Conference on the Essentials of Public Health Nursing Practice and Education, 1985).

◆ Specialization in the public health nursing is seen as a subset of community health nursing.

◆ Population-focused practice is the focus of specialization in public health nursing. This focus on community-based populations and the emphasis or health promotion and disease prevention are the fundamental factors that distinguish public health nursing from other nursing specialties.

◆ Population is defined as a collection of individuals who share one or more personal or environmental characteristics. The term population may be used interchangeably with the term aggregate.

Critical Thinking Activities

1. Define for your personal understanding (a) the essential functions of public health, (b) the specialist in public health nursing, and (c) the specialist in community health nursing.
2. State your opinion of the similarities and/or differences between a clinical nursing role and the population-focused role of the public health nursing specialist.
3. Review the models of Community Health Nursing Practice of the ANA and APHA as described in this chapter.
4. With three or four of your classmates, develop a plan for identifying two or three nurses in your community who are in an administrative role and discuss with them: (1) how they define the populations they are serving; (2) the strategies they use to monitor the population's health status; (3) the strategies they use to assure that the populations are receiving basic needed services; and (4) what initiatives they are taking to address problems.

Bibliography

Advisory Board Company: *Capitation 1: the new American medicine,* Washington, DC, 1994, Advisory Board Company.

Aiken LH, Salmon ME: Health care workforce priorities: what nursing should do now, *Inquiry* 31:318, 1994.

American Nurses Association, Division of Community Health Nursing: *Conceptual model of community health nursing,* Pub No CH-10, Kansas City, Mo, 1980, The Association.

American Public Health Association: *The definition and role of public health nursing in the delivery of health care: a statement of the public health nursing section,* Washington, DC, 1981, The Association.

Consensus Conference on the Essentials of Public Health Nursing Practice and Education, Rockville, Md, 1985, US Department of Health and Human Services, Bureau of Health Professions, Division of Nursing.

Council on Linkages Between Academia and Public Health Practice: The Guideline Development Project, *The Link,* Health Program Alliance, Johns Hopkins University, 7:2, 1995.

Institute of Medicine, Board on Health Promotion and Disease Prevention, Project on Public Health Performance Monitoring, Washington, DC, 1995.

Institute of Medicine: *The future of public health,* Washington, DC, 1988, National Academy Press.

Josten L, et al: Public Health Nursing Education: back to the future for public health sciences, *Fam and Community Health* 18:36, 1995.

Starr P: *The social transformation of American medicine,* New York, 1982, Basic Books, Inc.

US Public Health Service: *A Time for Partnership,* Prevention Report, Dec 1994/Jan 1995, Office of Disease Prevention and Health Promotion.

US Public Health Service: *The Core Functions Project,* 1993, Office of Disease Prevention and Health Promotion.

Williams CA: Beyond the Institute of Medicine Report: a critical analysis and public health forecast. *Fam Community Health* 18:12, 1995.

Williams CA: Population-focused community health nursing and nursing administration: a new synthesis. In McCloskey JC and Grace HK, editors: *Current issues in nursing,* ed 2, Boston, 1985, Blackwell Scientific Publications, Ltd.

Williams CA: Public Health Nursing: does it have a future? In Aiken LH, Fagin CM, editors: *Charting nursing's future: agenda for the 1990s,* Philadelphia, 1992, JB Lippincott.

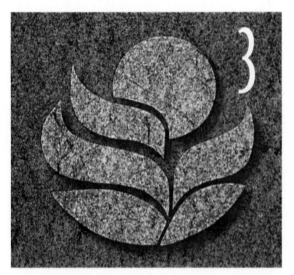

The Public Health and Primary Health Care Systems and Health Care Reform

Susan B. Hassmiller

Objectives

After reading this chapter, the student should be able to do the following:

- Describe three trends in the United States that are affecting health care.
- Define public health, primary care, primary health care, and community-oriented primary care.
- Differentiate between primary care and primary health care, including the workforce of each.
- Discuss the significance of Alma Ata as the basis for primary health care.
- Describe two of the most common health care systems that manage the personal care of Americans.
- Describe the current public health system in the United States.
- Compare and contrast the responsibilities of the federal, state, and local public health systems.
- Discuss community health nursing roles in selected governmental agencies.
- Analyze and discuss the major components of health care reform.
- Describe the steps of the community-oriented primary care (COPC) model.
- Compare and contrast COPC with primary care and public health.
- Discuss the importance of community participation in the COPC process or in any system of care.
- Define the nursing role in a COPC system of care.

Outline

Continued.

Outline—cont'd ▼

The American health care system has done a remarkable job in many ways in providing health care to the American people, particularly in technology development and skilled provider training. Today's health care facilities would defy the imagination of our predecessors. Although public and private health insurance programs protect most Americans from the financial ravages of illness, the system has some serious liabilities related to cost, quality, and access to care.

This chapter describes the current primary care and public health systems in the United States and the trends that affect these systems. A definition of terms used in this chapter can be found in the box at right. The systems will be compared and contrasted both with each other and with the concept of primary health care. Current concepts of health care reform are outlined in an effort to introduce a discussion of what an emerging health care system might look like. This chapter describes a reformed health care system as one that weaves primary care and public health into a single integrated system. The role of the community health nurse is presented in all of the systems . . . current and future.

THE CURRENT HEALTH CARE SYSTEM

Although the U.S. health care system can take credit for improving the lifespan of most Americans through advances in medical technology, science, and the pharmaceutical industry, the system is also plagued with issues related to cost, quality, and access to care. These issues, as described below, are at the center of health care debates around the United States.

Cost

In 1994 Americans spent $982 billion dollars, or nearly 14% of the gross domestic product (GDP), on health care (Shalala, 1994). This percentage is 40% higher than in Canada, the country that spends the next largest amount (Altman, 1992). By the year 2003 our health care costs will rise to $2.1 trillion, or 20% of our GDP, if we do nothing to halt this course (Sha-

lala, 1994). The cost containment efforts that have been instituted since 1983 have attempted to curb the growth of costs, but they have not solved this tremendous problem. (Chapter 5 gives details about the economics of health care.)

 Selected Health Care Definitions

Community-oriented primary care (COPC)—a community-responsive model of health care delivery that integrates aspects of both primary care and public health. It combines the care of individuals and families in the community with a focus on the community and its subgroups when services are planned, provided, and evaluated (Abramson, 1984).

Disease prevention—activities that have as their goal protecting people from the ill effects of actual or potential health threats.

Health—a state of complete physical, mental, and social well-being and not merely the absense of disease or infirmity (World Health Organization, 1986, p. 1).

Health promotion—activities that have as their goal developing human resources and behaviors that maintain or enhance well-being.

Primary care—personal health care services that provide for first contact, continuous, comprehensive, and coordinated care. Care is directed primarily at an individual's pathophysiological processes (Starfield, 1992).

Primary health care—essential care made universally accessible to individuals and families within a community, made available to them through their full participation, and provided at a cost that the community and country can afford (World Health Organization, 1978).

Primary prevention—actions designed to prevent a disease from occurring; reduces the probability of a specific illness occurring and includes active protection against unnecessary stressors or threats, that is, health promotion activities.

Public health—organized community efforts aimed at the prevention of disease and promotion of health. It links disciplines and rests on the scientific core of epidemiology (Institute of Medicine, 1988, p. 1).

Secondary prevention—early diagnosis and prompt treatment; includes activities such as screening for diseases, for example, hypertension, breast cancer, blindness, and deafness.

Tertiary prevention—treatment, care, and rehabilitation of people to prevent further progression of the disease (Pender, 1987).

Access

Increasing costs have been accompanied by another significant problem: poor access to health care. The American health care system is described as a two-class system: private and public. People with insurance or those who can personally pay for health care are viewed as receiving superior care compared with people whose only source of care depends on public funds. Within the second category there are working poor people who do not qualify for public funds, either because they make too much money to qualify or they are illegal immigrants. In 1994, 43 million Americans (or 14.7% of our total population) were uninsured (Shalala, 1994).

Other persons who are currently denied access to health care are those who are sick or at risk for getting sick with an illness that insurance companies consider too costly to cover. These persons are denied access to health care when insurance companies deny them coverage. An estimated 81 million Americans fall in this category (Shalala, 1994).

Finally, the access problem in the United States has been compounded by the gradual erosion of public health services. For example, funding to clinics in rural and heavily populated urban areas has been reduced, which means that many uninsured people seek care at the emergency room. To continue to care for uninsured clients, hospitals automatically charge more for their services to those who have insurance. This process of making up for lost revenue by charging more to those who are able to pay is called **cost shifting.** In 1992 the average shift was 31% (Shalala, 1994).

Quality

Quality of care is the third major concern in the United States. Although the United States is known for its sophistication in the areas of biomedical research and advanced lifesaving procedures, many Americans do not have access to these services. Instead, quality of care often depends on location (suburban, urban, rural), insurance status, and employment status. Even those individuals, however, who do have insurance, with easy access to medical care, lack adequate preventive care (Safriet, 1992).

TRENDS AFFECTING THE HEALTH CARE SYSTEM

Because of the national concern for the cost, access, and quality of health care, significant change is expected in the next decade. Several trends, including demography, technology, and economics, will have an impact on the way these changes will evolve.

Demographic Trends

The world's population is expected to double in the next 30 years as a result of two major factors: increased fertility and decreased mortality. The most explosive growth is occurring in Third World countries with a slowdown in the United States. Both the size of the population and the characteristics of its members are contributory influences.

Size of the Population

The Census Bureau reports that the U.S. population increased by 22 million between 1980 and 1990, an increase of 9.8%. Although this is the second lowest growth spurt in census history, the census predicts that the population will continue to grow until 2038, hitting a record high of 302 million before declining in the latter part of the next century. It is predicted that immigration (legal and illegal) will constitute almost half of all population growth in the United States in the next generation (Miller, 1991).

The U.S. birth rate has fluctuated greatly in the past 50 years, going from the baby boom between 1946 and 1964 to the baby bust of the 1970s, when the population reached its low point in 1976. The birth rate began rising again in the late 1970s when the baby boom women began having children. This will not continue since the baby boom women will no longer be of childbearing age (U.S. Bureau of the Census, 1989).

 Research Brief

Grumbach K, Keane D, Bindman A: Primary care and public emergency department overcrowding, A*m J Pub Health* 83(3):372-378, 1993.

A study conducted at the San Francisco General Hospital determined that many patients utilize emergency services as a substitute for accessible primary care providers. One-third of all patients surveyed did not consider their problem to be so serious that they could not have waited at least 1 to 3 days for a clinic appointment. Nurse-assigned acuity scores verified the patients' judgments in their own severity of illness and ability to wait.

Other than refusing to treat nonemergency patients or having them wait so long (through triage methods) that they eventually leave, the authors recommended the following:

1. Triage patients to determine who does not need emergency care. This select group of patients could be referred to primary care clinics in their own neighborhoods. Critical to this recommendation is the ability of the emergency room to maintain an ongoing relationship with neighborhood clinics in order to reserve appointments for emergency referrals. Access and availability of primary care providers are key to the success of this recommendation.

2. Develop a hospital-based urgent care clinic that would accept low-acuity new patients on a drop-in or next-day appointment basis.

This study points out the ineffective pattern of using emergency rooms for health problems that are not real emergencies.

Characteristics of the Population

The U.S. population is aging. Demographers predict a 74% increase in the number of people aged 50 years or older by the year 2020, whereas the number of people under 50 years will only grow by 1% (Exter, 1990). The elderly population will increase slowly during the next 20 years and then rapidly for the following 20 years. From 2010 to 2030, the number of people 65 years and older will increase substantially when the first baby boomer turns 65 years old in 2011. The over–85 years group is growing so rapidly that by 2050 this group will comprise approximately 24% of the elderly population.

The middle-aged population will also continue to increase since nearly one-third of Americans were born between 1945 and 1960. The entire baby boom generation will be over 35 years by the turn of the century.

Blacks are currently the largest minority group in the United States but will be surpassed by Hispanics by the year 2015 (Miller, 1991). Asian-Americans, although the smallest minority group in America, will wield the largest influence. They understand and blend in with the American way of life more quickly than any other minority, are more educated, and make more money per capita than other minorities and whites (Miller, 1991).

The U.S. household composition is also changing. Families constitute about 71% of all households, down from 81% in 1970 (U.S. Bureau of the Census, 1993). Three out of ten families are headed by single parents, usually the mother. Single-parent families constitute 24.5% of all white families with children, whereas 35% of Hispanic families with children and 63% of black families with children reside with only one parent.

In the past decade, mortality for both genders in all age groups has declined (Exter, 1990). As a result of medical progress, the leading causes of death have changed from infectious diseases to chronic and degenerative diseases. Substantial gains against infectious diseases resulted in steady declines of mortality among children. Mortality for older Americans also declined, especially during the 1970s and 1980s. However, people aged 50 years and older have higher rates of chronic illness, and they consume a larger portion of health care services than other age groups.

Social Trends

In addition to the size and changing age distribution of the population, other factors also affect the health care system. Several social trends that influence health care include changing life-styles, a growing appreciation of the quality of life, changing composition of families and living patterns, rising household incomes, and a revised definition of quality health care.

Historically, U.S. citizens have been driven by the American dream that emphasized hard work, getting a good education, and achieving a better life than the previous generation. However, the drive to achieve these goals has diminished, and major shifts in American values and life-styles have occurred. Replacing the work ethic is an increasing emphasis on an improved quality of life and the fulfillment of personal goals (Miller, 1991). This shift in values is reordering the relative importance of economic success.

In the future, Americans will spend more on health care, nutrition, and fitness (Miller, 1991). There will be a growing emphasis on the belief that people are responsible for their own health and an awareness that health is a valuable asset and efforts should be taken to improve it. Centers for promoting all aspects of health are developing in response to this movement.

Economic Trends

Sixty years ago income was distributed in such a way that a relatively small proportion of households earned high incomes; a somewhat larger portion of families were in the middle-income range; and the largest proportion of households were at the low end of the income scale. By the 1970s, household income had risen and income was more evenly distributed, both primarily resulting from two incomes coming into the family. There has always been and continues to be income disparity between whites and other minority groups, excluding Asian-Americans (Johnson, 1992; Miller, 1991).

Although the distribution of income has dramatically changed over time, more than 12 million families—about 20% of households—receive only 5% of the total income. In addition, high costs and lower real wages, especially for black women, continue to add to the difficulty of rising out of poverty (Johnson, 1992). This means that a sizable proportion of low-income Americans will continue to rely on public support to maintain a minimum standard of living. Chapter 5 provides a detailed discussion of the economics of health care and how financial constraints influence decisions about public health services.

Health Workforce Trends

The emphasis on physician specialization and specialists' tendency to charge more and order more tests than primary care physicians have added to the spiraling health care costs in this nation (Greenfield et al., 1992). A call for health care cost containment in the United States has demanded a work force that will help keep costs in line while maintaining quality and increasing accessibility. Current efforts are underway by government agencies, such as the Bureau of Health Professions of the U.S. Department of Health and Human Services, and private foundations, such as the Pew Health Professions Commission, to provide strategies for increasing a primary care work force in the United States. These strategies include increasing the number of primary care physicians (currently one-third of the total physician population), as well as increasing the number of advanced practice nurses, such as nurse practitioners and certified nurse midwives.

Historically, nursing care has been provided in a variety of settings, with the hospital being the dominant setting. Currently, two-thirds of all registered nurses are employed in hospitals; however, with an emphasis on cost containment and a greater orientation to community-based care, hospitals are downsizing their acute care facilities. Although it is estimated that by 2000 the need for nursing personnel will be about 1.8 million, it is predicted that many nurses working in acute care will face job loss or job uncertainty. One of the few exceptions will be those nurses working in the area of gerontology. The American Nurses' Association is currently working with the U.S. Department of Labor to develop strategies to train nurses to compete for jobs in primary care, public health, and critical care outside the hospital setting (*The American Nurse,* April 1994).

Increasing minority representation in nursing remains a priority. "Shortages of such individuals adversely affect access, quality of care, and costs" (U.S. Department of Health and Human Services [DHHS], 1993, p. 15). For example, persons from minority groups, especially where language is a barrier, are more comfortable with and more likely to access care from a provider of their own minority group. Although minorities comprised 22% of the U.S. population in 1991, minority nursing school enrollments accounted for only 14.2%. Nursing will have to compete with the other health care professions to recruit for the same pool of minorities.

Technologic Trends

Improved technology is rapidly changing the health care system and is having both positive and negative effects. On the positive side, technologic advances promise improved health care services and reduced costs. Reduced costs come from a more efficient means of delivering care as well as replacing people. Contradictory as it may seem, cost is also the most significant negative aspect of advanced health care technology. The more high-technology equipment and computer programs become available, the more they are utilized. High-technology equipment is expensive, quickly becomes outdated when newer developments occur, and often requires highly trained personnel.

Unquestionably, advances in medical technology will continue. However, it is anticipated that the emphasis will shift away from expensive diagnostic and therapeutic technologies. Efforts will focus on devising simpler, cheaper, and more mobile tests and procedures that are less oriented to tertiary care and can be used in nonhospital settings.

ORGANIZATION OF THE HEALTH CARE SYSTEM

An enormous number and range of facilities and providers make up the health care system. These include physicians' and dentists' offices, hospitals, health maintenance organizations (HMOs), nursing homes and other related inpatient facilities, mental health centers, ambulatory care centers, rehabilitation centers, and local, state, and federal official and voluntary agencies. In general, however, the American health care system is divided into two somewhat distinct components: a private or personal care component and a public health component, with some overlap, as will be discussed below. Although the personal care component is comprised of primary, secondary, and tertiary care, primary health care and primary care will receive the most elaboration in this chapter.

The Primary Health Care System

There is considerable controversy over what constitutes primary care and primary health care. Primary health care (PHC) can be distinguished from primary care in several important ways. **Primary health care,** generally defined more broadly than primary care, includes a comprehensive range of services, such as public health, prevention, and diagnostic, therapeutic, and rehabilitative services. PHC is essential care made universally accessible to individuals and families in a community. Health care is made available to them through their full participation and is provided at a cost that the community and country can afford (World Health Organization, 1978.) Full participation means that individuals within the community help in defining health problems and developing approaches to address the problems. The setting for primary health care is within all communities of a country and permeates all aspects of society.

PHC encourages self-care and self-management in health and social welfare aspects of daily life. People are educated to use their knowledge, attitudes, and skills in activities that improve health for themselves, their families, and their neighbors. The desired outcome from the PHC strategy is individual, family, and community self-reliance and competence.

The Primary Health Care Workforce

The primary health care workforce comprises a multidisciplinary team of health care providers. Team members include many professionals such as generalist and public health physicians, nurses, dentists, pharmacists, optometrists, nutritionists, community outreach workers, mental health counselors, and other allied health professionals. Community members are also considered important to the team.

| Did You Know? |

The cost of high-technology medical interventions for an early-term, low-birth-weight infant during the neonatal period alone can reach $200,000. Prevention measures in the form of early and effective prenatal education provided at a community nursing center can save this amount from the national health care budget (Lundeen, 1994).

The Primary Health Care Movement

The primary health care movement officially began in 1977 when the 30th World Health Organization (WHO) Health Assembly adopted a resolution accepting the goal of attaining a level of health that permitted all citizens of the world to live socially and economically productive lives. At the International conference in 1978 in Alma Ata, USSR, it was determined that this goal was to be met through PHC. This resolution became known by the slogan "Health for All (HFA) by the year 2000" and captured the official health target for all member nations of WHO.

In 1981 WHO established global indicators for monitoring and evaluating the achievement of HFA. In the *World Health Statistics Annual* (1986) these indicators are grouped into four categories: health policies; social and economic development; provision of health care; and health status. An important part of the global indicators is the emphasis on health as an objective of socioeconomic development (Mahler, 1981). In this context, health improvements are a result of efforts in many areas including agriculture, industry, education, housing, communications, and health care. Because PHC is as much a political statement as a system of care, each United Nations (UN) member country interprets PHC in the context of its own culture, health needs, resources, and system of government.

Finally, although the original definition of PHC has at times been misunderstood, it is important to understand the **Alma Ata declaration** as the basis for PHC and the global evolvement of this strategy over the past 10 to 15 years. For this reason the complete declaration is presented in Appendix B.

As a WHO member nation, the United States has endorsed primary health care as a strategy for achieving the goal of Health For All by the year 2000. However, PHC, with its emphasis on broad strategies, community participation, self-reliance, and a multidisciplinary health care delivery team, is not the primary strategy for improving the health of the American people. The national health plan for the United States focuses more on disease prevention and health promotion in the areas of most concern in the nation.

This focus is exemplified by the health objectives for the nation, *Healthy People 2000: National Health Promotion and Disease Prevention Objectives* (Healthy People 2000, 1991, p. 43). These objectives were published by the Public Health Service, Department of Health and Human Services, following a process of gathering data from health professionals and organizations throughout the United States.

The objectives focus on three overriding goals: increase the lifespan of healthy Americans; reduce health disparities among Americans and provide all Americans with access to preventive services; and decrease the race-based disparity in life expectancy.

Specific areas of concern for each of these goals include the following:

Table 3-1 Year 2000 Objectives and Public Health Service Elements

Eight essential elements (PHC)	Year 2000 objectives
Health education	Physical activity and fitness; tobacco, alcohol, and other drugs; mental health; surveillance and data systems; violence and abusive behavior
Proper nutrition	Nutrition
Maternal and child health care; family planning	Maternal and infant health; family planning
Safe water and basic sanitation	Environmental health
Immunization	Immunization and infectious diseases
Prevention and control of locally endemic diseases	HIV infection; chronic disorders; cancer; heart disease and stroke; sexually transmitted diseases; immunization and infectious diseases; clinical preventive services
Treatment of common diseases and injuries	Unintentional injuries; occupational safety and health
Provision of essential drugs	

Health promotion: nutrition; physical activity and fitness; consumption of tobacco, alcohol, and other drugs; family planning; violent and abusive behavior; mental health; and educational and community-based programs.

Health protection: environmental health, occupational safety and health, accidental unintentional injuries, food and drug safety, and oral health.

Preventive services priorities: maternal and infant health, immunizations and infectious diseases, human immune virus (HIV) infection, sexually transmitted diseases, heart disease and stroke, cancer, diabetes, other chronic disabling conditions, and clinical preventive services for these; also chronic disorders, and mental and behavioral disorders.

System improvement priorities: health education and preventive services, and surveillance and data systems (Healthy People 2000, 1991).

There is considerable overlap between the essential elements of PHC and the areas of concern stated in the *Year 2000 Objectives*. In Table 3-1 the eight essential elements of PHC are related to the U.S. priority areas, as defined by the Public Health Service.

The Primary Care System

Primary care, or what some refer to as primary medical care, is a personal health care system that provides for first contact, continuous, comprehensive, and co-

Table 3-2 Characteristics of Primary Care and Primary Health Care

Primary care	Primary health care
Individual-focused	Community-focused
Preventive, rehabilitative, with emphasis on curative	Curative, rehabilitative, with emphasis on preventive
Care provided by generalist physicians, nurse practitioners, nurse midwives, and physician assistants with help of ancillary team members	Care provided by a wide variety of health care team members such as physicians, community health nurses, community outreach workers, nutritionists, sanitation experts
Professional dominance	Self-reliance

ordinated care. It addresses the most common needs of clients within a community by providing preventive, curative, and rehabilitative services to maximize their health and well-being. Although primary care practitioners are encouraged to consider the client's social and environmental attributes in diagnosing, interventions are directed primarily at an individual's *pathophysiological* process (Starfield, 1992). Table 3-2 compares primary health care and primary care.

Primary care is an essential component of an overall primary health care system, so much so that the Institute of Medicine (IOM) is currently focusing its attention on a 24-month study to provide guidance for augmenting and improving primary care as an essential component of an effective and efficient health care system. Once published, the IOM's *Future of Primary Care* report will define primary care and the roles of primary care providers and will provide a comprehensive strategic plan of action for increasing the emphasis on primary care.

The Primary Care Delivery System

Primary care is delivered in a variety of accessible community settings such as physician offices, HMOs, community health centers, and **community nursing centers.** With the emphasis on cost containment the health care delivery system is focusing its efforts on **managed care** as an increasingly large segment of the primary care system. **Health maintenance organizations (HMOs)** and **preferred provider organizations (PPOs)** are two of the most common systems that manage the care for a specified population.

HMOs have been in existence for over 30 years. Each operates as an organized system of health care that, for a fixed fee, provides primary care services, emergency and preventive treatment, and hospital care to people who have agreed to obtain their medical care from the HMO for a specified period of time. Specialty care is received (and paid for) only on the recommendation of a staff HMO primary care provider. HMOs keep costs under control by encour-

aging prevention, keeping referrals to a minimum, and reducing unnecessary hospitalization.

A PPO is an organization of providers that contracts on a fee-for-service basis with third-party payers to provide comprehensive medical services to subscribers. The agreement between the PPO and the third-party payer allows subscribers to receive medical services at lower than usual rates (Roble et al., 1984). Physicians and other primary care providers can belong to several preferred provider plans. Other health care delivery organizations include community nursing centers and community health centers.

The Primary Care Workforce

Primary care developed in the 1960s as the need to re-examine the role of the general practitioner arose. The Millis Commission (1966) expressed concern that a knowledge explosion, development of new technologies, and an increasing number of new specialties were threatening the role of the general practitioner. The specialty of family practice and the arrival of nurse practitioners and physician assistants emerged in response to the need to provide primary care.

Currently, primary care providers include generalists who possess competencies in health promotion and disease prevention, assessment and evaluation of undiagnosed symptoms and physical signs, management of common acute and chronic medical conditions, and identification and appropriate referral for other needed health care services (U.S. Department of Health and Human Services, 1992). The health care personnel trained as **primary care generalists** include family physicians, general internists, general pediatricians, nurse practitioners, physician assistants, and nurse midwives. Some physicians with special training in preventive medicine/public health and obstetrics/gynecology also deliver primary care (U.S. Department of Health and Human Services, 1992).

Nurse practitioners (NPs) and certified nurse midwives (CNMs), both considered **advanced practice nurses,** are vital members of the primary care and primary health care team. Nurse practitioners receive advanced training usually at the master's level, with most taking a certification examination in a specialty area such as pediatrics, adult, gerontology, obstetrics/gynecology, or family. Training emphasizes clinical medical skills (history, physical, and diagnosis) and pharmacology in addition to the traditional psychosocial and prevention-focused attributes that are normally ascribed to nursing. Studies have shown that 60% to 80% of primary care, traditionally done by physicians, can be delivered by an NP for less money and with equal or better quality (Office of Technology Assessment, 1986).

Nurse midwifery is defined as "the independent management and care of essentially normal newborns and women antepartally, intrapartally, postpartally, and gynecologically, occurring within a health care system that provides for medical consultation, collaborative management, and referral. . ." (Rooks and

Haas, 1986, p. 9). The mother is the primary focus of care for nurse midwives, who spend the majority of their time on prenatal care, labor, delivery, and postpartum care, as well as family-planning services. Nurse midwives receive advanced training either at the master's level or by attending a school of nurse midwifery. All CNMs are certified by a national examination.

Physician assistants (PAs) operate under the license of a physician, which is different from NPs and CNMs, who operate as independent practitioners. The majority of PAs receive their training at the baccalaureate level and are able to sit for their certification boards once they have graduated. PAs assist or substitute for physicians in the performance of specific medical tasks. Like NPs, PAs are proficient in history, physicals, and the diagnosing and treating of uncomplicated medical conditions. Both groups are trained in prescribing a limited number of drugs, but the scope of their prescriptive authority depends on the state laws where they live. In the past CNMs and NPs have received considerable pressure to limit their practice to avoid infringing on what physicians perceive as their role. State practice laws are slowly being changed, with pressure from the federal government, NPs, CNMs, and consumers to practice independently, prescribe, and receive third-party reimbursement.

The Public Health System

Although the goal of the public health system is to ensure that the health of the community is protected, promoted, and restored, this system and the personal care system overlap. The overlap comes not only from the personal care system providing health promotion and disease prevention, but also through the public health system providing personal care services for those who cannot afford to receive their care elsewhere. For example, the U.S. Public Health Service provides a commissioned corps of uniformed health personnel, the **National Health Service Corps,** to serve residents of medically underserved areas.

The public health system is mandated through laws that are developed at the national, state, or local level. An example of public health laws instituted to protect the health of the community include mandatory immunizations for all children entering kindergarten and constant monitoring of the local water supply.

Organization of the Public Health System

The public health system is organized into multiple levels comprised of the federal, state, and local systems. Although not all local governmental units are involved in health care, most are. For example, school districts are responsible for health education and first aid, with many schools having on-site clinics that are responsible for a comprehensive array of the student's health, including mental health and family planning.

The Federal System

The **Department of Health and Human Services (DHHS)** is the agency most heavily involved with the health and welfare concerns of U.S. citizens. As mentioned earlier, the organizational chart of DHHS (Figure 3-1) depicts the office of the secretary and four principal operating components: the Social Security Administration, the Health Care Financing Administration, the Administration for Children and Families, and the Public Health Service. The Public Health Service is charged with regulating health care and overseeing the health status of Americans.

The U.S. Public Health Service

The **Public Health Service (PHS)** is the largest public health program in the world. Its mission is to protect and advance the health of the American people through the following areas:

◆ Medical research
◆ Disease tracking and identification
◆ Health care to American Indians, Alaska natives, and medically underserved populations
◆ Alcohol, drug abuse, and mental health programs
◆ Identification and correction of health hazards
◆ Promotion of exercise and healthy habits
◆ Protection of the U.S. food and drug supply
◆ Medical assistance after disasters (U.S. Public Health Service, 1994)

The major components of the PHS are shown in Figure 3-1. The PHS, directed by the assistant secretary for health, is organized into eight functional units: (1) the Centers for Disease Control and Prevention (CDC), (2) the Food and Drug Administration (FDA), (3) the Health Resources and Services Administration (HRSA), (4) the National Institutes of Health (NIH), (5) the Substance Abuse and Mental Health Services Administration (SAMHSA), (6) the Agency for Toxic Substances and Disease Registry (ATSDR), (7) the Agency for Health Care Policy and Research (AHCPR), and (8) the Indian Health Service (IHS). Ten regional offices are maintained to provide more direct assistance to the states (Table 3-3 for their locations). The Health Resources and Services Administration of the PHS contains the Bureau of Health Professions, which includes separate divisions for nursing, medicine, dentistry, and allied health professions.

The State System

Although state health departments vary widely in their roles, they have a substantial role in health care financing (such as Medicaid), providing mental health and professional education, establishing health codes, licensing facilities and personnel, and regulating the insurance industry (Brecher, 1990). They also have a substantial role in direct assistance to local health departments, including ongoing assessment of health needs.

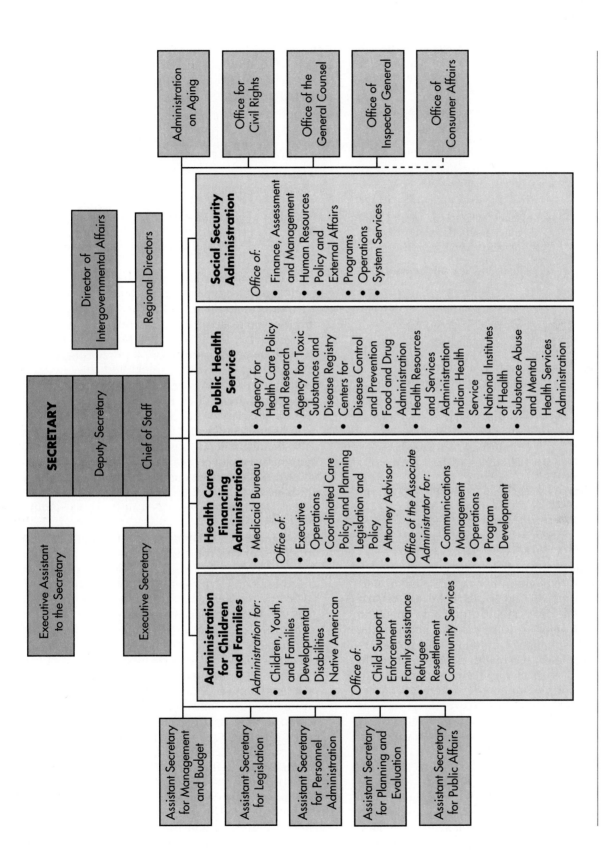

FIGURE 3-1

Organization of the U.S. Department of Health and Human Services. (From Office of the Federal Registry: *United States government manual* 1993/1994, Washington, DC, 1993, U.S. Government Printing Office.) Note: Effective March 31, 1995, the Social Security Administration was moved from the U.S. Department of Health and Human Services.

Table 3-3 Regional Offices of the U.S. Public Health Service

Region	Location	Territory
1	Boston	Connecticut, Maine, Massachusetts, New Hampshire, Rhode Island, Vermont
2	New York	New Jersey, New York, Puerto Rico, Virgin Islands
3	Philadelphia	Delaware, District of Columbia, Maryland, Pennsylvania, Virginia, West Virginia
4	Atlanta	Alabama, Florida, Georgia, Kentucky, Mississippi, North Carolina, South Carolina, Tennessee
5	Chicago	Illinois, Indiana, Michigan, Minnesota, Ohio, Wisconsin
6	Dallas	Arkansas, Louisiana, New Mexico, Oklahoma, Texas
7	Kansas City	Iowa, Kansas, Missouri, Nebraska
8	Denver	Colorado, Montana, North Dakota, South Dakota, Utah, Wyoming
9	San Francisco	American Samoa, Arizona, California, Guam, Hawaii, Nevada, North Mariana Islands, trust territories
10	Seattle	Alaska, Idaho, Oregon, Washington

The Local System

The local health department has direct responsibility to the citizens in its community or jurisdiction. Services and programs offered by local health departments vary greatly depending on the state and local health codes that must be followed, the needs of the community, and available funding and other resources. For example, one health department might be more involved with public health education programs and environmental issues, whereas another health department might emphasize direct patient care. Local health departments vary in their level of involvement with sick care or even primary care.

HEALTH CARE REFORM

The rising costs of health care in the United States, uneven access for consumers, and dissatisfaction of both consumers and health care professionals have created an atmosphere conducive to change. Consumers want lower costs, high-quality health care, and the ability to choose their provider. There has been significant debate about health care reform at the national level, but nothing definitive is expected in this century. It is

predicted that change will be incremental. Many states, unable and unwilling to wait for incremental changes, have initiated reform legislation including cost containment measures, insurance reform, and increased access for their medically indigent citizens. In addition, insurers, academic health centers, and managed care systems are also rapidly restructuring their services and systems.

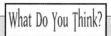

What Do You Think?

Mandating small business owners to purchase health insurance for their employees (employer mandates) is a reasonable way to help ensure that the health needs of the United States, especially working poor persons, will be taken care of.

Some common issues among the various legislative health care reform proposals include the following:

♦ Health care alliances. Some firms would be granted increased freedom to buy health care coverage directly from health insurers, set up their own insurance plan, or buy from a purchasing cooperative (Pearlstein, 1994).
♦ Guaranteed coverage. One suggested mandate would require that all insurance companies sell or renew policies for any buyer regardless of medical condition (Pearlstein, 1994). These measures would also include federal subsidies for small businesses to purchase employee health insurance, federal subsidies directly to low-income persons to help them purchase health insurance, and an increase in subsidies provided by the Medicaid program (Trafford and Rich, 1994).
♦ Managed care. Managed care is health care that manages or controls the amount and type of care a person receives for a set fee. This control mechanism is exactly what makes it so attractive to those who are concerned with containing health care costs and why managed care systems are on the rise. Examples of managed care are HMOs and PPOs (Pearlstein, 1994).
♦ Cost controls. All proposals are written with the promise of reducing the paperwork used in administering health programs, including a common electronic medical claims form. Increased price competition among health insurers will also be encouraged. A backup plan may be instituted to allow for government price controls if competition does not contain costs sufficiently (Firshein, 1994; Pearlstein, 1994).
♦ Primary and preventive care. Many policymakers have concluded that the health care system would benefit by increasing the primary care work force through effective use of generalist physicians, nurse practitioners, certified nurse midwives, and physician assistants. The goals are to emphasize preventive care and to create teams of generalist providers who can meet the needs of the population regard-

less of location (Curley et al., 1994). Disagreement exists about how the goal should be reached and to what extent the government should help (Firshein, 1994).

The Pew Health Professions Commission (O'Neil, 1993) has outlined several other general characteristics of the emerging health care system. They include an orientation toward health with an emphasis on the population as a whole. Also evident in these futuristic characteristics is the focus on the consumer in terms of encouraging and expecting patient partnerships in decision making. There will be more of a balance between the benefits and burdens of technology, and care will become more effective and efficient with the increased use of coordinated services and health provider teams. All of these characteristics are consistent with an emerging community health focus.

A NEW MODEL: THE INTEGRATION OF PUBLIC HEALTH AND PRIMARY CARE

What is needed to improve health care? First, delivery systems, as they strive to deliver the most cost-effective care possible, must also find ways to improve their access and quality in the communities they serve, especially to the underserved population. Second, students must be prepared to work together with other health professionals to understand the needs of the community and how to promote prevention. Third, *Healthy People 2000* (1991) and the World Health Organization's Health For All by the Year 2000 documents call for increased attention to population-based preventive activities as a means of increasing the health status of Americans. The systems must also become integrated as a means of controlling the cost of personal health care (Lee, 1994). In addition, there has been a call for all health professions' education to be more responsive in preparing students for a greater understanding of the needs of the community and prevention-oriented care (O'Neil, 1993). One model for integrating the public health and primary care systems is called community-oriented primary care.

Community-oriented Primary Care

Community-oriented primary care (COPC), a community-responsive model of health care delivery, integrates aspects of both primary care and public health. It combines the care of individuals and families in the community with a focus on the community and its subgroups when services are planned, provided, and evaluated (Abramson, 1984). This model contends that allocating more resources into community care will ultimately save money, increase access, and create better health outcomes in personal care (Hattis, 1993). As DHHS Assistant Secretary for Health Philip Lee, M.D., has emphasized, "When the public health system is not maintained and falls into disrepair, the health of the community suffers and, inevitably, the health risks, volume of care, and cost of care to the individual increases as well" (Ketter, 1994, p. 17).

Wright (1993), in speaking of health care reform and the evolving competitive marketplace, states that COPC is the most effective model for emphasizing prevention, utilizing a planning process that targets resources to high-priority needs, and for empowering communities to encourage individual responsibility. Wright (1993) describes the tools required to use the COPC model as follows:

1. A community-based primary care practice
2. An identifiable population or community for which the practice assumes responsibility for effecting change in health status
3. A planning, monitoring, and evaluation process for identifying and resolving health problems

Although COPC systems in the United States may attempt to invite and maintain **community participation,** this aspect of the plan cannot be overemphasized. The most effective and most sustainable individual and system changes come when there has been active participation from the people who live in the community. This was an important element in primary health care as well.

The W.K. Kellogg Foundation (1993), a foundation that financially supports efforts to improve the health of communities, states that a community-based practice must involve community members by allowing them to set their own priorities and solutions. Kellogg has found that when the right tools, such as power, information, and financial support, are shared with community members they become more actively involved in the process. Building a consensus among the many diverse community leaders who have a vested interest in the process will help to ensure a more accurate and comprehensive representation of the community's health needs as well as a wider array of solutions to these needs. In this context it must be remembered that health care cannot be separated from the broader scope of community development, such as housing and economic development. Consider the example of a young mother who has been scolded by a health professional for presenting her child with several infected insect bites, without ever addressing the issue of the unavailability of window screens in the family's apartment.

The strategies for using COPC are similar to the nursing process, using the community as the client. The steps are listed in the box on p. 46.

Role of the *Community Health Nurse in* COPC

Many public health nurses in the United States are practicing illness-oriented care as a result of public need and the revenue attached to these services (Miller et al., 1993). Salmon (1993) states this is a case of mistaken identity, because this role has diverted public health nurses away from their central roles in assessment, surveillance, policy, and health promotion and disease and injury prevention activities. Public health nurses move in and are trusted in the community like few other professionals. They can be found in schools, homes, and churches and on street corners developing relationships, collecting data, assessing needs, and providing care. In addition, with the knowledge that public health nurses have regarding community resources, they make excellent case managers (Bower, 1992). Public health nurses are ideally suited to practice using a COPC model. Although public health nurses will continue to be used for hands-on services, a generalist, prevention-oriented, public health background will allow them to bridge the gap between personal care and the health of the community.

Steps of the COPC Model

1. Define and characterize the community. Use personal knowledge (including observations) of the community in conjunction with data obtained from community leaders. Data should include morbidity and mortality, existing health care services and accessibility, transportation services, cultural diversity, and environmental issues.
2. Identify a list of community health problems and needs, and from that list formulate a community diagnosis. The process of formulating a diagnosis should develop as a consensus from key members of the delivery team and community leaders who truly represent the diverse needs and resources of the community.
3. Assist community leaders in the development of interventions corresponding to the community diagnosis. This would include personal care services as well as health promotion and disease prevention activities. Encourage interdisciplinary teamwork to gain maximum benefits from human resources. Maintain community input to determine feasibility and resources.
4. Coordinate and manage services. Work in partnership with social service agencies, health professionals, and community leaders to provide comprehensive care and encourage networking.
5. Evaluate the interventions with the input of community leaders. The system should allow for continuous feedback to allow for intermittent modification and redirection of resources.

Clinical Application

The goal of community health nursing is to promote and preserve the health of the population. The practice is general and comprehensive and is not limited to a particular age group. As a community health nurse it is important to guide and direct clients so they can seek the health care services that best meet their needs and resources. Guiding clients toward appropriate resources comes with the understanding that the community health nurse is familiar with characteristics specific to the community in which he or she is working.

During a well-child clinic visit, Jenna Wells, RN, met Sandra Farr and her 24-month-old daughter, Jessica. The Farrs had recently moved to the community. Mrs. Farr stated that she knew Jessica needed the last in a series of immunizations and because they did not have health insurance, she brought her daughter to the public health clinic. On initial assessment, Mrs. Farr told the nurse that her husband is newly employed and will not have any health care coverage for 30 days. The Farrs also need to decide which health care package they want. Mr. Farr's company offers a major medical plan and an HMO plan to all employees. Neither Mr. or Mrs. Farr has ever used an HMO, and they are not sure what services it provides. Almost under her breath, Mrs. Farr admits that she does not even know what an HMO is.

Recognizing that Mrs. Farr is sensitive about her lack of information about health care coverage but wants to make an informed decision, Nurse Wells continues with her initial assessment of the Farrs, completes the well-child assessment, and gives Jessica her immunizations. As Mrs. Farr dresses Jessica, the nurse collects several pamphlets and handouts on insurance and the type of health coverage each plan provides.

On returning to Mrs. Farr and Jessica, the nurse asks Mrs. Farr if she would like to look at some of the material on health insurance. Together, they review the information. Initially, Mrs. Farr looks confused and asks which choice the nurse would make. Nurse Wells says that she cannot really say which would work best for the Farrs, but she recommends that Mrs. Farr talk about the options with her husband. The nurse asks if she can call Mrs. Farr in 2 days to see if she has any questions about the insurance. Mrs. Farr looks pleased by this offer and comments that she will probably adjust better to the community once she chooses an insurance plan and finishes getting the immunizations for Jessica.

Two days later, the nurse telephones Mrs. Farr and learns that after carefully reviewing the information, the Farrs decided on the HMO. Both Mrs. Farr and Mr. Farr believe that health promotion is important, and this service is provided by the HMO. They also thought that since they did not know any of the local physicians or dentists, the HMO would give them enough choices to meet their needs.

Mrs. Farr reports that Jessica slept well on the night following the immunization and that there is no irritation around the site of the immunization nor any generalized discomfort. Before ending the conversation, the nurse asks Mrs. Farr if she would like the community welcome wagon to visit her. Following Mrs. Farr's enthusiastic response, the nurse contacts the local community service group that manages the welcome wagon and asks them to visit the Farrs.

Key Concepts

◆ Health care in the United States comprises a personal care system and a public health system, with overlap between the two systems.

◆ Primary care is a personal health care system that provides for first contact, continuous, comprehensive, and coordinated care.

◆ Primary health care is essential care made universally accessible to individuals and families in a community. Health care is made available to them through their full participation and is provided at a cost that the community and country can afford.

◆ Primary care is part of primary health care.

◆ Although primary care practitioners are encouraged to consider the client's biopsychosocial needs, interventions are directed primarily at the pathophysiological process.

◆ Public health refers to organized community efforts designed to prevent disease and promote health.

◆ Several important trends affecting the health care system are demographic, social, economic, political, and technological trends.

◆ There are 39 million uninsured people in the United States and many more who simply lack access to adequate health care.

◆ Many federal agencies are involved in government health care functions. The agency most directly involved with the health and welfare of Americans is the Department of Health and Human Services (DHHS).

◆ Most state and local jurisdictions have government activities that affect the health care field.

◆ Health care reform measures seek to make changes in the cost, quality, and access of our present system.

◆ Because of the current emphasis on community-based care, it is predicted that many nurses who are now working in acute care will soon face job loss and uncertainty.

◆ With an increasing emphasis on cost containment, the health care delivery system is focusing its efforts on developing managed care systems.

◆ Community-oriented primary care (COPC) is a model that emphasizes important aspects of both primary care and public health and in that respect is more consistent with the principles of primary health care.

◆ Strategies for using COPC can be likened to the nursing process, using the community as the client.

◆ The most sustainable individual and system changes come when there has been active participation from the people who live in the community.

◆ Building a consensus among the many diverse community leaders will help to ensure a more accurate and comprehensive representation of the community's health needs as well as the solutions to address the needs.

◆ Community health nurses are more than able to fill the gap between personal care and public health because of their skills in assessment, health promotion, and disease and injury prevention; knowledge of community resources; and ability to develop relationships with community members and leaders.

Critical Thinking Activities

1. Compare the local and state services where you live with those services presented in this chapter.

2. Debate the following: The major problem with the health care system is (choose one of the following topics) (1) escalating costs (including those from increased technology), (2) fragmentation, (3) access to care, or (4) quality of care.

3. Interview a nurse practitioner and physician assistant to determine any philosophic differences in their scope of practice.

4. If you were asked to plan a program designed for disease prevention in your community, what would you do? Describe the plan you would implement.

5. If there is an HMO in your community, interview three providers and three consumers to determine what each sees as the advantages and disadvantages of this type of care delivery system.

6. Visit your local health department and determine how its services fit into a primary care, public health, or community-oriented primary care model of care.

7. Determine whether any agency in your community is using the principles of COPC to deliver health care. Identify which principles they are using and those they could be using.

8. Describe three factors that might discourage the COPC approach to care in your community or in the United States.

Bibliography

Abramson JH: Application of epidemiology in community oriented primary care, *Pub Health Rep* 99(5):437-442, 1984.

Altman SH: *What can we learn from other countries about the mix and interrelationships of primary care and specialty care on access, quality, and cost?* Paper presented at the National Primary Care Conference, Washington, DC, March 1992.

Bower KA: *Case management by nurses,* Kansas City, Mo, 1992, American Nurses Publishing.

Brecher C: The government's role in health care. In Kovner AR, editor: *Health care delivery in the United States,* New York, 1990, Springer.

Curley T, Orloff TM, Tymann B: *Health profession's education linkages: community-based primary care training,* Washington, DC, 1994, National Governors' Association.

Division of Nursing: *Information booklet on the Division of Nursing,* Nov 1993, Rockville, Mo, Division of Nursing.

Exter T: Demographic forecast. *American Demographics* 12(2):55, 1990.

Firshein J: Countdown to health reform begins with differences galore, *J Am Health Policy* 4(2):3-5, 1994.

Greenfield S, Nelson EC, Zubkoff M, et al: Variations in resource utilization among medical specialties and systems of care: results from medical outcomes study. *JAMA* 267(12):1624-1630, 1992.

Hattis PA: Retooling for community benefit, *Health Progress* 74(7):38-41, 1993.

Havinghurst C: Countdown to health reform begins with differences galore. *J Am Health Policy,* 4(1):5-8, 1994.

Health Personnel in the United States: Eighth Report to Congress, 1991. *Primary care concerns,* (DHHS Pub No. HRS-P-OD-92-1). Washington, DC, Sept 1992, US Government Printing Office.

Healthy People 2000: national health promotion and disease prevention objectives, Washington, DC, 1991, USDHHS, Public Health Service.

Holmes A: States putting the brakes on comprehensive reforms, *J Am Health Policy,* March/April 1994; 4(2):4-6.

Institute of Medicine: *A manpower policy for primary health care,* (IOM pub no 78-2), Washington, DC, 1978, National Academy of Sciences.

Institute of Medicine: *The future of public health,* Washington, DC, 1988, National Academy Press.

Johnson T: Changing demographics in minority populations of the United States. In *Caring for the emerging majority: creating a new diversity in nurse leadership,* Rockville, Md, 1992, Division of Nursing and the Office of Minority Health.

Ketter J: Is there a cure for our ailing public health system? *Am Nurse* 26(6):1, 1994.

Lee P: *Shattuck lecture.* Delivered at the annual meeting of the Massachusetts Medical Society. Unpublished white paper, 1994.

Lundeen SP: Community nursing centers: implications for health care reform. In McCloskey JA, Grace HK, editors: *Current issues in nursing,* ed 4, St Louis, 1994, Mosby–Year Book.

Mahler H: The meaning of "Health for all by the year 2000," *World Health Forum* 2(1):5-22, 1981.

Miller CA, Moore K, Richards TN, et al: Longitudinal observations on a selected group of local health departments: a preliminary report, *J Pub Policy,* 13:34-50, Spring 1993.

Miller E: *Future vision,* Naperville, Ill, 1991, Sourcebooks Trade.

Millis JS, chairman: *The graduate education of physicians.* Report of the citizens commission on graduate medical education, Chicago, 1966, American Medical Association.

Office of Technology Assessment (OTA): *Nurse practitioners, physicians' assistants, and certified nurse-midwives: a policy analysis.* (Health Technology Case Study No 37), Washington, DC, 1986, US Government Printing Office.

O'Neil EH: *Health professions education for the future: schools in service to the nation,* San Francisco, 1993, Pew Health Professions Commission.

Pearlstein S: Health care reform bills caught in political labyrinth, *The Washington Post,* July 16, 1994, p A4.

Pender NJ: *Health promotion in nursing practice,* ed 2, Norwalk, Conn, 1987, Appleton & Lange.

Retraining programs benefit staff nurses. April *Am Nurs* 26(4):1, 1994.

Roble DT, Knowlton WA, Rosenberg GA: Hospital-sponsored preferred provider organizations, law, medicine, and health care. 12(5):204-209, 1984.

Rooks J, Haas JE, editors: *Nurse midwifery in America: a report of the American College of Nurse Midwives Foundation,* Washington, DC, 1986, American College of Nurse Midwives Foundation.

Safriet BJ: Health care dollars and regulatory sense: the role of the advanced practice nursing, *Yale J Regulation* 9(2):149-220, 1992.

Salmon ME: Public health nursing: the opportunity of a century, *Am J Pub Health* 83(12):1674-1675, 1993.

Shalala DE: Health care reform isn't dead, *The Washington Post,* Oct 10, 1994, p A23.

Starfield B: *Primary care: concept, evolution, and policy.* New York, 1992, Oxford University Press.

Trafford A, Rich S: Health care reform in congress? *The Washington Post,* Sept 20, 1994, pp 12-14.

US Bureau of Census: *Current population reports: population profile of the United States.* (Studies Series P-23 No 159) Washington, DC, 1989, US Government Printing Office.

US Bureau of Census: *Government organization, vol 1*(1), Washington, DC, 1992, US Government Printing Office.

US Bureau of Census: *Household and family characteristics.* P20-477, Washington, DC, March 1993, US Government Printing Office.

US Department of Health and Human Services: *Health personnel in the United States: eighth report to Congress 1991* (DHHS Pub No HRS-P-OD-92-1), Washington, DC, 1992, US Government Printing Office.

US Department of Health and Human Services: *An agenda for health professions reform,* Health Resources and Services Administration. 1993, Rockville, Md.

US Public Health Service: *Keeping America healthy,* Washington, DC, 1994, US Government Printing Office (brochure).

WK Kellogg Foundation: *Lessons learned in community-based health programming,* Battle Creek, Mich, 1993, The Foundation.

World Health Organization: *Primary health care,* Geneva, 1978.

World Health Organization: *Basic documents,* ed 36, Geneva, 1986, The Organization.

World Health Organization: *World health statistics annual,* Geneva, 1986.

Wright RA: Community-oriented primary care: the cornerstone of health care reform, *JAMA* 269(19):2544-2547, 1993.

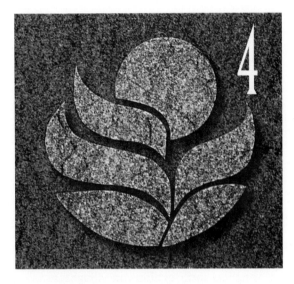

4 Perspectives on International Health Care

Kathleen Huttlinger

Objectives ▼

After reading this chapter, the student should be able to do the following:

◆ Identify the major aims and goals for world health that were presented at the International Conference on Primary Health Care at Alma Ata.
◆ Describe the role of community health nursing in international health.
◆ Describe the relationship between economic development and the status of health in developed and lesser developed countries.
◆ Identify at least five organizations that are involved in international health.
◆ Discuss some of the major health concerns that are present in developed and lesser developed countries.

Key Terms ▼

developed country
disability-adjusted life years (DALYs)
global burden of disease (GBD)
governmental organizations
health commodification
Health for All by the Year 2000 (HFA2000)
intergovernmental organizations
lesser developed country
Pan American Health Organization
philanthropic organizations
primary health care
private and commercial organizations
private voluntary organizations
professional and technical organizations
religious organizations
secular organizations
United Nations Childrens Fund (UNICEF)
World Bank
World Health Organization (WHO)

Outline ▼

This chapter provides a description of some of the major health problems of the world as they pertain to nurses who work in community settings. In particular, it discusses the role of primary health care in international health and presents examples of different health systems. Also discussed are ways that community health nurses are involved in world health. Lastly, it explains the relationship of economic development to health care throughout the world.

OVERVIEW OF INTERNATIONAL HEALTH

In 1977, attendees at the annual meeting of the World Health Assembly maintained that a major social goal for all of its member agencies should be "the attainment by all citizens of the world by the year 2000 a level of health that will permit them to lead a socially and economically productive life" (World Health Organization, 1986a, p. 65). The goal of **Health for All by the Year 2000 (HFA2000)** continued to be promoted by numerous other health-related conferences that were held around the world and was reinforced at the International Conference on Primary Health Care that was held in Alma Ata, Kazakhstan, in 1978 in what was then Soviet Central Asia. The conference was sponsored by the World Health Organization (WHO) and the United Nations Childrens Fund (UNICEF). The participants in this conference, who represented 143 countries and 67 organizations, adopted a resolution that proclaimed that the major key to attaining HFA2000 was the worldwide implementation of primary health care (Basch, 1990).

Since the conference at Alma Ata, the outgrowth and interest in world health and how best to attain it have been tremendous. This interest is reflected in a growing need among people around the world to know and understand the issues and concerns that affect health on a global basis. This is important in light of the fact that many countries have not yet experienced the technological growth in their health care systems that has been realized by more developmentally advanced countries such as the United States. Many terms are used to describe those nations that have achieved a high level of industrial and technological advancement (along with a stable market economy) and those that have not. For the purposes of this chapter, the term **developed country** is used to refer to those countries with a stable economy and a wide range of industrial and technological development. Examples of such countries are the United States, Canada, Japan, the United Kingdom, Sweden, and France. Countries that have not yet achieved stability with respect to their economy and technological development are referred to as a **lesser developed country.** A few countries considered lesser developed include Bangladesh, Zaire, Haiti, Guatemala, countries in sub-Sahara Africa, and the island nation of Indonesia. Both developed and lesser developed countries are found in all parts of the world and in all geographical and climatic zones (Evlo and Carrin, 1992).

Did You Know?

Indonesia is a country that has actively promoted the involvement of women in its health and economic development. *Posyandu*, or integrated health posts, have been established in villages throughout the country. Women are trained as community educators to address issues of water supply, sewage and garbage disposal, and the quality of house construction. They are also being taught the beneficial aspects of selling their handicrafts and other products on a commercial basis to enhance and develop the village's economic base.

All countries and regions of the world experience health problems of one kind or another. However, those countries that are lesser developed are often faced with a multiplicity of health care problems and concerns that often sound exotic and far removed to people in more developed nations. Some of the more exotic-sounding problems include such diseases as leishmaniasis, schistosomiasis, pediculosis, typhus, yellow fever, and malaria. Health problems that are still ongoing and in need of control in the lesser developed countries include measles, mumps, rubella, and polio, while the current health concerns of the more developed countries reflect ongoing struggles with hepatitis, the appearance of new viral strains such as the *hantavirus,* and larger social issues such as violence and substance abuse.

Beginning with the inception of HFA2000, most countries soon realized that they needed to improve their economic development and therefore requested monetary assistance and technological expertise from the wealthier countries (Collado, 1992; World Bank, 1992, 1993). Thus, as the economic agreements between countries removed financial and political barriers, growth and development were stimulated. Simultaneously, global health problems that once seemed very distant were now brought closer to people all over the world, political and economic barriers between countries fell, and the movement of population groups increased, as did the risk of exposure to numerous kinds of diseases and health risks (Basch, 1990). Not only did world travelers serve as hosts to various types of disease agents, but they also exposed themselves to diseases and environmental health hazards that were unknown or rare in their home country. Two examples of diseases from recent years that were once fairly isolated and rare but are now spread throughout the world are acquired immunodeficiency syndrome (AIDS) and drug-resistant tuberculosis (TB).

Despite efforts by individual governments and international health organizations to improve the general economy and welfare for all countries of the world, many health problems continue to exist, especially among the poor. Lesser developed countries still experience high infant and child mortality rates, with diarrheal and respiratory diseases considered to be the major contributory factors (World Bank, 1993). Other major worldwide health problems include nutritional deficiencies among all age groups, women's health and fertility problems, sexually transmitted diseases (STDs) and illnesses related to the human immunodeficiency virus (HIV), malaria, TB, drug-resistant diseases, occupational and environmental health hazards, and abuses of tobacco, alcohol, and drugs.

The importance of knowledge of the major problems and concerns of the world's health among community health nurses cannot be underestimated. Many of these concerns directly affect the health of individuals who reside in America. For example, with the recent passage of the North American Free Trade Agreement (NAFTA) between the United States, Canada, and Mexico, the borders between these countries have opened, allowing an increased movement of products and people. Along the United States/Mexico border, an influx of undocumented immigrants in recent years has raised concerns for the health of people who reside in these areas. Many immigrants have settled on unincorporated land, known as *colonias,* outside of the major metropolitan areas. For the most part, the *colonias* have no developed road, transportation, water, and electrical services. The result has been an increase in the appearance of numerous disease conditions that are associated with poverty, poor sanitation, and overcrowded conditions. These disease conditions include amebiasis, respiratory and other diarrheal diseases, and environmental health hazards (Cech and Essman, 1992).

Community health nurses play an active and participatory role in the international border areas where political and economic boundaries mesh. They often provide the only health care service in these areas. As such, they have contributed to the provision of reliable health care to the people in these areas and have served as valuable resources for identifying potential health risks.

INTERNATIONAL HEALTH AND THE ROLE OF PRIMARY HEALTH CARE

The role of **primary health care** in international health is associated with the worldwide conference that was held at Alma Alta and that proclaimed HFA2000 (WHO/UNICEF, 1978). The participants at this conference proposed that the delivery of primary health care should be made available to people throughout the world and that this care needed to be based on current technology and acceptable practice methods. It also proposed that members of communities needed to be involved in all aspects of the planning and im-

Research Brief

Corcega TF: Participatory research: getting the community involved in health development, *Int Nurs Rev* 39(6):185-188, 1992.

This participatory research project describes a mechanism by which individuals from communities are involved with the process of identifying and examining the health problems of their community and the potential ways to design solutions for them. A comparative analysis of program process and product from different settings around the world was used to determine the success and failures of such programs. Steps for undertaking the project are described, along with essential factors as entry point, mobilization approaches, problem issues, training, roles, and achievement of goals.

plementation of health services. (See Appendix A)

Recognizing that there would be differences among countries with respect to the implementation of primary health care because of local customs and environments, it was anticipated that several major components should be included in each plan. These components included (1) an organized approach to health education that involved professional health care providers and trained community representatives; (2) aggressive attention to environmental sanitation, especially food and water sources; (3) the involvement and training of community and village health workers in all plans and intervention programs; (4) the development of maternal and child health programs that would include immunization and family planning; (5) initiation of preventive programs that were specifically aimed at local endemic problems such as malaria and schistosomiasis; (6) accessibility and affordability of services for the treatment of common diseases and injuries; (7) the availability of chemotherapeutic agents for the treatment of acute, chronic, and communicable diseases; (8) the development of nutrition programs; and (9) promotion and acceptance of traditional medicine (WHO/ UNICEF, 1978).

The aim of participants of the Alma Ata conference was to emphasize universal access and participation and to encourage a reallocation of resources, if needed, to reduce the inequality of health care that existed among the nations of the world. They encouraged community participation in all aspects of health care planning and implementation and the delivery of health care that was "scientifically sound, technically effective, socially relevant and acceptable" (WHO/ UNICEF, 1978, p. 2).

The community health nurse can and does play an important role in the primary health care team throughout the world. In particular, nurses with community health experience can provide much needed knowledge and skill in those countries where nursing is not an organized profession and give guidance not only to the nurses, but also the auxiliary personnel who are participating as part of the primary health care team. In many settings throughout the world, community health nurses provide direct patient care and facilitate the educational and health promotional needs of the community. In contrast, in the more developed countries, nursing is often seen as one of the strongest advocates of the principles of primary health care through its social commitment to equality of health care and support of the concepts that are contained in the Alma Ata declaration.

MAJOR INTERNATIONAL HEALTH ORGANIZATIONS

The number of international health organizations continues to grow and reflects an increasing interest in the world's health. Basch (1990) classifies the organizations that participate and contribute to the world's health as (1) private voluntary, (2) philanthropic, (3) professional and technical, (4) commercial, (5) governmental, and (6) intergovernmental.

Private Voluntary

Private voluntary organizations include both religious and secular groups. **Religious organizations** consist of several denominations and religious interests and support many different kinds of health care programs, including the sponsorship of hospitals in rural and urban areas, refugee centers, orphanages, and leprosy treatment centers. For example, the Maryknoll Missionaries are sponsored by the Catholic Church and carry out health service projects around the world. The many Protestant and Evangelical groups function both as separate entities and as part of the Church World Service, which works jointly with **secular organizations** to improve efforts with health care, community development, and other needed projects. Some of the other private and voluntary groups that assist with the worldwide health effort include CARE, Oxfam, and Third World First. Most of these organizations receive funding from various countries, including the United States, the United Kingdom, Sweden, Canada, and countries in Western Europe.

Philanthropic

Philanthropic organizations are those that receive funding from private endowment funds. Some of the more active philanthropic organizations that are involved in health care throughout the world include the W.K. Kellogg Foundation, the Milbank Memorial Fund, the Pathfinder Fund, the Hewlett Foundation, the Ford Foundation, the Rockefeller Foundation, and the Carnegie Foundation. The purpose and programmatic goals of each organization widely differ with respect to funding, and this purpose may change as gov-

erning boards change. Some of the worldwide health care activities that have been sponsored throughout past years include projects in public and preventive health; vital statistics; medical, nursing, and dental education; family planning programs; economic planning and development; and the establishment of laboratories to investigate communicable diseases.

Professional and Technical

One of the most famous of the **professional and technical organizations** is the *Institut Pasteur,* which has been in existence since the 1880s. In particular, its laboratories have facilitated the development of sera and vaccines for many countries in need, have disseminated current health information, and have trained and provided fellowships for medical training and study in France.

Private and Commercial

Private and commercial organizations such as the Johnson & Johnson Company are those that provide financial and technical backing for investment, employment, and access to market economies and to health care. Several of these organizations have come under sharp criticism because of their promotion of infant formulas, pharmaceuticals, and medical supplies to lesser developed countries. For example, the health commodification of pharmaceuticals in Southern India has been criticized for not taking into consideration the cultural and social structure of the country and has thus interfered with a longstanding traditional medical system. **Health commodification** refers to the buying and selling of health and health care products such as pharmaceuticals. In Southern India, good health and prosperity are related to certain social parameters that have been bestowed to families and communities as a result of their conformity to the sociomoral order that was set down by their ancestors, gods, and patron spirits (Nichter, 1989). The taking of pharmaceutical agents thus disrupts the social and cultural order of things that have been addressed by more traditional practices. Similar controversies in other countries have involved infant formulas and oral rehydration therapies (ORTs).

Governmental

Various **governmental organizations** throughout the world enter into bilateral arrangements with other countries. Most of these arrangements are made between a lesser developed country and one that is more economically advanced. Some of the countries that have provided assistance include the United States, the United Kingdom, Japan, Sweden, Canada, and Germany. Incentives for engaging in formal arrangements may include economic enhancements for the benefit of both countries, national defense of one or both countries, or to enhance and protect the private investments that are being carried out by individuals in both nations. Lastly, countries with advanced medical systems and technology might want to enter into a collaborative effort with a lesser developed country to conduct medical research. For example, the Japanese government currently has an active collaborative arrangement with Indonesia to study ways to control the spread of yellow fever and malaria.

Intergovernmental

Four of the best-known **intergovernmental organizations** are the World Bank, the World Health Organization (WHO), the United Nations Childrens Fund (UNICEF), and the Pan American Health Organization (PAHO). These organizations collaborate with a number of governments, private foundations, and other health care efforts on an ongoing basis.

World Bank

The major aim of the **World Bank** is to facilitate significant interventions that are necessary to improve the health status of individuals who reside in areas where economical development is lacking. For example, it supports projects that enable communities to obtain safe and usable water and affordable housing, develop effective sanitation systems, and assist with numerous health care interventions such as family planning. It also provides financial assistance for those seeking careers as health providers. In addition, the World Bank has been involved in projects that focus on the development of economic growth and the improvement of internal infrastructures such as communication systems, roads, and electricity.

The World Bank has collaborated with the WHO from time to time, such as with the recent efforts to control the tropical disease onchocerciasis in West Africa. The World Bank will also lend money to governments and private foundations to develop specific projects that will advance the health status of their population.

World Health Organization

The history of the **World Health Organization (WHO)** can be dated to the mid-1880s, when the First International Sanitary Conference directed efforts at worldwide control of cholera (Basch, 1990). Continued efforts by this and other worldwide agencies culminated in the formation of the WHO in 1946 as an outgrowth of the League of Nations and the charter of the United Nations (UN). The UN charter provided for the formation of a special health agency to address the wide scope and nature of the world's health problems. The headquarters for the WHO is in Geneva, with six regional headquarters in Copenhagen, Alexandria, Brazzaville, New Delhi, Manila, and Washington, D.C. It is headed by a director general and five assistant generals.

The scope of the WHO is extremely broad and consists of more than 25 major functions with over 100 subfunctions. More than 1000 ongoing health-related projects are occurring at any one time. Some of these projects may be operated and funded by the WHO itself or in collaboration with other governments and health care agencies. However, most of the projects fall into those that are associated with technical services or services to governments. Requests for assistance are made directly to the WHO by a country for an individual project or as part of a larger, collaborative endeavor that involves many regions. Examples of collaborative endeavors include comparative family planning programs, applied research on communicable disease and immunization, or the project that investigates the role of midwifery in maternal and child health. However, a substantial number of the programs that are sponsored by the WHO involve individual countries, with emphasis placed on training medical personnel, development of health services, primary health care, and specific disease control programs.

United Nations Childrens Fund

The **United Nations Childrens Fund (UNICEF)** was formed shortly after World War II to assist children in the war ravaged countries of Europe. Shortly after the war, it became apparent that children throughout the world needed assistance. With financial assistance from the UN General Assembly, programs were developed to control yaws, leprosy, and TB. Other efforts have since been aimed at the provision of safe drinking water, education, and maternal and child health. UNICEF has worked closely with the WHO over the past years as an advocate for women's and children's health.

Pan American Health Organization

Founded in 1902, the **Pan American Health Organization** is one of the oldest continuously functioning international health organizations. This organization focuses its efforts on the countries of the Western Hemisphere, with particular emphasis on those in Latin America. It functions to distribute epidemiological information, to provide technical assistance with a wide range of health and environmental issues, to support fellowships, and to promote research and professional education.

INTERNATIONAL HEALTH AND ECONOMIC DEVELOPMENT

The issues and problems associated with world health are directly related to economic, industrial, and technological development. Even though several studies of the lesser developed countries have indicated that the general demand for health care is related to health production technology, little evidence shows how and under what circumstances this technology affects the use of actual health care services (Wouters, 1992). Access to services and the removal of financial barriers alone do not account for utilization patterns and availability of technology. In fact, in some cases, the introduction of health care technology from more developed countries to the lesser developed countries has led to less-than-satisfactory results. For example, during the 1980s in a country in the Eastern Mediterreanean area, two-thirds of the high-output x-ray machines were not in use because of a lack of qualified and trained individuals to carry out routine maintenance and repairs (Perry and Marx, 1992). In another example, a hospital in a Latin American country was given a high-technology neonatal intensive care unit by a wealthier and more technologically advanced country. However, 70% of the infants died after discharge because there were no follow-up nutritional and prevention services. Many of the infants experienced malnutrition and complications from dehydration on return to their home communities. More successful programs might have been developed for both of the previous examples, which focused on public health or more rudimentary kinds of health care technology (Perry and Marx, 1992).

Given the previous examples, the improvement in the overall health status of a population undoubtedly contributes to the economic growth of a country in several ways (World Bank, 1993):

1. A reduction in production loss that is caused by workers who are absent from work because of illness
2. An increase in the use of natural resources that may be inaccessible because of the presence of disease entities
3. An increase in the number of children who can attend school and eventually participate in their country's economic growth
4. The addition of monetary resources to the economic development of a country that has been otherwise spent on treating disease and illness

However, adequate health care coverage for individuals who reside in the lesser developed countries is often lacking because their governments reallocate financial resources from internal health needs and education and divert it to advance the country's market economy or to develop technology. Many countries also divert resources to develop the underlying infrastructure that they believe is needed for technological and industrial improvement. Unfortunately, when governments experience an economic crisis, household expenditures are affected adversely. Most often, the provision of health services in the lesser developed countries depends on the importation of drugs, vaccines, and other health care products. This provision depends on a network of foreign exchange that is influenced by economic and political factors. Often, the lesser developed countries have a difficult time maintaining a balance of payments, which leads to severe shortages of foreign exchange and subsequent reduction in the ability to import goods (Evlo and Carrin, 1992).

Because the economics of international development are complex, it is often difficult to convince governments to direct their resources away from perceived needs such as military and technology and instead place the resources in health and educational programs. Ideally, the role of the more developed countries is to assist the lesser developed countries in identifying internal needs and to support cost efficiency measures and share their technology and industrial expertise (Wouters, 1992).

It is important that nurses who work in international communities not only acknowledge the importance of technology and development but also recognize the political and economic ramifications as well. Provision of health services alone will not ease a country's health care plight.

HEALTH CARE SYSTEMS

The countries of the world present many different kinds of health care systems. However, most health care systems in place consist of several fundamental elements: (1) usership or who can utilize the system, (2) benefits or what kind of coverage a citizen might expect, (3) providers or who provides the health care, (4) facilities or where the provision of health care takes place, and (5) power or who controls access and usability of the system (Basch, 1990). The role of nursing in each of these countries is as diverse as the kind of health care system in which nurses are a part. To help illustrate these concepts, a brief description of several health systems is provided.

United Kingdom

The United Kingdom employs a health system that is owned and operated by the government, and services are available to all its citizens without cost or for a small fee. Administration of the services is conducted through a system of health authorities. Each health authority plans and provides services for $\frac{1}{4}$ to 1 million people. The services offered by each health authority are comprehensive in that health is available to all who want it and covers all aspects of general medicine, disability and rehabilitation, and surgery. Although physicians are the primary providers in this system, nurses and allied health professionals are also recognized and utilized. Services are made available through hospitals, private physicians and allied health professional clinics, health outreach programs such as hospice, boroughs, and environmental health services. Physicians are paid by the number of clients that they serve and not by individual visits. The system is financed by the government through individual and corporate taxation. Although the British system has come under criticism in past years, individual citizens maintain a high level of support for government funding and control of their health services.

One of the hallmarks of the system is a demonstrated reduction in infant mortality. This rate improved from 14.3 deaths per 1000 births in 1975 to

8.8 in 1988. Overall life expectancy for all of Great Britain's citizens also improved during the same time period (National League for Nursing, 1992).

Canada

The Canadian health care system is based on a national health insurance program that is operated by each provincial government. One notable feature of this system is that specialists are concentrated in centers, whereas primary care providers are evenly distributed throughout the Canadian provinces. Physicians are the primary providers, although nursing does play an active role in all aspects of health care delivery, including community and public health. Hospitals and other health care agencies have an annual budget that is set by the provincial government. Financing for the system is derived from provincial and federal governments, which receive monies through personal income taxes. Benefits are broad and cover every aspect of health care but limit certain kinds of elective surgeries as well as dental and eye care. As in Great Britain, infant mortality rates decreased during the past 10 years, and overall life expectancy has increased.

Sweden

Health care in Sweden is made available to all its citizens. The system is based on a national health service that is almost operately completely by the Swedish government. County councils hire physicians to operate the health systems on a local basis, with hospitals being run by either local or area agencies and with budgets determined by the area's medical needs. The role of nurses in the health care delivery system is not as pronounced as in the United States, Canada, or Great Britain, but there are indications that nurses are gaining in their professional role and autonomy. The financial basis for the Swedish health care delivery system is derived from a proportional wage tax of 13.5%, with 35% of the total costs generated by federal revenues. The remaining 4% is obtained through direct patient fees (National League for Nursing, 1992). The services that are provided for in this system are very comprehensive and range from all hospital expenses to preventive services, physician services, prescription drugs, dental and eye care, and psychiatric care. During the past 10 years, infant mortality has decreased and life expectancy rates have increased.

Cuba

In contrast to the previous systems, the medical system in Cuba is based on a nationalized medical care program similar to the one that was in operation in the former Soviet Union. The government organizes, plans, and controls all access and benefits that are provided. The Cuban government recognizes only physicians as primary providers of medical care. Because contact with the Cuban government and its people has been very sporadic and inconsistent during the past 30 years, very little is known about the role of nursing in Cuba. Traditional or folk healers known as *curanderos* have been forbidden to practice, but many individuals still seek them out for their medical care. Medical services are administrated and dispersed through urban polyclinics and rural health centers. In this system, all physicians must spend a large proportion of their time working for government service and only a small amount of time in private practice, for which they may charge a fee for service. Data with respect to infant mortality ratios and life expectancy have not been made available.

MAJOR WORLD HEALTH PROBLEMS AND THE BURDEN OF DISEASE

As indicated earlier, present indicators of world health demonstrate that critical health care needs still exist throughout the world despite very earnest attempts to attain good health for its populations. As world economies lagged during the late 1970s and 1980s, the amount of debt that was incurred by the lesser developed countries increased, and the money that was once used for health care was diverted to paying off the debt. Therefore, even though attempts have been made by lesser developed countries to address their health care needs, major health problems still exist. Communicable diseases that are often preventable are still common throughout the world but are more common in the lesser developed countries. In addition, both developed and lesser developed countries have to find ways to cope with the aging of their populations, which presents governments with a burden of providing care for people who become ill with more expensive noncommunicable and chronic forms of diseases and disabilities. Lastly, illnesses such as AIDS have emerged to raise new issues and concerns throughout the world, whereas some longstanding diseases such as TB and malaria still persist and add to a growing burden of overextended health care delivery systems throughout the world.

Mortality statistics do not serve to describe adequately the outlook of health in the world. The WHO and the World Bank (1993) have developed an indicator called the **global burden of disease (GBD).** The GBD combines losses from premature death and losses of healthy life that result from disability. *Premature death* is defined as the difference between the actual age at death and life expectancy at that age in a low-mortality population. People who have debilitating injuries or diseases must be cared for in some way, most often by family members, and thus no longer can contribute to the family's or community's economic growth (World Bank, 1993). The GBD represents units of **disability-adjusted life years,** or **DALYs**

(World Bank, 1993). In 1990, for example, 1.36 billion DALYs were lost worldwide, which equates to 42 million deaths of newborn children or of 80 million deaths of people who reach age 50. Following this, approximately 12.4 million children under age 5 died during the same year in developing countries, which represents a tremendous loss of future human potential. If these children could face the same risks as those in countries with developed market economies, the deaths would decrease by 90% to 1.1 million. This example serves to demonstrate the importance of having accessible and affordable health prevention programs for children around the world (World Bank, 1993). Thus, overall, premature deaths throughout the world during 1990 accounted for 66% of all DALYs lost, with debilitating injuries and diseases accounting for 34%.

As a comparison, in the lesser developed countries, 67% of all DALY loss in 1990 was attributed to premature death, whereas the more developed countries reported only 55% from this same cause. Communicable diseases still account for the greatest proportion of calculated DALYs worldwide for both males and females, followed by noncommunicable diseases and injuries. Research studies have indicated that infections and parasitic diseases remain a threat to the health of many population groups. The information from these studies demonstrate that there is still need for intervention with infectious and other kinds of communicable diseases. Conditions that contribute to one quarter of the GBD throughout the world include diarrheal disease, respiratory infections, worm infestations, malaria, and childhood diseases such as measles. In 1992, Sub-Sahara Africa demonstrated a GBD of 43% DALYs lost, largely because of preventable diseases among children. Other countries with comparable DALYs are India (28%) and the Middle Eastern crescent (29%). In adults, STDs and TB combine to account for 70% of the world's GBD (World Bank, 1993).

It is difficult to ascertain the total amount of loss even using the GBD because many consequences of disease and injury are difficult to measure. It is very difficult, for example, to measure the social and cultural impact of the disfigurements that are the result of accidents or debilitating diseases such as leprosy and river blindness. Likewise, it is very problematic to measure social conditions such as familial and marital dysfunction, war, and familial violence.

As already stated, communicable diseases still contribute substantially to the world's disease burden. The following sections describe those selected communicable diseases that still present problems worldwide: TB, AIDS, and malaria. Other health problems discussed include maternal and women's health, diarrheal disease in children, and nutrition.

Communicable Diseases

The long-term benefits of immunizing children against communicable disease are well documented. The successful campaign against smallpox during the 1960s and 1970s by the WHO is one example of how countries can work together to eradicate a major worldwide problem. Smallpox has been virtually eliminated throughout the world, with only occasional and incidental reportings. The systematic and planned smallpox program formed the basis for a series of worldwide efforts that are now being implemented to control and eradicate other infectious and communicable diseases. In 1974 the WHO formed the Expanded Programme on Immunization, which sought to reduce morbidity and mortality from diphtheria, pertussis, tetanus, TB, measles, and poliomyelitis throughout the world (Schild and Assad 1983; WHO, 1986b). The major aim of immunization is to induce an immunity to a disease without experiencing the actual disease.

Tuberculosis

It is estimated that 80 million new cases of TB will occur worldwide during the 1990s and that 8 million of these will be attributable to HIV. Predictions also indicate that 30 million people will die of TB during the same period, including 2.9 million individuals who are affected with HIV (Dolin et al., 1994). At present, TB represents the largest cause of death from a single infectious agent and strikes nearly 3 million people each year. This particular statistic represents 25% of adult deaths in the lesser developed countries that might have been prevented (WHO, 1992a). The growth of the world's population, including an increase in the number of aged individuals and the adverse effects of HIV, contributes to the large projected estimations of TB (Dolin et al., 1994).

A third of the world's population, or 1.7 billion people, harbor the TB pathogen *Mycobacterium tuberculosis*. Clinical manifestations of the disease include pulmonary TB, which is the most widespread form; TB meningitis, which is a leading cause of childhood mortality; and TB of a variety of other organs. The WHO (1992a) reported that of the 8 million new cases that were reported in 1992, 3.6 million were of the pulmonary TB form. Even through the disease is known in all age groups, the heaviest toll is among young adults.

The presence of disease-causing bacilli in sputum examination is not evident in all forms of pulmonary TB. About half the cases are detectable by sputum smear examination, and these are of the infectious pulmonary type. Chemotherapy undoubtedly reduces the numbers of individuals who die from TB. However, many of the lesser developed countries do not have organized treatment and prevention programs and therefore lose more people each year to TB than either malaria or measles (WHO, 1992a).

Although TB is known worldwide, the greatest number of cases are seen in sub-Sahara Africa, where the incidence is 260 cases per 100,000 people. This area is followed by the dense population centers in Southeast Asia and Western Pacific regions, with reportable cases of TB accounting for 60% of the new cases each year worldwide. As might be expected, the largest declining rates for TB are seen in the highly industrialized countries of the world. Worldwide, approximately 2.53 million deaths were attributable to TB in 1990, which exceeds the number of deaths that resulted from measles and malaria. The case fatality ratio for untreated TB is greater than 50%. Of these deaths, 1.1 million occurred in Southeast Asia and 0.6 million in the Western Pacific. Also in 1990, 116,000 TB deaths could be attributed to HIV infection, with most of these deaths occurring in sub-Sahara Africa (Dolin et al., 1994). Additional estimates have indicated that one-quarter of adult deaths that could be avoided in the lesser developed countries are caused by TB. This equates to a tremendous loss of social and economic potential for these countries.

Two factors are a threat to TB control and eradication. The first is the appearance of the HIV virus, which is one of the highest risk factors associated with latent TB. HIV-associated TB infections most often progress to an active disease. Information currently available suggests that 5% to 10% of these individuals infected with HIV and *M. tuberculosis* will develop TB each year. This can be compared with 2% of people infected with *M. tuberculosis* but not HIV who will develop TB (Dolin et al., 1994). The appearance of HIV has added to the difficulty of treatment programs in both developed and lesser developed countries. For example, in Africa, almost half of those individuals who are HIV seropositive are also infected with TB, and it is estimated that nearly 5% to 8% of these individuals will develop the clinical manifestations of TB. More importantly, the HIV-positive individuals with infectious TB increase the possibility of transmission of TB to their families and to the community, thus increasing the prevalence of this condition.

The second factor that poses a threat to the control and eradication of TB is the appearance of resistance of TB bacillus to isoniazid and rifampin, the two drugs that are currently being used to treat TB. Resistance to these drugs is already evident around the world, including the Mexico/Texas border communities (Quiroga, 1995). The WHO and other organizations maintain that a high priority needs to be given to TB control and eradication programs around the world. They advocate a short-term chemotherapy of smear-positive patients as being one of the most cost-effective health interventions available.

Bacille Calmette-Guérin (BCG) consists of a series of vaccines that induce active immunity and that are used to prevent TB and has been available since the 1920s. The effectiveness of BCG is still highly questionable, but research studies have demonstrated that it is effective in preventing the more lethal forms of TB, including meningitis and miliary disease in children (WHO, 1992a). These same studies have demonstrated that more than 80% of the infants in the lesser developed countries have been vaccinated with lesser coverage in sub-Sahara Africa. However, more studies are needed worldwide to determine the effect that BCG may have on the more infectious types of TB. Present indications are that BCG does not re-duce the transmission of infectious types of TB.

The standard chemotherapeutic treatments used in many countries for TB are isoniazid, thioacetazone, and streptomycin and are effective at reducing sputum-positive cases to noninfectious. Which drug and the combinations that are used vary from country to country. To be effective, however, treatment must be carried out on a consistent basis. Many of the lesser developed countries have difficulty getting patients to comply with any treatment regimen, and many of the TB intervention programs in these countries have been unable to carry out curative programs following standard treatment regimens (WHO 1992a). Therefore, the introduction of short-course chemotherapy (SCC) programs has been successful in several of the lesser developed countries, including Malawi, Mozambique, Nicaragua, and Tanzania, producing a cure rate of approximately 80%. The SCC program involves aggressive administration of chemotherapeutic drugs combined with short-term hospitalization. Short-term chemotherapy uses a combination of drugs over 6 to 8 months and costs about $50 to $80 (United States) per patient. The long-term program involves two to three drugs taken over 12 to 18 months for a cost of $10 to $15 (United States) per patient. However, only 30% of patients complete the 12 to 16-month program, whereas more than 60% complete the SCC program. The key to the program lies in a well-managed system with regular supply of anti-tuberculosis drugs to the treatment centers, follow-up care, and rigorous reporting and analysis of patient information (WHO, 1992a). Despite these efforts, however, little progress and international support have been given to place TB control programs as a number-one priority worldwide.

Acquired Immunodeficiency Syndrome

AIDS is rapidly becoming a major cause of morbidity and mortality throughout the world (Heyward and Curran, 1988; Kalibala and Anderson, 1993). Once infected, the HIV remains with individuals for the remainder of their lives. The virus may produce no symptoms for years, but risk increases with the threat of a breakdown of the immune system and the subsequent infections that may occur. Worldwide prevention programs are important because failing to control this virulent disease will result in damaging and costly consequences for all countries in the future.

In 1987, 100 countries reported the existence of HIV, which causes AIDS, with estimates of 5 to 10 million people who had already contracted the disease (Basch, 1990). Current estimates of the spread of AIDS indicate that more than 150 million people presently carry the virus throughout the world (Carrington, 1994). It is estimated that by the year 2000, AIDS will contribute to 3.3% of the global burden of disease and that 1.8 million people will die of AIDS each year (World Bank, 1993). This is particularly significant because recent reports indicate that infection rates for AIDS double rapidly in the lesser developed countries. The threat of AIDS doubling or tripling these projections by the year 2000 are realistic and frightening.

In the lesser developed countries, AIDS is associated with poverty. Approximately 80% of the individuals currently infected with HIV live in lesser developed countries. For example, countries in Sub-Sahara Africa lie in one of the areas of the world that is most affected by AIDS, and reports indicate that more than 8 million adults exhibit signs of infection. Based on population totals, this amounts to 1 in every 40 adults who are infected with HIV, with certain urban areas accounting for infection rates as high as 1 in every 3 adults. Unfortunately, this statistic is also evidenced by increases in childhood mortality when decreases were previously noted. UNICEF issued a report in 1990 that predicted that up to 5.5 million children would be orphaned during the 1990s in East and Central Africa as a result of parents with AIDS dying and leaving a child behind (Kalibala and Anderson, 1993).

Present efforts to control the spread of AIDS are directed toward prevention. AIDS spreads very rapidly in the absence of prevention, particularly among high-risk or core groups such as prostitutes (both male and female) and intravenous (IV) drug users. From these core groups, AIDS spreads in a slow but accelerated manner to the rest of the general population. Therefore, prevention and intervention programs that target core population groups are essential because their effectiveness diminishes as the infection moves out of high-risk and high-transmission core groups (World Bank, 1993).

The consequences of AIDS in terms of cost to the individual, family, community, and country are tremendous. AIDS affects adults in their most productive years. Since many of the AIDS victims are heads of households or major economic household contributors, a negative economic effect is experienced by families, communities, and countries. Those countries with the highest HIV infection and AIDS disease rates have discovered that their health systems quickly become overburdened. AIDS patients, with their related infection, tax even the most economically sound health care systems, let alone those striving to stay economically stable. If the spread of AIDS is left unchecked, many countries will experience an accelerated demand for health services that will infringe on the health care of noninfected HIV patients.

The WHO has established a program with collaborative governments that is directed at education at the individual and community levels, providing for safe blood transfusions and injections, and provision of care for those who have the disease (Basch, 1990). It is clear that many gaps are present in our understanding of AIDS and the HIV infectious process. Priorities to investigate more efficient and effective means by which to control the spread of HIV are being developed throughout the world, but much more needs to be done. Community health nurses can assist in this global effort by conducting research and intervention studies that address many of the identified problem areas involving AIDS, but particularly at the individual, family, and aggregate levels. Community health nurses are in opportune positions to develop intervention programs with target core populations, including young adults and women, and to participate in playing an active role in meeting this worldwide challenge.

Malaria

Malaria remains one of the most prevalent communicable diseases in the world, with 90 countries and areas considered to be malaria ridden (WHO, 1994). Countries where the disease is most endemic are those that lie in the tropical areas of Asia, Africa, and Latin America. It is estimated that 300 to 500 million people develop clinical cases of the disease each year, with more than 90% of these occurring in equatorial Africa (WHO, 1994). This current situation exists despite worldwide efforts to eradicate and control the spread of malaria over the past 50 years.

There are two primary modes of malarial control, vector reduction and chemotherapy (Basch, 1990). The methods of vector control vary widely, from the larvae-eating fish *Tilapia* to the use of insecticidal sprays and oils. Needless to say, the latter poses a potential threat to the environment, where other potential hazards such as lumbering and mining already threaten the delicate ecosystem of the tropical areas involved. Countries that do not have strict environmental laws continue to use DDT sprays to control mosquito populations despite DDT-resistant mosquitos having developed over time. The non-DDT insecticide sprays, such as malathion, are generally more costly to obtain and present an extra financial cost to the lesser developed countries. Other methods for control and eradication that are being considered by malaria-ridden countries are environmental management, reduction and control of the source, and elimination of the adult mosquito.

Chemotherapeutic agents can be used for both protection and treatment of the disease. Drugs for treatment and prophylaxis can be costly and often produce side effects. However, current evidence suggests that the *Plasmodium* sporozoites are becoming resistant to both treatment and preventive chemotherapeutic agents. Efforts are presently underway to develop an antimalarial vaccine, but so far the results have been less than successful.

Individuals who reside or travel to *Anopheles*-infected areas are urged to protect themselves with mosquito netting, clothing that protects vulnerable parts of the body, and various repellents.

Maternal and Women's Health

A recent study on women's health indicated that most deaths to women around the world are related to pregnancy and childbirth and that the majority of these occur in the lesser developed countries (AbouZahr and Royston, 1992). Throughout the world, women between ages 15 and 44 account for approximately one-third of the world's disease burden and one-fifth of the burden for women ages 45 to 59. This burden comprises diseases and conditions that are either exclusive or predominantly found among women, including maternal mortality and morbidity, cervical cancer, anemia, STDs, osteoarthritis, and breast cancer (World Bank, 1993). Although most of these conditions can be dealt with by cost-effective prevention and screening programs, most of the lesser developed countries have ignored women's health issues other than those directly related to pregnancy and childbirth. Emphasis for health programs appears to be directed to those that favor male children and adult males over adult females (Ganatra and Hirve, 1994).

What Do You Think?

There is a bias toward males and away from females in the delivery of health care in many countries of the world.

In addition to these facts, the lesser developed countries presently account for 87% of the world's births, but statistics from many of the lesser developed countries indicate that prenatal services and safe birthing services are unavailable, inaccessible, and unaffordable to women throughout the world, with the continent of Africa exhibiting the highest maternal mortality rates. An African woman's risk of dying from pregnancy-related causes is 1 in 20 (AbouZahr and Royston, 1992). Africa is followed by the countries of Bangladesh, Pakistan, and India. These three countries account for nearly half of the world's maternal deaths but only 29% of the world's births. In fact, these three countries have more maternal deaths each week than Europe has in a single year (Basch, 1990). Still, an accurate reporting of maternal death is difficult to obtain because many of the women who die live in remote areas of the world and are poor, and their deaths are considered by many to be unimportant (Kestler, 1993).

The primary causes of maternal mortality, particularly in lesser developed countries, are varied. Most of the causes that are directly related to maternal mortality include hemorrhage, infection, convulsions, and coma caused by eclampsia and obstructed labor and infections from unsanitary conditions and nonsterile and poorly performed abortions. Risk factors for maternal mortality include poor nutritional status, disease conditions, high parity, and age below 20 and above 35 years.

To date, very little attention has been paid to the problem of maternal mortality, even though the reported statistics are high throughout the world. There has been, however, a movement to address the issue by the WHO and by the UN Fund for Population Activities (UNFPA). These two organizations have called for government initiatives and actions to address direct obstetrical deaths as well as those that arise from indirect causes. The WHO and UNFPA have presented the rationale that their initiatives and their call for action for programs addressing maternal health are associated with the health of infants and children.

In support of the recommendations of the WHO and UNFPA, the World Health Assembly's Technical Discussions on Women, Health, and Development in 1992 presented several suggestions to the WHO. These suggestions included (1) assisting governments to initiate legislation that addresses women's health problems, (2) supporting research that addresses socioeconomic implications of diseases in women, and (3) developing proactive strategies to intervene and reduce health problems among women (WHO, 1992b). Even so, safe motherhood initiatives undoubtedly are drastically needed throughout the world. These initiatives need to include accessible family planning services, access of prenatal and postnatal health care services, ensuring access to safe abortion, and improving the nutritional status of all women.

Diarrheal Disease

Diarrhea is one of the leading causes of illness and death in children under 5 years of age throughout the world and is most prominent in the lesser developed countries. For example, Guerrant (1986) indicated that diarrheal disease accounted for more than half of all the causes of death among children in Brazil. The prevalence of diarrheal disease is so pervasive that in 1978 the World Health Assembly established a global program to reduce mortality and morbidity in infants and young children who suffer from all forms of the disease.

Diarrhea is a symptom of a variety of different illnesses, and the definitions and perceptions of it vary greatly from country to country. For example, in Bangladesh, diarrhea is defined as more than two watery or loose stools in 24 hours, while Indonesians define it as four loose stools in 24 hours (Basch, 1990). Definitions are complicated by the observable presence of blood, mucus, or parasites. The age of the individual who is experiencing the diarrhea also complicates definitions.

Causes of diarrhea are just as varied and diverse as its definitions and perceptions. Some of the causes include (1) viruses such as the rotavirus and Norwalk-like agents; (2) bacteria, including *Campylobacter jejuni*, *Clostridium difficile*, *Escherichia coli*, *Salmonella*, and *Shigella*; (3) environmental toxins; (4) parasites such as *Giardia lamblia* and *Cryptosporidium*; and (5) worms. Nutritional deficiencies can also cause diarrhea and are most often secondary to infectious agents.

Dehydration is an immediate result of diarrhea and leads to a loss of fluid and electrolytes. The loss of up to 10% of the body's electrolytes can lead to shock, acidosis, stupor, and failure of the body's major organs (kidney, heart, etc.). Persistent diarrhea often leads to loss of body protein and increased susceptibility to infection. Prevention and control of diarrheal disease, especially in infants and children, should therefore be a major aim of countries around the world.

In addition, many countries have developed diarrhea control programs that improve childhood nutrition. These programs focus on the promotion of breastfeeding, weaning practices, promotion of oral rehydration therapy (ORT), and supplementary feeding programs (Briscoe, 1984). However, all these programs must be considered in conjunction with improving the social and economic conditions that contribute to safe environmental, sanitary, and general living conditions of populations around the world (Basch, 1990).

Nutrition and World Health

Good nutrition is an essential part of good health. Poor nutrition by itself or that associated with infectious disease accounts for a large portion of the world's disease burden (World Bank, 1993). Those environmental and economic conditions that are related to poverty contribute to underconsumption of nutrients, especially those nutrients that are needed for protein building, such as iodine, vitamin A, and iron. Worldwide, women and children suffer disproportionately from nutrition deficits, especially of the micronutrients just mentioned (Humphrey et al., 1992).

One of the effects of poor nutrition is stunting or low height and weight for a given age. Stunting is most frequently the result of eating foods that do not provide enough energy and those foods that do not contain enough protein (World Bank, 1993). Since protein foods are usually more expensive than the nonprotein food sources, many households cut back or unconsciously eliminate protein-rich foods to save money. Several countries where populations are most affected by stunting are India (65%), Asia (50%, not including India and China), China (40%), and Sub-Sahara Africa (40%) (World Bank, 1993).

Iron deficiencies are also common in the lesser developed countries and severely affect women and children. A deficiency of iron in the diet reduces physical productivity and affects the capacity of children to learn in school. Iron deficiency in the diet also affects a person's appetite, causing many individuals and especially children to experience a lessened desire to eat, which in turn affects overall food intake and growth over a prolonged time.

Women are most susceptible to iron deficiency as a result of menstruation and child bearing. Women who experience iron deficiency can develop a severe shortage of iron in their blood that results in anemia. Anemia increases a woman's risk of hemorrhage during childbirth. A World Bank report (1993) indicated that 88% of all pregnant women in India were anemic, compared with 60% of the pregnant women in other parts of Asia. This statistic is compared with the developed, market economy countries, where only 15% of the population of pregnant women experience iron-deficiency anemia.

Other common dietary deficiencies observed throughout the world include iodine, vitamin A, and calcium deficiencies. The total impact of malnutrition and dietary deficiencies cannot be underestimated. Any malnourished condition among a population can increase susceptibility to illness. For example, the principal causes of death among malnourished persons are measles, diarrheal and respiratory disease, TB, pertussis, and malaria. The loss of life from these diseases can be measured as 231 DALYs worldwide, with one-fourth of the 231 being directly attributable to malnourishment and dietary deficiencies.

The worldwide initiatives that have been directed at overcoming nutritional deficits have included (1) control of infectious diseases, (2) nutritional education, (3) control of intestinal parasites, (4) micronutrient fortification of food, (5) food supplementation, and (6) food price subsidies (World Bank, 1993). In addition to contributions by individual governments, the organizations that have been most active in assisting with these initiatives have included the International Red Cross, the WHO, and many international religious and private foundations.

 ## Clinical Application

The role of community health nurses in international health varies dramatically from country to country, as does the role of professional nursing. It is not surprising to learn that nursing plays a more active role in health care delivery in the more technologically advanced countries such as the United States, Canada, Australia, New Zealand, the United Kingdom, and other countries in Western Europe. The more developed countries have a defined role for community health nurses, whereas the role is less defined, if at all, in lesser developed countries.

Many nurses who seek out international health experiences come from one of the more developed countries. Nurses may become employed by international agencies such as the WHO, UNICEF, and the Red Cross and often serve as consultants to nursing education programs, government agencies, and private health care agencies. In addition, large government and private hospitals such as those in Saudi Arabia and Kuwait frequently recruit American and Western European nurses to staff their hospitals, but they rarely seek out nurses to work in communities. However, the Peace Corps, Project Hope, and many private religious organizations have recruited nurses to work in health promotion and prevention projects in rural and isolated areas of the world. For example, Peace Corps and Hope nurses have been actively involved in community programs in Southeast Asia,

Clinical Application—cont'd

Africa, and Central and South America. The following application is an example of how community health nurses proved to be a valuable resource in the war-torn country of Nicaragua during the 1970s and 1980s.

Community Health and Nicaragua

Under the dictatorship of Somoza, health care was abysmal for the vast majority of Nicaraguans. The average life expectancy was 52 years of age for women and 54 for men. Malnutrition was rampant and affected 7 of every 10 children. Children between the ages of 1 and 2 years exhibited a mortality rate of 20%, with infant mortality comprising 120 of 1000 live births in the urban areas and 300 of 1000 live births in the rural areas. The chief causes of death among older children included tetanus, measles, and dehydration from gastroenteritis and diarrheal conditions, which are all preventable.

In July 19, 1979, the Sandinista government took control of Nicaragua after a very bitter and hard-fought revolution. One of the first postwar initiatives was the formation and implementation of country-wide health drives that were designed to provide universal access to primary, preventive, and community care services for all Nicaraguan residents. The Sandinista campaign promoted health education and the training of health care volunteers to promote personal and environmental cleanliness and good nutrition and to provide vaccinations against preventable diseases in local villages and communities. In addition, the government wished to initiate a plan to eradicate polio and malaria. All available nurses who were working in Nicaragua were engaged to assist in these activities. In addition, a call went out worldwide for nurses and physicians who were trained in primary care, community, and public health to assist the Sandinista government with their effort.

Nicaraguan nurses received special training in maternal and child health and were taught the principles of community and public health. They staffed many neighborhood and rural clinics and provided free prenatal care, medications, and food supplements. As part of this program, all infants and children were guaranteed free primary and disease preventive health care.

Unfortunately, the efforts of the Sandinistas were dissolved as a result of another bloody political revolution. Nicaragua has become one of the poorest countries in the Western Hemisphere and falls behind Haiti, which has held that distinction for decades. Universal access to primary and preventive care no longer exists. Neither polio nor malaria has been eradicated (McGuire, 1995).

Key Concepts

- Health for all the world's people is a collective goal of its nations and is being promoted by the major world health organizations.
- As the political and economic barriers between countries fall, the movement of people back and forth across international boundaries increases. This movement impacts the spread of various disease entities throughout the world.
- Community health nurses can and do play an active role in the identification of potential health risks at U.S. borders, with immigrant populations throughout the nation and as participants in international health care delivery.
- Primary health care is one of the major keys in the provision of universal access of health care for the world's populations.
- The major organizations that are involved in world health include (1) private voluntary, (2) philanthropic, (3) professional and technical, (4) commercial, (5) governmental, and (6) intergovernmental.
- The health status of a country is related to its economic and technical growth. The more technologically and economically advanced countries are referred to as developed, whereas those that are striving for greater economic and technological growth are termed lesser developed. Many lesser developed countries often divert financial resources from health and education to other internal needs such as defense or economic development that is not aimed at the poor.
- The global burden of disease (GBD) is a way to describe the world's health. The GBD combines losses from premature death and losses that result from disability. The GBD represents units of disability-adjusted life years, or DALYs.
- Critical world health problems still exist and include (1) communicable diseases such as tuberculosis, measles, mumps, rubella, and polio; (2) maternal and child health; (3) diarrheal diseases; (4) nutritional deficits; (5) malaria; and (6) AIDS.

Critical Thinking Activities

1. Divide into small groups and discuss how you might find out if there are immigrant communities in your area. You might want to contact your local health department, area social workers, or community social organizations and churches.
   a. Discuss how you might gain access to one of these immigrant groups. Once gaining access, how would you go about determining what specific health needs they may have? What are their beliefs about health and health care? What customs regarding health were followed in their country of origin? How does the American health care system differ from the health care system in their country?
   b. As a community health nurse, what kinds of interventions might you consider implementing with these immigrant populations?
2. Write to one of the major international health organizations and obtain their mission and goal statements. What kinds of health-related activities do they focus on? Find out if they use community health nurses in their efforts and how a nurse who is interested might become involved in their program and activities.
3. Pick a country or area of the world outside of the United States that interests you. Go to the library and obtain information about the following: (1) the status of health care in that country, (2) its major health concerns, (3) its GBD (global burden of disease), (4) if this country is developed or lesser developed, and (5) which, if any, international health care organizations are involved with the delivery of health care in that country.
4. Determine the role of primary health care in developed and lesser developed countries. Describe the role of community health nursing in primary health care in both types of countries.
5. Choose one or more of the following countries and find out from your local or state health department the health risks that are involved in visiting that country: (1) Indonesia, (2) Zaire, (3) Paraguay, (4) India, (5) Egypt, (6) Kenya, (7) Chile, (8) China, and (9) Haiti.

Bibliography

AbouZahr C, Royston E: Excessive hazards of pregnancy and childbirth in the Third World, *World Health Forum* 13:343-345, 1992.

Basch PF: *Textbook of international health,* New York, 1990, Oxford University Press.

Briscoe J: Water supply and health in developing countries, *Am J Public Health* 74:1009-1013, 1984.

Carrington T: AIDS pulls together the young and old in Ugandan villages, *Wall Street Journal,* Dec 29, 1994, pp 1A and 4A.

Cech I, Essman A: Water sanitation practices on the Texas-Mexico border: implications for physicians on both sides, *South Med J* 85(11):1053-1064, 1992.

Collado C: Primary health care: a continuing challenge, *Nurs Health Care* 13(8):408-413, 1992.

Crompton D, Savioli L: Intestinal parasitic infections and urbanization, *Bull World Health Organ* 71(1):1-7, 1993.

Dolin P. Raviglione M, Kochi A: Global tuberculosis incidence and mortality during 1990-2000, *Bull World Health Organ* 72(2):213-220, 1994.

Evlo K, Carrin G: Finance for health care: part of a broad canvas, *World Health Forum* 13:165-170, 1992.

Ganatra B, Hirve S: Male bias in health care utilization for under-fives in a rural community in western India, *Bull World Health Organ* 72(1):101-104, 1994.

Guerrant R: Unresolved problems and future considerations in diarrheal research, *Pediatr Infect Dis J* 5:S155-S161, 1986.

Heyward W, Curran J: The epidemiology of AIDS in the U.S., *Sci Am* October 1988, pp 72-81.

Humphrey J, West K, Sommer A: Vitamin A deficiency and attributable mortality among under-5-year-olds, *Bull World Health Organ* 70(2):225-232, 1992.

Kalibala S, Anderson S: AIDS in Africa: a family disease, *World Health* 6:8-10, 1993.

Kestler E: Wanted: better care for pregnant women, *World Health Forum* 14:356-359, 1993.

McGuire S: Personal communication, University of Texas at El Paso, 1995.

National League for Nursing: Comparison of national health care systems, *Nurs Health Care* 13(4):202-203, 1992.

Nichter M: Pharmaceuticals, health commodification, and social relations: ramifications for primary health care. In Nichter M, editor: *Anthropology and international health,* Boston, 1989, Kluwer Academic Publishers.

Perry S, Marx ES: What technologies for health care in developing countries? *World Health Forum* 13:356-362, 1992.

Quiroga M: Personal communication, director of nursing, El Paso City/County Health Department, 1995.

Schild GC, Assad F: Vaccines: the way ahead, *World Health Forum* 4:353-357, 1983.

World Bank: *World development report 1992: development and the environment,* New York, 1992, Oxford University Press.

World Bank: *World development report 1993: investing in health,* New York, 1993, Oxford University Press.

World Health Organization/United Nations Childrens' Fund: *Primary Health Care (WHO Alma Alta reaffirmed at Riga, Geneva, 1988),* Geneva, 1978, WHO.

World Health Organization: *Twelve yardsticks for health,* New York, 1986a, WHO.

World Health Organization: *WHO-CDD: research on vaccine development,* Geneva, 1986b, WHO Document CDD/IMV/86.1.

World Health Organization: Tuberculosis control and research strategies for the 1990's: memorandum from a WHO meeting, *Bull World Health Organ* 70(1):17-21, 1992a.

World Health Organization: Women, health and development, *Int Nurs Rev* 40(1):29-30, 1992b.

World Health Organization: World malaria situation in 1991, *World Health Bull* 72:160-164, 1994.

Wouters AV: Health care utilization in developing countries: role of the technology environment in "deriving" the demand for health care, *Bull World Health Organ* 70(3):381-389, 1992.

Part Two
Influences on Health Care Delivery and Community Health Nursing

In recent years the U.S. health care system has been under attack because of rapidly rising health care costs, inconsistency in the level of services provided from one area of the country to another, and a general inconsistency in the quality and accessibility of health services. With 43 million Americans uninsured and 12% of the remaining population underinsured, it has been recognized that equal access to health care services is not a right, as most Americans think it should be.

These factors have lead to major health care reform debates at the national level and in some states during the mid 1990s in an attempt to reorganize the health care system to provide universal access to cost-effective, quality care. Such debate is leading the health care delivery system into a managed care system in an arena of managed competition.

As a result of the debate legal, economic, ethical, social, cultural, political, and health policy issues have become extremely important. Now, more than any time in the history of community health nursing, it is essential for nurses to understand how these issues affect their practice and the outcomes of care.

In 1988 the Institute of Medicine study on the future of Public Health pointed out that the public health system has deteriorated as a major force for promoting the health of all people. The system was deemed to be unable to protect and improve the health of the most needy individuals and families.

In health care reform, public health is redefining its role in improving the nation's health. Community health nurses, as the largest public health provider workforce, will want to be a force in redefining the renewed public health system. Understanding the issues that affect decisions about health care priorities is imperative. Knowledge is power.

The chapters in Part Two provide the community health nurse with an understanding of the economical, ethical, cultural, environmental, and policy issues which affect nursing in general and community health nursing specifically.

Concern currently exists that the environment's effects on health and social conditions are causing an increase in the rate of infectious diseases. Community health nurses must be concerned with prevention, control, case-finding, reporting, and maintenance strategies as they relate to both communicable and infectious disease processes and to environmentally-related problems. Technological advances increasingly influence the environment and make it a potential threat to many aspects of health maintenance. Nurses must help others recognize how their actions as individuals, as well as in a composite group or community, are destroying vital parts of the environment. ▼

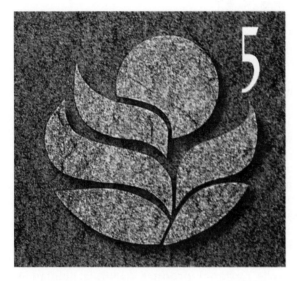

5 Economics of Health Care Delivery

Marcia Stanhope

Objectives

After reading this chapter, the student should be able to do the following:

◆ Define health economics.
◆ Identify levels of economic theories.
◆ Trace the evolution of the components of health care services.
◆ Identify the factors influencing health care economics.
◆ Trace the involvement of government and other third-party payers in health care financing.
◆ Discuss national health care reform, financing, and direct service delivery plans.
◆ Discuss proposed health care financing for the future.
◆ Analyze the impact of a primary prevention goal on health care economics.
◆ Discuss health care rationing.
◆ Describe the relationship between poverty and health care financing.

Key Terms

benefit schedule
capitation
cost-plus reimbursement
diagnosis-related groups (DRGs)
economics
efficiency
enabling legislation
fee screen system
gross domestic product (GDP)
gross national product (GNP)
health care rationing
health economics
Health Maintenance Organization Act
managed care
managed competition
Medicaid program
medical technology
medically indigent
Medicare program
population demography
price inflation
prospective cost reimbursement
prospective payment system
retrospective cost reimbursement
third-party payment

Outline

The health care delivery system of the 1960s and 1970s experienced vast expansions, unlimited financial resources, an open job market, and a nursing discipline that was expanding and broadening its responsibilities and influence. In contrast, the present health care delivery system is characterized by limited resources, regulatory restrictions, increased technological advances, increased competition, and more emphasis on health care delivery in the community, and health care reform.

Because of the preceding factors, the concerns of the twenty-first century will focus on examining the economics of health care delivery, limiting the continuous growth of the largest employing industry in the United States, and organizing and assigning priorities to use the available health care resources at the least cost. Nursing will be concerned with establishing its contribution to the health of the nation and ensuring its economic viability in the market as a major contributor in health care delivery.

With the current emphasis on cost consciousness in health care delivery, nurses are being challenged to implement changes in practice and participate in research and policy activities designed to reduce health care costs. These activities will require a basic understanding of economics, the economics of the delivery system, and how nurses can have a dramatic impact on cost and cost-effective care (Pew, 1993a).

This chapter provides an overview of the economic issues of the health care delivery system. Discussion focuses on factors influencing health care, methods for financing health care, economics of primary prevention, methods for financing health care, economics of primary prevention, methods for evaluating health and nursing costs, and the value of human life in health care spending. A brief view of health care financing and the impact of health care reform issues of accessibility, acceptability, affordability, and organization of the industry is also included. For community health nurses working with individuals and families, it is important to know how to provide quality care and control costs. For community health nurses working with communities and groups, one must be able to plan programs that are efficient and cost effective.

DEFINITIONS

To grasp the importance of the economics of health care and its significance to nursing, a basic understanding of key economic terms is essential.

Economics is the social science concerned with the problems of using or administering scarce resources in the most efficient way to attain maximum fulfillment of society's unlimited wants (Cleland, 1990). **Health economics** is concerned with the problems of producing and distributing the health care resources.

The goal of health economics is not unlike the *goal of public health*—to provide the most good for the most people, given available knowledge and resources.

The goal of health economics is to provide the best quality health care to the largest number of people, given available financial resources. The provision of health goods (services) requires money. Spending money on health goods limits the amount of money available for other goods, such as food, clothing, shelter, transportation, education, and recreation.

Society must begin to make tough decisions about how to use available resources. Today the United States allocates approximately 16% of the gross national product for health goods. This represented over $900 billion spent in 1994. Health care expenditures are projected to reach 20% of the gross national product by the year 2000 (Table 5-1). This means that $20 of every $100 will be spent on health care services.

The **gross national product (GNP)** is defined as the total value of all goods and services produced in the U.S. economy in 1 year (*Health: United States, 1993*, 1994). The GNP is the most comprehensive measure of a nation's total output of goods and services. For example, all cars, food, clothes, and houses that are made and sold are a part of the *goods* that help to describe the GNP. It is useful for comparing how much is spent in 1 year and tells people where society's values are. The value, or price, of a *service* is determined by using the consumer price index. The *consumer price index* is a shopping basket approach that compares prices of all consumed goods and services purchased by urban wage earners and their families on a monthly or quarterly basis. The medical care component of the consumer price index compares selected prices of hospital, medical, dental, and pharmaceutical products and services and gives a picture of how often the prices change for these services (*Health: United States, 1993*, 1994).

The **gross domestic product (GDP)** is a statistical measure that is used to compare health care spending between countries. The GDP defines the total value of all goods and services produced in the United States plus the value of services performed in the United States by foreign subjects minus the value of services performed in other countries by U.S. citizens (*Health: United States, 1993*, 1994). Whereas the GNP is used in the United States to compare costs of health care with other costs, such as defense, the GDP helps in comparing costs of health and nursing care in the United States with other countries such as Canada because it is a more exact measure of international comparisons than the GNP. Because today the United States is concerned about how much is spent for health care, it helps to compare with other countries to see if the United States is spending too much for the same services offered in those other countries.

ECONOMIC THEORIES

Two basic theories are applicable to the study and understanding of economics: microeconomic theory and macroeconomic theory.

Table 5-1 Gross National Product and National Health Expenditures in United States for Selected Years from 1929 to 1990

| Year | Gross national product in billions | National Health Expenditures | | |
		Amount in billions	Percent of gross national product	Amount per capita
1929	$ 103.9	$3.6	3.5	$29
1940	100.4	4.0	4.0	29
1950	288.3	12.7	4.4	80
1960	515.3	26.9	5.2	142
1970	1015.5	75.0	7.4	349
1980	2731.9	248.1	9.1	1055
1990	5487.8	675.0	12.3	2060

From Office of National Cost Estimates, Office of the Actuary: *Health Care Financing Rev* 14(2), 1991. HCFA Pub No 03335, Health Care Financing Administration, Washington, DC, US Government Printing Office, 1992.
NOTE: These data reflect Bureau of Economic Analysis, Department of Commerce, revisions to the gross national product as of December 1988 and Social Security Administration revisions to the population as of July 1992.

Microeconomic theory is concerned with the study of allocation and distribution of income. What should be produced and in what quantity? How should income be distributed among the members of society? The basic principles applied to the microeconomic theory are those of supply and demand. When the supply of a product or service increases, the demand decreases. This results in lower prices. Conversely, when demand goes up and supply goes down, the price goes up (Cleland, 1990).

An interesting point to remember is that to date the laws of supply and demand (microeconomic theory) have not worked in the health care industry because it is a monopoly with a captive consumer instead of a competitive market. Regardless of supply and demand, prices continue to go up. It remains to be seen whether the new spirit of competitiveness will have a positive effect on health care costs and if supply and demand will eventually work to control prices.

The primary objective of this level of theory is to explain the factors that determine prices, which affect resource allocation and result in income being distributed. This theory focuses on factors, including behaviors, related to individual clients and health care providers and agency and corporation administrators.

Macroeconomic theory concerns itself with the study of stability and growth of the total economy, the factors that determine levels of income and employment, general price levels, and the rate of economic growth. This theory is concerned with aggregate (group) variables that affect the total economy, such as cost, quality access to care, and health policies.

This theory is applicable to the following discussion in which global factors (macroeconomics) are examined that affect the health of the United States. Aggregate and organizational factors are examined in considering health care financing or a national health insurance, rationing, the new concept of managed care, and the poverty of health care (Cleland, 1990).

Community health nurses who work with individuals and families deal with microeconomic theory, because they are concerned with what services are available to their clients, at what cost, whether clients use the services, and how health providers and agency administrators respond to their clients' needs.

Community health nurses who work with aggregates (groups and communities) concern themselves with macroeconomic theory, because they are concerned with community health policy that makes the development of new programs possible, with budgets to offer programs, the client's ability to access services, and the total effect that services will have on improving the health of the community.

HEALTH SERVICES COMPONENTS: SYSTEM EVOLUTION

From the 1800s through the late 1900s, the U.S. health care delivery system experienced four developmental stages with differing emphasis on health care economics. The health services component framework is used to describe the evolution of the organization of health care delivery.

Four basic components provide the framework for health services delivery: *labor* (work force), *facilities, technology,* and *service intensity.* Historically, changes in these components have occurred concurrently with macro level (society) changes in morbidity, mortality, national health policy, and economic and social forces.

The *first developmental stage* of the health care delivery system occurred during the period 1800 to 1900. The period was characterized by epidemics of infectious diseases, such as plague, cholera, typhoid, smallpox, influenza, malaria, yellow fever, and gastric disorders. The health problems of the period were related to contaminated food and water supplies, inadequate sewage disposal, and poor housing conditions (Banta, 1995b; Pickett and Hanlon, 1990).

Minimal technology was available to aid in disease control. The doctor's black bag contained the few medicines and tools available for health care in the era, and hospitals were characterized by overcrowding, disease, and lack of cleanliness. Because sick persons, if cared for in a hospital, usually died because of hospital conditions, most people were cared for at home by family and friends.

During this period the labor force was composed of poorly trained physicians who attained their skills through apprenticeships with practicing physicians who were trained the same way. Nurses were typically volunteers recruited from the lower social strata or from religious orders. Their primary focus was to assist the clients with activities of daily living. In 1867 the first nurse training school was established at the New England Hospital for Women and Children to provide formal preparation for nursing in the United States; by 1877, organized district nursing (home nursing) had been established (Gardner, 1936; Kalish, 1986). In this first developmental phase the methods of financing were private pay for those who could afford health care, bartering with the physicians, or charitable contributions from individuals and organizations.

The *second developmental phase* of the health care delivery system, dating from 1900 to 1945, was marked by the control of acute infectious diseases. Environmental conditions began to improve, with major advances in water purification, sanitary sewage disposal, milk and water quality, and urban housing quality. The health problems of the era changed from mass epidemics to individual acute infections or traumatic episodes (Pickett and Hanlon, 1990).

The workers of the period were better educated. Physician education evolved from apprenticeships to scientifically based college education; the change occurred after the publication of the Flexner Report of 1910. Clinical medicine was in its "golden age" because of major advances in surgery and childbirth, identification of the cause of pernicious anemia, and such technologic discoveries as insulin in 1922 for control of diabetes, sulfa drugs in 1932 for treatment of infectious diseases, and antibiotics such as penicillin in the 1940s (Rice, 1994).

Nurses of the era were trained primarily in hospital schools of nursing, whose goal was to educate nurses in the dependent function of following physicians' orders. Hospitals and health departments were growing in numbers and strength. The public health departments' major emphasis was on quarantine and case finding. These tasks were delegated to the public health nurse. Also, 225 visiting nurse organizations were offering skilled attendance and were focusing on the teaching of cleanliness and the proper care of sick persons in the home. Thus health education was identified as a nursing function early in the development of the health care delivery system.

In addition to private and charitable financing of health care, city, county, and state governments were beginning to contribute through the provision of hospitals and clinics for poor persons, state mental institutions, and other specialized hospitals, such as tuberculosis hospitals.

The *third developmental stage,* from 1945 to 1984, showed a shift away from acute infectious health problems toward chronic health problems such as heart disease, cancer, and stroke as a recruit of lifestyles. Because of these changes in Americans' overall health, the focus of research and development also changed. Major technological advances of the era included the development of chemotherapeutic agents, immunizations, advances in anesthesia, advances in electrolyte and cardiopulmonary physiology, expansion of diagnostic laboratories and complex equipment such as the computed tomography (CT) scanner, organ and tissue transplants, radiation therapy, and specialty units for critical care, coronary care, and intensive care.

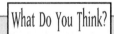

What Do You Think?

Although at one time Americans believed that theirs was the best health care system in the world, this is no longer true.

The numbers and kinds of health service facilities increased; health care providers constituted more than 5% of the total U.S. workforce. The three largest employers were hospitals, convalescent institutions, and physicians' offices. Between 1970 and 1984 alone the number of persons employed in the health care industry grew by 90%. The numbers of personnel employed in other sites, such as the community, also increased.

During this third developmental stage the system appeared to have unlimited resources for growth and expansion. The period was marked by the introduction of the health insurance industry and substantial growth of the federal government's role in financing health care.

Current problems and realities in the health care delivery system are reflected in a *fourth development stage* beginning during the Reagan presidential era, one of increasingly limited resources, restricted growth, and a reorganization of methods of financing and care delivery. Health care providers are being forced to be more introspective, to look at alternatives and options to the unlimited resources, growth, and services of previous decades. With substantial federal health policy changes, emphasis is slowly moving toward increased emphasis on preventive care.

This era is marked by ambulatory and community-based care, such as same-day surgical centers, health maintenance organizations (HMOs), expanded home health services, limited hospitalizations, and technologies of the era including MRI (magnetic resonance imaging), sonography, and telemedicine.

The numbers and kinds of health care providers also continued to increase in this period. Between 1989 and 1992 alone, employment increased by 13% although the total U.S. workforce only increased by 0.2% (*Health: United States, 1993,* 1994). Although in 1992 over 50% of all health providers worked in hospitals, nursing homes, and physicians' offices, with increasing emphasis on community-based care, this pattern is expected to change.

Unfortunately, a shift backward toward increases in communicable, infectious, and environmental illnesses is now occurring. Table 5-2 compares the leading causes of mortality from 1900 to 1992. Infant mortality is at a record low for the United States, whereas life expectancy is at a record high. Chronic illnesses resulting from environmental and life-style influences are increasing and, with the resurgence of communicable and infectious diseases, such as tuberculosis and acquired immunodeficiency syndrome (AIDS), promise to be the major health threats of the twenty-first century.

Health Care Providers

The types of health care providers and the number of practitioners of each type influence the economics of health care. Before 1940 there were fewer than 40 types of health care providers; in 1990 the number, as reported by the U.S. Department of Labor, had risen to more than 200. The increase in specialization led to changes in certification, qualifications, education, and standards of care in each professional area. The combination of these factors contributed to the increased number and kinds of providers to meet the demands of the health care system. As of 1992, there were approximately 603,400 physicians and 2.3 million nurses in the United States providing health care services to a population of 257 million. Of the practicing nurses, approximately 15% were employed in areas of community health. The above total represents approximately 236 physicians per 100,000 population and 697 registered nurses per 100,000 population. Since 1970 the physician population has grown by 84% and the nurse population by 134%. Table 5-3 shows the increase in the number of people employed in the health industry from 1970 to 1992 (*Health: United States, 1993,* 1994; USDHHS, 1994).

During the fourth developmental period the supply of specialty physicians has continued to increase, whereas the demand has declined, and now more primary care physicians are needed. This will lead to

Table 5-2 Leading Causes of Death in the United States, 1900 and 1992

Cause	Death rate per 100,000 population
1900	
Influenza and pneumonia	202.2
Tuberculosis	194.4
Diarrhea and enteritis	139.9
Heart disease	137.4
Cerebral hemorrhage	106.9
Nephritis	88.7
Accidents	72.3
Cancer	64.0
Diseases of early infancy	62.6
Diphtheria	40.3
Simple meningitis	33.8
Typhoid and paratyphoid	31.3
All causes	1173.8
1992	
Heart diseases	282.5
Malignant neoplasms	204.3
Cerebrovascular accidents	56.3
Chronic obstructive pulmonary disease	35.8
Unintentional injuries	33.8
Influenza and pneumonia	29.8
Diabetes mellitus	19.7
Suicide	13.2
Human immunovirus (HIV) infections	11.7
Homicide	10.4
All causes	697.5

more competition, different practice arrangements, and different payment mechanisms. Although the demand for nurses increased faster than the supply until 1994, the demand is subsiding and new nonlicensed assistive personnel (NLAPs) such as community health workers are being introduced into the system to take the place of the more expensive nurse. The primary reason for this increase was the change in the health care market philosophy from that of unlimited spending and care at any cost to one of the competitive and cost-driven market. Whereas the federal government and other payers are supporting the use of nurses and other health care workers to provide

Table 5-3   Persons Employed in Selected Health Service Sites, According to Place of Employment in United States from 1970 to 1992 (in thousands)

Site	1970*	1980	1992
Number of persons in thousands (all employed civilians)	76,805	99,303	117,598
All health service sites	4246	7339	10,271
Offices of physicians	477	777	1,434
Offices of dentists	222	415	583
Offices of chiropractors†	19	40	122
Hospitals	2690	4036	4,915
Nursing and personal care facilities	509	1199	1,750
Other health service sites	330	872	1,467

From U.S. Bureau of the Census: 1970 *Census of population: occupation by industry.* Subject Reports, Final Report PC, (2)-7C, Washington, DC, 1972, U.S. Government Printing Office, U.S. Bureau of Labor Statistics: Labor force statistics derived from: *Current population survey: a databook,* vol 1, Washington, DC, 1982, U.S. Government Printing Office: *Employment and earnings,* January *1983-93,* 37(1), 38(1), 39(1), 40(1), Washington, DC, 1983-1993, U.S. Government Printing Office; American Chiropractic Association: Unpublished data.
*April 1, derived from decennial census; all other data years are annual averages from the Current Population Survey.
†Data for 1980 are from the American Chiropractic Association; data for all other years are from the U.S. Bureau of Labor Statistics.
NOTES: Totals exclude persons in health-related occupations who are working in nonhealth industries, as classified by the U.S. Bureau of the Census, such as pharmacists employed in drugstores, school nurses, and nurses working in private households. Totals include federal, state, and county health workers. In the period 1983 to 1991, employed persons were classified according to the industry groups used in the 1980 Census of Population. Beginning in 1992, persons were classified according to the system used in the 1990 Census of Population.

care previously given by the more expensive physician, physicians and the hospital industry are promoting the use of NLAPs and cross training of respiratory therapists and others to do the work of nurses. Nurse-managed clinics, more emphasis on home care, community care, and preventive programs are being supported as less costly methods to provide quality care (micro level theory) and as the new frontier for nurse employment.

As *economic philosphy* on health care delivery has changed, other changes have included prospective payment, managed care (providing a given set of coordinated services to a client group at the best price), managed competition, industry self-insurance, decline in insurance benefits, nonphysician provider reimbursement, community-based services, a shift to profit health care, an emphasis on evaluating the effective-

ness of interventions and technologies, and health care reform.

Health Care Changes

This era will be noted as an era of vast changes in all sectors of health care delivery. Technologic advances of the era continue to focus on development of new biogenetic and drug therapies for problems such as AIDS, cancer, Alzheimer's and Parkinson's diseases, and fertility problems. Alternative health care delivery units are increasing and are community based. MRI and telemedicine are a few of the latest advances in technical equipment, whereas intrauterine fetal surgery exemplifies the latest surgical techniques. Meanwhile, however, the United States faces its first major epidemic in decades with the increasing number of AIDS cases. This epidemic, which is lifestyle related, cannot be controlled with modern technologies.

FACTORS INFLUENCING THE ECONOMICS OF HEALTH CARE

Four major factors are instrumental in influencing the economic growth of the health care system: price inflation, technology, intensity, and changes in population demography.

Price Inflation

Price inflation was the major overall economic problem between 1950 and 1980. General inflation affected the prices of all goods and services in the United States, including health care costs, which increased faster than the consumer price index, the inflation indicator. By 1990 inflation had slowed in the United States, but by 1993 health care costs showed twice the overall inflation rate of the United States (*Health: United States, 1993,* 1994).

Table 5-4 shows the changes in money spent for health care from 1950 to 1991. Note that this table shows a rise in health care expenditures from $12.7 billion in 1950 to $751.8 billion in 1991. Whereas the population had increased by 60% over this period, all health care costs had increased by 3400%. Thus the amount spent per person increased by approximately 2000%, or from less than $100 per person in 1950 to $2500 per person in 1991. Health services and supplies accounted for 92% to 97% of the total money spent, whereas research and construction costs decreased from 8% to 3%. Public health activities are reported to have increased by 11.5% although not reflected in Table 5-4 (*Health: United States, 1993,* 1994).

In 1985 inflation began to decline. With the decline in prices for other goods and services came the lowest annual increase in health care prices since 1960. Hospitals and physicians are the two major recipients of health care money, whereas government-sponsored

Table 5-4 National Health Expenditures and Percent Distribution According to Type of Expenditure in the United States for Selected Years from 1950 to 1991

Type of expenditure	1950	1960	1970	1980	1991
			Amount in billions		
Total	$ 12.7	$ 26.9	$ 75.0	$248.1	$751.8
			Percent distribution		
All expenditures	100	100	100	100	100
Health service and supplies	92	94	93	95	97
Personal health care	86	88	87	89	88
Hospital care	30	34	37	41	39
Physician services	22	21	19	19	19
Nursing home care	2	2	6	8	8
Home health	—	0.1	0.2	0.5	5
Drugs and medical sundries	14	14	11	8	8
Program administration and net cost of health insurance	4	4	4	4	6
Government public health activities	3	2	2	3	3
Research and construction	8	6	7	5	3
Noncommericial research	1	3	3	2	2
Construction	7	4	5	3	2

From Office of National Cost Estimates, Office of the Actuary: *Health Care Financing Rev* 14(2), 1991. HCFA Pub No 03335, Health Care Financing Administration, Washington, DC, 1992, U.S. Government Printing Office.
NOTE: Some numbers in this table have been revised and differ from previous editions of *Health: United States.*

public health care programs receive less than 3% of the total health care dollars.

Inflation in health care delivery remains the dominant factor in health economic issues today. By 1991 physician services almost doubled and hospital services almost tripled the overall inflation rate. Whereas the slowdown in price increases, especially in hospital care, may be attributed to the new *prospective payment system* (see p. 78), a number of assumptions have been made regarding reasons for price inflation in health care delivery:

1. As earnings increase and more people acquire health insurance, use of the system and the demand for services also increases.
2. Expenditures are rising in response to increased hospital wages, while lagging employee productivity is down, requiring more personnel.
3. Increases in supply, equipment, and salary expenditures result from the growth and the number of insurance plans (over 1500 today).
4. New and costlier methods of care force prices up.
5. Prices rise because of the building of costly, expensive-to-maintain hospital facilities that already exist in sufficient supply.
6. Changes in consumer life-styles and environmental hazards have created a new set of health problems that require services.
7. New kinds of health insurance coverage encourage increased use of services such as dental care and organ transplantation.
8. Increased community-based care services add to the overall costs.
9. Unnecessary care and defensive medicine are used to avoid lawsuits.
10. Clients are entering the system with more complex problems, such as AIDS clients, low-birth-weight infants, elderly persons with multiple chronic problems, and persons with drug-resistant tuberculosis (*Health: United States 1993,* 1994; Lee, 1994).

Although all factors mentioned have contributed to inflation in health care costs, some have had more effect than others. The availablity of insurance to cover health care costs and the development of new and costlier methods of health care technology appear to be the major contributors to increased costs. Increased wages for the new categories of health care personnel, such as nurse practitioners, physician assistants, and dental technicians, have also contributed to increased costs. The increased numbers of health care facilities and the vast duplication of services offered have contributed to the need for more employees, supplies, and equipment and thus to increased costs.

However, some change is occurring. For example, although hospitals have traditionally been the single largest employer of health personnel in the United States, the number of community-based employees has increased in 1994. Health care reimbursement schemes have changed and will cover the cost of more community-based care, such as home care, well child screening, and prenatal care, and eight states have passed health care reform laws to change how health care is delivered and provided.

Technology and Intensity

Medical technology has been defined by the Congressional Office of Technology Assessment as "the set of techniques, drugs, equipment, and procedures used by health care professionals in delivering medical care to individuals and the system within which such care is delivered" (Banta, 1995a). Included in any discussion of costs of technology is the cost of use of technology.

Intensity refers to the use of technologies, supplies, and health care services by or on behalf of the client. Intensity includes and is a partial measure of the use of technologies.

Health care professionals, such as physicians, have become dependent on technology for diagnosis and treatment. They have become the principal purchasing agents of technology for the client. Nurses, too, have become dependent on technologies to monitor client progress and make decisions about client care. The population, with an increasing sophistication about health and health care needs, demands the use of laboratory, radiological, diagnostic, palliative, and therapeutic services for treatment.

As new and more complex technology is introduced into the system, the trend toward increasing use and cost is evident. For example, between 1979 and 1988 there was a 400% increase in CT scans performed on hospital inpatients; meanwhile ultrasound diagnostic procedures and angiocardiography tripled (*Health: United States,* 1988, 1989).

One of the most significant examples of a technology contributing to increasing costs is that of renal dialysis. After a 1972 congressional amendment to the Social Security Act extended Medicare coverage to pay for renal dialysis, approximately 16,000 people received care under this program at a cost of $250 million. By 1979 costs had risen to $1 billion for 51,000 clients. Costs were projected to reach $2.8 billion by 1986. In 1987, 130,939 persons served by Medicare received renal dialysis, a 156% increase in 8 years.

Renal dialysis programs and other new technologies demand personnel and investments in equipment and facilities. They also add to administrative costs, especially when the federal government is involved in the financing and regulating of the technology. All clients

who qualify for health care financing through one of the federally funded programs qualify for the use of this and other technologies.

An example of a health care problem that has contributed to the cost of health care through medical care, research, development of new technologies and cash assistance to the clients is the recent AIDS epidemic. This is the first problem to reach epidemic proportions in recent memory. It is a prime example of a problem that will do much more than affect a growing number of people who will require a wide array of services (intensity), expensive treatments (technologies), and care. It will also exacerbate already existing concerns about health care financing. Expenditures by the federal government alone for the AIDS epidemic increased from $6 million to $5.2 billion between 1982 and 1993. Projections indicate a continuing rise in cost to care for the estimated 1.5 million people who are currently HIV seropositive on testing. In 1982 there were only 9000 cases; and in 1992 there were 230,179 AIDS cases (Centers for Disease and Prevention, Control, 1992, *Health: United States, 1993,* 1994).

The technologies and service intensity included in these figures are research, education and prevention,

Examples of Federal Regulatory Mechanisms Contributing to Technology Costs/Control

1906 Prescription drug regulation passes—Food, Drug, and Cosmetic Act; now Food and Drug Administration

1938 Manufacturers required to prove drug safety—Food, Drug, and Cosmetic Act

1952 Hill-Burton Act provides construction monies for new hospitals

1965 Amendments to Social Security Act providing Medicare and Medicaid result in increased use of technologies

1972 Social Security Act amendments extending coverage for end-stage renal disease provide payment for use of treatment technologies

1972 Social Security Act amendments provide for professional standards review organizations to review appropriateness of hospital care for Medicare and Medicaid recipients

1974 Health Planning and Resources Development Act introduces certificate-of-need authority to limit major health care expansion at local and state levels

1976 Medical devices amendments regulate safety and effectiveness of medical equipment, such as pacemakers

1978 Medicare End-Stage Renal Disease Amendment provides for home dialysis and for kidney transplantation

1978 Health Services Research, Health Statistics, and Health Care Technology Act establishes a national council on health care technology to develop standards for the use of medical technologies

1982 Tax Equity and Fiscal Responsibilities Act establishes prospective payment system for hospitalized Medicare patients by DRG category

1989 OBRA created a physician resource-based fee schedule to be implemented by 1992, with more emphasis on the "high tech" specialities of surgery

1989 OBRA created the Agency for Health Care Policy and Research to perform research on effectiveness of medical services, interventions, and technologies, including nursing

Table 5-5 Population Data, in Millions, for Selected Age Groups from 1950 to 1990

Age (yrs)	1950	1970	1990
Under 15	40.4	57.9	55.5
15-24	22.0	35.4	39.8
25-44	45.2	47.9	82.5
45-64	30.8	41.9	48.1
65 and over	11.1	20.0	31.0

veterans and Department of Defense medical care, Medicaid- and Medicare-funded medical care, and cash assistance. One medication alone was estimated to cost $6400 per year in 1989. The cost per individual case was approximately $85,000 per year in 1991 (Hellinger, 1991). The box on p. 72 lists a few federal regulatory mechanisms that have contributed to the control and cost of technology.

Changes in Population Demography

The fourth major contributor to rising health care costs is the changing **population demography.** The population of the United States is aging. It is projected that by the year 2000, 13% of the total population will be over 65 years of age, with the 85-year-old and older group growing at a rapid rate (Pew, 1993a). These population changes are summarized in Table 5-5.

This is expected to lead to pressure to spend more money, especially for long-term care, research, and prevention of chronic disease in this population group. Data indicate that the major increases in health care expenditures have been for the elderly population, whereas the least expenditures have been for people under 19 years of age.

Since the Social Security Amendments of 1965, the increase in Medicare expenditures for health care for elderly persons has been greater than the rate of increased expenditures for the remainder of the population. Reasons for the increased rate of expenditures are the rapid growth of the numbers of elderly persons in the United States, the increased number of elderly women who are heavier users of health services than men, the decline in family social support requiring elderly persons to seek care and assistance outside the family structure, the greater use of more complex medical and surgical services, and the increased ability of elderly persons to pay for services received.

In addition to the elderly population other demographic factors will add to increasing health care costs. The baby boom generation is becoming middle aged. This well-educated generation is more oriented to preventive health care and is moving into the time of life when long-term care will be needed. Just as this group increased the numbers of children requiring

health care in the 1950s, they now will increase the numbers of middle-aged persons requiring long-term care for chronic conditions (Pew, 1993a).

The declining younger population, usually the healthiest group requiring less health care service, or college-aged population will mean fewer persons to contribute to the cost of elder care. (Pew, 1993a).

Finally, there is an increase in the racial and ethnic groups in the United States who have traditionally entered the United States in poor health, lived in poverty, and had less access to health care services. As a result they will need and deserve to have their basic health care needs met. To provide access to such services adds to the overall health care costs (Pew, 1993a).

Table 5-6 depicts the distribution of the four factors affecting increased costs of health care delivery from 1967 to 1991. Clearly, population has been a significant contributor after inflation and technology. In 1967 prices and intensity had similar effects. In 1977 inflation began to outdistance all other factors influencing health care expenditures. In 1991 prices contributed 54% to the growth of all health care expenditures. From 1977 to 1991 intensity increased in contribution to overall costs while prices declined.

FINANCING OF HEALTH CARE: PRIVATE AND PUBLIC

Health care financing has evolved through the twentieth century from a system financed primarily by the consumer to a system financed by third-party payers, that is, private insurance companies and governments. This section discusses changes in government, private insurance, consumer, and public health funding of care.

Table 5-7 shows changes in the percentages of financing from various sources. From 1950 to 1990 direct consumer payment decreased, philanthropic payments increased, and third-party governmental and private insurance payments increased dramatically. The combined state and federal governments' contributions as third-party payers are currently higher than those of private payers. In 1990 third-party payers contributed 78% toward the total costs of health care for the consumer, leaving only 22% to be covered by out-of-pocket money.

Third-Party Payments

Medical insurance in the private sector was first offered in 1847 by a commercial insurance company. The purpose of the insurance was to defray financial losses from disability attributable to accidents and later to defray income losses caused by specific sicknesses attributable to catastrophic communicable diseases, such as smallpox and scarlet fever.

A comprehensive study in the 1920s by the Committee on the Costs of Medical Care showed that a small portion of the population was paying most of the costs of medical care for the majority of the peo-

Table 5-6   Average Annual Percent Change in Personal Health Care Expenditures and Percent Distribution of Factors Affecting Growth in United States

Period	Average annual percent change	Percent distribution of factors affecting growth			
		All factors	Prices	Population	Intensity*
1966-67	12.2	100	55	9	36
1976-77	12.3	100	64	7	29
1986-87	10.2	100	53	9	38
1990-91	11.6	100	54	9	37

From Office of National Cost Estimates, Office of the Actuary: *Health Care Financing Rev* 14(2), 1991. HCFA Pub No 03335, Health Care Financing Administration, Washington, DC, 1992, U.S. Government Printing Office.
*Represents changes in use and/or kinds of services and supplies.
NOTE: Some numbers in this table have been revised and differ from previous editions of *Health, United States.*

Table 5-7   Personal Health Care Expenditures and Percent Distribution, According to Source of Payment in United States for Selected Years from 1929 to 1990

Year	Total in billions*	Per capita	All sources	Direct payment	Private health insurance	Philanthropy and industry	Government		
							Total	Federal	State and local
1929	$ 3.2	$ 26	100.0	88.4†	‡	2.6	9.0	2.7	6.3
1940	$ 3.5	$ 26	100.0	81.3†	‡	2.6	16.1	4.1	12.0
1950	10.9	70	100.0	65.5	9.1	2.9	22.4	10.4	12.0
1960	23.9	126	100.0	55.9	21.0	1.7	21.4	8.9	12.5
1970	64.9	302	100.0	39.5	23.4	2.6	34.6	22.6	12.0
1980	219.7	934	100.0	27.1	29.7	3.5	39.7	28.9	10.8
1990	591.5	2279	100.0	21.9	31.7	3.6	42.9	30.9	12.0

From Office of National Cost Estimates, Office of the Actuary: *Health Care Financing Rev* 14(2), 1991. HCFA Pub No 03335, Health Care Financing Administration, Washington, DC, 1992, U.S. Government Printing Office.
*Includes all expenditures for health services and supplies other than expenses for prepayment and administration and government public health activities.
†Includes any insurance benefits and expenses for prepayment (insurance premiums less insurance benefits).
‡Figures are not separable from direct payment.
NOTE: Some numbers in this table have been revised and differ from previous editions of *Health, United States.*

ple. The Depression, rising medical costs, and the need to spread financial risk across communities spurred the development of the **third-party payment** system.

The system began as a major industry in the 1930s with the Blue Cross system, which initially provided prepayment for hospital care. It was modeled on the Baylor University prepayment plan established in 1929 to provide teachers with hospital coverage. In 1939 Blue Shield created plans to provide physician payment. The Blue Cross plans began as tax-free, non-profit organizations established under special **enabling legislation** in various states.

In the 1940s and 1950s hospital and medical-surgical coverage increased substantially. Employee group coverage appeared and profit-making commer-

cial insurance underwriters began offering health insurance packages with competitive premiums. The commercial insurance companies could offer lower premium rates because of the methods used to set rates. Blue Cross used a *community rate,* establishing a similar premium rate for all subscribers regardless of illness possibilities. In contrast, the commercial companies used an *experience rate* in which the premium was based on an estimate of the illness risk or the number of claims to be made by the subscriber.

The premium competition, the popularity of health insurance packages as a fringe benefit, and the use of health insurance as a negotiable collective bargaining item led to increased numbers of covered benefits, payment of higher portions of medical care expenses, and increased employer-paid premiums. These factors led to higher premium costs, higher health care costs, and plans that could economically cover high-risk segments of the population, such as aged, poor, or disabled persons. The average monthly cost for private health insurance increased 70% from 1988 to 1990, bringing the average employee's share of family health care insurance premiums to more than $200 per month. It is projected that continued health care inflation could increase the bill to $8000 per year for middle income workers by the year 2000 (Tokarski, 1989a; Pew, 1993a, Lee, 1994).

The needs of high-risk populations led to passage of Medicare and Medicaid legislation. These and other national health programs were authorized to provide health care coverage for specific population groups. These new programs, federal regulations, and insurance company reimbursement methods contributed to increased technological costs. Because money was available to be paid, physicians, hospital managers, and clients used more medical technology, and service intensity increased.

Three reimbursement methods have been or are currently used to pay agencies for health goods and services:

1. **Cost-plus reimbursement.** An agency may be reimbursed for the actual costs of treatment and care plus added allowable costs. These added costs include depreciation of costs of a building and equipment and administrative costs (e.g., administrative salaries, utilities, and office supplies).
2. **Retrospective cost reimbursement.** An agency may be reimbursed per unit of service, according to an agreed-on price usually predetermined by the state insurance departments or departments of health. In home health the unit of service is the home visit and the agreed-on price is a set amount of money paid for a home visit in the region of the United States in which the home care agency is located.
3. **Prospective cost reimbursement.** Based on previous experience and current rates for care, agencies and insurance companies attempt to predict an agency's costs for the year. The agency plans an annual budget with projected goals for services. The insurance company reimburses the agency based on predicted costs for services. For example, a home care agency may receive a check for 6 months to cover home care visits they predict they will make.

Positive and negative incentives were built into these reimbursement schemes. The cost-plus reimbursement scheme encouraged agencies to add depreciation and administrative costs that inflated actual treatment and care costs. The retrospective cost reimbursement method encouraged agencies to pad unit cost prices to cover unexpected cost increases, such as increased postal service. The prospective cost reimbursement scheme encouraged agencies to stay within budget limits and added an incentive for providing less service to contain or reduce costs.

Along with agency reimbursement, physician reimbursement is a key factor in the use and cost of technology and service intensity. The two primary methods for physician reimbursement have been:

1. **Benefit schedule**—a list of specific physician services that identifies the amount third parties must pay for them.
2. **Fee screen system**—a method that determines the usual, customary, and reasonable charge (UCR) for specific services, based on a regional evaluation of physician charges in all specialties. A maximum reimbursement limit by third parties is determined by the UCR for a specific service.

These fee-for-service reimbursement schemes were shown to be inflationary. Physicians controlled the numbers and kinds of services provided a client. As third-party reimbursement increased, physicians' fees increased. The consumer was responsible for the costs over and above the third-party coverage. Negative experience with fee-for-service physician reimbursement and the inflationary nature of the system have impeded progress toward third-party reimbursement for other health care providers, such as nurses.

The third-party pay system is often blamed for rising health care costs. Factors that support this belief include the following:

1. The cost-plus reimbusement scheme previously used to pay hospital care for Medicaid-Medicare and Blue Cross clients provided little incentive to control costs.
2. The third-party payers provided better coverage for the more expensive hospital services than for ambulatory care, home health care, or nursing home care. This encouraged consumer use of hospitals because more of the client's bill was paid by the insurer. If there was a choice between hospital and home care, hospital care was chosen.
3. Consumer demand for services increased and provider incentives to use less costly services were lacking, because government or private insurers paid most hospital and physician bills. The providers did not develop more ambulatory services because of the need for the consumer to pay out-of-pocket.
4. The UCR charge pay system encouraged physicians to charge maximum fees so they could boost the UCR charge schedule.
5. Third-party reimbursement for surgery, diagnostic procedures, and other technological interventions encouraged the provision of these services, regardless of their necessity.

Generally health care costs have risen faster than the cost of all goods and services.

Consumer Payments

Before 1930 and the beginning of Blue Cross, the consumer (client) had more influence over health care costs, because nearly all health care costs were paid out-of-pocket. However, the health care system has always been a seller's market, that is, the hospital, the physician, the HMO. Once the buyer (the client) makes the decision to enter the health care market, all goods and services are provided and controlled by the seller (the physician).

When the health care system was economically controlled by the consumer market, entrance into the system was restricted to those who could afford to pay or to those few who could find care financed by charitable and philanthropic organizations.

Today the consumer pays directly approximately 18% of all physician fees and 3% of all hospital bills. However, these figures do not reflect the amount of money the consumer pays in taxes to finance government-supported programs such as Medicare and Medicaid, the insurance premiums averaging $2500 per year that come from wages and therefore decrease the size of paychecks, or the direct insurance premiums paid for supplemental insurance to plug the gaps in the primary health insurance policy and Medicare (*Health: United States 1993*, 1994).

It is estimated that elderly persons pay approximately 20% of all health care costs directly and 74% pay private health insurance premiums (Rice 1994; U.S. House of Representatives, Select Committee on Aging, 1994). This is due to limits in coverage in Medicare and Medicaid programs, payment of premiums for Medicare, and the need to have additional insurance to cover these gaps. It is also caused by the limited number of physicians, hospitals, and other agencies who accept Medicare and Medicaid payment. Aged persons then are left to cover the difference between Medicare and Medicaid services and additional costs. In reality, the working consumer pays all health care costs directly or indirectly and should be more concerned about health care costs.

Until the mid-1980s, consumer demands increased and strengthened the benefits of private health insurance packages, the numbers of government programs available to aged and poor persons, and the availability and accessibility of health care services. These consumer demands contributed to health care inflation and caused a financial drain on the economic potential of the individual and the government. Beginning in the 1980s health insurance benefits were cut back. Medicare and Medicaid program benefits were reduced, prospective payment to hospitals was introduced, and more emphasis was placed on care in the home and community. To attempt to control physician costs, a new Medicare fee schedule, called a relative value scale, was adopted in 1991. This scale replaces the previously described methods of physician payment, placing more emphasis on payment of care received through primary care physicians in the community. It also places more value on prevention, health promotion, and evaluation with less value for surgery and the use of high technologies. This is an attempt to reduce inappropriate and unnecessary care (Lee et al., 1994).

Research Brief

Blandon R Donelon K, Hill C, Carter W, Beatric D, Altman D: Paying medical bills in the United States, *JAMA* 271(12):949-951, 1994.

A national survey of 1897 households, representative of the U.S. population, was conducted by the Harvard School of Public Health and the National Opinion Research Center for the Henry Kaiser Family Foundation. The purpose of the survey was to look at who in the United States reports problems paying medical bills, the insurance status of those surveyed, what other financial stresses they face, and how they cope with the realities of illness and disability.

The results showed that 19.4% (369) of those surveyed had a problem paying for medical bills: physician or hospital bills—15.6%; prescription medication bills—10.4%; nursing home bills—2.2%; and home health care bills—1.7%. The results also showed the following:

1. Three of four Americans who have problems paying medical bills have health insurance.
2. Financial worries about the cost of medical care frequently coincide with concerns about facing unemployment and meeting day-to-day household expenses.
3. Financial worries about health care services strike Americans when they are most vulnerable, while disabled, mentally ill, in fair or poor health, or caring for a sick family member.
4. Difficulty coping with medical bills affects all Americans regardless of income, age, gender, or race.

The authors recommended two solutions to the problem of paying medical bills:

1. Provide a comprehensive benefit package at a predictable cost.
2. Construct a new form of catastrophic insurance coverage that would protect people who face simultaneous loss of health and loss of income.

Government Payments

The federal government became involved in health care financing for population groups early in U.S. history. In 1798 the federal government created the Marine Hospital Service to provide medical service for sick and disabled sailors and to protect the nation's borders against the importing of disease through seaports. The Marine Hospital Service is considered the first national health insurance plan in the United States. The original plan cost each sailor 20 cents per month in a payroll deduction for illness care.

The National Health Board was established in 1879. The board was later renamed the United States Public Health Service (PHS). Within the PHS, the federal government developed a public health liaison with state and local health departments for the purpose of controlling communicable diseases and improving sanitation. Additional health programs were also developed to meet obligations to federal beneficiaries, including American Indians (Indian Health Service), the armed forces (Department of Defense), and veterans of wars (Veterans Administration).

Today, the federal government is involved in health care research, training, financing, and delivery and provides money for four aspects of public health: (1) broad national health interests, such as AIDS research; (2) special groups, such as mothers, infants, and the aged through WIC, Medicare, and Medicaid funds; (3) special problems or programs, such as food and drug safety through U.S. Food and Drug Administration (FDA) requirements and food inspection; and (4) international health through its affiliation with the World Health Organization.

Appendix A contains an overview of the major historical events depicting the federal government's increasing involvement in financing health care research, training, and delivery.

Public Health Care Funding

Most public governmental agencies operate on an annual budget and plan for costs by estimating salaries, expenses, and costs of services for a year. Public health agencies, such as the health departments and WIC programs, receive primary funding from tax revenues, with additional money for select goods and services through private third-party payers. Selected public health programs receive reimbursement for services as follows: through grants given by the federal government to states for prenatal and child health; through Medicare and Medicaid for home health, nursing homes, WIC programs, and early periodic screening and childhood development programs (EPSDT); and through collection of fees on a sliding scale for select client services, such as immunizations.

Only 3% of all health care–related federal funds are expended for government public health programs, such as mental health and WIC, as opposed to 97% for illness care in hospitals. Despite the 3% allotment, public health expenditures by states and territorial health agencies have increased at a rate of 11% per year between 1977 and 1991. Table 5-8 indicates the amount, source of funds, and program areas supported since 1976. Note an increasing emphasis on program areas. The effect of the fee-for-service issue is not as great in public health care as in private health care, because most providers are salaried. However, the increasing costs of health care goods and increasing salaries of providers have contributed to the rising costs of public health care as well.

National Health Care Plans

The **Medicare program,** Title XVIII of the Social Security Act of 1965, provides hospital insurance, Part A,

Table 5-8 Public Health Expenditures by State and Territorial Health Agencies, According to Source of Funds and Program Area: United States, Selected Fiscal Years 1976 to 1989

Funds and program area	1976	1980	1989
	Amount in millions		
Total	$2539.8	$4450.8	$9669
Source of funds			
Federal grants and contracts	796.9	1573.1	3503
State	1485.7	2513.3	5184
Local	96.1	114.0	154
Fees, reimbursements, and other	161.2	250.3	829
Program area			
WIC*	137.7	660.7	1938
Noninstitutional personal health other than WIC†	1079.0	1698.2	3972
State health agency–operated institutions	531.1	819.3	1459
Environmental health	199.2	298.0	520
Health resources	208.2	356.5	824
Laboratory	104.1	161.1	308
Other‡	280.6	457.0	649

From Public Health Foundation: *Public health agencies 1989: expenditures and sources of funds,* Washington, DC, 1989 (unpublished data).
*Supplemental Food Program for Women, Infants, and Children.
†Includes funds for maternal and child health services other than WIC, handicapped children's services, communicable disease control, dental health, chronic disease control, mental health, alcohol and drug abuse, and supporting personal health programs.
‡Funds for general administration and funds to local health departments not allocated to program areas.
NOTE: Data are reported for 55 health agencies in 50 states, the District of Columbia, and four territories (Puerto Rico, American Samoa, Guam, and the Virgin Islands).

and medical insurance, Part B, to elderly persons, permanently and totally disabled persons, and people with end-stage renal disease. Currently 36 million people are enrolled in Medicare, or more than 10% of the total U.S. population (*Health: United States 1993,* 1994).

The hospital insurance package, Part A, is available without cost to all elderly individuals who have paid Social Security taxes. Estimates indicate that 98% of the elderly population are covered by Part A. Part A provides payment for hospital services, home health services, and extended care facilities. This includes an

Table 5-9   Medicare Expenditures and Percent Distribution, According to Type of Service, in United States for Selected Years, from 1967 to 1992

Type of service	1967	1970	1980	1992
AMOUNT IN BILLIONS				
All expenditures	$4.7	$7.4	$36.8	$182.5
PERCENT DISTRIBUTION				
All services	100.0	100.0	100.0	100.0
Hospital care	69.1	71.0	72.6	68.1
Physician services	24.7	22.8	22.1	17.7
Nursing home care	5.4	3.7	1.4	4.5
Home health service	0.8	2.4	3.9	9.7

Data compiled by the Health Care Financing Administration.

annual deductible for the first 60 days of services and copayment for 61 to 90 days of service based on a rate equal to a 1-day stay in the hospital. That deductible has increased over the years as daily hospital costs have increased (Select, 1994).

The medical insurance package, Part B, is available to all people who wish to pay a monthly premium for the coverage. Approximately 96% of the elderly population is covered. The premium cost was $36.60 per month in 1994. Part B of Medicare provides coverage for services other than hospitalization, such as physician services, outpatient hospital care, outpatient physical therapy and speech therapy, home health care not covered by Part A, laboratory services, ambulance transportation, prostheses, equipment, and some supplies. After a deductible, up to 80% of reasonable charges are paid for these services. Part B resembles the major medical insurance coverage of private insurance carriers. Table 5-9 shows the increasing cost of the Medicare program from 1967 to 1992.

Since the passage of the Medicare amendments to the Social Security Act in 1965, the cost of Medicare has increased dramatically. Hospital care continues to be the major factor contributing to Medicare costs, however, with shorter hospital stays, home health and nursing home costs have increased dramatically.

As a result of the increasing costs, Congress passed a law in 1983 that radically changed Medicare's method of payment for hospital services. The Social Security amendments of 1983 (PL 98-21) mandated an end to cost-plus reimbursement by Medicare and instituted a 3-year transition to a **prospective payment system** (PPS) for inpatient hospital services. The purpose of the new hospital payment scheme was to shift the financial incentives away from the provision of more care, the use of more technology, and the use of more hospital care. Reimbursement is based on a fixed price per case for clients in 468 **diagnosis-related groups (DRGs)**. The objective of this system was to reduce hospital costs while maintaining an ac-

ceptable level of quality health care and access. Although this type of reimbursement was mandated for hospitals only, prospective payment for physicians, home health, long-term care, and ambulatory care continues to be considered. There is a possibility with health care reform that a capitated rate based on a DRG plan may occur.

The **Medicaid program,** Title XIX of the Social Security Act of 1965, provides financial assistance to states and counties to pay for medical services for the aged poor, the blind, the disabled, and families with dependent children. The Medicaid program is jointly sponsored and financed with matching funds from the federal and state governments. Currently, 32 million people are enrolled in Medicaid.

Full payment for five types of service was provided orginally: (1) inpatient and outpatient hospital care; (2) laboratory and radiological services; (3) physician services; (4) skilled nursing care, at home or in a nursing home, for people over 21 years; and (5) EPSDT services for those under 21 years (*Health: United States, 1993,* 1994). The 1972 Social Security Amendments added family planning to the list of full-pay services. Prescriptions, dental services, eyeglasses, intermediate care facilities, and coverage for the **medically indigent** are allowable program options. By law, the medically indigent are required to pay a monthly premium.

Any state participating in the Medicaid program is required to provide the six basic services to participants who are below state poverty income levels. The optional programs are provided at the discretion of each state.

In 1989 changes in Medicaid required states to provide care for children under 6 years and to pregnant women under 133% of the poverty level. For example, if the poverty level were $12,000, a pregnant woman could have a household income as high as $16,000 and still be eligible to receive care under Medicaid. These changes also provided for pediatric and family nurse practitioner reimbursement.

Federal government reorganization of the Medicaid program in the 1990s may include a requirement for states to begin prospective payment systems to reduce costs. Table 5-10 indicates the increased cost of the Medicaid program from 1967 to 1992.

In the past, the major contributor to costs in the Medicaid program has been nursing home care. When combined with hospital care, today it accounts for 57% of all costs to the program. Because of increasing emphasis on preventive care and community-based care, home health and other care, such as EPSDT, family planning, and clinics, are increasing in costs. See Table 5-11 for a comparison of Medicare and Medicaid programs.

With Medicare and Medicaid, the federal government purchases goods and services for population groups through independent health care systems such as private physicians and hospitals. In contrast, the *military medical care system* is a federal program that provides health care and insurance to military personnel and their dependents at no direct cost to the recipient.

Table 5-10   Medicaid Expenditures and Percent Distribution, According to Type of Service, in United States for Selected Years from 1967-1992

Type of service	1967	1970	1980	1992
AMOUNT IN BILLIONS				
All expenditures	$2.9	$5.2	$23.3	$91.5
PERCENT DISTRIBUTION				
All services	100.0	100.0	100.0	100.0
Hospital care	42.3	42.9	38.1	31.7
Physician services	10.9	13.3	9.7	6.7
Dentist services	4.4	3.2	2.0	0.9
Other provider services	0.9	1.4	2.2	0.6
Drugs and drug sundries	7.2	7.9	5.5	7.4
Nursing home care	31.7	27.2	38.1	25.7
Home health service	—	0.4	1.4	5.3
Other*	2.6	4.1	3.7	9.9

From Health Care Financing Administration.
*Other services include laboratory and radiological services, family planning services, EPSDT, clinics, and pro rated care.

The military medical system comprises hospitals and clinics, which provide military personnel with health care wherever they are located. This health care system has several important characteristics: (1) the system is all-inclusive and ever-present; (2) coverage is effective at all times; (3) prevention, early case-finding, and health promotion are emphasized; and (4) dependents and families are served by a subsystem that combines military and civilian health services (Sharfstein, 1990). This system places the federal government in the direct health service business.

The *Civilian Health and Medical Program of the Uniformed Services* (CHAMPUS) allows families and dependents to obtain private sector care if service is unavailable in the military system. The program is provided, financed, and supervised by the military system. In 1981 the CHAMPUS 1980-1992 program began direct, independent reimbursement of nurse practitioners and physician assistants for services to military dependents.

The *Veterans Administration health care system,* linked to the military health care system, operates within the United States for retired, disabled, and other specified categories of military service veterans. The system,

Table 5-11   Comparison of Medicare and Medicaid Programs

Feature	Medicare	Medicaid
Obtain information	Social Security Office	State welfare office
Recipients	Persons aged 65+ yr; disabled under 65 yr eligible after 2 yrs	Needy and low income, persons aged 65+ yr, blind, disabled, families with dependent children, some other children
Type of program	Insurance	Assistance
Government affiliation	Federal	Federal/state partnership
Availability	All states	All states
Hospital insurance	Financed by working persons; payroll contributions	Financed by federal and state government
Medical insurance	Monthly premiums paid by recipients (25%) and federal government (75%)	Federal and state government
Types of coverage	Inpatient and outpatient hospital care Posthospital skilled nursing facility Home health care Physician services Medical services and supplies Hospice care HMO Laboratory and radiological services	Inpatient and outpatient hospital care Skilled nursing facilities Home health care Physician services/dental services Other laboratory and x-ray services Screening, diagnosis, and treatment of children under 21 yr Family planning Health clinic services Supplements Medicare payments Services for mentally retarded persons Prescription drugs

Modified from Medicaid/Medicare: *Which is which?* USDHHS Pub No 02129, Washington, DC, 1984; National Health Care Financing Administration: *Health: United States, 1993,* DHHS Pub No (PHS) 94-1232, Washington, DC, 1994.

comprising 172 hospitals and more than 200 outpatient departments, is one part of a benefit package received by veterans. Eligibility for health care is often tied to other financial benefits within the system structure. Current cost of this program is $11 billion per year (*Health: United States, 1993,* 1994).

As with all other programs, military medical care systems' costs have increased. From 1980 to 1992, costs increased by 128% to $13 billion. This includes the Veterans Administration and the CHAMPUS program (*Health: United States, 1993,* 1994). The Indian Health Service provides direct care to native Americans living on reservations. This agency operates approximately 50 hospitals and 340 clinics to serve over 1 million native Americans. This service was established in 1911 through the Bureau of Indian Affairs in the Department of the Interior. This service, like the military service, provides a combination of public and private health care. Legislation passed in 1976 provides opportunity for tribes to assume responsibility of operating their own facilities. This service cost the Public Health Service $41 billion in 1988.

POVERTY AND HEALTH CARE FINANCING

In 1992, 73% of the U.S. population had health insurance provided through their employers. An additional 10% received insurance through public programs leaving 17% uninsured (43 million people). Of the 73.0% *insured*, 30 million, or 12% of the total population, were *underinsured*. These figures indicate that one in four citizens is not prepared for a health care crisis. This number includes 37 million Americans living in poverty (Grace, 1990; *Health: United States, 1993,* 1994; Rice, 1994).

The typical uninsured person is a member of a family (child or adult), whose adults do not work and therefore do not have access to insurance as an employment benefit. Others who are typically uninsured are young adults, minorities, or unmarried persons. These people may be in minimum wage jobs, and their employers may not offer health insurance as a benefit. Their salary levels are such that they cannot afford to purchase it on their own, or because of their age, they may not see the need for it. For these people a major illness can result in debt or disability that will keep them or place them at the poverty level. This may ultimately deny them access to health care. For those who are underinsured, poverty, homelessness, continuing ill health, disability, and loss of employment are but a few of the effects of a catastrophic illness.

Elderly persons, in spite of Medicare and sometimes private insurance supplements, pay a large portion of their health care bill out-of-pocket. Long-term care is the most common cause of catastrophic health care bills for this group. The cost of 1 year in a nursing home averaged $20,000 to $30,000 in 1989 (Korn et al, 1989). To receive Medicaid and certain Medicare benefits, elderly persons must "spend down" their life savings, including selling their homes, until they have only $1500 to $2000 left. It should be noted that long-term care is not used solely for elderly persons. In 1985, 12% of those in nursing homes were under 65 years, whereas 10% of all disabled persons were under 65 years. Therefore this issue is a concern to all ages. Although the majority of the elderly today are economically, physically, and socially sound, 13% live in poverty. The majority of these are women (Grau, 1988). Those in poverty are more likely to experience ill health, whereas others may experience age-related situational factors that put them at risk for poverty.

Poverty and health care funding are directly and indirectly related in three ways: (1) when an individual is impoverished and unable to qualify for public-supported programs, health care access may be denied; (2) when a person is underinsured, a catastrophic illness may lead to poverty; and (3) when a person is elderly and in poverty, illness is more likely to occur.

HEALTH CARE TRENDS

The economic viability of the health care delivery system is affected by a number of factors. Trends explored in this section include managed care, managed competition, health care rationing, health care financing schemes, health care reform, and payments for nursing services.

Managed Care

To spur the development of a comprehensive health care system for the entire U.S. population, the **Health Maintenance Organization Act** became law in 1972. As discussed in Chapter 2, health maintenance organizations (HMOs) are prepaid systems that provide comprehensive health care services to participants for a basic monthly premium or a *capitation fee:* one fee covering all services. Prepaid group practice plans existing in the United States since the 1940s served as models for the HMO Act. The intent of HMOs was to prevent costly hospitalization by educating consumers in illness prevention and health maintenance. A degree of success has been realized, as shown by up to 40% reduction in hospital use for HMO clients (Knickman and Thorpe, 1995).

HMO plans usually provide more coverage to an enrollee without copayment or deductible than is typical of other health insurance schemes. Federal and state governments continue to encourage the development of HMOs by providing grants and loans for planning and operation. Some states require employers to offer HMOs as health insurance options in benefit packages. There are more than 550 HMOs in the United States with 39 million enrollees, including 332 independent practice associations (IPAs), thereby offering a system that is competitive with other health insurance schemes (*Health: United States, 1993,* 1994).

Although an HMO may be a freestanding health care agency providing its own staff, the IPA is a type of HMO whereby a third-party payer contracts with a range of independent providers to give service to the HMO enrollees. Preferred provider organizations (PPOs) are arrangements using multiple physicians who agree to offer services to clients of a third-party payer at a discount rate. In 1993 15 million people enrolled in PPOs (*Health: United States, 1993,* 1994).

All of these schemes are called managed care programs, or services that organize and provide the type of care needed by the client. Some believe that this is not managed care but "utilization review: (see Chapter 22 or care based on selecting the least costly services to manage a problem. Managed care currently involves second surgical opinions, preauthorization of selected hospital admissions, concurrent review of care, outpatient surgery, and testing requirements to attempt to alleviate use of "inappropriate care" (Thorpe, 1995). Managed care should be a system of advocating for the client and obtaining a set of comprehensive services to meet client needs. In health care reform it has become a way of allocating services to the client to save money for the provider by controlling the costs of services the client receives (Iglehart, 1994).

Health Care Rationing

The crisis in health care financing has spurred a renewed effort to ration health care. With unsuccessful attempts at cost containment and cost reduction, new plans are being introduced to control use of services and technologies.

Rationing is not new to health care delivery. For decades the uninsured and those who do not qualify for governmental programs have been denied services or have been eligible for restricted services only. The absence of a universal health plan and the existence of federal program eligibility criteria are other examples of **health care rationing.**

With the introduction of new and limited technologies, "death committees" were formed and criteria established to determine who would benefit from the technology and who would be allowed to advance to terminal stages and death. Examples included committees, and in some instances one physician, who made decisions about which client would receive dialysis or organ transplantation.

In the mid-1970s, discussions were held about future policies to limit intensity of services and technologies, such as surgery for those who became ill because of personal life-styles, that is, smokers and lung cancer treatment, alcoholics and treatment for cirrhosis, the obese and treatment for cardiovascular disease. In fact, involvement in life-style risks today such as lack of seat belt use, drinking, and smoking habits often lead to increased insurance premiums. This concept of rationing is termed *blaming the victim* (Banta, 1995a).

By 1990 the Oregon State Health Plan had been passed to ensure basic health care to all state citizens.

This plan, recognized as a model health plan, required the use of managed care and ranking health services according to their effectiveness and benefit. The most effective and beneficial services were to be prioritized and paid for to the extent that the state legislature had the money to pay. These services were to be available to the poor and uninsured persons, who were also ranked, from those with the greatest need to those with the least need. Services that exceeded the state budget limit would not be included in the benefits, thus rationing services.

Other plans that preceded the Oregon Plan were Arizona's Medicaid plan to provide managed care to qualified recipients (1982) and Massachusetts Universal Health Plan (1988). Some plans have been successful in reducing overall costs, and others have not.

Several issues emerge as one considers the concept of rationing. Rationing implies limiting care that may be beneficial to the client's well-being. When resources become scarce, policymakers determine what will be rationed. Individual characteristics and effectiveness of technologies are most likely to affect a rationing decision. Elderly persons, whose life value may not be considered important, may be affected the most by such plans. Others who may be affected include women, minorities, and children in poverty. Children comprise 38% of those living in poverty. (*Health: United States, 1993,* 1994). The quality of care under rationing may be inferior to care received in a totally competitive market because of the restricted services offered.

Rationing of health care in any form implies reduced access to care and a potential decrease in acceptability, as well as quality, of services offered. There is the potential for more appropriate care through managed care and care that is better organized to meet the basic health care needs of the total population. Plans must include a mechanism for informed choice (Larkin, 1988; Williams, 1988; Enthoven and Kronick, 1989; Levine, 1989; Grace, 1990; Rooks, 1990).

One could argue that rationing restricts the individual's right of choice and thereby restricts total society's freedom. This response is opposite to that suggested by welfare economic theory. However, to allow continuing skyrocketing prices in health care restricts the monies available to spend on education, transportation, housing. The answer is not simple. Rand Corporation studies have shown that clients and providers will make choices based on who pays. The ability and willingness to pay through a fee-for-service system, or any cost sharing, such as an insurance deductible, decrease contact with the health care system (client self-rationing). "Free care" results in quicker decisions by clients to seek health care. Conversely when the client is paying, quicker decision are made by the provider to offer more complex care. Such provider decisions are often delayed in the managed care system, with set capitation payments, or in a free service, where the market controls rationing (Newhouse, 1985; Hahn, 1994).

Health Care Financing

Although the government and third-party payers continue to be the major source of funding, new trends in health care financing have emerged. Although prospective payment was introduced in 1983 to control government health care costs, private insurance has followed suit by requiring precontract arrangements and approval before the client can receive certain services, such as hospital admission or mammograms more than once per year. Also, reimbursement for selected services has been omitted or curtailed, or payment rates are set, routine chest x-rays, surgical procedures, air ambulance services, and number of hospital days.

A growth in competitive bidding for health care services, designed to create incentives for providers to compete on price, has also occurred. This concept was introduced in states to provide Medicaid services to eligible recipients. In this scheme hospitals and other health care agencies and providers who do not receive a contract with the state are not eligible to receive Medicaid payments for client care. The California program is highlighted as the greatest success in reducing overall Medicaid program costs (Brecher, 1995).

The reform of physician reimbursement, the first modern attempt to regulate and change physician fee structure, was introduced in 1990 in the Omnibus Reconciliation Act. After a study by the Physician Payment Review Commission established by Congress, the *resource-based relative value scale* was established, which is designed to shift physician fees toward increased reimbursement for such services as physical examinations, diagnostic services, teaching, and counseling, and decreased reimbursement for use of surgical procedures and technologies. This is an attempt to place more emphasis on prevention and promotion and lessen incentive to place clients in sick roles and to use unnecessary technologies (Knickman and Thorpe, 1995).

Although the prospective payment system was intended to reduce health care costs, costs were again on the increase after a reduction the first year. "Unbundling" of hospital services and an emphasis on community services shifted the costs from hospital to other agency services rather than reducing them. (For example, to "unbundle" services, hospitals separated laboratory, radiology, and outpatient surgery to cost units outside the hospitals.) Services on the increase included home health care, adult day care, ambulatory clinics, emergi-centers, nursing home care, and, in some instances, payment of a family member to care for the sick person in the home.

In addition to the comprehensive health care organizations, other alternative health care delivery services were emerging or expanding. These services represented a major change in the structure and pattern for delivering health care and reflected the increasing emphasis on direct out-of-pocket payment for health care services. Although the development of such health care alternatives provided ready access to a number of services to those who could pay, it encouraged fragmentation of care.

Insurance companies were beginning to reduce benefits while premiums and deductibles rose. Private insurers were moving more toward establishing experience rate premiums, placing a further burden on employers and employees.

While the federal government imposed taxes on a certain portion of insurance premiums paid by employers and employees, omitting the "free benefits" received as a result of employment, Medicare and Medicaid eligibility became more restrictive. These factors resulted in increased out-of-pocket expenses for all persons, regardless of age, if they chose hospitals or providers who were nonparticipants in Medicare, Medicaid, or private insurance programs. A non-participating provider or agency will not accept the usual, customary, and reasonable fees for services established by third-party payers; therefore the consumer must make up the difference. In some instances, nonparticipants will not accept Medicaid clients because of the fee structures of the governmental programs, thereby limiting access.

A major change that has had a positive impact for nurses is the growth in the number of self-insured or self-funded health plans. These funds are primarily found in major industries. When an industry or group of corporations bands together to self-insure, emphasis switches from sick care to prevention and health promotion. The purpose of the switch is to reduce sick care costs, increase productivity, reduce absenteeism, and enhance employee morale.

These programs use nurses to provide wellness programs, health assessment, and screening and monitoring of employees and their families. This change in health care provider emphasis results in savings to the company and has benefitted industry by reducing overall sick care costs (Christenson and Kiefhaber, 1988; Gillis, 1988; Knickman, and Thorpe, 1995).

The reported health care crisis of the 1980s and 1990s has led to increased emphasis on managed care and health care rationing. New health care financing plans are reflecting these changes.

Health Care Reform

Although there is no definitive answer to the questions of cost containment and cost reduction, it has been suggested that the only to provide health care for all persons is to reform the entire health care system.

In October 1993, President Clinton introduced the Health Security Act. This plan called for a major restructuring of the health care system and the financing of health care. The plan offered universal access to a basic benefit package of hospital, preventive, physician, and long-term care services. It supported the payment of services by requiring all employers to provide health insurance benefits for employees. All unemployed persons would receive benefits through a government-paid plan (Richardson, 1995).

Economics of Health Care Delivery **83**

Because of the President's requirement that all big and small businesses provide health insurance coverage, several Republican congressmen introduced health care reform bills that were similar to the President's but did not require universal coverage nor did they require employers to provide health insurance benefits. As a result of the national debates, health care reform legislation was not passed by 1995.

All of the debates, however, raised the awareness of society that something needed to be done. By 1994 eight states had introduced health care reform packages that encouraged **managed competition** as a way of controlling or reducing costs and **managed care** as a way of delivering services.

As previously discussed, managed care involves the marriage of the following types of service agencies into a unified network: HMO's, physicians' offices, hospitals, home health agencies, nursing homes, and support services, such as laboratories, radiology departments, same-day surgery centers, and perhaps public health departments. This network will then provide all services to clients with whom it contracts. Clients could be individuals, businesses, local and state governments, associations of retired persons (as an example of a group) and Medicaid clients in a certain geographical area. The managed care network provides client choice of providers within the system.

The managed care systems were to evolve using a managed competition approach. This approach creates market conditions in which the more efficient providers will thrive and the costly or inefficient will be put out of business.

Health care reform discussions offered three possible ways to finance and pay for health care: (1) the single-payer system; (2) the pay or play system; (3) and the current system. The *single-payer (all-payer) system* is a system whereby there would be one health insurance company to whom all premiums would be paid by clients and by whom all health bills would be paid to providers. By having only a one-payer system, administrative costs could be reduced, and client and provider paperwork would be reduced to completing a single-page form. In this instance the health insurance company could be a government or a private insurance company who received the contract to provide the services. Such a system would reduce competition in the health insurance industry, drastically reduce the number of companies, reduce jobs, and create unemployment in the industry.

The *pay or play system* of financing health care was a system introduced by the Health Security Act. This system would require all businesses and individuals (employer, employee, unemployed) to purchase health insurance through their business, job, or the government, that is, to be a "player." If one did not have health insurance then one would have to "pay" a penalty often greater than the cost of the health insurance premium. This system was proposed as a way of assuring that all persons would have health care coverage; thus universal access would be possible.

Businesses were not happy with this plan because it would require them to cover all players, increase their costs of health insurance, and reduce profits.

The *current system* involves 1500 private health insurance companies and state, local, and federal governments as the insurers and payers of health care bills. The health insurance industry is powerful and currently controls use of health care services, who can have health insurance, and costs. To reduce the size of this private industry and reduce its power would reduce overall health care costs. Currently one of every four health care dollars is spent on administrative costs, mostly paperwork, related to health insurance. To reduce government's role would reduce regulation of health care (Williams and Torrens, 1993). Which plan is best, no one really knows, but countries such as Canada and Great Britain, which have single payer systems, have lower health care costs (Reinhardt, 1994).

In 1991 many nursing organizations came together to support a reformed health care system. The box below shows what nursing thinks is needed.

Regardless of the health care reform plan chosen there is likely to be a two-tiered system. The first tier would provide a publicly financed health care program, funded primarily by a competitively bid, prepaid **capitation** plan with rationing of health care services. Social Security taxes, individual taxation, or taxation of employer health insurance contributions, and individual health insurance premiums may be used to finance this health care program. The government would pay health care providers a fixed fee to provide a basic level of health care to uninsured, poor, and elderly persons. The same basic package would be available to those with private health insurance.

The second tier would be a free market system in which individual health care could be purchased in excess of that provided by employers or government.

 Key Points in Nursing's Agenda for Health Care Reform

A restructured health care system emphasizing:
  Access; primary care; community based care
  Use of cost-effective providers
  Personal health and self-care
A standard package of essential health care services for all citizens
  A phase-in of essential services
  Planned health care services representing national demographics
  Steps to reduce health care costs based on managed care
  Case management
  Long-term care
  Insurance reforms
  No payment at point of care
  Establishing a public or private review to monitor the system

From American Nurses Association: 1991.

Care would be limited only by the amount of money a person is willing to pay.

The implications of the two-tiered system are many. The quality of care is of major concern. Quality of care in the first tier would depend largely on the ethics and expertise of the health care providers. If providers who are motivated by the need to help others are employed in the first tier, the quality of care may be higher than that currently offered to certain population groups, such as Medicaid and Medicare clients who will be a part of the first tier. If, on the other hand, first-tier providers are primarily those who cannot find positions in the second tier, quality may become an issue.

Access to care would become more equitable across population groups by such a system. The provider will not necessarily be able to distinguish the Medicaid client from the client with private insurance, because all clients in the first tier will have a similar insurance card. Costs and use would be controlled by the buyers of service—the government and corporations in the first level and the consumer in the second level (Estes, 1994; Lamm, 1994).

As changes in health care financing occur, nurses must plan for the future. They must be aware of the cost of nursing services and become more knowledgeable about economics and finance. They need to develop new interventions or methods of care that provide efficient quality care, take advantage of opportunities to play a leading role in the new alternative delivery systems, and assume a greater role in decision making and evaluating client care and nurse performance. Nurses can become entrepreneurs and bid to provide services in the managed care network.

Cost Applied to Nursing Care Delivery

Excessive and inefficient use of goods and services in health care delivery has been viewed by many as the major cause of rising costs in health care delivery. For this reason, in 1978 Congress established the Center for National Health Care Technology and mandated the center to define the safety, **efficiency,** and cost-effectiveness of medical procedures. Nursing is one service in the health care system, and landmark studies released by the center present a strong argument for the cost-effectiveness of nurse practitioners (Leroy and Solkowitz, 1981; *Nurse practitioners*, 1986). Many studies appear in the literature about the cost-effectiveness of nurse practitioners and cost benefit, efficiency, efficacy, and effectiveness of medical procedures and programs; however, data are becoming more available about the cost benefit, efficiency, and effectiveness of nurses generally (*Innovative Approach to Health Care for the Homeless*, 1990; OTA, 1990).

A recent statement issued by the American Nurses Association indicated that nurses should receive third-party reimbursement. The ANA recommended that nursing care should become a separate budget item in all organizations so that cost studies can show the efficiency and effectiveness of the nursing profession. At present, hospitals include nursing care costs in daily patient room charges. Other agencies, such as home health care agencies, include nursing care costs with administrative costs, supplies, and equipment costs. Major efforts have been underway that can be used by nurses to show actual costs of nursing care and their contributions to the system (Grimaldi et al., 1982; McKibbin et al., 1985; Thompson, 1984; *Innovative Approach to Health Care for the Homeless*, 1990).

At present, the United States provides third-party reimbursement for nurses. Medicare and Medicaid have provided *indirect nurse reimbursement* to agencies offering home health care services for a number of years. The Rural Health Clinic Services Act of 1977 provided for indirect reimbursement for the services of nurse practitioners in rural health clinics, with payment going to the clinics for nurses' salaries. In 1978 Maryland was the first state to provide direct reimbursement for nurse practitioners and nurse midwives; Maryland extended the legislation in 1979 to provide direct reimbursement for "any duly licensed health care providers" for services within their lawful scope of practice. Currently, 49 states provide direct reimbursement for nurse practitioner or nurse midwifery services and many others are pursuing reimbursement legislation.

The 1980 and 1989 Medicaid amendments to the Social Security Act provided for *direct reimbursement* of nurse midwives, pediatric nurse practitioners, and family nurse practitioners. The 1989 amendments allow these nurses to provide services without physician supervision. Today, over 100 nurse-managed clinics provide care to select client groups such as the elderly, homeless, and school children. In some states under Medicare and Medicaid nurses can be reimbursed for care given to these populations. Data show that nurses can care for 70% to 80% of all needs of these groups independently (*Innovative Approach to Health Care for the Homeless*, 1990). Beginning in 1990, under Medicare changes, nurse practitioners were allowed indirect reimbursement when, in collaboration with a physician, they provided services to nursing home residents.

In the 1990 Omnibus Budget Reconciliation Act, Medicare amendments included a provision for direct reimbursement of nurse practitioners and clinical nurse specialists, working in collaboration with a physician, for services provided in a rural area. Direct reimbursement may also be obtained under the Federal Employee Health Benefit Plan without physician supervision. All of these changes are moving toward more autonomous practice and are showing recognition of nurses' contributions to health care delivery.

COST-EFFECTIVENESS OF PRIMARY PREVENTION

An area in the health care delivery system that is beginning to show cost-effectiveness is primary prevention. Primary prevention has three major aspects: personal health services, such as immunization against infectious diseases; environmental services, such as adequate water and sewage treatment to prevent parasitic diseases or water fluoridation to prevent dental caries; and health behavior practices, such as non-smoking programs to prevent lung cancer, the use of seat belts to prevent accident fatalities, and good nutrition to prevent obesity and ensuing complications.

Benefits

Estimates indicate that 97% of health care dollars are spent on secondary and tertiary prevention. A growing body of evidence links personal health behaviors to leading causes of illness and death in the United States. For example, smoking results in one out of every six deaths from cancer, coronary artery disease, cerebrovascular disease, and chronic obstructive pulmonary disease. Failure to wear safety belts and driving while intoxicated result in injuries from motor vehicle accidents. Physical inactivity and poor diet are related to atherosclerosis, cancer, diabetes, and osteoporosis. Unsafe sexual practices cause unwanted pregnancy, sexually transmitted diseases, and AIDS (*Healthy People 2000,* 1991).

The principal reasons given for lack of emphasis on prevention in clinical practice and on spending less money for prevention include lack of third-party reimbursement, insufficient time to deal with client behaviors, and skepticism about clinical effectiveness of prevention techniques such as relaxation, exercise, and diet (Fischer, 1989). Preventive services produce dramatic reductions in morbidity and mortality. The major causes of mortality in our adult population have shown major decline since 1970. Several assumptions are made about the causes of the decline in mortality in the past 2 decades. These are improved life-stye, reduction in smoking, better diets, and use of seat belts.

Did You Know?

Infant mortality and life expectancy are indicators of the health of a nation. Although in the United States infant mortality is at a record low and life expectancy is at a record high, they do not indicate a better health care system but improved maternal and paternal health and nutrition and improved life-styles.

Reimbursement

Primary prevention measures could reduce care costs, as well as the risk of early death, disease, disability, and discomfort from disease. Why then have the federal and third-party payers not provided coverage for such measures? The answer is in the following discussion. In addition to the benefit of improved health status of the population, a focus on prevention could mean a reduction in the need for and use of medical, dental, hospital, and health provider services. This would mean that the health care system, the largest employer in the United States, would be reduced in size and become more controlled by the client than by the seller of these services. However, with the increasing costs of health care, consumer demand, and changes in financing mechanisms, there is a new trend toward financing more preventive care services. Today, the third-party payers are beginning to cover preventive services, recognizing that the growth of the health care system can no longer be supported.

Preventive Services

The *goal* of public health is to provide activities to improve and protect the well-being and health of the nation. Preventive community health services include health planning, disease prevention and control, consumer safety, and occupational safety and health. National health priorities are set by the federal government, and financial support through block grants is provided to the 55 state and territorial health agencies and to the over 3000 local health departments. These health departments use funds to provide direct community services, such as public health nursing, home health care, immunizations, venereal disease control, chronic disease screening, and consumer protection.

Resources allocated to public health funding will likely be influenced by the following current issues: the possible increases in communicable disease; an increased awareness of measures to prevent chronic diseases, mental illnesses, suicide, accidents, substance abuse, homicide, and sexually transmitted diseases; and the emphasis of health care reform on prevention. More emphasis on prevention and social issues through public health measures will enhance the health of culturally diverse populations (Miller, 1994).

Federal Recommendations

In 1979 the Surgeon General of the United States published a report entitled *Healthy People.* The report called for a renewed preventive health care commitment through the identification of priorities and specific goals. The central theme of the report was that the health of the nation could be significantly improved through actions taken by individuals and by policymakers to promote a safer, healthier environment for all at home, at work, and at play.

The report suggested that most people could improve their personal health by observing the following practices:
- Elimination of cigarette smoking
- Reduction of alcohol abuse

◆ Moderate dietary changes to reduce intake of excess calories, fat, salt, and sugar
◆ Moderate exercise
◆ Periodic screening for major causes of morbidity and mortality, such as blood pressure and cancer
◆ Adherence to speed laws and usage of seat belts

The report also emphasized the link between physical and mental health and the need to maintain strong family ties, the assistance of supportive friends, and the use of community support systems.

For the policymakers, the report suggested a need to recognize the relationship between health and the physical environment, which could lead to the reduction of morbidity, and mortality caused by air, water, and food contamination; accidents; radiation exposure; excessive noise; occupational hazards; dangerous consumer products; and unsafe highway design.

Subsequently, in 1980 the Secretary of DHHS presented a report, *Promoting Health/Preventing Disease—Objectives for the Nation,* that outlined the national health status and objectives to be attained by the health care system by 1990. The following target areas were identified in the report: control of high blood pressure; pregnancy and infant health; immunization; sexually transmitted diseases; toxic agents; occupational health; flouridation and dental health; surveillance of infectious disease; smoking; misuse of alcohol and drugs; nutrition; physical fitness and exercise; and stress. The objectives of the report were aimed at reducing death rates and related measures of poor health, reducing measurable risks, increasing public and professional awareness of risk and reduction possibilities, and improving services (*Health: United States, 1980,* 1981). Preliminary data indicate progress toward achieving the national goal of reduction of mortality at every life stage (*Prevention, 89/90,* 1990).

In 1990 the Office of Disease Prevention and Health Promotion released the report *Healthy People 2000.* The new national health objectives are designed to build on the 1990 objectives, setting targets to improve health status, reduce risk, and improve services. The priorities of the year 2000 objectives appear in the box. Three overall goals are to be met by the year 2000: (1) increase span of healthy life for Americans, (2) reduce health disparities among Americans, and (3) achieve access to preventive services for all Americans (see Appendix A).

Reducing the burden of avoidable illness and disability will reduce the human and economic costs imposed on the U.S. population. To accomplish the goals of prevention, changes will have to occur in environmental protection, life-styles, and orientation of health providers and institutions toward health promotion. Support is being gained from employers, schools, product designers and manufacturers, food distributors, and the insurance industry for preventing injury and promoting healthier life-styles, thereby reducing the overall economic burden of health care delivery in the United States.

 Priorities of *Healthy People 2000*

Healthy People 2000 is a national public-private initiative led by the U.S. Public Health Service (PHS) to reduce preventable death, disease, and disability by the year 2000. The cornerstone of this initiative, the National Health Promotion and Disease Prevention Objectives, was developed through a 3-year, broad-based effort involving groups and individuals in the health care system, business and industry, voluntary organizations, communities, and federal, state, and local agencies.

The new health objectives, which build on the 1990 objectives established in 1980, set targets to improve Americans' health status, reduce risks, and improve services. Many will challenge the nation to confront such issues as quality of life and health disparities among our citizens. Priorities are emerging in the areas of health promotion, health protection, and preventive services. Special sections also summarize needs related to specific age groups and data collection systems.

PRIORITIES

Health Promotion
Physical activity and fitness
Nutrition
Tobacco
Alcohol and other drugs
Family planning
Mental health
Violent and abusive behavior
Educational and community-based programs

Health Protection
Unintentional injuries
Occupational safety and health
Environmental health
Food and drug safety
Oral health

Surveillance and Data System

Preventive Services
Maternal and infant health
Heart disease and stroke
Cancer
Other chronic and disabling conditions
HIV infection
Sexually transmitted diseases
Immunizations and infectious diseases
Clinical preventive services

Age Related
Healthy babies
Healthy children
Healthy adolescents and youth
Healthy older people

Healthy People 2000: national health promotion and disease prevention objectives, Washington, DC, 1991, USDHHS, Public Health Service.

The Value of Human Life

The concept of *human capital* has evolved in economics as a way of measuring the value society places on the worth of the individual. The value is quantified and expressed in dollar amounts, and it constitutes a

Table 5-12 Years of Potential Life Lost Before Age 65 Yr for Selected Causes of Death: United States, 1980 and 1990 (data based on national vital statistics system)

Cause of death	Years lost per 1000 population under 65 yrs of age	
	1980	1990
All causes	64.2	56.2
Diseases of the heart	8.4	6.3
Cerebrovascular diseases	1.4	1.2
Malignant neoplasms	9.1	8.5
Chronic obstructive pulmonary diseases	0.6	0.6
Pneumonia and influenza	1.0	0.8
Chronic liver disease and cirrhosis	1.5	1.1
Diabetes mellitus	0.6	0.6
Accidents and adverse effects	13.7	9.8
Motor vehicle accidents	8.4	6.1
Suicide	3.1	3.1
Homicide and legal intervention	3.7	3.7
Human immunodeficiency virus infection	—	3.3

From National Center for Health Statistics: *Vital statistics of the United States*, vol II. Mortality, part A, for data years 1970-91, Public Health Service, Washington, DC, US Government Printing Office; data computed by the Division of Analysis from data compiled by the Division of Vital Statistics and from Table I of the Division of Vital Statistics. NOTE: For data years shown, the code numbers for cause of death are based on the International Classification of Diseases, Ninth Revision, described in Appendix II, Table V.

real limit on how much money either people or society will pay for personal health care.

A major goal of the health care delivery system today is to preserve and maximize human capital by offering health-preserving and social practices that result in avoidance of disease (primary prevention) and by offering diagnosis, treatment, and rehabilitation services for existing diseases (secondary and tertiary prevention). The past goal of the health care delivery system has been to emphasize the "sickness system." DHHS health goals suggest that a higher value should be placed on primary prevention. Table 5-12 shows the potential life lost for those who died prematurely from the leading causes of death. Although over 1.4 million years of potential life were lost, the years lost were twice as great for the black male population as for the white.

An example of the costs of life-style–related illness to the health care system can be found by looking at the cost of HIV. In 1993 the cost to the nation was $5.2 billion, whereas alcoholic drug abuse cost $1.8 billion. Costs of lung cancer were $1.5 billion by 1990.

The outcome of health care goals should be the provision of a quality of life that will promote happiness, productivity, efficiency, and the capacity to engage in and enjoy life activities. Quantifying life is meaningless to the person unless the quality of life is good and unless functional days become more valuable than dollars spent. An emphasis on primary prevention may hold the key to reducing dollars spent while increasing the quality of life.

FACTORS AFFECTING HEALTH LEVELS

The goal of health economics is quality care leading to health and wellness of the population. Four major factors are known to affect health levels: personal behavior, environmental factors, human biology, and the health care system.

Society's investment in the *health care system* has been based on this premise: more health services equal better health. The increasing investment society has made in health care delivery is shown in Table 5-1. Although the investment has been a major one, medical services are said to have the least effect on health (McKinlay and McKinlay, 1977; McKeown, 1981; Pickett and Hanlon, 1990).

As first documented in England and Wales in the nineteenth century, health has improved throughout history, resulting in an increased life expectancy for infants and children. The reductions in deaths from the early nineteenth century causes of death—infectious diseases—were attributed to improved nutrition from increased food supplies. Major advances in hygiene and safe food and water contributed to continuing declining death rates after the 1850s. The World Health Organization contends that experience in Third World countries today supports the premise that adequate diet reduces risk of infection, thereby leading to decreased morbidity.

Health problems of the twentieth century are being attributed primarily to *personal behavior* and *environmental* factors. Although these two factors are coming to the forefront as major influences on health, answers to the question of genetic, or human biological, influence on health are still being explored. For instance, risk factors for heart disease and stroke are being related to life-style influences such as smoking, diet, and exercise and to genetic influences such as family history of heart disease, stroke, and hypertension. The federal health goals of the 1990s focus on control of *behavioral influence* thought to be the major determinants of health, such as alcohol and drug abuse, smoking, nutrition, exercise, and stress, and *environmental influences* thought to be the major determinants of illness, such as pollution of air, water, noise, and foods. The goals also address control of and risk reduction from human *biological influences* and the improvement of *health care services*. The remainder of the text will focus on the personal, environmental, and biological influences affecting the nation's health.

Clinical Application

The goal of health economics is to provide maximum benefit to the clients of health care services. Thus the goal of a community health nursing service should be to provide a program that will provide quality of care and meet the needs of the clients served. The amount of money the client, the community, and the agency spend in offering a service is beneficial if the client is satisfied and if there are enough clients in the community to justify the employment of nurses to provide the service.

Connie, a community health nursing student, has identified a caseload of five families in a home health nursing program offered by the local health department. She is interested in *assessing* the costs of care to her clients and to the agency. Connie approaches the appropriate administrator or director of nurses and asks the following questions: how is the agency reimbursed for home care visits and how much does each visit cost? Who pays? Also, she asks if nursing care costs are known. When she finds that the agency is primarily a Medicare-financed agency and that the cost of a home visit is determined by a regional standard of the Health Care Financing Administration, she knows that her families must be eligible for Medicare, unless they have private insurance that will cover home visits or Medicaid eligibility for their children.

When she finds that nursing costs are known, she asks why the visit costs are so high. The administrator shares with Connie that lights, water, nurse supplies, buying cars for the nurses to drive, and secretarial and administrative salaries are a part of the per visit costs. Although Connie's work occurs in the client's home, support services through a central office must be available to help Connie with her work, accounting for the cost of the visit.

Connie then asks about the criteria clients must meet to be able to use the service. She wants to determine for herself if the service is rationed. Connie learns that Medicare, Medicaid, and private insurance limit the services her clients are able to receive. When they reach the limits of the criteria they must seek care through private payments, hospitals, nursing homes, or family support.

The stated goal for offering a service is to provide nursing care in the home to reduce the need for clients to be hospitalized. Unless clients have someone at home to care for them between nurse visits, they may need to go to the hospital or nursing home.

Connie inquires at the local hospital about the room cost per client day. She divides the number of nursing visits by the home health program into the total cost of visits the client received for the year. She then recognizes the differences between the costs of staying at home and staying the same number of days in the hospital. This sample formula provides Connie with some data to compare cost of care per day in the hospital to the cost of care per visit in the home.

In one of her families, the Smiths, the husband has died and the wife can no longer be cared for at home. Connie is informed that the client will need to be admitted to a nursing home for a period of time. In *planning* for the transition from home care to nursing home, Connie contacts social services to consult with the client about the "spend down" process, so the client may be eligible for Medicare and Medicaid coverage of nursing home costs.

As Connie *implements* her nursing care plan for her families, she knows, for the three families covered by Medicare within the limited criteria, all costs of care are paid, except for certain medicines, homemaker services, and some supplies and equipment. For the client going to the nursing home, Connie recognizes that this move will deplete most of her financial assets. Connie talks with the director of nurses about implementing a homemaker/aide service that can be covered by third-party payers to reduce the possibility that others may need nursing home placement.

Connie discharged the second family, after the number of visits covered by private insurance was depleted, and on *evaluation* it was determined that Mr. Jones could be assisted by his wife until he returned to work. She recognized that a safety program in the factory in which Mr. Jones worked could have prevented the back injury he received from a fall. This fall required nursing care and physical therapy as follow-up to hospitalization.

Connie then asked her clients for permission to perform a client or family satisfaction survey. An example of the satisfaction survey Connie used appears in Appendix J. Connie performed the client satisfaction survey and tallied her results as an *evaluation* of the care she had given them. The clients were satisfied with the home health service, and the cost of visits to the clients was lower than that of a hospital day. Connie considered the service appropriate.

NOTE: In this example it is assumed that the care received in one home visit will equal the care needed one hospital day, that hospital nursing care costs are included in the room charge, and that the home nursing visit cost includes other agency charges, such as administrative overhead.

Key Concepts

◆ From 1800 to the 1980s the U.S. health care delivery system experienced three developmental stages, with different emphasis on health care economics. Since 1985, the health care delivery system appears to have entered a fourth developmental stage.

◆ Four basic components provide the framework for health care delivery: labor (work force), facilities, technology, and intensity.

◆ Four major factors have been instrumental in influencing the growth of the health care delivery system: price inflation, technology, intensity, and changes in population demographics.

◆ Health care financing has evolved through the twentieth century from a system financed primarily by the consumer to a system financed primarily by third-party payers.

◆ To solve the problems of rising health care costs, a number of plans for future payments of health care are being considered; all include rationing.

◆ Excessive and inefficient use of goods and services in health care delivery has been viewed as the major cause of rising health care costs.

◆ The concept of human capital has evolved in economics as a way to measure the value society places on the worth of an individual.

◆ The goal of health economics is maximum benefits from services of health providers, leading to health and wellness of the population.

◆ Economics is concerned with use of resources including money to fulfill society's unlimited wants.

◆ Health economics is concerned with the problems of producing services and programs and distributing them to clients.

◆ The goal of public health is providing the most good (works) for the most people.

◆ Nurses need to understand basic economic principles so as not to contribute to rising health care costs.

◆ The GNP is a measure of events in the United States.

◆ The GDP compares events in the United States to other countries.

◆ Microeconomics theory shows how the economic "laws" of supply and demand do not work in the health care system.

◆ Macroeconomic theory helps one to look at national and community issues that affect health care.

◆ Social, economic, and communicable disease epidemics mark the problems of the twenty-first century.

◆ Medicare and Medicaid are two government-funded programs that help to meet the needs of high-risk populations in the United States.

◆ Health care reform focused primarily on health insurance reform will change the way health care is delivered and financed in the twenty-first century.

◆ Eighty-three percent of the U.S. population has health insurance. The 12% uninsured represents 43 million people, mostly elderly persons and children.

◆ Poverty has a detrimental effect on health.

◆ Managed care networks are the way most persons will receive health care in the twenty-first century.

◆ Managed competition will keep costs down.

◆ Health care rationing is now and always has been a part of the health care system.

◆ Nurses are cost-effective providers and must be an integral part of managed care networks.

◆ *Healthy People 2000* is a document that has established U.S. health objectives.

◆ Human life is valued in health economics, like money. An emphasis on changing life-styles and preventive care will reduce the unnecessary years of life lost to early and preventable death.

Critical Thinking Activities

1. Define in your own words the following terms: economics, health economics, gross national product, consumer price index, human capital, gross domestic product.

2. State the goal of health economics and compare to the goal of public health.

3. Review Chapter 6, "Ethics in Community Health Nursing Practice." Debate in the class the ethical implications of the goal of rationing. Focus your debate on the implications for community health nursing practice.

4. Invite a community health nurse administrator to meet with your class or clinical conference group. Ask how inflation, changes in population, and technology have changed the community health care delivery system and community health nursing.

Bibliography

An innovative approach to nursing care of the homeless/very poor, Washington, DC, 1990, TSNI.

Arno P, et al: Economic and policy implications of early intervention in HIV diseases, *JAMA* 262(11):1493, 1989.

Banta HD: Technology assessment in health care. In Kovner A, editor: *Health care delivery in the United States,* New York, 1995a, Springer.

Banta HD: What is health care? In Kovner A, editor: *Health care delivery in the United States,* New York, 1995b, Springer.

Becker E, et al: Refinement and expansion of the Harvard resource-based relative value scale: the second phase, *Am J Pub Health* 80(7):799, 1990.

Blendon R, Donelan K: The public and emerging debate over national health insurance, *N Engl J Med* 323(3): 208, 1990.

Brecher C: The government's role in health care. In Kovner A, editor: *Health care delivery in the United States,* New York, 1995, Springer.

Caplan R: The commodification of American health care, *Soc Sci Med* 28(11): 1139, 1989.

Carney K et al: Hospice costs and medicare reimbursement: an application of break-even analysis, *Nurs Econ* 7(1):41, 1989.

Centers for Disease Control and Prevention: National Center for Infectious Diseases, Division of HIV/AIDS: Atlanta, 1992.

Christenson G, Kiefhaber A: Highlights from the national survey of worksite health promotion activities, *Health Values* 12(2):29, 1988.

Cleland V: *The economics of nursing,* Norwalk, Conn, 1990, Appleton & Lange.

Congress of the United States, Office of Technology Assessment: *Health care in rural America,* Washington, DC, 1990, US Government Printing Office.

Congress of the United States, Office of Technology Assessment: *Medicare's prospective payment system: strategies for evaluating cost, quality, and medical technology,* OTA-H-263, Washington, DC, 1985, US Government Printing Office.

Congress of the United States, Office of Technology Assessment: *Nurse practitioners, physician assistants, and certified nurse midwives: quality, access, cost and payment issues,* Health Program, 1986 (unpublished report).

Cook A: Comparable worth: an economic issue, *Nurs Management* 21(2):28, 1990.

Cummings S, et al: The cost effectiveness of counseling smokers to quit, *JAMA* 261(1):75, 1989.

Curtin L: *Economics and nursing care: nursing practice in the 21st century,* Kansas City, Mo, 1988, American Nurses' Foundation, Inc.

Enthoven A, Kronick R: A consumer choice health plan for the 1990s, *N Engl J Med* 320(1):30, 1989.

Estes C: Privatization, the welfare state, and aging: the Reagan-Bush legacy. In Lee P, Estes C, editors: *The nation's health,* ed 4, Boston, 1994, Jones & Bartlett.

Fischer M, editor: *Guide to clinical preventive services: an assessment of effectiveness of 169 interventions. Report of the United States preventive services task force,* Baltimore, 1989, Williams & Wilkins.

Frank K: Rationally rationing health care: effectiveness research by another name? *Nurs Econ* 7(6):289, 1989.

Gardner M: *Public health nursing,* New York, 1936, MacMillan.

Gillis D: Employers ally with nursing in the war on health care costs, *Nurs Health Care* 9(4):173, 1988.

Ginzberg E: Health care reform—why so slow? *N Engl J Med* 322(20):1464, 1990.

Goldsmith J: National health insurance catches corporate attention, *Modern Healthcare* 89:33, 1989.

Grace H: Can health care costs be contained? *Nurs Health Care* 11(3):125, 1990.

Gram L: Illness gendered poverty among the elderly, *Women's Health* 12(3/4):103, 1988.

Green J, Arno P: AIDS: the cost and financing of care, *Caring* 15, 1989.

Grimaldi P: New Medicare rates for ambulatory surgery, *Nurs Management* 21(4):20, 1990.

Grimaldi P, et al: RIMs and the cost of nursing care, *Nurs Management,* 13, 1982.

Haddon R: The final frontier: nursing in the emerging health-care environment, *Nurs Econ* 7(3):155, 1989.

Haddon R: An economic agenda for health care, *Nurs Health Care* 11(1):21, 1990.

Hahn B: Health care utilization: the effect of extending insurance to adults on Medicaid or uninsured medical care, *J Med Care* 32(3):227-239, 1994.

Hamm-Vida D: Cost of nonnursing tasks, *Nurs Management* 21(4):46, 1990.

Harrington C, Culbertson R: Nurses left out of health care reimbursement reform, *Nurs Outlook* 38(4):156, 1990.

Harris M: The changing scene in community health nursing, *Nurs Clin North Am* 23(3):559, 1988.

Havas S, et al: Report of the New England Task Force on reducing heart disease and stroke risk, *Pub Health Rep* 104(2):134, 1989.

Hawken P, Hillestad A: Promoting nursing's health care agenda through collaboration, *Nurs Health Care* 11(1):17, 1990.

Health care financing administration statistics, Washington, DC, 1989, Bureau of Data Management and Strategy.

Health United States, 1980, USDHHS Pub No (PHS) 81-1232, Hyattsville, Md, 1981, Department of Health and Human Services.

Health: United States, 1985, DHEW Pub No (PHS) 86-1232, Washington, DC, 1985, Department of Health and Human Services.

Health: United States, 1989 and prevention profile, USDHHS Pub No (PHS) 90-1232, Hyattsville, Md, 1990, Department of Health and Human Services.

Health: United States, 1993, DHHS Pub No (PHS) 94-1232, Washington, DC, 1994, U.S. Government Printing Office.

Healthy People: the Surgeon General's report on health promotion and disease prevention, DHEW Pub No (PHS) 79-55071, Washington, DC, 1979, Department of Health, Education, and Welfare.

Healthy People 2000: national health promotion and disease prevention objectives, Washington, DC, 1991, USDHHS, Public Health Service.

Hellinger F: Forecasting the medical care costs of the HIV epidemic, *Inquiry* 28:213-225, 1991.

Higgins C: The economics of health promotion, *Health Values* 12(2):38, 1988.

Hoyer R: Private insurance: where does long-term care fit in? *Caring* 12, 1989.

Huey F: To the president and Congress: nurses know that US citizens can get better access to better health care at affordable costs: are you ready to change the system? *Am J Nurs* 1483, 1988.

Iglehart J: The American health care system: managed care. In Lee P, Estes C, editors: *The nation's health,* ed 4, Boston, 1994, Jones & Bartlett.

Iglehart J: Managed competition. In Lee P, Estes C, editors: *The nation's health,* ed 4, Boston, 1994, Jones & Bartlett.

Ives J, Kerfoot K: Pitfalls and promises of diversification, *Nurs Econ* 7(4):200, 1989.

Jones K: Evolution of the prospective payment system: implications for nursing, *Nurs Econ* 7(6):299, 1989.

Kalish P, Kalish B: *The advance of American nursing,* Boston, 1986, Little Brown & Co.

Kelley M: The omnibus budget reconciliation act of 1987, *Nurs Clin North Am* 24(3):791, 1989.

Kelly L: Nursing's velvet revolution, *Nurs Outlook* 38(1):15, 1990.

Kenkel P: HMO profit outlook begins to brighten, *Modern Healthcare* 28, 1989.

Kenkel P, Morrissey J: Enthoven's proposal: managed-care solution to plight of uninsured, *Modern Healthcare* 28, 1989.

Kenkel P, Morrissey J: Managing to survive: it may come down to size or entrenchment, *Modern Healthcare* 21, 1989.

Kinzer D: Why the conservatives gave us universal health care: a parable, *Health Services Administration* 34(3):299, 1989.

Knickman J, Thorpe K: Financing for health care. In Kovner A, editor: *Health care delivery in the United States,* New York, 1995, Springer.

Korn K et al: The need to reform the long-term care system, *Caring* 42, 1989.

Kovner A: *Health care delivery in the United States,* New York, 1995, Springer.

Lamm R: The brave new world. In Lee P, Estes C, editors: *The nation's health,* ed 4, Boston, 1994, Jones & Bartlett.

Larkin H: Will the public support health care rationing? *Hospitals* 79, 1988.

LaRochelle D: The moral dilemma of rationing nursing resources, *J Prof Nurs* 5(4):173, 1989.

Lawrence R, Mezey A: Ambulatory care. In Kovner A, editor: *Health care delivery in the United States,* New York, 1995, Springer.

Lee P, Solfel D, Luft H: Costs & coverage: pressures toward health care reform. In Lee P, Estes C, editors: *The nation's health,* ed 4, Boston, 1994, Jones & Bartlett.

Lee P, Estes C, editors: *The nation's health,* ed 4, Boston, 1994, Jones & Bartlett.

Leroy L, Solkowitz S: *The implications of cost-effectiveness analysis of medical technology,* Congress of the United States, Office of Technology Assessment, Case Study No 16, Washington, DC, 1981, US Government Printing Office.

Levine M: Ration or rescue: the elderly patient in critical care, *Crit Care Nursing Q* 12(1):82, 1989.

Loucine D, Huckabay R: Identification of issues in determining the cost of nursing services, *Nurs Admin Q* 13(1):72, 1988.

Lyons J: AIDS: what are the costs? Who will pay? *Nurs Econ* 6(5):241, 1988.

Mahoney M, et al: Years of potential life lost among a native American population, *Pub Health Rep* 104(3):279, 1989.

Markus G: Considered approaches to physician payment in the '90s. *Nurs Econ* 6(2):63, 1988.

McCombie S: Politics of immunization in public health, *Soc Sci Med* 28(8):843, 1989.

McGivern D: Teaching nurses the language of the marketplace, *Nurs Health Care* 9(3):127, 1988.

McKeown T: Determinants of health. In Lee P, Brown N, Red I, editors: *The nation's health,* San Francisco, 1981, Boyd & Fraser.

McKibbin R, et al: *DRGs and nursing care,* HCFA grant No 15-C-98421/7-02, Kansas City, Mo, June 1985, Center for Research, American Nurses' Association.

McKinlay JB, McKinlay SM: The questionable contribution of medical measures to the decline of mortality in the United States in the twentieth century, *Milbank Mem Fund Q* 55(3):405-H428, 1977.

McMahon L: A critique of the Harvard resource-based relative value scale, *Am J Pub Health* 80(7):793, 1990.

Melnick G, Mann J: Are Medicaid patients more expensive? A review and analysis, *Med Care Rev* 46(3):229, 1989.

Miller S: Race in the health of America. In Lee P, Estes C, editors: *The nation's health,* ed 4, Boston, 1994, Jones & Bartlett.

Navarro V: Why some countries have national health insurance, others have national health services, and the United States has neither, *Soc Sci Med* 28(9):887, 1989.

Nemes J: Health care stocking up on ESOPS, *Modern Healthcare* 89:24, 1989.

Newhouse J, et al: Are fee-for-service costs increasing faster than HMO costs? *Med Care* 23(8):960, 1985.

Newswatch: Catastrophic legislation provides new dose of SNF, home health, and spouse benefits, *Geriatr Nurs* 260, 1988.

Pallarito K: Managed care reaches for access to capital, *Modern Healthcare* 89:68, 1989.

Pepper C: Long-term care insurance, *Caring* 4, 1989.

Pew Health Professions Commission: *Contemporary issues in health professions, education and workforce reform,* San Francisco, 1993a, UCSF Center for the Health Professions.

Pew Health Professions Commission: *Resource book for health professions, education strategies, planning and policy development,* San Francisco, 1993b, UCSF Center for the Health Professions.

Pfaff M: Differences in health care spending across countries: statistical evidence, *J Health Polit Policy Law* 15(1):1, 1990.

Phillips B: Epidemiological issues in health promotion and cost containment, *Health Values* 12(2):31, 1988.

Phillips E, et al: DRG ripple and the shifting burden of care to home health, *Nurs Health Care* 10(6):324, 1989.

Pickett G, Hanlon J: *Public health administration and practice,* St Louis, 1990, Times Mirror/Mosby College Publishing.

Pillar B, et al: Technology, its assessment, and nursing, *Nurs Outlook* 38(1):16, 1990.

Polich C: Financing long-term care: the role of the federal government, *Caring* 16, 1989.

Popp R: Health care for the poor: where has all the money gone? *J Nurs Admin* 18(1):8, 1988.

Prevention 89/90: federal programs and progress, Washington, DC, 1990, Department of Health and Human Services, US Government Printing Office.

Redman B, et al: Policy perspectives on economic investment in professional nursing education, *Nurs Econ* 8(1):27, 1990.

Reinhardt U: Providing access to health care and controlling costs: the universal dilemma. In Lee P, Estes C, editors: The nation's health, ed 4, Boston, 1994, Jones & Bartlett.

Relman A: Economic incentives in clinical investigation, *N Engl J Med* 320(14):933, 1989.

Rhodes A: EPSDT: the law, *MCN* 17:261, Sept/Oct 1992.

Rice D: The health status and national health priorities. In Lee P, Estes C, editors: *The nation's health,* ed 4, Boston, 1994, Jones & Bartlett.

Richardson H: Long-term care. In Kovner A, editor: *Health care delivery in the United States,* New York, 1995, Springer.

Rodwin V: Comparative health systems. In Kovner A, editor: *Health care delivery in the United States,* New York, 1990, Springer.

Rooks J: Let's admit we ration health care—then set priorities, *Am J Nurs* 90(6):39, 1990.

Rubin R et al: Private long-term care insurance; simulations of a potential market, *Med Care Rev* 27(14):182, 1989.

Safriet B: Health care dollars and regulatory sense: the role of advanced practice nursing, *Yale J Regulation* 9(2):417-497, 1992.

Schell E: Lessons from the Canadian health care system, *Nurs Econ* 7(6):306, 1989.

Scitovsky A, Rice D: Estimates of the direct and indirect costs of acquired immunodeficiency syndrome in the United States, 1985, 1986, and 1991, *Pub Health Rep* 102(1):5, 1987.

Sherfstein S: In Kovner A, editor: *Health care delivery in the U.S.,* New York, 1990, Springer.

Sofaer S, Kenney E: The effect of changes in the financing and organization of health services on health promotion and disease prevention, *Med Care Rev* 46(3):313, 1989.

Smith D: Health promotion for older adults, *Health Values* 12(2):46, 1988.

Theilheimer L: Aging and long-term care: a consumers' view, *Caring* 25, 1989.

Thompson J: The measurement of nursing intensity. In *USDHHS health care financing review: 1984 annual supplement,* Baltimore, 1984, Health Care Financing Administration.

Thorpe K: Health care cost containment. In Kovner A, editor: *Health care delivery in the United States,* New York, 1995, Springer.

Tokarski C: Employees' insurance costs jump 70%, *Modern Healthcare* 89:20, 1989a.

Tokarski C: Health care costs mount an assault on defense department, *Modern Healthcare* 89:28, 1989b.

Tokarski C: Vet group wants health systems of the VA and defense to boost sharing efforts, *Modern Healthcare* 89:19, 1989c.

Ulin P: Global collaboration in primary health care, *Nurs Outlook* 37(3): 134, 1989.

US Department of Health and Human Services: *The registered nurse population, 1992,* Washington, DC, Feb 1994, US Government Printing Office.

US House of Representatives, Select Committee on Aging: Medicare and Medicaid's 25th anniversary—much promised, accomplished, and left unfinished. In Lee P, Estes C, editors: *The nation's health,* ed 4, Boston, 1994, Jones & Bartlett.

Wagner L: AIDS forecast update, *Modern Healthcare* 89:4, 1989a.

Wagner L: HCFA revises rules on home-care claims, *Modern Healthcare* 89:4, 1989b.

Wagner L: Rules on home-care training rapped as vague, expensive, *Modern Healthcare* 89:4, 1989c.

Wagner L: Shift in mortality seen as evidence of PPS efficiency, *Modern Healthcare* 89:4, 1989d.

Warner S: Third-party payments for nurses: untangling the web, *Nurs Health Care* 9(4):181, 1988.

Washington focus: Political trends and health care reform, *Nurs Health Care* 10(4): 178, 1989.

Wedig G: Health status and demand for health, *J Health Econ* 6:151, 1988.

Williams A: Priority setting in public and private health care, *J Health Econ* 6:173, 1988.

Williams S, Torrens P: Managed care: restructuring the system. In *Introduction to health services,* ed 4, Albany, NY, 1993, Delmar Publishers, Inc.

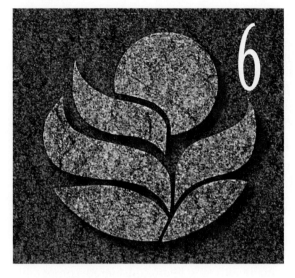

6

Ethics in Community Health Nursing Practice

Sara T. Fry

Objectives ▼

After reading this chapter, the student should be able to do the following:

- ◆ Describe professional responsibilities in community health care.
- ◆ Identify the relationship of ethical rules, principles, and theories in community health nursing decisions.
- ◆ Discuss the application of ethical principles, including their potential conflicts, in community health nursing practice.
- ◆ Apply the concept of accountability to CHN.
- ◆ Discuss client's rights in today's health care system.
- ◆ Develop a community health nursing care plan that takes into account a theory of distributive justice.

Key Terms ▼

advance directives
advocacy
autonomy
beneficence
caring
clients' rights
Code for Nurses
codes of ethics
coercive health measures
confidentiality
egalitarian theory
entitlement theory
ethical decision making
informed consent
justice
maximin theory
moral accountability
Patient's Bill of Rights
principles
public health ethic
right to health
right to health care
rule of utility
rules
theories
utilitarian theory
veracity

Outline ▼

Clients' Rights and Professional Responsibilities in Community
    Health Care
    Clients' Rights
    Societal Obligations
    Professional Responsibilities
Ethical Principles in Community Health
    Relationship of Ethical Rules, Principles, and Theories
    Principle of Beneficence
    Principle of Autonomy
    Principle of Justice
Application of Ethics to Community Health Nursing Practice
    The Priority of Ethical Principles
    Accountability in Community Health Nursing
    Future Directions

Community health nurses experience many ethical conflicts in today's health care delivery system. The nursing profession has traditionally upheld the rights and needs of the individual client. Today, however, this focus is difficult to maintain when nurses have the additional goal of maximizing the health of populations at risk. The traditional focus is also difficult to maintain when nursing resources are influenced by legislation and funding for specific population groups. One result of this latter difficulty is that other populations identified as being at risk are not adequately served by community health nursing efforts because of the lack of funds. Nurses who experience this conflict between the individualistic focus of the professional ethic and the aggregate focus of community health recognize the dilemma of professional nursing in community health settings.

The purpose of this chapter is to analyze traditional ethics of professional nursing and apply these principles to the practice of community health nursing. Since the client is the focus of all nursing actions, clients' rights are discussed first.

Not all nursing actions are simply correlative to clients' rights. General ethical principles, moral rules, and the various theories of social justice also influence health care delivery and nursing services. These principles, their definitions, and applications in community health nursing are presented, and their priority in community health nursing is discussed. Accountability—being answerable to someone for what has been done in the nursing role—is a strong value in nurs-ing, directing the nurse to practice professional skills and expertise in a certain way. Thus the development of methods to measure accountability is also a high priority in community health nursing. It is a priority because community health nursing not only must demonstrate the cost effectiveness of its services in promoting health and preventing illness, but also must show how it meets normal requirements for professional practice. If community health nursing can demonstrate its ability to increase the community's health while meeting requirements for accountability to clients, great gains will be made in the name of community health nursing services.

CLIENTS' RIGHTS AND PROFESSIONAL RESPONSIBILITIES IN COMMUNITY HEALTH CARE

Clients' Rights

One of the earliest recognitions of **clients' rights** concerning health was made by the National Convention of the French Revolution in 1793. Underscoring the theme of basic human rights, the leaders of the revolution declared that there should be only one patient to a bed in hospitals and that hospital beds should be placed at least 3 feet apart (Annas, 1978). This kind of

direction by a legislating body has continued to be prominent in making the rights to health and health care extensions of basic human rights. However, the recognition of other clients' rights, such as rights to informed consent, to refusal of treatment, or to privacy, have apparently been aided by consumer groups and health care providers such as the American Hospital Association (AHA) (Annas, 1978).

Right to Health

A **right to health** has been historically recognized as one of the basic human rights. When introducing the Public Health Act of 1875 to the British Parliament, Prime Minister Disraeli noted that "the health of the people is really the foundation upon which all their happiness and all their powers of state depend" (Brockington, 1956, p. 47). In modern times, the right to health has been considered comparable to the rights of life and liberty. The right to health obligates "the State to prevent individuals from depriving each other of their health" (Szasz, 1976, p. 478).

In the United States, early nineteenth-century public health measures such as sanitation and water supply regulations to control the spread of disease demonstrate early protective laws concerning human health and hygiene. However, most of these measures protected a negative right to health: the right to not have one's health endangered by the actions of others.

Positive obligations to provide services may seemingly "flow from negative rights" (Beauchamp and Faden, 1979, p. 124): The negative right to be free to enjoy good health may lead to the positive right to obtain certain services or community health safeguards. For example, the negative right not to have one's health endangered by others led to public health measures concerning sewage disposal, water supplies, and the regulation of prostitution (Brockington, 1956). This negative right has even led to regulations concerning housing and measures protecting children's health. More recently, it has encouraged some community health advocates to propose broad, federally supported programs and services to protect citizens against preventable diseases and disability (in particular, alcoholism and smoking-related illness) caused, in part, by social conditions (Beauchamp, 1976, 1980, 1985).

Thus, advocacy—in the guise of protecting a negative right to health—has helped open the door to consideration of the right to health as a positive right. It has been aided by documents such as the Universal Declaration of Human Rights of the United Nations Assembly. This document acknowledges the right of all persons to a standard of living adequate to provide for health and well-being and the right "to food, clothing, housing, and medical care" (UNESCO, 1949). Thus, this document suggests that persons have not only a strong negative right to health, but also a strong positive right to health care as well. It suggests that persons are entitled to certain services, programs, and goods to maintain or achieve health as a basic human right.

Right to Health Care

Even though one may think that the "right to health" is an elliptical term for the "right to health care" (Daniels, 1979), the two terms denote different kinds of rights. The right to health is a negative right to a natural human good, which can be of various degrees. It is a right not to have one's health interfered with by others. However, the **right to health care** is a positive right to goods and services to maintain and improve whatever state of health exists. It is a rights claim against the state or its agencies to provide specific health care services. For example, immunization programs, kidney dialysis services, home health services for Medicare and Medicaid recipients, and federally funded prenatal and family planning services all recognize the positive right to specific health care services.

The distinction between the two terms is often blurred for two reasons. First, the World Health Organization (WHO) defines *health* as "a state of complete physical, mental, and social well-being and not merely the absence of disease or infirmity" (Who, 1958). The emphasis on complete physical, mental, and social well-being in this definition suggests that one is unhealthy without complete well-being. However, we know that persons experience varying degrees of health but are not necessarily "unhealthy." Services must be provided to bring about physical, mental, and social well-being for one to possess complete health. Thus, in recognizing a right to health, the right to health care services to achieve *complete* health must also be recognized.

This is obviously a mistake. The WHO definition of health should merely be considered an ideal state of health—one that very few persons actually possess or maintain over a long time. As a definition of an ideal state of health, it has no bearing on the provision of health care services as a right of all persons and should not be construed as a state that must, in fact, exist.

A second reason why the distinction between the terms "right to health" and "right to health care" has become blurred stems from the recent advancements of modern medicine and the willingness of government to subsidize medical treatment for specific disorders such as renal disease (P.L. 92-603, 1972) and some genetic disorders (P.L. 92-278, 1976). This tendency has created an escalation of expectations in terms of services to achieve optimal health. It seems as if government, in recognizing a right of citizens to be as healthy as possible, must necessarily recognize a right of citizens to those services to achieve optimal health. Therefore, by subsidizing treatment of some diseases and genetic disorders,

Requirements of the Patient Self-Determination Act (PSDA)

◆ Provide written information to adult clients about their rights to make medical decisions, including the right to accept or refuse treatment and the right to formulate advance directives.
◆ Document in each client's record whether the client has previously executed an advance directive.
◆ Implement written policies regarding the various types of advance directives.
◆ Ensure compliance with state laws regarding medical treatment decisions and advance directives.
◆ Refrain from discriminating against individuals regarding their treatment decision specified in an advance directive.
◆ Provide education for staff and the community on issues and the law concerning advance directives.

From Omnibus Budget Reconciliation Act of 1990, sections 4206 and 4751, PL 101-508, Nov 5, 1990.

government has created the idea that the right to health means a right to good health, a state that can only be achieved through the provision of specific health care services.

Yet this is clearly wrong. In an analysis of Szasz's position (1976), Bell points out that "the right to health does not entail a right to health care because it does not entail a right to good health (only a right to good health if I already have it)" (Bell, 1979, p. 162). Recognition of the right to health does not mean simply that the state is obligated to initiate health ser-vices to maintain health or improve it. Although there may be other reasons why the differences between the right to health and the right to health care are not clear, these two reasons are certainly pertinent.

Other Rights

The rights to health and health care are not the only basic human rights of clients recognized by the health care delivery system.

The basic human right of all clients to refuse treatment was formally legislated by the Omnibus Budget Reconciliation Act (OBRA) of 1990. The Patient Self-Determination Act (PSDA) became effective Dec. 1, 1991. This act requires all health care institutions receiving Medicare or Medicaid funds to inform clients that they have the right to refuse medical and surgical care. Clients also have the right to initiate a written **advance directive,** that is, a written or oral statement by which competent persons make known treatment preferences and/or designate a surrogate decision-maker in the event they should become unable to make medical decisions on their own behalf.

Home health care agencies and managed care organizations are required to make this information avail-

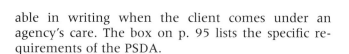

Did You Know?

In 1972 the AHA issued its study entitled *The Patient's Bill of Rights*. Soon, health care facilities began to use this document for health care providers to communicate rights to their clients. The bill affirmed the basic human rights of all clients who seek health care services (AHA, 1973). It included the rights to (1) receive considerate and respectful care, (2) obtain complete medical information, (3) receive information necessary for giving informed consent, (4) refuse treatment, (5) request services, (6) refuse participation in research projects, (7) expect reasonable continuity of care, (8) be informed of institutional regulations, (9) have privacy, (10) have personal information and medical records treated confidentially, (11) be provided with information on other institutions and individuals related to care and treatment, and (12) examine and obtain explanations of financial charges.

Ethical Framework of the President's Commission

The Commission concludes that:

Society has an ethical obligation to ensure equitable access to health care for all.

The societal obligation is balanced by individual obligations.

Equitable access to health care requires that all citizens be able to secure an adequate level of care without excessive burdens.

When equity occurs through the operation of private forces, there is no need for government involvement, but the ultimate responsibility for ensuring that society's obligation is met, through a combination of public and private sector arrangements, rests with the federal government.

The cost of achieving equitable access to health care ought to be shared fairly.

Efforts to contain rising health care costs are important but should not focus on limiting the attainment of equitable access for the least well served portion of the public.

From President's Commission for the Study of Ethical Problems in Medicine and Biomedical and Behavioral Research: *Securing access to health care*, vol 1, Washington, DC, 1983, US Government Printing Office.

able in writing when the client comes under an agency's care. The box on p. 95 lists the specific requirements of the PSDA.

Societal Obligations

The issue of client rights is a problem in health care delivery because society does not articulate its obligations to citizens regarding health. As a result, health care providers fail to recognize and protect clients' basic rights. To correct this problem, health professionals need to ask: What are societal obligations to citizens regarding health? What kind of responsibilities do health care providers have in response to client rights?

Discrepancies in availability of health services according to income or place of residence were reported in a lengthy document entitled *Securing Access to Health Care* (1983) by the President's Commission for the Study of Ethical Problems in Medicine and Biomedical and Behavioral Research. The commission reached several conclusions concerning current patterns of access to health care and made significant recommendations for changes.

The cornerstone of these conclusions is that "society has an ethical obligation to ensure equitable access to health care for all" (President's Commission, 1983, p. 4). Commission members noted that this obligation "rests on the special importance of health care and is derived from its role in relieving suffering, preventing premature death, (and) restoring functioning" (p. 29). Considering these obligations, the commission recommended that costs for health care for those unable to pay ought to be spread equitably at the national level and that costs should not be "allowed to fall more

heavily on the shoulders of residents at different localities" (p. 30). The commission further recommended that the federal government assume ultimate responsibility for ensuring that equitable access to health care for all is achieved "through a combination of public and private sector arrangements" (p. 29). These conclusions and recommendations are summarized in the box above, right.

Professional Responsibilities

In response to clients' rights, health care professionals have particular duties or responsibilities, as illustrated in Figure 6-1. Some of these duties are supported by professional codes of ethics and correlate with the client's basic liberty rights.

Code Duties

Professional **codes of ethics** are statements encompassing rules that apply to persons in professional roles. Two questions generally arise concerning the importance of these codes in health care delivery: (1) What is their relation to universal moral principles? and (2) What is their relation to legal requirements for professional practice? (Beauchamp and Walters, 1978).

In answering the first question, we should consider the rules contained in professional codes of ethics for nurses to be specific applications of more universal moral principles. Some professional codes of ethics are merely statements about professional etiquette or conduct between professional groups and have no relation to external principles. This is not the case in nursing. The professional code of ethics for nurses

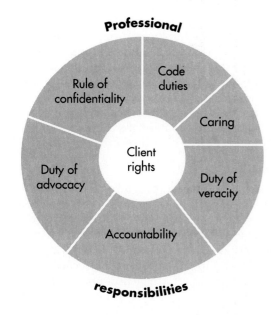

Professional

Rule of confidentiality

Code duties

Caring

Client rights

Duty of veracity

Duty of advocacy

Accountability

responsibilities

FIGURE 6-1

Client rights and professional responsibilities.

prescribes moral behavior and actions based on moral principles (Fry, 1982). Thus the professional nurse has a moral obligation to follow the rules in a code of ethics such as the *Code for Nurses with Interpretive Statements* of the American Nurses Association (ANA) (1985).*

In answering the second question, some of the rules in the **Code for Nurses** have legal ties to licensure requirements concerning professional acts. For example, the rules of respecting client confidentiality and accountability are mentioned in the *Code for Nurses* as both morally obligatory and legally required.

Codes of ethics also prescribe duties that are required of the professional in response to clients' rights (Fry, 1994). The duties of veracity and advocacy are specifically mentioned in the *Code for Nurses* as correlating with clients' rights.

Veracity

Truthfulness has long been regarded as fundamental to the existence of trust among human beings. Persons have a duty of **veracity**—a duty to tell the truth and not lie or deceive others. In health care relationships, several arguments are usually given in support of a duty to tell the truth (Beauchamp and Childress, 1994).

One argument claims that telling the truth and not lying or deceiving is part of the respect we owe other persons. We respect persons because they are self-determining, or autonomous, individuals with all the rights and privileges of autonomous persons. These include the right to be told the truth and not be lied to or deceived. Because we respect persons and their autonomy, we have a duty of veracity. An example is be-

ing truthful to clients regarding the nature of the care they are receiving.

A second argument claims that the duty of veracity is derived from, or is a way of expressing, the duty of keeping promises (Ross, 1930). Communicating with the client creates an implicit contract to tell the truth and not lie or deceive. The contract between client and community health nurse creates the expectation that nurses will, in interacting with the client, speak truthfully.

A third argument claims that relationships of trust are necessary for cooperation between clients and health care professionals. After all, not to tell the truth or to deceive clients will, in the long run, undermine relationships and cause undesirable consequences for future relationships with clients. Thus the community health nurse has a responsibility to maintain truthful relationships with clients to protect and strengthen other health care relationships in general.

However, community health nurses often have difficulty heeding or observing a duty of veracity. The truth is sometimes withheld or filtered because a nurse may think certain information will cause a client anxiety. This tendency is illustrated in a 1975 survey in which more than 15,000 nurses were asked how knowledge of the client's condition should be handled by the nurse: "When a patient who has a terminal illness bluntly asks you if he is dying and his physician does not want him to know, what do you usually do?" Of those surveyed, 1% said that they would tell him; 1% would avoid the question or try to distract him; 1% would reassure him that he was just ill, not dying; 2% would lie, saying they did not know; 14% would tell him that only the physician could answer the question; and the majority (81%) would ask why he brought up the question or would try to get him to talk about his feelings (Popoff, 1975).

Nurses also withhold information because they think that clients, particularly if very sick or dying, do not really want to know the truth about their conditions. However, this belief is not substantiated by surveys of sick and dying clients. In a survey of 100 clients with cancer, 89% preferred knowing their condition; in a survey of 100 clients without cancer, 82% said they preferred knowing; in a survey of 740 clients being diagnosed in a cancer detection center, 98.5% said they wanted to know their condition (Veatch, 1978).

Regardless of the reasons for not telling the truth to clients or withholding information, it is clear that community health professionals have a duty of veracity. As the *Code for Nurses*† notes, "Clients have the moral right . . . to be given accurate information, and all the information necessary for making informed judgments" (ANA, 1985, p. 2). In fact, the duty not to lie or deceive is a stronger moral duty than the duty

---

*Hereafter referred to as Code for Nurses.

†Quotations from *Code for Nurses* reprinted with permission of the ANA.

to disclose information.* The duty of veracity correlates with the client's right to know and includes a strong moral obligation not to lie or deceive.

Confidentiality

In general social interaction, certain information is regarded as confidential. Regarding information as confidential enables us to control the disclosure of personal information and to limit the access of others to sensitive information (Fry, 1984).

In community health care relationships, **confidentiality** of information is maintained for several reasons. First, if health care professionals did not follow a rule of confidentiality, clients might not seek help when they needed it. They would not reveal necessary information that would facilitate treatment. For example, family planning clients might not reveal information about their reproductive history that would facilitate appropriate and safe nursing care and follow-up treatment. Maintaining confidentiality helps protect the functioning of nurse-client relationships.

A second reason for maintaining confidentiality is that privacy is recognized as a basic human right. Because persons are self-determining moral agents, they have a right to determine how personal information, especially health information, is communicated. As the *Code for Nurses* points out, "The nurse safeguards the client's right to privacy by judiciously protecting information of a confidential nature" (ANA, 1985, p. 4). Because of respect for persons, nurses respect clients' rights to privacy by maintaining the moral rule of confidentiality.

In health care relationships, however, the duty to observe the rule of confidentiality is not always absolute. It is merely a *prima facie* duty; that is, it may be overridden when in conflict with other duties that are morally stronger. The duty to observe confidentiality may be overridden for several reasons:

1. *When in conflict with other duties toward the client.* For example, the duty to preserve life may outweigh the duty to respect confidential information concerning self-destructive wishes of the client.
2. *When in conflict with duties toward identified others.* For example, if a mental health client tells the nurse of intent to harm or kill another member of the community, the nurse's duty to protect others by warning the intended victim will override the duty of confidentiality. This action may even be required by law (Tarasoff, 1976).
3. *When in conflict with duties toward unidentified others or the rights and interests of society in general.* For example, the law requires communicable diseases such as tuberculosis or venereal disease to be reported regardless of the confidential nature of that infor-

mation. Another example includes health records used for epidemiological research without the client's knowledge. Of course, stringent constraints are placed on the use of this information by epidemiologists in health research (Gordis and Gold, 1980; Kelsey, 1981). In general, however, the duty to increase or protect the health of the community through research outweighs the duty to respect the confidentiality of health records.

Advocacy

The nursing profession recognizes a strong duty of **advocacy** where the care or safety of clients is concerned. As the *Code of Nurses* states, ". . . the nurse must be alert to and take appropriate action regarding any instances of incompetent, unethical, or illegal practice by any member of the health care team or the health care system, or any action on the part of others that places the rights or best interests of the client in jeopardy" (ANA, 1976, 1985, p. 6). In the role of advocate, the nurse speaks for or in support of the best interests of the individual client or vulnerable client populations.

The role of advocate can be difficult for the community health nurse. First, clients should always determine what is in their best interests. Doing what the nurse thinks is in the best interests of clients can lead to paternalism when the wishes of clients are never ascertained.

Second, the duty of advocacy extends to populations at risk, which may bring the community health nurse into conflict with health policy or established professional practices within a community or institution. Nurse advocates who have experienced this kind of conflict have sometimes found their jobs and other professional relationships in jeopardy (Smith, 1980). Positions of advocacy can be difficult to maintain when they conflict with accepted professional practices.

Third, does the duty of advocacy require community health nurses to put their own job, health, or professional standing at risk on behalf of advocacy for the client? According to Beauchamp and Childress (1994), this is not a moral requirement of the principle of beneficence. The nurse must fulfill the primary commitment to client care and safety by protecting the client from harm. The implicit contract of the nurse-client relationship does, in general, require positive acts of benefiting from care rendered. However, strictly speaking, this contract does not extend to the role of advocate. Thus, the community health nurse is only required, in the role of advocate, to protect, speak for, and support the interests of the client *not* to be harmed in the provision of health care services.

Caring

The value of **caring** is widely recognized as important to the nurse-client relationship (Fry, 1988). Caring behavior is expected of the nurse and is generally considered fundamental to the nursing role. Leininger (1984), for example, argues that caring has a direct re-

---

*The duty to disclose information evolves from special relationships between agents. In such relationships, one agent can claim a right to information that the other agent would not be obligated to provide to a stranger. The duty not to lie, however, does not depend on special relationships. Lying threatens any relationship because lying is telling something false to deceive a person.

lationship to human health. Her research demonstrates that all cultures and communities practice caring behaviors that reduce intercultural stresses and conflicts and protect human survival.

Recent feminist interpretations of human caring relate it to ethical behaviors and choices. Noddings (1984) states that "... to care may mean to be charged with the protection, welfare, or maintenance of something or someone" (p. 9). Nurse caring is specifically directed toward the protection of the health and welfare of clients in the community. When caring is valued as important to the nursing role, it indicates a commitment toward the protection of human dignity and the preservation of human health as well.

Pellegrino (1985) also characterizes caring as a moral obligation or duty among health professionals. He believes that one is obligated to promote the good of another with whom a special relationship exists. Since nurses have special relationships with their clients, they are called on and expected to provide caring behaviors to those who have health needs. Caring is a form of involvement with others that is directly related to concern about how other individuals experience their world (Benner and Wrubel, 1989). Caring is therefore always practiced within some context, and its significance is interpreted in terms of the special duties or obligations between individuals within that context (Fry, 1994).

Accountability

The need within the nursing practice for **moral accountability** in response to basic human rights has long been recognized. Even Florence Nightingale reputedly made strong objections to the overriding of a person's will for the benefit of others in the performance of nursing care (Palmer, 1977).

Even as nurses promote progress in health care delivery, they must simultaneously protect the rights of the individual (Gortner, 1974). In the *Code for Nurses,* accountability is defined as "being answerable to someone for something one has done" (ANA, 1985, p. 8). Accountability includes providing an explanation to one's self, the client, the employing agency, and the nursing profession for what one has done in the role of nurse. It is an obligation that has both moral and legal components and implies a contractual agreement between two parties. When a community health nurse enters into a contractual agreement to perform a service for a client, the nurse will be held answerable for performing this service according to agreed-on terms, within an established time period, and with stipulated use of resources and performance standards. The nurse as contractor is responsible for the quality of the services rendered and is accountable to the individual client, the health service agency, the nursing profession, and even his or her own conscience for what has been done (Fry, 1983a).

The moral obligation of accountability corresponds to the client's right to an accepted level of competent nursing care and the right to self-determination in health care. As a moral obligation, accountability directs the professional to act in a particular way according to moral norms (Fry, 1981, 1986b).

In nursing, and especially in community health nursing, accountability appears to be what defines the kinds of relationships among client, nurse, other professionals, and the public at large that form the moral foundations of the professional ethic (Fry, 1994). Furthermore, since accountability correlates to clients' rights to competent levels of nursing care, it is responsive to the humanistic traditions that permeate nursing's history. Accountability enables the nurse to achieve the protection of the client's human dignity and right to self-determination in health matters.

 Research Brief

Duncan SM: Ethical challenge in community health nursing, J *Adv Nurs* 17:1035-1041, 1992.

Community health nurses frequently face situations involving ethical conflicts. In a descriptive study of 30 practicing community health nurses, Duncan (1992) found that typical ethical conflicts often involved clients' rights, nurse interactions with colleagues and the system, and nurses' rights.

The most disturbing ethical conflicts, however, involved high-risk parenting situations. High-risk parenting was defined as any situation in which the health and safety of parents and children were at risk or there were problems with some aspects of parenting. Because community health nurses had contact with the families in their homes, they were usually the first persons to recognize the degree of risk and the need for preventive care or child-protective interventions.

These situations were ethically troubling because the signs of inadequate parenting and safety risks to children were often unclear or unprovable. Therefore, nurses had difficulty determining the focus of their care: the health of the child or the long-term health of the family. They also found that these situations often involve a delicate balancing of children's and parents' rights. The community health nurses identified a great need to develop their knowledge of and skills for working with high-risk families and for using ethical decision-making strategies.

Duncan's research is important because it describes ethical conflicts in community health nursing practice and the ethics education and skill development needs as perceived by practicing nurses.

ETHICAL PRINCIPLES IN COMMUNITY HEALTH
Relationship of Ethical Rules, Principles, and Theories

In making moral decisions, we usually appeal to various rules, principles, or theories (Figure 6-2). **Rules** state that certain actions should (or should not) be

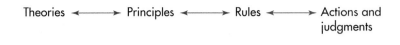

FIGURE 6-2

The relationship of ethical theories, principles, and rules.

performed because they are right (or wrong). An example would be that "nurses ought to always tell the truth to clients." **Principles** are more abstract than rules and serve as the foundation of rules. For example, the ethical principle of autonomy is the foundation for such rules as "Always support the right to informed consent," "Tell the truth," and "Protect the privacy of the client." Likewise, the principle of justice serves as the foundation of rules such as "Treat equals equally" and "Divide your time on the basis of needs." **Theories,** however, are collections of principles and rules. They provide theoretical foundations for deciding what to do when principles or rules conflict. Examples of a few major theories are *utilitarianism, deontologism,* and *natural law.*

Within theories, the various moral rules and principles are arranged according to their importance or justifiability. For example, in utilitarianism the principle of beneficence often carries more weight than the ethical principles of autonomy or justice.

However, ethical principles are not absolute. Each ethical principle is always morally significant but may not always prevail when in conflict with other principles. Ethical theories simply suggest which ethical principles will more likely prevail when moral decisions have to be made.

But what makes some judgments moral and others nonmoral? Moral judgments are evaluations of what is good or bad, right or wrong and have certain characteristics that separate them from nonmoral evaluations such as personal preferences, beliefs, or matters of taste. The difference between the evaluations lies in the reasons for or the characteristics of the judgments themselves (Frankena, 1973). Moral judgments are generally made concerning human actions, institutions, or character traits.

Community health nurses frequently make moral judgments. When the nurse decides to arrange a home visiting schedule on the basis of need or seriousness of illness, a moral judgment is made. When the nurse decides to refer a client to a physician for further evaluation based on the expressed wishes of the client and his or her condition, a moral judgment is made. When in response to a request for an abortion a nurse decides, regardless of personal beliefs, to inform the client of all the options available, a moral judgment is made. When a nurse, resisting pressure from other individuals, decides not to participate in political activities that might lessen health care coverage for vulnerable populations, a moral judgment is made.

Principle of Beneficence

Definition

The principle of **beneficence** is that "we ought to do good and prevent or avoid doing harm" (Frankena, 1973, p. 45). Beneficence is a duty to help others gain what is of benefit to them but does not carry the obligation to risk one's own welfare or interests in helping others. Some theorists maintain that beneficence does not morally require us to always benefit others even when we can do so. Rather, we are only morally required to prevent harm, which may be true in general social interactions among persons. However, the implicit contract underlying the nature of the nurse-client relationship seems to indicate that positive benefiting or acts of beneficence should take place.

The need for health care forms the basis of the relationship between community health nurse and client and imposes a moral duty on the nurse to benefit the client through nursing actions. However, there may be limits on the amount of beneficial nursing care a client should expect. Certainly nurses should not be expected to provide nursing care to individual clients or client populations if they are putting themselves at risk. Care also should not be expected if clients' needs infringe either on nurses' personal lives or on their responsibilities to other clients or their own families. Although the duty to prevent harm to clients is a stringent one, the claim to positive benefiting is limited.

Applications in Community Health

In community health nursing, the principle of beneficence can be applied in (1) balancing harms and benefits to client populations and (2) the use of cost-benefit analyses in decisions affecting client populations.

Balancing Harms and Benefits. Service that brings about the greatest balance of good over evil, or benefit over harm, is in accordance with a **rule of utility.** This rule is derived from the principle of beneficence and includes a moral duty to weigh and balance benefits against harms to increase benefits and reduce the occurrence of harms (Beauchamp and Childress, 1994).

In community health a rule of utility may be the basis for deciding whether to fund certain health programs more than others, conduct screening programs for communicable diseases, or conduct research projects in which individual rights to privacy may be concerned. In each example, the decision is made by balancing the possible harms and benefits of several alternative courses of action. The community health nurse should accurately assess the known benefits and harms to clients from the point of view of nursing care and should present them with other relevant facts that might enter into the decision-making process.

Cost-Benefit Analysis. Cost-benefit analysis is a specific application of the principle of beneficence. It measures the harms and benefits of various health programs while also figuring the costs of potential trade-offs in certain courses of actions. Examples of factors taken into consideration include lives saved, costs averted, taxes saved, and illness prevented. All these are eventually converted into one common unit, usually money, to measure the benefits and costs of alternative approaches to a problem or to decide how to distribute health program funds.

Problems and Conflicts

Decision making in community health settings on the basis of a principle of beneficence and of weighing harms and benefits raises moral questions concerning (1) paternalism in health care decisions and (2) the extent of the rule of utility in decision making.

Paternalism. Paternalism is a liberty-limiting principle that is frequently invoked to override people's actions or expressed wishes for their own good or best interests. Parents may override a child's desire to play with the interesting knobs on a stove because they do not want the child to get burned. Community health nurses may override clients' expressed wishes "not to hear any bad news" by telling them the results of laboratory testing so that their health status can be treated and improved. Nurses do this because they feel it is in clients' best interests to know the status of their health.

It is morally justified to restrict a person's liberty when not doing so could cause possibly life-threatening physical harm. However, it is more difficult to justify paternalistic actions for perceived psychological harms. For example, it might seem morally justified to override a teenager's desire to participate in a research project that poses a potential health risk. However, it is not morally justifiable to withhold information of a defective fetus from a woman who is 6 months' pregnant because it might cause her psychological harm and grief during the remaining months of pregnancy.

It is also difficult to justify paternalistic actions for benefiting the person whose liberty is restricted. For example, it is difficult to morally justify forcibly giving medication to a mental health client who has refused chemotherapy simply because the medication will benefit him by reducing this paranoia or irrational fears. However, health care practitioners often carry out paternalistic actions. Are there some acts of paternalism that are morally justified, and if so, what are the criteria for justified paternalism in community health decisions?

Since paternalism always violates the moral principle of autonomy and the moral rule to treat persons as self-determining moral agents, justified paternalism is a very limited area. According to Gert and Culver (1979), paternalism is justified only if (1) the evils that would be prevented are much greater than the evils, if any, that would be caused by the violation of the moral rule and (2) we would be willing to universally allow the violation of the moral rule in these same circumstances and be able to publicly advocate this kind of violation. Thus, justified paternalism seems to be limited to those acts that prevent persons from committing some grave bodily harm to themselves— self-mutilating or self-destructing behaviors and acts committed out of ignorance, such as unknowingly ingesting harmful substances. Beyond these and similar acts, it is difficult to justify paternalism in community health.

Extent of the Rule of Utility. Attempting to bring about the greatest possible balance of benefit over harm in community health may lead to two problems. The first is the potential overriding of individual liberties and values for the common good (Fry, 1985). For example, in calculating the benefits of a health policy in terms of tax savings and other economic benefits, the health needs of individual citizens may be overlooked or simply not deemed as important. Human needs and wants that cannot be easily or accurately converted into monetary units may simply be left out in deciding on the greatest amount of overall benefit. As MacIntyre (1979) pointed out, cost-benefit analysis in particular cannot truly represent the value choices of individuals. Thus, policy decisions based on the rule of utility as expressed in cost-benefit analysis may be inaccurate and irrelevant to the health needs of individuals.

A second problem arises when the rule of utility is applied in health policy decisions having long-term effects. For example, it is often unclear how short-term harms and benefits ought to be weighed against long-term consequences in cost-benefit analysis. If the benefits and harms to individual health or economic savings in the future are judged more important than present savings or health conditions, individual and collective interests in health may be sacrificed for future benefits.

Principle of Autonomy
Definition

Autonomy refers to freedom of action that an individual chooses. Persons who are autonomous are capable of choosing and acting on plans they themselves have selected.

To respect persons as autonomous individuals is to acknowledge their personal rights to make choices and act accordingly (Fry, 1994). They are respected as self-determining moral agents or persons. Thus, when nurses respect persons as moral agents, they are acting in accordance with the requirements of the moral principle of autonomy.

Applications in Community Health

The principle of autonomy is applied in community health through (1) respect for persons; (2) protection of privacy; (3) provision of informed consent; (4) freedom of choice, including treatment refusal; and (5) protection of diminished autonomy.

Respect for Persons. In community health, clients are respected because they are persons and have the right to determine their own plan of life. Community health nurses acknowledge respect by seriously considering the opinions and choices of clients and not obstructing their actions unless they are harmful to themselves or others. Denying clients freedom to act on their own judgments or withholding information necessary to make judgments demonstrates a lack of respect for clients.

Elderly clients provide an example. Community health nurses often find it easier and quicker to communicate with family members than with the clients themselves. They may simply tell the client what treatment has to be performed, not giving them choices or even involving them in deciding on the treatment plan. Age, however, does not render a client less worthy of our respect (Figure 6-3). Elderly persons have the right to determine their life and health plans insofar as they have the capacity to do so. To deny them the opportunity to choose according to their capacities demonstrates a lack of respect for persons and is an infringement of the principle of autonomy.

Protection of Privacy. Community health nursing care involves close observation of clients, physical touching, and access to personal health and economic information about clients and their families. All these aspects of nursing care may invade the privacy of clients or threaten their right to control personal information.

Since the relationship between nurse and client is built on trust, the nurse has a responsibility to protect the privacy of clients and their families insofar as their health is concerned. Personal information gathered in the home assessment of clients must be recorded in a manner that acknowledges respect for clients' privacy and is communicated only to those directly concerned with client care.

When personal economic information must be shared with third parties for payment of nursing care, clients have the right to authorize or withhold disclosure of information. Even though the information may be essential for continuity of nursing care services, the client retains control of all information.

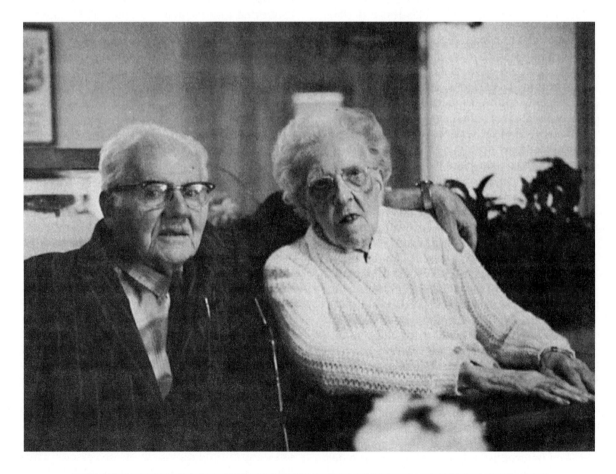

FIGURE 6-3
Age does not render clients less worthy of our respect.

When clients' records are examined for quality assurance purposes, or when notes about home or clinic visits are included in research studies, the protection of privacy may be a genuine problem. Using health records in determining funding levels for community health nursing services does not justify using nurse-generated information about the client without the client's knowledge and permission. Health record information can only be used for quality assurance purposes or research studies. This information can be shared with others only under clearly defined policies and written guidelines protecting client privacy. Community health nursing services are also responsible for making sure that policies and guidelines appropriately protect client privacy. These services must ensure that clients are informed of this protection *before* their personal information is released to any source. Only then can an agency meet the requirements of the ethical principle of autonomy.

Provision of Informed Consent. The principle of autonomy requires that clients be given "the opportunity to choose what shall or shall not happen to them" (National Commission, 1978, p. 10). Clients are provided this opportunity when adequate disclosure standards for **informed consent** are included in the contract for community health nursing services. Three elements are essential for adequate informed consent: information, comprehension, and voluntariness.

1. *Information.* The nurse must disclose information about treatment procedures, their purposes, any discomforts and anticipated benefits, alternative procedures for therapy, and options for questioning procedures or ending the contract at any time. Clients should also be adequately informed about how confidentiality of their health records will be maintained.

2. *Comprehension.* The manner and context in which information is conveyed to clients is also important for informed consent requirements. Clients must be allowed time to consider information provided by the community health nurse, as well as time to ask questions. If the client is unable to comprehend because of a language barrier, the nurse must provide an interpreter. The client must be competent to understand and make decisions rationally. Competent clients can understand a treatment procedure or proposed care plan, weigh its discomforts and benefits, and then make decisions about undertaking the procedure or plan.

3. *Voluntariness.* Any contract or agreement with the client constitutes valid consent only if it is given voluntarily and is free of coercion or undue influences. Voluntariness includes the freedom to choose one's own health goals without the controlling influence of another person or certain conditions, such as debilitating disease, psychiatric disorders, and drug addictions (Beauchamp and Childress, 1994). Again, the principle of autonomy is the main ethical principle guiding this provision.

These three elements—information, comprehension, and voluntariness—constitute informed consent in community health nursing practice. Informed consent is not valid without all elements, and no contract between client and nurse is ethically acceptable without valid informed consent.

Individual Freedom of Choice. Respecting the client's right to self-determination includes respecting a decision to refuse treatment. Factors the nurse must weigh include the client's personal freedom, the potential harm to the client or other citizens, the cost of treatment refusal, and the values of society (Capron, 1978). As long as a client is judged competent to make this kind of decision, however, it is difficult to infringe on autonomy by not allowing treatment refusal. The right of the patient to refuse treatment and the right to initiate written advance directives are protected by the Patient Self-Determination Act (1990).

Some of the most interesting and difficult legal cases involving treatment refusal have involved the exercise of religious beliefs (*In re estate of Brooks,* 1965). Others have involved the autonomy of the teenage minor to refuse lifesaving treatment such as kidney dialysis (Veatch, 1976). More recent cases affecting the values of entire communities have involved the right of parents to refuse lifesaving treatment for their defective newborns (Lyons, 1985; Will, 1982) and the right of the terminally ill to refuse life-sustaining food and water (Annas, 1985; Fry, 1986b; Lynn and Childress, 1983).

In community health nursing, respect for the client's or guardian's right to refuse treatment may hinge on the nurse's judgment of the client's decision-making ability. The physical competency of the elderly or severely ill client, the psychological competency of former mental clients, and the maturity or legal competency of minors may, in part, rely on the assessment of client abilities by the community health nurse. In some situations the nurse may need to assess whether an advance directive is an accurate statement of what the client wants, whether a client has fully taken into account the consequences of a treatment decision before completing an advance directive, and whether a surrogate decision maker is inappropriately making decisions for a client with intact decision-making capacity (Mezey et al., 1994).

In situations of questionable competency, decisions have generally opted for the preservation of life (Beauchamp and Childress, 1994). In situations in which competency to make decisions has been established, other factors such as obligations to others (e.g., dependent children) may determine whether autonomy of choice will be respected. No hard-and-fast rule on treatment refusal can be made. Yet community health nurses should recognize that respect for persons may involve allowing clients and their legal guardians to make decisions concerning their lives and health that may be very difficult for the nurses to accept.

Protection of Diminished Autonomy. The principle of autonomy is generally applied only to persons capable of autonomous choice. Factors such as immaturity or physical or psychological incapacities may diminish one's autonomy. In such cases, it is sometimes considered justifiable to interfere with the actions of these individuals to protect them from harmful results of their choices and actions. This interference, however, requires appeals to other principles, such as beneficence.

The community health nurse may have difficulty recognizing when diminished capacities render clients incapable of self-determination. The capacity for self-determination is relative to maturity, chronological age, the presence or absence of illness, mental disability, or social factors. However, respect for the principle of autonomy requires that practitioners recognize when persons lack the capacity to act autonomously and therefore are entitled to protection in health care delivery (Figure 6-4).

Problems and Conflicts

Respecting the ethical principle of autonomy can be difficult in community health nursing practice. Those areas creating the most conflict for nurses have included (1) carrying out **coercive health measures** and (2) invasions of privacy for health reasons.

Coercive Health Measures. Clients consulting a community health agency may have a communicable disease that not only is harmful to themselves if untreated but also may affect the health of family members, neighbors, or co-workers. The client may not want to receive treatment and may even refuse to take medications or attend follow-up care recommended for the illness. For example, many areas of the United States still require clients diagnosed with active tuberculosis to be confined until their disease is no longer considered active or communicable to others. Clients have no choice in the matter. They must be admitted and must take treatment, regardless of their own wishes, choices, or life plans.

The community health nurse may be the one to enforce these regulations or be the agent to override a client's expressed wishes in this matter. Thus, nurses may find themselves forced to choose between individual rights to self-determination in health matters and the protection of the community's health.

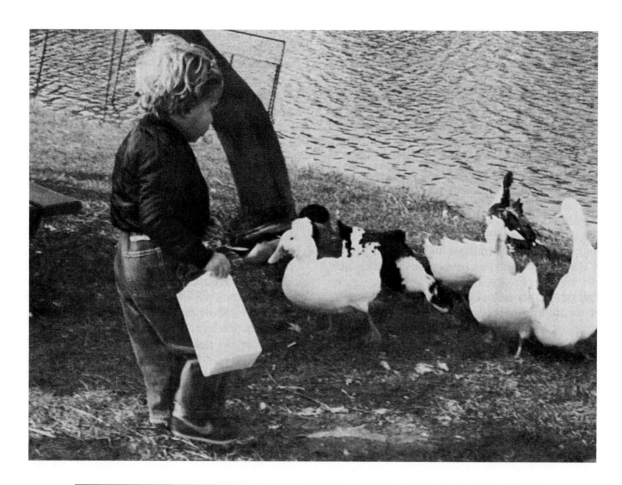

FIGURE 6-4

Children have diminished autonomy and are entitled to protection in health care delivery.

Invasions of Privacy. In protecting the health of vulnerable populations, the community health nurse may infringe on rights to privacy by actively gathering private information. For example, a sharp rise in the incidence of venereal disease among a high-school population may require interviewing teenagers diagnosed with the disease and accurately following up with all named contacts. This action may lead to invasions of individual privacy through discussion of sexual habits and preferences and potential disclosures to adults, including parents.

All these actions infringe on self-determining behavior but are considered justifiable because of potential harm to others. Nonetheless, it is the nurse's responsibility to inform those whose privacy is invaded that information will be recorded and communicated in a way that does not infringe on their future privacy.

Privacy may also be invaded by the assessment and recording of personal client information. For example, the community health nurse may record information about the social habits and life-styles of pregnant women. Subsequently, that information may be used in research studies correlating neonatal mortality and morbidity with social habits during pregnancy. This type of personal information is often freely communicated because of the trust relationship between nurse and client. It may also be recorded in the client's record without full understanding of the potential impact of this information if, in fact, a child is born with anomalies related to social habits or life-styles during pregnancy. The presence of this information in prenatal records means that it might eventually be shared with other health professionals and members of the client's family, constituting further invasions of the client's right to privacy of personal information.

In community health, these invasions of privacy may be justified because they prevent harm to innocent third parties. However, communicating this information while remaining sensitive to the client's right to privacy may create conflicts of interest for the nurse.

Principles of Justice

Definition

The formal principle of **justice** holds that equals should be treated equally and that those who are unequal should be treated differently according to their differences (Beauchamp and Childress, 1994). In considerations of a community's health, we appeal to material principles of justice (i.e., need, merit, contributions to society) to determine which social burdens and benefits, including health goods, should be distributed among all individuals in the community.

Applications in Community Health

Different theories of justice may be considered in deciding how to distribute health care resources. These theories include the (1) entitlement theory, (2) utilitarian theory, (3) maximin theory, and (4) egalitarian theory. Each theory has its advantages and disadvantages in distributing health goods in the community.

Entitlement Theory. The **entitlement theory** claims that everyone is entitled to whatever they get in the natural lottery at birth. The theory assigns no responsibility to government or its agencies to improve the lot of those less fortunate than others. If people are healthy and rich and have been able to acquire possessions by purchase, gift, or legitimate exchange, they are entitled to what they have. They may also increase their possessions in any way possible, as long as they do not cheat others (Nozick, 1974).

It is unfortunate that some people are mentally or physically disabled, but others have no obligation to give money to those with disabilities to make their lives more comfortable. Aiding the unfortunate is simply an act of charity of community members.

In this theory, inequalities between individuals in health, position, and wealth are tolerated. Only aggression or harm against others and the unjust acquisition of goods are prohibited. Thus the actual distribution of goods seems more in line with a principle of autonomy of right to liberty than a principle of justice (Veatch, 1981).

Utilitarian Theory. The **utilitarian theory** of justice holds that the best way to distribute resources among citizens is to decide how expending or using resources will achieve the greatest good and serve the largest number of people (Mill, 1957). In times of limited resources, when all that is needed or wanted cannot be provided in the community, this method of distribution is appealing. Although it does tend to overlook the needs and wants of individuals, it manages to maximize net benefits over costs and serves the greatest number of people.

In this theory the needs and wants of some individuals will not be satisfied, and they may, indeed, be harmed in the process. This is unfortunate. Still, by distributing limited resources so that "the greatest good for the greatest number" is achieved, government and its agencies would fulfill their obligations to citizens. It is easy to see that the principle of beneficence dominates other considerations in utilitarianism. Justice is served by benefiting the greatest number at the least cost.

Maximin Theory. The **maximin* theory** of justice first identifies the least advantaged members of the community and decides how they might be benefited rather than deciding on greatest net aggregate benefit. It then permits free exercise of liberty by all citizens. At the same time, it allows social and economic inequalities to evolve so that these inequalities benefit the least advantaged or least well-off members of society (Rawls, 1971). Many kinds of inequalities in

---

*Maximin is an abbreviation for "maximizing the minimum position in society."

health, health care resources, and possession of economic benefits will be tolerated and considered, just as long as the position of the least advantaged is improved or benefited. For example, health professionals can charge high fees or receive substantial salaries as long as they also serve the interests of disadvantaged persons. In a similar manner costly health care resources such as kidney dialysis, magnetic resonance imaging (MRI) scans, and artificial hearts can be developed and purchased by those who can afford them, as long as the lot of the least advantaged persons is also improved in the process.

Obviously, distributing health goods according to this theory will create problems in times of limited resources. Providing benefit first to the least advantaged persons is a constraint on the expansion of health care resources and technological advancement. Thus, it is possible that technological advancement and the development of more sophisticated health care goods cannot be made widely available to the public in times of limited economic resources. The result is that interests and needs in matters of health may not be satisfied within this system of justice.

Egalitarian Theory. The **egalitarian theory** of justice holds that justice requires the "equality of net welfare for individuals" (Veatch, 1981, p. 265). In this theory the distribution of goods in the community takes the needs of all citizens into account equally. Thus, everyone would have a claim to an equal amount of all goods and resources, including health care.

Clearly, this is a goal that cannot be achieved. It would be virtually impossible for any system of justice to guarantee equality of goods and resources for everyone, let alone equal health care. At least with respect to health care, the egalitarian theory must be amended. Instead of health care being a good that everyone should have in equal amounts, basic health care should be viewed as a good to which all should have equal access. Everyone should have equal access to those basic health goods and resources to improve their health according to need (Green, 1976; Veatch, 1981).

This system respects the autonomy of individuals to seek the health services they need or want and gives equal consideration to the positive benefiting of individuals in improved health. Most important, it is just because it follows the dictates of a principle of justice while, at the same time, not limiting the liberty of anyone in terms of basic health needs. It treats equals equally and unequals unequally and provides a just manner for the distribution of health resources in the community.

Problems and Conflicts

The application of a principle of justice in community health nursing creates conflicts in two areas. First, it generates considerable challenges about establishing priorities for the distribution of basic goods and health services in the community. Second, it creates conflicts in determining which population or individuals shall obtain available health goods and nursing services.

Distributing Basic Goods and Services. In deciding how to distribute basic health care assets or resources within a community, the first decision is to set the priorities. Should the protection and promotion of health be the main consideration? Or should a major portion of resources be set aside for other social goods, such as housing or education? If community leaders agree that everyone has a right to equal access to basic health care according to need and that this right must be satisfied for justice to be served, then enough community assets and financial resources will be allotted to meet the requirements of this basic right (Milio, 1975).

A second decision concerns the most effective and efficient methods of meeting this basic right while preventing catastrophic events needing immediate and more concentrated attention. Such events may lead to death or disability. Should the emphasis be placed on direct health care services (e.g., clinics, programs) to care for illness, or should indirect services (e.g., health education, transportation services) to prevent illness or promote health receive equal emphasis?

Third, decisions will have to be made for the appropriate relationship between rescue services and preventive services. Is it more effective to concentrate on kidney dialysis and terminal cancer services, or should concentrated effort and economic resources be devoted to prevention of disease and disability through, for example, hypertension and diabetes screening?

Fourth, decisions will need to be made about whether certain diseases or categories of illness receive more emphasis than others. For example, should the prevention and treatment of coronary heart disease take precedence over the prevention and treatment of venereal disease? Decisions in this area may result in allocating money and services to certain socioeconomic or racial groups. Such delicate decisions will require careful consideration to avoid conflicts of interest.

Fifth, in establishing certain priorities, it is necessary to ascertain whether these priorities will compromise important values or principles. For example, preventive strategies aimed at discouraging alcohol consumption or smoking may involve emphasis on behavioral change or the altering of life-styles. The nurse might question whether these preventive strategies would have a substantial impact on the autonomy of community members, particularly regarding their choice to engage in behaviors that are health risks.

Clearly, acting on certain priorities may create conflicts of interest among health care providers, with subsequent influence on the actual delivery of needed nursing care. These conflicts of interest continue into the next area of decision making.

Distributing Nursing Resources. Once the priorities for health are designated, community health nursing services need to decide how to deliver health care equally according to client needs.

One strategy may be to focus services on those who have the most reasonable chance of benefiting from services; examples are children and childbearing families. This is a utilitarian approach to distributing services aimed at providing the greatest overall benefit. It is questionable whether this strategy meets the moral requirements of a principle of justice, which holds that everyone has a claim of equal access to basic health care services according to need. Certainly a strategy that focuses on one age group in the community will overlook many individual needs and cannot be considered just.

A second strategy is to provide basic services in all categories in limited amounts and accommodate requests for nursing care services on a first-come, first-served basis. This approach may certainly cost more in terms of services provided. It may even overlap with similar services provided in the community through health maintenance organizations (HMOs) or group practices of private family physicians. It does meet the basic requirement of providing the opportunity for everyone to have equal access to services, even though they may have to wait a long time to be served. However, it may not be the most efficient means of disbursing nursing resources according to the needs of clients.

A third strategy is to focus nursing services on those who are most able to pay for services, an approach that is all too frequently used in today's health care delivery system. This approach has been fostered by legislation and funding by government and its agencies. Unfortunately, this approach may have limited relevance to the needs of a particular community. For example, focusing the majority of nursing resources on a home health care program because of Medicare reimbursements would be unjust to other community health needs if the community had only a small elderly population.

A fourth approach is to categorize those in the community according to health needs and decide who should receive first priority. Those who cannot survive without nursing resources (those receiving kidney dialysis or respiratory therapy at home) would have first priority. Those who can be assisted to prevent long-term disability (e.g., populations at high risk, the preeclamptic client, children with minor cardiac anomalies) would come next. Last priority would be given to those who do not have an acute disabling illness or are not at risk of long-term disability (e.g., school-age children, the elderly, or some persons with chronic diseases). Other groups who may be given a high priority include those whose health needs can be easily met and who can benefit the health of others (e.g., women with uncomplicated pregnancy, mothers with children under 2 years of age).

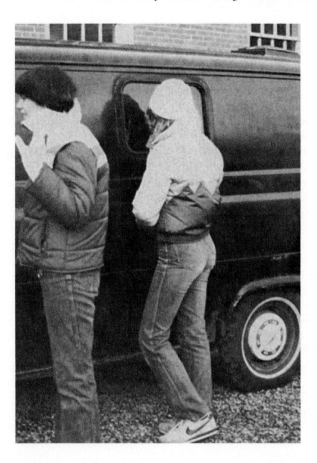

FIGURE 6-5

Teenage populations have a low priority in the allocation of health and nursing services.

This approach has a decidedly utilitarian twist, and it limits the access of some groups to nursing services according to their priority (Figure 6-5). While it does distribute nursing resources according to who can benefit the most, some clients (e.g., dying cancer clients) would have no access to the system at all. This can hardly be considered just if we adopt the principle of justice (rather than a utilitarian principle of beneficence) as the guiding principle for distributing health goods.

As can be demonstrated by all of these various approaches to distributing nursing care resources, the moral requirements of justice create numerous conflicts of interest for health practitioners when they face specific choices.

APPLICATION OF ETHICS TO COMMUNITY HEALTH NURSING PRACTICE
The Priority of Ethical Principles

In community health nursing, ethical principles direct and guide nursing actions with individuals and aggregate groups. The professional ethic in most nursing actions places a greater emphasis on the observance of the principles of autonomy and beneficence than on the principle of justice (Fry, 1982). For example, in the *Code for Nurses,* respect for the principle of autonomy is emphasized by such statements as "the nurse provides services with respect for human dignity and the uniqueness of the client," that "clients have the moral right to determine what will be done with their own person," and that "the nurse's respect for the worth and dignity of the individual human being applies irrespective of the nature of the health problem" (ANA, 1976, 1985, pp. 2, 3). All these statements indicate a high respect for client autonomy or claim that the nurse has a strong, primary duty to respect the client's right to self-determination.

The ethical principle of beneficence is given slightly less emphasis in the *Code for Nurses.* For example, the code claims that "the nurse's primary commitment is to the health, welfare, and safety of the client"; that "the nurse safeguards the client's right to privacy by judiciously protecting information of a confidential nature"; and that "nurses are responsible for advising clients against the use of products that endanger the client's safety and welfare. . . . The nurse may use knowledge of specific services or products in advising an individual client, since this may contribute to the client's health and well-being" (ANA, 1976, 1985, pp. 4, 6, 15). Acts of beneficence may even include overriding the autonomy of individuals in the interests of other clients. The *Code for Nurses* justifies this action whenever "the nurse recognizes those situations in which individual rights to autonomy in health care may temporarily be overridden to preserve the life of the human community" (ANA, 1976, 1985, pp. 2, 3).

However, the principle of justice is not strongly emphasized in the professional code of ethics. The *Code for Nurses* notes in passing that nursing practice is not influenced by age, sex, race, color, personality, or other personal attributes or individual differences in customs, beliefs, or attitudes. The code states that "nursing care is delivered without prejudicial behavior"; that "the nurse adheres to the principle of nondiscriminatory, nonprejudicial care in every situation and endeavors to promote its acceptance by others"; and that "the setting shall not determine the nurse's readiness to respect clients and to render or obtain needed services" (ANA, 1976, 1985, pp. 3, 4). Clearly, these statements related to the moral requirements of the principle of justice are not as strong as those related to the moral requirements of the principles of autonomy and beneficence.

In community health nursing, nursing actions are guided not only by the professional ethic and its priority of ethical principles, but also by the **public health ethic,** which has a different priority of principles. This ethic is strongly modeled on the priority of the principle of beneficence and follows the rule of utility in disease detection and prevention and in health maintenance (Beauchamp, 1976; Shindell, 1980). This emphasis certainly influences the practice of community health nursing, as is evidenced by the statement of the definition and role of public health

nursing from the Public Health Nursing Section, American Public Health Association (1980). It describes public health nursing's role in identifying aggregates (or groups) moving "away from solely meeting the needs of consumers as individually presented and toward practicing public health nursing for the 'sum' of individuals or families within the program" (American Public Health Association, 1980, p. 9).

This statement indicates an orientation in community health nursing toward following a rule of utility in matters of health. The needs of aggregates are determined for providing population groups with net benefit over possible health harms (Fry, 1985). This emphasis on the moral requirements of the principle of beneficence does not align with the highly individualistic approach of the *Code for Nurses,* with its emphasis on respect for client autonomy.

Accountability in Community Health Nursing

Moral accountability in nursing practice means that nurses are answerable for how they promote, protect, and meet the health needs of clients while respecting individual rights to self-determination in health care. In community health nursing, where the greater emphasis is on aggregates rather than individual clients, moral accountability means being answerable for how the health of aggregate groups has been promoted, protected, and met (Figure 6-6).

What Do You Think?

Meeting accountability requirements in community health nursing will be different from meeting accountability requirements in other spheres of nursing practice.

For example, the professional ethic clearly indicates that nurses are morally accountable for how they respect the client's right to self-determination and provide health services with respect for "the uniqueness of the client." However, the application of this ethic in community health nursing indicates that community nurses are morally accountable for how they provide health services to maximize total net health in population groups. This ethic further holds that nurses are accountable for demonstrating, through research, the increased health of aggregate groups while containing costs (Schlotfeldt, 1976). This is the meaning of accountability in community health nursing. Rather than being primarily accountable for how the moral requirements of the principle of autonomy are met, the community health nurse is primarily accountable for how the moral requirements of the principle of beneficence are met by nursing services.

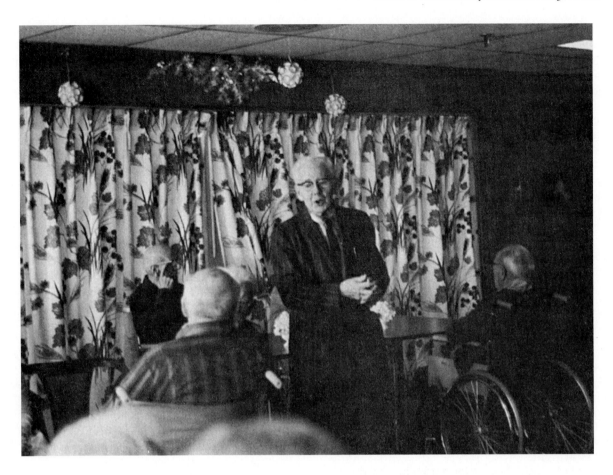

FIGURE 6-6
Community health nurses are accountable for the health of aggregate groups, such as elderly clients in a nursing home.

The moral requirements of the principles of autonomy and justice are still important in community health nursing, but they are less important than the requirements of the principle of beneficence. In community health nursing, the emphasis of the professional ethic is slanted toward benefit to aggregates, which implies following a rule of utility in planning, implementing, and evaluating community health nursing services.

Future Directions

The emphasis on the moral requirements of a principle of beneficence in community health nursing has two implications. The first is heralded by the position paper *The Definition and Role of Public Health Nursing in the Delivery of Health Care*. This document holds that public health nursing derives its theoretical direction from both public health services and professional nursing theories. Its goal is to "improv[e] the health of the entire community" (American Public Health Association, 1980, p. 4). If community health nursing is defined in this way, it is important that the planning, implementation, and evaluation of nursing services in the community be clearly differentiated from the pro-

vision of nursing services in other spheres of health care delivery. Community health nursing is a synthesis of the sciences of both public health and nursing (Archer, 1982). However, there must be a clear understanding of how the ethical components of professional practice, including the observance of clients' rights and professional responsibilities, are considered in the provision of nursing services. Clarity and agreement on the priority of ethical principles in community health nursing are also necessary. Improving the health of the entire community by identifying aggregates and directing resources to them indicates an orientation toward meeting health needs according to the rule of utility. Is the ethical principle of beneficence the principle that should primarily guide community health nursing practice? The moral underpinnings of community health nursing clearly need to be given careful consideration in any statement defining the role of the discipline.

The second implication concerns the evaluation of accountability in community health nursing practice. Certainly, community health nursing has been affected by changes in both the health care delivery system and nursing practice in recent years. Accountability requirements have likewise been affected by changes in public and professional expectations and the scope of nursing practice (Cushing, 1983; Warren, 1983). For example, the expanded role of the nurse has increased the legal accountability of the nurse practitioner, who is certified to function as an independent caregiver. Thus, there is a current and future need for periodic assessment of the moral and legal requirements of accountability in community nursing services.

One must also determine how accountability will be measured in community health nursing and how existing programs and services will be evaluated to determine the effectiveness of various nursing services in meeting accountability requirements. This task has yet to be accomplished by today's community health nursing leaders.

 ## Clinical Application

Ethical decision making in the clinical area involves many variables. It can be enhanced by an orderly process that considers ethical principles, client values, and professional obligations. The need for this orderly process is demonstrated by the increasing use of ethical decision-making frameworks in nursing practice (Thompson and Thompson, 1985). Although such frameworks should not be used as foolproof formulas for ethical decision making, they help individual nurses to explore moral issues and relevant values to arrive at specific decisions (Fry, 1989, 1994).

Jameton's Method for Resolving Nursing Ethics Problems is a representative framework that can be used in community health nursing practice (1984). His framework involves six steps and is summarized in the box at right.

The use of ethical decision-making frameworks can assist the community health nurse in situations laden with conflicting values. They are not used to "solve" the moral conflict, but they do provide an orderly means for considering the issues involved.

The following are typical case situations encountered in community health nurse practice. Use Jameton's Method for Resolving Nursing Ethics Problems to analyze the issues and clarify the decision-making process. The questions after each case will help you apply the moral concepts and ethical principles in this chapter to the nurse-client relationship in community health nursing practice.

Case 1: What Are Society's Obligations to the Client?

Mr. H is a 48-year-old man referred to the visiting nurse association for evaluation and treatment of stasis ulcers on his legs and for maintenance of a weight reduction program for both Mr. H and his wife. Mr. H is 6 feet tall and weighs more than 380 pounds. The Hs have a 27-year-old mentally retarded son.

When she visited the home, Karla Lowe, the VNA nurse, found large, oozing, sticky areas of raw tissue on Mr. H's legs. Ms. Lowe cleaned and dressed the ulcers and continued visiting the Hs every other day for the next 3 months. As the ulcers began to heal, Ms. Lowe attempted to engage the Hs in discussion about nutrition and hygiene and to encourage them to start a weight reduction program. Mr. and Mrs. H were not interested and chose not to participate in any type of weight reduction program.

 Jameton's Method for Resolving Nursing Ethics Problems

1. *Identify the problem.* The nurse should clarify what is at issue: values, conflicts, and matters of conscience.
2. *Gather additional information.* The nurse should decide who is the main decision maker and what the clients or their surrogate decision makers want.
3. *Identify all the options open to the decision maker.* All possible courses of action and their outcomes should be considered. The likelihood of whether future decisions might have to be made should also be evaluated.
4. *Think the situation through.* Consider the basic values and the professional obligations involved. Explore the ethical principles and relevant rules.
5. *Make the decision.* The decision maker should choose the course of action that reflects his or her best judgment.
6. *Act and assess the decision and its outcomes.* The nurse should compare the actual outcomes of the situation with the projected outcomes. Can the process of decision making be improved for further situations having similar characteristics? Can this decision be generalized to other patient care situations?

Summarized from Jameton A: *Nursing practice: the ethical issues*, Englewood Cliffs, NJ, 1984, Prentice-Hall.

Several months went by and Mr. H's ulcers stopped healing. When they began to deteriorate, he was hospitalized. Within a few weeks, they had healed enough that he could return home. Ms. Lowe visited his home to change dressings as before, but despite her efforts the ulcers deteriorated once again. It was too soon for him to return to the local hospital under his SSI benefits, so it was arranged to have him admitted to the state hospital. Two days later he signed himself out of this hospital. "It was too far away, and I didn't know anybody. Besides, they were too rough on me," he stated.

Angered by Mr. H's decision, his physician refused to continue treating him, and Ms. Lowe was left without any current physician orders. This meant that she could no longer give Mr. H physical care or receive reimbursement for her visits. Mr. H's unwillingness to cooperate in the development of "healthy behaviors" made him ineligible for the agency's health mainte-

Clinical Application—cont'd

nance program. When Ms. Lowe explained the situation to her patient, Mr. H said that Mrs. H could wash his legs and apply the medicine that Ms. Lowe had been applying. Besides, he did not think that his physicians had really helped him, and he had no intention of ever going to one again. He would miss Ms. Lowe's visits but thought he would manage. Ms. Lowe left the VNA number to call if they ran into any unforeseen problems.

Nearly a year passed. One summer day Mrs. H called Ms. Lowe. She said that Mr. H was "awful sick" and had been in bed for nearly a month. VNA policy allowed a one-time evaluation visit, so Ms. Lowe visited the home. She found Mr. H's legs alive with the larvae of the summer flies attracted to the steamy bedroom. She urged Mr. H to seek hospitalization. He would not be turned away, even if he no longer had a physician. Mr. H agreed, an ambulance was called, and Mr. H was transported to the local hospital. Because of the condition of his legs, a bilateral leg amputation was performed.

When news of Mr. H's general condition got out (he had created quite a sensation in the emergency room of the local hospital), the people of the small town were aghast. How could a man be allowed to rot away? Where were all the services? Who was responsible? The mayor appointed a special task force to investigate the matter. Months (and endless newspaper columns) later "no fault" was found, and it was announced that the town's health services "had sufficient mechanisms to prevent such a thing from ever happening again." Mr. H recovered, obtained prostheses, and moved to another state where he had family to help him.

Yet Ms. Lowe was not satisfied. Didn't the system fail clients such as Mr. H? Did clients have an obligation to accept the services offered to them and the recommendations of health workers who took care of them? If they refused to follow recommendations, did it mean that health care services should be totally withdrawn? Couldn't the amputations have been prevented if Ms. Lowe had at least continued her visits and prevented the extreme condition of Mr. H's legs before his last hospitalization?

Discussion Questions

1. What are society's health care obligations to Mr. H?
2. What are the VNA's obligations to Mr. H according to the Patient Self-Determination Act?
3. Can the conclusions in the report of the President's Commission, *Securing Access to Health Care*, help Ms. Lowe?
4. Is it reasonable for clients such as Mr. H to refuse treatments in advance by executing a written advance directive? Why or why not?

Case 2: The Visiting Nurse and the Obstinate Client: Are Professional Responsibilities Ever Limited?*

Mr. Jeff Williams, team leader in Home Health Care Services at the county health department, was preparing to visit Mr. Rufus Chisholm, a 59-year-old client recently diagnosed as having emphysema. Well known to the health department, Mr. Chisholm was unemployed because of a farming accident several years earlier. Hypertensive and overweight, he was also a heavy long-term cigarette smoker despite his decreased lung function. Mr. Williams visited Mr. Chisholm to find out why the client had missed his latest chest clinic appointment. He also wanted to find out if the client was continuing his medications as ordered.

As Mr. Williams parked his car in front of his client's house, he could see Mr. Chisholm sitting on the front porch smoking a cigarette. A flash of anger made him wonder why he continued trying to teach Mr. Chisholm reasons for not smoking and why he took the time from his busy home care schedule to follow up on Mr. Chisholm's missed clinical appointments. This client certainly did not seem to care enough about his own health to give up smoking.

During the home visit, Mr. Williams determined that Mr. Chisholm had discontinued the use of his prophylactic antibiotic and was not taking his expectorant and bronchodilator medication on a regular basis. Mr. Chisholm's blood pressure was 210/114, and he coughed almost continuously. Although he listened politely to Mr. Williams's concerns about his respiratory function and the continued use of his medications, Mr. Chisholm simply made no effort to take responsibility for his health care. Even so, another clinic appointment was made, and Mr. Williams encouraged the client to attend.

As he drove to his next home visit, Mr. Williams wondered to what extent he was obligated as a nurse to spend time on clients who took no personal responsibility for their health. He also wondered if there was a limit to the amount of nursing care a noncooperative client could expect from a community health service.

Discussion Questions

1. What are Mr. Williams's professional responsibilities for Mr. Chisholm's rights to health care?
2. Is there a limit to the amount of care nurses should be expected to give to clients?
3. What authority defines the moral requirements and moral limits of nursing care to clients?

Case 3: When the Family Asks the Nurse Not to Tell the Truth

Ralph Bradley, a recently widowed man in his midsixties, was discharged from the hospital following

*Cases 2 through 7 modified from Veatch RM, Fry ST: *Case studies in nursing ethics*, Philadelphia, 1987, Lippincott.

Continued.

Clinical Application—cont'd

exploratory surgery that disclosed colon cancer with metastasis to the lymph nodes. His physician referred him to a community health agency for nursing care follow-up. In reading the referral, the nurse learned that Mr. Bradley had been living with a married daughter and her family since his wife's death. An unmarried daughter apparently lived nearby, visiting him regularly and helping with his daily care. The referral did not explain what, if anything, the client had been told by his physician concerning his condition.

During the first home visit, it became apparent that Mr. Bradley did not know that the tumor removed from his body had been diagnosed as cancerous or that it had metastasized to the lymph nodes. He did not realize the seriousness of his condition, but he did express concern about his health. He complained of vague pain in the abdomen, asked for information about the results of the tests performed before discharge from the hospital, and wanted to know how soon he would be able to return to his work as a cabinetmaker. When the nurse avoided a direct answer to these questions, Mr. Bradley asked directly, "Is everything all right?" The married daughter, who was present when her father was asking these questions, assured him that everything was all right and that he would soon be up and around.

Walking the nurse to her car when the visit was over, the married daughter confided that it was the family's wish that their father not be told how serious his condition was. She said that her mother's recent death had been very difficult for him to accept. They did not want him to be further burdened with the knowledge of his condition. The nurse listened, acknowledging the difficulties posed by the wife's recent death and the father's serious condition. She told the daughter, however, that it would be very difficult, if not impossible, for anyone from her agency to continue to provide nursing care to Mr. Bradley without his knowledge of his condition.

When she returned to her office, the nurse discussed Mr. Bradley's situation with her supervisor. The nurse did not want to continue visiting the client knowing he was being deceived by the physician and family. The supervisor suggested that she consult with the attending physician as soon as possible and explain that Mr. Bradley was asking questions about his condition. Luckily, the nurse was able to reach the physician before it was time to make the next home visit. She asked the physician what the client had been told about his condition. The physician said that at the family's request, Mr. Bradley had not been told that he had cancer. He said he agreed with the family that Mr. Bradley could probably not withstand the anxiety of knowing he had a terminal illness so soon after his wife's death. The physician also expressed concern about Mr. Bradley's daughters who, as he put it, "need a little time to accept the mother's death, as well as accept the impending death of the old man." The physician said that he would consider any act of

disclosure on the nurse's part at this time to be inappropriate to her role as a visiting nurse and inconsistent with the well-being of the client and his family.

Discussion Questions
1. What is the professional duty of veracity?
2. What reasons might the community health nurse give for telling the truth to Mr. Bradley?
3. What reasons might the community health nurse give for *not* telling Mr. Bradley the truth?
4. How does not telling the truth constrain nursing care in the community?

Case 4: The Nurse Who Could Not Protect the Client's Right to Confidentiality

Jane Sanborn was the occupational health nurse in a federal health agency. Among her responsibilities was the completion of the health status section of a form that included both personal and health history for periodic health examinations of the facility's employees. The physician completed the medical portion of the health report, recorded a decision about the employee's fitness for work, and returned the report to Ms. Sanborn, who maintained a confidential file for employees' health reports and records. Employees were asked to sign a statement on the health report that information in the report relating to employee fitness for the job could be shared with the employer as necessary.

One day Ms. Sanborn received a memo directing her to send a copy of an employee's health report to Washington, D.C., for filing in a centralized data bank. Ms. Sanborn questioned the request and asked for an explanation of the purpose of the centralized file. No explanation was provided, and the original request was repeated. Ms. Sanborn responded that she would send the health record as soon as she obtained the consent of the employee. The employee's original consent was to share information only with his immediate employer. Before she could contact the employee, however, Ms. Sanborn was again asked to send the health record immediately; additional consent from the employee was not required. When she discussed the matter with the physician and the administrator of the health facility, Ms. Sanborn was told that she should comply with the request—it was the accepted practice to send any requested employee health records to the centralized file without obtaining consent from employees. Under pressure from both the physician and the administrator, she sent the health record to the centralized data bank.

Discussion Questions
1. Why did Jane Sanborn break confidentiality in this situation?
2. Is there a morally justifiable reason to override the employee's right to confidentiality in this case situation?

Clinical Application—cont'd

3. Why is following the rule of confidentiality important in community health nursing?

Case 5: The Nurse Epidemiologist and Newborn Morbidity Statistics

Sharon Smith was the community health nurse responsible for interpreting mortality and morbidity statistics for her county health department. Based on a preliminary listing of figures, she initiated a comparative study of newborn morbidity from the death certificates of infants delivered at five county hospitals. The study revealed that one hospital had a high rate of newborn deaths. On closer look, the nurse found that the interns and residents of this hospital were using a particular kind of instrument-assisted delivery. When she presented her findings to the county health officer, he shelved the report. She persisted and eventually went public with her findings. Despite eventual investigation into the matter and a change of the procedures at the hospital in question, Ms. Smith was labeled "a traitor" by officials at her health department, and she lost the support of nurse colleagues employed by the county health agency. After several months of this treatment, she resigned her position.

Discussion Questions
1. What does the duty of advocacy mean in this case situation?
2. What is the appropriate action for the nurse in protecting the health, welfare, and safety of the client?
3. Does the duty of advocacy override personal concerns of the nurse? Why or why not?

Case 6: The Client Who Did Not Want to be Clean

Marion Downs, a community health nurse, must decide whether or not to refer her patient, 72-year-old Sadie Jenkins, to the community fiduciary for consideration of conservatorship and guardianship. Miss Jenkins has no living relatives and lives alone in a one-room apartment furnished with a bed, refrigerator, table, chair, lamp, and small sink. Since she does not have a stove, two meals per day are supplied by her landlord. With the support of her Social Security check and food stamps, she has adequate money for her needs and has lived for more than 10 years in these arrangements. She is also in good physical health.

Marion has made four home visits to Miss Jenkins to check her vital signs and medication routine following recent treatment in the Health Center's Hypertension Clinic. Although Miss Jenkins has made excellent progress and no longer requires visits from the community health nurse, her landlord, the other residents of her small apartment building, and her immediate neighbors are urging the nurse to "do something" about Miss Jenkins. Admittedly, Miss Jenkins's apartment has a strong odor from the long-term accumulation of dust, dirt, and mold. There are visible cockroaches in the apartment, and an unemptied bedpan is often sitting next to Miss Jenkins's bed (it is "too much trouble," Miss Jenkins stated, to walk to the hall bathroom shared by Miss Jenkins and two other tenants). Marion has noticed that Miss Jenkins has worn the same soiled clothes every time she has been to her apartment. It is also obvious that Miss Jenkins has not bathed for a long time, her hair is unwashed, and she apparently does not clean her nails and dentures. In addition, her toenails are so long that they have perforated the canvas of her tennis shoes, apparently the only shoes that she likes to wear.

However, Miss Jenkins is comfortable with her lifestyle and does not want to change her living arrangements. Although Marion has offered to contact agencies to help Miss Jenkins—homemaker service, counseling, and senior citizens—Miss Jenkins says that she is comfortable and does not want or need help from anyone.

Discussion Questions
1. Should Marion use her role of community health nurse to create an arrangement by which Miss Jenkins would lose the right to control her person, her financial resources, and her environment?
2. Can an individual in the community be forced to be clean and to live in a clean environment?
3. How far should a nurse go in providing "good" for a client, and who determines what is "good"?

Case 7: When Aging Parents Can No Longer Live Independently

Joyce Fisher, a home health agency nurse, has just received a telephone call from the daughter of a client, 82-year-old Mr. Sims, whom she had visited some months before. The daughter was very distraught, telling Joyce that her father had fallen at home but refused to be seen by a physician. Ms. Sims's mother had called her at her place of business and pleaded with her to come to the home and stay with them. The daughter was exasperated by the frequency of these types of phone calls from her parents in recent weeks and was appealing to Joyce for help in making some long-term decisions for the care and safety of her parents.

Joyce clearly remembers the conversations that she had with Mr. and Mrs. Sims and their daughter several months ago after Mr. Sim's last hospitalization. Mr. and Mrs. Sims live alone in a small home and are frequently visited by the daughter, who buys their groceries and takes them to their various health appointments. Mr. Sims has always been the decision maker of the family but allows this amount of assistance from the daughter "for Mama's sake." Another daughter lives in a nearby city but has chronic health problems that prohibit her active involvement in the affairs of her parents. A son lives on the West Coast

Continued.

Clinical Application—cont'd

and travels constantly in his line of business. He supports his parents by sending money for their expenses to his sister (Mr. Sims has refused direct financial aid from any of the children). All three children are concerned about the future welfare of their parents but have been unsuccessful in persuading them to change their mode of living.

The present problem exists because Mr. and Mrs. Sims are losing their ability to live independently and make their own decisions. Mr. Sims's unexplained falls are also increasing, a continued source of worry for Mrs. Sims and a genuine concern for their daughter. They all look toward Joyce Fisher as the person who can help them make and support a decision that will preserve some autonomy for the aging parents and respect their choices and life-style. Yet Joyce

doubts that what is best for all concerned can avoid infringing on the choices and self-respect of the parents.

Discussion Questions

1. What is the role of the home health nurse in assisting individuals to reach a decision with which they can live?
2. What does it mean to respect Mr. and Mrs. Sims as autonomous individuals?
3. Do clients really have the right to refuse services or treatment from the community health nurse? Does such refusal limit future treatment? Why or why not?
4. Is there any happy medium for aging parents when they can no longer live independently?

Key Concepts

♦ Because clients have rights, health care professionals have responsibilities to tell the truth, respect confidentiality, function as client advocates, and accept accountability for providing proper health care.

♦ The development of methods to measure accountability is a high priority in community health nursing.

♦ A right to health has been historically recognized as a basic human right.

♦ The negative right to be free to enjoy good health may lead to the positive right to obtain certain services or community health safeguards.

♦ "Right to health" and "right to health care" are different kinds of rights and should be kept separate.

♦ Use of the *Patient's Bill of Rights* has been how many health care providers communicate rights to their clients. However, the *Patient's Bill of Rights* has been criticized for several reasons.

♦ Clients have the right to accept or refuse treatment and the right to formulate advance directives.

♦ According to a recent presidential commission, "society has an ethical obligation to ensure equitable access to health care for all."

♦ The professional code of ethics for nurses prescribes moral behavior and actions based on moral principles.

♦ The need for moral accountability within nursing practice has been recognized ever since Florence Nightingale began her nurse training program.

♦ The ethical principles operable in community health nursing are beneficence, autonomy, and justice.

♦ The four major theories of justice used to decide the allocation of health are resources are the entitlement theory, the utilitarian theory, the maximin theory, and the egalitarian theory. The moral requirements of justice create numerous conflicts of interest for health practitioners when specific choices must be made.

♦ The professional ethic generally places a greater emphasis on observance of the principles of autonomy and beneficence than on the principle of justice in most nursing actions.

♦ In community health nursing, moral accountability means being answerable for how the health of aggregate groups has been promoted, protected, and met.

♦ Clients' rights to equal access to health care and the aggregate's needs and interests in health matters will often compete for the attention and services of the nurse.

Critical Thinking Activities

1. Hold a conference among two or three nursing students and two or three practicing community health nurses. Discuss how community health nurses assume responsibility and accountability for individual nursing judgments and actions in their areas of practice. Be sure to distinguish moral accountability from legal accountability.

2. Suggest three ways by which community health nursing might extend the scope of accountability for nurses in delivering nursing care services to aggregate groups in the community.

3. Select an aggregate group at risk in your community. Formulate a plan of nursing care delivery in response to a health care need using a specific theory of distributive justice.

4. Determine how client's rights to privacy are respected and protected in a community health care agency. To what extent do community health nurses contribute to the protection of client privacy? Are client records used in research studies? If so, how is personal information about the client protected? Suggest two methods by which client privacy could be more adequately protected. What would be the relative costs and benefits of your proposed methods?

5. Discuss the role of nurses in discussing and implementing advance directives in community health settings.

Bibliography

American Hospital Association: Statement on a patient's bill of rights, *Hospitals* 47:41, 1973.

American Nurses' Association: *Code for nurses with interpretive statements*, Kansas City, Mo, 1976, 1985, The Association.

American Public Health Association, Public Health Nursing Section: *The definition and role of public health nursing practice in the delivery of health care: a statement of the public health nursing section*, Washington, DC, 1980, The Association.

Annas GJ: Patients' rights movement. In Reich WT, editor: *Encyclopedia of bioethics*, vol 3, New York, 1978, Free Press.

Annas GJ: Fashion and freedom: when artificial feedings should be withdrawn, *Am J Public Health* 75:685-688, 1985.

Archer SE: Synthesis of public health science and nursing science, *Nurs Outlook* 30:442-446, 1982.

Beauchamp DE: Public health and social justice, *Inquiry* 13:3-14, 1976.

Beauchamp DE: Public health and individual liberty, *Ann Rev Public Health* 1:121-136, 1980.

Beauchamp DE: Community: the neglected tradition of public health, *Hastings Center Rep* 15:28-36, 1985.

Beauchamp TL, Childress JF: *Principles of biomedical ethics*, ed 4, New York, 1994, Oxford Press.

Beauchamp TL, Faden RR: The right to health and the right to health care, *J Med Philos* 4:118-131, 1979.

Beauchamp TL, Walters L: Patients' rights and professional responsibilities. In Beauchamp TL, Walters L, editors: *Contemporary issues in bioethics*, Belmont, Calif, 1978, Wadsworth.

Bell NK: The scarcity of medical resources: are there rights to health care? *J Med Philos* 4:158-169, 1979.

Benner P, Wrubel J: *The primacy of caring: stress and coping in health and illness*, Menlo Park, Calif, 1989, Addison-Wesley.

Brockington C: *A short history of public health*, London, 1956, Churchill.

Capron AM: Right to refuse medical treatment. In Reich WT, editor: *Encyclopedia of bioethics*, vol 4, New York, 1978, Free Press.

Cushing M: Expanding the meaning of accountability, *Am J Nurs* 83:1202-1203, 1983.

Daniels N: Rights to health care and distributive justice: programmatic worries, *J Med Philos* 4:174-191, 1979.

Feinberg J: *Social philosophy*, Englewood Cliffs, NJ, 1973, Prentice-Hall.

Frankena WK: *Ethics*, Englewood Cliffs, NJ, 1973, Prentice-Hall.

Fry ST: Accountability in research: the relationship of scientific and humanistic values, *Adv Nurs Sci* 4:1-13, 1981.

Fry ST: Ethical principles in nursing education and practice: a missing link in the unification issue, *Nurs Health Care* 3:363-368, 1982.

Fry ST: Dilemma in community health ethics, *Nurs Outlook* 31:176-179, 1983a.

Fry ST: Rationing health care: the ethics of cost containment, *Nurs Econ* 1:165-169, 1983b.

Fry ST: Confidentiality in health care: a decrepit concept? *Nurs Econ* 2:413-418, 1984.

Fry ST: Individual vs. aggregate good: ethical tension in nursing practice, *Int J Nurs Studies* 22:303-310, 1985.

Fry ST: Ethical aspects of decision-making in the feeding of cancer patients, *Semin Oncol Nurs* 2:59-62, 1986a.

Fry ST: Ethical inquiry in nursing: the definition and method of biomedical ethics, *Periop Nurs Q* 2:1-8, June 1986b.

Fry ST: The ethic of caring: can it survive in nursing? *Nurs Outlook* 36:48, 1988.

Fry ST: Ethical decision making. Part I. Selecting a framework, *Nurs Outlook* 37:248, 1989.

Fry ST: *Ethics in nursing practice: a guide to ethical decision making*, Geneva, 1994, International Council of Nurses.

Gert B, Culver CM: The justification of paternalism. In Robinson WL, Pritchard MS, editors: *Medical responsibility: paternalism, informed consent, and euthanasia*, Clifton, NJ, 1979, Humana Press.

Gordis L, Gold E: Privacy, confidentiality, and the use of medical records in research, *Science* 207:153-156, 1980.

Gortner SR: Scientific accountability in nursing, *Nurs Outlook* 22:764-768, 1974.

Green R: Health care and justice in contract theory perspective. In Veatch RM, Branson R, editors: *Ethics and health policy*, Cambridge, Mass, 1976, Ballinger.

In re estate of Brooks, 32 Ill, 2d 361, 205 NE 2d 435, 1965.

Jameton A: *Nursing practice: the ethical issues*, Englewood Cliffs, NJ, 1984, Prentice-Hall.

Kant I: *Groundwork of the metaphysic of mortals*, New York, 1964, Harper & Row. (Translated by HJ Paton, originally published in 1785.)

Kelsey JL: Privacy and confidentiality in epidemiological research involving patients, *IRB* 3:1-4, 1981.

Leininger MM: *Care: the essence of nursing and health*, Detroit, 1984, Wayne Sate University Press.

Lynn J, Childress J: Must patients always be given food and water? *Hastings Center Rep* 13:17-21, 1983.

Lyons J: *Playing god in the nursery*, New York, 1985, Norton.

MacIntyre A: Utilitarianism and cost-benefit analysis. In Beauchamp TL, Bowie NE, editors: *Ethical theory and business*, Englewood Cliffs, NJ, 1979, Prentice-Hall.

Mezey M, Evans LK, Golub ZD, Murphy E, White GB: The Patient Self-Determination Act: sources of concern for nurses, *Nurs Outlook* 42:30-38, 1994.

Milio N: *The care of health in communities: access for outcasts,* New York, 1975, Macmillan.

Mill JS: Utilitarianism, New York, 1957, Bobbs-Merrill. (Edited by O Priest, originally published in 1863).

National Commission for the Protection of Human Subjects of Biomedical and Behavioral Research: *The Belmont report: ethical principles and guidelines for the protection of human subjects of research,* DHEW Pub No (OS) 78-0012, Washington, DC, 1978.

Noddings N: *Caring: a feminine approach to ethics and moral education,* Berkeley, 1984, University of California Press.

Nozick R: *Anarchy, state, and utopia,* New York, 1974, Basic Books.

Omnibus Budget Reconciliation Act of 1990, sections 4206 and 4751, PL 101-508, Nov 5, 1990.

Palmer LS: Florence Nightingale: reformer, reactionary, researcher, *Nurs Res* 26:84-89, 1977.

Pellegrino E: The caring ethic: the relation of physician to patient. In Bishop AH, Scudder JR, editors: *Caring, curing, coping: nurse, physician, patient relationships,* Birmingham, 1985, University of Alabama Press.

Popoff D: What are your feelings about death and dying? Part 1, *Nursing* 5:15-24, 1975.

President's Commission for the Study of Ethical Problems in Medicine and Biomedical and Behavioral Research: *Securing access to health care,* vol 1, Report on the ethical implications of differences in the availability in health services, Washington, DC, 1983, US Government Printing Office.

Public Law 92-603, Social Security amendments of 1972, 92nd Congress, Oct 30, 1972.

Public Law 92-278, The national sickle cell anemia, Cooley's anemia, Tay-Sachs and Genetic Disease Act, Title IV, 90 stat, Section 410, 1976.

Rawls J: *A theory of justice,* Cambridge, Mass, 1971, Harvard University Press.

Rosen G: *Preventive medicine in the United States: 1900-1975,* New York, 1975, Science History Publishers.

Ross WD: *The right and the good,* Oxford, 1930, Oxford University Press.

Schlotfeldt RM: Accountability: a critical dimension of health care, *Health Care Dimen* 3:137-148, 1976.

Shindell S: Legal and ethical aspects of public health. In Last JM, editor: *Maxcy-Rosenau public health and preventive medicine,* ed 11, Norwalk, Conn, 1980, Appleton-Century-Crofts.

Smith CS: Outrageous or outraged: a nurse advocate story, *Nurs Outlook* 28:624-625, 1980.

Szasz T: The right to health. In Gorovitz S, et al, editors: *Moral problems in medicine,* Englewood Cliffs, NJ, 1976, Prentice-Hall.

Tarasoff v. Regents of The University of California, 131 Cal Rptr 14, 551 P2d 334, 1976.

Thompson JB, Thompson HO: *Bioethical decision making for nurses,* Norwalk, Conn, 1985, Appleton-Century-Crofts.

UNESCO: *Human rights, a symposium,* New York, 1949, Allan Wingate.

Veatch RM: *Death, dying, and the biological revolution,* New Haven, Conn, 1976, Yale University Press.

Veatch RM: Truth-telling: attitudes. In Reich WT, editor: *Encyclopedia of bioethics,* vol 4, New York, 1978, Free Press.

Veatch RM: *A theory of medical ethics,* New York, 1981, Basic Books.

Veatch RM, Fry ST: *Case studies in nursing ethics,* Philadelphia, 1987, Lippincott.

Warren JJ: Accountability and nursing diagnosis, *Am J Nurs Admin* 13:34-37, 1983.

Will GF: The killing will not stop, *Washington Post,* April 22, 1982, p A-29.

Williams C: Community health nursing: what is it? *Nurs Outlook* 25:250-252, 1977.

World Health Organization: *The first ten years of the World Health Organization,* New York, 1958, WHO.

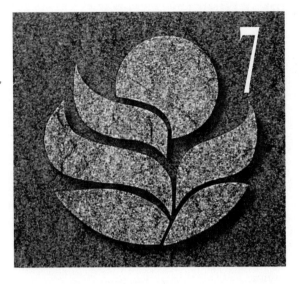

7

Cultural Diversity and Community Health Nursing Practice

Cynthia Degazon

Objectives ▼

After reading this chapter, the student should be able to do the following:

◆ Discuss the relevance of cultural competence to community health nursing.
◆ Describe at least four barriers to developing cultural competence.
◆ Conduct a cultural assessment of a person from a cultural group other than one's own.
◆ Implement nursing interventions to help people achieve health using cultural competence.

Key Terms ▼

cultural awareness
cultural blindness
cultural competence
cultural conflict
cultural encounter
cultural imposition
cultural knowledge
cultural shock
cultural skill
culture
culture brokering
ethnicity
ethnocentrism
prejudice
race
racism
stereotyping

Outline ▼

Caring for culturally diverse groups has been a focus of community health nursing since its inception. As early as 1893, public health nursing was started by nurses in New York City, who provided home care to immigrants, particularly recent arrivals (Denker, 1994). These nurses were not from the same cultural background as the immigrants and had to deal with the cultural differences between themselves and the persons in their care.

The United States has always been a multicultural society. Recent changes in immigration laws have stimulated migration and increased the volume of cultural groups entering the United States. (Thornton, 1992). The 1965 amendment to the Immigration and Nationality Act changed the quota system that discriminated against individuals from Southern and Eastern Europe, and the Refugee Act of 1980 provided opportunities to immigrate for those who needed to escape political persecution, such as Cubans, Vietnamese, Laotians, Cambodians, and Russian Jews. Table 7-1 summarizes the immigration patterns of these groups over the past 30 years.

If the current migration trend continues, the United States will consist of a wider variety of cultural groups, with 51.1% of the total projected population being of various ethnic minority groups (Statistical Abstracts, 1992). Based on physical or cultural characteristics and lack of power within the dominant system, many people are members of minority groups. In this chapter, emphasis is on traditional minority groups, which include African-Americans, Asians, Hispanics, and Native Americans, because they have more economic difficulties, poorer health, and less accessibility to health care than other groups. The homeless, migrant workers, refugees, and people living in poverty are discussed within the context of their culture.

There is great diversity among the cultural groups in expectations and experiences. In turn, their perceptions of health and illness also differ. Hence, the workplace offers enormous challenges for community health nurses who want to understand perceptions of health and illness of clients as they provide interventions that promote wellness.

In many instances, especially in home care, community health nurses must assist ill persons from various cultures over a period of weeks or months to adjust to alterations in health status, adopt individual and family behaviors to improve health status, and, overall, to develop health-promoting patterns. In addition, there is an insufficient number of ethnic minority nurses who work in communities to help other nurses understand the experiences of diverse cultural groups (Bernal, 1993).

The purpose of this chapter is to explore cultural competence among community health nurses. Nurses who care for clients (individuals, families, and communities) that are culturally different from themselves will be able to apply strategies for developing cultural competence.

CULTURE, ETHNICITY, AND RACE

The concepts of culture, ethnicity, and race play a strong role in understanding cultural behavior. In every day living, these three concepts are often used incorrectly, but a culturally competent nurse would be expected to understand the meaning of each.

Culture

Culture is a set of ideals, values, and assumptions about life that are widely shared among a group of people (Brislin, 1993). Each individual has a culture with traditions that provide guidance toward solutions to life's problems (Leininger, 1978, 1991, 1993). Culture provides the organizational structure for what members of the cultural group determine as acceptable behavior.

Learning the characteristics of a culture occurs through frequent or continuous contact with persons from that culture (Brookins, 1993; Leininger, 1993). Parents and family are the most important sources for the transfer of traditions from one generation to another. The transfer process begins at an early age during child rearing when the child is taught both explicit and implicit behaviors of the culture (Payne, 1986). The explicit behaviors, such as language, are observable and allow the child to identify the self with other persons of the culture. Such identification allows the child to experience and share traditions, customs and life-styles with others. The implicit behaviors are less visible and include the way individuals think about others who are not a part of their culture. These behaviors are subtle and difficult for persons to articulate and explain, yet they are very much a part of the culture.

It is the organization of each culture that distinguishes one culture from another. Such organizational elements include language and the arts, child-rearing practices, religious practices, family structure and values, and attitudes (Locke, 1992). In the case of language, there are idiomatic expressions unique to each language (Phillips et al., 1994). Similarly, humor differs among cultures—what one culture thinks of as funny may not be funny at all to another culture. The organizational elements of various cultures have been described by Andrews and Boyle (1995), Giger and Davidhizar (1995), Kavanagh and Kennedy (1992), Spector (1991), and Leininger (1991). It is important that nurses know these organizational elements in order to provide appropriate care to persons of diverse cultures. This does not mean, however, that we should overlook or fail to incorporate the individuality of any person within any culture when generating a plan of care. Just as all cultures are not alike, all individuals within a culture are not alike. Each individual should be viewed as a unique human being with differences that are respected. The box on p. 120 summarizes factors that may contribute to individual differences within cultures.

Table 7-1 Immigrants by Country of Birth: 1971 to 1992 (In thousands, for fiscal years ending in year shown)

Country of birth	1971-80	1981-90	1991-92	Country of birth	1971-80	1981-90	1991-92
All Countries	4,493.3	7,338.1	2,801.2	**North America***	1,645.0	3,125.0	384.0
Europe*	801.3	705.6	280.6	Canada	114.8	119.2	28.7
France	17.8	23.1	5.8	Mexico	637.2	1,653.3	1,160.0
Germany	66.0	70.1	16.4	Caribbean*	759.8	892.7	237.5
Greece	93.7	29.1	4.0	Barbados	20.9	17.4	2.6
Ireland	14.1	32.8	17.0	Cuba	276.8	159.2	22.1
Italy	130.1	32.9	5.2	Dominican Republic	148.0	251.8	83.4
Poland	43.6	97.4	44.7	Haiti	58.7	140.2	58.5
Portugal	104.5	40.0	7.2	Jamaica	142.0	213.8	42.7
Romania	17.5	38.9	14.6	Trinidad and Tobago	61.8	39.5	15.4
Soviet Union (former)†	43.2	84.0	100.6	Central America*	132.4	458.7	168.7
Armenia	NA	NA	6.1	El Salvador	34.4	214.6	73.6
Azerbaijan	NA	NA	1.6	Guatemala	25.6	87.9	36.0
Belarus	NA	NA	3.2	Honduras	17.2	49.5	18.1
Moldova	NA	NA	1.7	Nicaragua	13.0	44.1	26.7
Russia	NA	NA	8.9	Panama	22.7	29.0	7.0
Ukraine	NA	NA	14.4				
Uzbekistan	NA	NA	1.7	**South America***	284.4	455.9	135.2
Spain	30.0	15.8	3.4	Argentina	25.1	25.7	7.8
United Kingdom	123.5	142.1	33.9	Brazil	13.7	23.7	12.9
Yugoslavia	42.1	19.2	5.3	Chile	17.6	23.4	4.7
				Colombia	77.6	124.4	32.9
Asia*	1,633.8	2,817.4	715.5	Ecuador	50.2	56.0	17.3
Afghanistan	2.0	26.6	5.6	Guyana	47.5	95.4	20.8
Cambodia	8.4	116.6	5.9	Peru	29.1	64.4	26.1
China: Mainland	202.5‡	388.8‡	71.9				
Taiwan	‡	‡	29.6	**Africa***	91.5	192.3	63.3
Hong Kong	47.5	63.0	20.9	Egypt	25.5	31.4	9.2
India	176.8	261.9	81.9	Ethiopia	NA	27.2	9.7
Iran	46.2	154.8	32.8	Nigeria	8.8	35.3	12.5
Iraq	23.4	19.6	5.6				
Israel	26.6	36.3	9.3	**Other Countries§**	37.3	41.9	11.5
Japan	47.9	43.2	15.0	Australia	14.3	13.9	3.9
Jordan	29.6	32.6	8.3				
Korea	272.0	338.8	45.9				
Laos	22.6	145.6	18.7				
Lebanon	33.8	41.6	11.8				
Pakistan	31.2	61.3	30.6				
Philippines	360.2	495.3	124.6				
Syria	13.3	20.6	5.7				
Thailand	44.1	64.4	14.5				
Turkey	18.6	20.9	5.0				
Vietnam	179.7	401.4	133.0				

Data from *Statistical Abstract of the United States: 1994*, ed 114, Washington, DC, US Bureau of the Census.
NA: Not available.
*Includes countries not shown separately.
†Includes other republics and unknown republics, not shown separately.
‡Data for Taiwan included with China: Mainland.
§Includes New Zealand and unknown countries.

Factors Influencing Individual Differences within Cultural Groups

Age
Religion
Language and dialect spoken
Gender-identity roles
Socioeconomic background
Geographical location in the country of origin
Geographical location in the current country
History of the subcultural group with which clients identify in their current country of residence
History of the subcultural group with which clients identify in their current country of origin
Amount of interaction time among older and younger generations
The degree of assimilation in the current country of residence.
Immigration status*
Conditions under which migration occurred*

Except where noted,* factors are from Orque M: In Orque MS, Bloch B, Monrroy LSA, editors: *Ethnic nursing care: a multi-cultural approach*, St Louis, 1983, Mosby, pp 5-48.

Ethnicity

Ethnicity is the shared feeling of peoplehood among a group of individuals (Gordon, 1964). It is based on individuals sharing similar cultural patterns, such as values, beliefs, customs, behavior, and traditions, that over time create a common history. Ethnicity is sustained by race, religion, national origin, or some combination of these factors and is influenced by education, income level, location, and association with other than one's own ethnic group. Hence, there are intraethnic variations, and not all individuals of a particular ethnic group express the same level of ethnicity.

Race

Race is primarily a social classification that relies on physical markers, such as skin color, to identify group membership (Spickard, 1992). Individuals may be of the same race, but differ in ethnic affiliations. Those people who are classified as African-American may have been born in Africa, North America, or the Caribbean. Although the group is heterogeneous, they are often viewed as ethnically and racially homogeneous. A frequent consequence of this is that the many cultural differences and ethnic identifications of individuals are obscured or suppressed in favor of their racial characteristics (Snowden and Holschuh, 1992). This often blurs understanding of this culturally diverse group. Another factor highlighting race's diminishing importance in comparison to ethnic identity is the interracial family. Physical changes in biracial and multiracial generations lead to changes in physical appearances of individuals and make race less important in ethnic identity (Hall, 1992).

CULTURALLY COMPETENT BEHAVIORS

Cultural competence is an ongoing life process that results from an interplay of factors that motivate persons to develop knowledge, skill, and ability to care for individuals, families, and communities (Frei et al., 1994; Orlandi, 1992). It reflects a higher level of expertise than cultural sensitivity, which once was thought to be all that was needed for nurses to effectively care for culturally different clients.

The goal of culturally competent nursing care is to provide care consistent with the client's cultural needs. It includes four principles (AAN Expert Panel Report, 1992): (1) care is designed for the specific client; (2) care is based on the uniqueness of the person's culture and includes cultural norms and values; (3) care includes empowerment strategies to facilitate client decision making in health behavior; and (4) care is provided with sensitivity to the cultural uniqueness of clients.

Cultural Competence

Many of us are socialized by and have familiarity with the dominant culture (Brislin, 1993). As long as we are operating within that culture, we respond automatically to a variety of situations and do not have to examine the cultural content of our behavior. However, in today's climate of increased diversity, nurses are caring for a greater number of culturally diverse clients than ever before. Cultural competence is needed to provide nursing care that meets the needs of these persons.

Community health nurses must be culturally competent because (1) the nurse's culture often differs from that of the client, (2) care that is not culturally competent may further increase the cost of health care and decrease opportunities for positive outcomes, and (3) specific objectives for persons of different cultures need to be met as delineated in *Healthy People 2000* (1991). A discussion of these reasons follows.

First, nurses come from a variety of cultural backgrounds and are steeped in their own cultural traditions. Each nurse has a unique set of cultural experiences that gives meaning and understanding to his or her behavior. Since the nursing profession is a subsystem of the U.S. health care system, many nurses also bring a biomedical perspective to the practice environment that may differ from clients' beliefs and values. With such incongruence of beliefs and values, when the client and community health nurse interact they may have a different understanding about the meaning of problems, and different expectations on what to do to promote and protect health. In these circumstances, cultural competence enables nurses to engage strategies that respect clients' values and expectations without diminishing the nurses' own values and expectations.

Second, in the current health care climate of economic constraints, the health care industry has moved toward cost effectiveness. Cost effectiveness means that there is a balance between cost and quality. Quality of care means that positive health outcomes are achieved. Care that is not focused on the clients' values and ideas is likely to increase cost and diminish quality (Anderson, 1990). For example, when clients are using both folk and biomedical Western medicine and nurses fail to elicit and integrate this information in their teaching, the clients may not derive the full benefits of the treatment protocol. This suggests that positive outcomes, which are indicators of quality, may not be met. When quality is compromised, additional resources may be needed to achieve the health care outcomes. Increased use of resources means that cost is increased.

Third, achievement of the *Healthy People 2000* objectives (Healthy People 2000, 1991) requires that clients' life-styles and personal choices be considered. For example, the American health care system views excessive drinking as a sign of disease. In 1987, 52.2 per 100,000 Native Americans died of alcohol-related motor vehicle accidents. The national goal is to reduce these deaths to 44.8 per 100,000 by the year 2000, a rate significantly higher than the nation's overall goal of 5.8 per 100,000. However, many Native Americans view excessive alcohol consumption as a legitimate way of participating in community ceremonies (Orlandi, 1992). It is viewed as a sign of rejection to refuse to drink with family. Although in Western culture alcoholism is viewed as a mental illness, in the Native American culture, it may be viewed as a disharmony between the individuals and their spirit world and treated as such through traditional medicine. West (1993) asserts that "if the government sends Indians to a health clinic where personnel do not understand the holistic health practices of Indians and where young white people serve as caregivers and as authority figures, failure is likely to result." To have successful outcomes, nurses who develop community health programs to reduce alcohol-related deaths must respect the cultural uniqueness of American Indians. Table 7-2 gives examples of health promotion objectives for selected minority groups who are at risk.

Developing Cultural Competence

Nurses develop cultural competence in different ways, but development occurs mainly through experiences with clients of other cultures and through the nurses' receptivity to these experiences (Frei et al., 1994). Since there are varying degrees of cultural competence, not all nurses may reach the same level of development.

As summarized in Table 7-3, Orlandi (1992) suggests a three-stage process for developing cultural competence: cultural incompetence, cultural sensitivity, and cultural competence. Each stage is conceptualized based on four dimensions of cultural compe-

Table 7-2 Selected Risk-Reduction Objectives for Target Groups

Objectives	1987 Baseline	2000 Target
1. Reduce coronary heart disease deaths to no more than 100 per 100,000 people Target group: African-Americans	163	115
2. Reduce deaths caused by alcohol-related motor vehicle crashes to no more than 8.5 per 100,000 people Target group: Native American men	52.2	44.8
3. Reduce homicides to no more than 7.2 per 100,000 people. Target groups: African-American men between 15-34 years of age Hispanic men between 15-34 years of age	90.5 53.1	72.4 42.5
4. Increase years of healthy life to at least 65 years. (Baseline estimated 62 years in 1980) Target groups: African-Americans Hispanics	56 62	60 65
5. Reduce cigarette smoking to a prevalence of no more than 15% among people 20 years of age and older (Baseline: 29% in 1987, 32% for women and 27% for men) Target population: Southeast Asian men	55%	20%

Healthy People, 2000: national health promotion and disease prevention objectives, Washington, DC, 1991, USDHHS, Public Health Service.

tence. *Stop now and describe your cultural competence with persons of a culture different from your own by staging each of these four dimensions.*

Campinha-Bacote (1991) expands the development of cultural competence to include (1) cultural awareness, (2) cultural knowledge, (3) cultural skill, and (4) cultural encounter. **Cultural awareness** is an appreciation of and sensitivity to the client's values, beliefs, practices, life-styles, and problem-solving strategies (Campinha-Bacote, 1991). To be aware suggests that nurses are receptive to learning about the cultural dimensions of the client. Nurses who are culturally aware understand the basis for their own behavior and how it inhibits or facilitates the delivery of competent care to persons from cultures other than their own (AAN Expert Panel Report, 1992). For example, culturally aware nurses know of cross-cultural differences in the meaning of health. While being aware of the value of health to clients, they do not become angry with themselves or clients when clients do not follow instructions; rather, they evaluate the clients' be-

Table 7-3   The Cultural Competence Framework: Stages of Competence Development

	Culturally incompetent	Culturally sensitive	Culturally competent
Cognitive dimension	Oblivious	Aware	Knowledgeable
Affective dimension	Apathetic	Sympathetic	Committed to change
Skills dimension	Unskilled	Lacking some skills	Highly skilled
Overall effect	Destructive	Neutral	Constructive

From Orlandi MA: In Orlandi MA, editor: *Cultural competence or evaluators*, Washington, DC, 1992, US Department of Health and Human Services, pp 293-299.

haviors within a cultural context and do not impose their own values of health on clients. The box below identifies a number of questions that nurses may focus on as they try to understand their own culture and its implication in who they are.

Cultural knowledge is another component that is essential to caring for a multicultural society. **Cultural knowledge** provides nurses with organizational elements of cultures and current information on what is necessary to provide effective nursing care. Nurses who do not have basic cultural knowledge may have difficulty in interpreting clients' behaviors and, as a consequence, develop feelings of inadequacy and helplessness (Leininger, 1989). In a study of community health nurses (*N* = 150), Bernal and Froman

(1987) found that the nurses indicated they did not feel confident in caring for African-Americans, Puerto Ricans, and Southeast Asians. Nurses with more education were not more culturally competent than those with less education. A missing link in the nurses' education may have been knowledge of cultures surveyed. When knowledge of the client's culture is missing or inadequate, it also can lead to negative situations, such as misinterpretation of client situations, lack of cooperation of clients with the health care regimen, and/or inadequate use of health services (Jezewski, 1990; Leininger, 1991). It is unrealistic to expect that community health nurses have knowledge of all cultures and cultural influences. Instead, they should be aware of, or know how to obtain knowledge of those influences that affect groups with whom they interact.

The third component to developing cultural competence is cultural skill. **Cultural skill** reflects the integration of cultural awareness and cultural knowledge to meet clients' needs. An example of cultural skill is effective communication with persons of differing cultures. When interacting, culturally skillful nurses use appropriate touch during conversation, modify the physical distance between self and others, and use strategies to avoid cultural misunderstandings while meeting mutually agreed upon goals.

Early Cultural Awareness

Think about the first time you had contact with someone you realized was culturally different from you.
Briefly describe the situation/event.
How old were you?
What were your feelings?
What were your thoughts?

What did your parents and other significant adults say about those who were culturally different from your family?
What adjectives were used?
What attitudes were conveyed?

As you got older what messages did you get about minority groups from the larger community or culture?

As an adult how do others in the community talk about culturally different people?
What adjectives were used?
What attitudes were conveyed?
How does this reinforce or contradict your earlier experience?

What parts of this cultural baggage make it difficult to work with clients from different cultural groups?

What parts of this cultural baggage facilitate your work with clients?

From Randall-David E: *Culturally competent HIV counseling and education*, McLean, Va, 1994, The Maternal and Child Health Clearinghouse.

Did You Know?

Nurses may assist clients to develop cultural encounters with clients of other cultures who are recovering from similar illnesses. In these educational groups, clients come into contact with other clients of diverse cultures, who are interested in survival, new adjustment strategies, and integrating themselves back into families, community, and workplace.

The fourth component to developing cultural competence is cultural encounter. During **cultural en-**

counters with clients, nurses learn directly from clients about their experiences and the significance of these experiences for health (Leininger, 1991). Cultural encounters involve all interactions, not only those that are health related discussions of clients' lives (Jezewski, 1990). A successful encounter may be evaluated based on four aspects: (1) nurses should feel successful with established relationships with the client; (2) clients feel that the interactions were warm, cordial, respectful, and cooperative; (3) the tasks are accomplished efficiently; and (4) both nurses and clients experience minimal stress (Brislin, 1993).

In some communities, nurses may have few opportunities to develop cultural competence by working directly with persons of other cultures. When nurses have new encounters with persons who are culturally different from themselves, they should adapt general cultural concepts to the situations until they are able to learn directly from clients about their cultures.

Cultural competence development is facilitated by an open environment, (i.e., one that encourages discovery and questioning). In addition to exposure to individuals from other cultures, development can occur from reading about other cultures, taking courses about other cultures, and discussing the cultural meaning of health behavior. Nurses should be aware that having cultural competence is not synonymous with being a cultural expert on a group that is different from your own.

Increasing cultural competence is a slow process because it takes time to break old ways of thinking and performing (Frei et al., 1994). Since the development process is challenging, nurses should expect to experience difficulty but not to allow the difficulty to discourage them in developing cultural competence.

Dimensions of Cultural Competence

Data from the Sunrise model (Leininger, 1991) suggests three modes to direct nursing decisions and actions that are based on negotiations between the client and nurse. They are preservation, accommodation, and repatterning that guide in delivering culturally competent care. Nurses integrate their professional care knowledge with the client's care knowledge and practices to negotiate and promote care for clients that reflect the client's values. When these decisions and actions are used in conjunction with cultural brokering, the nurse is able to fulfill the various roles vital to providing holistic care for culturally diverse clients.

Cultural Preservation

When nurses use culture preservation they are able to support clients to use those aspects of the client's culture that promote healthy behaviors. For example, the nurse allows a client, whose culture is based on an extended-family network, time to discuss a health matter with family members and refrains from influencing the client to make a unilateral decision quickly.

Cultural Accommodation

In using culture accommodation, nurses recognize that even though they believe that a particular practice has no scientific utility for health promotion or disease prevention, they would recognize the cultural relevance of the practice and help clients to integrate it with the planned treatment protocol. Nurses may accommodate the oral tradition of African-Americans when educating them about AIDS. This requires greater use of dialogue and other forms of verbal communication while decreasing the emphasis on written material. Such a teaching strategy would reflect the importance of oral networks in meeting the needs of the African-American community.

Research Brief

Parker JG: The lived experience of Native Americans with diabetes within a transcultural nursing perspective, J *Transcult Nurs* 6:5-11, 1994.

The purpose of this qualitative study was to discover, document, and analyze the lived experiences of Native Americans diagnosed with non-insulin dependent diabetes mellitus (NIDDM). The sample consisted of 10 Native Americans, who were at least 25 years of age and who were diagnosed with NIDDM for at least 5 years. Data were gathered through clinical observations and nonstructured, taped interviews, which took place in the clients' homes, mainly around the kitchen table.

Themes and patterns of statements were put into six categories: (1) characteristic reactions to NIDDM, (2) characteristic responses to loss of health, (3) identification with others, (4) fear associated with the disease process, (5) peace associated with diagnosis of NIDDM and self-care, and (6) grieving associated with diagnosis of NIDDM.

Findings suggest that NIDDM had become a way of life for Native Americans who expected that at some time during the course of living, they would develop NIDDM. They made modifications in their daily behavior that allowed them to participate in traditional lifeways while at the same time living with the disruptions of the disease. The value of sharing cultural traditions with family and community was often more important to them than maintaining dietary control. When participants made these choices, they did so knowing the negative consequences of their actions on health. Results of this study underscore the need for community health nurses to understand the Native American's view of diabetes as it affects quality-of-life issues. Moreover, it supports the need to develop diabetes education programs that are compatible with the Native American's perspective, even if it is different from the dominant Anglo American Culture.

Cultural Repatterning

Cultural repatterning focuses on nurses' actions to help clients make changes in culture behaviors when these behaviors are harmful, negative, or maladaptive to the clients' well-being. Since diabetes is positively correlated with obesity (Kumanyika and Ewart, 1990), culturally competent nurses would discuss and integrate cultural foods and religious practices in weight reduction and diabetes management strategies. The nurse also would teach diabetic clients how to make adjustments in cultural eating patterns to minimize diabetes complications.

Culture Brokering

Culture brokering is another action used by culturally competent nurses to ensure that clients receive culturally appropriate care (Jezewski, 1990). **Culture brokering** is advocating, mediating, negotiating, and intervening between the health care culture and the client's culture on behalf of clients. Culturally competent community health nurses are in a position to understand both cultures and may use knowledge to resolve or minimize problems that may have resulted from individuals in either culture not understanding the other person's culture. Nurses should understand the impact of occupational mobility, poverty, and formal education on migrant workers' use of preventive health care, and that they may only seek health care when they are ill and unable to work. When nurses care for them, they teach about such issues as environmental sanitation, nutrition, and preventive maintenance because it may be the only opportunity that the nurse will ever have with those particular migrant workers.

INHIBITORS TO DEVELOPING CULTURAL COMPETENCE

When nurses fail to provide culturally competent nursing care, it may be because they have had minimal opportunity for learning about transcultural nursing, pressure from community health agencies to increase productivity with increases in case loads, or pressure from colleagues and community who are not knowledgeable about cultural concepts (Sands and Hale, 1987). A combination of any of these factors may result in nurses' behaviors, such as stereotyping, prejudice and racism, ethnocentrism, cultural imposition, cultural conflict, and cultural shock.

Stereotyping

Stereotyping is the basis for ascribing certain beliefs and behaviors to groups without recognizing individual differences within the groups (Toupin and Son, 1991). It is a common practice used by all people at one time or another. Stereotyping blocks the willingness of people to be open and learn about specific individuals or groups. In the absence of information and time to observe and judge, nurses make generaliza-

tions about clients that allow for quick decision making. This is problematic in that with added information, people who stereotype are often not receptive to changing these ideas. New information may be distorted to fit with preconceived ideas and may not reflect the facts. Stereotypes can be positive or negative. Nurses use negative stereotypes when they label individuals by diagnosis, such as labeling a Native American who complains of gastric symptoms as an alcoholic before assessing the source of his problem or labeling a young, African-American woman with abdominal pain as having a sexually transmitted disease. Asians are stereotyped as the "model" minority group; as such, there is the expectation that they will always behave in ways that reinforce this stereotypical notion. Other groups are stereotyped as "industrious and hard working." To minimize the use of stereotypes, nurses should consider the interplay of culture, economics, and individual choice on behavior as they interact with clients.

Prejudice and Racism

Prejudice is the emotional manifestation of deeply held beliefs about other groups (Brislin, 1993). It usually denotes negative attitudes. Some individuals believe that persons of a particular race, skin color, cultural practice, or social standing are inferior and cannot benefit fully from society's offerings of education, good jobs, and community activities (Brislin, 1993). To justify these beliefs, individuals may then deny persons who are different from themselves the opportunity to benefit from societal offerings.

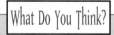

| What Do You Think? |

A 90-year-old South American woman refuses to have her nursing care provided by an African-American nurse. Should a nurse from another racial group be assigned to provide the care or should the client be transferred to another community health agency?

Racism, a form of prejudice, refers to the belief that persons who are born into a particular group are inferior in intelligence, morals, beauty, self-worth, and so forth (Brislin, 1993). The Tuskegee Syphilis Study is a well-known example of racism directed at a specific cultural group (Thomas and Quinn, 1991). This study was conducted by the Public Health Service (PHS) to observe the effects of syphilis on African-American men over a period of 40 years. African-American men with syphilis were recruited for the study but were not told that they had syphilis. These men were told that they were being treated for "bad blood," and yet treatment for syphilis was being withheld. As a result, hundreds of men lost their lives because of the effects of syphilis. The consequence of such racism is that not only do some African-Americans believe that research might be designed to harm them, but that all care might be a part of a research study designed to harm, especially government programs.

Prejudice and racism can be understood using a two-dimensional matrix: overt versus covert and intentional versus unintentional, (Locke and Hardaway, 1980). There are four types of prejudice/racism that result from this matrix and that exist in society. Since nurses are members of society, they too can exhibit prejudice. The following examples are behaviors of nurses that reflect each type of racism.

1. *Overt Intentional.* A nurse does not explain community resources to minority clients because he or she believes that minorities receive too much government assistance.

2. *Overt Unintentional.* Two clients attend the neighborhood health care center. The nurse develops an extensive teaching plan that provides the nonminority client with information on the effects of sodium on kidney functioning. The nurse feels that the minority client is not capable of understanding such complex information and does not develop a teaching plan for the client. At the end of the client's visit, the nurse says to the client, "Take care of yourself. I will see you next time."

3. *Covert Intentional.* The nurse provides clients with information about hypertension and does not discuss with them their cultural diet practices but expects them to engage in behavioral modification.

4. *Covert Unintentional.* A nurse makes a home visit to see an Hispanic family with seven children. Because the client does not volunteer information, the nurse assumes that she is an illegal immigrant who does not have health insurance and cannot afford nursing care services.

Ethnocentrism

Ethnocentrism or cultural prejudice is the belief that your cultural group determines the standards for behavior by which all other groups are to be judged (Locke, 1992). This is in contrast to **cultural blindness** in which differences between cultures are ignored, and the person acts as though they do not exist (Andrews and Boyle, 1995). Persons with ethnocentric beliefs devalue behaviors that differ from their own and judge other behaviors to be inferior. Nurses who have an ethnocentric approach devalue clients' experiences because they are unfamiliar and make the nurse uncomfortable; the nurse may treat the client's behavior with suspicion or hostility (Andrews and Boyle, 1995).

Cultural Imposition

The belief in one's own superiority, or ethnocentrism, may lead to cultural imposition. **Cultural imposition** is the process of imposing one's values on others.

Nurses are imposing their values on clients when they forcefully promote Western medical traditions while ignoring the clients' value of non-Western treatments, such as acupuncture, herbal therapy, or spiritualistic rituals.

Cultural Conflict

Cultural conflict is a perceived threat that may arise from a misunderstanding of expectations between clients and nurses when either group is not aware of cultural differences (Andrews and Boyle, 1995). Although cultural conflicts are unavoidable, the goal for nurses should be to manage conflicts so that they do not impede the delivery of culturally competent nursing care (Brislin, 1993).

Cultural Shock

Cultural shock may occur when nurses interact with clients whose culture is different from their own, especially cultures of which they have little knowledge or exposure (Friedman, 1992). Cultural shock may be a normal reaction to beliefs and practices of clients' cultures that are disallowed or disapproved of in the nurse's own culture (Andrews and Boyle, 1995). When in clients' homes nurses may find that the differences between cultures may be more obvious to them than in some other settings than others because of feelings of powerlessness in an environment where their control is drastically reduced. Being aware of their own cultural beliefs and having knowledge of other cultures may help nurses to be less judgmental and more accepting of cultural differences.

CULTURAL NURSING ASSESSMENT

A cultural nursing assessment is "a systematic appraisal or examination of individuals, groups, and communities as to their cultural beliefs, values, and practices to determine specific needs and interventions within the cultural context of the people being evaluated" (Leininger, 1978, pp. 85-86). It is a component of data collection that nurses use to help them identify and understand clients' perspectives of health and illness. By adopting a relativistic approach, nurses avoid judging or evaluating clients' beliefs and values in terms of their own culture.

A nonjudgmental perspective toward the client's cultural dimensions is facilitated through such skills as listening explaining, acknowledging, recommending, and negotiating (Berlin and Fowkes, 1982). It is vital that nurses listen to clients' perceptions of their problems and, in turn, that nurses explain to clients their own perceptions of problems discussed. Nurses and clients should acknowledge and discuss similarities and differences in the two perceptions in order to develop recommendations for management of problems. Finally, nurses must negotiate with clients on nursing care actions to meet clients' needs.

A variety of tools are available to assist nurses in conducting cultural assessments (Andrews and Boyle, 1995; Fong, 1985; Leininger, 1991; Tripp-Reimer et al., 1984). The focus of such tools varies, and selection is determined by the dimensions of culture to be assessed.

During initial contacts with clients, nurses should perform a cultural assessment, which may be brief or the beginning of an in-depth assessment (Tripp-Reimer et al, 1984). In a brief cultural assessment, nurses ask clients about their ethnic background, religious preference, family patterns, food patterns, and health practices. Such basic information would help nurses to understand the client from the client's perspective and to recognize the uniqueness of the client and thus avoid stereotyping. Data from a brief assessment help to determine the need for an in-depth cultural assessment.

Data for an in-depth cultural assessment should be conducted over a period of time and not be restricted to the first encounter with the client. This gives both clients and nurses time to get to know each other and, especially for clients, to perceive nurses in helping relationships. Tripp-Reimer and her colleagues (1984) suggest that an in-depth cultural assessment should be conducted in two phases: a collection phase and an organization phase. The data collection phase consists of three stages. First the nurse collects self-identifying data similar to that which was collected in the brief assessment. In the next stage the nurse raises a variety of questions that would elicit information on clients' perception of what brings them to the health care system, the illness, and treatments expected. In the third stage, which occurs after the nursing diagnosis is made, nurses identify cultural factors that may influence the effectiveness of nursing care actions.

In the organization phase, data are systematically examined, and areas of incongruence between the client's cultural needs and the goals of Western medicine are identified. Nurses may utilize Leininger's (1991) three actions (as discussed on page 123) to guide them in selecting and discussing culturally appropriate interventions with clients.

Members of minority groups may distrust and fear the Western medical health care system of which nurses are a part. Persons from these cultures initially may have difficulty discussing their beliefs, values, and practices with nurses. This would be especially so when they do not know how nurses will receive the information.

The key to a successful cultural assessment lies in nurses being aware of their own culture. Randall-David (1989) developed a variety of principles that may be helpful as nurses conduct cultural assessments. Nurses should

1. Always be cognizant of their environments. They should look around them and listen to what is being said and understand nonverbal communications before asking questions or taking action.

2. Know about community social organizations, such as schools, churches, hospitals, tribal councils, restaurants, taverns, and bars.
3. Know the specific areas that they want to focus on before they begin the cultural assessment.
4. Select a strategy to help them gather cultural data. Strategies may include in-depth interviews, informal conversations, observations of everyday activities or specific events of the client, survey research, and a case-method approach to study certain aspects of a client.
5. Identify a confidante that will help "bridge the gap" between cultures.
6. Know the appropriate questions to ask without offending the clients.
7. Interview other nurses or health care professionals who have worked with the specific client to get their input.
8. Talk with formal and informal community leaders to gain a comprehensive understanding about significant aspects of community life.
9. Be aware that all information has both subjective and objective aspects and they should verify and cross check the information that is collected before acting on it.
10. Avoid pitfalls in making premature generalizations.
11. Be sincere, open, and honest with themselves and the clients.

Using a Translator

Communication with the clients or families is required for a cultural assessment. When nurses do not speak or understand the client's language, they should make every effort to obtain assistance from a translator. Hatton's (1992) research findings suggest that nurses should be aware of the powerful role translators play in determining information shared between clients and nurses. Translators may emphasize their personal preferences by influencing both nurses' and clients' decisions to select and participate in treatment modalities. Nurses may minimize this by learning basic words and sentences of the most commonly spoken language(s) in the community. In addition, nurses should consider the following when they use translators:

1. When feasible, select translators who have knowledge of health-related terminology.
2. Observe the client for nonverbal messages, such as facial expressions, gestures, and other forms of body language (Giger and Davidhizar, 1995). If the client's responses do not fit with the question, the nurse should check to be sure that the translator understands the question.
3. Accuracy in transmission of information may be increased by asking the translators to translate the client's own words and asking the client to repeat the information that was communicated.

4. Family members as translators should be used with caution because it may not be culturally appropriate to discuss intimate health matters with certain family members (Tripp-Reimer and Afifi, 1989).
5. Gender of the translator may be of concern particularly when asking questions about sexuality or child birth (Brown, 1990; Tripp-Reimer et al., 1984).
6. Differences in socioeconomic status and educational level between the client and the translator may lead to problems in interpretation of information. Confidentiality also may be threatened if the client and the translator are from the same community.
7. Birth origin and language or dialect spoken should be identified before selecting a translator. For example, Chinese clients speak different languages depending on the region in their homeland in which they were born.
8. Avoid using professional jargon, colloquialisms, abstractions, idiomatic expressions, slang similes, and metaphors (Randall-David, 1989). Nurses should speak slowly and use words that are common in the client's culture.
9. Clarify roles with the translator and review the situation and information to be translated prior to and at the end of each health care encounter (Hatton, 1992).

VARIATIONS AMONG CULTURAL GROUPS

Although all cultures are not the same, all cultures have the same basic organizational factors (Giger and Davidhizar, 1995). These factors should be explored in a cultural assessment because of their potential for differences among groups. They are (1) communication, (2) space, (3) social organization, (4) time, (5) environment control, and (6) biological variations. Some of these differences among cultural groups are presented in Table 7-4.

Communication

Verbal and nonverbal patterns of communication vary across cultures, and if nurses do not understand the client's cultural rules in communication, the client's acceptance of a treatment regimen may be jeopardized (Price and Cordell, 1994). An example of this occurred when a nurse gave instructions to Asian clients on taking antituberculin drugs. The clients smilingly responded with "yes, yes." The nurse interpreted this response to mean that the clients understood the instructions and that they were accepting of the treatment protocol. One week later, when the clients returned for a follow-up visit, the nurse discovered that the medications had not been taken. The nurse knew that acceptance by and avoidance of confrontation or disagreement with those in authority are important behaviors in the Asian culture; interventions were ad-

justed accordingly. The nurse repeated the medication instructions, gave the clients an opportunity to raise questions and concerns and to repeat the instructions that were given. The nurse also discussed the cultural meaning and treatment of tuberculosis.

Space

Personal space is the area that persons need between themselves and others in order to feel comfortable. Findings from Hall's (1963) research indicate that Anglo American nurses have the following specific spatial preferences that may be observed when they care for clients.
1. *An intimate zone* (0 to 18 inches) is used when performing specific aspects of a physical assessment, such as an eye, ear, or nose examination. Entering this zone may be discomforting for both clients and nurses when they have not had time to establish a trusting relationship with each other.
2. *Personal distance* (18 inches to 4 feet) is used when performing other aspects of the physical examination
3. *Social distance* (4 to 12 feet) is used for small-group interaction when no touching is required.
4. *Public distance* (12 or more feet) is used during impersonal interaction, such as conducting workshops and community meetings.

Other cultural groups also have spatial preferences. To illustrate, Hispanics tend to be comfortable with less space because they like to touch persons with whom they are speaking. Asians may view touching strangers as inappropriate; therefore, nurses may stand further away from Asian than from Hispanic clients. Community health nurses should take cues from clients in order to place themselves in the appropriate spatial zone and avoid misinterpretation of clients' behavior as they handle their spatial needs.

Social Organization

Social organizations, especially that of the family, also are defined differently across cultural groups. In the African-American culture, for example, family may include individuals who are unrelated or remotely related. Members of families depend on the extended family and kinship networks for emotional and financial support in times of crises. Mothers and grandmothers play significant roles in African-American households and should be included in health care decisions. The significance of family also varies across cultures. This is particularly so in the Hispanic and Asian cultures. Members of these groups tend to believe that the needs of families come before those of individuals. In the Native American cultures, members honor and respect their elders and look to them for leadership, believing that wisdom comes with increasing age (West, 1993). When working with clients from these cultures, nurses should be aware that it

Table 7-4   Variations among Selected Cultural Groups

	African-Americans	Asians	Hispanics	Native Americans
Verbal communication	Asking personal questions of some one that you have met for the first time is seen as improper and intrusive.	High respect for others, especially those in positions of authority.	Expression of negative feelings is considered impolite.	Speaks in a low tone of voice and expects that the listener will be attentive.
Non-verbal communication	Direct eye contact in conversation is often considered rude.	Direct eye contact among superiors may be considered disrespectful.	Avoidance of eye contact is usually a sign of attentiveness and respect.	Direct eye contact is often considered disrespectful.
Touch	Touching another's hair is often considered offensive.	It is not customary to shake hands with persons of the opposite sex.	Touching is often observed between two persons in conversation.	A light touch of the person's hand instead of a firm handshake is often used when greeting a person.
Family organization	Usually have close, extended family networks. Women play key roles in health care decisions.	Usually have close, extended family ties. Emphasis may be on family needs rather than individual needs.	Usually have close, extended family ties. All members of the family may be involved in health care decisions.	Usually have close, extended family ties. Emphasis tends to be on family rather than on individual needs.
Time	Often present oriented.	Often present oriented.	Often present oriented.	Often present oriented.
Perception of health	Harmony of mind, and spirit with nature.	When there is a balance between the "yin" and "yang" energy forces.	Balance and harmony among mind, body, spirit, and nature.	Harmony of mind, body, spirit, and emotions with nature.
Alternative healers	"Granny," "root doctor," voodoo priest, spiritualist.	Acupuncturist, acupressurist, herbalist.	Curandero, espiritualista, yerbero.	Medicine man, shaman.
Self-care practices	Poultices, herbs, oils, roots.	Hot and cold foods, herbs, teas, soups, cupping, burning, rubbing, pinching.	Hot and cold foods, herbs.	Herbs, corn meal, medicine bundle.
Biological variations	Sickle cell anemia, mongolian spots, keloid formation, inverted "T" waves, lactose intolerance, skin color.	Thalassemia, drug interactions, mongolian spots, lactose intolerance, skin color.	Mongolian spots, lactose intolerance, skin color.	Cleft uvula, lactose intolerance, skin color.

From Giger JN, Davidhizar RE: *Transcultural nursing,* ed 2, St Louis, 1995, Mosby; Spector RE: *Cultural diversity in health and illness,* ed 3, Norwalk, Conn, 1991, Appleton & Lange; Payne KT: In Taylor OL, editor: *Nature of Communication disorders in culturally and linguistically diverse populations,* San Diego, 1986, College Hill Press.

may be futile to exclude family involvement in decision making. At the same time, nurses should advocate for the individual, so that when families make decisions, the individual's needs also are being considered.

Time Perception

The perception of time also differs across cultures. Some cultures are considered future oriented, others present oriented, and still others past oriented (Brink, 1984). In the American middle-class culture, time takes on a future orientation and individuals are willing to delay immediate gratification until future goals are accomplished. Clients valuing longevity may moderate their dietary intake and engage in exercise activities to minimize future health risks. In contrast, poorer families may place greater value on quality of life and view present time as being more important than future time. They may ignore dietary restrictions so that they enjoy closeness with family in cultural celebrations. When nurses discuss health-promotion and disease-prevention strategies with persons from a present time orientation, they should focus on the immediate benefits these clients would derive rather than on future outcomes. In cultures that focus on a past orientation, for example, the Vietnamese culture, individuals may focus on wishes and memories of their ancestors and look to them to provide direction for current situations (Giger and Davidhizar, 1995). In this culture, time is viewed as being more flexible than in the American culture. It has less of a fixed point and individuals are not offended by being late or early for appointments. Along with culture, socioeconomic status influences perception of time, and nurses should clarify the clients' perception in order to avoid misunderstanding.

Environmental Control

Environmental control refers to the relationships between humans and nature. Some groups perceive man as having mastery over nature, others perceive humans to be dominant by nature, while others see harmonious relationships between humans and nature (Brink, 1984). Individuals who perceive mastery over nature believe that they can overcome the natural forces of nature. Such individuals would expect curative results for malignancy through the use of medications, antibiotics, surgical interventions, radiation, and chemotherapies. In contrast, in the subjugation-to-nature view, which is held by many African-Americans and Hispanics, individuals believe that they have little or no control over what happens to them. They may not adhere to a cancer treatment protocol because of the belief that nothing will change the outcome because it is their destiny. These individuals are less likely than those of other world views to engage in imagery or meditation activities. Persons who hold the harmony-with-nature view, such as

Asians and Native Americans, may perceive that illness is a disharmony with other forces and that medicine is only able to relieve the symptoms rather than cure the disease. These groups are likely to look to naturalistic solutions, such as herbs and hot and cold treatments to resolve or cure a cancerous condition.

Biological Variations

Biological variations distinguish one racial group from another. They occur in areas of growth and development, skin color, enzymatic differences, and susceptibility to disease (Andrews and Boyle, 1995; Giger and Davidhizar, 1995). For example, Western-born neonates are slightly heavier at birth than those born in non-Western cultures. Another biological variation is mongolian spots that are present on the skin of African-American, Asian, Mexican, and Native American babies. These are bluish discolorations that may be mistaken for bruises. Other common and obvious variations include skin color, eye shape, hair texture, adipose tissue deposits, shape of ear lobes, thickness of lips, and body configuration. Variations in growth and development may be influenced by environmental conditions, such as nutrition, climate, and disease.

DIETARY PRACTICES AND CULTURAL ORIENTATION

Dietary practices are an integral part of the assessment process for all families, especially since they play a prominent role in health problems of some groups (Healthy People 2000, 1991). Efforts to understand dietary patterns of clients need to go beyond relying on membership in a defined group. Knowing clients' assimilative practices makes it possible to develop treatment regimens that would not conflict with their cultural food practices. The box below identifies a number of questions that nurses would want to ask when conducting a dietary assessment.

In mutual goal setting with the client and nutritionist to change harmful dietary practices, the nurse might need to consult culturally oriented magazines.

 Assessment of Dietary Practices and Food Consumption Patterns

What is the social significance of food in your family?
What foods are most frequently bought for family consumption?
Who makes the decision to buy the food?
What foods, if any, are taboo or prohibited for the family?
Does religion play a significant role in food selection?
Who prepares the food? How is it prepared?
How much food is eaten, when is it eaten, and with whom?
Where does the client live, and what types of restaurants do they frequent?
Has the family adopted foods of other cultural groups?
What are the family's favorite recipes?

Table 7-5   Selected Food Preferences and Associated Risk Factors among Selected Cultural Groups

Cultural group	Food preferences	Nutritional excess	Risk factors
African-Americans	Fried foods, greens, bread, lard, pork, and rice.	Cholesterol, fat, sodium, carbohydrates, and calories.	Coronary heart disease, and obesity
Asians	Soy sauce, rice, pickled dishes, and raw fish.	Cholesterol, fat, sodium, carbohydrates, and calories.	Coronary heart diease, liver disease, cancer of the stomach, and ulcers.
Hispanics	Fried foods, beans and rice, chili, carbonated beverages	Cholesterol, fat, sodium, carbohydrates, and calories.	Coronary heart disease and obesity.
Native Americans	Blue corn meal, fruits, game and fish.	Carbohydrates and calories.	Diabetes, malnutrition, tuberculosis, infant and maternal mortality.

Data from Andrews and Boyle: *Transcultural concepts in nursing,* ed 2, Philadelphia, 1995, JB Lippincott; Giger and Davidhizar: *Transcultural nursing,* ed 2, St Louis, 1995, Mosby; Jackson and Broussard: Cultural challenges in nutrition education among American Indians, *Diabetes Educator* 13(1): 47-50, 1987.

A number of popular magazines, such as *Essence* and *Ebony,* have created new dishes from old family recipes using healthier ingredients. These dishes are very tasty and resemble old traditions, yet, they are not as harmful.

Table 7-5 lists various dietary practices that are prevalent among some cultural groups in American society. Many of these practices may have their origin in religious, as well as cultural, traditions. Religion may become a medium for creating additional tensions in the nurse-client relationship as nurses negotiate with clients to meet their health needs.

SOCIOECONOMIC FACTORS AND CULTURE

Socioeconomic factors contribute significantly to understanding perceptions of health and illness among minority groups. These groups usually do not have similar opportunities for education, occupation, income earning, and property ownership as the dominant group. Consequently, members of minority groups are disproportionately represented on the lower tiers of the socioeconomic ladder. Poor economic achievement is also a common characteristic found among populations at risk, such as those in poverty, the homeless, migrant workers, and refugees.

Nurses should be able to distinguish between culture and socioeconomic class issues and not misinterpret behavior as having a cultural origin when in fact it should be attributed to socioeconomic class (Payne, 1986). Data suggest that when nurses and clients come from the same social class, it is likely that they operate from the same health belief model, consequently, there is less opportunity for misinterpretation and communication problems.

There is also danger in believing that certain cultural behaviors, such as folk practices, are restricted to lower socioeconomic classes. Roberson (1987) found that health professionals, such as nurses and physicians, also used folk systems in conjunction with the biomedical system to promote their health and prevent disease. Hence, there is the necessity for community health nurses to conduct a cultural assessment for all individuals when they first come in contact with them.

Community health nurses should have guidance in integrating cultural concepts with other aspects of patient care to meet their clients' total health care needs. The last section of this chapter provides illustrations of the principles of cultural diversity in community health nursing practice.

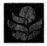 **Clinical Application**

Case 1: Nurse-Client Interaction

The first case study illustrates a nurse-client interaction where the nurse skillfully negotiates with the client and family to improve the family's health within the context of their culture.

Mr. Nguyen, a 64-year-old man, from rural Vietnam, entered the United States with his family 3 years ago through the displaced persons program. Mr Nguyen was a farmer in his homeland, and since his arrival he has been unable to obtain a stable job that would allow him to adequately care for his family. His finan-

cial resources are limited and he has no insurance. He speaks enough English to interact directly with people outside his family and community. His oldest daughter, Shu Ping, is enrolled in a 2-year program to become a registered nurse.

The Nguyen family attends the neighborhood church where there are other Vietnamese families. Mr. Nguyen also has been attending the clinic at the hospital but refuses to discuss with his family, even with Shu Ping, the reason for these visits. Shu Ping became increasingly concerned because she observed her fa-

Clinical Application—cont'd

ther to have insomnia, retarded motor activity, an inability to concentrate, and weight loss. But Mr. Nguyen denied that he was not well. Shu Ping decided to discuss her concerns with a nurse, with whom she had developed an attachment at the church. She invited the nurse to her home for lunch on a Saturday so she could meet her father and validate her impressions.

After several visits with the family, the nurse was able to establish a close enough relationship with Mr. Nguyen to engage him in a discussion of his health. Because of her extensive work with other Vietnamese immigrants, the nurse was familiar with themes of loss and decided to focus her conversation with Mr. Nguyen on his adjustment to the new community living, gains and losses as a result of immigration, and coping strategies. After several discussions with Mr. Nguyen, he confided in the nurse that he feared that he was dying because he had been diagnosed with cancer of the small intestine. He further revealed that he did not share the diagnosis with the family because he did not want them to know of his "bad news." Mr. Nguyen had refused treatment because he knew that people never got better after they had gotten cancer; they always died.

The following are considerations that should be taken in providing culturally competent nursing care:
1. Assess the degree of acculturation to the new environment.
2. Discuss the meaning of health to the client.
3. Discuss the prognosis for a person with cancer in Vietnam.
4. Discuss the prognosis for a person with cancer in the United States.
5. Discuss the medical treatment and surgical interventions for cancer of the intestines.
6. Discuss how the nurse may involve the family in his care and decision making.
7. Discuss how the nurse may act as a culture broker to change the client's expected outcome.
8. Assess the family's coping skills and ability to support the client's diagnosis and treatment.
9. Assess the family's support systems.

Case 2: Health Beliefs

This second case study illustrates the nurse acknowledging and respecting the client's health beliefs about illness, even though these beliefs may be different from the nurse's own. The nurse is able to understand multiple world views, to explain illness, to seek symptom relief for the client, and to judge the efficacy of health care outcomes.

Ms. Lopez brought her 18-month-old daughter, Maria, to the pediatric clinic at the community health center. Ms. Lopez reported that Maria had diarrhea of 48-hours' duration, loss of appetite, and bloated abdomen that was tender to touch. A review of health systems by the physician revealed no abnormalities, and vital signs were within normal limits for Maria's age. Based on these findings, the physician told Ms. Lopez that she found nothing wrong with Maria and if the appetite did not improve in 2 days, she should bring the baby back to see her.

Ms. Lopez then went to the nurse's office and requested that the nurse review the physician's findings with her. The nurse observed that Ms. Lopez still seemed very concerned about the baby and did not appear to be relieved to hear that Maria was well. The nurse shared with Ms. Lopez her observations and asked for validation. In talking with Ms. Lopez, the nurse found out that she had changed the baby's formula 3 days ago and her mother-in-law had diagnosed Maria as having *empacho*. Her mother-in-law was insisting that she take Maria to see a *sobadora*. Ms. Lopez too felt that something was wrong with the baby, but she was unsure what to do since the physician said that the baby was fine. Ms. Lopez also shared that when she was a child in Mexico she had *empacho* and was treated by a *sobadora* who performed an abdominal massage with warm oil and prepared herbal teas for her.

The nurse made an appointment for the mother to return to the clinic the next day where the baby could be examined in her presence by a sobadora. Because of the number of Hispanic mothers who use folk practices, the nurse had incorporated into her weekly schedule consultations with a reputable sobadora who understood modern medicine and folk practices.

The following considerations should be taken in providing culturally competent nursing care:
1. Demonstrate sensitivity to variations in beliefs and behavior.
2. Have knowledge about commonly held beliefs for cultural groups in your community and for whom you frequently care.
3. Know the resources within the community.
4. Use brokering techniques to successfully negotiate between different world views.
5. Conduct an accurate nursing assessment.
6. Incorporate other treatments into nursing management.

Case 3: Communication

The third case study exemplifies in one interaction how communication difficulties can develop when a nurse is oblivious to the client's culture, and how a nurse can enhance communication and shorten the cultural distance between herself and the client.

Ms. Jones, a 25-year-old Jamaican mother of a 3-month-old baby, currently is residing in a transitional homeless shelter for abused women. She has been a housewife for 4 years, but has 2 years of college, suggesting marketable skills. One morning, Ms. Jones became very upset and loud, screaming that her baby was crying, and her comfort measures were not consoling the baby. The nurse had interacted with Ms. Jones on previous occasions and found her

Continued.

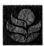

Clinical Application—cont'd

to have a very quiet and caring demeanor and asked her why she was upset. The client responded that she was upset for two reasons. First, she did not have access to "gripe water," a common home remedy used for babies with perceived gastrointestinal distress. Secondly, and more significantly, she heard a nurse refer to her as "woman," rather than calling her by her name. The client interpreted the nurse's behavior as disrespectful and felt that because she lived in a shelter, she was not being treated with dignity.

The following considerations should be taken in providing culturally competent nursing care:

1. Explore with the client why she is upset.
2. Discuss with the client what "woman" means in her culture.
3. Explain the generic meaning of "woman" in the American Culture.
4. Offer to act as a mediator and express the client's feelings to her nurse colleague.
5. Offer the client an opportunity to participate in the mediation process.
6. Increase one's knowledge on "gripe water" and explore ways that the client may obtain it.
7. Discuss comforting techniques and, if necessary, offer additional ones.
8. Evaluate whether or not the client's problems were resolved or minimized through accepting and integrating the client's culture values in the treatment protocol.

Key Concepts

♦ Learning about different cultures helps to prepare community health nurses to competently care for clients from diverse cultures.
♦ Culturally competent nursing care means that the negotiated treatment protocol reflects clients' experiences.
♦ Nurses may use cultural preservation, cultural accommodation, cultural repatterning, and cultural brokering to provide culturally competent care.

♦ The needs of clients vary based on variables, such as age, education, religion and socioeconomic status; each client should be assessed to determine his/her specific cultural needs.
♦ Nurses should complete a cultural assessment on every client with whom they interact.
♦ Cultural competence means that the nurse has attained cultural awareness, has cultural knowledge, uses cultural skills, and has cultural encounters with culturally diverse clients.

Critical Thinking Activities

1. Discuss the pros and cons of cross-cultural preparation for community health nurses.
2. Visit the local Health Department to identify cultural groups in your local area. Indicate the percentage of each group.
3. Conduct an interview with a person of a different culture. Determine the cultural meaning of illness, time, and religion for that individual.
4. Describe what it has felt like to be put in an inferior position or have disparaging remarks made about you.
5. Identify some positive and negative stereotypes that are used to describe groups in your community. Discuss the implication for these stereotypes in health teaching and for these groups.
6. Discuss how socialization in your community has influenced your selection of friends and colleagues.
7. Interview an older person. Discuss his or her use of folk practices in health promotion and disease prevention.
8. Interview a health professional. Discuss his or her use of folk practices in health promotion and disease prevention.
9. Identify the major values of the dominant culture. Discuss how they differ from other cultural groups.
10. Discuss strategies that you could use when caring for clients who do not speak your language and for whom no translator is readily available.

Bibliography

AAN Expert Panel on Culturally Competent Health Care: Culturally competent health care, *Nurs Outlook* 40:277-283, 1992.

Anderson JM: Health care across cultures, *Nurs Outlook,* 38:136-139, 1990.

Andrews MM, Boyle JS: *Transcultural concepts in nursing care,* ed 2, Philadelphia, 1995, JB Lippincott.

Berlin E, Fowkes W: A teaching framework for cross-cultural health care, *West J Med* 139:934-938, 1982.

Bernal H: A model for delivering culture-relevant care in the community, *Public Health Nurs* 10(4):228-232, 1993.

Bernal H, Froman R: The confidence of community health nurses in caring for ethnically diverse populations, *Image* 19:201-203, 1987.

Bowser BP: Cross-cultural medicine: a decade later, *West J Med* 157:286-289, Sept, 1992.

Brink PJ: Value orientations as an assessment tool in cultural diversity, *Nurs Res* 33:198-203, 1984.

Brislin R: *Understanding culture's influence on behavior,* Fort Worth, Tex, 1993 Harcourt Brace College Publishers.

Brookins GK: Culture, ethnicity, and bicultural competence: implications for children with chronic disease and disability, *Pediatrics* 92:1056-1062, 1993.

Brown BJ: A world view of nursing practice. In Chaska NL, editor: *The nursing profession,* St Louis, 1990, Mosby, pp 406-414.

Buchwald D, Panwala S, Hooton T: Use of traditional health practices by Southeast Asian refugees in primary care clinic, *West J Med* 156:507-511, 1992.

Campinha-Bacote J: *The process of cultural competence,* Wyoming, Ohio, 1991, Transcultural CARE Associates.

Caudle P: Providing culturally sensitive health care to Hispanic clients, *Nurse Pract* 18(12):40, 43-47, 1993.

Center for Disease Control: *Diabetes in the United States: a strategy for prevention,* Public Health Service, Washington, DC, 1992, Government Printing Office.

Crow K: Multiculturalism and pluralistic thought in nursing education: Native American world view and the nursing academic world view, *J Nurs Ed* 32(5):198-204, 1993.

Degazon CE: A contrast in ethnic identification, social support, and coping strategies among three cultural groups of African elders, *J Cultural Diversity* 1(4):79-85, 1994.

Degazon CE: Coping, diabetes and the older African American, *Nurs Outlook* (in press).

Denker EP, *Healing at home: Visiting Nurse Service of New York, 1893-1993,* Dalton, Mass, 1994, Studley Press.

DeSantis L, Thomas JT: The immigrant Haitian mother: transcultural nursing perspective on preventive health care for children, *J Transcul Nurs* 2(1):2-15, 1990.

Eliason MJ: Ethics and transcultural nursing care, *Nurs Outlook* 41(5):225-228, 1993.

Fong CM: Ethnicity and nursing practice, *Top Clin Nurs* Sci 7(1): 1-11, 1985.

Frei F, Hugentobler M, Schurman S, Duell W, Alioth A: *Work design for the competent organization,* Westport, Conn, 1994, Quorum Books.

Friedman MM: *Family nursing,* ed 3, Norwalk, Conn, 1992, Appleton & Lange.

Geissler EM: *Pocket guide to cultural assessment,* St Louis, 1994, Mosby.

Giger JN, Davidhizar RE: *Transcultural nursing,* ed 2, St Louis, 1995, Mosby.

Giger JN, Davidhizar R, Cheery B: Biological variations in the Black patient, *Imprint* 32(2):95-105, 1991.

Gordon, MM: *Assimilation in American life,* New York, 1964, Oxford University Press.

Hall CCI: Please choose one: ethnic identity choices. In Root MPP, editor: *Racially mixed people in America,* Newbury Park, Calif, 1992, Sage Publications, pp 250-264.

Hall E: Proxemics: the study of man's spacial relations. In Gladston I, editor: *Man's image in medicine and anthropology,* New York, 1963, International Press.

Hatton DC: Information transmission in bilingual, bicultural contexts, *J Community Health Nurs* 9(1):53-59, 1992.

Healthy people 2000: national health promotion and disease prevention objectives, Washington, DC, 1991, USDHHS, Public Health Service.

Hodnicki DR: Homelessness: health-care implications, *J Community Health Nurs* 7(2):50-67, 1990.

Hodnicki DR, Horner SD: Homeless mothers' caring for children in a shelter, *Issues Ment Health Nurs* 14:349-356, 1993.

Jackson LE: Understanding, eliciting, and negotiating clients' multicultural health beliefs, *Nurse Pract* 18(4):30-43, 1993.

Jackson MM, Broussard BA: Cultural challenges in nutrition education among American Indians, *Diabetes Educator* 13(1):47-50, 1987.

Jezewski MA: Culture brokering in migrant farm worker health care, *West J Nurs Res* 12:497-513, 1990.

Jezewski MA: Culture brokering as a model for advocacy, *Nurs Health Care* 14(2):78-85, 1993.

Kavanagh KH, Kennedy PH: *Promoting cultural diversity,* Newbury Park, Calif, 1992, Sage Publications.

Kumanyika SK, Ewart CK: Theoretical and baseline considerations for diet and weight control of diabetes among Blacks, *Diabetes Care,* 13:1154-1161, 1990.

Lapierre ED, Padgett J: How can we become more aware of culturally specific body language and use this awareness therapeutically? *J Psychosoc Nurs* 29(11):38-41, 1991.

Leininger MM: *Transcultural nursing: concepts, theories, and practices,* New York, 1978, John Wiley & Sons.

Leininger MM: Transcultural nursing: a worldwide necessity to advance nursing knowledge and practice. In McCloskey J, Grace H, editors: *Nursing issues,* Boston, 1989, Little, Brown, & Co.

Leininger MM: *Culture care diversity & universality: a theory of nursing,* New York, 1991, National League for Nursing.

Leininger MM: Culture care theory: the comparative global theory to advance human care nursing knowledge and practice. In Gaut DA, editor: *A global agenda for caring,* New York, 1993, National League for Nursing, pp 3-18.

Lipson JG: Afghan refugee mental health issues, *Issues Ment Health Nurs* 14:411-423, 1993.

Locke DC: *Increasing multicultural understanding,* Newbury Park, Calif, 1992, Sage Publications.

Locke DC, Hardaway YV: Moral perspectives in interracial settings. In Cochrane D, Manley-Casimir M, editors: *Moral education: practical approaches,* New York, 1980, Praeger, pp 269-285.

Mollica RF, Lavelle J: Southeastern Asian refugees. In Comas-Diaz L, Griffith EEM, editors: *Clinical guidelines in cross-cultural mental health,* New York, 1987, John Wiley & Sons.

National Coalition of Hispanic Health and Human Services Organizations (COSSMHO): *Delivering preventive health care to Hispanics: a manual for health providers,* Washington, DC, 1988, COSSMHO.

Orlandi MA editor: *Cultural competence for evaluators,* Washington, DC, 1992, US Department of Health and Human Services.

Orque M: Orque's ethnic/cultural system: a framework for ethnic nursing care. In Orque MS, Bloch B, Monrroy LSA, editors: *Ethnic nursing care: a multi-cultural approach,* St Louis, 1983, Mosby, pp 5-48.

Pachter LM: Culture and clinical care, *JAMA* 71(9):690-694, March 2, 1994.

Parker JG: The lived experience of Native Americans wit diabetes within a transcultural nursing perspective, *J Transcult Nurs* 6:5-11, 1994.

Payne KT: Cultural and linguistic groups in the United States. In Taylor OL, editor: *Nature of communication disorders in culturally and linguistically diverse populations,* San Diego, 1986, College-Hill Press, pp 19-45.

Pellegrino E, Mazzarella P, Corsi P, editors: *Transcultural dimensions in medical ethics,* Federick, Md, 1992, University Publishing Group.

Phillips LA, Luna de Hernandez I, Torres de Ardon E: Focus on psychometrics: strategies for achieving cultural equivalence, *Res Nurs Health* 17:149-154, 1994.

Place BE: Understanding the meaning of chronic illness: a prerequisite for caring. In Gaut DA, editor: *A global agenda for caring,* New York, 1993, National League for Nursing, pp 281-291.

Price JL, Cordell B: Cultural diversity and patient teaching, *J Cont Ed Nurs* 25:163-166, 1994.

Randall-David E: *Strategies for working with culturally diverse communities and clients,* Bethesda, Md, 1989, Association for the Care of Children's Health.

Randall-David E: *Culturally competent HIV counseling and education,* McLean, Va, 1994, The Maternal and Child Health Clearinghouse.

Roberson MHB: Folk health beliefs of health professionals, *West J Nurs Res* 9:257-263, 1987.

Sands RF, Hale SL: Enhancing cultural sensitivity in clinical practice, *J Black Nurses Assoc* 2(1):54-63, 1987.

Seideman RY Williams R, Burns P, Jacobson S, Weatherbyn F, Primeaux M: Culture sensitivity in assessing urban Native American parenting, *Pub Health Nurs* 22(2):98-103, 1994.

Simmons RC: A simple defense of western biomedical explanatory schemata, *Med Anthropol* 15:201-208, 1993.

Snowden LR, Holschuh J: Ethnic differences in emergency psychiatric care and hospitalization is a program for the severely mentally ill, *Community Men Health J* 28:281-291, 1992.

Spangler Z: Generic and professional care of Anglo-American and Philippine American nurses. In Gaut DA, editor: *A global agenda for caring,* New York, 1993, National League for Nursing, pp 47-61.

Schwartz D: Caribbean folk beliefs and Western psychiatry. *J Psychosoc Nurs* 23(11):26-30, 1985.

Spector RE: *Cultural diversity in health and illness,* ed 3, Norwalk, Conn, 1991, Appleton & Lange.

Spickard PR: The illogic of American racial categories. In Root MPP, editor: *Racially mixed people in America,* Newbury Park, Calif, 1992, Sage Publications, pp 12-23.

Thomas SB, Quinn SC: The Tuskegee syphilis study, 1932 to 1972: implications for HIV education and AIDS risk education programs in the Black community, *AJPH* 8(11):1498-1505, 1991.

Thornton MC: The quiet immigration: foreign spouses of U.S. citizens, 1945-1985. In Root MPP, editor: *Racially mixed people in America,* Newbury Park, California, 1992, Sage Publications, pp 64-76.

Toupin E, Son L: Preliminary findings on Asian Americans: the "model minority" in a small private East Coast college, *J Cross-Cult Psychol* 22:403-417, 1991.

Tripp-Reimer T, Afifi LA: Cross-cultural perspectives on patient teaching, *Nurs Clin North Am* 24:613-619, 1989.

Tripp-Reimer T, Brink PJ, Saunders JM: Cultural assessment: content and process, *Nurs Outlook* 32(2):78-82, 1984.

Uba L: Cultural barriers to health care for Southeast Asian refugees, *Pub Health Rep* 107(5):544-548, 1992.

US Department of Commerce: *Statistical abstract of the United States,* ed 114, Washington, DC, 1994, US Government Printing Office.

Wali A: *Multiculturism—An anthropological perspective.* Report from the Institute of Philosophy and Public Policy, 12(1):6-8, 1992.

Wenger AFZ: Cultural meaning of symptoms, *Holist Nurse Pract* 7(2):22-35, 1993.

West EA: The cultural bridge model, *Nurs Outlook* 41:229-237, 1993.

Wilk RJ: The Haitian refugee: concerns for health care providers, *Soc Work Health Care* 11(2):61-74, 1985-1986.

Wuest J: Removing the shackles: a feminist critique of noncompliance, *Nurs Outlook* 41(5):217-224, 1993.

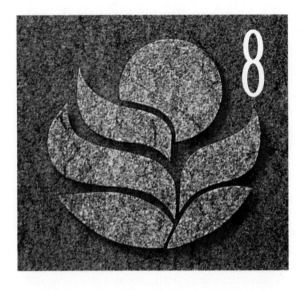

8

Environmental Health

Max R. Lum ◆ Beth F. Hibbs ◆ Lynelle Phillips ◆ Diane M. Narkunas*

Objectives ▼

After reading this chapter, the student should be able to do the following:

◆ Identify and characterize environmental health problems through community or client assessment.
◆ Discuss how to prevent or mitigate potential or actual environmental toxic exposures through primary, secondary, and tertiary interventions.
◆ Define the principles of exposure pathway analysis and toxicologic analysis.
◆ Identify key environmental health information resources.
◆ Develop an interdiscplinary (or team) approach to address environmental health threats.
◆ Describe how to effectively communicate environmental health risks to community members.
◆ Describe inherent ethical, social, and legal implications for environmental health issues and nursing practice.
◆ Describe the role of the community health nurse as a concerned citizen and health provider.
◆ Develop an intervention plan that addresses an environmental issue of concern in your community.

Key Terms ▼

adverse health effects
Agency for Toxic Substances and
    Disease Registry (ATSDR)
air pollution
biomarker
contaminated
environmental exposures
environmental health
environmental justice
environmental pollution
Environmental Protection Agency (EPA)
exposure history
exposure pathways
food chain
hazardous waste
health hazards
health history
health risks
pollutants
risk communication
Superfund
toxicity

Outline ▼

Continued.

*The contributors would like to acknowledge Jeanne A. Bucsela, MS, M Lib, for her editing contribution in the preparation of this chapter, and Mary Ellen Simpson, RN, MS, CNS, for reviewing the content.

Outline–cont'd ▼

The scope of **environmental health** is difficult to define. In the broadest sense, it includes all aspects of the relationship between host and health and the effect of hazardous biological and chemical agents on human health. The current popular concept of environmental disease is related to illness or injury caused by external chemical and physical agents. For this chapter, environmental health excludes a discussion of adverse health effects caused by nicotine, alcohol, diet, or other life-style factors and by workplace exposure because these topics are discussed in other chapters. In short, this chapter's use of the term environmental health refers to the care of individuals exposed to **environmental pollution** in their homes, and neighborhoods through such media as contaminated soil, water, air, and the **food chain.**

Community health nurses are often called upon to address environmental health problems. The impact of changing ecosystems on human health, particularly relative to infectious diseases, is evident. Hazardous

Model Standards for Environmental Health

Air Quality
Food Protection
Noise Control
Radiological Health
Sanitation in Facilities (General)
Sanitation in Facilities (Child Care)
Sanitation in Facilities (Mobile Home Parks)
Sanitation in Facilities (Public Buildings: Governmental and Nongovernmental)
Sanitation in Facilities (Recreational Areas)
Sanitation in Facilities (Schools)
Solid Waste Management
Toxic and Hazardous Substances
Vector and Animal Control
Wastewater Management
Water (Safe Drinking)
Housing Services
Institutional Services
Community Surveillance

(Adapted from *Healthy Communities 2000: model standard guidelines for community attainment*, Washington, DC, 1991, American Public Health Association.)

substances, such as lead-based paint, also affect human health, particularly children's health. Thousands of health professionals, representing many academic disciplines in partnership with consumers, have contributed to producing a set of measurable targets in various areas to be achieved by the year 2000. The report in *Healthy People 2000* goes a long way toward setting priority objectives in the area of environmental health (Healthy People 2000, 1991). The report identifies three priority objectives for environmental health, as shown in the box below: (1) Eliminate blood levels above 25 μg/dl in children under age 5; (2) Increase protection from air pollutants so that at least 85% of people live in counties that meet **Environmental Protection Agency (EPA)** standards; and (3) Increase protection from radon so that at least 40% of people live in homes tested by homeowners and found to be (or made to be) safe (Lum, 1995).

THE ROLE OF COMMUNITY HEALTH NURSES

Historical Perspective

Florence Nightingale, the founder of modern nursing, was famous for her concern about santitation in the human environment. Nightingale focused on developing sanitary codes for military hospitals. She recognized that environmental contamination of army hospitals resulted in **health hazards** for ailing soldiers. Due to her administrative efforts in sanitation, the mortality rate of hospitalized soldiers dropped from 42.7% to 2.2% in 6 months (Donahue, 1985). Nightingale went on to found the Nightingale School of Nurses where she taught her students to be sure that patients always had clean air to breathe and safe water to drink (Nightingale, 1946).

The industrial age brought new problems of hazardous substance pollution. Many methods used to dispose of wastes were not considered harmful and were not regulated. The effects of environmental pollution and the need to regulate the use and disposal of hazardous substances first came to public attention in the 1960s when Rachel Carson wrote *Silent Spring,* a book about the dramatic effects of pesticides on wildlife. Health professionals became increasingly aware of the effects of pollution on health, and some health departments began tracking its effects. In

1966, 80 persons died in New York City from air pollution-related causes during a 4-day atmospheric inversion.

Toxic gas (methyl isocyanate) that leaked from a Union Carbide plant in Bopal, India, in 1984 resulted in the mortality and morbidity of thousands of persons. The release of radiation from a nuclear power plant at Chernobyl in the Soviet Union (1986) contaminated large areas of northern Europe. In the United States during the 1970s, the discovery of widespread distribution of a hazardous substance at Love Canal in New York state led to major concerns regarding chemical dump sites and **hazardous waste.** National incidents like Love Canal and others that followed led to the creation of new regulatory agencies and legislation charged with protecting citizens from hazardous substance exposure.

In response to a growing environmental health problem, the U.S. Food and Drug Administration (FDA) expanded its role, and the following agencies were established: The National Institute of Environmental Sciences (NIEHS) in 1966, the EPA in 1970, the Consumer Product Safety Commission (CPSC) in 1972, and the **Agency for Toxic Substances and Disease Registry (ATSDR)** in 1980.

Hazardous Substances in the Home and Environment

Indoor Air Pollution

Most people today spend 80% to 90% of their time indoors. EPA studies show that many important **pollutants** are far more concentrated inside the home and workplace (Tarcher, 1992). Because young children spend so much time in the home, they may be at particular risk. Air pollution is truly a global problem. Crossing national boundaries often distant from emission sources, it poses immediate and long term human health and environmental concerns.

Tobacco Smoke

Environmental tobbacco smoke is a mixture of more than 4700 compounds. Second-hand smoke also contains carcinogenic hydrocarbons and respirable particles. Increased public concern regarding second-hand smoke has resulted in new laws restricting smoking in public facilities.

Wood Stoves and Gas Ranges

Thirteen million wood stoves are in use in the United States, and 800,000 are sold annually. When not properly maintained or vented, wood stoves emit noxious gases, including carbon monoxide, oxides of nitrogen, particulates, and hydrocarbons.

Building Materials

Building materials used in the home may cause health effects in certain sensitive populations. For example, some building and household materials, such as particle board, insulation, carpet, and carpet adhesives, contain formaldehyde that volatilizes into the air.

Asbestos

From 1950 to early 1970, asbestos was widely applied as a spray in areas requring soundproofing, thermal proofing, or durability. Inhalation of asbestos fibers released into the air has been associated with the development of lung cancer.

Radon

Radon, a colorless, odorless gas, is a product of the uranium decay chain and is found in earth minerals (Amdur et al., 1991). Radon can enter homes through cracks in basement walls and floors. Radon-contaminated well water is another source of human exposure. Radon progeny can enter the body through inhalation of air or ingestion of water contaminated with radon. Radon can also attach to airborne particulates, such as cigatette smoke, and can be inhaled. Radon injures tracheobronchial cells, thereby causing lung cancer (ATSDR, 1990). The EPA estimates that approximately 14,000 lung cancer deaths per year are attributable to radon (Radford, 1985; USEPA, 1993).

Common Household Products

A 1987 EPA study found 12 common organic pollutants from household products at concentrations approximately 2 to 5 times higher in air inside homes than in outdoor air (EPA, 1987). Commonly used compounds that can have serious adverse effects are methylene chloride (found in paint strippers and thinners and adhesive removers), tetrachloroethylene (used in dry cleaning of clothes), and paradichlorobenzene (found in room air fresheners, toilet bowl deodorizers, and moth crystals).

Hazards in External Environment

Pesticide and Lawn Care Products

Pesticides and lawn care products are potentially hazardous, especially to agricultural workers and children. At least 1400 active ingredients are found in more than 34,000 available preparations. Estimated annual use of these chemicals is 2.6 billion pounds. Pesticide exposure can occur through dermal contact, inhalation, or ingestion. Worldwide, intoxications attributed to pesticides have been estimated to cause as many as 500,000 annual illnesses, with as many as 20,000 deaths. Naphthalene, a common household pesticide, is found in mothballs and some air fresheners (for toilets or diaper pails). Naphthalene can damage red blood cells, causing hemolytic anemia in infants who have glucose-6-phosphate dehydrogenase (G6PD) deficiency (ATSDR, 1993a).

Childhood lead poisoning is the number one environmental health problem in the United States (ATSDR, 1988).

Research Brief

Sargent JD, et al: Childhood lead poisoning in Massachusetts communities—its association with sociodemographic and housing characteristics, Am J Public Health 85(4):528-33, 1995.

In 1991, the Centers for Disease Control (CDC) recommended that blood lead levels in children be below 10 μg/dl. Because of the frequency with which lead is found in the environment, many communities have instituted childhood lead-screening programs. The purpose of this study was to look at the incidence of lead poisoning in communities with various sociodemographic and housing characteristics.

The incidence of lead poisoning in Massachusetts communities was correlated with sociodemographic and housing characteristics. Children living in communities that have low rates of home ownership and high rates of poverty, single-parent families, and pre-1950s housing were 7 to 10 times more likely to show evidence of lead poisoning.

Additional biological variables in black children may increase their risk for lead poisoning. For example calcium is known to block the absorption of lead from the gastrointestinal tract, and an examination of The National Health and Nutrition Examination Survey (1976-1980) data showed that black children had significantly lower calcium intakes than did white children.

Implications for community health nursing practice are as follows:

1. In states similar to Massachusetts that do not have resources for obtaining widespread environmental lead-screening data, this model may help the nurse target community lead-screening programs.
2. A priority nursing intervention might include community nutritional counseling that focuses on the importance of dietary calcium. This intervention might be targeted specifically toward black children living in rented homes in older neighborhoods.

Lead Products and Waste

Childhood lead poisoning may be the number one environmental health problem in the United States (ATSDR, 1988). In school children, lead exposure at low levels has been associated with lower class ranking and higher absenteeism, poor eye-hand coordination, slow reaction time, and lower vocabulary test scores. In 1991, the Centers for Disease Control and Prevention (CDC, 1991) recommended lowering the childhood blood lead level at which health intervention should occur from 25 μg/dl to 10 μg/dl.

Although lead was banned in 1972 from paint used in homes, millions of homes, particularly those built before 1950, still contain high amounts of lead paint. Some homes have water pipes made from lead or ones containing lead solder. Significant exposures have occurred in children who play in lead-contaminated soil. Acidic foods stored in imported pottery may leach lead from ceramic glazes. Parents who are exposed occupationally can bring lead home on their clothing and shoes. Some folk medicines, such as Greta and Azarcon, that contain high percentages of lead, are used in the Latin culture to treat diarrhea or gastrointstinal upset. Other folk remedies containing lead include Alarcon, Alkohl, Bali Goli, Coral, Ghasard, Liga, Pay-loo-ah, and Rueda (CDC, 1991).

Recreational Hazards

Recreational areas and products can pose hazards to health. Polluted lakes and streams can expose persons who swim or fish in them to toxins, including naturally occurring red tide (seawater discolored by a high density of dinoflagellates that are toxic to many forms of marine life). Wooden playground structures may be treated with protective sealants that have arsenic-containing compounds, pentachlorophenol, and creosote. Some play sands and clays have been reported to contain asbestos-like fibers. Materials used in arts and crafts may contain potentially hazardous silica and talc dust, solvents, vapors, or heavy-metal fumes.

Water Supply

Drinking water can contain various environmental pollutants. Pollutants found in underground water are usually water-soluble chemicals that are easily carried with rain through the soil. Surface water and groundwater sources are both vulnerable to industrial solvents, heavy metals, pesticides, fertilizers, and runoff and leaching from hazardous waste sites. An EPA groundwater survey detected trichloroethylene in approximately 10% of the wells tested. An estimated 25% of all water supplies have detectable levels of tetrachloroethylene (ATSDR, 1993). Nitrates frequently found in fertilizers are common contaminants of rural, shallow, private wells.

Soil Contamination

Ingestion of **contaminated** soil poses a risk of toxicity, especially for children under age 6 because of their tendency to put things in their mouths. Some chemicals, such as lead and dioxin, bind tightly with soil. Certain heavy metals, such as lead, and pesticides, such as chlordane, remain in soil for years.

Hazardous Waste

About 275 million tons of hazardous waste are generated every year in the United States, or 1900 pounds per citizen. More than 64,000 areas are contaminated by hazardous waste nationwide. Of these, approximately 1300 to 1400 sites have been placed on or are proposed for the National Priorities List (NPL), a list of the worst waste sites in the United States. An estimated 41 million U.S. residents live within 4 miles of hazardous waste sites and may be at risk for exposure (NRC, 1991).

Physical Agents

Physical hazards can also present dangerous environmental threats to public health. Children are especially attracted to these hazards by curiosity and a quest for adventure. Examples of physical hazards include sharp objects, uncovered holes or tanks, mud or sludge pits, and abandoned materials, equipment, and structures. The community health nurse can identify potential physical hazards in the community and bring these to the attention of proper city or state officials for removal or for installation of a fence to isolate the hazard from the public.

Biological Agents

Biological agents, such as bacteria and viruses, can contaminate foods, soil, and water. Some also infect blood-sucking insects, such as mosquitos, ticks, and fleas. Infected animals can also transmit disease to humans.

One of the most common agents identified in water-borne illness is giardia lambia. Other agents found in potable water include *shigella,* campylobacter, hepatitis, *yersinia, V. cholerae,* and rotovirus. Transmission of some agents can also occur during recreational bathing in swimming pools, whirlpools, and saunas. One very common agent reported in food-borne illnesses is *salmonella.* Other agents commonly found in food include shigellosis, hepatitis A, and campylobacter. Soils can carry tetanus *bacillus.* Some insects and other arthropods can also carry disease. Mosquito-borne diseases include malaria, yellow fever, dengue, equine encephalitis, and filariasis. Fleas can carry plague and endemic typhus. Ticks can transmit Lyme disease and Rocky Mountain spotted fever. Some more commonly reported diseases transmitted primarily from animals to humans include, rabies, anthrax, brucellosis, leptospirosis, and trichinosis (Last and Wallace, 1992).

Plant and Animal Toxins

Plant and animal toxins also have the ability to adversely affect human health. Bites from poisonous snakes, spiders, bees, and wasps found in many parts of the country require prompt medical assessment and treatment, especially for individuals who are sensitive to these toxins. Some outdoor and indoor plants and fungi can also produce toxic effects if ingested. The nurse should become familiar with common plant and animal toxins in their living and working areas. Specific first aid treatment and other medical guidelines may be obtained from local or regional poison control centers.

Outdoor Air Pollution

Air pollution is often a mixture of gases and particulates. Frequently, the gases include carbon monoxides, nitrogen oxides, sulfur oxides, and hydrocarbons. Other toxic pollutants of concern are volatile organic compounds, metals, asbestos, and partially or incompletely burned compounds.

Radiation

Radiation is usually classified as either ionizing (containing enough energy to release electrons) or nonionizing (having insufficient energy to release electrons (e.g., microwaves and radar). The **adverse health effects** of ionizing radiation are well known. Humans are continuously exposed to ionizing radiation from the environment. The body can tolerate some exposure to ionizing radiation, and adverse health effects depend on the total dose, the rate at which the dose is received, the kind of radiation, and the organs and tissues affected. Health effects may be related to the ionization process that destroys the capacity of cells to reproduce and divide. Tissues, such as some skin cells, the lining of the digestive tract, and bone marrow (which contains blood-forming cells), are more sensitive to radiation than are muscle, nerves, and the bone itself (Mettler and Moseley, 1985).

Nonionizing radiation in the ultraviolet range presents a health hazard and is associated with development of skin cancer. As the protective atmospheric ozone layer is depleted, nonionizing radiation in the atmosphere increases. Waste from nuclear power plants can also pose dangerous risks if not properly handled and stored. Environmental radiation also comes from man-made power sources. The potential effects of electric and magnetic fields are not well understood and are currently under active investigation.

Linking Environmental Exposure to Disease
Key Definitions
Epidemiology

As discussed in Chapter 11, epidemiology, the investigation of the occurrence of disease in human populations, is one of the first techniques used in assessing the relationship between an agent and a disease. Epidemiology is a powerful tool in addressing the causality and resulting adverse health effects associated with chemical and physical exposures (Lilienfeld, 1978; WHO, 1983). However, epidemiologic evidence is often difficult to obtain because (1) the latency period between exposure and disease may be extended, (2) small groups of exposed persons make statistical results uncertain, and (3) analysis of complex life styles and other factors is difficult.

Toxicologic Studies

Assessing the **toxicity** of hazardous substances is the primary purpose of toxicologic studies. Animal studies provide the major source of information about adverse health effects, including the development of pathologic changes in affected organs (Klaassen et al., 1991). Human case studies of hazardous substance exposure are difficult to quantify because the exact amount of exposure is rarely known. Frequently, a recommended level for protecting public health is based on animal studies. Then uncertainty factors are applied to reduce the exposure level further and assure that it is protective of human health. The primary resource for conducting experimentally based toxicity testing in the United States is the National Toxicology Program, which was established in 1978 (Rall et al., 1987).

Clinical Observation

The importance of professional judgment in well-trained and alert nurses should not be underestimated. The adverse health effects of such agents as diethylstilbestrol (DES), kepone, polyvinyl chloride (PVC), thalidomide, and others were recognized, not by research programs, epidemiological studies, or computer modeling, but by state clinicians in the course of their practice (Creech and Johnson, 1974; Jackson, 1979; Miller, 1981). Early observations are immediately useful for clinical interventions and can also provide impetus and direction for epidemiological laboratory and controlled clinical studies.

Dose Response

For most **environmental exposures,** the type and severity of adverse health effects are dependent on dose. For many chemicals, a threshold dose can be determined through animal studies. Exposures above the threshold dose result in health effects; exposures below the threshold dose result in no observed adverse health effects. Thresholds are absent or unknown for certain chemicals, especially carcinogens, and for ionizing radiation (Beaumont and Breslow, 1981; Upton, 1988). For substances that produce hypersensitivity or allergic reactions which are immunologic in nature, a previous sensitization is necessary. After sensitization, allergic reactions develop from exposure to low doses of the inciting agent.

Latency

Health effects from environmental pollution may occur long after an exposure event. This is especially true of chemicals that cause cancer. The longer this latency period is between exposure and the onset of health effects, the more difficult it is to confirm a causal association. Thus, the health professional must be alert to exposures that may have occurred weeks, months, or even years before.

Risk Assessment

Although many techniques are available for assessing environmental health, the method currently advocated by the EPA is Quantitative Risk Assessment. Risk assessment is not mandated by law but is an integral part of what focuses and shapes environmental rules and regulations. Basically, risk assessment is an attempt through statistical or biological modeling to give a numerical estimate of the probability of **health risks** in a given population (see box below). Risk assessments are used primarily to facilitate remediations

(cleanup) or other risk management actions usually focused on a particular site.

Risk assessment depends on data from clinical studies, epidemiological studies, toxicological studies, and in-vitro testing.

Goals for Nursing Action

Given the environmental health issues confronting communities today, the community health practitioner should be able to identify environmental exposures and conditions, take appropriate preventive and treatment measures, and make appropriate referrals for follow-up. To carry out this standard of care, community health nurses must do the following:

1. Conduct exposure assessments and take histories of individual clients, families, and communities.
2. Understand the relationship to illness or injury of environmental pollution commonly found in contaminated air, water, and soil.
3. Call known or suspected hazards to the attention of local, state, and federal public health agencies or other entities as indicated by information from the client or community environmental history.
4. Be alert to opportunities for preventive and protective activities to limit or interdict exposure.
5. Communicate appropriate health risk information to persons concerned about environmental hazard exposure.
6. Be sensitive to the ethical, social, and legal implications of appropriate interventions for environmental disease.

ENVIRONMENTAL HEALTH INFORMATION RESOURCES*

Often communities are confused by media stories related to a toxic waste site or incident. Clients may show symptoms of illness with no apparent cause. Clients may not know they have been exposed to chemicals or to what chemicals, if they have been exposed, or they may know only trade names or slang terms for these substances. A child may become ill and the parents suspect ingestion of a household toxic substance, but household products may have inadequate labeling for proper identification. In today's world, nurses faced with such situations must know where to go for toxic substance information. Some key resources for environmental health information are shown in the box on p. 141.

Thus, identifying and accessing environmental health information is an important component of the nurse's process for assessing the client and community. Data sources in environmental health are

Key Steps in the Assessment Process

- ◆ EXPOSURE ASSESSMENT. Determining what environmental exposures are occurring or are anticipated to occur for relevant populations.
- ◆ HAZARD IDENTIFICATION. Establishing whether the exposure causes the adverse effect.
- ◆ DOSE-RESPONSE ASSESSMENT. Relating dose to the toxicologic response.
- ◆ RISK CHARACTERIZATION. Determining the relationship among exposure, target dose, and adverse health consequences.

*Use of trade names is for identification only and does not imply endorsement by the Agency for Toxic Substances and Disease Registry, the Public Health Service, or the U.S. Department of Health and Human Services.

Key Environmental Health Information Resources

Federal, state, and local environmental health agencies
Regulatory environmental agencies
Community action groups
Poison control centers
Occupational/environmental clinics
Environmental organizations
Universities/health science education programs
Hotlines
Consumer information bureaus
Occupational health and safety agencies
Emergency response teams
Computerized information services

important tools for providing an environmental health assessment and analysis at the client and community level. By knowing how to access the best scientific data available and then being able to discuss how exposure can impact human health, the nurse can provide an important community health service.

The clinician is encouraged to build a network of occupational and environmental medical specialists for information, consultation, and referral. Consultants are important sources of environmental information. These consultants can be medical or environmental specialists, such as clinicians specializing in occupational and environmental health, industrial hygienists who are often employed by state health departments or industry, or county environmental health scientists who often receive the first call from concerned citizens about exposures in the environment. Occupational health nurses, often employed at clients' worksites, also have expertise and experience that may be valuable to the clinician (see Appendix B.1 and B.4).

Referral resources, such as occupational or environmental clinics or education centers, should be considered. The Association of Occupational and Environmental Clinics (AOEC) is a network of clinics that provides professional training, community education, exposure and risk assessment, clinical evaluations, and consultative services (see Consultation Resources, Appendix B.1 and B.4). Your state or local poison control center is an example of an important information resource in an emergency situation (see Certified Regional Poison Control centers, Appendix B.2).

Community activist groups are another important source of environmental information, especially if community environmental issues of concern exist. Although national community groups are important, local community activists should be the first line of contact. Some groups to consider are the Chamber of Commerce, the League of Women Voters, Physicians for Social Responsibility, and the local chapter of the Sierra Club.

Finally, printed reference sources, including books and journals, Material Safety Data Sheets (MSDS), publications, and electronic information systems contain a wealth of information.

Data Sources for Community Assessment and Analysis

Local Governmental Resources

A leading resource for environmental health information is the local health department and environmental agencies. Local government resources can help nurses find the source of exposure, identify **exposure pathways,** and provide information related to disrupting the exposure. They can also provide information for existing screening diagnosis and treatment programs related to environmental exposure, for example, lead screening and treatment programs for children. Local health department sanitarians or other environmental professionals can also provide valuable data. Birth, death, and other records filed at local health departments are useful sources of information. Unusual trends in cancer or birth outcomes may indicate environmental health problems that require further investigation.

State Government Resources

Three important environmental agencies are the state health, environmental, and poison control centers. The state health agency provides information on reported health concerns in the vicinity of the problem facility, health databases, health advisories, disease registries, epidemiological studies or surveys, and public meetings related to specific environmental concerns. State agencies have information on hazardous waste sites with state-level priority; active facilities that use, dispose, or transport hazardous substances; emergency chemical spills; lakes and streams with fishing advisories or bans; air quality for metropolitan areas; and locations of sanitary and hazardous waste landfills.

The state environmental agency provides technical consultations and responds to public inquiries about harmful health effects related to exposure to chemical contaminants, radon, lead, and other environmental hazards. It also identifies resources available for screening, environmental sampling, and environmental monitoring data. The state poison control center maintains a resource and information center about acute and chronic toxic effects of toxic substances. It also provides clinical information, including antidotes, treatment, and referral to a toxicologist. Some state health agencies maintain cancer and birth-defect registries and can provide rates for counties and districts and sometimes even for zip code or census-tract areas.

Federal Government Resources

Federal agencies are comprehensive sources for public health and environmental information. A variety of agencies can help the public health nurse. The EPA has information about high-priority hazardous waste sites for cleanup or environmental remediation and health hazard data. It maintains lists of NPL hazardous waste or **Superfund** sites and environmental data. The ATSDR, funded by Superfund legislation, is a public health agency that is mandated to prevent exposure and adverse human health effects associated with exposure to hazardous substances from waste sites, unplanned releases, and other sources of pollution present in the environment. Its regional offices, located within the EPA regional offices, have information about community health risks, how to prevent exposures associated with specific sites, and possible health effects related to exposure to toxic substances at sites. The Consumer Protection Agency and the Fish and Wildlife Commission can provide health and environmental risk data on issues such as fish contaminated with mercury. Environmental information related to federal legislation, such as the EPA Clean Air Act, Clean Water Act, and the Safe Drinking Water Act, can be accessed by telephone. Federally funded hotlines are available on topics such as radon, lead, emergency response, and toxicology. (See State/Federal/National Resources, Appendix B.2.)

The Toxic Chemical Release Inventory database (TRI) is another federal source of environmental health information. TRI data are submitted to the EPA by industrial facilities. This database lists all reported releases of hazardous substances within a city, zip code area, county, or state and is available to the public. By using the TRI database, community health nurses can determine potential sources of environmental contamination in their city or county and perhaps identify areas of concern. Data are available for any part of the United States (USEPA, 1989).

Electronic Information Systems

The development of electronic databases has revolutionized the retrieval of up-to-date, accurate, and comprehensive information on environmental health issues. On the plus side, accessing environmental health information electronically provides a wide range of available knowledge and decreases the amount of research time. The challenge is to determine available resources, how to use them, their cost, and how useful they are. Database information ranges from bibliographical or descriptive to detailed information on toxic exposure and health effects. Databases or data systems are commonly accessed through on-line databases, Compact Disk-Read Only Memory (CD-ROM), and electronic bulletin boards and mail systems (see computerized information Resources, Appendix B.3).

ENVIRONMENTAL HEALTH ASSESSMENT

A variety of clues may link environmental exposures to illness or injury of clients or the community. Investigating possible environmental health causation begins with awareness and is followed by assessment. Two approaches are available for environmental health assessment: community-wide health assessment and individual and family assessment.

Community-Wide Health Assessment

The community-wide assessment is designed to provide a framework in which information and health-related data can be collected from the community.

This information can then be evaluated using an interdisciplinary team of health professionals.

As discussed in Chapter 15, the initial assessment of environmental health in a community can be effectively completed through (1) windshield surveys (seeing a community by driving through it and making observations through the car windshield), and (2) gathering existing information from government agencies and from interviewing community members. *(Government agency data sources for community asssessment and analysis are described in the Environmental Health Information Resources section of this chapter.)* Completing these two steps will identify possible sources of environmental pollutants and bring potential community health threats into focus.

Sources of pollution can be industrial facilities, farms, golf courses, or even residential areas with heavy pesticide or herbicide use, all of which can cause air, soil, or groundwater pollution. Areas with heavy traffic flow may be sources of air pollution. Homes built before 1960 may have been painted with lead-based paint or have lead pipes or solder in their plumbing. Airports and railroad yards may have fuel leaks that contaminate groundwater. A partial checklist of common sources of environmental pollutants is presented in Figure 8-1.

Exposure Pathways Analysis

Once an area of possible environmental health concern has been identified, another windshield survey should be conducted and local health officials should be contacted to determine all posssible routes of environmental pollutant exposure for the community. Figure 8-2 presents a checklist that may help guide the survey. Basically, the survey should identify all possible routes by which environmental pollution can migrate off the site and the points at which residents may contact those pollutants. The assessment includes all environmental media: groundwater, surface water, soil, air, and the food chain. When assessing a source, it is important to note whether access to the site is restricted by fences or warning signs. Experienced environmental health professionals require special training from the Occupational Safety and Health Administration (OSHA), appropriate personal protective equipment, and detailed safety plans before investigating a hazardous waste site. *Do not go along to investigate a potential hazardous waste site.* Inexperienced individuals could unknowingly expose themselves to very dangerous levels of toxic substances (ATSDR, 1992b).

Groundwater. Groundwater can be the most significant pathway of exposure, especially if community members are using contaminated groundwater as a drinking water source. "Groundwater is contained in a geological layer, which may also be called an aquifer. Aquifers are composed of permeable or porous geological materials, and may either be unconfined (and thereby most susceptible to contamination) or confined by relatively impermeable material" (Chivian et al., 1993). Twenty percent of Americans receive their wa-

	Present?	Operational?
Waste storage and treatment activities		
Landfill-Municipal wastes		
Landfill-Industrial/medical wastes		
Incinerator-Municipal wastes		
Incinerator-Industrial/medical wastes		
Wastewater (sewage) treatment facility		
Other waste storage/treatment/disposal		
Waste recycling activity		
Battery recycling		
Drum/container recycling		
Tire storage/recycling		
Waste oil recovery		
Solvent recovery		
Other recycling/recovery		
Government activity		
DOE/DOD Ordnance-Nuclear		
DOE/DOD Ordnance-Conventional		
Military equipment production/maintenance		
Other government activities		
Mining activity		
Subsurface mining		
Surface mining		
Metal ore processing/refining/smelting		
Oil/gas extraction refinery		
Other mining		
Manufacturing activity		
Chemical processing/production		
Agricultural (fertilizers/pesticides)		
Machinery production		
Textiles		
Dry cleaning/laundry operation		
Wood preserving		
Paper production		
Other manufacturing/fabricating/processing		
Other activities		
Areas of heavy pesticide/herbicide use		
Heavy traffic areas (highways, urban areas)		
Neighborhoods with homes built before 1960		
Railroad yards		
Airports		

FIGURE 8-1
Windshield survey checklist for potential sources of environmental pollutants.

Source of environmental pollution:
Location:

Regulatory status: [ ] Federal ____
　　　　　　　　　　[ ] State ____
　　　　　　　　　　[ ] Local ____
　　　　　　　　　　[ ] Unregulated ____
(Assess by contacting EPA or state environmental department)

Closest resident/residential area:

Closest school/daycare/youth club:

	past	present	future
Groundwater use (within a mile)			
[ ] Private well use/number:			
[ ] Drinking/cooking			
[ ] Outdoor/yard			
[ ] Irrigation			
[ ] Industrial			
[ ] Abandoned			
[ ] Public/municipal well			
Surface water use (within a mile)			
Description:			
[ ] Swimming/recreation			
[ ] Drinking water source			
[ ] Health advisories			
[ ] Fishing			
[ ] Water contact			
Soil use (within a mile)			
[ ] Parks/play areas for children			
[ ] Trespassing in restricted areas			
[ ] Gardening			
Ambient air quality (within a mile)			
Prevailing wind direction:			
[ ] Frequent air inversions			
[ ] Odors			
[ ] Visual emission			
Food chain use (withing a mile)			
[ ] Game animal hunting			
[ ] Farming			
[ ] Gardening			
[ ] Fishing			
[ ] Subsistence			
[ ] Sport			

Physical hazards (on or near the site)

[ ] Equipment ____　　　　　[ ] Confined spaces ____　　[ ] Unstable structures ____
[ ] Storage containers ____　　[ ] Asphyxiation ____　　　　[ ] Waste piles ____
[ ] Debris ____　　　　　　　 [ ] Acid conditions ____　　　 [ ] Mine shafts ____
[ ] Fire ____　　　　　　　　 [ ] Caustic conditions ____　　[ ] Explosive conditions ____
[ ] Lagoons, ponds, impoundments ____　　　　　　　　　　 [ ] Pits ____

FIGURE 8-2
Site assessment checklist.

ter from small suppliers, including private wells, surface water, cisterns, and springs. At least one-third of them have either never had their water tested or the tests indicate levels of chemicals above the EPA's maximum contaminant level (NRC, 1977-1989).

Private wells, which may be the sole source of water for a household, often tap unconfined aquifers. The importance of having clean water is also recognized in the Public Health Service publication, *Healthy People 2000* (1991). By identifying potentially contaminated private wells, community health nurses can help meet the goal of verified clean water for 85% of the public.

Surface Water. Surface water includes anything from drainage ditches to rivers or even a shoreline. Surface water bodies may be a point of exposure for the community, or they may facilitate the transport of environmental pollutants from a site to a residential area. The direction and type of surface water drainage should be observed during the survey. Also, note any reported fishing or water-contact advisories listed by the state environmental agency (ATSDR, 1992b).

Air. Ambient air quality may be assessed during the survey. Peculiar or unpleasant odors should be noted. If a plume or discharge from a stack is evident, the color and wind direction should be noted. The presence of air inversions should also be assessed because they may act to concentrate air pollution. Air inversions occur when air closest to the ground is cooler than the air above and thus cannot rise (Blumenthal, 1985). Air inversions frequently occur in valleys or "basins." A haze or fog is sometimes created during an air inversion. Because ambient air conditions may be highly variable, it may be necessary to contact the local sanitarian or state air quality department for more background information on ambient air quality.

If this is a municipal community, check with the state environmental department or local air pollution control authority to determine whether the community is in compliance with the National Ambient Air Quality Standards (NAAQS). Pollutants covered by NAAQS criteria include ozone, carbon monoxide, nitrogen dioxide, sulfur dioxide, particulate matter, and lead. In 1988, approximately 50% of Americans lived in counties that exceeded the NAAQS. Tropospheric ozone, which can be a potent respiratory irritant, was exceeded most frequently (Tarcher, 1992). Community health nurses who are aware of ambient air quality can help protect members of their community who are vulnerable to harmful effects of air pollution, including persons who have asthma or chronic obstructive pulmonary disease.

Food Chain. Some hazardous substances can bioaccumulate in the food chain. For example, concentrations of polychlorinated biphenyls (PCBs) may be as much as 660,000 times higher in fish than in the surrounding water (ATSDR, 1993b). Because of possible bioconcentration, the potential for exposure through human consumption of foods grown or raised near a hazardous site should be noted.

Physical Hazards. Assessing the existence of potential physical hazards on a site may be important if frequent trespassing is evident (ATSDR, 1992b). The use of such areas for play or exploration by children should be especially noted. For example, a landfill may be an attractive play area for children. But landfills may often be riddled with physical hazards, such as sharp metal objects, sink holes, and rusted drums. Note such physical hazards whenever assessing a potential hazardous waste site.

Human Exposure Analysis

A human exposure analysis must be conducted to determine whether the client or community has actually been exposed to an environmental hazard. Environmental health scientists use a method called exposure pathway analysis. An exposure pathway is the process by which an individual is exposed to contaminants that originate from some source of contamination (ATSDR, 1992b). Understanding how exposure occurs is the key to protecting a community or client. Residents will not get sick simply living near a source of environmental pollution. They must be exposed and absorb environmental pollutants into their systems. Thus, a completed exposure pathway must exist.

An exposure pathway consists of five elements:
1. A source of contamination
2. An environmental medium: air, soil, surface water, groundwater, or food chain
3. A point of exposure: human contact with the contaminated medium
4. A route of exposure: inhalation, ingestion, or dermal exposure
5. A receptor population: people who are exposed or potentially exposed to contaminants of concern at a point of exposure.

When all five elements are present, the pathway is called a completed exposure pathway. If one or more of the pathway elements is unconfirmed but could exist, the pathway should be characterized as a potential exposure pathway (ATSDR, 1992b).

Individual and Family Assessment

Community assessment is an important part of the nurse's preparation for intervening in the community. Individual and family assessment provides a basis for the nursing care plan for individuals and families. Taking a thorough environmental exposure history is critical in determining a nursing diagnosis and intervention. The following factors should be considered as part of the history assessment of a situation involving hazardous substance exposure.

An environmental **exposure history** has three components: (1) exposure survey, (2) environmental history, and (3) health history. The components of an exposure history (listed in box on p. 146) will be

Components of an Environmental Exposure History

1. EXPOSURE
Location
Name of hazardous substance(s)
Form (solid, powder, liquid, vapor)
Route into body (inhalation, ingestion, dermal, injection)
Contact time (how long)
Contact frequency (how often)
Dose (amount)
Who knows, who needs to know about the exposure

2. ENVIRONMENT
A. Home
Water source (private well, city water)
Fertilizer use (farm)
Pesticide use
Home insulating, heating and cooling
Recent renovation/remodeling
Air pollution (indoor/outdoor)
Hobbies
Home cleaning agents
Proximity to heavy industry or hazardous waste site(s)

B. Work
Company
Job task
Names of hazardous substances worked with
Protective equipment recommended (is it used?)

3. HEALTH HISTORY
A. Host Factors
Health conditions currently experienced
Physical
Psychological/emotional
Chronic Conditons
Developmental
Children
Pregnancy
Lactating
Personal Habits
Smoking
Drinking
Hygiene

B. Cultural
Beliefs
Folk medicines
Dietary practices
Language barriers
Reading and writing skills

---

elicited through the exposure form (see resources pages). Although a positive response to any question on the form indicates the need for further inquiry, a negative response to all questions does not necessarily rule out a toxic exposure etiology or significant previous exposure. Refer to the listing of hazardous substances in the Home and Environment section above.

Exposure Survey

In an exposure survey, first determine the specific location of the hazardous substance exposure and the boundaries or size of the contaminated area. Question whether others were exposed or are at risk of exposure. Determine the source and status of an exposure, that is, did the hazardous substance come from an ongoing industrial activity or work process that should be discontinued or from an accidental spill that has already occurred.

Identify the name(s) and correct spelling(s) of all hazardous substances involved. Some hazardous substances are known by many names, and the spelling of completely different substances may differ by only one letter. Confirm the name(s) by checking a written source, such as a label. When possible, obtain the Chemical Abstract Service (CAS) number of the hazardous substance so that the health effects can be more easily researched (through computer databases). Identify physical characteristics of the hazardous substance. Determining the form a substance takes (i.e., solid, powder, liquid, vapor from liquid, fumes from

metals, gas) is important because this may indicate how the substance moves in the environment and how it may move into the body.

Toxic substances can enter the body through skin contact, inhalation, ingestion, and injection. Understanding how the substance enters the body will help focus the physical assessment. This information can also indicate what protective measures may be necessary to prevent future exposures. Vehicles, such as cigarettes, food, and water, can help transfer the substance into the body and should also be considered. Drawing a vapor through a burning cigarette can change the chemical components of the vapor as it is inhaled into the lungs. Food and water extensively contaminated with toxic substances may have priority public health implications because of the potentially large number of persons who could become exposed.

Contact time and frequency of exposure are two important factors in helping to determine how much exposure a client has experienced. Determine the length of time in minutes, hours, or days that the exposure lasted and the frequency of exposure—once only, once a week, or every day.

Try to determine the highest dose or amount of substance the client has been exposed to. This will often be difficult to measure unless chemical monitoring records are available. In some cases, post-exposure environmental sampling may be obtained and can be used to help estimate possible exposure dose scenarios.

Recognize which possible health effects can result from a given exposure. Clients may be convinced they have contracted a specific medical condition from exposure to a specific substance. Yet if nurses know that the medical condition is not associated with that substance, they can counsel and educate their clients. Remember, not everyone exposed to a toxic substance will experience health effects.

Check the toxicity of the substance; know what dose is needed for a health response to occur. Look up possible federal (OSHA, EPA, ATSDR, and National Institute for Occupational Safety and Health [NIOSH]) and state regulatory levels or advisories for information about the toxic substance in question. Know how rapidly the substance acts and remember that exposure to carcinogens may show delayed effects on a client's health.

Assess who is aware of the exposure and who needs to know about it. Identify persons who may need to be notified inside and outside the community. Also, consider where and from whom information or assistance can be obtained to implement interventions that affect groups of individuals, cost money, or affect work practices.

Environmental History

Home. Environmental factors such as temperature, humidity, and ventilation can contribute to the hazards of some substances. Solvents can evaporate quickly if left uncovered in a hot environment. Such evaporation in any enclosed air space will quickly elevate contaminant levels to unsafe concentrations. Humidity can be a protective factor with toxic dust. In a high-humidity environment, dust consolidated with moisture in the air will quickly become heavy and fall to the ground. The direction and forcefulness of air currents can determine whether dust and toxic vapors are blown by fans or outdoor breezes into or away from a client's breathing zone. Vapors and gases can also be trapped and may build to unsafe levels in rooms or enclosed spaces that lack or have poor ventilation.

Hobbies that include toxic substances can compound exposures. For example, an industrial lead welder may be exposed at work to lead levels that will not affect his health. However, if he is remodeling a home that contains lead-based paint, he could be exposed to unsafe levels when his home and work exposures are combined.

Work. The community health nurse should compile a comprehensive inventory of a patient's occupations, employers, and current and potential exposures in the workplace. The nurse should note every job the client had, regardless of duration. Recent changes in work processes or routines and the details of job functions may reveal exposures unexpected from job titles. Determine whether protective equipment is recommended and whether the client actually uses it. Military service with potential toxic exposure should also be ascertained.

Health History

Host Factors. Obtain a thorough **health history** from the client who is concerned about toxic substance exposure. Evaluate health factors that may place the client at higher risk for adverse health effects from toxic exposures. A history of chronic health conditions that affect a person's absorption, metabolism, and excretion of toxic substances is important to consider. For example, a person with a compromised liver, the body's main detoxification organ, may be affected at lower doses than are healthy individuals. Inhalation of toxic dusts may be life threatening for persons who have chronic obstructive pulmonary disease. Personal habits such as smoking, drinking, and personal hygiene should be considered.

Developmental factors, such as those present in growing children and pregnant or lactating women, require special considerations with certain hazardous substances. Lead is absorbed and stored more easily in the body of a child than in an adult. A pregnant woman's fetus may be sensitive to some toxic substances that are able to cross the placenta. Lactating women may excrete toxic substances in their breast milk (Guzelian et al., 1992).

Some persons are more sensitive than others to chemical exposures. These individuals may have become sensitized through past exposures to a particular chemical or family of chemicals. Sensitized individuals then experience health effects at lower doses than do persons who are not sensitized. Multiple chemical sensitivity syndrome is a diagnosis attributed to exposures to multiple environmental chemicals at very low levels.

Psychological impact and stress are not uncommon in individuals and families who are going through environmental contamination crises. Sometimes, in addition to concerns about their health and well-being, families must also deal with reporters and attorneys.

Cultural Factors. Inquire about cultural beliefs and practices (e.g., folk medicines that contain lead), language barriers, and dietary practices. A Southeast Asian family whose main food staple is fish from a contaminated creek, might have significant exposure if fish in the creek bioconcentrate contaminants. A good understanding of cultural beliefs and language barriers will help determine the nursing intervention needs and strategies.

Physical Examination of Individuals Concerned about Hazardous Substance

Exposure. While performing an examination, consider the following: Know how the substance gets into the body. Understand how long it stays in the body and if it is metabolized (into more- or less-toxic substances). Know how it is distributed by the body; is it stored in fat, bone, or breast milk? Understand how it leaves the body; is this mainly through urine, feces, or exhaled breath?

A **biomarker** is a change—physical or chemical—that can be measured in a functioning biological system. A biomarker of exposure is present when the substance or its metabolite can be detected in body tissue without any apparent health effect. Assess the status of target systems the substance is known to affect. Changes in these systems are sometimes referred to as biomarkers of effect. Examples of toxic substances associated with biomarkers of effect include asbestos, which can cause a rare cancer (mesothelioma); vinyl chloride, which is associated with liver cancer; and lead, which is associated with impaired learning in children. Lead can also be a biomarker of exposure when it is detected in blood and other tissues before an effect occurs.

Assess the impact of health risk factors (identified on the environmental health history) that could be magnified if a significant exposure exists. These might be present in persons who have preexisting health conditions, in pregnancy and lactating women, and in children.

Testing for exposure levels is not always easy, cost-effective, or convenient. Some substances leave the body rapidly, and if testing is not performed within the first several hours after exposure, the test will show nothing. Other tests need special equipment and special laboratories to collect and analyze the samples. Remember, a positive test for a biomarker of exposure may only confirm what is already known, that an exposure has taken place. Also, detectable levels of a hazardous substance in a client's body do not necessarily mean health effects will result from the exposure.

ADVERSE HEALTH EFFECTS

For most chemical and physical agents in the environment, the health effects are unsuspected, undetected, or poorly understood. As might be expected, a causal relationship between exposure and illness or injury is difficult to show. If the practitioner is to intervene successfully, a basic understanding of the relationship between toxic exposure and an adverse health effect is essential. For clinical purposes, an adverse health effect is a response that either impairs an organ function at the subclinical level or results in illness, injury, or death. An acute effect develops rapidly; chronic effects are long-lasting.

NURSING DIAGNOSIS, PLANNING, AND INTERVENTION

Diagnosis

After analyses for exposure and toxicity are completed, nursing diagnoses for individuals can be very specific (Carpenito, 1995). Because high doses of chemicals can affect the renal and hepatic systems, consider using nursing diagnoses associated with these conditions, especially in cases of severe chemical exposures. Other possibilities include diagnoses of "risk" based on the vulnerability of the client, family, aggregate, or community. An individual may be at risk because of age, underlying health status, or intensity of exposure. For example, someone with chronic obstructive pulmonary disease may be at higher risk for health effects from air pollution than a healthy person would be. Children are at risk for lead poisoning because of their increased hand-to-mouth behaviors and increased absorption of lead in their digestive and neurological systems. Determining the exposure pathway and completing the toxicological analyses will identify who may be at risk by identifying who has been most exposed and who is most susceptible to adverse effects from the chemical.

Community-based nursing diagnoses identify aggregates and population responses. Examples of these include "ineffective community coping" and "ineffective community management of therapeutic regimen." An environmental hazard may be sensationalized, cause outrage among community members, and result in prolonged uncertainty about the severity of the hazard and its long-term health effects. Consider a diagnosis of "ineffective community coping" for any community that undergoes this type of stress. A diagnosis of "ineffective community management of therapeutic regimen" may be considered when barriers exist to providing needed health screening programs or environmental remediation.

Nursing diagnoses of "possible" are appropriate when the community health nurse needs additional data to rule out or confirm problems. In an exposure pathway analysis, one or more of the elements (i.e., source, media, exposure point, route, or receptor population) may be suspected but not confirmed. In this case, a nursing diagnosis of "possible" is appropriate to reduce the risk of harm to the community. For example, history has shown that children living near smelters have high exposures to heavy metals such as lead. Any smelter community could have a nursing diagnosis of "possible" even before environmental contamination of heavy metals is confirmed. For a summary of steps in making an environmental health nursing diagnosis, see Table 8-1.

The community health nurse may proactively communicate with and provide information for the client and community and also for other health care providers, public health officials, and state and federal officials. Facilitating a good communication web will strengthen the nurse's information base and that of others and help reduce inconsistent, inaccurate, and confusing messages about the exposure scenario. (See Health Risk Communication later in this chapter.)

After developing a nursing diagnosis for the target population or client, the nurse can identify needs, set goals, and plan interventions.

Planning: Setting Goals and Objectives

The goals for preventive health interventions are achieved by two actions: (1) removing the contamina-

Table 8-1 Summary of Steps in Formulating an Environmental Health Nursing Diagnosis

Step	Function	Question to answer
From the assessment	Identify target group or community aggregate who have been exposed and are at high risk for health effect (EXPOSURE ANALYSES)	Who in the community has been exposed?
1	Identify the unhealthful response or the risk for unhealthful response (TOXICOLOGICAL ANALYSES)	Is there a risk for injury or has an actual injury occurred?
2	Identify the related host and environmental factors	Host: What characteristics of the target group influence the risk for injury? Environment: What characteristics of the environment influence the risk for injury?
3	Identify any existing data that may substantiate the nursing diagnosis	Are there any epidemiological or other health outcome data that correlate injury risk with environmental contamination?

tion and (2) educating the population at risk. Thus, protecting the public from environmental pollution focuses on environmental remediation or community health education.

Community health nurses possess unique skills in community-wide and family interventions, synthesized by combining the nursing process with public health science (Clemen-Stone et al., 1995). These skills prepare them to collaborate with other disciplines in identifying environmental hazards and planning for their removal and to develop community health education activities for families or communities at risk (Salmon, 1993).

Intervention Strategies

Team Approach

Whether the goal of separating community members from the environmental hazard is achieved through cleanup or education, a team approach will be needed for success. For cleanup, regulatory agencies will be important players. The EPA and state environmental agencies are responsible for enforcing environmental laws. Contacting advisory agencies, such as ATSDR, may also help influence cleanup activities.

In addition to the community health nurse, other members of the team might include sanitarians, industrial hygienists, engineers, safety officers, primary care providers, health educators, fire fighters, toxicologists, and chemists. Elected government officials, ranging from local to federal officials, may also be key players in negotiating a cleanup activity. Critical to cooperation from government officials or agencies is a sound public health basis for recommending cleanup, and effective communication.

A basic assumption in community health education is that *people are more eager to adopt changes when they play a role in determining what the changes will be and how they will be effected* (Dignan and Carr, 1987). This statement indicates the need for community members to be part of the team.

Local television stations and newspapers may also be helpful, especially in community health education. Providing reporters with fact sheets or other written materials that are in "lay" terms often improves the accuracy of reported issues.

Community meetings, existing community groups, schools, and churches can also be effective in identifying community leaders and potential team players.

Types of Intervention

Nursing interventions are action plans for addressing the needs identified in the nursing diagnosis. They include the following:

Preventive Actions. Preventing exposure of clients to potentially dangerous hazardous substances is a priority. Isolate the hazard from the client. Intervene to change the environment to prevent or reduce the hazard or exposure.

Communication. Work with community leaders; local, state, and federal health officers; and school officials to identify ways to reduce or prevent exposures. Assess plans for long-term involvement by these officials and individuals. Suggest that public health officials conduct follow-up community health screening, education programs, and community health studies.

Referral. Refer clients experiencing health effects related to an exposure to a primary care provider (preferably skilled in chemical exposure assessment) for testing and treatment. Refer the following categories of clients for appropriate medical follow-up.

♦ Clients who experience health effects that are believed to be related to the hazardous substance exposure.
♦ Persons at high risk for experiencing complications due to preexisting health conditions (i.e., affecting lungs, liver, kidneys).

◆ Women who have had significant exposure and are pregnant or lactating; check the condition of the fetus and the quality of breast milk.

◆ Persons who have been exposed to carcinogens; document the incident on the medical record and counsel for appropriate periodic health screening.

◆ Concerned, anxious clients, in a confirmed or questionable hazardous substance exposure situation, who may need to validate their health status (Hibbs, 1994).

Education. Provide information and recommend actions that can be or have been taken to prevent exposure. Provide information on dose, frequency, route of exposure, environmental pathways, substance toxicity, and health effects. Provide information on potential, delayed health effects and reinforce the importance of periodic health screening for these effects.

Reassure and reinforce the concept that not everyone exposed to hazardous substances will experience adverse health effects (explain the concept that response varies with dose).

Treatment. Consider evaluating, recommending, and implementing ongoing health screening programs for persons exposed to hazardous substances that cause delayed health responses. Intervene to support rehabilitative or protective activities. Provide counseling and referral for psychological trauma. Periodically assess client capabilities and revise care plan as needed.

Enforcement of Public Health Guidelines. Provide information regarding public health protective guidelines and off-limit areas in the community. Assess and intervene in instances where these guidelines are not followed. Oversee or organize, as needed, community supervision of restricted areas, especially those near children's play areas. Check the effectiveness of **risk communication,** especially in bilingual communities.

Timing of Intervention

The nurse can also implement several specific intervention actions (Hibbs, 1994) with the individual and the community under the concepts of primary, secondary, and tertiary prevention as described by Leavell and Clark (1965). Primary, secondary, and tertiary interventions are distinguished by whether they are initiated before, during, or after exposure.

Primary Intervention. Primary intervention is preventive in focus and generally occurs before an exposure takes place. Primary intervention also focuses on intervening to relieve fears and anxiety regarding toxic substances in nonexposure situations.

Secondary Intervention. Secondary intervention generally occurs once an exposure pathway to a client has been identified. The nurse focuses on protecting the client from further exposure or preventing repeated exposure. Secondary intervention also focuses on recognizing and reducing adverse health effects. The nurse targets persons who have been exposed to hazardous substances and who may or may not be experiencing adverse health effects, including clients who could be at future risk for developing delayed health effects.

Tertiary Intervention. Tertiary intervention generally occurs after an exposure has been discontinued and the client experiences long-term adverse health effects. Interventions are rehabilitative or protective in focus. Tertiary intervention is targeted to clients who have experienced exposure that either resulted in or exacerbated long-term or chronic health conditions.

HEALTH RISK COMMUNICATION
Overview: Defining the Need

Often the public does not agree with the experts' assessment of environmental risk. Experts define risk in terms of probability of illness, injury, or exposure occurring to a specific segment of the population (Hance et al., 1988). The public, on the other hand, is concerned about being personally affected by a given hazard.

To understand community health concerns, it is necessary to appreciate the major role that human nature plays in the public's assessment of risk. Human judgment of risks is also affected by psychological and cultural factors and by the manner in which health information is communicated. However, successful health risk communication must begin with the realization that risk perception is, to a significant extent, predictable. The public reacts to certain sorts of risks and ignores others, and it is often possible to know in advance whether the health communication problem will be panic or apathy or something in between. Differences between risk perceptions are real and relevant, and they must be recognized as such. Appreciating human nature, the lens through which people perceive information about health risks, will help. Doing something to remedy the unfamiliarity, the feeling of being controlled by others, or the sense of unfairness will help us to more effectively make personal and public decisions that affect us and our communities.

However, understanding and appreciating human nature and personal feelings are not the total answer. Health risk communication involves a certain amount of control, and control affects how people perceive risk and how they receive information about their health risks and quality of life. The solution is obvious but difficult to implement. Community involvement or public participation in the health assessment process should begin early and continue throughout the health assessment process. This means the community nurse must be willing to begin communicating with the public before the experts begin the assessment process, even before policy-development decisions have been concluded.

Primary Goal of Health Risk Communication

The goal of communication is simply to involve concerned citizens in your community assessment and care plan. Communities and experts working together can determine the level of environmental health risk and what to do about it. Success depends partly on the nurse's belief that health risk communication is an integral part of the primary caregiver's role.

Nurses will be faced with clients who worry about their exposure to chemicals. These clients will ask many questions: What can a particular chemical do to me? Are my symptoms due to hazardous substance exposure? Do my symptoms come from an unknown exposure? Have I been exposed? How do I know? In answering such questions, a community health nurse will need to possess the skills discussed earlier, that is, an ability to perform a community, client, or family assessment about the nature of exposure to environmental pollution; knowledge of the health hazard of the substances involved; the ability to communicate the effect of the health risk to the client; and a willingness to assist in activities that prevent further exposure or the development of disease.

FUTURE TRENDS IN ENVIRONMENTAL HEALTH

Evaluating Causation

Evaluating the nonspecific and often delayed health effects of exposure to environmental chemicals frequently presents a challenge to health care providers. For many chemical mixtures in commercial use, the possible health effects are poorly understood. One perplexing and disabling condition is known as multiple chemical sensitivity. Persons suffering from this disorder believe they are sensitive to low levels of chemicals commonly present in the environment.

New research has only begun to provide tools that will help in studying questions relating to causation. For example, the use of positron emission tomography (PET) to visualize glucose metabolism (illustrating specific parts of the brain affected by chemicals), may

some day give important clues into neurological and psychological effects. Research has also provided new understanding of the importance of genetic makeup and its influence on individual susceptibility to various chemicals.

Factors, such as concomitant exposures, lifestyle, underlying health, age, gender, and nutritional status, may all act in concert to modify the body's response to a particular exposure. Thus, all potential risk factors should be considered in cases suspected of having environmental origins. The importance of host factors in combination with exposure is of major concern in the increased susceptibility of the fetus and very young children (Tarcher, 1992).

> ### What Do You Think?
>
> Environmental health, as it relates to the phrase, "The greatest good for the greatest number," poses particular problems for minorities who live near hazardous waste sites. Some individuals find it politically expedient to confine environmental wastes only to communities that are already affected, but other persons see this as neither fair nor just (Paehlke, 1994).

Environmental Justice

New efforts have focused on reaching out to include minority communities in discussions about environmental health issues. Thus, citizens as well as local health professionals and other officials are involved in community assessment and education. In bilingual communities, addressing specific translation needs, both verbal and written, has also been helpful. If a minority population affected by hazardous waste feels separated from the decision-making process, its members are understandably outraged about the substantive issues and believe **environmental justice** has not been served.

Clinical Application

At the county health department, a 3-year-old boy named Billy presents with gastric upset and behavior changes. These symptoms have persisted for several weeks. Billy's parents report that they have been renovating their home to remove lead paint. They had been discouraged from routinely testing their child because their insurance did not cover testing and they could not find information on where to have the test done. Their concern has heightened with the persistent symptoms in their child.

You test Billy's blood-lead level and find 45 µg/dl. You research lead poisoning and discover that children are at great risk because of their proclivity for absorbing lead into their central nervous systems. You also find that chronic lead poisoning may have long-term effects, such as developmental delays and impaired learning ability. You refer Billy to his primary care physician. On further investigation, you find that Billy's home was built before 1950 and is still under renovation. The sanitarian tests the interior

Continued.

Clinical Application—cont'd

paint and finds a high lead content. Copious amounts of sawdust from sanding are noted in various rooms of the home. You determine that a completed exposure pathway exists.

Source:	lead paint
Environmental media:	paint chips/dust
Exposure point:	inside the home
Exposure route:	ingestion, inhalation of dust
Receptor:	Billy

Because of the neurologic effects of lead, you assess Billy's development using the Denver II test and find delays in several areas. Synthesizing results of the Denver II, and the pathway and toxicologic analyses, you develop the following nursing diagnosis for Billy:

Altered growth and development related to compromised physical ability, and dependence secondary to neurologic impairment as evidenced by a blood lead level of 45 μg/dl and abnormal Denver II results.

Working with Billy's pediatrician, parents, and local school system, you enroll Billy in Head Start. You share information about lead poisoning and Billy's exposure and health history with the Head Start teachers and develop ways that his teachers and parents can stimulate his development.

Community-Wide Intervention

During your home visits, you note several other old homes in Billy's neighborhood that are under renovation. Billy's parents report that several friends are asking them questions about lead poisoning. You are concerned about the difficulty Billy's parents had in testing his blood-lead level. You make the following nursing diagnoses: (1) Children exposed to homes built before 1950 are at high risk for poisoning due to lack of environmental hazard awareness. (2) Ineffective community management of therapeutic regimen due to lack of availability of lead-screening programs.

Primary Prevention

The community health nurse launches a community-wide lead poisoning prevention program. This includes educational material about where lead is found in the home environment and how to test for lead (test kits are available in many stores).

The community health nurse targets parent-group leaders, local newspapers, and the school system to distribute educational materials.

Secondary Prevention

As recommended by CDC, you implement a blood-lead screening program. Your target population is children under 6 years of age who live in homes built before 1950 (CDC 1991).

During follow-up visits to homes where elevated lead levels have been confirmed, you educate parents on methods to reduce lead exposure:

1. Restrict children's play areas away from window sills and window wells.
2. Advise parents to plant grass and groundcover near the home to keep children away from soil where chipped paint has fallen throughout the years.
3. Wash children's hands and faces before meals and snacks.
4. Wash toys and pacifiers frequently.
5. Counsel parents of children who have elevated lead levels about the need for a diet high in iron and calcium.
6. Refer other children in the home, who have not been tested, for blood-lead testing.
7. Educate parents about wet-mopping the floors weekly with a cleaning solution high in phosphorus (5% to 8%).
8. Use washable rugs in entryways.

Tertiary Prevention

The initial blood-lead screening results indicate several children with blood-lead levels over 40 μg/dl. A follow-up protocol is developed in which these children are referred for treatment to a pediatrician and evaluated by community health nurses and a sanitarian. Developmental delays in the children and sources of lead exposure are assessed with referral and follow-up to appropriate programs.

Evaluation

One year later, all high-risk children (living in homes built before 1950) are enrolled in the blood-lead screening program. Children who have elevated blood-lead levels have been identified and treated successfully. Through cooperation with the state health department, local media, and area schools, the community demonstrates a good understanding about the hazards of lead exposure for children and the methods for mitigating that exposure.

Key Concepts

- Broadly defined, environmental health includes all aspects of the relationship between host and health and the effect of hazardous biological and chemical agents on human health. For this chapter, environmental health refers to the care of individuals exposed to environmental pollution in their homes and neighborhoods through such contaminated media as soil, water, air, and the food chain.

- Industrialization and advances in technology provide an improved quality of life and conveniences that were unimaginable a century ago. However, the industrial age also brought new problems of environmental pollution and toxic human exposures. In recent history, environmental public health problems have been addressed by legislation and establishment of public health and regulatory agencies.

- Nurses should be able to identify and characterize environmental health threats by community or client assessment.

- Community health nurses are in an ideal position to detect environmental health hazards and to use primary, secondary, and tertiary interventions to prevent or mitigate potential or actual toxic environmental exposures.

- For help in understanding environmental health threats, it is important to recognize other disciplines that are available to provide information and expertise. Examples include the environmental health scientist at your local government agency or the industrial hygienist at a company suspected of polluting the environment. These professionals can provide current environmental data that could affect nursing intervention.

- Nurses should have an understanding of the biological, physical, chemical, and psychosocial hazards affecting all segments of the community they serve, particularly individuals at risk such as children and elderly clients.

- The sciences of environmental health, exposure assessment, toxicology, epidemiology, and health education provide important skills to help public health nurses recognize potential environmental health threats to their clients and communities.

- Community health nurses must be able to communicate environmental health risks and prevention strategies clearly and effectively by developing messages that are easily understood and appropriate for each client and community.

- To protect public health, nurses must recognize the ethical, social, and legal implications of environmental health issues at the national and local levels and recognize how these can affect nursing practice.

- As health professionals and community members, nurses can play important roles in supporting a healthy environment. Knowing how to identify and access current scientific environmental health resources is necessary to identify hazards in the community, to help individuals understand potential environmental exposure, and for nursing diagnosis.

Critical Thinking Activities

1. Strengthen the bond between your academic or clinical setting and your community by sponsoring an environmental health outreach activity at your local library to answer or identify environmental problems of concern.

2. Encourage scientific literacy in your community by writing at least one letter to the editor or a think piece for the "op-ed" page of your local newspaper. The article should focus on praising or correcting factual representation of health data.

3. Familiarize yourself with the Toxic Release Inventory and its relevance to your community. Inform local health and political officials of its utility and limitations.

4. Perform a "windshield survey" of environmental health-related issues of concern in your community. Prepare an action plan to accomplish goals. Address what can be accomplished with varying levels of fiscal and human resources.

5. Review and determine what the number one environmental hazard is in your community. Indicate the scientific support for your decision and discuss three potential long-range consequences and how they might be successfully prevented.

Bibliography

Agency for Toxic Substances and Disease Registry (ATSDR): *The nature and extent of lead poisoning in children in the United States: a report to Congress,* Atlanta, 1988, US Department of Health and Human Services, Public Health Service.

Agency for Toxic Substances and Disease Registry (ATSDR): *Toxicological profile for radon,* Atlanta, 1990, US Department of Health and Human Services, Public Health Service.

Agency for Toxic Substances and Disease Registry (ATSDR): *Taking an exposure history: case studies in environmental medicine,* (26), Atlanta, 1992a, US Department of Health and Human Services, Public Health Service.

Agency for Toxic Substances and Disease Registry (ATSDR): *Public health assessment guidance manual,* Chelsea, Michigan, 1992b, Lewis Publishers.

Agency for Toxic Substances and Disease Registry (ATSDR): *Toxicological profile for tetrachloroethylene,* Atlanta, 1993, US Department of Health and Human Services, Public Health Service.

Agency for Toxic Substances and Disease Registry (ATSDR): *Toxicological profile on naphthalene: draft for public comment,* Atlanta, 1993a, US Department of Health and Human Services, Public Health Service.

Agency for Toxic Substances and Disease Registry (ATSDR): *Toxicological profile for selected polychlorinated biphenyls (PCBs),* Atlanta, 1993b, US Department of Health and Human Services, Public Health Service.

Amdur MO, Doull J, Clausen CD, editors: *Casarett and Doulls toxicology: the basic science of poisons,* ed 4, New York, 1991, Pergamon.

Beaumont JJ, Breslow N: Power considerations in evaluation of epidemiology studies of vinyl chloride workers, *Am J Epidemiol* 114:725, 1981.

Blumenthal DS: *Introduction to environmental health,* New York, 1985, Springer.

Burger R: *National disaster medical system (NDMS): national response team emergency planning guide,* Washington, DC, 1987, US Government Printing Office.

Carpenito LJ: *Nursing diagnosis: application to clinical practice,* Philadelphia, 1995, JB Lippincott.

Centers for Disease Control (CDC): *Preventing lead poisoning in young children: a statement by the Centers for Disease Control,* Atlanta, 1991, US Department of Health and Human Services, Public Health Service.

Chivian E, McKally M, Hu H, et al: *Critical condition: human health and the environment,* Cambridge, Mass, 1993, MIT.

Clemen-Stone S, Eigsti DG, Mcguire SL: *Comprehensive community health nursing,* ed 4, St Louis, 1995, Mosby.

Creech JL, Johnson MN: Angiosarcoma of the liver in the manufacture of polyvinyl chloride, *J Occup Med* 16:150, 1974.

Dignan MB, Carr PA: *Program planning for health education and health promotion,* Philadelphia, 1987, Lea & Febiger.

Donahue MP: *Nursing: the finest art,* St Louis, 1985, Mosby.

Guzelian PS, Henry CJ, Olin SS, editors: *Similarities and differences between children and adults: implications for risk assessment,* Washington, DC, 1992, International Life Sciences Institute.

Hance BJ, Chess C, Sandman PM: *Improving dialogue with communities: a risk communication manual for government,* Trenton, NJ, 1988, New Jersey Department of Environmental Protection, Division of Science Research.

Healthy Communities 2000: model standard guidelines for community attainment, Washington, DC, 1991, American Public Health Association.

Healthy People 2000: national health promotion and disease prevention objectives, Washington, DC, 1991, USDHHS, Public Health Service.

Hibbs BF: Chemical exposure evaluation and intervention, *J Am Assoc Occup Health Nurs* 284-9, June 1994.

Jackson RS: Early testing and subsequent evaluation of the insecticide kepone, *Ann NY Acad Sci* 392:318, 1979.

Klaassen CD, et al: Evaluation of safety: toxic evaluation. In Amdur MO, Doull J, Clausen CD, editors: *Casarett and Doulls toxicology: the basic science of poisons,* ed 4, New York, 1991, Pergamon.

Last JM, Wallace RB, editors: *Maxcy-Rosenau-Last: Public health and preventive medicine,* ed 13, Norwalk, Conn, 1992, Appleton and Lange.

Leavell HR, Clark EG: *Preventive medicine for the doctor in his community: an epidemiologic approach,* ed 3, New York, 1965, McGraw-Hill.

Lilienfeld DE: Definitions of epidemiology, *Am J Epidemiol* 107:87, 1978.

Lum MR: Environmental public health: future direction, future skills, *Fam Community Health* 18(1):24-35, 1995.

Mettler FA Jr, Moseley RD: *Medical effects of ionizing radiation,* Orlando, Fla, 1985, Grune and Stratton.

Miller RW: Areawide chemical contamination: lessons from case histories, *JAMA* 245:1548, 1981.

National Research Council (NRC): *Safe Drinking Water Committee: drinking water and health,* vol 1-9, Washington, DC, 1977-1989, National Academy Press.

National Research Council (NRC): *Risk assessment in the federal government: managing the process,* Washington, DC, 1983, National Academy Press.

National Research Council (NRC): *Environmental epidemiology: public health and hazardous wastes,* vol 1, Washington, DC, 1991, National Academy Press 20-1, 114-5.

National Response Team (NRT): *Hazardous materials emergency planning guide,* NRT-1, Washington, DC, 1987, US Environmental Protection Agency, Pub. No. WH-56A.

Nightingale F: *Notes on nursing,* London, 1859, Haris and Sons (republished Philadelphia, 1946, Lippincott).

Paehlke RC: Environmental values and public policy. In Vig NC, Kraft ME, editors: *Environmental policy in the 1990s,* Washington, DC, 1994, CQ.

Radford EP: Potential health effects of indoor radon exposure, *Environ Health Perspect* 62:218, 1985.

Rall DP, et al: Alternative to using human experience in assessing health risk, *Annu Rev Public Health* 8:355, 1987.

Salmon ME: An open letter to public health nurses, editorial, *Public Health Nurs* 10(4):211-212, 1993.

Sargent JD, Brown MJ, Freeman JL, et al: Childhood lead poisoning in Massachusetts communities—its association with sociodemographic and housing characteristics, *AM J Public Health* 85(4):528, 1995.

Slovic P, Lichtenstein S, Fischoff B: *Acceptable risk,* Cambridge, 1981, Cambridge University.

Sparks PJ, Daniell W, Black DW, et al: Multiple chemical sensitivity syndrome: a clinical perspective, *J Occupat Med* 36(7):718-37, 1994.

Tarcher AB, editor: *Principles and practices of environmental medicine,* New York, 1992, Plenum Medical Book.

Upton AC: Are there thresholds for carcinogenesis? The thorny problem of low level exposure. In Maltoni C and Selikoff IJ, editors: *Living in a chemical world: proceedings of an international conference on the occupational and environmental significance of industrial carcinogens,* New York, 1988, NY Academy of Sciences.

US Environmental Protection Agency (USEPA): *Study on household organic pollutants,* Washington, DC, 1987, US EPA.

US Environmental Protection Agency (USEPA): *The toxic release inventory,* Washington, DC, 1989, US EPA Pub No 560/4-900017.

US Environmental Protection Agency (USEPA): *Citizens' guide to radon,* Washington, DC, 1993, US EPA Pub No BG-004.

World Health Organization (WHO): *Guidelines on studies in environmental epidemiology,* Environmental criteria document 27, Geneva, 1983, WHO.

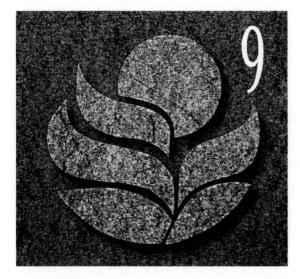

9

Policy, Politics, and the Law: Influences on the Practice of Community Health Nursing

Marcia Stanhope*

Objectives

After reading this chapter, the student should be able to do the following:

◆ Describe the trends and roles of several levels of government.
◆ Identify the impact of changing governmental roles and structures on health care.
◆ Describe the major governmental functions in health care.
◆ Discuss community health nursing roles in selected governmental agencies.
◆ Shape health policy by participating in the regulation-making process and the political arena.
◆ Describe selected laws that affect community health nursing practice, both generally and in special areas of practice.
◆ Conduct a brief exercise in legal research as one means of staying informed about current law.

Outline

*The author acknowledges the contribution of Cynthia Northrop to this chapter's content.

Community health nurses are affected significantly by the political system of the United States, as well as other governmental and institutional influences responsible for implementing health policy. This chapter provides descriptions of the institutions, including organization and primary functions of governments, governmental regulation, and the influence of politics on nursing practice. The chapter concludes with an overview of laws affecting community health nursing practice.

DEFINITIONS

To understand the relationship between health policy, politics, and laws, one must first understand the definitions of the terms. **Policy** is a settled course of action to be followed by a government or institution to obtain a desired end. *Health* policy then is simply a set course of action to obtain a desired *health* outcome, either for an individual, family, group, community, or society. Policies are made not only by governments but also by such institutions as a health department or other health care agency, a family, or a professional organization.

Politics plays a role in the development of such policies. One finds politics in families, in professional and employing agencies, and in governments. **Politics** is the art of influencing others to accept a specific course of action. Therefore one employs political activities to arrive at a course of action (the policy). **Law** is a system of privileges and processes by which people solve problems based on a set of established rules; it is intended to minimize the use of force. Laws govern the relationships of individuals and organizations to other individuals and to government. Through political action a policy becomes a law. As one will find in reading this chapter, after a law is established, regulations further define the course of action (policy) to be taken by organizations or individuals in reaching an outcome. **Government** is the ultimate authority in society and is designated to enforce the policy whether it be related to health, education, economics, social welfare or any other societal issue. The following discussion explains government's role in health policy.

GOVERNMENTAL ROLE IN HEALTH CARE

In the United States, the federal and most state governments are composed of three branches: the executive branch is composed of the President (or governor), cabinets, and regulatory units, such as the Department of Health and Human Services; the legislative branch is made up of two houses of Congress: the Senate and the House of Representatives; and the judicial branch is composed of the Supreme Court. Each of these branches plays a significant role in development and implementation of health policy. The executive branch administers and regulates policy, for ex-

ample, the Division of Nursing of the Department of Health and Human Services writes criteria to fund nursing education. The legislative branch passes laws that become policy, for example, the Medicare Amendments of the 1966 Social Security Act. The judicial branch interprets laws and the meaning of policy, as in its interpretation of states' rights to grant abortions.

One of the first constitutional challenges to congressional legislation in the area of health and welfare came in 1937, when Congress established unemployment compensation and old-age benefits. Although Congress had created other health programs, its legal basis for doing so had never been challenged before. The Supreme Court interpreted the meaning of the Constitution and decided that such federal government action was within congressional powers to promote the general welfare. Most legal bases for congressional action in health care are found in Article I, Section 8 of the U.S. Constitution. They include the following:

1. Provide for the general welfare
2. Regulate commerce among the states
3. Raise funds to support the military
4. Provide spending power

These statements have been interpreted by the Court to include a wide variety of federal powers and activities.

State power concerning health care is mostly **police power.** This means that states may act to protect the health, safety, and welfare of their citizens. Such police power must be reasonably exercised, and the state must demonstrate that it has a compelling interest in taking actions, especially actions that might infringe on individual rights.

Examples of a state exercising its police powers include requiring immunization of children before school admission and requiring casefinding, reporting, follow-up care, and treatment of tuberculosis. These activities protect the health, safety, and welfare of state citizens.

Trends and Shifts in Governmental Roles

Governmental involvement in health care at both the state and federal levels began gradually. Many historical events correspond closely with the role that has developed. Wars, economic instability, depressions, different viewpoints, and political parties all have shaped the governmental role. The New Deal, Roosevelt's post-Depression plans to revive the country, established major precedents for government spending on health care for Americans. In 1930 federal laws were passed to promote the public health of merchant seamen and the Native Americans. The Social Security Act of 1935 was a substantial piece of legislation, which has grown to include not only the aged and unemployed but also survivors' insurance for widows and children, child welfare, health department grants, and maternal and child health projects, Medicare an

Medicaid. In 1934 Senator Wagner of New York initiated the first national health insurance bill. Debate still continues on the extent of governmental responsibilities in health care. The most recent debate was responsible for the proposal of the National Health Security Act of 1993 by President Clinton.

Before the 1930s the only major governmental action relating to health was the creation in 1798 of the Public Health Service. The **Department of Health and Human Services (DHHS),** a regulatory agency known until 1980 as the Department of Health, Education, and Welfare (DHEW), was not created until

 Research Brief

Schlesinger M, Lee TK: Is health care different? Popular support of federal health & social policies, J *Health Polit Policy Law* 18(3 part 2):551-628, Fall 1993.

The purpose of this study was to determine whether there has been a shift in popular attitudes toward federal policies that corresponds with an increasing political interest in health care reform.

Survey data collected between 1975 and 1989 were used to answer the following questions:

1. Who supports and who opposes an active federal role in health care reform?
2. How do those who support such policies differ from those who oppose them?
3. How do patterns of public support for health care compare with patterns of support for social policy?
4. How are these differences changing over time?

This study concluded that there is a higher level of popular support for government action in health care, and is distributed among population groups differently than for other federal policies.

Support for federal health policy has grown over time. The gaps in support between rich and poor, educated and uneducated, old and young are reduced for health policy. Characteristics that make a difference in how one responds to federal policies are age, gender, race, education, marital status, income level, employment status, and rural vs. urban community. Gaps in support for antipoverty programs and general domestic policies still exist.

There is some evidence that growing support for health policy may be a result of the political ideology of the Reagan and Bush administrations. Support for such policy does not translate into a willingness to pay for new health programs.

Community health nurses can use this study to form strategies for promoting health care reform. Community health nurses will want to show others (clients, communities, legislators) how health care reform is an investment in society by improving the health of the nation; that health care reform promotes equal opportunity for all citizens to have health care; and that supporting investments in health care for all will eventually reduce the cost of health care for every citizen.

1953. It had a small predecessor that had been established in 1939, the Federal Security Agency. In 1946 Congress enacted a mental health bill and the Hospital Survey and Construction Act and created the National Institutes of Health in 1948. These legislative acts created entities that became part of the executive branch, now within the DHHS (see Chapter 3).

In a democracy the role of government in the area of health care depends on the beliefs of its citizens. Strong beliefs of self-determination and self-sufficiency mixed with beliefs about social responsibilities are hallmarks of a multiple approach to solving society's problems. Political party platforms demonstrate how different beliefs yield different approaches to problems.

A good example of this is the current debate between the Democratic and Republican parties over health care reform. The Democratic platform called for a health care system that was universally accessible and affordable. The Republican platform supports a continuation of the current system and a reduction in government's role in health care delivery, through cuts in Medicare and Medicaid benefits. Nurses are becoming more aware of the influence of political parties on health care delivery.

In 1991 the American Nurses Association, the National League for Nursing, the American Association of Colleges of Nursing and more than 60 nursing specialty organizations published nursing's agenda for health care reform (see Chapter 5). This "white paper" was a response to the political party's attempts to reform health care, indicating the direction organized nursing wanted to see the new policy develop.

Prior to the current response to reform, a major effort of the Reagan administration was to shift federal government activities to the states. In addition, passage in 1985 of the Gramm-Rudman Act, which was designed to decrease the federal budget deficit, not only promoted the continued shift of federal programs to states but also resulted in significant cutbacks in health and social programs. This effort continues in 1995 as the Republican controlled congress wants to cut maternal and child health programs and school lunch programs at the federal level. They want to give a sum of money to the states in the form of block grants to continue the programs as the state governments want.

The public is concerned about this approach because the states will not have to spend the money, for example, on the school lunch program but can spend the money instead on other programs that may not be as beneficial to children in poverty.

This discussion has focused primarily on trends and shifts within and among different levels of government. An additional aspect of governmental responsibilities is the relationship between government and individuals. Freedom of individuals must be balanced with government powers. Citizens express their views on the amount of governmental interference that will be tolerated. For example, the issue of sex education in public schools shows at least two viewpoints on the government-individual relationship:

1. Ever since the legislative branch of government established a system of education, some citizens believe that education should include content on sex.
2. Some citizens believe sex education belongs in the family and should not be interfered with by public schools, which are governmentally established.

These are only two of the views expressed in the literature. There are strong feelings about this issue, and the example shows how opinions about governmental versus individual responsibilities can be divided.

Governmental Health Care Functions

Federal, state, and local governments all carry out four general categories of health care functions: (1) direct services, (2) financing, (3) information, and (4) policy setting.

Direct Services

Federal, state, and local governments provide direct health services to certain individuals and groups. For example, the federal government provides health care to Native Americans, members and dependents of the military, veterans, and federal prisoners. State and local governments employ community health nurses to deliver services to individuals and families, usually based on financial need. State and local governments also may provide direct, specific services to all individuals, such as hypertension or tuberculosis screening, immunizations for children, and primary care for inmates in local jails or state prisons.

Financing

Governments pay for some health care services, training of personnel, and research. Financial support in these areas has significantly contributed to and affected consumers and health care providers. State and federal governments finance the direct care of clients through the Medicare, Medicaid, and Social Security programs. Many nurses have been educated with government funds; schools of nursing have been built and equipped through federal capitation funds. Other health care providers also have been financially supported by governments. Monies in the form of grants have been given by governments for specific research and demonstration projects. One of the best-known centers of medical research is the federally funded National Institutes of Health. In 1993 the National Institute of Nursing Research was established by Congress to promote nursing research. This will provide a substantial sum of money to the discipline of nursing for the purpose of defining the knowledge base of nursing.

Information

All branches and levels of government at one time or another have collected, analyzed, and made available

Table 9-1 International and National Sources of Data on the Health Status of the U.S. Population

Organization	Data source
INTERNATIONAL	
United Nations	Demographic Yearbook
World Health Organization	World Health Statistics Annual
FEDERAL	
Public Health Service	National Vital Statistics System
	National Survey of Family Growth
	National Health Interview Survey
	National Health Examination Survey
	National Health and Nutrition Examination Survey
	National Master Facility Inventory
	National Hospital Discharge Survey
	National Nursing Home Survey
	National Ambulatory Medical Care Survey
	National Morbidity Reporting System
	U.S. Immunization Survey
	Surveys of Mental Health Facilities
	Estimates of National Health Expenditures
	AIDS Surveillance
	Abortion Surveillance
	Nurse Supply Estimates
Department of Commerce	U.S. Census of Population
	Current Population Survey
	Population Estimates and Projections
Department of Labor	Consumer Price Index
	Employment and Earnings

data about health care and health status in the United States. An example is the annual report, *Health: United States,* compiled by the DHHS. Collection of vital statistics, including mortality and morbidity data, gathering of census data, and sponsoring health care status surveys are all government activities. Table 9-1 lists examples of available international and federal government data sources on the health status of the total U.S. population. These sources are available in the government documents sections of most large libraries. This information is especially important to community health nurses because it can help nurses understand the major health problems in the United States, as well as those in their own state.

Policy Setting

Policy setting relates to all government functions. Decisions about health care are made by governments at all levels and within all branches. Governments often show preference between groups when giving financial support. Such decisions affect the health care resources of each group and show the influence of government policy setting. Health policy decisions, or courses of action, usually have broad implications for economic growth, resource use, and development in the health care field. Examples of policy setting include the passage of amendments to the Social Security Act that established Medicare and the Professional Standards Review Organization (PSRO) in 1972 to monitor the quality of care given to hospitalized Medicare clients. The law that has had the most significant impact on the development of public health policy, public health nursing, and social welfare policy in the United States is the Sheppard-Towner Act of 1921.

In 1912 the Child Health Bureau was established as part of the U.S. Public Health Service. In 1917 the Bureau published a report, "Public Protection of Maternity and Infancy," to highlight findings of studies on infant and maternal mortality and consequently on the plight of women and children in the United States. In 1918 the first congresswoman, Jeanette Rankin, introduced a bill that later became the Sheppard-Towner Act. This act made public health nurses available to provide health services for women and children; offered well-child and child-development services; provided adequate hospital services and facilities for women and children; and provided grants-in-aid for the establishment of maternal and child welfare programs.

The Sheppard-Towner Act helped to establish precedent and set patterns for the growth of modern-day public health policy. It established the federal government's involvement in health care and the system for federal matching grants-in-aid awarded to states. The Act set the role of the federal government in creating standards to be followed by states in conducting categorical programs such as today's Women, Infants, and Children (WIC) and Early Periodic Screening and Developmental Testing programs (EPSDT). Also established were the position of the consumer in influencing, formulating, and conducting public policy; the government's role in research; a system for collecting national health statistics; and the integration of health and social services (Pickett and Hanlon, 1990). This policy established the importance of prenatal care, anticipatory guidance, client education, and nurse-client conferences, all of which are viewed today as essential community health nursing responsibilities.

ORGANIZATION OF GOVERNMENTAL AGENCIES

Community health nurses are actively involved with many levels of international and national government. This section discusses international organizations and roles of community health nurses in different national governmental agencies.

International Organizations

In June, 1945 many national governments joined together to create the United Nations. Aims and goals described in its charter include several dealing with human rights, world peace, security, and promotion of economic and social advancement of all people. The United Nations is headquartered in New York City and is made up of six principal subgroups. Several other subgroups and many specialized agencies and autonomous organizations are also within the system. One of the special autonomous organizations is the **World Health Organization (WHO)** (see Chapter 3).

Established in 1946, WHO relates to the United Nations through the Economic and Social Council to attain its goal of the highest possible level of health for all. Headquartered in Geneva, Switzerland, WHO is composed of three main branches: the World Health Assembly, the Executive Board, and the Secretariat (Figure 9-1). The organization has six regional offices. The office for the Americas is located in Washington, D.C., and is known as the Pan American Health Organization (PAHO).

The World Health Assembly, to which all United Nations members belong, meets annually and is the policy-making body of WHO. WHO provides worldwide services to promote health, cooperates with member countries in their health efforts, and coordinates biomedical research. Its services, which benefit all countries, include a day-to-day information service on the occurrence of internationally important diseases; publication of the international list of causes of disease, injury, and death; monitoring of adverse reactions to drugs; and establishment of world standards for antibiotics and vaccines. Assistance available to individual countries includes support for national programs to fight disease, train workers, and strengthen health services. An example of biomedical research collaboration is a special program to study six widespread tropical diseases: malaria, leprosy, "snail fever," filariasis, leishmaniasis, and "sleeping sickness."

The number of community health nursing roles in international health is increasing. Besides offering direct health services, nurses serve as consultants, educators, and program planners and evaluators. They focus their work on a variety of community health concepts, including environment, sanitation, communicable disease, wellness, and primary care. At least two of the contributors to this text have been WHO consultants, Dr. Beverly Flynn and Dr. Carolyn Williams.

In 1978 the International Conference on Primary Health Care sponsored by WHO and held in Alma-Ata, USSR, declared that the world community's goal should be the attainment of a level of health by the year 2000 that would permit all peoples to live socially and economically productive lives (WHO, 1978). The conference resolved that primary health care was the key to attaining this goal (see Appendix A-4).

At about the same time, the WHO Expert Committee on Community Health Nursing convened and out-

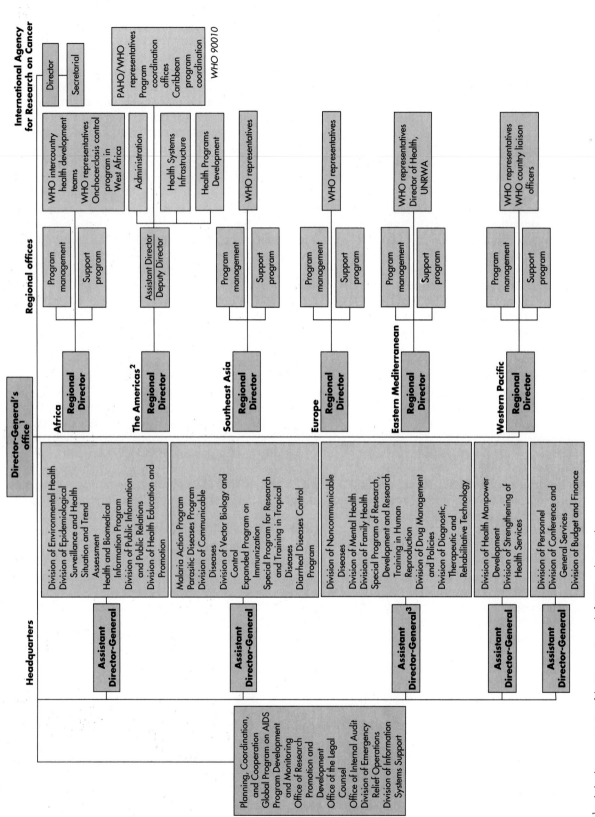

FIGURE 9-1

Structure of the World Health Organization. (Used with permission of the Office of Publication, Geneva, 1990, WHO.)

lined the broad role of community health nurses in primary health care. WHO is encouraging strengthened regulation of nursing education and practice related to primary health care, and it is in support of nurses in their efforts to become forces in attaining the goal of "health for all" (Mahler, 1985; WHO, 1986). This is an example of an international organization and policy that is certain to affect the future of nursing education and community health nursing practice.

Federal Agencies

Many federal agencies are involved in governmental health care functions. Legislation passed by Congress may be delegated to any regulatory agency within the executive branch for implementation, surveillance, regulation, and enforcement. Congress decides which agency will monitor specific laws. For example, most health care legislation is delegated to the Department of Health and Human Services (DHHS); however, legislation concerning the environment or occupational health would probably be monitored by the Environmental Protection Agency or the Labor Department. Examples of those departments most involved with health care are included in the following discussion.

Department of Health and Human Services (DHHS)

DHHS is the agency most heavily involved with the health and welfare concerns of U.S. citizens. It touches more lives than any other federal agency. As mentioned earlier, the organizational chart of DHHS (Figure 3-1, p. 43) depicts the office of the Secretary and four principal operating components: the Social Security Administration, the Health Care Financing Administration, the Administration for Children and Families, and the Public Health Service. The Public Health Service is charged with regulating health care and overseeing the health status of Americans.

Public Health Service

The major components of the **Public Health Service (PHS)** are shown in Figure 3-1, p. 43. The PHS has been a longstanding, significant contributor to the improved health status of Americans. The Health Resources and Services Administration of the PHS contains the Bureau of Health Professions, which includes a Division of Nursing, as well as Divisions of Medicine, Dentistry, and Allied Health Professions.

The Division of Nursing has these specific goals (USDHHS, HRSA, Division of Nursing, 1995):
- Enhancing nursing's contribution to primary health care and public health.
- Developing and promoting innovative practice models for improved and expanded nursing services.
- Enhancing racial and ethnic diversity and cultural competency in the nursing workforce.
- Promoting improved and expanded linkages between education and practice.
- Improving and expanding nursing services to high-risk and underserved populations.
- Enhancing nursing's contributions to achieving the *Healthy People Year 2000* objectives and health care reform.
- Capacity building for meeting the nursing service needs of the nation.

In late 1985 Congress overrode a Presidential veto, allowing the creation of the **National Center for Nursing Research,** within the National Institutes of Health. The research and research-related training activities previously supported by the Division of Nursing were transferred to this new Center. The Center is the focal point of the nation's nursing research activities. It promotes the growth and quality of research in nursing and patient care, provides important leadership, expands the pool of experienced nurse researchers, and serves as a point of interaction with other bases of health care research. (In 1993 the Center became one of the National Institutes of Health and was renamed the National Institute of Nursing Research.)

A significant addition to the PHS in 1990 was the creation of the Agency for Health Care Policy and Research (AHCPR). This agency is charged with conducting research on effectiveness of medical services, interventions, and technologies, including research related to nursing interventions and outcomes that contribute to the improved health status of the nation. Currently AHCPR is conducting focus groups to look at research showing positive outcomes of care for specific client problems, that is, incontinence, pain management.

The AHCPR has published protocols for care of clients with a variety of health problems. These protocols will become the future standards of health care delivery. In addition, AHCPR has a project called "Put Prevention Into Practice" to promote the use of standardized protocols for primary care delivery for clients across the age span. (See Protocols, Appendix A-2). These protocols can be used by community health nurses in planning disease prevention and health promotion activities for their clients.

Other Federal Goverment Agencies

DHHS has primary responsibility for federal health functions. The cabinet departments of the federal government carry out certain other functions. Those departments include Commerce, Defense, Labor, Agriculture and Justice.

Department of Commerce. Within the Department of Commerce (DOC) is the Bureau of the Census, which carries out an information function in health care. Established in 1902, this bureau conducts a census of the population every 10 years. The most recent was in 1990. Also a part of the DOC is the National Oceanic and Atmospheric Administration, which provides special services in support of controlling urban air quality, a major factor in community health today.

Department of Defense. The Department of Defense (DOD) delivers health care to members of the military and their dependents. The Assistant Secretary of Defense for Health Affairs administers the Civilian Health and Medical Program of the Uniformed Services (CHAMPUS). Each department within Defense (Army, Navy, Air Force, and Marines) has a surgeon general. Health services, including community health services for members of the military, are delivered by a Health Services Command in each department. In each command, nurses of high military rank, including brigadier general, are part of the administration of health services.

Department of Labor. The Department of Labor has two agencies with health functions: the Occupational Safety and Health Administration and the Mine Safety and Health Administration. Both are charged with writing safety and health standards and ensuring compliance in the workplace. This includes conducting inspections, investigating complaints, and issuing citations if necessary. Each agency coordinates its activities with state departments of labor and health.

Department of Agriculture. The Department of Agriculture is involved in health care primarily through administering the Food and Nutrition Service. Although plant, product, and animal inspection by the Department of Agriculture is also related to health, the Food and Nutrition Service oversees a variety of food assistance activities. This service collaborates with state and local government welfare agencies to provide food stamps to needy persons to increase their food purchasing power. Other programs include school breakfast and lunch programs; the Supplemental Food Program for Women, Infants, and Children (WIC); and grants to states for nutrition education and training. These programs are ones that will be negatively affected if Congress decides that states will administer these programs rather than the federal government. Monies will be given to the states as **block grants.** A block grant is a sum of money given to a state or local government whereby the federal government states a general purpose for the use of the money but allows the state or local area to spend the money without meeting specific conditions. A general purpose might be nutrition. The state could then determine where the nutrition money would go. It may not go to the programs just mentioned, which have been successful (Grad, 1990).

Department of Justice. Health services to federal prisoners are administered within the Department of Justice. The Medical and Services Division of the Bureau of Prisons includes medical, psychiatric, dental, and health support services. It also administers environmental health and safety, farm operations, and food service, along with commissary, laundry, and other personal services for inmates.

State and Local Government Departments

Most state and local (county and city) jurisdictions perform governmental activities that affect the health care field. At the state level, three executive branch departments are described: health, education, and corrections. The organization of a local health department also is outlined, and community health roles are discussed.

Selected Health Departments

Selected programs within a typical state health department are as follows:

Legal services
Services to the chronically ill and aging
Juvenile services
Medical assistance: policy, compliance, operations
Mental health and addictions
Mental retardation and developmental disabilities
Environmental programs
Departmental licensing boards
Division of vital records
Health services cost review
Health planning and development
Preventive medicine and medical affairs

In most state health departments, community health nurses serve in many capacities. These capacities are similar to those in international and federal agencies: consultation, direct services, research, teaching, supervision, planning, and evaluation of health programs. Most health departments have a division or department of community health nursing.

Every state has a board of examiners of nurses. The board may be found either in the department of licensing boards of the health department or in an administrative agency of the governor's office. Created by legislation known as a *state nurse practice act*, the examiner's board is made up of nurses and consumers. A few states have other providers or administrators as members. The functions of this board are described in the **practice act** of each state and generally include licensing and examination of registered nurses and licensed practical nurses; approval of schools of nursing in the state; revocation, suspension, or denial of licenses; and writing of regulations about nursing practice and education. Nurse practice acts will be discussed later in a section on the scope of nursing practice.

State Education Departments

Some state departments of education coordinate health curricula and services provided within local school systems. Other state legislatures mandate coordination of services solely within the health department or jointly between the health and education departments. Often liaison groups or councils are formed to facilitate joint coordination. These councils develop policy and guidelines for school health services and health education. Community health nurses often represent health and education departments at these councils and help shape health policy. Community health nurses also serve in departments of education in capacities similar to those in health departments.

State Departments of Corrections

Community health nurses work in state departments of corrections as planners and coordinators and sometimes as supervisors of health and nursing services for inmates in state prisons. Community health nurses in such state positions also may coordinate the health service efforts of local jails. Local jails may hire nurses directly or use the services of community health nurses in local health departments.

Local Health Departments

Depending on funding and other resources, programs offered by local health departments vary greatly. A fairly comprehensive list of such programs, taken from an urban-suburban county health department in a mid-Atlantic state, is shown in the box below. At the local level, as at the state level, coordination of health efforts between health departments and other county or city departments is essential. For example, local boards of education and departments of social services are an integral part of activities of local governments. More often than at other levels of government, community health nurses at the local level provide direct services. Some community health nurses

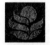 Examples of Programs Provided by Local Health Departments

Addictions and alcoholism clinics
Adult health
Birth and death records
Child day care and development
Child health clinics
Crippled children's services
Dental health clinic
Environmental health
Epidemiology and disease control
Family planning
Geriatric evaluation
Health education
Home health agency
Hospital discharge planning
Hypertension clinics
Immunization clinics
Information services
Maternal health
Medical social work
Mental health
Mental retardation and developmental disabilities
Nursing
Nursing home licensure
Nutrition division
Occupational therapy
Physical therapy
School health
Speech and audiology
Vision and hearing screening

deliver special or selected services, such as follow-up of contacts in cases of tuberculosis or venereal disease, or providing child immunization clinics. Other community health nurses have a more generalized practice, delivering services to families in certain geographical areas. This method of delivery of community health nursing services involves broader needs and a wider variety of nursing interventions.

Social Welfare Programs

In addition to health programs, federal, state, and local governments also provide social welfare programs. Generally these programs provide monetary benefits to the poor, elderly, disabled, and unemployed.

The federal Social Security Act established a number of programs, which include the social insurance programs, Social Security, unemployment insurance, and welfare programs.

The Social Security Administration, which is within the DHHS, administers the following programs:
1. Old Age Survivors and Disability Insurance (OASDI)
2. Aid to Families with Dependent Children (AFDC) and
3. Supplemental Security Income (SSI).

OASDI provides monthly benefits to retired and disabled workers, their spouses and children, and to survivors of insured workers. AFDC, which is a federal and state program, helps needy families with children. AFDC subsidizes children deprived of the financial support of one of their parents as a result of death, disability, absence from the home, or, in some states, unemployment.

SSI is a federal program for the aged, blind, and disabled that may be supplemented by state support. The funds for these programs are provided by contributions from employees, employers, and self-employed individuals. These contributions are pooled into a special trust fund that is paid upon a worker's retirement, death, or disability as partial replacement of the earnings the family has lost.

In 1965, amendments to the Social Security Act created Medicare and Medicaid. These programs are administered by the Health Care Financing Administration (HCFA) within the DHHS; in the case of Medicaid the administration is done in conjunction with state governments. (See Chapter 5 for additional discussion of Medicare and Medicaid programs.)

In addition, there are human development services coordinated by the Division of Administration for Children and Families within DHHS. Programs are focused on the aging, children, youth and families, Native Americans, and the developmentally disabled. For example, the Older Americans Act is designed to promote the welfare and needs of older people. Through this act the federal government promotes the development of state-administered community-based systems of comprehensive social services for the elderly.

Social programs focused on children and families include programs on adoption opportunities, Head Start services, runaway-youth facilities, child-abuse prevention and treatment, juvenile justice, and delinquency prevention. Other programs promote the social and economic development of Native Americans.

The Administration for Developmental Disabilities in this division assists states in increasing the provision of quality services to persons with developmental disabilities. Grants are administered that support projects aimed at removing physical, mental, social, and environmental barriers for these disabled individuals.

Social welfare policies and programs affect community health nursing practice. Community resources that improve the quality of life for specific populations help nurses to assist clients in attaining optimal health.

Impact of Governmental Health Functions and Structures on Community Health Nursing

The variety and range of functions of government agencies has had a major impact on the practice of community health nursing. Funding in particular has shaped roles and tasks of community health nurses. The designation of money for specific needs has led to special, more narrowly focused community health nursing roles. For example, funds assigned to communicable disease programs or family planning usually will not support home care services. Therefore nurses develop specialty roles related to these funded programs (e.g., immunization nurses, family planning nurses).

Training grants from the DHHS, Division of Nursing for nurse practitioners in primary care have provided incentives to individual nurses to attend programs and develop new community health nursing roles within the health care system. Finally, school, adult, and pediatric nurse practitioners emerged primarily because of the funding provided by government agencies.

Other health policy information, funding, and direct services functions of government have influenced community health nursing. Legislatures have identified special needs and programs to meet the needs of special populations, such as migrant workers, pregnant women, homeless persons, or at-risk children. Often community health nurses are called upon to implement these programs. Vital statistics and other epidemiological data collected by government agencies have influenced the location, work force, planning, and evaluation of community health nursing services.

According to the evolving policies of the federal government and administrations of the 1980s, federal money given to the states was in the form of block grants. The block grant had a great impact on community health nursing. Having less money in special programs resulted in a shift of community health nursing roles toward more generalized practice. Whether community health nursing should be a specialty or a generalized practice is an age-old debate.

The purpose of mentioning the debate here is to show how government funding has shaped the functions of community health nurses within all levels of government. When governments give money to special programs, community health nursing roles become specialized and take care of the needs of certain clients only, such as the immunization of children. When governments give money to states to spend as they wish, community health nursing roles become generalized, and the nurse takes care of all client needs; for example, pregnant mothers, sick children, and a homeless men's health assessment are all provided in one clinic.

COMMUNITY HEALTH NURSES' ROLE IN THE POLITICAL PROCESS

The number and type of laws influencing health care are increasing. Because of this, involvement in the political process at all possible points is most important to community health nursing. The community health nurse's basic understanding of this political process should include knowing who the lawmakers are, how bills become law, the regulation-writing process, and methods of influencing the process and shaping health policy. (See Figure 9-2 on how a bill becomes law.)

The federal and state legislatures are composed of two houses: an assembly, or house, and a senate. Representatives and senators are elected by the people within geographic jurisdictions. Each state has two federal senators and one or more representatives, depending on the state's population. Each state has its own rules for deciding on the numbers of senators and representatives within the state for the state legislature.

Although Congress meets throughout the year, state legislatures have sessions of varying lengths. Each legislature has its own leadership, usually dominated by either the Democratic or Republican party. Roles include the presiding officer, party floor leaders, and committee chairpersons.

An important part of this **legislative process** is the work of the staffs of the legislatures. These individuals do the legwork, research, paperwork, and other activities that move policy ideas into bills and then into law. In addition to the individual legislators' staffs, committee staffs are also important. Both of these can provide valuable information for constituents and their legislators. Nurses often serve as staff to legislators, or are constituents of a legislator and will want to give to or get information from that legislator about health policy.

The legislative process begins with ideas that are developed into bills. After a bill is drafted, it is introduced to the legislature, given a number, read, and assigned to a committee. Hearings, testimony, lobbying, education, research, and informal discussion follow. If the bill is passed from the committee, the entire house hears the bill, amends it as necessary, and votes on it.

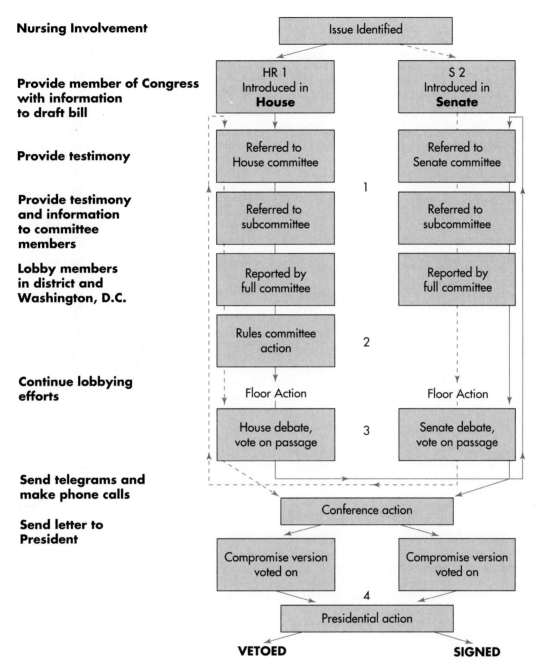

The Federal Level

Nursing Involvement

Issue Identified

HR 1 Introduced in **House**

S 2 Introduced in **Senate**

Provide member of Congress with information to draft bill

Referred to House committee

Referred to Senate committee

Provide testimony

1

Referred to subcommittee

Referred to subcommittee

Provide testimony and information to committee members

Reported by full committee

Reported by full committee

Lobby members in district and Washington, D.C.

Rules committee action

2

Continue lobbying efforts

Floor Action

Floor Action

House debate, vote on passage

3

Senate debate, vote on passage

Send telegrams and make phone calls

Conference action

Send letter to President

Compromise version voted on

Compromise version voted on

4

Presidential action

VETOED

SIGNED

[1] A bill goes to full committee first, then to special subcommittees for hearings, debate, revisions, and approval. The same process occurs when it goes to full committee. It either dies in committee or proceeds to the next step.

[2] Only the House has a Rules Committee to set the "rule" for floor action and conditions for debate and amendments. In the Senate, the leadership schedules action.

[3] The bill is debated, amended, and passed or defeated. If passed, it goes to the other chamber and follows the same path. If each chamber passes a similar bill, both versions go to conference.

[4] The President may sign the bill into law, allow it to become law without his signature, or veto it and return it to Congress. To override the veto, both houses must approve the bill by a 2/3 majority vote.

FIGURE 9-2

How a bill becomes law. (From Mason DJ, Talbott SW, Keavitt JK: *Policy and politics for nurses: action and change in the workplace, government, organizations, and community,* ed 2, Philadelphia, 1993, WB Saunders.)

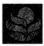

The How-To's of Communication

BUILD A PROFESSIONAL IMAGE

What images do you have of yourself: strong, assertive, confident, competent, powerful? To be politically influential requires that we are effective image shapers. What images do you convey in the workplace, the community, the government, and professional organizations? The following checklist will help you identify some of your messages.

◆ In your daily encounters with clients and their families, do your verbal and nonverbal behaviors convey your professional pride and confidence?

◆ Do you carry business cards to facilitate contacts with persons you meet?

◆ Do you share your expertise through the local and national media?

◆ Do you thoroughly document your nursing care?

◆ Do you spend time every day teaching and listening to the concerns of your patients and their families?

◆ At staff meetings, do you set the tone for serious collaboration by asking questions and giving your opinions?

◆ Do you regularly communicate your ideas, concerns, and suggestions to your supervisors, public officials, and organizational leaders?

◆ Do you vote in every national and local election?

◆ What does your body language communicate?

From Mason DJ, Talbott SW, Keavitt JK: *Policy and politics for nurses: action and change in the workplace, government, organizations, and community,* ed 2, Philadelphia, 1993, WB Saunders.

◆ Do you call or write to supervisors, community people, public officials, and organizational leaders to thank them when they have helped you with a problem or issue?

◆ Does your attire communicate that you are a serious, businesslike professional?

REFINE YOUR COMMUNICATION SKILLS

Since communication is a key aspect of political activity and policy development, it is imperative to possess finely honed skills:

◆ Get assistance in developing your writing and speaking; they are indispensable in sending messages that will be taken seriously.

◆ Attend continuing education sessions on public speaking, writing, and media training.

◆ Volunteer to speak at programs in your workplace, at nursing association meetings, and in the community.

◆ Testify at public hearings.

◆ Write short articles in your areas of expertise for your local newspapers and workplace newsletters.

◆ Team up with colleagues when you visit legislators, write an article, testify, or speak on a radio show or at a workshop. You will learn from the shared experience and bolster each other's confidence.

◆ Learn invaluable influence skills through committee work and involvement in nursing organizations, work-related committees, political action committees, multidisciplinary and consumer groups, and political clubs.

◆ Vote and get others to vote.

Tips for Writing to Legislators

1. Use your own stationery, not hospital or agency stationery. A letter is better than a postcard or telegram. Use your own words; form letters are not as effective as original ones.

2. Identify your subject clearly. State the name (and bill number if possible) of the legislation you are writing about.

3. Be brief, giving the reasons that you are for or against the legislation. Explain how the issue would affect you, the nursing profession, patients, and/or your community.

4. Know what committees your legislators serve on and indicate in the letter if the bill will be brought before any of those committees. Know the current status of the bill (where it is in the legislative process).

5. Sign your name with "R.N." after it. Be sure your correct address is on the letter and the envelope. (Envelopes sometimes get thrown away before the letter is answered.)

6. Be courteous. A rude letter neither makes friends nor influences the legislator. Be sure to express your appreciation for work well done, a good speech, a favorable vote, or fine leadership in committee or on the floor.

7. Timing is important. Try to write your positions on a bill while it is in committee. Your legislators will usually be more responsive to your appeal at that time rather than later, when the bill has already been dealt with by a committee.

8. Limit your letter to one issue.

9. Keep a copy of all correspondence for your files. Send a copy of your letter, and any response from the legislator, to the government relations staff at your professional nursing organization.

10. Address written correspondence as follows:

U.S. Senator	U.S. Representative
Honorable Jane Doe	Honorable Jane Doe
United States Senate	House of Representatives
Washington, DC 20510	Washington, DC 20515
Dear Senator Doe:	Dear Representative Doe:

The same general format applies to state and local officials.

11. Mailgrams, which take two days, and telegrams, which are faster, can be ordered through Western Union's toll-free number: 1 (800) 325-6000.

12. You may be able to send a facsimile transmission (fax) to your legislator if you both have the necessary technology. This technique offers speed and conveys a sense of urgency. If you choose this method, follow up by sending the original letter through the mail.

From Mason DJ, Talbott SW, Keavitt JK: *Policy and politics for nurses: action and change in the workplace, government, organizations, and community,* ed 2, Philadelphia, 1993, WB Saunders.

Tips for Visiting Legislators

1. Call ahead to make an appointment to meet with the legislator. If the legislator is unavailable, ask to meet with the staff person who handles health issues.
2. Prepare. Know the background of the legislator and the history of the bill or issue you are discussing. Contact the government relations staff at your professional nursing organization to let them know about the visit. They may be able to provide important information about the issue, the political climate, your legislator's previous record on this issue, and the overall lobbying strategy on this issue.
3. At the beginning of the visit, introduce yourself and state what you want to discuss. Specify the issues and bills.
4. Ask the legislator what her or his position is on the issue or bill.
5. Many legislators and staff may not be familiar with nursing practice or legislative concerns. Be prepared to discuss them in basic terms. If possible, be prepared with facts about nursing practice in your state or district.
6. Ask if she or he has heard from others who support this issue or bill. Ask what the supporters are saying.
7. Ask if she or he has heard from opponents. Ask who the opponents are and what their arguments are.
8. Offer to provide additional information if you do not have data at hand—but do not make promises you cannot keep. It is better to admit you do not know than to promise and not deliver or to convey erroneous information.
9. Follow up with a thank-you note, and share your reflections on the visit.
10. Keep a written record of your visit. Notify government relations staff of your professional nursing organization so that they can follow up with the legislator.
11. Spend more time with your legislators even if their position is not in agreement with yours. You might lessen the intensity of their positions and maintain contact for subsequent issues.
12. Invite legislators to meet you and your colleagues at your work site to help expand their understanding of nursing and health care issues.

From Mason DJ, Talbott SW, Keavitt JK: *Policy and politics for nurses: action and change in the workplace, government, organizations, and community,* ed 2, Philadelphia, 1993, WB Saunders.

Tips for Action

◆ Get to know your legislators and the chair of your state board of nursing. Make sure you meet the governor and know the governor's chief executive aide (the person who really runs the show).
◆ Apply the problem-solving and negotiation skills you have developed in nursing to the process of making and implementing laws. They are the same skills you use to convince a diabetic patient to let you help him or her develop a care plan.
◆ Cultivate relationships with people who make the rules or pass the laws.
◆ Run for office.
◆ Develop a bipartisan nurse advisory council to assist your local legislator. (One state organized a statewide advisory group for a U.S. Senator. This group previewed U.S. health legislation for the Senator, and several nurses testified before the U.S. Senate Appropriations Subcommittee on Health and Human Services.)
◆ Spend an hour or two a week to upgrade your knowledge of political developments, health policy initiatives, legislators, and state government executives.
◆ Learn how health care funds are allocated through the political process.

From Mason DJ, Talbott SW, Keavitt JK: *Policy and politics for nurses: action and change in the workplace, government, organizations, and community,* ed 2, Philadelphia, 1993, WB Saunders.

A majority vote moves the bill to the other house, where it is read, amended, and voted on.

Community health nurses can be involved in this process at any point. Many professional nursing associations have professional lobbyists, legislative committees, and political action committees (PACs) to shape health policy.

Common methods of lobbying include face-to-face encounters, personal letters, mailgrams, telegrams, telephone calls, testimony, petitions, reports, position papers, fact sheets, letters to the editor, news releases, speeches, coalition-building, demonstrations, and law suits. Depending on the issue, each of these can be equally effective. The boxes on pages 166 and 167 offer tips on communication, writing to and visiting legislators, as well as general tips on political action.

Behind the scenes of this process lies the political party activity in which community health nurses should be involved. A wide variety of activities are available, including voting, participating in the party organization, registering voters, getting out the vote, fundraising, building networks or communication links, and participating in political action committees.

The passage of the National Health Research Extension Act of 1985 is an example of how nurses can use their influence. This act included the establishment of the National Center for Nursing Research. The Center began as the idea of a small group of nurses who worked to gain the support of colleagues and major national nursing organizations. Individual nurses provided testimony to Congress on the importance of nursing research. Some visited their congressional representatives to lobby for the bill. Many wrote letters and provided position papers and fact sheets to help legislators understand the need for the Center. Although the process took several years, the idea became a reality. Both the nursing profession and the consumer will benefit from the research and the knowledge base developed through the Center, now a National Institute of Health.

PRIVATE SECTOR INFLUENCE ON REGULATION AND HEALTH POLICY

In each level of government the executive branch can, and in most cases must, prepare regulations. These regulations are detailed, and they establish, fix, and

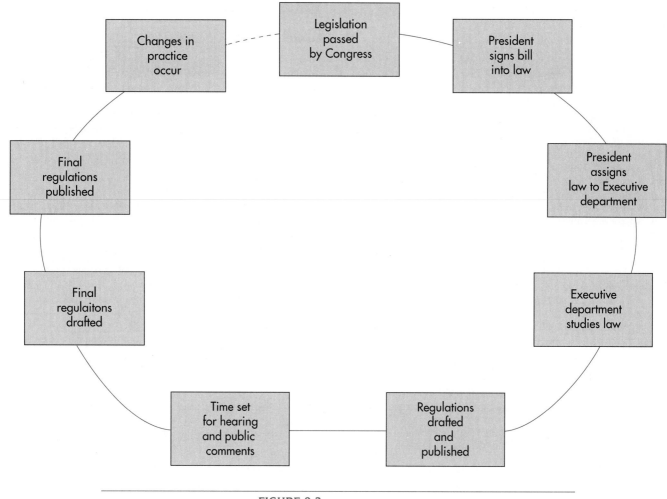

FIGURE 9-3

The regulation writing process.

control standards and criteria for carrying out certain laws. Figure 9-3 shows the steps in the typical regulation-writing process.

When the legislature passes a law and delegates its administration to an agency, it gives that agency the power to make regulations. Because regulations flow from legislation, they have the force of law.

The **private sector,** which includes everyone that is not part of the government or **public sector,** can influence and shape legislation through many means. Through the same means, the private sector also influences the writing of regulations. This part of the chapter will describe the process of regulation writing and ways to influence it. Community health nursing students and clinicians are members of the private sector and are influenced by regulations that affect nursing practice.

Process of Regulation

After a law is passed, the appropriate executive department begins the process of regulation by studying the topic or issue. Advisory groups or special task forces, including nondepartmental members, are sometimes formed to provide the content of the regulations. As the work of the groups or individual department members progresses, initial drafts of the proposed regulations are written. Community health nurses, including students, can influence these regulations by writing letters to the regulatory agency in charge or by speaking at public hearings.

After refinement, the proposed regulations are put into final draft form and printed in the legally required publication. At the federal level the legally mandated channel is the *Federal Register.*

Similar registers exist in most states where regulations from state departments, including state health departments, are published. The publication of proposed regulations includes notice about a time period within which public comment will be accepted. Public comment in this situation is usually in written form. The notice also may give a date, time, and place for a hearing that is open to the public. Anyone may attend; if one wishes to speak at the hearing, published rules for that procedure must be followed. This usually involves notifying the agency of one's intent to speak and limiting the length of testimony as specified by the agency.

Revisions made to the proposed regulations are based on public comment and public hearing. Depending on the amount and content of the public reaction, final regulations are prepared or more study of the area and issues is conducted. Final published regulations carry the force of law. The date when regulations become effective also is published. It is at this point that practice is changed to conform to the new regulations.

Close monitoring by, and participation of, the private sector in regulation writing can begin as soon as a law is passed and delegated to an executive branch agency. Government manuals, updated at least yearly, list names and phone numbers of individuals within the executive branch. Early contact and expression of interest in how a particular law gets administered may result in membership on a task force or advisory board. The membership of such groups is public information, and one can contact these members to determine their thoughts on the direction the regulations will take.

Regular surveillance of the *Federal Register* or state registers is essential. Once proposed resolutions are published and members of the private sector may influence regulations by attending the hearings, providing comments, testifying, and engaging in lobbying aimed at individuals involved in the writing. Concrete, written suggestions for revision submitted to these individuals are usually persuasive.

Final regulations, published in a ***Code of Regulations*** (both federal and state), usually lead to changes in practice. Regulations need to be made available to all individuals whose practice is affected. This dissemination can be helped effectively by private sector involvement. Regulations need to become included in manuals of policies and procedures of the agencies affected by them. For example, Medicare regulations setting standards for nursing homes and home health are incorporated into these agencies' manuals.

LAWS AFFECTING COMMUNITY HEALTH NURSING PRACTICE

Community health nursing combines nursing practice and public health practice. The community health nurse is subject to the laws relating to nursing practice and public health practice.

This part of the chapter will discuss the various types of laws, how they affect community health nurses, and the legal resources available.

Types of Laws

Several definitions of laws are available. However, many of these tend to describe what law is *not* rather than what it is. Definitions of law include the following:

1. A rule established by authority, society, or custom
2. The body of rules governing the affairs of people within a community or among states; social order; the common law
3. A set of rules or customs governing a discrete field or activity; e.g., criminal law, contract law
4. The system of courts, judicial process, and legal officers, or lawyers giving effect to the laws of a society

These definitions reflect the close relationship of law to community and to society's customs and beliefs. Since community health nursing reflects society's beliefs and customs, law has had a major impact on this practice. Although community health nursing practice emerged from individual voluntary activities, society soon recognized the need for it. Through legal mandates, positions and functions for nurses in community settings were created. These functions in many instances carry with them the "force of law." For example, if the community health nurse discovers a person with smallpox, the law directs the nurse and others legally designated in the community to take specific action. This is just one example of how the law has shaped community health nursing practice.

There are three types of laws in the United States: (1) constitutional law, (2) legislation and regulation, and (3) judicial and common law.

Constitutional Law

Constitutional law emerges from federal and state constitutions. From this type of law community health nurses can get answers to questions in selected practice situations. For example, on what basis can the state require quarantine or isolation of individuals with tuberculosis? The answer to this question can be found in constitutional law.

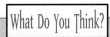
What Do You Think?

The community's rights are more important than the individual's rights when there is a threat to the health of the public.

The U.S. Constitution specifies explicit and limited functions of the federal government. All other powers and functions are left to the individual states. The major power of the states relating to community health nursing practice is the right to intervene in a reasonable manner to protect the health, safety, and welfare of the citizenry. As described earlier in this chapter, the state's "police power" is not without limitation. First, it must be a "reasonable" exercise of power. Second, if the power interferes or infringes on individual rights, the state must demonstrate that there is a "compelling state interest" in exercising its power. Hence, isolating an individual or separating one from a community because he has a communicable disease has been deemed an appropriate exercise of state powers. The state can isolate an individual even though it infringes on individual rights (freedom, autonomy), under the following conditions:

1. If the isolation is done in a reasonable manner
2. If there is a compelling state interest in the prevention of an epidemic
3. If the isolation is necessary to protect the health, safety, and welfare of individuals in the community or the public as a whole.

The legal, and medical community's, and AIDS activists' rejection of the social quarantine of individuals with AIDS is an example of how individual freedom and autonomy of the individual come before "compelling state interest."

Legislation and Regulation

Legislation is the type of law that comes from the legislative branches of federal, state, or local government. Much legislation has an impact on community health nursing. **Regulations** are very specific statements of law that relate to individual pieces of legislation.

Community health nurses often are employed by the executive branch through the state or local health department. Hence, nursing interventions are often directed at implementing legislation and regulations. Nurses employed in other community settings—those with no governmental responsibilities or legal mandates—are nevertheless often subject to legislation and regulations. For example, community health nurses employed by private agencies who are rendering home health care must deliver care according to federal Medicare legislation and regulations or state Medicaid legislations and regulations in order for the agency to be reimbursed for those services. Private and public health care services rendered by community health nurses are subject to many government regulations.

Judicial and Common Law

Judicial and **common law** is the last group of laws having an impact on community health nursing. Judicial law is based on court or jury decisions.

The opinions of the courts are judicial opinions and are referred to as "case law." The court uses other types of laws to make its decision, including previous court decisions or cases. **Precedent** is one principle of common law. Judges are bound by previous decisions unless they are convinced that the "old law" is no longer relevant or valid. This process is called "distinguishing" and usually involves a demonstration of how the currently disputed situation differs from the previously decided situation. Other principles of common law are part of a court's rationale and the basis of making a particular decision. Such principles include justice, fairness, respect for individuals, autonomy, and self-determination. These play an important role in decisions made by courts (see Chapter 6).

General Community Health Nursing Practice and the Law

Despite the broad nature and varied roles of community health nursing practice, two legal aspects apply to most practice situations. The first aspect is **professional negligence,** or malpractice; the second is the **scope of practice** defined by custom and state practice acts.

Professional Negligence

Professional negligence or malpractice is defined as an act or failure to act on behalf of a client which leads to injury of that client. To prove that a nurse was negligent, the client must prove *all* of the following:

1. The nurse owed a duty to the client, or was responsible for the client's care.
2. The duty to act as a reasonable, prudent nurse, or as another community health nurse would act under the circumstances, was breached or not fulfilled.
3. The failure to be reasonable under the circumstances led to the alleged injuries.
4. The injuries provided the basis for a monetary claim through the legal system.

Reported cases involving negligence and community heath nurses are almost nonexistent. As one example, a case involving an occupational health nurse is discussed. Although occurring some years ago, this example clearly represents the four criteria which must be present to prove negligence. Since nurses still use standing orders, a similar problem could happen to a nurse today.

The California case of *Cooper versus Motor Bearing Co.,* 288P 2d 581, involved an occupational health nurse who negligently implemented standing orders on an injury involving a puncture wound. The nurse, by her own testimony, did not examine or probe the wound, nor did she refer the worker to a physician; she simply swabbed and bandaged it. Only after 10 months, in which time there were many documented visits to the dispensary and the worker complained that the wound was not healing, did the nurse refer him to the company doctor. On referral, basal cell carcinoma was found and surgery followed.

The fact that the nurse was employed by the industry to render first aid established the first element of negligence: a duty was owed the worker. The nurse acknowledged that it was her duty to refer any unfamiliar or questionable condition or injury to the doctor for diagnosis. The standard of good nursing care in the community was to examine the wound for the presence of foreign bodies. The nurse knew the normal healing time was 1 to 2 weeks. If a wound persisted and did not heal, proper nursing care would indicate referral to a physician. Testimony was given that the practice of an occupational health nurse in this particular type of industry is to probe wounds for foreign bodies. According to the nurse's education and experience, she should have been aware of the possibility of foreign objects being present in such a wound.

In this case the nurse's failure to detect the foreign body was the proximate cause of the basal cell carcinoma. The pain, suffering, lost time and wages, and bodily disfigurement were all injuries that could be calculated and totaled as a monetary amount. The nurse and the company were found negligent by the California Court.

An integral part of negligence suits is the question of who should be sued. Obviously, those who made the mistakes should be sued, but part of the consideration has to do with who can best compensate for the injuries. When a nurse is employed and functioning within the scope of that employment, the employer is responsible for the nurse's negligent actions. This is referred to as the doctrine of **respondeat superior.** By directing a nurse to carry out a particular function, the employer becomes responsible for negligence, along with the individual nurse. The scope of employment is usually more inclusive than a job description but does not include criminal activities. Because employers are usually better able to compensate for the injuries suffered, they are sued more often than the nurses themselves.

Community health nurses employed by government agencies need to ascertain whether that agency has **sovereign immunity.** Under this doctrine the agency may be exempt from suit for particular kinds of actions, such as negligence. However, sovereign immunity will not protect nurses who are acting under the auspices of the government when the negligence occurs. Individual public health nurses may have personal immunity for particular practice areas, such as giving immunizations. In some states the legislature has granted personal immunity to community health nurses to cover all aspects of their practice.

Community health nursing students need to be aware that they are governed by the same laws and rules governing the graduate nurse. Students are expected to meet the same standard of care of any licensed nurse practicing under the same or similar circumstances. Lower standards of care by students are not acceptable. Students are expected to be able to perform all tasks and make clinical decisions based on the knowledge they have gained or been offered, according to their progress in their educational programs. If a faculty member gives a student an assignment based on the student's progress in the program, the faculty member is not considered liable for the student's actions.

Scope of Practice

The issue of **scope of practice** involves differentiating between the practices of physicians, nurses, and other health care providers. Scope of practice is assessed by (1) examining the usual and customary practice of a profession, and (2) taking into account how legislation defines the practice of a particular profession in a jurisdiction. The issue is especially important to community health nurses who have traditionally practiced in a wide scope.

The usual and customary practice of community

health nursing can be determined through a variety of sources, including the following:

1. Contents of community health nursing educational programs, general and special
2. Experience of other practicing nurses (peers)
3. Activities and statements, including standards, of community health nursing professional organizations
4. Policies and procedures of agencies employing nurses
5. Needs and interests of the community
6. Literature, including books, texts, and journals.

All these sources can describe and help determine the scope of the usual practice of a community health nurse.

Every community health nurse should know and follow closely the proposed changes in practice acts in nursing, medicine, pharmacy, and other related professions. These pieces of state legislation define the scope of practice for professionals in these areas. The nurse always should examine *all* definitions related to nursing practice. For example, a review of the Pharmacy Act will let the nurse know whether to question the right to "dispense" medications in a methadone clinic in a local health department, when following physician prescription and preparing several identical doses for the client to take between clinic visits. Defining scope forces one to clarify both independent and dependent community health nursing functions. The failure to know one's limitations could lead, for example, to charges of practicing as a pharmacist without a license, with subsequent fines and possible suspension or revocation of license. Just as practice acts vary, so do the issues of scope of practice. It is best to refer directly to practice acts for a particular state code.

Because of the variety of legal aspects, the following section deals with areas of practice having special focuses.

Special Community Health Nursing Practice and the Law

Legal aspects of community health nursing vary, depending on (1) the setting where care is delivered, (2) the clinical specialty, and (3) the functional role. Four special areas of community health nursing practice and their respective legal aspects will be discussed to illustrate how the law affects specific practice areas. Those four areas are school and family health, occupational health, home care and hospice services, and correctional health. Examples of legislation and judicial opinions affecting community health nurses within these selected areas are included.

School and Family Health

School and family health nursing may be delivered by community health nurses employed by health departments or boards of education. School health legislation establishes a minimum of services that must be provided to children in public and private schools. For example, most states require that children be immunized against certain communicable diseases before entering school. Children must have had a physical examination by that time, and most states require at least one physical at a later time in their schooling. Legislation also specifies when and what type of health screening will be conducted in schools; examples are vision and hearing testing.

Legislation treating child abuse and neglect makes a large impact on community health nursing practice within schools and families. Most states require nurses to notify police or a social service agency of any situation in which they suspect a child is being abused or neglected. This is one instance in which society permits a professional to breach confidentiality to protect someone who may be in a helpless and vulnerable position. There is civil immunity for such reports, and the nurse may be called as a witness in any subsequent hearing. In fact, the majority of legal cases involving community health nurses concern child abuse.

Other examples of federal legislation affecting community health nursing practice with regard to schools and families are Head Start, early diagnostic screening programs, nutritional programs, services for the handicapped, and special education. Most of this legislation, although written by the U.S. Congress, requires cooperative federal and state funding, planning, and implementation. Each nurse working within a service based on legislation should be oriented to the legislation. It is advisable that the legislation and its regulations be included in the nursing agency's manual of policies and procedures so that the nurse may refer to it.

Occupational Health

Occupational health is another special area of practice that is affected greatly by state and federal laws. The **Occupational Safety and Health Act (OSHA)** imposes many requirements on industries. These requirements shape the functions of community health nurses and the types of services given to workers. OSHA also establishes a reporting system for workers exposed to toxic agents in the workplace. A record-keeping system required by OSHA greatly affects health records in the workplace. Each state has an agency similar to OSHA that also monitors and inspects industries, as well as the health services rendered to them by nurses. Most states have a "worker's right to know" law requiring employers to provide employees with information concerning the nature of toxic substances they may encounter in the workplace during their employment. In addition, all states have workers' compensation statutes that provide a legal opportunity for claims of workers injured on the job. Access to records, confidentiality, and the use of standing orders are legal issues of great significance to nurses employed in industries.

Home Care and Hospice

Home care and hospice services rendered by community health nurses are affected greatly by state laws that require licensing and certification. Compliance with these laws is directly linked to the method of payment for the services. For example, a service must be licensed and certified to obtain payment for services through Medicare. Federal regulations implementing Medicare have an effect on much of community health nursing practice, including how nurses record details of their visits.

Many states have passed laws requiring nurses to report elder abuse to the proper authorities. Legislation affecting home care and hospice services has related to such issues as the right to death with dignity, rights of residents of long-term facilities and home-health clients, definitions of death, and the use of living wills, specifically advanced directives that now must be given to and signed by all clients of community health nurses. The legal and ethical dimensions of community health nursing practice are particularly important in this area of practice. Individual rights, such as the right to refuse treatment, and nursing responsibilities, such as the legal duty to render reasonable and prudent care, may often be in conflict in delivering home and hospice services. Much case discussion, sometimes including outside consultation, is required when rights and responsibilities are in conflict and a decision must be made to resolve that conflict.

Correctional Health

Nursing practice in correctional health systems is controlled by federal and state laws and regulations and by recent Supreme Court decisions. The laws and decisions relate to the type and amount of services that must be provided for incarcerated individuals. For example, physical examinations are required of all prisoners after they are sentenced. Regulations specify basic levels of care that must be provided for prisoners, and care during illness is particularly addressed. Court decisions requiring adequate health services are based on constitutional law. If minimum services are not provided, it is a violation of a prisoner's right to freedom from cruel and unusual punishment. Such decisions provide a framework that strongly influences the setting of nursing priorities. For example, providing sick calls would take priority over nutritional classes.

Did You Know?

Persons with communicable diseases such as tuberculosis may be confined to a prison hospital if they are considered a threat to their community by failing to follow their treatment regimen.

Each of the preceding areas of special community health nursing practice is shaped significantly by legislation and judicial opinion. Those nurses responsible for setting and implementing program priorities need to identify and monitor laws related to each special area of practice.

Legal Resources

In addition to seeking legal counsel, community health nurses can actively remain current with respect to nursing-related laws and regulations. There are many resources in public libraries and law libraries, including the following:

State bar association publications
State code
State annotated code
Indexes to codes
Supplements to codes and indexes
Federal Register and state registers
Codes of regulations (federal and state)
Administrative agency rules and decisions
Case law
Opinions of attorney generals
Legal dictionaries
Legislative histories
Legal periodicals

In using these legal resources, begin by reviewing the topical index to each source. As the headings are reviewed, several can be identified as relating to the content areas of practice (such as immunizations or family planning) and the types of clients (e.g., minors, adolescents, and children) served by the community health nurse. Computer search tools are often available. One legal computerized search tool is called **Lexis.** The Library of Congress has a service called **Scorpio.** Both services will search not only books and journals but also recent case laws, bills, amendments, and legislation. One of the best ways to stay informed is to read the area newspaper.

 ## Clinical Application

Larry was in his final rotation in the bachelor of science in nursing program at State University. He was anxious to complete his community health nursing course because upon graduation he would begin a position as a staff nurse specializing in school health at the local health department. His wife was expecting their first child, and she had been receiving prenatal care at the health department.

Larry was aware that a few years ago the federal government had, by law, provided block grants to states for primary care, maternal child health programs, and other health care needs of states. He had read the Federal Register and knew that the regulations for these grants had been written through DHHS departments. He was aware that these regulations did not require states to fund specific programs.

Larry read in the local paper that the health department was closing its prenatal clinic at the end of the month. When this state had received its block grant, they decided to spend its money for programs other than prenatal care.

The next day Larry began the process of *assessing* the situation. He knew that his wife and others like her were in jeopardy of losing their prenatal care, placing them at risk for premature delivery, low birth weight, or other such complications. In the law library, he reviewed the state register to see if regulations for the block grants had been finalized. He also checked state health statistics, which included vital statistics providing the current infant and maternity mortality rates in the state. In addition to comparing these data with national statistics, he reviewed the literature for research that would show the relationships between prenatal care, normal deliveries, and complications of pregnancy and delivery.

To his surprise, Larry found that a 3-year study in his own state showed improved pregnancy outcomes as a result of prenatal care. The results were further improved when the care was delivered by community health nurses.

Larry was concerned that, as a student, he would have little influence. However, he decided to call his classmates together to *plan* a course of action. After some discussion, a representative contacted the local nurses' association and found that the association was also extremely concerned about the problem. Together the groups contacted their local senators and representatives and asked for a meeting to discuss the issue. Larry also contacted the legal aid society. He found a lawyer interested in consulting with them in preparing written and oral testimony. The testimony was to be presented to the state health department during the process of preparing the regulations for the block grants.

Since Larry had been the leader in rallying support for the issue, he was asked to present this testimony. To *implement* the planned action, he used the national and state statistics, his literature review, and his own family situation to present his argument for the needed support for prenatal care.

Because his own senators and representatives were sympathetic to the issue, he was able to get their support for his testimony. The regulatory process took approximately 180 days. Larry wanted to *evaluate* the outcome of lack of prenatal care and found that during this time the infant mortality rate in the state was already on the rise. This incident, the support of the nursing organization, and congressional influence led to changes in the state Medicaid law, increasing the number of women in the state who could obtain prenatal care through the health departments.

Key Concepts

- Many historical events have been significant in developing the role of government in health care.

- The legal basis for most congressional action in health care can be found in Article I, Section 8 of the U.S. Constitution.

- The four major health care functions of the federal government are direct service, financing, information, and policy setting.

- The goal of the World Health Organization is the attainment by all people of the highest possible level of health.

- Many federal agencies are involved in government health care functions. The agency most directly involved with the health and welfare of Americans is the Department of Health and Human Services (DHHS).

- Most state and local jurisdictions have government activities that affect the health care field.

- The variety and range of functions of government agencies have had a major impact on community health nursing. Funding in particular has shaped the role and tasks of community health nurses.

- The private sector can influence legislation in many ways, especially through influencing the process of writing regulations. Nurses are a part of the private sector.

- The number and types of laws influencing health care are increasing. Because of this, involvement in the political process is most important to community health nurses.

- Professional negligence and the scope of practice are two legal aspects particularly relevant to nursing practice.

- Community health nurses must consider the legal implications of their own practice in each clinical encounter.

- The federal and most state governments are comprised of three branches: the executive, the legislative, and the judicial.

- Each branch of government plays a significant role in health policy.

- The first national health insurance bill was introduced in Congress in 1934.

- The U.S. Public Health Service was created in 1798.

- The political party platforms are good sources of information to find out how a government will respond to a health policy issue.

- *Health: United States* is an important source of data about the nation's health care problems.

- In 1912 the Child Health Bureau was established.

- In 1921 the Sheppard-Towner Act was passed and had important influence over child health programs and community health nursing practice.

- The Division of Nursing, the National Institute of Nursing Research, and the Agency for Health Care Policy and Research are governmental entities important to nursing.

- Community health nurses through state and local health departments function as consultants, direct care providers, researchers, teachers, supervisors, and program managers.

- The state governments are responsible for regulating nursing practice within the state.

- Federal and state social welfare programs have developed to provide monetary benefits to the poor, elderly, disabled, and unemployed.

- Social welfare programs affect community health nursing practice. These programs improve the quality of life for special populations, thus making the nurse's job easier in assisting the client with health needs.

- The community health nurse's scope of practice is defined by legislation and by standards of practice within the specialty.

Critical Thinking Activities

1. Conduct an interview with the local health officer. Ask for information from a 10-year period. See if you can see trends in population size and needs and corresponding roles and activities of government that were implemented to meet these changes.

2. Examine a current health department budget and compare it with a budget from previous years. Has there been any impact on health care because of changes in government spending?

3. Select a community health nursing role you would like to examine more closely. Interview a person in that role, asking questions about job function, organizational structure, agency goals, salary, mobility within the agency, and potential contributions of this role to the health of the community.

4. Locate your state register or other documents, such as newspapers, that publish proposed regulations. Select one set of proposed regulations and critique them. Submit your opinion in writing as public comment, or attend the hearing and testify on the regulations. Be sure to submit something in writing. Evaluate your participation by stating what you learned and whether the proposed regulations were changed in your favor.

5. Find and review your state nurse practice act and define your scope of practice.

6. Contact your local public health agency to discuss the state's official powers in regulating epidemics, such as the recent AIDS outbreak. Explore the state's right to protect the health, safety, and welfare of the citizens. Ask about the conflict between the state's rights and individual rights and how such issues are resolved. Ask about the standards of care that apply to this issue and how it is decided which services offered to clients should be mandatory and which should be voluntary. Explore how the role of public health differs in these epidemics compared with the past epidemics of smallpox and tuberculosis.

Bibliography

American Nurses Association: *A conceptual model of community health nursing,* Kansas City, Mo, 1982, The Association.

American Nurses Association: *Code for nurses,* Kansas City, Mo, 1985, The Association.

American Nurses Association: *Standards of community health nursing practice,* Kansas City, Mo, 1986, The Association.

American Public Health Association: *The definition and role of public health nursing in the delivery of health care,* Washington, DC, 1981, The Association.

Aroskar M: Legal and ethical issues: politics and ethics in nursing—implications for education, *J Prof Nurs* 10(3):129, May-June, 1994.

Chaney E: Personal and vicarious liability, *J Pediatr Nurs* 2(2):132, 1987.

Chapman E: Putting the case for the nurse: handling and avoiding clinical negligence claims, *J Prof Nurs* 9(7):443-4, 446-7, Apr, 1994.

Cohen W, Milburn L: Political action, *Nurs Health Care* 9(6):294, 1988.

Creighton H: *Law every nurse should know,* ed 5, Philadelphia, 1986, WB Saunders.

Creighton H: Legal implications of home health care, *Nurs Manage* 18(2):14, 1987.

Creighton H: Legal implications of policy and procedure manual, part 1, *Nurs Manage* 18(5):22, 1987.

Cushing M: Million-dollar errors, *Am J Nurs* 4:435, 1987.

Cushing M: Keeping watch, *Am J Nurs* 8:1021, 1987.

Cushing M: A strong defense, *Am J Nurs* 10:1278, 1987.

Cushing M: Perils of home care, *Am J Nurs* 4:441, 1988.

Dahl R: *Democracy in the United States: promise and performance,* ed 2, Chicago, 1972, Rand McNally & Co.

Davis A and Aroskar M: *Ethical dilemmas and nursing practice,* ed 2, New York, 1983, Appleton-Century-Crofts.

Division of Nursing, Bureau of Health Professionals, Health Services and Resources Administration, Public Health Service: *The division of nursing,* Hyattsville, Md, 1993, The Division.

Feutz S: The expansiveness of liability to third parties, *J Nurs Adm* (4):9, 1987.

Fiesta J: The nursing shortage: whose liability problem? Part 1, *Nurs Mgt* 21(1):24, 1990.

Fiesta J: The nursing shortage: whose liability problem? Part 2, *Nurs Mgt* 21(2):22, 1990.

Gittler J: Controlling resurgent TB, *J Health Polit Policy Law* 19(1), 107-47, Spring, 1991.

Gittler J, Bayer R: Public health policy and TB, *J Health Polit Policy Law* 19(1), 149-54, Spring, 1994.

Gittler J, Boubjer R: The importance of public health for the 21st century, *J Health Polit Policy Law* 19(1), 155-63, Spring, 1994.

Grad F: *The public health law manual,* ed 2, APHA, 1990, Washington, DC.

Green J: The $147,000 misunderstanding: repercussions of overestimating the costs of AIDS, *J Health Polit Policy Law* 19(1), 69-90, Spring, 1994.

Halpern S: Government involvement in maternal and child health care: a learning resource for the nurse-midwife, *J Nurse Midwifery* 32(1):34, 1987.

Health: United States, 1993, DHHS Pub No (PHS) 1232, Hyattsville, Md, 1994, US Department of Health and Human Services.

Hinshaw A: The impact of nursing science on health policy, *Commun Nurs Res* 25:15-26, Spring, 1992.

Hudson-Rodd N: Public health: people participating in the creation of healthy places, *Public Health Nurs* 11(2), 119-26, April, 1994.

Jacobs LR: Health reform impasse: the politics of American ambivalence toward government, *J Health Polit Policy Law* 18(3 part 2):629-55, Fall, 1993.

Leavitt J, Barry C: Learning the ropes—developing political expertise, *Imprint* 40(4):58-61, Sept-Oct, 1993.

Luquire R: Six common causes of nursing liability, *Nursing* 88(1):61, 1988.

Malher H: Nurses lead the way, *WHO features,* No 97, June 1985.

Manke K: Politics and the nurse manager, *Nurs Manage* 24(12):35-7, Dec, 1993.

Marks D: Legal implications of increased autonomy, *J Gerontol Nurs* 13(3):26, 1987.

Martin F: Documentation tips to help you stay out of court, *Nursing* 24(6):63-4, June, 1994.

Martin J, White J, Hansen M: Preparing students to shape health policy, *Nurs Outlook* 37(2):89, 1989.

Mason DJ, Talbott SW, Keavitt JK: *Policy and politics for nurses: action and change in the workplace, government, organizations, and community,* ed 2, Philadelphia, 1993, WB Saunders.

Nagelkerk J: Policy-making, *J Nurs Adm* 24(5), 14-5, 64, May, 1994.

Northrop C, Kelly M: *Legal issues in nursing,* St Louis, 1987, Mosby.

Northrop C: Filling in charting gaps . . . in court, *Nursing* 87(9):43, 1987.

Northrop C: Adequate staffing . . . whose problem is it? *Nursing* 87(6):43, 1988.

Northrop C: Legal content in the nursing curriculum: what students need and how to provide it, *Nurs Outlook* 37(4):200, 1989.

Office of Federal Register: *United States government manual,* Washington, DC, 1990, US Government Printing Office.

Painter S: Shield yourself from liability, *Nursing* 87(5):47, 1987.

Parsons M: Five common legal risks: could these stories have happened to you? *Nursing Life* (6):26, 1986.

Patton C, Sawicki D: *Basic methods of policy analysis and planning,* ed 2, Englewood Cliffs, NJ, 1993, Prentice Hall.

Pickett G, Hanlon J: *Public health administration and practice,* St Louis, 1990, Times Mirror/Mosby College Publishing.

Primary health care needs. Conclusion and recommendations of a WHO study group, *Int Nurs Rev* 34(2):52, 1987.

Rogge M: Nursing and politics: a forgotten legacy, *Nurs Res* (1):26, 1987.

Rothman D: A century of failure: health care reform in America, *J Health Polit Policy Law* 18(Part I):271-86, Summer, 1993.

Scearse P: Public policy and the conservatives, traditionals, and influentials, *J Prof Nurs* 3(3):132, 1987.

Scearse P: Disease, debts, and the political process, *J Prof Nurs* 4(4):239, 1988.

Schanz S: Health care provider liability: traditional principles, *Nurs Econ* 5(6):311, 1987.

Schlesinger M, Lee TK: Is health care different? Popular support of federal health and social policies, *J Health Polit Policy Law* 18(3 part 2): 551-628, Fall, 1993.

Sharp N: Nurses in public policy—legislature effects: what's next? *Nurs Manage* 24(11):22-3, 26, Nov, 1993.

Sharpe N: All politics is local and other rules, *Nurs Manage* 25(3):22, 24-5, Mar, 1994.

Smith C: Patient teaching: it's the law, *Nursing* 87(7):67, 1987.

Smith G: Using the public agenda to shape PHN practice, *Nurs Outlook* 37(2):72, 1989.

Sullivan G: Home care: more autonomy, more legal risks, *RN* 57(5):1 63-4, 67-9, May, 1994.

Szasz A: The labor impacts of policy change in health care: how federal policy transformed home health organizations and their labor practices, *J Health Polit Policy Law* 15(1):191, 1990.

Thomas PA: Teaching students to become active in public policy, *Public Health Nurs* 11(2):75-9, Apr, 1994.

USDHHS, HRA, BHPR Division of Nursing, 1995, Washington D.C.

United Nations: *Basic facts about the UN,* New York, 1990, The UN.

WHO & UNICEF: *Primary HealthCare: a joint report,* Geneva, World Health Organization, 1978.

World Health Organization: *The work of WHO, 1988-1990: biennial report of the Director-General,* Geneva, 1990, WHO.

World Health Organization: *Technical report series,* 738, Geneva, 1986, WHO.

Part Three Conceptual Frameworks Applied to Community Health Nursing

In 1988 the National Center for Nursing Research (NCNR) was established under the National Institutes of Health for the purpose of facilitating nursing research. In 1993 the U.S. Congress expanded the scope and functions of NCNR and made it one of the National Institutes of Health and renamed it the National Institute of Nursing Research (NINR). The NINR is crucial to the profession's movement to build a stronger base for practice. Though no conceptual or theoretical model will meet the needs of all community health nurses, several nursing and public health models serve as frameworks for organizing educational programs and for making practice decisions.

In 1988 the Institute of Medicine report on the *Future of Public Health* identified three primary functions of public health: assessment through data collection and sharing of information; policy development for family, community and state level health policies; and assurance of the availability of necessary health services for clients. These are called the Core Public Health Functions and are important to the practice of all public health providers including nurses. In 1993 the Public Health Nursing Directors of Washington State developed a model showing how public health/community health nurses perform the three core functions with all clients: individuals, families, and communities.

The scientific base provided by public health as a specialty continues to lay a useful foundation for community health nursing. In Part Three, five chapters provide information about how to use conceptual models, epidemiology, research, and principles of education to organize community health practice to meet the core functions of public health. Each chapter provides both theory and practical application of the specific topic to the clinical area. The goal of this section is to provide readers with a helpful set of tools that can be used to influence public health and community health nursing practice.

It has been estimated that the effect of the medical care system on usual indexes for measuring health is about 10%. The remaining 90% is determined by factors over which health care providers have little or no direct control, such as life-style and social and physical environmental conditions. This text focuses on the processes and practices for promoting health, principally by the community health nurse, who is considered an ideal person to personally demonstrate and teach others how to promote health. To be effective, health promotion requires that people cease focusing on how to "fix" themselves and others only when they detect physical and emotional disequilibriums and that they, instead, assume personal responsibility for health promotion. Such a change in emphasis requires that health care providers incorporate health promotion techniques into their practice. ▼

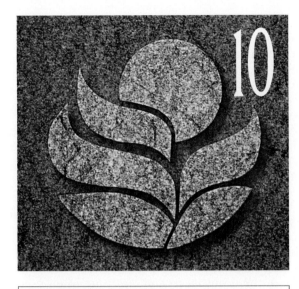

10

Organizing Frameworks Applied to Community Health Nursing

Jeanette Lancaster ◆ Lois W. Lowry ◆ Karen S. Martin

Key Terms

boundary
client problem
concept
conceptual model
construct
data management
documentation
entropy
equifinality
evaluation
feedback
flexible line of defense
general systems theory
hypothesis
intervention
lines of resistance
model
negentropy
Neuman Systems Model
normal line of defense
nursing diagnosis
nursing intervention
nursing practice
nursing process
Omaha Intervention Scheme
Omaha Problem Classification Scheme
Omaha Problem Rating Scale for
    Outcomes
Omaha System
openness
organization
proposition
theory
wholeness

Objectives ▼

After reading this chapter, the student should be able to do the following:

◆ Define the terms *theory, model, concept,* and *conceptual model.*
◆ Differentiate between conceptual model and theory.
◆ Identify at least three uses of conceptual models in nursing.
◆ Differentiate between the ANA and the APHA models of community health nursing.
◆ Describe key components of the Neuman Systems Model and the Omaha System.
◆ Apply the Neuman Systems Model to community health practice.
◆ Apply the Omaha System to community health practice.

Outline ▼

Community health nursing is the specialty area that blends nursing and public health theory into a population-focused practice designed to promote and preserve the health of communities. "The focus of community health nursing practice is the community as a whole, with nursing care of individuals, families and groups being provided within the context of promoting and preserving the health of the community as a whole" (Association of Community Health Nursing Educators [ACHNE], 1990, p. 1)

This chapter provides two detailed examples of how concepts, models, and theories guide community health nursing practice. First, theory and theory development are discussed, followed by a description of the competencies and essential functions of community health nursing. Next, two models for organizing data and guiding community health nursing practice are presented in detail. These models are the Neuman Systems Model and the Omaha System. Over the last decade, these two models have demonstrated usefulness in community health nursing. This in no way implies that these are the only two models that effectively guide community health nursing practice; however, they are frequently used and with good results. At present, both models are used to guide curriculum design in schools of nursing, the conduct of nursing research, and nursing practice in service agencies.

DEFINING CONCEPTS, MODELS, AND THEORIES

What is a theory? A **theory** is a construct that accounts for or organizes phenomena. A nursing theory explains or describes a specific phenomenon of nursing (Barnum, 1994). A theory focuses on one or more concrete, specific concepts and statements; it is clearly stated and operationally defined; and hypotheses can be established and tested through research.

Models are ways of viewing real phenomena. Models can be either physical, symbolic, or mental. A physical model is a specific, observable replica of the real structure. For example, when a new health department building is about to be constructed, the architect may assemble a small replica that is simply a scaled version of the proposed new structure. Symbolic models have a higher level of abstraction than do physical models. For example, signs within a health department have symbolic meaning to those who read them. That is, a "no smoking" sign signifies that the readers should refrain from certain actions. Likewise, a sign that states "do not use the elevator in case of fire" conveys a specific message of what not to do in a certain situation by using symbolism. Mental models have an even greater level of abstractness than do both physical and symbolic models in that they convey a mental image, not a real picture. For example, the term *nursing* has different meanings to each person.

A **conceptual model** is a set of images and thought patterns that are conveyed by language. In nursing,

conceptual models convey meaning to four core concepts: person, environment, health, and nursing. Conceptual models represent an early stage in theory development by providing focus and identifying relevant variables that can then be tested through theory analysis.

Conceptual models provide a frame of reference for members of a discipline to guide their thinking, observations, and interpretations. In those conceptual models with the greatest usefulness in community health nursing, people are seen as being in continuous interaction with a dynamic environment. Because the focus is the community, nursing care of individuals, families, and groups is considered within the context of the community (ACHNE, 1990). Table 10-1 defines several key terms useful in understanding concepts, models, and theories.

Although the terms *model* and *theory* are often used interchangeably, they differ in several ways. One main difference is in the level of abstraction. A conceptual model is a highly abstract system of global concepts and propositional statements. In contrast, a theory focuses on one or more concrete, specific concepts and statements. A second difference involves the ability to test the model or theory. A conceptual model cannot be tested directly because the concepts are not operationally defined and the relationships are not observ-

Table 10-1   Key Terms to Understanding Frameworks for Community Health Nursing

Term	Definition
Conceptual model	A set of concepts that provides a frame of reference for members of a discipline to guide their thinking, observations, and interpretations; propositions of a conceptual model are abstract and general.
Concepts	The building blocks of theory; they describe mental images of phenomena and can be concrete (chair) or abstract (body temperature).
Constructs	Concepts that describe phenomena that are not directly observable, such as society, intelligence, and age.
Propositions	Statements that describe the relationship between concepts; for example, "persons and their environment are in constant interaction" is a proposition.
Theory	A set of interrelated constructs (concepts), definitions, and propositions that present a systematic view of phenomena by specifying relationships among variables, with the purpose of explaining and predicting phenomena.

Kerlinger F: *Foundations of behavioral research*, ed 3, 1973, New York, Holt, Rinehart & Winston.

able. On the other hand, a theory is clearly stated and operationally defined, and **hypotheses** are formulated so they can be tested through research. Conceptual models constitute a key stage in theory development by providing focus, identifying relevant variables, and ruling out other variables as unrelated.

USING CONCEPTUAL MODELS

Conceptual models with the greatest application to community health nursing view people as being in continuous interaction with the environment. The environment is dynamic and can be either positive or negative. The unique feature of community health nursing is the emphasis on assisting individuals, families, groups, and communities to maintain their highest possible level of health. To accomplish this, the community is viewed from a holistic perspective as a motivator or disrupter of health. The nursing goal is to assess, plan, implement, and evaluate ways to make the community a healthier place to live.

To some extent, everyone has developed a conceptual model because all people have assumptions and beliefs about how the world operates. Everyone has a unique set of concepts guiding how ideas and information are categorized and how situations are viewed and responses selected. A person's conceptual models influence behavior either consciously or unconsciously. In particular, models direct one's world view. The *world view* refers to philosophical assumptions about the nature of person-environment interactions. That is, a person's conceptual models determine what is considered relevant, what is eliminated, which concepts or constructs are identified, and how they are defined. For example, Orem's world view claims that an environment "promotes personal development in relation to becoming able to meet present or future demands for action" (1985, p. 138). On the other hand, Rogers' (1980) world view of person and environment regards them as irreducible wholes, changing continuously, mutually, creatively, and inseparably. Each model states unique assumptions about the world view it represents.

In addition to reflecting diverse world views, conceptual models of nursing can be classified according to their origins, such as systems theory, human development, interaction, human needs, or outcomes (Marriner-Tomey, 1994; Meleis, 1991). Most nursing models fall within these classifications because each suggests a way to interpret and link the four meta-paradigm concepts of the discipline of nursing—person, environment, health, and nursing—according to a specific school of thought. That is, all models identify person as an integrated biopsychosocial being but may use different definitions. For instance, a *person* may be defined as an adaptive system (Roy, 1984), an energy field (Rogers, 1980), or a behavioral system (Johnson, 1980). *Environment* is often identified as all internal and external influences that surround persons. *Health* may be presented as a continuum from illness to wellness or a value or a dichotomy of stability versus instability. The concept of *nursing* is also defined, and nursing actions are described to represent a specific viewpoint of the model (Fawcett, 1989). A nursing model often reflects more than one viewpoint; it is then classified within the most dominant category.

Many nurses use one particular nursing model to guide practice; others merge more than one model into a unique guide for practice; and still others integrate theories borrowed from other disciplines, such as psychology, sociology, and the biological sciences. Conceptual models are useful in nursing education, research, administration, and practice. Later in this chapter, the Neuman Systems Model is applied to the development of an undergraduate nursing curriculum and to nursing practice.

In nursing, specific theories are employed to describe, explain, and predict client manifestations of actual or potential health problems (Fawcett, 1989). Whereas a model, like a blueprint for building a house, describes the structure of how parts are related, a theory moves beyond description to the more complex level of prediction by describing the relationships among the parts. In nursing practice, models incorporate three essential components: the client, the goal of the nursing intervention, and the activities that the nurse employs to attain the goal. By using models in practice, nurses can identify problems from which hypotheses can be generated. These hypotheses can then be tested in practice and education.

The ANA Conceptual Model and Standards of Community Health Nursing Practice

The definition of community health nursing included in the American Nurses Association (ANA) Conceptual Model of Community Health Nursing emphasizes health promotion and consumer involvement and considers health as being influenced by multiple factors within people and by the environments in which people live (ANA, 1980). The definition in the ANA Standards of Community Health Nursing Practice is as follows (ANA, 1986, p. 1):

Community health nursing practice promotes and preserves the health of populations by integrating the skills and knowledge relevant to both nursing and public health. The practice is comprehensive and general, and is not limited to a particular age or diagnostic group; it is continual, and is not limited to episodic care.

This definition like the previous definition in the 1980 Conceptual Model document encompasses both direct and indirect services to individuals, families, groups, and communities. Its scope is concerned with both wellness and illness in providing, as well as facilitating, the delivery of services. This definition uses the terms community health nursing and public health nursing synonymously. In addition, as shown in the box on p. 182, standards of practice have been

Standards of Community Health Nursing Practice

1. The nurse applies theoretical concepts as a basis for decisions in practice.
2. The nurse systematically collects data that are comprehensive and accurate.
3. The nurse analyzes data collected about the community, family, and individual to determine diagnoses.
4. At each level of prevention, the nurse develops plans that specify nursing actions unique to client needs.
5. The nurse, guided by the plan, intervenes to promote, maintain, or restore health; to prevent illness; and to effect rehabilitation.
6. The nurse evaluates responses of the community, family, and individual to interventions in order to determine progress toward goal achievement and to revise the data base, diagnoses, and plan.
7. The nurse participates in peer review and other means of evaluation to ensure the quality of nursing practice. The nurse assumes responsibility for professional development and contributes to the professional growth of others.
8. The nurse collaborates with other health care providers, professionals, and community representatives in assessing, planning, implementing, and evaluating programs for community health.
9. The nurse contributes to theory and practice in community health nursing through research.

American Nurses Association: *Standards of Community health nursing,* Kansas City, 1986, The Association.

developed to guide both generalist practice and specialist practice in community health (ANA, 1986).

The focus of community health nursing is on the prevention of illness and the promotion and maintenance of health. Nursing activities to achieve these goals include client education, counseling, advocacy, and management of care. The major emphasis in community health nursing is on primary care and begins when the client enters the health care system and continues throughout the duration of the client's care. Secondary care and tertiary care are emphasized less. With clients considered a part of the team, the goal of care is to help clients assume self-responsibility for health care.

The major goal of the community health nurse, as pointed out in Chapter 1, is the preservation and improvement of the community's health. This overall objective is accomplished in two major modes, or ways. The first way is through direct primary care to individuals, families, and groups within a designated community. Practicing in the first mode, community health nurses work directly with clients to promote optimal health and, where health has been disrupted, to assist in restoration and stabilization of chronic conditions. The pattern of practice takes place through clinics, home health care, and group work with clients having common health needs. Practice is collaborative with other members of the health care team, is holistic in orientation, and emphasizes the evaluation of

nursing care to individuals, families, and the community. Specific ways in which community health nurses provide direct primary health care include:

- ◆ Immunizing children and conducting well-child clinics
- ◆ Providing nursing care to clients with diseases such as tuberculosis, acquired immunodeficiency syndrome (AIDS), and sexually transmitted diseases
- ◆ Conducting primary care clinics in locations such as migrant camps, school-based clinics, work sites, shelters, and correctional facilities

Practice in the second mode focuses directly on the health of the total population and considers how community health problems and issues affect individuals, families, and groups. The goal of population-based practice is to enable communities to be healthy. Goal achievement requires a collaborative, interdisciplinary process of assessment, policy development, and assurance activities. Examples of community *assessment* would include evaluating the potential health risk factors and disease indicators in a community. For example, the problem of improper waste disposal or stagnant water near a residential area would be considered a community health nursing problem in terms of how this environmental condition influences the morbidity and mortality of the residents. Community health nurses would engage in *policy development* to establish partnerships with other agencies to reduce the identified problem of environmental pollution, that is, improper waste disposal or the presence of stagnant water. The nurse would advocate for the health needs of the residents and serve as a catalyst to effect change in the community.

Assurance activities refer to monitoring access to health services, determining the effectiveness of the services provided in relation to the needs of the people, and working to improve continually the quality of the health services. In the second mode, population-based practice versus service to individuals, families, and groups, the focus is on the community as client, and the goal is to assist communities to identify health needs, establish priorities, plan and implement actions, and identify and intervene in factors affecting the health of the community. This mode emphasizes the ongoing interaction between people and their environment in which each is affected by the other.

A strong and effective public health system must be population-focused with an orientation toward primary care.

The APHA Definition of Public Health Nursing

The Public Health Nursing Section of the American Public Health Association (APHA) has defined public health nursing as follows (1981, p. 4):

Public health nursing synthesizes the body of knowledge from the public health sciences and professional nursing theories for the purpose of improving the health of the entire community. This goal lies at the heart of primary prevention and health promotion and is the foundation for public health nursing practice. To accomplish this goal, public health nurses work with groups, families, and individuals as well as in multidisciplinary teams and programs. Identifying the subgroups (aggregates) within the population which are at high risk of illness, disability, or premature death and directing resources toward these groups is the most effective approach for accomplishing the goal of public health nursing. Success in reducing the risks and in improving the health of the community depends on the involvement of consumers, especially groups experiencing health risks, and others in the community, in health planning, and in self-help activities.

Public health nursing, or community health nursing, is population-focused practice, and the goal is to promote healthy communities. This is the central feature that differentiates community health nursing from all other specialty areas. Promotion of population-focused practice requires "the collaborative, interdisciplinary process of assessment, policy development, and assurance activities to promote healthy outcomes in a community" (APHA, 1994, p. 4). Specific competencies include:

1. Community assessment to determine health risk factors and disease indicators
2. Policy development to reduce health problems
3. Assurance activities to promote the effective implementation of policy at the service delivery level
4. Personal health care practices to enable individuals to assume responsibility for their own health and to participate as members of the community as a whole. This personal care system occurs at the work site, school, home, farm, barrio, shelter, and correctional facility with multiracial and multiethnic populations. The public health nurse teaches and evaluates individuals, families, and communities to facilitate utilization of primary health care (APHA, 1994).

Both the ANA and the APHA definitions emphasize the blending of nursing and public health knowledge as a foundation for determining the scope of practice. They both acknowledge that community health nursing efforts are directed toward *all* people, whether they are cared for as individuals, as part of a family, in a community, or as a community at large. Each definition emphasizes a multidisciplinary role for the successful implementation of public health practice, and they both focus on the increasing priority of health

promotion. The APHA definition emphasizes primary care more than the ANA definition. It also clearly points out the need to determine within a community those groups at greatest risk for health disruption so that nursing interventions can target them to prevent the onset of disease.

Systems Models in Community Health Nursing

As mentioned, a variety of conceptual models can be used to guide nursing actions. However, community health nursing as defined by both the ANA and the APHA can be logically understood from a systems perspective. Systems theory can be used to describe and explain the behaviors of individuals, groups, and communities. It emphasizes how each isolated variable affects the whole and how the whole affects each part. Conceptual models based on systems theory, known as systems models, are especially useful in community health nursing. Communities, made up of multiple subsystems and groups that interface and influence each other, can be analyzed, interpreted, and understood from a systems theory perspective.

Systems models focus on the "organization, interaction, interdependency and integration of parts and elements" (Chin, 1980, p. 24). Systems models are based on **general systems theory** as described by von Bertalanffy (1952, p. 11), who wrote that "every organism represents a system, by which term we mean a complex of elements in mutual interaction." Concepts frequently discussed in relation to general systems theory are wholeness, organization, openness, boundary, entropy, negentropy, and equifinality. **Wholeness** refers to that condition in which a collection of parts responds as an integrated single part. The arrangement of the elements and their relationship to each other represent their **organization.**

The **openness** of a system refers to the extent to which it exchanges energy with the environment. An open system is affected by the environment (receives input) and in turn affects the environment by its output. In an open system, a continuous give-and-take occurs with the environment. In contrast, in a closed system, no energy is exchanged and no interaction occurs with the environment. All living systems are open; the use of the term "closed system" actually indicates a relative expression, since at present it is impossible to demonstrate a totally closed system.

Boundary refers to a line or border that defines what elements constitute the system. In biological terms the cell membrane is a boundary encompassing the contents of a cell. In social systems the boundary is more like an imaginary line that groups certain individuals together. Thus a boundary can be physical or may be designated by roles and expectations. Simply stated, a boundary is similar to a fence around the system. Another way to view boundary is to consider it as a filter that permits the exchange of elements, information, or energy between the system and its environment. The more porous the filter is, the greater the

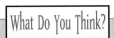

degree of interaction that is possible between the system and its environment.

Each system requires a specific form of energy to continue functioning. **Entropy** is a concept based on the second law of thermodynamics, which states that elements in a closed environment will proceed toward greater randomness or less order. Entropy is also described as disordered energy, or energy that is bound and cannot be converted to work. **Negentropy** is the energy that is "free," can be used for work, and tends toward order. Because living systems are open systems, they make use of negentrophy rather than entropy. In systems theory, **equifinality** means the end state of the open system is independent of the beginning state.

Feedback is the process whereby the output of the system is redirected as the input to the same system. The body, as a physiological system, uses feedback to regulate temperature, heart rate, and respiration. All open or living systems have input, output, and feedback.

Communities can be understood from a systems perspective in the following way. According to systems theory, the *community* is an open system that exchanges materials such as energy, goods and services, values, and ideals with the environment inside and outside the community. The community as a system has boundaries, the most obvious being geographical lines. The imaginary boundary is one that encompasses all the subsystems in the community and identifies what is inside and outside the community. En-

tropy can be compared to landfill garbage dumps, which disintegrate and the results of which may not be converted to something useful. Negentropy can be compared to the resources, health, wealth, and altruistic values of the people. Equifinality indicates the community's attempt to attain or maintain balance and beauty. Communication is the means within the community that subsystems relate to each other and to the entire community.

The community is a social system made up of interrelated and interdependent subsystems. The subsystems are economics, education, religion, health care, politics, welfare, law enforcement, energy, and recreation. When any one of the subsystems is affected, it affects the community as a whole. One subsystem that immediately affects the whole community is the economic system. If a major employer in the community lays off workers, the entire community, including its economic, social, educational, and health care institutions, will be affected.

Systems thinking, popularized in the 1960s, remains relevant in today's world. Four nurse theorists, Johnson (1980), King (1981), Roy (1984), and Neuman (1989), formulated conceptual models of nursing based on systems theory. Table 10-2 summarizes the definitions of person (client), environment, health, and nursing according to these theorists and others. Although all these models are applicable to community health nursing, the Neuman Systems Model is particularly suited to community health nursing and is discussed in detail.

Table 10-2 Definitions of Person, Environment, Health, and Nursing

Person or client	Environment	Health	Nursing
Roy			
An adaptive system (Roy, 1984, p. 28) can be a person or group.	"All conditions, circumstances, and influences surrounding and affecting the development and behavior of persons or groups" (Roy, 1984, p. 39).	"A state and a process of being and becoming an integrated and whole person. Integrity means soundness or an unimpaired condition that can lead to completeness or unity" (Roy, 1984, p. 269).	The science that observes, classifies, and relates the processes by which persons positively affect their health status, and the practice discipline that uses this particular scientific knowledge in providing a service to people (Roy, 1984, p. 4).
Rogers			
"Unitary man—a four-dimensional, negentropic energy field identified by pattern and organization and manifesting characteristics and behaviors that are different from those of the parts and which cannot be predicted from knowledge of the parts" (Rogers, 1980, p. 332).	A four-dimensional, negentropic energy field identified by pattern and organization and encompassing all that is outside any given human field (Rogers, 1980, p. 332).	Health not specifically defined; however, disease and pathology are value terms (Rogers, 1980, p. 336) and since values change, phenomena perceived as disease (e.g., hyperactivity) may change over time and not be perceived as disease.	Goal of nursing is that individuals achieve their maximum health potential through maintenance and promotion of health, prevention of disease, nursing diagnosis, intervention, and rehabilitation (Robers, 1970, p. 86).

Table 10-2   Definitions of Person, Environment, Health, and Nursing—cont'd

Person or client	Environment	Health	Nursing
Johnson Behavioral system (Johnson, 1980, p. 207).	Malfunctions in behavioral systems are frequently caused by "sudden internal or external environmental change" (Johnson, 1980, p. 212; refers to human interaction with environment, p. 209).	"It seems reasonable to assume that health would be considered behavior that is orderly, purposeful, predictable, and functionally efficient and effective" (Johnson, 1980, p. 209).	Goal of nursing is to "restore, maintain, or attain behavioral system balance and stability at the highest possible level for the individual" (Johnson, 1980, p. 214).
Orem "A receiver of care, someone who is under the care of a health professional at this time, in some place or places" (Orem, 1985, p. 49).	Although not explicitly defined, speaks to the role of the nurse in providing a developmental environment (Orem, 1985, p. 141) that may be physical or psychosocial; is the total environment.	"The state of wholeness of developed human structures and of bodily and mental functioning" (Orem, 1985, p. 179).	"Deliberate action to bring about humanely desirable conditions in persons and their environments" (Orem, 1985, p. 15).
Neuman "A composite of the interrelationship of the five variables (physiologic, psychologic, sociocultural, developmental and spiritual) that are always present" (Neuman, 1989).	"All internal and external forces that could affect life and development" (Neuman, 1983, p. 246); "consists of the internal and external forces surrounding man at any point in time. Created environment represents an open system exchanging energy with both the internal and external environments" (Neuman, 1989, p. 32).	"Health or wellness is the condition in which all parts and subparts (variables) are in harmony with the whole of man." Disharmony "reduces the wellness state" (Neuman, 1983, p. 246). Health is equated with system stability. The wellness-illness continuum implies energy flow is continuous between client system and environment (Neuman, 1989).	"Nursing can use this model to assist individuals, families, and groups to attain, retain and maintain a maximum of total wellness by three modes of prevention as intervention" (Neuman, 1989, p. 35).
King "A social, sentient, rational, reacting, perceiving, controlling, purposeful, action-oriented, and time-oriented being (King, 1981, p. 143).	Writes about environment, but does not define it; "the internal environment of human beings transforms energy to enable them to adjust to continuous external environmental changes..." (King, 1981, p. 5).	"Dynamic life experiences of a human being, which implies continuous adjustment to stressors in the internal and external environment through optimum use of one's resources to achieve maximum potential for daily living" (King, 1981, p. 5).	"Nursing is perceiving, thinking, relating, judging, and acting vis-à-vis the behavior of individuals who come to a nursing situation" (King, 1981, p. 2). "Nursing is a process of human interactions between nurse and client whereby each perceives the other and the situation; and through communication, they set goals, explore means, and agree on means to achieve goals."

THE NEUMAN SYSTEMS MODEL

Betty Neuman developed the Health Care Systems Model as an organizing framework for graduate students to facilitate their understanding of client needs within a holistic viewpoint (Neuman and Young, 1972). Neuman defines, describes, and links together the four concepts of nursing's metaparadigm (person, environment, health, nursing) within the model from world views of organism and change. Neuman uses the systems approach in her model to provide organization while maintaining the potential to accommodate change in the system. Neuman believes that as nursing becomes more complex and comprehensive, a broad, flexible, expansive structure is required. Systems thinking enables nurses to focus on clients, themselves, and their surrounding environments in an interactive, creative way. The system provides an organizational structure that maintains relative stability during the process of change (Neuman, 1989).

The **Neuman Systems Model** depicts an open system in which persons and their environments are in dynamic interaction (Neuman, 1989). The client system is composed of five interacting variables: physiological, psychological, sociocultural, developmental, and spiritual. These variables have a basic core structure unique to the individual, but with a range of responses common to all human beings. Client systems may be individuals, families, groups, or communities.

The model, as seen in Figure 10-1, shows the client system as concentric rings surrounding the basic core. The outer ring is a broken circle indicating an open system that exchanges energy with the environment. This ring, called the **flexible line of defense,** protects the system in a dynamic way, expanding when more protection is provided and contracting when less protection is available. The second ring, the **normal line of defense,** represents the usual wellness level of the client system. This line of defense is the result of previous system behavior and defines the stability and integrity of the system. As with the flexible line of defense, the normal line of defense is dynamic and may expand or contract when under the influence of stressors in order to maintain system stability. A series of inner circles between the normal line of defense and the basic core, known as **lines of resistance,** contain factors that support the defense lines and protect the basic structure. The lines of resistance are activated when stressors invade the system to assist the system in reconstituting. If lines of resistance are ineffective in their efforts, system energy is depleted and death of the system may occur (Neuman, 1989).

In the model, environment is defined as all internal and external influences surrounding and affecting the client system. The client may influence or be influenced by environmental forces, either positively or negatively, at any given point in time. The processes of input, output, and feedback between the client and environment are circular and reciprocal. Stressors occurring within and outside the client system can create instability. Thus the lines of resistance and defense are activated to defend the system in the presence of stressors. When system stability is attained, maintained, or retained, the result is a healthy system. Figure 10-1 shows stressors invading the lines of defense and classifies stressors as intrapersonal, interpersonal, or extrapersonal factors.

Optimal system stability is the best possible health state at any given time when all system variables are in balance within the client system. Variance from wellness occurs when the system gets out of balance (Neuman, 1989). For example, client system energy levels are affected by actual or potential stressors that can increase energy with positive stress *(eustress)* or decrease energy with distress or negative stress. High-level wellness is evidenced by abundant energy within a client system. When more energy is generated than used, the client system moves toward negentropy; conversely, when more energy is required than generated, movement is toward entropy or illness.

The major goal of nursing in the Neuman Systems Model is to keep the client system stable through accurate assessment of actual and potential stressors, followed by implementation of appropriate interventions. Three intervention modalities are suggested: *primary prevention* strategies are implemented to strengthen the lines of defense by reducing risk factors and preventing stress; *secondary prevention* begins after the occurrence of symptoms to strengthen the lines of resistance by establishing relevant goals and interventions to reduce the reaction; and *tertiary prevention* can be initiated at any point after treatment when some degree of system stability has occurred. Reconstitution at this point depends on the successful mobilization of client resources to prevent further stressor reaction or regression (Neuman, 1989). Figure 10-1 depicts the three intervention strategies targeted toward the client system.

The three prevention-as-intervention modalities can be used separately or simultaneously to direct nursing actions. Within the systems perspective, all modalities lead back toward primary prevention in a circular fashion. Health promotion, therefore, becomes a specific goal for nursing action in the Neuman model. For example, before or after stressor invasion, intervention goals include education and mobilization of support resources to bolster lines of defense, reduce the effect of a stressor, and increase client resistance. Health promotion efforts support secondary and tertiary goals to promote optimal wellness.

Health promotion within the Neuman Systems Model makes the model useful in meeting the objectives of *Healthy People 2000* (1991). Specifically, *Healthy People 2000* emphasizes the prevention of suffering and disease and the reduction of costs associated with treatment of illness as the declared goals for the decade of the 1990s.

Further, the Neuman Systems Model has been adopted by nurses in 14 countries to guide curriculum development and nursing practice with individuals,

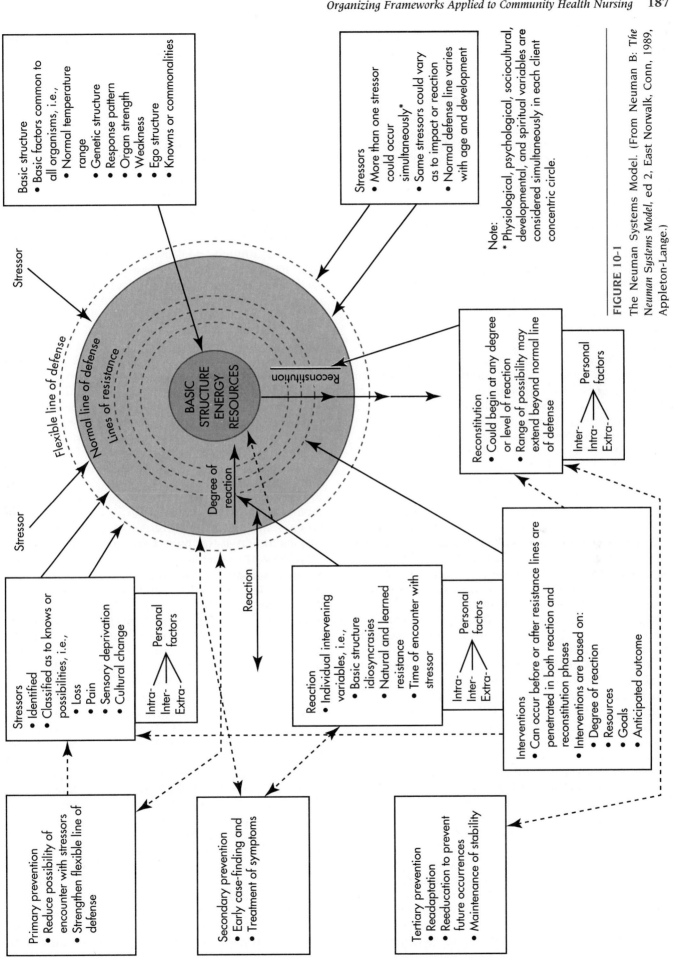

FIGURE 10-1

The Neuman Systems Model. (From Neuman B: *The Neuman Systems Model*, ed 2, East Norwalk, Conn, 1989, Appleton-Lange.)

families, and communities. Recently, several community nursing centers have adopted the model as their framework. The familiar vocabulary of the model, its systems perspective, and the integration of multiple psychosocial theories increase the usefulness of this model. The comprehensive nature of the model encourages utilization by other health care disciplines as well, such as physical therapy, social work, and public health. Indeed, the Neuman Systems Model facilitates a multidisciplinary approach to providing quality care at an efficient cost.

APPLICATION OF THE NEUMAN SYSTEMS MODEL TO EDUCATION

As mentioned, the Neuman Systems Model is used frequently and successfully by community health nurses in the United States, Canada, and some European countries. In some cases, the community health nurses consider clients or families in their own settings within the community as the focus of care. In other instances, the community itself is the client. As described in Chapter 15, the community is considered the client only when nursing practice is community oriented and emphasizes healthful change for the whole community's benefit.

Community-as-client goals frequently emphasize health promotion and health maintenance of the community as a whole or of groups of associated individuals in the community referred to as *aggregates* (Beddome, 1989). Further, when community is the focus of service, the nurse and community must form a partnership to achieve their goals. In community partnerships the members and professionals who have vested interests in the success of the effort actively participate in collaborative decision making (Goeppinger and Shuster, 1992). Assessment, diagnoses, planning, intervention, and evaluation are targeted toward the community rather than individuals within the community. (For more information on community as client, refer to Chapter 15.)

In the Neuman Systems Model the community is seen as a system of interfacing subsystems. Optimal functioning within and between the subsystems will result in optimal functioning of the whole system. Conversely, dysfunction within or between any of the subsystems will compromise the function or health of the entire system. Stressors that affect any subsystem and create instability for the community must be assessed so that appropriate interventions can be designed to reduce these stressors and promote health. This process is interactive and collaborative between the nurses and the community.

Three types of prevention can be used. Primary prevention is appropriate to identify community risk factors and to plan mutually for health education programs with the community leaders. Secondary prevention interventions are initiated when one or more normal defenses of the community have been invaded, resulting in the development of specific health problems. At this point, the community health nurse would assist the community in identifying the stressors and would begin treatment to correct the problem as well as initiate interventions to strengthen the lines of resistance to prevent further dysfunction within the community system.

Tertiary prevention, the third intervention strategy, is most appropriate within a community that has become chronically dysfunctional over time. For example, a major disaster such as a hurricane or flood (external stressor) or an influenza epidemic (internal stressor) can create multiple health problems for the community and leave it severely compromised. The community losing a major source of employment (e.g., coal mining, steel manufacturing) or having a high incidence of heart disease are other examples. Over time, chronic health problems develop because of these stressors and lead to poor nutrition, postponement of medical care, depression, and ultimately to a chronically ill community. Through tertiary prevention the community health nurse assists the community to readapt and reeducate to prevent further instability. The nurse also initiates primary intervention to reduce the possibility of further encounters with stressors and to strengthen lines of defense. The three types of interventions may be initiated individually or concurrently after the stressors have been identified, the degree of reaction assessed, and the resources and goals established between the community and health care professionals.

As seen in Figure 10-1, the core or basic structure of the community as client represents the energy resources and basic factors common to the infrastructure of the community. These can be classified as physiological, psychosocial, sociocultural, developmental, and spiritual variables (Neuman, 1989). Table 10-3 provides a definition and example of each variable; for instance, physiological community variables are the structure (e.g., geographical boundaries, rural or urban) and functions (e.g., local government, police and fire protection) of the community. Each of the five variables is interdependent with the other variables; flexible boundaries exist between them. In fact, examples of some factors could be categorized under more than one variable, such as health beliefs (sociocultural and spiritual) or aging (developmental and physiological). The purpose of categorization under variables is to provide a comprehensive framework for assessment, thereby eliminating the possibility of overlooking any community area. Understanding that the variables are interactive and interdependent supports the notion of a community gestalt and wholeness, as proposed in the Neuman Systems Model.

As with people, however, communities do not function optimally all the time. Stressors, either positive or negative, affect one or more subsystems within the community, thus affecting the whole. As systems theory indicates, a change in one subsystem will affect the entire system. Stressors can be defined as *intracommunity* (originating from within one or more sub-

Table 10-3   Definitions and Examples of Community Variables

Variable	Definition	Examples
Physiological	Structures and functions of community	Urban, rural, suburban Geographical boundaries/location Water, sewage systems Safety systems (police, fire) Government Transportation system
Psychological	Cognitive, affective, and communication characteristics	Happy/depressed town Intelligence level Communication patterns Liberal vs. conservative Isolation vs. sensory overload
Sociocultural	Pattern of social, economic, demographic, political, recreational, and health characteristics	Poor/middle class/affluent Race, ethnicity Type of industry Day care for elderly/children Ambulance service Clinics/hospitals
Spiritual	Moral, religious, and value systems of community	Churches Health beliefs Burial practices X-rated bookstores
Developmental	History, stage, and evolution of subsystems and aggregates in community	National registry of homes Aging/adolescent population Deteriorating city

systems or the whole), *intercommunity* (originating from adjacent areas) or *extracommunity* (imposed from structures outside the community). For example, a hazardous waste dump adjacent to an elementary school would be an intracommunity stressor, whereas racial tension between in-town residents and out-of-town residents would be an intercommunity stressor. Examples of extracommunity stressors could be new industries encroaching on farm lands surrounding the community, an interstate highway system planned through town, or decreased federal funding for community health services. Table 10-4 provides further examples of stressors within each variable of community as client.

Community health nurses create linkages between subgroups within the community and intracommunity and extracommunity resources to assist the community in maintaining health. Communication is the medium by which information is exchanged and plans formulated to raise health standards. Sometimes the nurse must motivate the community to change and must provide the leadership for implementing change. The community health nurse begins the change process by becoming familiar with the basic structure of the community and developing a data base of community variables. Assessment of the infrastructures that protect the community is paramount. For example, police and fire protection, health and illness services, and the penal system represent the lines of re-

sistance within the community established to protect, stabilize, and maintain a steady state for the community. These are depicted as broken lines in concentric circles surrounding the core in the Neuman Systems Model (see Figure 10-1).

Neuman's normal line of defense represents the usual range of responses developed over time that mark the unique aspects of any community. These could include the type of politics and government structure, ways of doing business to maintain a stable economy, and communication lines within and among groups and organizations. The normal line of defense could also be viewed as the usual coping behaviors the community uses to maintain balance. The normal line of defense is protected by the flexible line of defense, which acts as a buffer zone so that the normal state of community wellness is maintained. If the community is stable, the flexible line of defense can expand to provide more services for citizens, greater economic opportunities for industry, or more recreational parks within the community. On the other hand, if the community experiences a minor emergency, such as a fire or disease outbreak, the flexible line of defense contracts to protect the community. The lines of resistance then mobilize to protect the infrastructure of the community.

Using the Neuman Systems Model perspective as just described, the community health nurse can develop a mental image of the community as client that

Table 10-4   Stressors Affecting Community-as-Client Variables

Physical	Psychological	Social/cultural	Developmental	Spiritual
INTRACOMMUNITY				
Increased infant mortality	Insufficient health education about AIDS	Homes crowded in downtown	High teen pregnancy rate	Many sect churches
Hazardous waste dump	Increased divorce rate	Park land bought by developer	Potential need for more child care centers	Health beliefs influenced by folk wisdom
Water supply contaminated	Potential for decreased emotional health in public housing areas	Decreased family income	Deteriorating inner city community	
INTERCOMMUNITY				
Poor roads connecting town or regional medical center	Anger between political parties	Racial tension between migrants and townspeople	Historical significance of town	Diverse value system between rural and urban sectors
Distribution of physicians uneven	Potential for isolation of elderly rural persons	Bussing students grades 4-6	Age of community	
	Inadequate communication system between rural and urban areas			
EXTRACOMMUNITY				
Interstate highway system planned through town	Belief system of national political party in opposition to community's beliefs	Potential for unemployment related to industrial plant closing	New industry encroaching on farm land	New morality in opposition to community values
Nuclear power plant site outside town	Fear of environmental contamination	Influx of ethnic groups	Potential for increase in young families to support new industry	Community selected as headquarters site for national denomination
Flu epidemic			Potential growth in schools	
Decreased state funding for services				

includes variables that represent its structure and the lines of defense. A data base can be established at this point.

The next step is to identify community stressors and to assess the degree of community reaction to the stressors. The selection of appropriate interventions follows stressor identification and depends on the aim of the intervention. For example, primary prevention might include giving immunizations, supporting positive coping strategies, and providing health education seminars. Early case finding followed by appropriate referrals, counseling about high-risk behaviors, and the use of medications illustrate secondary interventions. Assisting the community to readapt after a major epidemic or period of debilitation would constitute tertiary intervention. Common to all three models of intervention are client advocacy, coordinating health resources, and providing information to maintain or regain system stability.

Examples of the use of the Neuman Systems Model in community health nursing education and practice follow. In the first example, the faculty at Lander University in Greenwood, SC, developed a senior community health nursing course to illustrate how the model is used to assess an industrial community client (Freese, 1994).

In this course the Community-as-Client Model, as adapted from Neuman by Anderson et al. (1986), pro-

vided the conceptual basis for community analysis in a project that involved faculty and student collaboration to identify and meet the health needs of one plant's industrial workforce. Three course objectives were addressed:

1. Assess a community from a theory-based perspective. Students completed a class activity to apply each component of the Community-as-Client Model to the target workforce as a system. For example, the system core was viewed as the industrial plant's 500 employees, and flexible lines of defense were viewed as the industry's response to stressors, such as a program to prevent back injuries.

2. Develop a theory-based community health care plan. Based on assessment of the industry as a community/client, students identified health problems, stated each problem as a community nursing diagnosis, and planned strategies to address them. For example, workers were experiencing knowledge deficit in four areas: protecting sensory modalities (vision and hearing), managing stress, preventing injuries, and preventing heart disease. The health care plan for this industrial community identified planned teaching for each area of knowledge deficit.

3. Address a community health problem using nursing theory. Students conducted teaching sessions

for employees to address each of the four areas of knowledge deficit using a teaching plan for each area. For example, teaching to prevent injuries focused on strengthening the flexible lines of defense through proper body mechanics for lifting and carrying and instructions for back exercises, as well as on strengthening the normal line of defense by avoiding body positions that can cause injury. Throughout each phase of the project, faculty and students collaborated as colleagues to translate theory into practice by applying the model to a local industrial plant as community/client.

The Neuman Systems Model can also be used by nurses who work with transcultural populations to identify stressors unique to that cultural community. In a second example, Freese and Hassell (1994) used the Neuman Systems Model with Hispanic worker populations, including migrants and laborers in the rural South. Beddome (1989) and Anderson et al. (1995) state that the community system is composed of 8 interdependent subsystems that interact with the basic core of the community: its people, their values, beliefs, culture, and religion. Physiological, psychological, sociocultural, developmental, and spiritual variables identified by the Neuman Systems Model affect the basic core and subsystems, as detailed next for the Hispanic worker population.

The Basic Core

Freese and Hassell (1994) describe how the basic core is affected by the eight subsystems. However, in the example that follows they have combined communication and transportation into a single subsystem as well as health and safety.

Hispanic workers comprise a vulnerable aggregate community defined by a common Hispanic value and belief system, a common language (Spanish as the primary or only language), and similar occupations that include migrant and menial employment. The shared Hispanic culture is a strong cohesive factor within the basic core. Commitment to family ties strengthens the normal line of defense. However, the male-dominant culture may adversely influence women's health related to contraception, self-esteem, and passivity. Values related to time orientation may adversely affect access to health care because of a wider frame of reference to time; appointment times are not observed or appointments are missed (Spector, 1991).

Communication and Transportation Subsystem

Significant language barriers exist. Despite a common Spanish basis, dialect differences among Mexican, Puerto Rican, and Guatemalan languages and dialects create intracommunity stressors. Intercommunity stress results from lack of bilinguality in interfacing communities, especially among health care providers, public officials, and law enforcement officers. Phone access is limited.

Lack of transportation limits access to employment, recreation, and health care. In some areas, however,

local migrant health program grants include funding for vans to transport community members to clinics and specialists.

Health and Safety Subsystem

The normal line of defense of the community is adversely affected by lack of access to medical and dental services, communication problems related to language differences, poor health records systems, lack of immunizations, poor nutrition, and substandard housing. Lines of resistance related to the reliance on folk remedies and healers may create intercommunity communication problems between Western medical practitioners and community members.

Safety issues extend beyond merely substandard housing to lack of adequate sanitation and proper waste disposal. Occupational exposure to pesticides, sunlight, allergens, and work-related injuries places Hispanic workers at significant risk. Violence in migrant work camps, aggravated by ethnic differences, drugs, and alcohol, is a serious safety issue.

Economics Subsystem

The normal and flexible lines of defense are adversely affected by pervasive poverty that extends to every level and system. Effects of poverty include lack of education, poor nutrition, and lack of environmental sanitation. Lack of transference of health care benefits represents a significant extracommunity stressor related to federal and state legislation. Public debate on health care responsibility for illegal aliens has not been completed.

Education Subsystem

Lack of formal education is a common stressor contributing to inadequate employment skills, poor health and life-style choices, and poor interface with the dominant Anglo culture. As a result, Hispanic workers are prone to exploitation by employers and crew bosses.

Law and Politics Subsystem

Most persons of the Hispanic community are of Mexican origin; because of their transient nature or illegal status, they have no political voice. Although many heads of households have work permits or are legal residents, family members are often illegal aliens. Services designated for residents of the county or state may be denied to nonresident workers. Nurses, acting as advocates to obtain services for clients, must be sensitive to the legal resident status of Hispanic workers, a serious potential stressor if the worker is an illegal alien.

Religion Subsystem

Ninety percent of the community members are Catholic. The spiritual nature of the mind and body is integral to the Hispanic culture. However, the underlying fatalism of the culture predisposes many to apathy, hopelessness, and powerlessness. Lack of birth control contributes to high birth rate and high incidence of sexually transmitted disease.

Providing transcultural health care for Hispanic workers requires nurses to attune to actual and potential culture-based stressors so that they do not become barriers to effective care (Freese and Hassell, 1994).

APPLICATION OF THE NEUMAN SYSTEMS MODEL TO PRACTICE

The third example of the Neuman Systems Model involves service delivery in Canada. Recently, the model was introduced for consideration in the province of Ontario, Canada as the organizing framework for the delivery of long-term care services (Smith, 1994). An analysis of the existing long-term care services found them to be fragmented, duplicative, inequitably accessible, and lacking in some areas. The proposed long-term care reform in Canada will target seniors, adults with disabilities, family caregivers, and individuals of any age who need health and support services. A primary goal of the new system is to provide consumers with easier access to long-term care services in their homes and communities. Current not-for-profit, long-term service agencies will be brought together with a single point of entry to simplify access for consumers. Multiservice agencies (MSAs) that deliver community-based services that meet standards and are funded by and accountable to the government will be developed across Ontario to achieve this goal (Ministry's of Health Community of Social Services and Citizenship, 1993).

The Canadian government encouraged the provinces to develop creative designs for their MSA model. The Neuman Systems Model was presented as a structure for the delivery of MSA services in Huron County, Ontario (Smith, 1994). Neuman's model fits with the Ministry's guidelines for MSAs because it focuses on illness prevention and health promotion. Consumers' participation in their care and collaboration with professional and non-professional members in the system are encouraged.

Figure 10-2 demonstrates how the Neuman Systems Model provides a framework for organizing the structure and function of an MSA. The open lines in the diagram depict open communication and interaction among the various levels in the system. For example, the core represents seniors, adults with disabilities, and caregivers, who may discuss concerns with administrators as well as service providers, and vice versa. The model core includes those individuals identified by the Ministry's who need long-term care services. According to the Neuman Systems Model, this is the aggregate community. The internal services, which include emergency response teams, relief, and short-stay beds in long-term care facilities (lines of resistance), help defend the core against external and internal stressors. Potential stressors include loss of funding, provincial policy change, limited number of beds available in long-term care facilities, and limited

human resources for the provision of care. This network of professional resources, who can respond to the needs of service providers and to individuals receiving services, assists the core (seniors, etc.) in remaining in the community. In Figure 10-2 the emergency quick-response teams and palliative pain management team may temporarily step in to educate the service providers on pain management and provide symptom relief to individuals in pain. The service providers (normal line of defense) in Figure 10-2 address the steady state of service delivery to the core. These include nurses, physiotherapists, occupational therapists, volunteers, and transportation and meal service personnel. Service providers help maintain the core in the community to prevent or delay institutionalization (Smith, 1994).

The administrative level (flexible line of defense) in Figure 10-2 represents a buffer that protects and supports individuals involved in the day-to-day care of the core and ultimately protects and supports the core itself. The administrative level can utilize all three modes of prevention—primary, secondary, and tertiary—to reduce stressors. The primary prevention mode is used by the administration to communicate health care changes and community needs that may affect the system. Secondary prevention is exercised by managing the day-to-day concerns that may affect both the core and the service provider's ability to cope with stressors. Tertiary prevention focuses on long-range planning by coordinating system goals and ensuring availability of short-stay beds in long-term care facilities.

As stated, the government of Ontario encouraged creativity in designing the MSA model. Figure 10-3 depicts the MSA model with four satellites in Huron County to meet local community needs and ensure accessibility. The MSA with the only governing body that facilitates administrative streamlining is centrally located in the town of Clinton. The four satellite offices are geographically located in the north, south, west, and east of the county and do not require an administration level but do have three board members. The board members in each of the five MSAs include a consumer, volunteer, and service provider representing the communities they serve. In all, a total of 15 board members discuss funding needs for the overall county. Figure 10-3 is shown as a pie, with each local community having a "piece" of that pie. Having the satellites in the five local communities promotes use of local experience, provides equitable access, and ensures consumers that their needs will be met.

Utilizing the Neuman Systems Model as the MSA model is both creative and cost-effective. A system that streamlines administration through stressor identification and identifies any need for program development or additional services promotes effective and appropriate use of resources. The Neuman Systems Model facilitates a system that is planned in partnership with communities and provides a way to measure outcomes. A process for measuring service satisfaction

ADMINISTRATION

- Board of Directors
- Executive Director
- Total quality management
- Volunteer Coordinator
- Education/training
- Finance

SERVICE PROVIDERS

- Case manager
- Professional staff
- Personal support workers
- Volunteers
- Meals
- Transportation
- Adult day programs

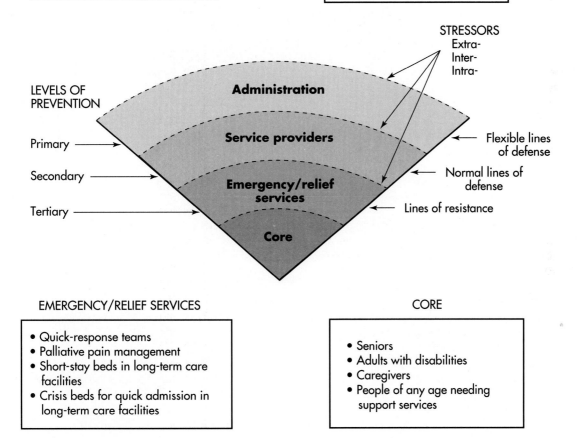

STRESSORS
Extra-
Inter-
Intra-

LEVELS OF
PREVENTION

Administration

Service providers

Emergency/relief
services

Core

Primary

Secondary

Tertiary

Flexible lines
of defense

Normal lines of
defense

Lines of resistance

EMERGENCY/RELIEF SERVICES

- Quick-response teams
- Palliative pain management
- Short-stay beds in long-term care facilities
- Crisis beds for quick admission in long-term care facilities

CORE

- Seniors
- Adults with disabilities
- Caregivers
- People of any age needing support services

FIGURE 10-2

The Neuman Systems Model adapted to design a fully developed multiservice agency (MSA) model. Broken lines represent open interrelationships among subsystems, facilitating collaboration and participation.

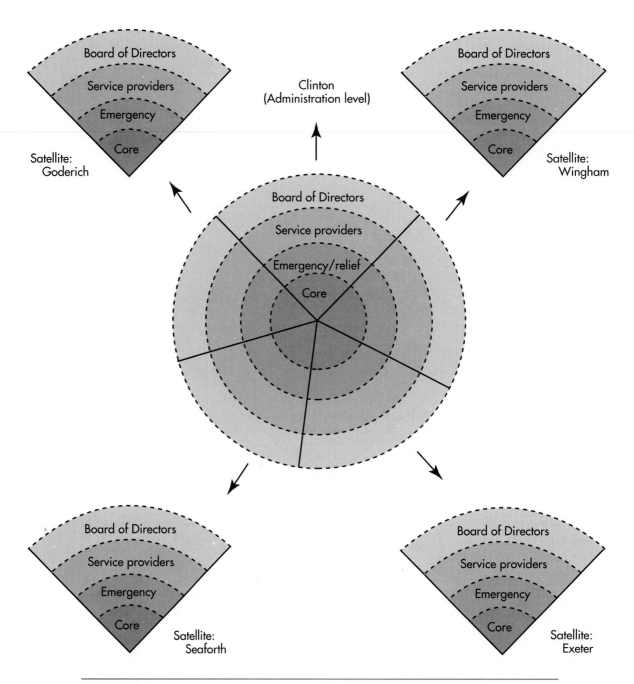

FIGURE 10-3

The Neuman Systems Model adapted as the multiservice agency model (MSA) in Huron County, Ontario, Canada. The model includes satellites in five communities. The MSA satellite centrally located in Clinton includes the administrative level. Each MSA satellite has three board members representing the five local communities.

will be developed, and individuals using the services can evaluate service accessibility and equitability.

THE OMAHA SYSTEM

Nurses and administrators in community-based settings face urgent practice, documentation, and data management challenges (Martin and Scheet, 1992a). The scope of community health nursing practice has always been complex, diverse, and independent. However, because of the magnitude and speed of current health care system changes, community health nurses and administrators have critical needs in three areas:

1. Timely, valid, and reliable data that describe clients' demographic characteristics, severity and acuity of their illnesses, type and location of services, and reimbursement issues.
2. Timely, valid, and reliable data that quantify the clients receiving care, the services they receive, and the costs and outcomes of that care.
3. Verbal and written methods for collaboration among nurses and between nurses and other professionals.

According to Clark and Lang (1992), "If we cannot name it, we cannot control it, finance it, teach it, research it or put it into public policy." Counting data must be added to naming data in Lang's statement to address urgent practice, documentation, and data management challenges.

The ANA established a Steering Committee on Data Bases in 1991 to explore interrelated concerns involving changing nursing practice, standardized nursing language, and automation. The ANA committee decided to (1) recognize four diverse classification systems that met their research, practice, and information system criteria, (2) publicize the systems and the related issues in a monograph, and (3) collaborate with the National Library of Medicine to include the systems in the Metathesaurus, a data base that is available internationally (ANA, 1993; Zielstorff et al.,

1993). The four systems are North American Nursing Diagnosis Association (NANDA), the Omaha System, the Iowa Nursing Interventions Classification, and the Home Health Care Classification. NANDA consists of nursing diagnoses that have been used most frequently in acute care settings (Carroll-Johnson and Parquette, 1994). The **Omaha System** comprises nursing diagnoses, interventions, and an outcome rating scale; it is used most frequently in community-based settings (Martin and Scheet, 1992a, 1992b). Because the Iowa Nursing Interventions Classification was designed for use with NANDA, it is also used in many acute care settings (McCloskey and Bulechek, 1992). The Home Health Care Classification focuses on interventions generated by home health care agencies and includes some of the NANDA nursing diagnoses (Saba et al., 1991). Table 10-5 compares the four systems. The Omaha System's Problem Classification Scheme, Intervention Scheme, and Problem Rating Scale for Outcomes are described in detail later in this section. The references just cited offer information about the other three systems.

Definitions

Although the following concepts have been defined in various ways, their similarities involving evolution and interchangeable use are emphasized in this chapter. The concepts are nursing diagnosis and client problem; nursing interventions, actions, and activities; and evaluation and outcome measurement. All concepts can be adapted to apply to divergent situations and populations. The concepts can be incorporated into community health programs as well as acute and long-term care programs. The concepts are applicable to the client as a single individual, family, group, or community.

Nursing diagnosis is a clinical judgment about individual, family, or community responses to actual and potential health problems and life processes. It

Table 10-5 Comparison of Classification Systems

Systems and origins	Taxonomic structure and organization	Settings where especially applicable
North American Nursing Diagnosis Association (NANDA) (early 1970s)	Nursing diagnoses with nine human response patterns	Hospitals, ambulatory care, nursing homes
Iowa Nursing Interventions Classification (mid-1980s)	Nursing interventions with six domains	Hospitals, ambulatory care, nursing homes
Home Health Care Classification (1987)	Some NANDA nursing diagnoses; nursing interventions with four categories	Home care
Omaha System (early 1970s)	Nursing diagnoses/client problems with four domains; interventions with four categories; rating scale with three concepts and Likert-type scale	Community, including home care, public health, schools, nursing centers, emerging health delivery settings

provides the basis for selection of nursing interventions to achieve outcomes for which the nurse is accountable (Carroll-Johnson, 1990). **Client problem** is a matter of difficulty or concern that historically, presently, or potentially adversely affects any aspect of the client's well-being; accurate problem identification enables the professional to focus interventions (Martin and Scheet, 1992a).

Intervention describes activity that follows a thought process or written exercise usually referred to as planning. It is an action or activity implemented to address a specific client problem and to improve, maintain, or restore health or prevent illness (Martin and Scheet, 1992a). A **nursing intervention** is any direct care treatment that a nurse performs on behalf of a client. These treatments include nurse-initiated treatments resulting from medical diagnoses and performance of the daily essential functions for the client who cannot perform these activities (Bulechek and McCloskey, 1989).

Evaluation is a process designed to determine a value or amount or to compare accomplishments with some standards. Donabedian's (1966) structure, process, and outcome framework is considered classic and has provided nurses with an evaluation model. Evaluation based on client outcomes assumes that changes in client health status and behavior result from or are consequences of care. Evaluation has been defined as measurement of client progress by comparing client knowledge, behavior, and status ratings at admission, regular intervals, and dismissal (Martin and Scheet, 1992a).

Concepts of the Nursing Process

Nursing diagnosis is an essential, even pivotal, component of the **nursing process**. Nursing diagnosis follows the data collection or assessment phase. The identification of accurate nursing diagnoses or client problems is critical to the success of nursing care. Plans and interventions, the next phases of the nursing process, reflect the art and science of nursing. The nurse's skill in selecting and implementing optimal interventions is crucial to achieving the best possible outcomes. The final phase of the nursing process, evaluation, often receives little attention from clinicians or administrators in the practice setting. Without examining the results of care during and at the end of nursing service, accurate conclusions about the efficiency and effectiveness of care are not possible. Fortunately, heightened interest in evaluation and measurement of client outcomes is occurring because of new accreditation and federal regulations, legislation, escalating health care costs, and increasingly vocal consumers.

It is important for the community health nurse to recognize that the nursing process exists within a larger perspective. In addition to nursing, other disciplines that require logical, scientific thinking and systematic nomenclature also employ a problem-solving

Table 10-6　Relationship of nursing process to problem-solving and medical diagnostic processes

Problem-solving process	Medical diagnostic process	Nursing process
Information gathering	History and physical examination	Data collection
Problem	Diagnosis	Nursing diagnosis
Plan	Plan	Plan
Action	Treatment	Intervention
Evaluation	Evaluation	Evaluation

approach. The problem-solving process includes generalized information gathering, problem identification, and analysis, as well as decision making based on fact, intuition, and experiences. Physicians employ a medical diagnostic process that is similar to the nursing process and the problem-solving approach. Table 10-6 illustrates the relationship of the nursing process to the medical diagnostic and problem-solving processes.

 Research Brief

Martin KS, Scheet NJ, Stegman MR. Home health clients: characteristics, outcomes of care, and nursing interventions, Am J *Public Health* 83(12): 1730-1734, 1993.

A 1989-1993 study was designed to provide descriptive data about the characteristics of home health clients, the services that nurses provide to those clients, and the outcomes of those services. Few similar studies have been conducted. The study examined 2403 home health clients served by four agencies in Nebraska, New Jersey, and Wisconsin. Demographic, health history, and clinical data were analyzed. The Omaha System was used as the model for describing and measuring data specific to clients' health-related problems, nursing interventions, and outcomes of care. Results of the study included the following: (1) the median age of the clients was 68.6 years; (2) nurses conducted 70% of all home visits, identified 9107 client problems, and provided more than 96000 interventions; and (3) clients' knowledge, behavior, and status improved on problem-specific outcome subscales. These data depict important characteristics of home health clients in a large national sample and suggest that community health services do make a difference. Findings also support the usefulness of the Omaha System in describing and quantifying nursing practice in community-focused settings.

Description and Application to Practice

The staff and administrators of the Visiting Nurse Association (VNA) of Omaha, Neb, began addressing **nursing practice, documentation,** and **data management** concerns as early as 1970. They began the process of converting a narrative method of documentation to a problem-oriented approach. At that time, no systematic nomenclature or classification of client problems existed that could be used with a problem-oriented record system. This realization provided the impetus for initiating research at the VNA of Omaha.

With the assistance of community health nursing educators, the first project was conducted in 1975 and 1976 and was funded through a contract with the Division of Nursing, U.S. Department of Health, Education, and Welfare. The Problem Classification Scheme resulted from that first research. It was designed to produce a valid and reliable scheme of client problems or nursing diagnoses applicable in home care, public health, school health, nursing centers, ambulatory care, and emerging health delivery settings.

The VNA of Omaha staff conducted three more projects. The goal of the research funded by the Division of Nursing was to develop an Intervention Scheme and Problem Rating Scale for Outcomes using an approach similar to that used for the Problem Classification Scheme. The validity and reliability of the three schemes were established during these two projects (Martin and Scheet, 1992a, 1992b). The fourth research project was funded by a 1989-1993 grant from the National Center for Nursing Research, National Institutes of Health. It was designed to collect and analyze data about relationships within the Omaha System, suggest needed revisions, and explore the potential for implementation in diverse settings (Martin et al., 1992, 1993). Since federal funding provided for the development of the Omaha System, it exists in the public domain and is available for general use.

Concepts included in the nursing process and clinical judgment provide the theoretical framework for the Omaha System. As depicted in Figure 10-4, when the three Omaha System schemes are considered collectively, they are equivalent to the nursing process. The client as an individual, family, or community appears at the center of the model to illustrate the range of the Omaha System's applicability and the pivotal nature of the client in the delivery of service.

Staff from the VNA and seven test agencies located in Iowa, Delaware, Texas, Indiana, New Jersey, Wisconsin, and Nebraska participated in the research projects to develop and refine the three interrelated components of the Omaha System. An inductive approach was used throughout the research projects. Empirical data generated by practicing community health nurses provided the basis for the development and refinement processes. Approximately 600 nurses were directly involved in generating data and evaluating the system.

The Omaha System is the only system developed *by* practicing community health nurses *for* practicing community health nurses. Nurses who practice in diverse

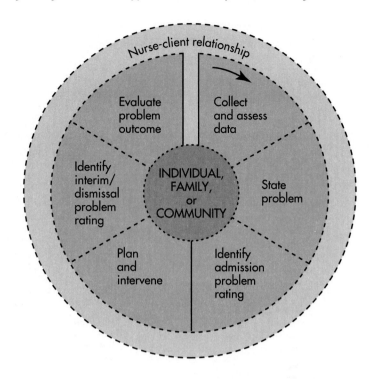

FIGURE 10-4

Conceptualization of the family nursing process. (Modified from Martin KS, Scheet NJ: *The Omaha System: applications for community health nursing*, Philadelphia, 1992, Saunders.)

community-focused settings need comprehensive tools to manage client data. Nurses, however, are not the only members who make up community-focused health care delivery teams. The goals of the Omaha System research were (1) to develop a structured and comprehensive system that could be both understood and used by members of various disciplines and (2) to foster collaborative practice. Therefore, the Omaha System was designed to guide practice decisions, sort and document pertinent client data uniformly, and provide a framework for an agency-wide, interdisciplinary clinical data management information system capable of meeting the needs of clinicians, supervisors, and administrators (Martin, 1994).

When Omaha System surveys were conducted nationally, approximately 250 sites indicated they were users. Their number of employees using the Omaha System ranged from one to 600 persons (Martin and Scheet, 1992a). Users included nurses and members of many disciplines: home care and public health agencies, nursing centers, clinics, schools, ambulatory care centers, correctional facilities, and nursing education programs. Since the Omaha System books were released in 1992, the number of users has dramatically increased, but no systematic survey has been conducted to count them.

Problem Classification Scheme

The **Omaha Problem Classification Scheme** is a client-focused taxonomy of nursing diagnoses com-

Domains and Problems of the Omaha Problem Classification Scheme

I. Environmental Domain
- 01. Income
- 02. Sanitation
- 03. Residence
- 04. Neighborhood/workplace safety
- 05. Other

II. Psychosocial Domain
- 06. Communication with community resources
- 07. Social contact
- 08. Role change
- 09. Interpersonal relationship
- 10. Spirituality
- 11. Grief
- 12. Emotional stability
- 13. Human sexuality
- 14. Caretaking/parenting
- 15. Neglected child/adult
- 16. Abused child/adult
- 17. Growth and development
- 18. Other

III. Physiological Domain
- 19. Hearing
- 20. Vision
- 21. Speech and language
- 22. Dentition
- 23. Cognition
- 24. Pain
- 25. Consciousness
- 26. Integument
- 27. Neuro-musculo-skeletal function
- 28. Respiration
- 29. Circulation
- 30. Digestion-hydration
- 31. Bowel function
- 32. Genito-urinary function
- 33. Antepartum/postpartum
- 34. Other

IV. Health Related Behaviors Domain
- 35. Nutrition
- 36. Sleep and rest patterns
- 37. Physical activity
- 38. Personal hygiene
- 39. Substance use
- 40. Family planning
- 41. Health care supervision
- 42. Prescribed medication regimen
- 43. Technical procedure
- 44. Other

---

prised of simple and concrete terminology. The language of the scheme is organized at four discrete levels of abstraction, a characteristic that increases its power. The vocabulary of each of the four levels is consistent and parallel. Because the scheme is not intended to be exhaustive, terms that are consistent with the scheme's classification rules can be added where the place-holder term, "Other," appears. The levels of the scheme are (1) domains, (2) problems, (3) modifiers, and (4) signs and symptoms. The content and relationship of the domain and problem levels are depicted in the box above and further illustrated by a case example (see Clinical Application).

The four domains, the first levels of the scheme, define the scope of community-focused practice. These domains are (1) Environmental, (2) Psychosocial, (3) Physiological, and (4) Health Related Behaviors. Understanding the meaning of and relationship among the domains is a prerequisite to implementing the scheme accurately.

The 40 client problems are the second level of the Problem Classification Scheme (40 excludes "Other" term in each domain; see the box above). These client problems or nursing diagnoses are the most critical portion of the scheme. Problems identified by the nurse are always documented in the client record. Two sets of modifiers represent the third level of the scheme and are used in conjunction with each client problem. Modifiers selected by the community health nurse are (1) Family or Individual

Categories of the Omaha Intervention Scheme

I. Health Teaching, Guidance, and Counseling

Health teaching, guidance, and counseling are nursing activities that range from giving information, anticipating client problems, encouraging client action and responsibility for self-care and coping, to assisting with decision making and problem solving. The overlapping concepts occur on a continuum with the variation due to the client's self-direction capabilities.

II. Treatments and Procedures

Treatments and procedures are technical nursing activities directed toward preventing signs and symptoms, identifying risk factors and early signs and symptoms, and decreasing or alleviating signs and symptoms.

III. Case Management

Case management includes nursing activities of coordination, advocacy, and referral. These activities involve facilitating service delivery on behalf of the client, communicating with health and human service providers, promoting assertive client communication, and guiding the client toward use of appropriate community resources.

IV. Surveillance

Surveillance includes nursing activities of detection, measurement, critical analysis, and monitoring to indicate client status in relation to a given condition or phenomenon.

Second Level of the Omaha Intervention Scheme: Targets

01. Anatomy/physiology	33. Medication administration
02. Behavior modification	34. Medication set-up
03. Bladder care	35. Mobility/transfers
04. Bonding	36. Nursing care, supplementary
05. Bowel care	37. Nutrition
06. Bronchial hygiene	38. Nutritionist
07. Cardiac care	39. Ostomy care
08. Caretaking/parenting skills	40. Other community resources
09. Cast care	41. Personal care
10. Communication	42. Positioning
11. Coping skills	43. Rehabilitation
12. Day care/respite	44. Relaxation/breathing techniques
13. Discipline	45. Rest/sleep
14. Dressing change/wound care	46. Safety
15. Durable medical equipment	47. Screening
16. Education	48. Sickness/injury care
17. Employment	49. Signs/symptoms—mental/emotional
18. Environment	50. Signs/symptoms—physical
19. Exercises	51. Skin care
20. Family planning	52. Social work/counseling
21. Feeding procedures	53. Specimen collection
22. Finances	54. Spiritual care
23. Food	55. Stimulation/nurturance
24. Gait training	56. Stress management
25. Growth/development	57. Substance use
26. Homemaking	58. Supplies
27. Housing	59. Support group
28. Interaction	60. Support system
29. Lab findings	61. Transportation
30. Legal system	62. Wellness
31. Medical/dental care	63. Other
32. Medication action/side effects	

and (2) Actual, Potential, or Health promotion. Using two modifiers with a problem enhances application across the health-illness continuum and adds an important degree of specificity and precision. Some nurses have expanded the Individual and Family modifiers to include groups and communities.

The fourth level of the Problem Classification Scheme involves a cluster of signs and symptoms specific to each problem. Clues and cues are produced as the nurse gathers, sorts, and prioritizes data. These suggest signs and symptoms that, in turn, suggest the presence of actual client problems.

Intervention Scheme

The **Omaha Intervention Scheme** is a systematic arrangement of nursing actions or activities designed to help nurses and other health care professionals document both plans and interventions. The scheme is intended for use with nursing diagnoses. Using the same taxonomic principles as described for the Problem Classification Scheme, the language is organized into three levels of abstraction or specificity: (1) categories, (2) targets, and (3) client-specific information. The content and relationship of the category and target levels are depicted in the box on p. 198, bottom

right and further illustrated with a case example (see Clinical Application on p. 202).

The four intervention categories represent the essence of community health practice. When viewed collectively, the categories describe the clinician's primary functions in relation to importance and time. The categories are (1) Health Teaching, Counseling, and Guidance, (2) Treatments and Procedures, (3) Case Management, and (4) Surveillance.

The second level of the Omaha Intervention Scheme is an alphabetical listing of 62 targets (excludes "Other;" see box above). *Targets* are the objects of nursing interventions. The targets are used to delineate a problem-specific intervention category by offering a more specific level of detail.

The third level of the Intervention Scheme is designed for client-specific information. Pertinent, concise words or short phrases are generated by clinicians as they develop plans or document care provided to a specific client. Although not part of the research projects, VNA of Omaha Staff organized their suggestion into care planning guides specific to each of the 40 problems of the Problem Classification Scheme (Martin and Scheet, 1992b). The box on p. 200 gives select examples of problems and the signs and symptoms which help to identify the problem.

Examples of Problems, Modifiers, and Signs/Symptoms from the Omaha Problem Classification Scheme

01. Income

Health promotion
Potential deficit
Deficit
    01. low/no income
    02. uninsured medical expenses
    03. inadequate money management
    04. able to buy only necessities
    05. difficulty buying necessities
    06. other

33. Antepartum/postpartum

Health promotion
Potential impairment
Impairment
    01. difficulty coping with pregnancy/body changes
    02. inappropriate exercise/rest/diet/behaviors
    03. discomfort
    04. complications
    05. fears delivery procedure
    06. difficulty breast-feeding
    07. other

08. Role change

Health promotion
Potential impairment
Impairment
    01. involuntary reversal of traditional male/female roles
    02. involuntary reversal of dependent/independent roles
    03. assumes new role
    04. loses previous role
    05. other

35. Nutrition

Health promotion
Potential impairment
Impairment
    01. weighs 10% more than average
    02. weighs 10% less than average
    03. lacks established standards for daily caloric/fluid intake
    04. exceeds established standards for daily caloric/fluid intake
    05. unbalanced diet
    06. improper feeding schedule for age
    07. nonadherence to prescribed diet
    08. unexplained/progressive weight loss
    09. hypoglycemia
    10. hyperglycemia
    11. other

Table 10-7 The Omaha Problem Rating Scale for Outcomes

Concept	1	2	3	4	5
KNOWLEDGE					
The ability of the client to remember and interpret information	No knowledge	Minimal knowledge	Basic knowledge	Adequate knowledge	Superior knowledge
BEHAVIOR					
The observable responses, actions, or activities of the client fitting the occasion or purpose	Not appropriate	Rarely appropriate	Inconsistently appropriate	Usually appropriate	Consistently appropriate
STATUS					
The condition of the client in relation to objective and subjective defining characteristics	Extreme signs/symptoms	Severe signs/symptoms	Moderate signs/symptoms	Minimal signs/symptoms	No signs/symptoms

Problem Rating Scale for Outcomes

The **Omaha Problem Rating Scale for Outcomes** is a five-point Likert-type scale that offers a systematic, recurring way of measuring client progress throughout the time of service. It was designed for use with any client problem in the Problem Classification Scheme. In addition, the scale provides both a guide for practice and a method of documentation. When establishing the initial ratings for client problems, the nurse creates an independent data baseline, capturing the condition and circumstances of the client at a specific point in time. This admission baseline is used for comparison with the client's ratings at later intervals and at dismissal. The content and relationship of the concepts and numerical ratings are depicted in Table 10-7 and further illustrated by a case example (see Clinical Application).

The Problem Rating Scale for Outcomes comprises three summated or Likert-type ordinal scales for Knowledge, Behavior, and Status. Knowledge involves what a client knows and understands about a specific health-related problem. Behavior involves what a client does—the client's practices, performances, and skills. Status involves what a client is and how the client's conditions or circumstances improve, remain stable, or deteriorate. Although the three concepts are interrelated, they represent three distinct dimensions of client outcomes. The three dimensions of the scale are equal in importance, although they may not be equally important when used with a specific client.

The ratings have characteristics of ordinal scales: (1) mutually exclusive classes or categories, (2) each continuum collectively exhaustive, and (3) categories that fit into a specific order or sequence. Each scale has a continuum of five categories or degrees for response; very positive and negative categories are located at the ends of each continuum.

Clinical Application

The following case example illustrates the use of the Omaha System and the relationship between the system and the nursing process. The case example, although fictitious, is a composite of many clients served by the staff of the Polk County Health Department, Balsam Lake, Wis. Data collection, data assessment, problem identification, interventions, and outcome measurement are illustrated for a typical admission visit by a community health nurse. Systematic and comprehensive data can be obtained from an individual and family by using the three components of the Omaha System and then can be sorted, collated, and analyzed. This process is also applicable to the group and community levels. Individual, family, group, and community data that are aggregated can provide meaningful information about the degree of health or illness within a specific population.

Julie Bear came to the County WIC Clinic for food and information about available resources. Julie was a 15-year-old Native American who lived with her mother, two brothers, and one sister. She had no source of personal income and was unsure about how to access tribal health services. Julie was 5 months pregnant and a primipara. She had no visible edema but had proteinuria. She had just seen a family practice physician, who diagnosed nephrotic syndrome and prescribed a low-sodium, high-protein diet. Based on her diagnosis, prenatal questionnaire scores, and financial status, she qualified for WIC and the agency's public health nursing program for case management and home visits.

The community health nurse, Lucy Benson, could not call to schedule a visit because Julie's family did not have a phone. When Lucy arrived, Julie's mother said that Julie was living with her grandmother. Lucy called the grandmother and found out that Julie was not home. After repeated calls to the grandmother, Lucy was able to make the admission visit 2 days later.

During the visit, the nurse collected objective and subjective data according to the Environmental, Psychosocial, Physiological, and Health Related Behaviors domains of the Problem Classification Scheme. Data were examined to identify signs, symptoms, and problems. The nurse was sensitive to Julie's heritage and cultural values and recognized that pregnancy and parenting are culturally defined processes.

Julie's blood pressure was 140/88, her temperature 99.0° F, and her pulse 88. She had 4+ pitting edema in her feet and ankles, generalized puffiness, and some rales in her lungs. Julie also reported genital edema. Lucy reported these data immediately to Julie's physician, who indicated that Julie needed to return for an examination as soon as possible.

Julie was 5 feet, 6 inches tall. Her weight before pregnancy was 170 pounds; she had gained 20 pounds since becoming pregnant. When Lucy asked about her eating patterns, Julie described an unbalanced diet that was high in sodium and included many canned government commodity foods. Although Julie thought that her low-sodium diet was a form of punishment, she said that she knew she must change her eating patterns and agreed that she would eliminate potato chips and french fries. She was willing to have a registered dietitian visit later that week.

Julie planned to keep her baby even though she had not wanted to become pregnant. She indicated that she was frightened about labor and delivery. She had made no preparations for her newborn; she was considering breast-feeding. She did not want to talk about becoming pregnant other than to say that she was intoxicated when she conceived and did not know who had fathered her baby. Julie said that she was moving back to her mother's home tomorrow.

During the admission visit, Lucy identified five problems in the Bear family: Income, Role change, Antepartum/postpartum, Nutrition, and Health care supervision. Four of the problems, modifiers, and signs and symptoms are shown in the box and further

Continued.

Table 10-8   Case Example of the Bear Family Using the Omaha System

Domain	Client data	Problems and signs/symptoms	Ratings*	Interventions
Environmental	Julie—no income; family—low income. No phone. Uncertain about tribal health services. PH home visits approved.	01. Income: actual/family 01. low/no income 05. difficulty buying necessities	K = 2 B = 3 S = 3	
Psychosocial	Unplanned pregnancy; conceived while intoxicated. 15-year-old Native American. Lives with mother and grandmother.	08. Role change: potential/Julie		
Physiological	5 months pregnant. Primipara. BP 140/88. 4+ pitting edema feet & ankles; vaginal edema; generalized puffiness. T 99.0, P 88, elevated proteinuria. Frightened about labor and delivery. Plans to breast-feed. No baby supplies yet.	33. Antepartum/postpartum: actual/Julie 02. inappropriate exercise/rest/diet/ behaviors 04. complications	K = 2 B = 2 S = 1	I 01, 49, 50 III 50 IV 50
Health Related Behaviors	5'6", AP 170 lb, gained 20 lb. Diet: high Na and canned commodity foods. Referred to low-Na diet as punishment.	35. Nutrition: actual/Julie 01. weighs 10% more than average 04. exceeds established standards for daily caloric/fluid intake 05. unbalanced diet 07. nonadherence to prescribed diet	K = 3 B = 2 S = 2	I 23 III 37
	Serious problems require complex services and many appointments.	41. Health care supervision: potential/Julie		

*K, Knowledge; B, Behavior; S, Status. See also Table 10-7 and text boxes for Omaha Scheme.

Clinical Application—cont'd

illustrated in Table 10-8. When Lucy considered these problems in relation to the modifiers, she recorded family as the modifier for Income and individual as the modifier for the other four problems. She then considered the problems in relation to the second set of modifiers. One or more signs and symptoms were identified for the three actual problems: Income, Antepartum/postpartum, and Nutrition. Supporting data indicated risk factors for the potential problems: Role change and Health care supervision. Lucy did not identify any health promotion problems, the third option available in the Omaha Problem Classification Scheme. As an experienced community health nurse, Lucy considered more problems than the five she identified and documented on the first visit. These included Communication with community resources, Interpersonal relationship, Human sexuality, Abused child/adult, Genito-urinary function, and Substance use. Lucy recognized, however, that insufficient data were available at the admission visit to document further problems. She planned to monitor Julie closely, make numerous subsequent visits, and collect more

objective and subjective data that would lead to documenting or ruling out other problems.

As Lucy thought about the problems she was identifying as she conducted the admission visit, she decided that three were priority problems: Income, Antepartum/postpartum, and Nutrition. Therefore, she identified admission Knowledge, Behavior, and Status ratings for these three problems (Table 10-8). The decisions about priority problems and ratings helped guide her interventions during that visit and her plans for the future.

During the first visit, Lucy's interventions for Antepartum/postpartum involved (1) Health Teaching, Guidance, and Counseling; (2) Case Management; and (3) Surveillance. Her interventions for Nutrition included (1) Health Teaching, Guidance, and Counseling and (2) Case Management. Table 10-8 depicts the Intervention Scheme targets and client-specific information as well as the categories for the admission visit.

When Julie saw the family practice physician several days later, she had gained 5 more pounds and

Clinical Application–cont'd

continued to exhibit proteinuria. The physician referred her to a nephrologist, who inserted a long-term cuffed Groshong catheter for giving albumin. The community health nurse was to use the catheter to give Julie 25 g 25% albumin by intravenous infusion at 2 ml/minute twice weekly. Julie was to receive her third weekly dose at the physician's office, where she would be examined and have laboratory work, including hemoglobin, hematocrit, serum protein, and electrolytes. Lucy would document the changes in Julie's status by adding Genito- urinary function as an Actual, Individual, priority problem with the symptom, proteinuria. From the Intervention Scheme, Lucy would use Surveillance (category) and targets such as Screening and Signs/symptoms—physical to monitor and document Julie's weight gain, edema, lung sounds, cuffed catheter site, and other signs and symptoms closely. On the days Lucy gave the albumin, she would use the Intervention Scheme Treatment and Procedures (category), Medication administra-

tion (target), and describe the medication, dose, route, and reaction.

The case example and the tables were written to depict the data collection, data assessment, problem identification, intervention, and problem rating process that occurred during the first home visit. Use of the Omaha System increased the meaning of that process and the potential to communicate it accurately to others. Table 10-8 depicts:

1. The four domains listed in the Domain column.
2. Pertinent subjective and objective data in the Client data column. Less pertinent data obtained during the visit are not recorded.
3. Sorted and collapsed data used to generate pertinent problems and signs and symptoms in the Problems and signs/symptoms column.
4. Numerical ratings for the priority problems in the Ratings column.
5. Categories and targets in the Interventions column.

Key Concepts

◆ Models can be physical, symbolic, or mental ways of viewing real phenomena.

◆ Conceptual models guide members of a discipline in their thinking, observing, and interpreting.

◆ Community health nursing is population focused, and the goal is to improve the health of the community.

◆ Community health nursing practice is interdisciplinary and includes assessment, policy development, and a wide range of actions designed to promote healthy outcomes in a community.

◆ Systems models have particular usefulness for guiding education, practice, and research in community health nursing.

◆ The Neuman Systems Model can be effectively used to guide community health nursing education and practice.

◆ The Neuman Systems Model depicts an open system where people are in dynamic interaction with the environment in regard to physiological, psychological, sociocultural, developmental, and spiritual variables.

◆ The Neuman Systems Model includes primary, secondary, and tertiary intervention modalities, which make it especially useful in community health.

◆ The Omaha System was developed and refined through a process of research. Reliability and validity were established for the entire system.

◆ The Omaha System is unique in that it is the only complete system of nursing language developed inductively *by* practicing community health nurses *for* practicing community health nurses.

◆ The Omaha System was designed to follow taxonomic principles. The system consists of a Problem Classification Scheme, Intervention Scheme, and Problem Rating Scale for Outcomes. The system includes language and codes for nursing diagnoses, nursing interventions, and client outcomes.

◆ The Omaha System offers benefits in three principal areas: practice, documentation, and data management. These areas are of concern to community health educators and students, as well as community health clinicians and administrators.

Critical Thinking Activities

1. Identify several concepts in nursing that you think are related and that guide actions. Using the concepts, try to construct a conceptual framework for your practice.
2. Debate one of these issues: (a) conceptual models should (should not) guide nursing practice, or (b) conceptual models help (hinder) community health nursing practice.
3. Choose a clinical experience where you have visited a family in their home, or think of a fictitious family. Analyze their situation, including your nursing care plan, using the Neuman Systems Model.
4. Accompany an experienced home health, public health, or school health nurse on a home, clinic, or school visit. Observe and discuss if that nurse uses a nursing diagnosis, intervention, or outcome measurement system/framework.
5. Work with a partner or in a small group. Select a community health client whom you have visited or think of a fictitious client. List typical referral and first visit data. Independently apply the three parts of the Omaha System to the client data. Compare each portion of your selections with your partner or group members. Discuss.

Bibliography

American Nurses Association: *A conceptual model of community health nursing practice*, Kansas City, Mo, 1980, The Association.

American Nurses Association: *Standards of community health nursing practice*, Kansas City, Mo, 1986, The Association.

American Nurses Association: Nursing classifications recognized by National Library of Medicine, *Am Nurse* 25:9, 1993.

American Public Health Association: *The definition and role of public health nursing in the delivery of health care*, Washington, DC, 1981, The Association.

American Public Health Association, Public Health Nursing Section Legislative Committee: *Guidelines for talking points: a public health nursing perspective on health care reform*, Washington, DC, 1994, The Association.

Anderson E, McFarlane J, Helton A: Community-as-client: a model for practice, *Nurs Outlook* 34(5):220-224, 1986.

Association of Community Health Nursing Educators: *Essentials of baccalaureate nursing education for entry level practice in community health nursing*, Louisville, Ky, 1990, The Association.

Barnum BJS: *Nursing theory: analysis, application, evaluation*, ed 3, Philadelphia, 1994, Lippincott.

Beddome G: Application of the Neuman Systems Model to the assessment of community-as-client. In Neuman B, editor: *The Neuman Systems Model: application to nursing education and practice*, ed 2, East Norwalk, Conn, 1989, Appleton & Lange.

Bulechek GM, McCloskey JC: Nursing interventions: treatments for potential nursing diagnoses. In Carroll-Johnson RM, editor: *Classification of nursing diagnoses*, Philadelphia, 1989, Lippincott.

Carroll-Johnson RM: Reflections on the 9th biennial conference, *Nurs Diagn* 1(1):49-50, 1990.

Carroll-Johnson RM, Parquette M, editors: *Classification of nursing diagnoses: proceedings of the tenth conference*, Philadelphia, 1994, Lippincott.

Chin R: The utility of systems models and developmental models for practitioners. In Riehl JP, Roy SC, editors: *Conceptual models for nursing practice*, ed 2, New York, 1980, Appleton-Century-Crofts.

Clark J, Lang N: An international classification for nursing practice, *Int Nurs Rev* 39(4):109-111, 1992.

Donabedian A: Evaluating the quality of medical care, *Milbank Memorial Fund Q* 44(2):166-206, 1966.

Fawcett J: *Analysis and evaluation of conceptual models of nursing*, ed 2, Philadelphia, 1989, Davis.

Freese BT: Health in the workplace: assessment of community-as-client, 1994. (Unpublished manuscript.)

Freese BT, Hassell JS: Hispanic community as client, 1994. (Unpublished manuscript.)

Goeppinger J, Shuster GF: Community as client: using the nursing process to promote health. In Stanhope M, Lancaster J, editors: *Community health nursing*, ed 3, St Louis, 1992, Mosby.

Healthy People 2000: national health promotion and disease prevention objectives, Washington, DC, 1991, USDHHS, Public Health Service.

Johnson DE: The behavioral system model for nursing. In Riehl JP, Roy SC, editors: *Conceptual models for nursing practice*, ed 2, New York, 1980, Appleton-Century-Crofts.

Kerlinger FN: *Foundations of behavioral research*, ed 2, New York, 1973, Holt, Rinehart & Winston.

King I: *A theory for nursing: systems, concepts, process*, New York, 1981, Wiley.

Kuhn MA: *Pharmacotherapeutics: a nursing process approach*, Philadelphia, 1994, Davis.

Marriner-Tomey A: *Nursing theorists and their work*, ed 3, St Louis, 1994, Mosby.

Martin KS: How can the quality of nursing practice be measured? In McCloskey JC, Grace HK, editors: *Current issues in nursing*, ed 4, St Louis, 1994, Mosby.

Martin KS, Leak GK, Aden CA: The Omaha System: a research-based model for decision making, *J Nurs Adm* 22(11):47-52, 1992.

Martin KS, Scheet NJ, Stegman MR: Home health clients: characteristics, outcomes of care, and nursing interventions, *Am J Public Health* 83(12):1730-1734, 1993.

Martin KS, Scheet NJ: *The Omaha System: applications for community health nursing*, Philadelphia, 1992a, Saunders.

Martin KS, Scheet NJ: *The Omaha System: a pocket guide for community health nursing*, Philadelphia, 1992b, Saunders.

McCloskey JC, Bulechek GM, editors: *Nursing interventions classification*, St Louis, 1992, Mosby.

Meleis AI: *Theoretical nursing*, ed 2, Philadelphia, 1991, Lippincott.

Ministry's of Health, Community and Social Services and Citizenship: *Partnership in long-term care: a new way to plan, manage and deliver services and community support*, Toronto, 1993.

Neuman B: Family intervention using the Betty Neuman Health care. In Clements IW, Roberts FB, editors: *Family health: a theoretical approach to nursing care*, New York, 1983, Wiley.

Neuman B: *The Neuman Systems Model: application to nursing education and practice*, ed 2, East Norwalk, Conn, 1989, Appleton & Lange.

Neuman B, Young RJ: A model for teaching total person approach to patient problems, *Nurs Res* 21:264, 1972.

Orem D: *Nursing: concepts of practice*, ed 3, New York, 1985, McGraw-Hill.

Rogers ME: *An introduction to the theoretical basis of nursing*, Philadelphia, 1970, Davis.

Rogers ME: Nursing: a science of unitary man. In Riehl JP, Roy CS, editors: *Conceptual models for nursing practice*, New York, 1980, Appleton-Century-Crofts.

Roy C: *Introduction to nursing: an adaptation model*, ed 2, Englewood Cliffs, NJ, 1984, Prentice-Hall.

Saba VK, O'Hare PA, Zuckerman AE, Boondas J, Oatway DM: A nursing intervention taxonomy for home health care, *Nurs Health Care* 12(6):296-299, 1991.

Smith NE: *Neuman Systems model adapted as the model for a fully developed multi-service agency in Huron County.* Paper presented at the meeting of the Long-Term Care Planning Committee, Clinton, Ontario, 1994a.

Spector R: *Cultural diversity in health and illness,* ed 3, East Norwalk, Conn, 1992, Appleton & Lange.

von Bertalanffy L: *Problems of life: an evaluation of modern biological and scientific thought,* New York, 1952, Harper.

Zielstorff RD, Hudgings CI, Grobe SJ, NCNIP: *Next-generation nursing information systems,* Washington, DC, 1993, American Nurses Association/National League for Nursing.

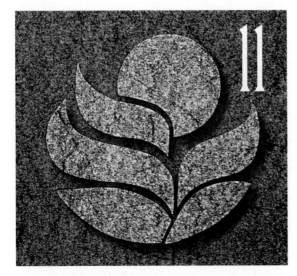

11

Epidemiological Applications in Community Health Nursing

Robert E. McKeown ◆ Carol Z. Garrison

Objectives ▼

After reading this chapter, the student should be able to do the following:

◆ Define epidemiology and describe its essential elements and approach.
◆ Describe the history of epidemiology and how its scope and methods have evolved.
◆ Discuss the elements and interactions of the epidemiologic triangle.
◆ Outline the relation of the natural history of disease to the various levels of prevention and to the design and implementation of community interventions.
◆ Understand and interpret basic epidemiologic measures of morbidity and mortality.
◆ Understand and illustrate descriptive epidemiologic parameters of person, place, and time.
◆ Recognize and describe the features of common epidemiologic study designs.
◆ Describe essential characteristics and methods of evaluating a screening program.
◆ Understand the most common sources of bias in epidemiologic studies.
◆ Understand and interpret epidemiological research and apply findings to community health nursing practice.

Key Terms ▼

agent
analytic epidemiology
attack rate
bias
case-control study
causality
cohort study
confounding
cross-sectional study
descriptive epidemiology
determinants
distribution
ecological fallacy
ecological study
environment
epidemic
epidemiology
host
incidence
levels of prevention
natural history of disease
negative predictive value
point epidemic
positive predictive value
prevalence
rates
reliability
risk
screening
secular trends
sensitivity
specificity

Outline ▼

Definition and Description
History
Basic Concepts in Epidemiology
    Epidemiologic Triangle: Agent, Host, and Environment
    Stages of Health and Intervention
Basic Methods in Epidemiology
    Sources of Data
    Measures of Morbidity and Mortality
    Comparison Groups
Descriptive Epidemiology
    Person
    Place
    Time

Continued.

Continued.

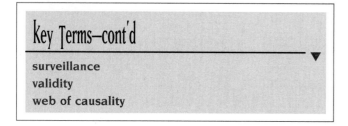

An outbreak of a deadly pneumonia after a 1976 American Legionnaires convention in Philadelphia, a rare cancer striking a select California population in 1981, and declining mortality from cardiovascular disease (CVD) are all subject matter for epidemiology. Epidemiologists determined the disease distribution and the causal agent of Legionnaire's disease; they characterized the syndrome and determined the major risk factors for AIDS; and they continuously study CVD morbidity and mortality trends.

DEFINITION AND DESCRIPTION

Epidemiology has been defined as "The study of the *distribution* and *determinants* of health-related states or events in specified populations, and the application of this study to control of health problems" (Last, 1988). As the scope of epidemiology has broadened in this century, so the definition has undergone transformation. The term originally referred to epidemics that were primarily infectious in origin, but now it includes chronic diseases, such as cancer and cardiovascular disease, and, more recently, mental health and other health-related events, such as accidents, injuries and violence, occupational and environmental exposures and their effects, and positive health states. In addition, epidemiologic methods now are used to study health-related behaviors, such as physical activity and in health services research. Epidemiologic methods are used extensively to determine to what extent the goals of *Healthy People 2000* (1991), the nation's health objectives, are accomplished.

Epidemiology is the science of health events affecting populations, investigating the distribution and determinants of those events, and focusing on characterizing a health outcome in terms of what, who, where, when, and why. The **distribution** of health

events has to do with the patterns of those events in populations, that is: What is the disease? Who is affected? Where are they? When do events occur? The **determinants** of health events are those factors, characteristics, and behaviors that determine (or influence) the patterns: How does it occur? Why are some affected more than others? The results of these investigations are used to guide or evaluate policies and programs that improve the health of the community.

The first step in the epidemiologic process is to define a health outcome (the case definition, usually cases of disease, but also of injuries, accidents, or even wellness). Epidemiology has played important roles in the refinement of the case definition for AIDS and in the development of precise diagnostic criteria for psychiatric disorders. Epidemiologic methods are then used to quantify the frequency of occurrence and characterize both the case group and the population from which they come (i.e., describing the distribution, the who, where, and when) and to search for factors that explain the pattern or risk of occurrence (i.e., determinants, the why and how). These two foci suggest the two major categories of epidemiology: **descriptive epidemiology,** which seeks to describe a disease entity according to person, place, and time and **analytic epidemiology,** which is directed toward understanding the etiology (or origins and causal factors) of the disease.

The World Health Organization defines health as "a state of complete well-being, physical, social, and mental, and not merely the absence of disease or infirmity" (Institute of Medicine, 1988, p. 39). The Institute of Medicine's (IOM) 1988 study *The Future of Public Health* defined the mission of public health as "the fulfillment of society's interest in assuring conditions in which people can be healthy" and noted "the *substance* of public health [is]: organized community efforts aimed at the prevention of disease and promotion of health" (IOM, 1988, pp. 40-41). This definition implies establishment of public policies and programs and the delivery of specific services to individuals. Public health activity is channeled in three directions: community prevention (proactive), disease control (reactive), and personal health (proactive and reactive) services. The IOM report notes that epidemiology is "the mother science of public health," which is described as a constellation of disciplines with a common mission: optimal health for the whole community.

Epidemiology, therefore, builds on and draws from other disciplines and methods, including clinical medicine and laboratory sciences, quantitative methods, especially biostatistics, and public health policy and goals. It should be clear, however, that epidemiology differs from clinical medicine, whose focus is on the diagnosis and treatment of disease in *individuals.* The focus of epidemiology, on the other hand, is the study of *populations* in order to understand the causes of disease and to influence and evaluate the development of effective interventions to prevent disease and maintain health. Effective community health nursing bridges these disciplines in its focus on individual clients and services provided for them and also in its appropriation of epidemiologic methods and findings in community health programs and preventive measures.

HISTORY

Some writers cite Hippocrates in the fourth century BC as an ancient precursor of epidemiology (Timmreck, 1994; Winkelstein and French, 1972). He maintained that to understand health and disease in a community one should look to geographic and climatic factors, the seasons of the year, the food and water consumed, and the habits and behaviors of the people. His approach does anticipate in a general way the major categories of descriptive epidemiology: namely the distribution of health states by personal characteristics, place, and time. However, modern epidemiology only emerged within the last two centuries, and developed as a discipline with a distinctive identity and method in this century (Susser, 1985).

Notable events in the history of epidemiology are listed in Table 11-1. This section highlights a few major developments. It was in the nineteenth century that germ theory developed with the isolation of organisms, including a number of infectious agents, induction of disease in susceptible hosts, and development of the idea of specificity in the relation of organism and outcome. These successes led to increased emphasis on the role of the agent in the genesis of disease. Yet Pasteur also recognized the role of personal characteristics, such as immunity and host resistance, in explaining differential susceptibility to disease (Susser, 1973; Vandenbroucke, 1990). Further, the accomplishments of the sanitary movement in reducing disease contributed to the acceptance of germ theory while emphasizing the importance of the environ-

mental influences for disease rates and variability by person, place, and time (IOM, 1988).

Two refinements in research methods in the eighteenth and nineteenth centuries were critical for the formation of epidemiologic methods: use of a comparison group and the development of sophisticated quantitative techniques (numeric measurements or counts). One of the most famous examples of use of a comparison group is found in the pivotal mid-nineteenth century investigation of cholera by John Snow, whom some call the "father of epidemiology" (Lilienfeld and Stolley, 1994; Susser, 1973; Timmreck, 1994). By mapping cases that clustered around a single public water pump in one outbreak, Snow laid the foundation for showing a connection between water supply and cholera. He later observed that cholera rates were higher in areas supplied by water companies whose water intakes were downstream and subject to greater sewage contamination than in those whose water came from further upstream. In several areas, two water company lines were overlapping so that households in the same neighborhood were served by different companies. Because households in close proximity to each other had different sources of water, differences observed in rates of cholera could not be attributed to location or economic status. Snow showed that households receiving water from a company whose intake had been moved away from sewage contamination had rates of cholera substantially lower than those supplied by a company whose intake was still in a contaminated section of the river (Table 11-2). Snow realized this was an example of what is called a "natural experiment," which gave added credibility to his argument that foul water was the vehicle for transmission of the agent that caused cholera.

Another of what Abraham Lilienfeld called the "threads of epidemiology" (Lilienfeld and Lilienfeld, 1980) is found in the increased emphasis on a quantitative approach. One prominent example of the use of quantitative methods to study large public health problems was Edwin Chadwick's 1842 "Report on the Sanitary Conditions of the Laboring Population of Great Britain," in which mortality (vital statistics) and morbidity data demonstrated the association between mortality and environmental conditions: poor sanitation, overcrowding, contaminated water (Chadwick, 1842). Chadwick recognized that mortality was an indicator of larger morbidity, that is, the number who die from a disease is but "an indication of the much greater number" who suffer from the disease but survive (Lilienfeld, 1984).

In this century, development and application of epidemiologic methods were stimulated by changes in society brought on by such factors as the Great Depression, World War II, a rising standard of living for many but abject poverty for others, improved nutrition, new vaccines, better sanitation, the advent of antibiotics and chemotherapies, and declines in infant and child mortality, as well as in the birth rate. The re-

Table II-I   Significant Milestones in the History of Epidemiology

1662	John Graunt	Used Bills of Mortality (forerunner of modern vital records) to study patterns of death in various populations in England. Published early form of life table analysis.
1747	James Lind	Study of scurvy using observation and comparison of response to various dietary treatments. Early precursor of clinical trial.
1760	Daniel Bernoulli	Used life-table technique to demonstrate that smallpox inoculation conferred lifelong immunity.
1775	Percival Pott	First "cancer epidemiologist." Noted high proportion of patients presenting with cancer of scrotum were chimney sweeps. Inferred the exposure to soot was the cause. (Lack of a comparison group would reduce validity of inference by today's standards.)
1798	Edward Jenner	Demonstrated effectiveness of smallpox vaccination.
1798	Marine Hospital Service	Forerunner of U.S. Public Health Service (1912).
1836	Pierre Charles-Alexandre Louis	Comparative observational studies to demonstrate ineffectiveness of bloodletting. Emphasized the importance of statistical methods ("*la méthode numerique*"). Influenced many of the pioneers in epidemiology in England and the United States.
1836		Establishment of Registrar-General's Office in England as registry for births, deaths, marriages.
1840s	William Farr	Developed forerunner of modern vital records system in Registrar-General's Office. Study of mortality in Liverpool led to significant public health reform. Pioneered mortality surveillance and anticipated many of the basic concepts in epidemiology. His data provided much of the basis for Snow's work on cholera.
1850		Founding of London Epidemiological Society. Known for influential reports on smallpox vaccination and studies of cholera.
1850	Lemuel Shattuck	Report on sanitation and public health in Massachusetts.
1850s	John Snow	Epidemiologic research on transmission of cholera. Used mapping and natural experiment, comparing rates in groups exposed to different water supplies.
1870-1880s	Robert Koch	Discovery of causal agents for anthrax, tuberculosis, and cholera; development of causal criteria.
1887	Joseph Kinyuon	Founded "Laboratory of Hygiene," forerunner of the National Institute of Health (1930).
1921	Wade Hampton Frost	Founded first U.S. academic program in epidemiology at Johns Hopkins.
1942		Office of Malarial Control in War Areas established; became Communicable Disease Control (CDC) in 1946; then Centers for Disease Control (1973); now Centers for Disease Control and Prevention.
1948		Framingham cohort study of cardiovascular disease begins.
1950s	A. Bradford Hill Richard Doll	Pioneering studies on smoking and lung cancer.

From IOM: *The future of public health*, Washington, DC, 1988, National Academy Press; Lilienfeld DE, Stolley PD: *Foundations of epidemiology*, ed 3, New York, 1994, Oxford University Press; *Public Health Service Fact Sheet*, Washington, DC, 1984, USDHHS, Public Health Service; Susser M: *Epidemiol Rev* 7:147-173, 1985; Timmreck TC: *An introduction to epidemiology*, Boston, 1994, Jones and Bartlett.

| Table 11-2 | Household Cholera Death Rates by Source of Water Supply in John Snow's 1853 Investigation |

Company	Number of houses	Deaths from cholera	Deaths per 10,000 households
Southwark and Vauxhall Company	40,046	1,263	315
Lambeth	26,107	98	37
Rest of London	256,423	1,422	59

From Snow J: In *Snow on Cholera*, New York, 1855, The Commonwealth Fund, p. 86.

sult of these changes was increased longevity and a shift in the age distribution of the population, which meant an increase in age-related diseases: coronary heart disease, stroke, cancer, and senile dementia (Susser, 1985). Figure 11-1 shows the 10 leading causes of death in the United States in 1990 and in 1992 with the percentage of all deaths attributed to each.

There was a concomitant shift from looking for single agents, such as the infectious agent that causes cholera, to seeking multifactorial etiology (i.e., many factors or combinations of factors contributing to disease, such as the complex of factors that cause cardiovascular disease). The possibility that behavioral and environmental causes existed for many conditions formerly thought to be degenerative diseases of aging raised the possibility of prevention or delay of onset (Susser, 1985). In addition, the development of genetic and molecular techniques (such as genetic markers for increased risk of breast cancer and sophisticated tests for antibodies to infectious agents or for other biological markers of exposures to environmental toxins, such as lead or pesticides) have markedly enhanced the epidemiologist's ability to classify persons in terms of exposures or inherent susceptibility to disease.

In recent years, new infectious diseases, such as Lyme disease, Legionnaire's disease, and HIV/AIDS, as well as new forms of old diseases, such as resistant strains of tuberculosis, have once again placed infectious disease epidemiology in the spotlight, with renewed emphasis on incorporating the latest molecular techniques along with advances in epidemiologic methods and analysis (CDC, 1994; IOM, 1988; Lederberg et al., 1992). As noted above, epidemiologic methods also have been applied to a broader spectrum of health-related outcomes, including accidents, injuries and violence, occupational and environmental exposures, psychiatric and sociological phenomena, health-related behaviors, and in health services research. This demonstrates again the collaborative and multidisciplinary nature of epidemiologic investigations (Susser, 1985).

BASIC CONCEPTS IN EPIDEMIOLOGY
Epidemiologic Triangle: Agent, Host, and Environment

Epidemiologists understand that disease results from complex relations among causal agents, susceptible persons, and environmental factors. These three elements—**agent, host, environment**—are called the epidemiologic triangle (Figure 11-2, *A*). Changes in one of the elements of the triangle can influence the occurrence of disease by increasing or decreasing a person's risk for disease. Risk is understood as the probability an individual will become ill (Last, 1988). As Figure 11-2, *B* suggests, both agent and host, as well as their interaction, are influenced by the environmental context in which they exist, while the environment itself may be influenced by them. Some examples of these three components are listed the box below.

Causal relationships are often more complex than the epidemiologic triangle conveys. It is more common today to speak of a **web of causality,** recognizing the complex interrelationships of numerous factors interacting, sometimes in subtle ways, to increase (or decrease) risk of disease. Further, associations are sometimes mutual with lines of causality going in both directions. Fortunately, effective interventions to disrupt causal pathways and prevent disease are often possible without a complete understanding of all causal elements in their interrelations. A common example of complex factors in a causal web is depicted for cardiovascular disease in Figure 11-3. There is further discussion of causality later in this chapter.

Stages of Health and Intervention

The goal of epidemiology is to understand causal factors well enough to devise interventions to prevent

 Examples of Agent, Host, and Environmental Factors in the Epidemiologic Triangle

AGENT

Infectious agents (bacteria, viruses, fungi, parasites)
Chemical agents (heavy metals, toxic chemicals, pesticides)
Physical agents (radiation, heat, cold, machinery)

HOST

Genetic susceptibility
Immutable characteristics (age and gender)
Acquired characteristics (immunologic status)
Life-style factors (diet and exercise)

ENVIRONMENT

Climate (temperature, rainfall)
Plant and animal life (may be agents or reservoirs or habitats for agents)
Human population distribution (crowding, social support)
Socioeconomic factors (education, resources, access to care)
Working conditions (levels of stress, noise, satisfaction)

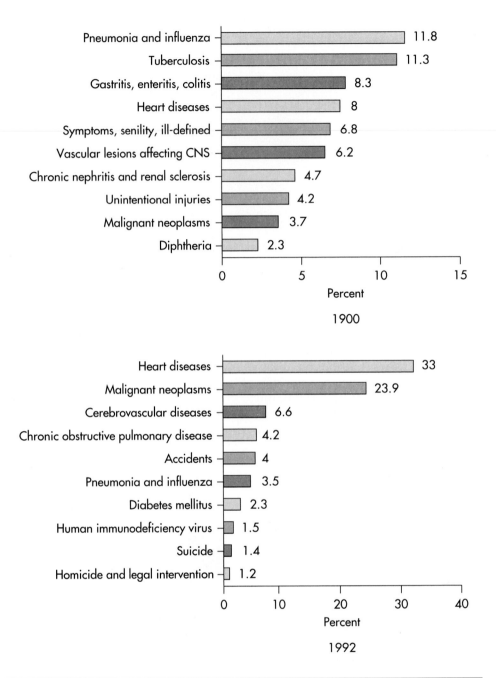

FIGURE 11-1

Ten leading causes of death as a percent of all deaths, United States, 1900 and 1992. (From Kochanek KD, Hudson BL: *Monthly Vital Statistics Report Suppl* 43(6), Hyattsville, Md, National Center for Health Statistics, 1995; Brownson et al: *Chronic disease epidemiology and control*, Washington, DC, 1993, American Public Health Association.)

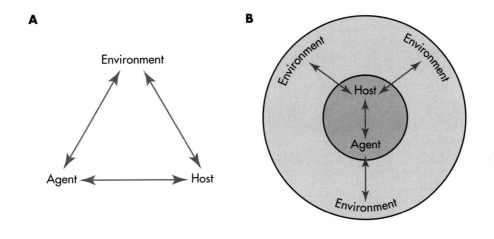

FIGURE 11-2

Two models of the Agent-Host-Environment interaction (the "epidemiologic triangle").

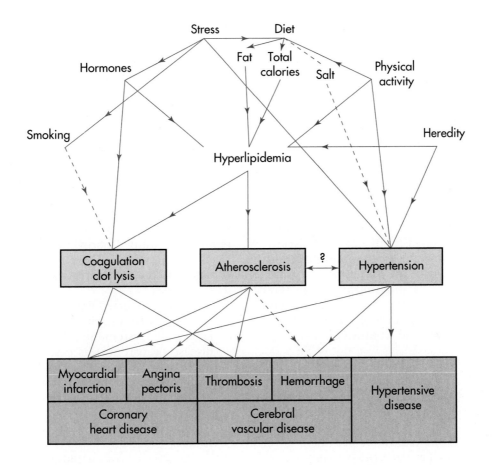

FIGURE 11-3

An example of a web of causality for cardiovascular disease. (From Stallones RA: In *Cerebrovascular disease epidemiology: a workshop*, Public Health Monograph No 76, 1966, US Public Health Service, Pub No 1441).

Table 11-3   Relation of the Stages of Disease to Levels of Prevention

STAGE OF DISEASE PROCESS

Prepathogenesis	Pathogenesis		Resolution
↓	↓	↓	↓
Susceptibility	Preclinical	Clinical	Death, disability, recovery

LEVELS OF PREVENTION

Primary prevention	Secondary prevention	Tertiary prevention

EXAMPLES OF INTERVENTION

Immunization	Pap smear	Physical therapy
Diet and exercise	Screening for HIV	Surgery, medical treatment

adverse events before they start (prevent initiation of the disease process or prevent injury). Where primary prevention is impossible or has failed, intervention must occur at later stages. Public health professionals speak of three levels of prevention tied to specific stages in the **natural history of disease.** The natural history of disease is the course of the disease process from onset to resolution (Last, 1988). Table 11-3 illustrates the relation among the stages of disease and **levels of prevention.** Community health nurses have the potential for playing a leading role in understanding and implementing primary and secondary preventive measures, as well as supplying tertiary prevention services.

Primary Prevention

Primary prevention involves interventions that promote health and prevent disease processes from developing. These activities are aimed at individuals who are susceptible to disease but have no discernable pathology (prepathogenesis). Community health nurses often play an important role in primary prevention programs, such as immunizations, general health education, programs for improving diet and physical activity, parenting education, and provision of and training in use of barrier contraceptives.

Secondary Prevention

Secondary prevention aims to detect disease in the early stages (early pathogenesis) before clinical signs and symptoms manifest in order to intervene with early diagnosis and treatment. The goal is to reverse or reduce the severity of the disease or provide a cure. Screening programs, such as Pap smears to detect cervical dysplasia or blood pressure checks, are often used to detect early disease in symptom-free persons. Family counseling might be viewed as another form of secondary prevention, designed to intervene before problems become serious. Because of the important role that community health nurses play in secondary prevention, a more detailed discussion of screening programs is presented later in the chapter.

Tertiary Prevention

Tertiary prevention is directed toward persons with clinically apparent disease. The aim is to ameliorate the course of disease, reduce disability, or rehabilitate. Examples include the use of physical therapy to prevent contractures in patients with stroke or head or spinal cord injuries or rehabilitating an injured worker to return to work. Rehabilitative job training with counseling for juvenile offenders would be another form of tertiary prevention. Community health nurses often play a critical role in monitoring compliance and in providing services that contribute to recovery or enhanced quality of life for persons affected by disease or injury.

BASIC METHODS IN EPIDEMIOLOGY
Sources of Data

One of the first issues to be confronted in any epidemiologic study is how the data will be obtained (Kelsey et al., 1986). There are three major categories of data sources commonly used in epidemiologic investigations:

1. Routinely collected data, such as census data, vital records (birth and death certificates), and surveillance data (systematic collection of data concerning disease occurrence) as carried out by the Centers for Disease Control and Prevention (CDC);
2. Data collected for other purposes but useful for epidemiologic research, such as medical and insurance records; and
3. Original data collected for specific epidemiologic studies.

The census is conducted every 10 years in this country, and provides population data, including distribution by demographic features (age, race, sex), as well as geographic distribution and additional information concerning economic status, housing, and education. These data provide denominators for various rates (discussed in the following text).

Vital records are the primary source of birth and mortality statistics. Although registration of births and deaths is mandated in most countries, providing one of the most complete sources of health-related data, the quality of specific information varies. For example, on birth certificates, sex and date of birth are fairly reliable, whereas gestational age, level of prenatal care, or smoking habits of the mother during pregnancy are less reliable. On death certificates, the quality of the cause of death information varies over time and from place to place, dependent on diagnostic capabilities and custom. Vital records are readily available in most areas; they are inexpensive, convenient, and allow study of long-term trends. Mortality data, however, are only informative for fatal diseases.

Hospital, physician, and insurance records provide information on morbidity, as do **surveillance** systems for specific diseases, such as those reported to CDC and regional disease registries, which solicit reports of all cases of a particular disease within a geographic region, such as cancer registries. The National Center for Health Statistics also sponsors periodic health surveys and examinations in carefully drawn samples of the U.S. population. These surveys provide information on the health status and behaviors of the population. Other information, such as occupational exposures, may be available from employer records. For many studies, however, the only means of obtaining the needed information is to collect the required data in a study specifically designed to investigate a particular question. The design of such studies is discussed below.

Measures of Morbidity and Mortality

Rates in Epidemiology

Epidemiology is interested in the distribution of health events. Since people differ in their probability or *risk* of disease, the primary concern is how they differ. Mapping cases of a disease in an area, as John Snow mapped cases of cholera in one area of London, and as many epidemiologists now map various health-related events, can be instructive, especially if other factors, such as industrial development, show similar patterns. However, mapping cases only is limited in what it can reveal. A higher *number* of cases may simply be the result of a larger population, more people who are potential cases. Any description of disease patterns should take into account the size of the population at risk for the disease (i.e., we should look not only at the numerator, the number of cases, but also at the denominator, the number of people in the population at risk). For examples, 50 cases of influenza might be viewed as a serious epidemic in a population of 250, but would indicate a rather low rate in a population of 250,000.

There is no specific value of incidence or prevalence that indicates that an epidemic exists. An **epidemic** occurs when the rate of disease, injury, or other condition is clearly in excess of the usual (endemic) level of that condition. Since smallpox has been eradicated, even one case of smallpox anywhere in the world might be considered an epidemic by this definition. In contrast, given the high rates of ischemic heart disease in this country an increase of many cases would be needed before an epidemic was noted, though some might argue that the very high rates that exist compared to earlier periods already indicate an epidemic.

For that reason, epidemiologic studies usually rely on **rates,** a measure of the frequency of a health event in a defined population during a specified period of time (Last, 1988). Most rates have three common factors: a numerator, consisting of the number of persons who experienced the event of interest (e.g., deaths, cases of disease); a denominator, which is the population at risk of the event; and an indication of the time period during which the events were enumerated.

The Concept of Risk

Risk refers to the probability an event will occur within a specified time period, and a population at risk is the population of persons for whom there is some finite probability (even if small) of that event. For example, though the risk of breast cancer in men is very small, a few men do develop breast cancer and therefore could be considered part of the population at risk. There are some outcomes for which certain people would never be at risk (e.g., men cannot be at risk of ovarian cancer, nor can women be at risk of testicular cancer). A high risk population, on the other hand, would include those persons who, because of exposure, life-style, family history, or other factors, are at greater risk of disease than the population at large. For example, so far as we know, all persons are susceptible to HIV infection and subsequent development of AIDS. Therefore, everyone is in the population at risk for HIV/AIDS. Persons who have multiple sexual partners without adequate protection or who use IV drugs would be in the high-risk population for HIV infection.

What Do You Think?

Should HIV testing be anonymous (no one but the person tested knows the test result) or confidential (selected laboratory or public health personnel know the results but are bound to protect the identity of persons tested and the results)? Who needs to know? If an HIV positive child attends school, who, if anyone, should be informed of the child's HIV status?

Mortality Rates

There are a number of mortality rates with which the student should be familiar and which are provided in the box on p. 216. Although measures of mortality re-

Common Mortality and Morbidity Rates

PROPORTIONS AND RATES

Proportion
A ratio in which the numerator is included in the denominator. Ex: the proportion of the population that is age 65 or older. In 1991, there were 31,753,000 persons 65 or older in a total population of 252,177,000:

$$\frac{31,753,000}{252,177,000} = 0.126 \text{ or } 12.6\%$$

Rate
A proportion that indicates the portion of a population who experience an event during some specified period of time, e.g., the annual infant mortality rate. In 1991 there were 36,766 deaths under one year of age and 4,110,907 live births:

$$\frac{36,766}{4,110,907} = 0.0089 \text{ or } 8.9 \text{ deaths per 1000 live births.}$$

Crude mortality rate
Usually an annual rate, it represents the proportion of a population who die from any cause during the period.
Ex: In 1991 there were 2,169,518 deaths in a total population of 252,177,000.

Age-specific rate

$$\frac{\text{No. of deaths among persons of given age group}}{\text{Midyear population of that age group}}$$

Ex: 1991 Age-specific rate for 15 to 24 year olds

$$\frac{36,452}{36,399,000} = 100.1 \text{ deaths per 100,000 15 to 24 year olds}$$

Cause specific rate

$$\frac{\text{No. of deaths from a specific cause}}{\text{Midyear population}}$$

Ex: 1991 Cause-specific rate for HIV

$$\frac{29,555 \text{ HIV deaths}}{252,177,000} = 11.7 \text{ per 100,000}$$

Case-fatality rate

$$\frac{\text{No. of deaths from a specific disease in a given period}}{\text{No. of persons diagnosed with that disease}}$$

Ex: If 87 of every 100 persons diagnosed with lung cancer dies within 5 years, the 5-year case fatality rate is 87%. The five-year survival rate would then be 13%.

Proportionate mortality ratio

$$\frac{\text{No. of deaths from a specific disease}}{\text{Total number of deaths in the same period}}$$

Ex: In 1991 720,862 deaths from diseases of the heart out of 2,169,518 deaths from all causes.

$$\frac{720,862}{2,169,518} = 0.332 \text{ or } 33.2\% \text{ of all deaths were due to heart disease}$$

Infant mortality rate

$$\frac{\text{No. infant deaths under one year of age in a year}}{\text{No. of live births in the same year}}$$

Ex: In 1991 there were 36,766 deaths under one year of age and 4,110,907 live births:

$$\frac{36,766}{4,110,907} = 0.0089 \text{ or } 8.9 \text{ deaths per 1000 live births}$$

Neonatal mortality rate

$$\frac{\text{No. infant deaths under 28 days of age in a year}}{\text{No. of live births in the same year}}$$

Ex: In 1991 there were 22,978 neonatal deaths and 4,110,907 live births.

$$\frac{22,978}{4,110,907} = 5.59 \text{ per 1000}$$

Postneonatal mortality rate

$$\frac{\text{No. infant deaths from 28 days to 1 year in a year}}{\text{No. of live births in the same year}}$$

Ex: In 1991 there were 13,788 postneonatal deaths and 4,110,907 live births:

$$\frac{13,788}{4,110,907} = 3.35 \text{ per 1000}$$

From the National Center for Health Statistics: *Health, United States, 1993,* Washington, DC, 1994, Public Health Service.

flect serious health problems and changing patterns of disease, they are limited in their usefulness. They are only informative for fatal diseases and do not provide direct information about either the level of existing disease in the population or the risk of getting any particular disease. Further, it is not uncommon for a person to die *with* one disease (e.g., prostate cancer) but *from* a different cause (e.g., stroke).

Since the population changes during the course of a year, the convention is to take an estimate of the population at midyear as the denominator for annual rates. The crude mortality rate is interpreted as the risk of death for a person in this population for that year. These rates are multiplied by a scaling factor, usually 100,000, to avoid small fractions. The result is then expressed as the number of deaths per 100,000 persons. Although a crude mortality rate is calculated easily and represents the true rate of death for the total population, it has certain limitations. It does not reveal specific causes of death, which change in relative importance over time. Also, it is affected by the age distribution of the population, since older people are at much greater risk of death than younger people.

Mortality rates also are calculated for specific groups (e.g., age-, gender-, or race-specific rates). In these instances, the number of deaths occurring in the specified group is divided by the population at risk, now restricted to the number of persons in that group. This rate may be interpreted as the risk of death for persons in the specified group during the period of observation.

The cause-specific mortality rate is an estimate of the risk of death from some specific disease in a population. It is the number of deaths from a specific cause divided by the total population at risk, usually multiplied by 100,000. Two related measures should be distinguished from the cause-specific mortality rate. The case fatality rate (CFR) is the proportion of persons diagnosed with a particular disorder (i.e., cases) who die within a specified period of time. The CFR may be interpreted as an estimate of the risk of death within that period for a person newly diagnosed with the disease (e.g., the proportion of persons with breast cancer who die within 5 years). Since the CFR is the proportion of diagnosed persons who die within the period, 1 minus the CFR yields the survival rate. For example, if the 5-year CFR for lung cancer is 87%, then the 5-year survival rate is only 13% (Brownson et al., 1993). Persons diagnosed with a particular disease often want to know the probability of surviving. These rates provide that information.

The second measure to be distinguished from the cause-specific mortality rate is the proportionate mortality ratio (PMR), the proportion of all *deaths* that are due to a specific cause. The denominator is not the population at risk of death but the total number of deaths in the population; therefore, the PMR is not a rate, nor does it estimate the risk of death. The magnitude of the PMR is a function of both the number of deaths from the cause of interest *and* the number of deaths from other causes. If deaths from certain causes decline over time, deaths from other causes that remain fairly constant may have increasing PMRs. For example, motor vehicle accidents accounted for 5.2 deaths per 100,000 persons aged 5 to 14 in the United States in 1992. This was 23% of all deaths in this age group (the PMR). By comparison, motor vehicle accidents caused 21.9 deaths per 100,000 persons 65 years of age and older in 1992, which was less than 0.5% of all deaths in the older age group (Kochanek and Hudson, 1995). This demonstrates that, although the *risk* of death from a motor vehicle accident was over four times as great in the older group (based on the rates), such accidents accounted for a far greater proportion of all deaths in the younger group (based on the PMR). The reason has to do with the much greater risk of death from other causes in the older group.

Health professionals also are interested in measures of infant mortality since they are used around the world as an indicator of overall health and availability of health care services. The most common measure, the infant mortality rate, is the number of deaths to infants in the first year of life divided by the total number of live births. Because the risk of death declines rather dramatically during the first year of life, neonatal (literally, "newborn") and postneonatal mortality rates are also of interest. These and related rates are shown in the box on p. 216. The neonatal mortality rate is calculated as the number of infant deaths up to 28 days of life divided by the number of live births, whereas the postneonatal mortality rate is found by dividing the number of deaths occurring to infants from 28 days to one year of age by the number of live births.

Rate Adjustment

The previous section discussed the importance of rates in epidemiologic studies. However, rates can be misleading when compared across different populations. For example, the risk of death increases rather dramatically after 40 years of age, so a higher crude death rate is expected in a population of older people compared to a population of younger people (Mausner and Kramer, 1985). One can divide populations into homogeneous age groups (called strata) and compare mortality rates within each age group. However, this method proves cumbersome if the comparison involves several populations with multiple-age strata. Instead, age-adjustment methods are used to permit fair comparison of overall death rates. Age adjustment is based on the fact that two factors determine a population's overall mortality rate: the *age distribution* of the population and the *age-specific mortality rates* within each age stratum.

Age adjustment can be performed by two methods: *direct* or *indirect*. Both methods require a set of "standard population" data. The standard population can be an external population, such as the U.S. population for a given year, a combined population of the groups under study, or some other standard chosen for relevance or convenience. Using the *direct* method of age adjustment, we ask the question, "If the study population had the same age distribution as the standard population, what would be its hypothetical death rate?" In calculating a directly adjusted rate, we apply the age-specific death rates from the study population to the age distribution of the standard population.

In the *indirect* method of age adjustment, the question is "If the people in the study population were dying at the same age-specific rates as people in the standard population, what would be the hypothetical death rate?" In calculations, we apply the standard population age-specific death rates to the study population's age distribution. The indirect method is often preferable when the age-specific death rates for the study population are unknown or unstable (i.e., based on relatively small numbers).

Although this discussion has focused on age-adjustment because age is the strongest predictor of risk of death, this process can be used to adjust for any factor that might vary from one population to another. For example, birth weight is the most important predictor of infant mortality. To compare infant mortality rates across populations with differing birth weight distributions, these methods may be used to produce birth-weight-adjusted infant mortality rates. However, all adjusted rates are fictitious rates. They may resemble crude rates if the distribution of the study sample is similar to the distribution of the standard population. The magnitude of adjusted rates is dependent on the standard population used. Choice of a different standard would produce a different adjusted rate.

Measures of Morbidity

Prevalence Rate. Epidemiologists and other health professionals are interested in measures of morbidity, especially *prevalence* and *incidence* rates, which provide information concerning the levels of disease in a population, the rate of disease development, and the risk of disease. The **prevalence** rate is a measure of existing disease in a population at a particular time (i.e., the number of *existing* cases divided by the current population). One also can calculate the prevalence of a specific risk factor or exposure. For example, in a survey of 4000 high school students, 920 reported smoking cigarettes on a regular basis. The prevalence of cigarette use in this population would be:

$$\frac{920 \text{ smokers}}{4000 \text{ students}} = 0.23 \text{ or } 23\%$$

A prevalence rate is not an estimate of the risk of *developing* disease because it is a function of both the rate at which new cases of the disease develop and how long those cases remain in the population. In this example, the prevalence of smokers in a high school is a function of how fast students are beginning to smoke and how long they continue once started. The duration of a disease is affected by case fatality, cure, or migration. A disease with a short duration (e.g., an intestinal virus) may not have a high prevalence even if the rate of new cases is high, because cases do not accumulate. A disease with a long course will have a higher prevalence than a rapidly fatal disease that has the same rate of new cases.

Incidence Rate. The **incidence** rate reflects the number of *new* cases developing in a population at risk during a specified time. It estimates the risk of developing the disease in the observed population within a specified time. The population at risk is considered to be persons without the disease of interest but who are at risk of acquiring it. Note that existing (or "prevalent") cases are excluded from the population at risk for this calculation, since they already have the condition and are no longer at risk of developing it. Incidence counts new cases in a disease-free group (or *cohort*) of persons who are followed for some period. The risk of disease is a function of both the rate of new disease development and the length of time the population is at risk. To continue with the example above, one could follow the 3080 nonsmoking students and note the number who began smoking during the follow-up period. If 250 students began smoking during a 1-year follow-up, the 1-year incidence of cigarette smoking in this population would be:

$$\frac{250}{3080} = 0.081 \text{ or } 8.1\%$$

Incidence and Prevalence Compared. Because the prevalence rate measures existing cases of disease, and is roughly proportional to the incidence times the duration of disease it is affected both by factors that influence risk and by factors that influence survival or recovery. In mathematical notation

$$P \approx I \times D$$

where P = prevalence
I = incidence
D = duration

For that reason, prevalence measures are less useful when looking for factors related to disease etiology. Because prevalence rates reflect duration in addition to the risk of getting the disease, it is difficult to sort out what factors are related to risk, and, indeed, these risk factors may be masked by differences in survival or cure. Incidence rates, on the other hand, are the measure of choice for such considerations, since incidence is affected only by factors related to the risk of developing disease and not to survival or cure. Prevalence is useful in planning health care services, since it is an indication of the level of disease existing in the population and therefore of the size of the population in need of services.

Attack Rate. One final measure of morbidity, often used in infectious disease investigations, is the **attack rate,** a form of incidence rate defined as the proportion of persons exposed to an agent who develop the disease. Attack rates are often specific to an exposure; food-specific attack rates, for example, are the proportion of persons becoming ill after eating a specific food item.

Comparison Groups

The use of *comparison groups* is at the heart of the epidemiologic approach. Incidence or prevalence rates in groups that differ in some important characteristic must be compared to gain clues about which factors influence the distribution of disease (disease determinants or risk factors). Observing the rate of disease only among persons exposed to a suspected risk factor will not show clearly that the exposure is associated with increased risk until the rate observed in the exposed group is compared with the rate in a group of comparable unexposed persons. To illustrate, one might investigate the effect of smoking during pregnancy on the rate of low birth weight by calculating the rate of low-birth-weight infants born to women who smoked during their pregnancy. However, the hypothesis that smoking during pregnancy is a risk factor for low birth weight is supported only when the low-birth-weight rate among smoking women is compared to the (lower) rate of low-birth-weight infants born to nonsmoking women.

DESCRIPTIVE EPIDEMIOLOGY

Descriptive epidemiology describes the *distribution* of disease, death, and other health outcomes in the population according to person, place, and time, providing us a picture of how things are or have been—the who, where, and when of disease patterns. *Analytic epidemiology,* on the other hand, searches for the *determinants* of the patterns observed, the how and why. That is, epidemiologic concepts and methods are employed to discern what factors, characteristics, exposures, or behaviors might account for differences in the observed patterns of disease occurrence. Descriptive and analytical studies are observational, meaning the investigator merely observes events as they are or have been and does not intervene to change anything or to introduce a new factor. *Experimental* or intervention studies, on the other hand, include interventions to test preventive or treatment measures, techniques, materials, policies, or drugs.

Person

Personal characteristics of interest in epidemiology include race, gender, age, education, occupation, income (and related socioeconomic status), and marital status. The single most important characteristic for overall mortality is age. The mortality curve by age drops sharply during and following the first year of life to a low point in childhood, then begins to increase through adolescence and young adulthood, until after about 40 years of age when the curve begins to increase exponentially (Mausner and Kramer, 1985).

There are also substantial differences in mortality and morbidity experienced by gender. Female infants have lower mortality than comparable male infants, and the survival advantage continues throughout life: life expectancy for women is greater than for men (Kochanek and Hudson, 1995; NCHS, 1994). However, the patterns for specific diseases may vary. Women have lower rates of coronary heart disease until menopause, after which the gap narrows. For other diseases, such as rheumatoid arthritis, the prevalence among women is greater than among men (Brownson et al., 1993).

Though the concept of race as a variable for public health research has come under scrutiny (CDC, 1993), there are clear differences in morbidity and mortality by race in the United States (Kochanek and Hudson, 1995; NCHS, 1994). For example, the 1992 age-adjusted death rate for African-Americans was 1.6 times higher than for white Americans. Death rates were also higher among blacks for 13 of the 15 leading causes of death in 1992. The infant mortality rate for African-American infants, though declining, is still more than twice as high as the rate among whites. A recent CDC workshop report notes that the significance of race in epidemiologic research "is mainly derived from social arrangements. Thus, race should be viewed within public health surveillance as a sociological phenomenon" (CDC, 1993).

Place

When considering the distribution of a disease, one thinks of geographic patterns: does the rate of disease differ from place to place (e.g., with local environment)? If there were no effects of geography on disease occurrence, we might expect to see random geographic patterns. That is often not the case. For example, at high altitude there is a lower oxygen tension, which may result in smaller babies. Other diseases reflect distinctive patterns by place, for example Lyme disease is more likely to be found in areas where there are reservoirs of the disease, a large tick population as the vector for transmission to humans, and contact between the human population and the tick vectors (Benenson, 1990).

In general, one expects variations by geographic location (place) to be due to differences in the chemical, physical, or biological environment. However, variations by place also may result from differences in population densities or customary patterns of behavior and life-style or other personal characteristics. For example, one might find variations by place because of high concentrations of a religious, cultural, or ethnic group who practice certain health-related behaviors. The high rates of stroke found in the southeastern United States are likely a result of a number of social and personal factors that may have little to do with geographic features per se.

Time
Secular Changes

The third component of descriptive epidemiology is time: Is there an increase or decrease in the frequency of the disease over time or are other temporal patterns evident? Long-term patterns of morbidity or mortality (i.e., over years or decades) are called **secular trends.** Secular trends may reflect changes in social behavior or practices. For example, the increase in lung cancer mortality that has been observed in recent years is a delayed effect of increases in smoking in prior years, and the decline in gastric cancer may be due to less reliance on cured foods (Brownson et al., 1993).

Some apparent secular trends may be the result of increased diagnostic capability or changes in survival (or case fatality) rather than in *incidence.* For example, case fatality from breast cancer has decreased in recent years while the incidence of breast cancer has increased. Some, though not all, of the increased incidence is due to improved diagnostic capability. These two trends result in a breast cancer mortality curve that is flatter than the incidence curve (Brownson et al., 1993; Holleb et al., 1991). Relying on the mortality data alone does not accurately depict the true situation.

A third factor affecting secular trends is the effect of changes in case definition or revisions in the coding of a disease according to *International Classification of Diseases* (ICD), now in its tenth edition. Either changes in case definition or other changes in coding and classification can produce an artificial change in the rate (Kochanek and Hudson, 1995).

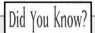

Did You Know?

Lung cancer has now surpassed breast cancer as the leading cause of cancer mortality among women. The rapidly rising rate of lung cancer deaths in women mirrors the patterns of increased rates of smoking among women and increased cigarette advertising directed toward women.

Point Epidemic

One temporal and spatial pattern of disease distribution is the **point epidemic.** This time-related pattern is particularly important in infectious disease investigations, but also it is recognized as a significant indicator for toxic exposures in environmental epidemiology. A point epidemic is most clearly seen when the frequency of cases is graphed against time. The sharp peak characteristic of such graphs indicates a concentration of cases about some point or period of time. It often indicates the response of the population to a common source of infection or contamination to which they were all simultaneously exposed. Knowledge of the incubation or latency period (the time between exposure and development of signs and symptoms) for the specific disease entity can help in determining the probable time of exposure. A common example of a point epidemic is an outbreak of gastrointestinal illness from a food-borne pathogen.

Cyclical Patterns

In addition to secular trends and point epidemics, there are also cyclical time patterns of disease. One common type of cyclical variation is seasonal fluctuation in a number of infectious illnesses. Seasonal changes may be influenced by changes in the agent itself, changes in population densities or behaviors of animal reservoirs or vectors, or changes in human behaviors resulting in changing exposures (being outdoors in warmer weather and indoors in colder months). There also may be artificial seasons, created by calendar events, such as holidays and tax-filing deadlines, which may be associated with patterns of stress-related illness. Patterns of accidents and injuries also may be seasonal, reflecting differing employment and recreational patterns. Some disease cycles, such as influenza, evidence patterns of smaller epidemics every few years, depending on strain, with major pandemics occurring at longer intervals (Benenson, 1990).

Event-Related Clusters

A third type of temporal pattern are nonsimultaneous, event-related clusters. These are patterns in which time is not measured from fixed dates on the calendar but from the point of some exposure, event, or experience presumably held in common by affected persons, though not occurring at the same time. An example of this pattern would be postpartum depression, with time measured from the birth of the infant to onset of symptoms. Clearly, if births occur on a regular basis, one might see depressive symptoms spread across the calendar, making identification of a cluster related to the births difficult. If, however, the cases are plotted against time since birth, postpartum depression is likely to show up as a peak in the number of cases at some period after the births.

ANALYTIC EPIDEMIOLOGY

Whereas descriptive epidemiology deals with the *distribution* of health outcomes, *analytic* epidemiology seeks to discover the *determinants* of outcomes, the how and the why (i.e., the factors that influence ob-

Table 11-4   Comparison of Major Epidemiologic Study Designs

Study design	Advantages	Disadvantages
Ecological	1. Quick, easy, and inexpensive first study 2. Uses readily available existing data 3. May prompt further investigation, suggest other/new hypotheses.	1. Ecological fallacy—the associations observed may not hold true for individuals 2. Problems in interpreting temporal sequence (cause and effect)
Cross-sectional (Correlational)	1. Gives general description of scope of problem, provides prevalence estimates 2. Often based on population (or community) sample, not just those who sought care 3. Useful in health service evaluation and planning 4. Data obtained at once; less expense and quicker than cohort because no follow-up 5. Baseline for prospective study or identify cases and controls for case-control study	1. No calculation of risk-prevalence, not incidence 2. Temporal sequence unclear 3. Not good for rare disease or rare exposure unless large sample size or stratified sampling 4. Selective survival can be major source of selection bias; surviving subjects may differ from those who are not included (death, institutionalization, etc.) 5. Selective recall or lack of past exposure information can bias.
Case-control (Retrospective, Case Comparison)	1. Less expensive than cohort, smaller sample required 2. Quicker than cohort, no follow-up 3. Can investigate more than one exposure 4. Best design for rare diseases 5. If well designed, can be important tool for etiologic investigation 6. Best suited to diseases with relatively clear onset (timing of onset can be established so that incident cases can be included)	1. Greater susceptibility than cohort studies to various types of bias (selective survival, recall bias, selection bias in choice of both cases and controls) 2. Information on other risk factors may not be available resulting in confounding 3. Antecedent-consequence (temporal sequence) not as certain as in cohort 4. Not well suited to rare exposures 5. Gives only an indirect estimate of risk 6. Limited to a single outcome because of sampling on disease status
Prospective Cohort (Concurrent Cohort, Longitudinal, Follow-up)	1. Best estimate of disease incidence 2. Best estimate of risk 3. Fewer problems with selective survival and selective recall 4. Temporal sequence more clearly established 5. Broader range of options for exposure assessment	1. Expensive in time and money 2. More difficult organizationally 3. Not good for rare diseases 4. Attrition of participants can bias estimate 5. Latency period may be very long, may miss cases 6. May be difficult to examine several exposures
Retrospective Cohort (Nonconcurrent Cohort)	1. Combines advantages of both prospective cohort and case-control 2. Shorter time (even if follow-up into future) than prospective cohort 3. Less expensive than prospective cohort because relies on existing data 4. Temporal sequence may be clearer than case-control	1. Shares some disadvantages with both prospective cohort and case-control 2. Subject to attrition (loss to follow-up) 3. Relies on existing records, which may result in misclassification of both exposure and outcome 4. May have to rely on surrogate measures of exposure, such as job title, and vital records information on cause of death

served patterns of health and disease, and increase or decrease the risk of adverse outcomes). This section will deal with analytic study designs and the related measures of association derived from them. Table 11-4 summarizes the advantages and disadvantages of each design.

Ecological Studies

An epidemiologic study that is a bridge between descriptive epidemiology and analytic epidemiology is the **ecological study.** The descriptive component involves examining variations in disease rates by person, place, or time. The analytic component lies in the effort to determine if there is a relation of disease rates to variations in rates for possible risk (or protective) factors or characteristics. The identifying characteristic of ecological studies is that only aggregate data, such as population rates, are used rather than data on individuals' exposures, characteristics, and outcomes. For example, information on per capita cigarette consumption might be examined in relation to lung cancer mortality rates in several countries, or several groups of people, or in the same population at different times. Other examples include comparison of rates of breast feeding and of breast cancer, average dietary fat content and rates of coronary heart disease, or unemployment rates and level of psychiatric disorder.

Ecological studies are attractive because they often make use of existing, readily available rates, and are therefore quick and inexpensive to conduct. They are subject, however, to **ecological fallacy** (i.e., associations observed at the group level may not hold true for the individuals that comprise the groups, or associations that actually exist may be masked in the grouped data. This may be the result of other factors operating in these populations for which the ecological correlations do not account. For that reason ecological studies may be suggestive, but require confirmation in studies using individual data (Lilienfeld and Stolley, 1994; Mausner and Kramer, 1985).

Uncertainty concerning the temporal sequence of events is a disadvantage of ecological studies shared with cross-sectional study designs (discussed below). For example, in the study of unemployment rates and psychiatric disorder, it is unclear whether unemployed persons are at higher risk for psychiatric problems or persons with existing psychiatric problems are more likely to be unemployed. Though determining whether one event precedes or succeeds another may seem at first to be a simple matter, in practice it may be difficult to confirm.

Cross-Sectional Studies

The **cross-sectional study** provides a snap shot, or cross-section, of a population or group (Lilienfeld and Stolley, 1994; Mausner and Kramer, 1985). Information is collected on current health status, personal characteristics, and potential risk factors or exposures all at once. The cross-sectional study is characterized by the *simultaneous* collection of information necessary for the classification of exposure and outcome status, though there may be historical information collected (e.g., on past diet, or history of radiation exposures). The question asked is: Do the characteristics or exposure factors coexist with the health problem of interest?

Cross-sectional studies are sometimes called prevalence studies because they provide the frequency of existing cases of a disease in a population. One way cross-sectional studies evaluate the association of a factor with a health problem is to compare the prevalence of the disease in those with the factor (or exposure) to the prevalence in the unexposed. The ratio of the two prevalence rates is an indication of the association between the factor and the outcome. For example, a prevalence ratio of 2 means that the disease is found two times more often in persons with the characteristic or exposure than in those without. If there is no association, the prevalence in the two groups should be similar and the prevalence ratio will be close to 1. A value less than 1 may suggest a protective association, that is those with the factor or exposure are *less* likely to have the disease than those without the factor. For example, the prevalence of coronary heart disease (CHD) is lower among those who are physically active than among sedentary persons, so the prevalence ratio for the association between physical activity and CHD will be less than 1. Prevalence ratios require caution in interpretation because the prevalence measure is affected by cure, survival, and migration and does not estimate the risk of *getting* the disease.

Cross-sectional studies are subject to bias resulting from selective survival, that is existing cases who have survived to be in the study may be different from cases diagnosed about the same time who have died and are not available for inclusion. Suppose physical activity not only reduced the risk of heart disease, but also markedly improved survival among those with heart disease. Sedentary persons with heart disease would then have higher fatality rates than physically active persons who did develop heart disease. One might observe higher rates of physical activity in a group of persons surviving with heart disease than in a general population without heart disease, both because of the survival advantage and participation of survivors in cardiac rehabilitation programs. It would erroneously appear that physical activity was a risk factor for heart disease.

Case-Control Studies

In the **case-control study** design subjects are enrolled *because* they are known to have the outcome of interest (these are the cases) or they are known *not* to have the outcome of interest (these are the controls). Case-control status is verified using a clear case definition and some previously determined method or protocol (e.g., by an examination, laboratory test, or medical chart review). Information is then collected on the exposures or characteristics of interest, frequently from existing sources, subject interview, or questionnaire (Armenian, 1994; Breslow and Day, 1980; Schlesselman, 1982). The question in a case-control study is "Do persons with the outcome of interest (cases) have the exposure characteristic (or a history of the exposure) more frequently than those without the outcome (controls)?"

Given the way subjects are selected for a case-control study, neither incidence nor prevalence can be calculated directly. In a case-control study, an odds ratio tells us how much more (or less) likely the exposure is to be found among cases than among controls. The odds of exposure among cases (a to c in the table below) are compared to the odds of exposure among controls (b to d). The ratio of these two odds provides us with an estimate of the relative risk (discussed below).

Suppose a research group wanted to study risk factors for suicide attempts among adolescents. They were able to enroll 100 adolescents who had attempted suicide and selected 200 adolescents from the same community with no history of suicide attempt. One of the factors they want to investigate is a history of substance abuse (SA). Through a questionnaire and other medical records they were able to determine that 68 of the 100 adolescents who had attempted suicide had a history of substance abuse, while 36 of the 200 adolescents with no suicide attempt had such a history. The information could be presented as follows:

	Suicide attempt	No attempt
History of SA	68 a	36 b
No history of SA	32 c	164 d
	100	200

The odds of a history of substance abuse among suicide attempters is a/c or 68/32, while the odds of substance abuse among controls is b/d or 36/164. The odds ratio (equivalent to ad/bc) is

$$\frac{68 \times 164}{36 \times 32} = 9.68$$

This would be interpreted to mean that adolescents who attempted suicide are almost 10 times more likely to have a history of substance abuse than adolescents who have not attempted suicide. Note that, as with the prevalence ratio, an odds ratio of 1 is indicative of no association (i.e., the odds of exposure are similar for cases and controls). An odds ratio less than 1 suggests a protective association, that cases are *less* likely to have been exposed than controls.

Because the number of cases is known or actively sought out or recruited, case-control studies do not demand large samples or the long follow-up time that are often required for prospective cohort studies. That is

why many of the influential cancer studies have been of the case-control design.

On the other hand, case-control studies are prone to a number of biases. (*Bias*, a systematic deviation from the truth, is discussed below.) Because these studies begin with existing cases, differential survival can produce biased results. The use of recently diagnosed (or "incident") cases may reduce this bias. Since exposure information is obtained from subject recall or past records, there may be errors in exposure assessment or misclassification. As a result of the sampling on disease status, case-control studies are limited to a single outcome, though they may investigate a number of potential risk factors.

Cohort Studies

In epidemiology, the term cohort is used to describe a group of persons who is born at about the same time, or, in analytic studies, a group of persons, generally sharing some characteristic of interest, who is enrolled in a study and followed over a period of time to observe some health outcome. Because of this ability to observe the development of new cases of disease, **cohort study** designs allow for calculation of incidence rates and therefore estimates of risk of disease. Cohort studies may be prospective or retrospective (Breslow and Day, 1987).

Prospective Cohort Studies

In a prospective cohort study (also called a longitudinal or follow-up study), subjects determined to be free of the outcome under investigation are classified on the basis of the exposure of interest at the beginning of the follow-up period. The subjects are then followed for some period of time to ascertain the occurrence of disease in each group. The question is "Do persons with the factor (or exposure) of interest develop (or avoid) the outcome more frequently than those without the factor (or exposure)?"

For example, one might recruit a cohort of subjects, who would be classified as physically active ("exposed") and sedentary ("not exposed"). One might further quantify the amount of the "exposure" if there were sufficient information. These subjects would then be followed over time to determine the development of coronary heart disease. This study design avoids the problem of selective survival seen in the earlier example of a cross-sectional study of physical activity and CHD. The cohort study also has the advantage of allowing us to estimate the *risk* of acquiring disease for those who are exposed compared to those who are unexposed (or less exposed). This ratio of incidence rates is called the relative risk.

For example, suppose 1000 physically active and 1000 sedentary middle-aged men and women were enrolled in a prospective cohort study. All were free of CHD at enrollment. Over a 5-year follow-up period, regular examinations detect CHD in 120 of the sedentary men and women and in 48 of the active men and women. Assuming no other deaths or losses to follow-up, the data could be presented as follows:

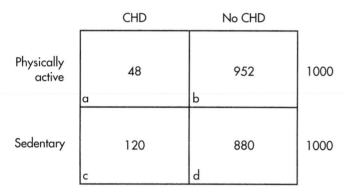

The incidence of CHD in the active group is [a/(a + b)] = 48/1000, and the incidence of CHD in the sedentary group is [c/(c + d)] = 120/1000. The *relative risk,* is

$$\frac{48/1000}{120/1000} = 0.4$$

Note that because physical activity is protective for CHD, the relative risk is less than 1. The interpretation for this hypothetical example is that, over a 5-year period, persons who are physically active had about 0.4 the risk of CHD compared to sedentary persons. If the risk were greater for those exposed, the relative risk would be greater than 1. For example, if the relative risk of CHD for smokers compared to nonsmokers were 3.5, it would be interpreted to mean that the risk of CHD among smokers is 3.5 times the risk among nonsmokers. The null value indicating no association is 1, since the incidence rates and thus the risk would be equal in the two groups if there were no association.

Because subjects are enrolled prior to disease onset, the cohort design is able to study more than one outcome, calculate incidence rates and estimate risk, establish the temporal sequence of exposure and outcome with greater clarity and certainty, and may avoid many of the problems of the earlier study designs with selective survival or exposure misclassification. On the other hand, large samples are often necessary to insure that enough cases are observed to provide statistical power to detect meaningful differences between groups. This is complicated by the long period required for some diseases to develop (the latency period). Also, the number of subjects required to observe sufficient cases make longitudinal studies unsuitable for very rare diseases unless they are part of a larger study of a number of outcomes.

Research Brief

Lieberman E, Gremy I, Lang JM, Cohen AP: Low birthweight at term and the timing of fetal exposure to maternal smoking, Am J Public Health 84(7):1127-1131, 1994.

This research describes a study of over 11,000 term live births at a Boston hospital to determine if rates of small for gestational age (SGA) births are associated with level and timing of maternal cigarette smoking during pregnancy. Data were collected from interviews and medical record reviews. Women were classified as nonsmokers, smokers throughout pregnancy, smokers first trimester only, smokers first and second trimesters only, or smokers second and third trimesters or third trimester only. Infants with birthweights less than the tenth percentile for their gestational age were classified as SGA. There was a significantly increased risk of delivering a SGA infant for women who smoked throughout pregnancy and those who began smoking in the second or third trimester, even after controlling for confounding variables. Compared to nonsmokers, the risk was not significantly greater for those women who quit smoking by the end of the second trimester. There was also a dose-response relation between the number of cigarettes smoked during the third trimester and the risk of SGA.

This research confirms that the greatest effect of smoking on fetal growth retardation occurs in the third trimester of the pregnancy, though other adverse outcomes may be associated with smoking earlier in pregnancy. It provides further support for the importance and value of smoking cessation programs during pregnancy, and underscores the importance of interventions that encourage women not to relapse.

Retrospective Cohort Studies

Retrospective cohort studies combine some of the advantages and disadvantages of case-control studies and prospective cohort studies. One relies on existing records, such as employment, insurance, or hospital records, to define a cohort who is classified as having been exposed or unexposed at some time in the past. The cohort is followed over time using the records to determine if the outcome occurred. Retrospective cohort studies (also called historical cohort) may be conducted entirely using past records, or may include current assessment or additional follow-up time after study initiation. The obvious advantage of this approach is the savings in time, since one does not have to follow the cohort forward to wait for new cases of disease to develop. The disadvantages are largely related to the reliance on existing historical records. Retrospective cohort studies frequently are used in occupational epidemiology where industrial records are available to investigate work-related exposures and health outcomes.

EXPERIMENTAL STUDIES

The study designs discussed so far are called observational studies because the investigator observes the association between exposures and outcomes as they exist, but does not intervene to alter the presence or level of any exposure or behavior. In intervention studies the investigator initiates some treatment or intervention that may influence the risk or course of disease. Experimental studies are designed to test whether interventions or treatments are effective in preventing disease or improving health. Like observational studies, experimental studies generally use comparison (or control) groups, but unlike observational studies there is the possibility of randomly allocating persons to a particular treatment or intervention group. Intervention studies are of two general types: clinical trials and community trials (Lilienfeld and Stolley, 1994; Meinert, 1986).

Clinical Trials

In clinical trials, the research issue is generally the efficacy of a medical treatment for disease, such as a new drug or existing drug used in a new or different way, surgical technique, or other treatment. The preferred method of subject allocation in clinical trials is randomization (i.e., assigning treatments to patients so that all possible treatment assignments have a predetermined probability but neither subject nor investigator determines the actual assignment of any participant). Randomization avoids the bias that may result if subjects self-select into one group or the other or if the investigator or clinician chooses subjects for each group.

A second aspect of treatment allocation is the use of masking or "blinding" treatment assignments. The optimal design for most situations is the double-blinded study in which neither subject nor investigator knows who is receiving which treatment. The aim of blinding is to reduce differential misclassification (i.e., the tendency to overestimate therapeutic benefit for the experimental treatment when it is known who is receiving it).

Clinical trials generally are thought to provide the best evidence of causality because of the assignment of treatment and the greater control over other factors that could influence outcome. Like cohort studies, clinical trials are prospective in direction and provide the clearest evidence of temporal sequence.

However, clinical trials are generally conducted in a contrived situation, under very controlled conditions, and in very select patient populations. That means that efficacious treatment may not be so effective when applied under more realistic clinical conditions in a more diverse patient population. There are also ethical considerations in experimental studies which go beyond those that apply to observational studies. Finally, clinical trials tend to be very costly in time, personnel, facilities, and other factors.

Community Trials

Community trials are similar to clinical trials in that an investigator determines the exposure or intervention, but in this case the issue is often health promotion and disease prevention rather than treatment of existing disease. The intervention is usually undertaken on a large scale, with the unit of treatment allocation being a community, region, or group rather than individuals. Although a pharmaceutical product may be involved in a community trial, such as fluoridation of water or mass immunizations, community trials often involve educational, programmatic, or policy interventions. Studying the effect on birth outcomes of altered requirements for Medicaid eligibility for pregnant women compared to the birth outcomes in areas that retain existing requirements would be an example of a community trial.

Although community trials provide the best means of testing whether changes in knowledge or behavior, policy, programs, or other mass interventions are effective, they are not without problems. For many interventions, it may take years for the effectiveness of the intervention to be evident. In the meantime, other factors also may influence the outcome either positively (making the intervention look more effective than it really is) or negatively (making the intervention look less effective than it really is). Comparable community populations without similar interventions for comparative analysis are often difficult to determine. Even when comparable comparison communities are available—especially when the intervention is improved knowledge or changed behavior—it is difficult and unethical to prevent the control communities from making use of generally available information, effectively making them less different from the intervention communities. Finally, because community trials are often undertaken on a large scale and over long periods of time, they can be very expensive, requiring large staff, complicated logistics, and extensive communication resources.

SCREENING

Screening is defined as the application of a test to people who are as yet asymptomatic for the purpose of classifying them with respect to their likelihood of having a particular disease. Screening was cited earlier in the chapter as a component of secondary prevention efforts. From a clinical perspective, the aim of screening is early detection, before development of symptoms, when there is a more favorable prognosis because treatment can be begun before the disease becomes clinically manifest. From a public health perspective, the objective is to sort out efficiently and effectively those who *probably* have the disease from those who *probably* do not, again in order to ascertain early cases for treatment or initiate public health prevention and control programs. Note that a screening test is *not* a diagnostic test. Persons who are positive on

Characteristics of a Successful Screening Program

1. Valid (accurate); there is a high probability of correct classification of persons tested.
2. Reliable (precise); gives consistent results from time to time, place to place, and person to person.
3. Capable of large group administration;
   a. fast, in both the administration of the test and obtaining the results, and
   b. inexpensive in both personnel required and in the materials and procedures used.
4. Innocuous; there are few if any side effects and the test is minimally invasive
5. High yield; the test is able to detect enough new cases to warrant the effort and expense. Yield is defined as the amount of previously unrecognized disease that is diagnosed and treated as a result of screening.

a screening test (i.e., who probably have the disease) must be evaluated by follow-up diagnostic procedure to determine whether they actually have the disease. Screening programs, therefore, require provision for follow-up and referral for diagnostic confirmation and treatment of those who are determined to be true cases.

Successful screening programs have several characteristics that depend on both the tests and population screened. Characteristics of an effective screening program are listed in the box above. Among the desirable traits are the availability of reliable and valid screening tests (Mausner and Kramer, 1985).

Reliability and Validity
Reliability

In any measurement there is concern for the precision or **reliability** of the measure (its consistency or repeatability) and the accuracy of the measure (Is it really measuring what we think it is and how closely?). Suppose you want to do a blood pressure screening in a community. You will take blood pressures on a large number of people, perhaps following up with repeated measures for individuals with higher pressures.

If the sphygmomanometer used for the screening varies in its readings so that one does not get the same reading twice in a row, then it lacks precision. The instrument would be unreliable even if the overall mean of repeated measurements were close to the true overall mean for the persons measured. The problem would be that the readings would not be reliable for any individual, which is what a screening program requires.

On the other hand, suppose the readings are reproducible, but, unknown to you, tend to be about 10 mm Hg too high. This instrument is producing precise and reliable readings. However, the uncorrected (or uncalibrated) instrument lacks accuracy (does not

give a valid reading). In short, a measure can be consistent without producing valid results.

There are three major sources of error affecting the reliability of tests:
1. Variation inherent in the trait itself (e.g., blood pressure that changes with time of day, activity, level of stress, and other factors);
2. Observer variation, which can be divided into intraobserver reliability (consistency by the same observer) and interobserver reliability (consistency from one observer to another);
3. Inconsistency in the instrument, which includes the internal consistency of the instrument (e.g., do all items in a questionnaire measure the same thing) and the stability (or test-retest reliability) of the instrument over time.

Validity: Sensitivity and Specificity

Validity in a screening test is measured in terms of the probability of correctly classifying an individual with regard to the disease or outcome of interest. It is usually measured by sensitivity and specificity. **Sensitivity** quantifies how accurately the test identifies those *with* the condition or trait. In other words, sensitivity represents the proportion of persons with the disease whom the test correctly identifies as positive (true positives). High sensitivity is needed when early treatment is important and when identification of every case is important.

Specificity indicates how accurately the test identifies those *without* the disease (i.e., the proportion of persons without the disease whom the test correctly identifies as negative [true negatives]). High specificity is needed when rescreening is impractical and when reducing false positives is important.

The sensitivity and specificity of a test are determined by comparing the results obtained from applying the test to a population with results obtained from a definitive diagnostic procedure used in that same population (sometimes called the "gold standard"). For example, the Pap smear is a common screening procedure for detection of cervical dysplasia and carcinoma. The definitive diagnosis of cervical cancer, however, requires a biopsy. Histological confirmation of malignant cells is the common "gold standard" in screening for cancer. The ideal for a screening test is 100% sensitivity and 100% specificity, meaning that the test identifies 100% of those who actually have the disease according to the definitive diagnostic procedure, and the test is negative for all those whom the definitive procedure demonstrates do not have the disease. In practice, sensitivity and specificity are often inversely related. That is, if the test results are such that one can choose some point beyond which a person is considered positive (a "cutpoint"), as in a blood pressure reading to screen for hypertension or a serum glucose reading to screen for diabetes, then moving that critical point to improve the sensitivity of the test will result in a decrease in specificity, or an improvement in specificity can be made only at the expense of sensitivity.

Table 11-5 Classification of Subjects According to True Disease State and Screening Test Results for Calculation of Indices of Validity.

Result of screening test	Disease state	
	Disease	**No disease**
Positive	True positive (TP)	False positive (FP)
Negative	False negative (FN)	True negative (TN)

Sensitivity 5 TP/(TP 1 FN)
Specificity 5 TN/(TN 1 FP)
False-negative "rate" 5 1 2 Se 5 FN/(FN 1 TP)
False-positive "rate" 5 1 2 Sp 5 FP/(TN 1 FP)
Positive predictive value 5 TP/(TP 1 FP)
Often multiplied by 100 and expressed as percentage.

Table 11-5 shows a typical table for classification and calculation of sensitivity and specificity. Some writers refer to a false-positive rate, which is 1 minus the specificity, and a false negative rate, or 1 minus the sensitivity. These "rates" are simply the proportions incorrectly classified among nondiseased and diseased subjects, respectively.

A third measure associated with sensitivity and specificity is the predictive value of the test. The **positive predictive value** is the proportion of persons with a positive test who actually have the disease, interpreted as the probability that an individual with a positive test has the disease. Less often used is the corresponding measure for persons with negative tests, the **negative predictive value,** which is the proportion of persons with a negative test who are actually disease-free. Although sensitivity and specificity are relatively independent of the prevalence of disease, predictive values are affected by the level of disease in the screened population, as well as by the sensitivity and specificity of the test. When the prevalence is very low, the positive predictive value will be low, even with tests that are sensitive and specific. Additionally, lower specificity produces lower positive predictive values because of the increase in the proportion of false-positive results.

Factors to consider in setting cutpoints include the cost (both human and economic costs) of missing true cases (false negatives) by lowering the sensitivity versus the cost of falsely classifying noncases (false positives) by lowering the specificity. Factors include the importance of capturing all cases, the likelihood the population will be rescreened, the interval between screenings relative to the rate of disease development, and the prevalence of the disease. A low prevalence typically requires a test with high specificity, otherwise the screening will produce too many false positives in the large nondiseased population. On the other hand, a disease with a high prevalence usually requires high sensitivity, otherwise too many of the real cases will be missed by the screening (false negatives).

Two or more tests can be combined to enhance sensitivity or specificity. They may be combined in *series* or in *parallel*. In series testing one is considered positive only if positive on *all* tests in the series, and one is considered negative if negative on *any* test. Series testing enhances specificity, producing fewer false positives, but sensitivity may be low. In series testing sequence is important: one often uses a very sensitive test first to pick up all cases plus false positives, then a second test which is very specific to eliminate false positives.

In parallel testing one is considered positive if positive on *any* test and is considered negative only if negative on *all* tests. Parallel testing enhances sensitivity, leaving fewer false negatives, but specificity may be low.

CAUSALITY
Statistical Associations

One of the first steps in assessing the relation of some factor with a health outcome is determining whether a statistical association exists. For instance, ask whether the presence or severity of a disease (say lung cancer) is influenced by the presence or amount of some potential risk factor (say smoking). If the probability of disease seems unaffected by the presence or level of the factor, as evaluated by a statistical test, no association is apparent. If, on the other hand, the probability of disease does vary according to whether the factor is present, then there is a statistical association. The earlier discussion of null values is pertinent at this point. When an observed measure of association (such as a relative risk) does not differ by a statistically significant amount from the null value, we may not assume there is an association between the factor and outcome under investigation.

For example, we want to know if gender is related to the risk of a disease. If there is no association, the proportion of females with the disease should be about the same as the proportion of males with the disease. With no association, the proportion in each gender group should be approximately the same as the overall proportion in the population studied. If, however, the proportion in one group is greater or less than expected, based on the overall proportion with the disease, there may be an association. For this situation, we would evaluate whether the association is statistically significant by a chi-square test statistic, which is calculated from the actual number observed in each cell of the table compared to the number expected based on both the overall proportions with and without disease and the overall proportions of males and females in the population.

To say a result is statistically significant means that the observed result is unlikely to be due to chance. Note that statistical significance is also determined by sample size. In other words, the difference between 34.3% and 35.9% in a study group of 1000 is not statistically significant at $\alpha = 0.05$. However, in a much larger sample, a difference of this amount would be significant.

Bias

One also may observe a statistically significant result because of **bias,** a systematic error due to the study design. For example, if there were a gum ball machine with colors randomly mixed, and I got three red ones in a row, that would be due to chance. If, however, the person loading the gum ball machine had poured in a bag of red ones first, then green ones, then yellow, it would not be surprising to get three red ones in a row, because of the way the machine was loaded. In epidemiologic studies, we sometimes see results because of the way the study was "loaded" (i.e., the way the study was designed or subjects were selected or information collected and subjects classified). Although the types of bias are numerous, there are three general categories of bias.

Bias attributable to the way subjects enter a study is called *selection bias.* It has to do with selection procedures and the population from which subjects are drawn. It may involve self-selection factors as well. For example, are teenagers who agree to complete a questionnaire on alcohol, tobacco, and other drug use representative of the total teenage population?

Bias attributable to misclassification of subjects in the study is information or *classification* (or misclassification) bias. It is related to how information is collected, including the information that subjects themselves supply or how subjects are classified.

Bias resulting from the relation of the outcome and study factor with some third factor not accounted for is called **confounding.** For example, there is a well-known association between maternal smoking during pregnancy and low-birth-weight babies. There is also an association between alcohol consumption and smoking that is not due to chance nor is it causal. (That is, drinking alcohol does not cause a person to smoke, nor does smoking cause a person to drink alcohol.) If one were to investigate the association of alcohol consumption and low birth weight, smoking would be a confounder since it is related to both alcohol consumption and low birth weight. Failure to account for smoking in the analysis would bias the observed association between alcohol use and low birth weight. In practice we can often identify potentially confounding variables in order to adjust for them in analysis.

Criteria for Causality

The existence of a statistical association does not necessarily mean there is a causal relation. As the previous sections have shown, the observed association may be a random event (due to chance) or may be due to bias from confounding or in the study design or execution. Statistical associations, although necessary to an argument for **causality,** are not sufficient proof. The criteria for causality, originally established to evaluate the link between an infectious agent and a disease, have been revised and elaborated to apply also to other outcomes. While various lists of criteria have

 Criteria for Causality

1. Strength of association. A strong association between a potential risk factor and an outcome supports a causal hypothesis (i.e., a relative risk of 7 provides stronger evidence of a causal association than a relative risk of 1.5).
2. Consistency of findings. Repeated findings of an association with different study designs and in different populations strengthen causal inference.
3. Biological plausibility. Demonstration of a physiologic mechanism by which the risk factor acts to cause disease enhances the causal hypothesis. Conversely, an association that does not initially seem biologically defensible may later be discovered to be so.
4. Demonstration of correct temporal sequence. For a risk factor to cause an outcome it must precede the onset of the outcome. (See the discussion of this issue in the section on study designs.)
5. Dose-response relation. The risk of developing an outcome should increase with increasing exposure (either in duration or quantity) to the risk factor of interest. For example, studies have shown that the greater the amount a woman smokes during pregnancy, the greater the risk of delivering a low-birth-weight infant.
6. Specificity of the association. The presence of a one-to-one relationship between an agent and a disease (i.e., a disease is caused by only one agent and that agent results in only one disease lends support to a causal hypothesis, but its absence does not rule out causality). This criterion grows out of the infectious disease model, where it is more often, though not always, satisfied and is less applicable in chronic diseases.
7. Experimental evidence. Experimental designs provide the strongest epidemiologic evidence for causal associations, but they are not feasible or ethical to conduct for many risk factor-disease associations.

been proposed, there is fairly general agreement on seven criteria which are listed in the box above (Lilienfeld and Stolley, 1994).

Although no single epidemiologic study can satisfy all criteria, epidemiology relies on the accumulation of evidence, as well as the strength of individual studies, to provide a basis for effective public health interventions and policies.

APPLICATIONS OF EPIDEMIOLOGY IN COMMUNITY HEALTH NURSING*

Community health nurses work in a range of settings and agencies providing direct services and interaction with individual clients and their families, including visiting nurse associations, community-based maternity and child health or mental health centers, alcohol

---

*This section and the following clinical application are taken, with modifications, from Chapter 9 of the previous edition, The epidemiological model applied in community health nursing, by Linda Shortridge and Barbara Valauiso.

and drug intervention programs, health maintenance organizations, and nursing centers. Nursing in occupational health settings must consider family resources and needs in planning care even when contact is limited to the individual worker. Nurses employed in administrative positions, such as the director of a visiting nurse association or the nursing administrators in a health department, may be involved in planning and evaluating services of the agency, or in coordinating the services of a variety of community agencies. Similarly, nurses serving on community boards will need to be concerned with coordination of existing services and planning to meet currently unmet needs. Regardless of the agency or the nurses' position, epidemiologic methods provide essential resources for planning, conduct, and evaluation of their work.

Care of patients and families is based on the following steps of the nursing process: (1) assessment; (2) planning; (3) implementation; and (4) evaluation. The same process is used in providing care for communities. In both instances, epidemiology furnishes the baseline information for assessing needs, identifying problems, formulating appropriate strategies for study of the problems, setting priorities in development of a plan of care, and evaluating the effectiveness of care.

Agencies that provide care to communities relate to agencies whose primary pupose is the provision of direct services to clients through referrals, required reporting, and feedback mechanisms. If such information is available at all levels with a common basis of understanding and interpretation, then the referral and reporting system within a community will be facilitated and the system should respond effectively to a need. To assess needs, the nurse providing direct care requires data on the presence or absence of risk characteristics, including family composition and relationships, socioeconomic and cultural factors, environmental factors, and medical and health history. The nurse involved in planning services for the community requires parallel data—including the presence and distribution of risk characteristics, population composition by age, race, and socioeconomic and cultural factors, environmental factors, and medical and health histories.

Assessment of health needs based on sound quantitative and qualitative measurement (descriptive epidemiology), understanding factors that influence health and disease (analytic epidemiology), and evaluation of treatment interventions and program and policy implementation (analytic and experimental epidemiology) are essential for nurses at all levels to plan and provide appropriate care. Epidemiologic concepts, such as the web causality, the natural history of disease, and primary, secondary, and tertiary prevention, provide a unifying approach for studying and understanding disease processes and interventions. Measures of morbidity and mortality provide a standard means of quantifying both the extent of health problems and the risk of specific outcomes. Study design methods provide the tools for extending our understanding of factors that place persons at increased risk or, conversely, provide protection from adverse outcomes. These examples represent some of the ways the practice of community health nursing is enhanced by the understanding and application of epidemiologic concepts and methods.

 # Clinical Application

The following hypothetical situation illustrates the use of epidemiologic data by nurses providing direct services and involved in planning at the community level:

A nurse in the Visiting Nurse Service received a referral for a home visit to a 15-year-old mother whose premature infant has just been discharged from the hospital. The mother of the infant lives with her 40-year-old mother and her 45-year-old father. On her way from the bus stop to the house, the nurse passes overturned trash cans with garbage strewn in the street and numerous teenagers lounging on the doorstep of a neighboring house. When she arrives, she notes that the apartment is hazy with cigarette smoke but appears clean and tidy. Upon assessing the infant, she finds that the baby has a temperature of 39° C and diarrhea but no signs of upper respiratory infection. The grandmother reports that the temperature was normal when the infant was discharged from the hospital late the previous day. The baby's mother has returned to school. The grandmother has quit a part-time job so she can take care of the baby. She reports that they can just scrape by on her husband's salary of $16,000 a year. The baby's mother is doing poorly in school, and the family has decided that when she turns 16 she should quit school and obtain a part-time job to help with family expenses and caring for the baby. The nurse learns that the baby's mother is continuing to see the baby's father and that she is irritable and impatient when the baby cries.

The nurse relies on information from epidemiology to assess and interpret the situation and plan appropriate nursing care. For example, the baby has an elevated temperature accompanied by diarrhea. He was fed once during the night and once in the morning with bottles of milk sent home from the hospital. Only the afternoon feeding was from formula mixed in the home. The nurse makes use of her knowledge of the natural history of infectious diseases: (1) an elevated temperature and diarrhea in the absence of respiratory symptoms suggest a milk-borne infection or some other infection transmitted by oral-entry. Since the temperature is elevated, the symptoms are probably caused by an infection rather than a toxin. (2) Gastrointestinal infections often have an incuba-

Continued.

Clinical Application—cont'd

tion period longer than 24 hours, though some food-borne intoxications have very short incubation periods (a few hours), and all but the last feeding were from hospital-supplied formula. The nurse concludes that the infection may have originated in the hospital and initiates a referral of the baby to a pediatrician for culture and treatment. Because of the nature of community health nursing, the care by this nurse does not stop at this individual level but continues with a report to health department nurses of a possible hospital-related infection in the premature nursery. These personnel will need to follow up on other recent discharges and to work with hospital epidemiologists to identify the source of infection.

The nurse also applies principles of epidemiology in the assessment of the high-risk factors present in this family. Teenage pregnancies are at increased risk for low birth weight and perinatal and infant mortality. Close spacing of pregnancies increases the risks to physical health of both the mother and the fetus. This teenage mother appears to be at risk of becoming pregnant again. Such a pregnancy has a higher probability of complications. Additional infants in this family would increase pressures on the mother and her parents and disrupt family interactions, creating an environment conducive to child abuse. Nursing interventions include counseling the mother regarding birth control options and referral to a family-planning center. Plans should encompass teaching the mother about normal behaviors and growth and development of the infant.

In a broader sense, the nurse is also concerned for the need for accessible community services to support this family and others with similar needs. For example, the referral for family-planning services should be made to a facility that is accessible, affordable, and sensitive to the special needs of adolescents. If these types of facilities are not available for referral, the community health nurse acts as an advocate for the teenage population by participating in health boards responsible for the planning of community health services.

The mother's plan to terminate her education is another indication of a high-risk situation. Epidemiologic data provide evidence of the long-term impact of educational level on the health of the teenage mother and infant. The teenager experiences a developmental crisis when the tasks of parenthood are superimposed on the normal development processes of the adolescent. The nurse counsels the mother regarding the need to continue her education, continues to act as an advocate for the client by contacting the school nurse for counseling with the mother, and refers the mother to a community teen mothers' group for support. If programs are not available in the schools or community to support teenage mothers, then many clients will be faced with the same dilemma occurring in this family. The nurse assesses the need for such services and plans appropriate community-based interventions to provide them to the teenage population.

Given the hazards of both first- and second-hand smoke for childhood respiratory infections and the development of lung cancer and emphysema, the presence of high levels of cigarette smoke is also of concern. The nurse should work with both the mother and other family members to quit or reduce smoking, especially in the baby's presence.

In this clinical situation the nurse is providing individual care to the teenage mother and family. These interventions will bring the mother into contact with nurses in other community agencies—the health department nurse, the family-planning clinic nurses, and the school nurse. If appropriate services are not available to meet the needs of the client, the nurse plans interventions directed to other clients with similar needs. Facilities, such as family-planning centers and adolescent mothers' groups, are available for referrals because nurses and other professionals engage in health planning. This process includes monitoring births in the community. If the rate of births to unmarried women is increasing, particularly among adolescents, family-planning centers in high-risk neighborhoods may be established. The health planning process also includes monitoring rates of school dropout, including high-risk groups such as teenage mothers. In high-risk communities, school-based services may be indicated that can provide educational counseling, information on growth and development, and, in some cases, assistance with child care. When nurses monitor appropriate epidemiologic indicators and participate in the health planning process, the services needed for appropriate intervention with young clients will be available and the nurse providing direct services can make appropriate referrals. Ongoing monitoring of these indicators provides feedback as to the effectiveness of the services.

Key Concepts

♦ Epidemiology is the study of the distribution and determinants of health-related events in human populations, and the application of this knowledge to improving the health of communities.

♦ Epidemiology is a multidisciplinary enterprise that recognizes the complex interrelationships of factors that influence disease and health at both the individual and community level and provide basic tools for the study of health and disease in communities.

♦ Epidemiologic methods are used to describe health and disease phenomena and investigate the factors that promote health or influence the risk or distribution of disease. This knowledge can be useful in planning and evaluating programs, policies, and services, and in clinical decision making.

♦ Basic concepts important to epidemiology are the interrelations of agent, host, and environment (the "epidemiologic triangle"); interactions of factors, exposures, and characteristics in a causal web affecting risk of disease; and levels of prevention corresponding to stages in the natural history of disease.

♦ Primary prevention involves interventions to reduce the incidence of disease by promoting health and preventing disease processes from developing. Secondary prevention includes programs (such as screening) designed to detect disease in the early stages before signs and symptoms are clinically evident in order to intervene with early diagnosis and treatment. Tertiary prevention provides treatments and other interventions directed toward persons with clinically apparent disease, with the aim

of ameliorating the course of disease, reducing disability, or rehabilitating.

♦ Basic epidemiologic methods include use of existing data sources to study health outcomes and related factors, and the use of comparison groups to assess the association of exposures or characteristics to health outcomes.

♦ Epidemiologists rely on rates to quantify levels of morbidity and mortality. Prevalence rates give a picture of the level of existing cases in a population at a given time. Incidence rates measure the rate of new case development in a population and provide an estimate of the risk of disease.

♦ Descriptive epidemiologic studies provide information on the distribution of disease and health states according to personal characteristics, geographic region, and time. This knowledge enables community health practitioners to target programs and allocate resources more effectively, and provides a basis for further study.

♦ Analytic epidemiologic studies investigate associations between exposures or characteristics and health or disease outcomes, with a goal of understanding the etiology of disease. Analytic studies provide the foundation for our understanding of disease causality, as well as for developing effective intervention strategies aimed at primary, secondary, and teritary prevention.

♦ Epidemiologic methods also are used in the planning and design of screening (secondary prevention) and community health intervention (primary prevention) strategies and in the evaluation of their effectiveness.

Critical Thinking Activities

1. Look at a recent issue of the *Final Mortality Statistics* from the National Center for Health Statistics or the most recent issue of *Health: United States*. Examine the trends in cause-specific mortality and choose one or two of the leading causes of death.

   a. On the basis of current epidemiologic evidence, what factors have contributed to the observed trend in mortality for this disease? Changes in survival? Changes in incidence?

   b. Are the changes due to better (or worse) primary,

   secondary, or tertiary prevention? Are there modifiable factors, such as health behaviors, that lend themselves to better prevention efforts? What would they be?

2. Examine the leading causes of death for infant mortality in the United States.

   a. What differences in intervention approaches are suggested by the various causes of death?

   b. How would you design an epidemiologic study to examine risk factors for specific causes of neona-

Continued.

Critical Thinking Activities—cont'd

tal and postneonatal mortality? What types of epidemiologic measures would be useful? What study design(s) would be appropriate?

c. How would you use the information from your study to develop an intervention program and to define the target population for your intervention?

3. Find a report of an epidemiologic study in one of the major public health, nursing, or epidemiology journals. How do the findings of this study, if valid, affect your nursing practice? How do you incorporate the results of epidemiologic research into your nursing practice?

Bibliography

Armenian HK, editor: Applications of the case-control method, *Epidemiol Rev* 16(1):1-164, 1994.

Benenson AS: *Control of communicable diseases in man,* ed 15, Washington, DC, 1990, American Public Health Association.

Breslow NE, Day NE: *Statistical methods in cancer research: vol I—the analysis of case-control studies,* Lyon, 1980, International Agency for Research on Cancer, p 13-40.

Breslow NE, Day NE: *Statistical methods in cancer research: vol II—the design and analysis of cohort studies,* Lyon, 1987, International Agency for Research on Cancer, p 1-46.

Brownson RC, Remington PL, Davis JR: *Chronic disease epidemiology and control,* Washington, DC, 1993, American Public Health Association, p 85f, 291.

Centers for Disease Control and Prevention (CDC): Use of race and ethnicity in public health surveillance. Summary of the CDC/ATSDR workshop, *MMWR* 42(No. RR-10), 1993.

Centers for Disease Control and Prevention (CDC): Addressing emerging infectious disease threats: a prevention strategy for the United States (Executive Summary), *MMWR* 43(No RR-5): 1-18, 1994.

Chadwick E: *Report on the sanitary conditions of the laboring population of Great Britian,* Edenburgh, 1842, University Press.

Fox SH, Koepsell TD, Daling JR: Birth weight and smoking during pregnancy—effect modification by maternal age, *Am J Epidemiol* 139:1008-1015, 1994.

Healthy People 2000: national health promotion and disease prevention objectives, Washington, DC, 1991, USDHHS, Public Health Service.

Holleb AI, Fink DJ, Murphy GP: *American Cancer Society textbook of clinical oncology,* Atlanta, 1991, American Cancer Society.

Institute of Medicine (IOM): *The future of public health,* Washington, DC, 1988, National Academy Press, p 58-65.

Kelsey JL, Thompson WD, Evans AS: *Methods in observational epidemiology,* New York, 1986, Oxford University Press, p 46-76.

Kochanek KD, Hudson BL: Advance report of final mortality statistics, 1992, *Monthly Vital Statistics Report Suppl* 43(6), 1995, Hyattsville, Md, National Center for Health Statistics.

Last John M: *A dictionary of epidemiology,* ed 2, New York, 1988, Oxford University Press.

Lederberg J, Shope RE, Oaks SC, and the Institute of Medicine, editors: *Emerging infections: microbial threats to health in the United States,* Washington, DC, 1992, National Academy Press.

Lieberman E, Gremy I, Lang JM, Cohen AP: Low birthweight at term and the timing of fetal exposure to maternal smoking, *Am J Public Health* 84(7):1127-1131, 1994.

Lilienfeld AM: Epidemiology and health policy: some historical highlights, *Public Health Reports* 99(3):237-241, 1984.

Lilienfeld AM, Lilienfeld DE: The 1979 Heath Clark Lectures: the epidemiologic fabric—weaving the threads, *Int J Epidemiol* 9(3):199-205, 1980.

Lilienfeld DE, Stolley PD: *Foundations of epidemiology,* ed 3, New York, 1994, Oxford University Press, p 28-30.

Mausner JS, Kramer S: *Epidemiology—An introductory text,* ed 2, Philadelphia, 1985, WB Saunders.

Meinert CL: *Clinical trials: design, conduct and analysis,* New York, 1986, Oxford University Press.

National Center for Health Statistics (NCHS): *Health, United States, 1993,* Hyattsville, Md, 1994, Public Health Service.

Public Health Service Fact Sheet, Washington, DC, 1984, USDHHS, Public Health Service.

Schlesselman JJ: *Case-control studies: design, conduct, analysis,* New York, 1982, Oxford University Press, p 69-104.

Shortridge L, Valanis B: The epidemiological model applied in community health nursing. In Stanhope M, Lancaster J, editors: *Community health nursing: process and practice for promoting health,* ed 3, St Louis, 1992, Mosby.

Snow J: *On the mode of communication of cholera,* ed 2, 1936. In *Snow on Cholera.* New York, 1855, The Commonwealth Fund.

Stallones RA: Prospective Epidemiologic Studies of Cerebrovascular Disease. In *Cerebrovascular disease epidemiology: a workshop,* Public Health Monograph No 76, 1966, US Public Health Services, Pub No 1441.

Susser M: *Causal thinking in the health sciences,* New York, 1973, Oxford University Press, p 54-59.

Susser M: Epidemiology in the United States after World War II: the evolution of technique, *Epidemiol Rev* 7:147-173, 1985.

Timmreck TC: *An introduction to epidemiology,* Boston, 1994, Jones and Bartlett, p 70-73.

Vandenbroucke JP: Epidemiology in transition: a historical hypothesis, *Epidemiology* 1(2):164-166, 1990.

Winkelstein W, French FE, editors: *Basic readings in epidemiology,* ed 3, New York, 1972, MSS Educational Publishing.

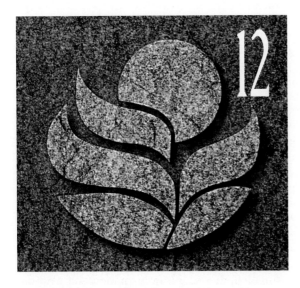

12 Research Applications in Community Health Nursing

Beverly C. Flynn ◆ Joyce S. Krothe

Objectives ▼

After reading this chapter, the student should be able to do the following:

◆ Discuss priority areas for research in community health nursing with consideration for primary health care and health promotion.
◆ Describe the stages of the research process and methodological considerations.
◆ Describe roles and issues in research.
◆ Cite several community health nursing research studies employing both quantitative and qualitative methods.
◆ Identify ways the practicing community health nurse can participate in the research process.

Key Terms ▼

assumptions
health promotion
human subjects review committees
limitations
national health objectives
practice-based research
primary health care
qualitative methods
quantitative methods
research process

Research for community health nursing has increased over the years. However, community health nurses must continue to expand the scientific knowledge base unique to their practice to provide high-quality services and creative, scientifically oriented solutions to today's health problems.

How can we best structure such research? Primary health care, as defined by the World Health Organization (WHO, UNICEF, 1978), is proposed as an appropriate framework to guide research and to develop concepts in community health nursing. **Practice-based research** questions and the key concepts of primary health care and health promotion, as defined by the World Health Organization (*Ottawa Charter*, 1986; WHO, UNICEF, 1978), also form an appropriate research framework This chapter also focuses on selected research issues, the roles and functions of the researcher and collaborators, and examples of research from community health nursing practice.

RELATIONSHIP OF COMMUNITY HEALTH NURSING TO PRIMARY HEALTH CARE

All countries that sent representatives to a world conference in Alma Ata, Russia, endorsed **primary health care** as the best approach for reaching the goal of "health for all by the year 2000" (WHO, UNICEF, 1978 p. 16):

Primary health care is essential health care based on practical, scientifically sound and socially acceptable methods and technology made universally accessible to individuals and families in the community through their full participation and at a cost that the community and country can afford to maintain at every stage of their development in the spirit of self-reliance and self-determination.

Health promotion further supports primary health care. **Health promotion** is "the process of enabling people to increase control over, and to improve, their health" (*Ottawa Charter*, 1986, p. 1). Five major aspects of health promotion, in order of priority, are: building health-promoting public policy, creating supportive environments, strengthening community action, developing personal skills, and reorienting health services.

Community health nursing, primary health care, and health promotion are linked to each other. Each incorporates community-based practice, involvement of the community in health care decisions and goal setting, a focus on disease prevention and health promotion, and use of an interdisciplinary and multisectoral approach in planning and implementing appropriate solutions to health problems. Because community health nursing, primary health care, and health promotion are complementary, research conducted by community health nurses can make a significant contribution to primary health care practice.

In response to the complex issues in health care reform, Buhler-Wilkerson (1993) suggests that commu-nity health nurses revisit Lillian Wald's vision of the role of community-based nursing. Community-based nursing should provide care responsive to clients' needs while "encouraging public responsibility, and providing a unifying structure for the delivery of comprehensive, equally available health care" (Buhler-Wilkerson, 1993, p. 1785). This focus on individual needs within a social and economic context—a multi-sectoral approach—is consistent with the philosophy of primary health care and serves as a conceptual framework for research.

Although the past decade has witnessed a renewed emphasis on research-based nursing practice, the roots of nursing research can be traced to Florence Nightingale. Her early emphasis was on careful observation of clients and adaptation of nursing care based on systematic observation, as opposed to trial and error. Nightingale's methodology provided the foundation for the evolution of nursing science and a unique body of research-based nursing knowledge (Brockopp and Hastings-Tolsma, 1994).

THE RESEARCH PROCESS

The nursing process, epidemiological process, and **research process** are all problem-solving methods of scientific inquiry. Each involves assessment, planning, implementation, evaluation, and action. The action phase leads to ongoing reassessment, followed by additional planning and implementation. The epidemiological and research processes develop knowledge. The nursing process uses knowledge in providing health and health-related services to individual clients, families, groups, and communities.

The nursing process and the epidemiological processes as applied to community health nursing are discussed elsewhere in this text. The stages of the research process are summarized in the box on p. 235.

Although the listing is sequential, the researcher actually works back and forth between the various stages of the research process. Decisions made in any one stage must be consistent with decisions made in other stages. All stages are viewed as part of the total study and are arrived at logically and systematically. To clarify each stage of the research process, the researcher presents examples from nursing practice.

Assessment/Conceptual Stage

The assessment or conceptual stage involves translating a hunch or curiosity about a clinical problem into a question that can be researched. For example, a community health nurse may be curious about why some elderly people in the community can live independently while others enter a nursing home. The nurse conducts an initial review of related research literature to gain an overview of the situation and its current stage of research. This initial literature review helps the nurse select a purpose and scope for the study. In the example given, the community health

Stages of the Research Process

ASSESSMENT/CONCEPTUAL STAGE

Identifying a problem for study
Initial review of related literature
Identifying the purpose of the research
Delineating the population to be studied

PLANNING/DESIGN STAGE

Formulating and delimiting the research problem
Continuing review of related literature
Selecting a conceptual framework
Selecting a research design and appropriate methodology
Designing the data collection plan
Finalizing and reviewing the research plan
Human subjects approval process
Pilot studies and revisions in design

IMPLEMENTATION/EMPIRICAL STAGE

Inviting potential participants to participate
Implementing data collection plan
Preparing data for analysis

EVALUATION/ANALYTICAL STAGE

Analyzing the data
Interpreting the results
Drawing conclusions

ACTION/DISSEMINATION STAGE

Communicating the research findings
Using the findings in practice
Informing health policy makers
Taking action for social change
Planning additional research

Selected stages of the research process are modified from Polit DF, Hungler BP: *Essentials of nursing research: methods, appraisal, and utilization,* Philadelphia, 1993, Lippincott.

nurse would decide that the purpose of the study is to determine how community health nursing services are assisting elderly persons to live in the community. Next, characteristics of the study population are clearly defined. For example, the study population may include elderly people within a specific age range and who live within a specified geographical area served by a particular community health nursing agency.

Planning/Design Stage

Once a relevant purpose, scope, and study population are selected, the researcher enters the planning or design stage. This is a logical, organized process that proceeds consistently step by step. Planning involves critical thinking and communicating ideas in a clear and logical way, consistent with the format required by potential funding sources.

Designing a research project is a problem-solving process. After identifying a problem for study and formulating a question about the problem, the researcher

must continue to review related literature, decide on a methodology consistent with the research question, and write a clear proposal. Tornquist and Funk (1990) provide a helpful resource for writing a research proposal. Brink and Wood (1994) point out that not all questions can or need to be answered by research. They define a researchable question as "an explicit query about a problem or issue that can be challenged, examined, and analyzed and that will yield useful new information" (p. 2). Potential topics for research stem from the thoughts, observations, and practice experiences of the community health nurse.

In planning, the specific research focus is stated. In the previous example, the community health nurse decides that the problem to be investigated is a lack of information about the relationship between community health nursing services and the ability of elderly people to live independently in the community.

Next, key terms are defined. In the example, the nurse decides that for the purpose of the study, elderly people will be defined as persons 75 years of age or older who live in the geographical area served by a specific community health nursing agency. Reviews of the literature can be used to define terms and assist in further developing a scientific body of knowledge for nursing practice. In addition, through an extensive literature review, the nurse identifies conceptual frameworks and analyzes how research and data analyses were carried out in previous research studies. Of particular concern is what has and has not worked in practice based on findings of previous research studies.

The nurse also must select a conceptual framework that is appropriate for the problem to be investigated. In the example, the nurse selects an ecological conceptual framework that can be adapted from the health services research field. This framework incorporates environmental concerns, health services, and client characteristics that are congruent with the basic premise of primary health care.

Next, the nurse delineates specific research questions or hypotheses for the research. These statements include the key variables of the study. The **national health objectives** may be helpful in specifying and defining key variables (Healthy People 2000, 1991). The national health objectives indicate major health concerns for different age groups and provide specific standards that researchers can use to evaluate program progress.

In our example, the nurse questions whether the range of community health nursing services for elderly people will preserve independence. The national health objectives specify that independence is preserved when there are no more than 90 per 1000 people aged 65 or older who have difficulty performing two or more personal care activities. It is hypothesized that the greater the range of community health nursing services available, the more elderly people are able to live independently in the community. The key variables are the range of community health nursing services and elderly people's performance of personal care activities.

The nurse next selects a research approach appropriate to the phenomenon being investigated; it may be historical, survey, or experimental. Each approach creates different requirements for a research design. Considerations include whether the data will be collected at one point in time or longitudinally and whether the data will be collected cross-sectionally or across various groups in the population. In the example, the nurse decides that a historical approach, or a review of past information, will not adequately address the problem. An experimental approach is not feasible because the study cannot be conducted under controlled conditions. Instead, the nurse decides that a survey is the most appropriate approach for comparing elderly people living independently in the community with use of community health nursing services. This approach permits a research design for collecting data during one time period.

Planning also should include consideration of methodologies appropriate to the research question. **Quantitative methods** have been the dominant methodologies in nursing research. However, there is a growing acceptance of nursing science as a composite of different perspectives and varied research methodologies. Although recognition of **qualitative methods** as a tool of science is rather recent in the nursing literature, its tradition in the United States began during the late 1800s. "At that time, qualitative strategies were used to disclose the rapidly developing social problems in cities pursuant to industrialization, urbanization, and mass immigration. Qualitative descriptions encouraged social change by making urban problems visible to the public" (Munhall and Boyd, 1993 p. 72).

Traditional scientific inquiry is usually referred to as quantitative research. This method advocates objectively gathering data that can be verified by another researcher and generalized to other populations. These methods are characterized by deductive reasoning, objectivity, quasi-experiments, statistical techniques, and control.

Although many nursing research questions are amenable to traditional methodologies, others require a different approach. Qualitative methods may be more compatible with a particular phenomenon being studied. They are characterized by inductive reasoning, subjectivity, discovery, description, and the meaning of an experience to the individual (Brockopp and Hastings-Tolsma, 1994).

Munhall and Boyd (1993) suggest that nurse researchers will find a congruence between nursing's philosophical embrace of humanism and holism and qualitative methodologies. At the same time, "not every research interest can be accommodated by the qualitative perspective, nor should nursing . . . adopt a single method for developing knowledge about . . . the multi-dimensional world of nursing" (Munhall and Boyd, 1993).

> ## Did You Know?
>
> Although the dominant methodology used in nursing research has been quantitative, there is a growing acceptance of nursing science as a composite of different perspectives and thereby of quantitative and qualitative research methodologies (Munhall and Boyd, 1993).

During the 1980s, Sarter (1988) noted that the paths to nursing knowledge were broadening to include qualitative methods. This broadening affords the nurse scholar access to human experience. Many nurse theorists have embraced the importance of understanding the clients' perspective as central to providing appropriate nursing care.

Once the researcher has considered methodological options, the next stage involves selecting a data-gathering method, such as observing, measuring, or interviewing. The researcher identifies specific techniques or instruments that are consistent with the research design. For example, if a questionnaire is considered for data collection, a specific instrument could be selected, such as picture questionnaires, instead of print, for subjects who cannot read.

Decisions need to be made about a data-gathering method for each of the major variables in the research study. The researcher may decide to use more than one instrument. In the example, the nurse decides to use both observing and interviewing methods. The nurse will observe community health nurses who provide services to elderly people to delineate the scope and range of services provided. To avoid making nurses and clients feel uncomfortable about being observed, the nurse researcher plans to use qualitative methodology and participant observation in working with the community health nurses. Thus the nurse researcher will participate in a natural situation for data collection. In addition to observation, a quantitative method, such as an interview questionnaire, may be used to determine the level of physical functioning of elderly people.

The plan for data analysis is guided by the research questions and methodologies employed. It is useful to identify the computer software available to assist with data analysis and also to decide how findings will be presented. For example, the researcher may want to design sample tables for the data once they are collected. These tables will help ensure that all the data necessary to answer the research questions have been collected.

The research questions and plan for data analysis guide sample selection. The research method to be used directs the sample size. There are many methods of sample selection, but two will be considered here: random and deliberate sampling. Random sampling means that every case or participant has an equal opportunity of being included in the study. Deliberate sampling means that specific persons are invited to participate in the study. Choice of research methodologies will determine the characteristics of the sample population.

In the example the nurse decides to study elderly persons within the geographical boundaries served by a community health nursing agency. After consultation with a statistician, the nurse decides that the sample should consist of 100 elderly persons over 75 years of age living in the community. This figure is based on an estimated sample size required for the statistics selected. The researcher may use power analysis software that can help to determine sample size. Of course, it is impossible to know the exact number of elderly people living in the community, so the nurse estimates the total elderly population based on census data. A deliberate sample of persons 75 years of age and older is selected, until 100 are included in the sample.

Important in the design phase is research approval by the institutional **human subjects review committees.** These are groups of representatives of various related disciplines or departments brought together to review research proposals. Their major concerns are protecting human research participants from physical or mental harm, as well as protecting the researcher from undue complaints. This process also satisfies a number of funding agencies and federal, state, and institutional regulations.

In the example, the local health department has a committee that reviews research proposals involving health department services. The nurse researcher must obtain approval from the committee before the research begins. The first step is to communicate clearly in writing to the review committee what is planned, how participants will be involved in the research, and whether or not their participation will put them at risk for physical or mental harm. The researcher is ethically responsible for carrying out these plans as directed or approved by the committee. Changes that occur in the plans need to be reported to the committee for further sanctioning.

Pilot studies can be used to test data-gathering methods and to apply the data analysis plan. A pilot study is especially important when the data-gathering technique is unfamiliar to the researcher: the instrument may be new, it may not have been used with the population under study, or the study may be conducted in an unfamiliar environment. The nurse researcher in the example decides to pilot test the study with five elderly clients from a neighboring county after obtaining permission from both the nurse and the clients.

Next, the assumptions and limitations of research need to be identified. **Assumptions** are characteristics of the research situation that are not explored, usually because they have been well demonstrated in previous research. An assumption of the fictitious study is

that some community services enable elderly people to live independently in the community.

The **limitations** are uncontrollable elements of the research. They limit the certainty of the findings or their applicability to the population in general. In this study, a limitation is that deliberate sampling does not ensure that all elderly people are equally represented. As a result, the study findings may not be applicable beyond the study sample.

Implementation/Empirical Stage

The implementation or empirical stage of the research plan refers to the carrying out of the research procedures. This stage includes inviting the sample group members to participate, obtaining their informed consent, collecting and verifying the data, and analyzing the data. The nurse researcher may send a letter to potential participants inviting them to participate. After a follow-up phone call, an appointment is arranged with the client and the community health nurse. At this meeting the participants, both the client and the nurse, are asked to give their signed informed consent to participate in the study.

The nurse researcher then collects data through observation and interviews. Any conflicting information is validated with the participants, and consensus is reached. Depending on methodological choices, data analysis occurs concomitantly with data collection (qualitative methodology) or at the conclusion of the data collection phase (quantitative methodology).

Regardless of methodological considerations, data collection and analysis follow specified guidelines. "Like empirical method, each qualitative approach requires certain steps, in a certain order, according to certain rules, and is thus subject to certain measures of the value of research findings. Merely interviewing people does not place a study in the qualitative paradigm" (Munhall and Boyd, 1993 p. 90). The researcher must be aware of the strict guidelines of all methodologies used.

Evaluation/Analytical Stage

The evaluation or analytical stage includes analyzing the findings and comparing them with previous research results. Conclusions are then drawn, building on a body of previous knowledge. Research reports should provide clear documentation of what was done and when. The results of the research for the specific problem, research questions, or hypotheses under study are presented. If the research design is quantitative, hypotheses that were not supported also need to be reported. Recommendations for future research should be clear and consistent with the study results. The need for replication studies should be specified. Replication studies with other populations are useful because recommendations for practice should be based on more than one set of study results. The research findings are presented to professional colleagues; to persons in decision-making positions, such as administrators, policy makers, and legislators; and to the general public, which might be affected by any decisions made.

In the hypothetical research example, the study findings indicated that the greater the range of community health nursing services, the greater the ability of elderly people to live independently. Future research should include information regarding severity of health problems. The nurse researcher presented the findings to the administrators and staff at the local health department, to the county-wide senior citizen organization, to professional colleagues at their annual meeting, to a reporter for an article in a local paper, and to the state legislative committee responsible for formulating policy for community-based care.

Action/Dissemination Stage

The results of nursing research should be used in practice. Nurses must make specific recommendations based on research findings to improve the health of the community. By applying research results in practice, nurses can institute social change. Policy makers, other professionals, and the community learn that the research findings are relevant and applicable to practice.

In the example, the nurse may discover that the presence of a support person is a significant factor in enabling an elderly person to live independently in the community. Clients who are regularly visited by a community health nurse may be able to maintain independent living for a longer time.

The results of such a study could support the expansion of community health nursing services. The economic difference between maintaining elderly clients in their homes versus placing them in an institution could be a compelling argument in support of expanded home health care services. Research documenting the cost effectiveness of nursing care is vitally needed. Such effectiveness is measured in many ways beyond cost, including quality of care and client satisfaction.

The results of research can assist agencies in developing research programs within their organizations. The results should be presented to clinical audiences (Tornquist et al., 1989): research experiences can mobilize staff nurses to build a program of research around common clinical problems. Reporting the results of research outcomes in professional journals and at professional meetings also facilitates the growth and use of nursing knowledge (Brockopp and Hastings-Tolsma, 1994).

Relevant research findings must also be reported to community groups. This information can become part of the community's educational experience and help the community to make appropriate decisions based on local needs.

Most important, data-based information from nursing research should be communicated to policy makers at the local, state, and national levels. Research findings thus inform health policy makers and create responsive policy formulation (Flynn et al., 1991).

PRACTICE-GENERATED QUESTIONS FOR RESEARCH

Significant questions for reserach can be generated from community health nursing practice in response to everyday observations in the field. Brink and Wood (1994) identify that point at which observation ceases to be an everyday occurrence and becomes genuine research: "It stops being a normal part of everyday life and becomes research if it is systematically planned and recorded. This makes the difference between simply observing the world around you and collecting research data through observation" (p. 147).

Novice community health nurses often have difficulty identifying potential questions for research that arise from their practice. The following discussion focuses on examples of questions for research that are generated in practice. These questions are grouped by the concepts of primary health care: accessibility, community involvement, disease prevention and health promotion, appropriate technology, and multisectoral approach.

Accessible Health Care

Accessibility of health services refers to the extent to which community health nursing services reach people who need them the most and how equitably these services are distributed throughout the population. A question for research related to this concept is whether community health nursing services are accessible to those in greatest need. For example, are the services available to groups of people most in need of them in terms of time, location, and personnel? Are these services available in both urban and rural areas? Who uses and who does not use the community health nursing services? What are the health care needs of the people who use the service compared with those who do not? What are the barriers to the use of services? Are the costs too high? Are the services relevant to consumers' perceived needs? Are community health nurses sensitive to the concerns of consumers? Do consumers have transportation to reach the services? Are services offered at times when those most in need of them are able to access them?

Community Involvement

Community involvement is concerned with the level of participation of community residents in health care decision making. To promote community development and self-reliance, residents themselves need to participate in decisions about the community health. Residents and health providers need to work together to identify problems and to seek solutions.

Questions for research generated from practice relate to the level and mechanism of community involvement in health decision making. For example, to what extent is the community involved in the various stages of assessing health care needs, planning, management, and monitoring community health nursing services? What mechanisms and processes can people use to be actively involved and to take joint responsibility, along with community health nurses, for decisions? In particular, what decisions involving the community have been implemented? Are the community health nursing services better used as a result?

Disease Prevention and Health Promotion

Community health focuses on health promotion and prevention of disease rather than on curative services. Examples are activities that include physical exercise, seat belt use, smoking cessation, and other healthful life-style changes.

Priority questions for research include the following: What are the major preventable health problems

 Research Brief

Long KA, Boik RJ: Predicting alcohol use in rural children: a longitudinal study, Nurs Res 42(2):79-85, 1993.

Rural adults are at high risk for alcohol abuse. Use among rural children follows national trends of earlier age for onset of alcohol-abusing behavior. The purpose of this study was to describe the prevalence and correlates of alcohol use, to evaluate risk factors, and to examine the ability to predict alcohol use among rural sixth- and seventh-grade children.

A total of 625 sixth- and seventh-grade children from six rural schools participated in the study. They completed questionnaires that assessed various demographic, attitudinal, and psychometric measures known to be reliable predictors of alcohol use. This was a follow-up study that initially collected data from the students as third and fourth graders. Results indicated that 58% of the participants reported using alcohol. Findings indicated that negative self-concept and negative school attitudes in third and fourth grades correlated most highly with alcohol use in the sixth and seventh grades.

Implications for community health nursing include the following: (1) assessing predictors of alcohol use in young children can identify those at high risk for later use and abuse, and (2) nurses working in schools can intervene to prevent the development of alcohol use in elementary school-age children.

in the community? For example, are there high rates of automobile accidents or heart disease in a particular community? Are problems being addressed by preventive and health-promoting measures? What measures are being taken to reduce or control these problems? Do the community health nursing services include recommendations for infant car seat use, programs to reduce alcohol intake among drivers, smoking cessation programs, and programs that promote health in schools?

Appropriate Technology

Appropriate technology refers to health care that is both relevant and acceptable to people's health needs and concerns. It includes issues of cost and affordability of services within the context of existing resources, such as the number and type of health professionals and other providers, equipment, and supplies and their pattern of distribution throughout the community. The National Science Foundation's definition (1979) of appropriate technology summarizes these considerations: "Appropriate technologies are defined as those which are decentralized, require low capital investment, conserve natural resources, are managed by their users, and are in harmony with the environment" (p. 1).

The overriding questions to be answered include the following: Do the services use the simplest and least costly technology available? Are the services acceptable to the community? Are they affordable initially and over time? What is the cost effectiveness of alternative approaches or strategies for community health nursing services? Are family home visits as effective as working with families in groups? Are nonprofessionals, such as home health aides, effective in providing some aspects of community health nursing services? What are the most effective management and supervisory techniques for nonprofessionals and professionals within a community health nursing agency?

Multisectoral Approach

The health of a community cannot be improved by intervention only within the health sector. Other sectors are equally important in promoting the community's health and self-reliance. For example, education, environment, industry, housing, and nutrition are interrelated with health. Therefore, these sectors need to work together to coordinate their goals, plans, and activities to ensure that they contribute to the health of the community and to avoid conflicting or duplicating efforts.

Relevant questions for research include the following: What mechanisms exist that promote or hinder multisectoral collaboration? Do the committees or task forces that address community-wide concerns represent various fields, such as education, industry, housing, transportation, and health? What are examples of multisectoral efforts in seeking solutions to community problems? How were successful solutions derived in the past? What factors contributed to their success? What conflicts exist across sectors? How are conflicting activities across the various sectors resolved? What are the gaps in efforts across the various sectors in solving community health problems?

ROLES AND ISSUES IN RESEARCH

Although some of the roles of the community health nurse researcher and issues related to research are presented in other sections of this chapter, additional aspects are worthy of consideration.

Relationships

The practicing community health nurse may conduct research or work with a researcher within an organization in carrying out a study. The practicing nurse, the administrator of nursing services, and the researcher are partners in a joint endeavor. Partners each have their own areas of expertise, but they benefit from the expertise of the others. The community health nurse, as an expert in practice, can identify problems that must be researched and the feasibility of various research designs. The administrator can help identify policy issues related to the research and can provide organizational support. The researcher can help develop practice problems into researchable questions, suggest appropriate research methods, and design data collection and analyses.

The nurse may also work with the community group concerned with the research problem. Citizens, professionals, and other persons interested in community health may identify a priority problem for research. In this case, persons in the group have expertise about the community, and the researcher and the community health nurse work as resources to the group in conducting the research.

Involving others in the research process is not without problems. Perhaps the most difficult aspect for researchers is sharing activities that usually fall under their domain, such as involving others in identifying the important questions to be researched. Because community health nursing research often takes place in a dynamic setting in which the chief responsibility is health care (e.g., a neighborhood clinic), priority may be given to clinical commitments rather than to research. For example, access to records and files may be controlled by others, and client information may be withheld by the agency. As a result, the research itself may become part of the politics of the situation. Researchers need to be aware of these dynamics and use their expertise to ensure that the research is conducted with proper attention to sound principles. Skills in communication and collaboration are essential to the process.

Communication

Communication with participants, co-researchers, community health nursing practitioners, administrators, community residents, and policy makers is important throughout the research process. Communication can take many forms. The researcher needs to consider the appropriateness of verbal, written, and visual aids in clarifying information being presented. Often the researcher has an academic background and appointment and has been educated differently from practitioners and community citizens. Because researchers in nursing are often practitioners first, this gap may be closed. Even so, the researcher must carefully consider how the information is presented, including the level of understanding of the reader or listener, and be attentive to issues of concern to the audience being addressed. The format of presentation will vary depending on whether the audience is a group of academic researchers, practicing community health nurses, policy makers, or community citizens.

Information must be disseminated about the research early in the study and throughout the project. Negative findings, such as the discovery that nursing intervention did not reduce costs, must be presented along with positive results. A focus on concepts rather than on the specific program being studied may facilitate the acceptance of negative findings.

Ethics and the Researcher Role

Ethical issues need careful attention when research of any type is conducted. Ethical issues arise out of conflicting social pressures between the profession and the larger society. For example, should one publish the results of research when the findings reflect negatively on a particular group? This information may be taken out of context and used to limit government funding of services to a particular group.

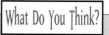

What Do You Think?

The nurse researcher has an ethical responsibility to report both positive and negative results of research regardless of the consequences to community health nursing programs being studied.

Ethical issues also must be considered in designing a study. For example, community health nurses may wish to evaluate the effectiveness of the home health agency's policies for the care of clients with acquired immunodeficiency syndrome (AIDS). It would be unethical to assign a group of clients with AIDS as a control group if that meant withholding information about the diagnosis from the community health nurses providing nursing services to these clients.

Dilemmas may arise over ensuring the confidentiality of responses, disclosing the actual purpose of the research to the respondents, or even disseminating results of the research to the respondents. As noted earlier, research plans are under close scrutiny by human subjects review committees in institutions today. The researcher is ethically responsible for carrying out these plans as directed or approved by the committee. Changes that occur in research plans must be reported to the committee for further sanctioning.

There are also ethical considerations in data reporting. Fraudulent research data and results of health-related research have been published. This issue is important in nursing research because few replication studies exist. The effects of publishing false findings can be widespread, affecting not only the profession but also, more important, persons in the community and policy formulation.

Position of Researcher in Employment Setting

Who employs the researcher and potential uncertainties about the authority structure are often major sources of concern for the nurse researcher. In an academic setting the researcher may be a faculty member who also has responsibilities for classroom teaching, clinical supervision of students, academic advising, and committee work. To be involved in a major research effort, the faculty member typically will need to be relieved of some of these responsibilities. Consideration can be given to a semester of full-time research, a reduction in teaching responsibilities and committee work, or some combination of these for the duration of the project.

It may be possible to establish more innovative employment opportunities in research: status as a visiting scholar or visiting researcher within a community organization or university, shared positions between universities and other organizations, or the promotion of sabbatical leave opportunities between service and academic institutions. When researchers are hired by community organizations, they should clarify their research role. Questions should include the following: What are the other expectations for this position, for example, service, administration, or other research? How will the results be disseminated if they reflect negative features of a service program or a professional group? If the organization chooses not to disseminate a research report, what happens to the researcher's work? Does the researcher have continued access to the data? Can the researcher prepare papers for presentation at professional meetings and in the professional literature? Researchers need to establish a clear understanding with their employers and administrators about the organization of and expectations for their work, as well as the organization's authority in relation to publication and the researcher's access to data for professional purposes.

Another aspect that needs to be reemphasized relates to the action phase of the research process. For example, after completing an investigation, the results are found to be significant for community health nursing practice. The researcher must use the results in practice. He or she also must see that the findings are clearly understood by relevant others, such as administrators, community health nurses, legislators, or citizens in the community. The community health nurse researcher may need to communicate research findings to legislators so that appropriate policies and legislation are enacted. At this point, the link between research and practice can best become reality.

Funding of Research

A final issue is obtaining funds for research. Some federal funding is available for nursing research through agencies such as the National Institute of Nursing Research and the Agency for Health Care Policy and Research. However, obtaining money for research, especially federal funding, is increasingly competitive. For this reason, the pursuit of funding from voluntary foundations and organizations should not be overlooked. Private foundations, such as the Robert Wood Johnson Foundation or the W.K. Kellogg Foundation, offer program funding that can include evaluation research.

State and local funding sources include community foundations, local chapters of Sigma Theta Tau, regional nursing research societies, the March of Dimes, the American Heart Association, the American Cancer Society, hospitals, and corporations. Universities may offer small grants for faculty to initiate research. Local and state health departments offer program grants through maternal child health or various preventive block grants that have evaluation research components. Finally, employers can sometimes grant release time from work so that educators, administrators, consultants, and practitioners can conduct research.

Table 12-1 provides a summary of selected examples of funding sources. Researchers need to explore alternative funding sources, be aware of new funding initiatives, and design creative financing options.

Mechanisms for collaborative research also need to be established and funded. Research institutes and centers with connections between community groups, health care organizations, industries, and universities can facilitate research in community health nursing. Such institutes can promote interdisciplinary collaboration to study community health problems and practice issues. The institutes also provide a unique environment for the delineation and articulation of the various research roles. The institutes afford collaborative opportunities for community residents, students, educators, and service personnel to seek solutions to community health problems. Joint financing could be arranged between a community group, a service agency, and a university for research.

Table 12-1   Examples of Funding Sources for Research

Level of funding	Funding source
NATIONAL	
Federal	National Institutes for Health
	National Institute for Nursing Research
	National Cancer Institute
	Agency for Health Care Policy and Research
Private/voluntary	W.K. Kellogg Foundation
	Robert Wood Johnson Foundation
	Pew Charitable Trusts
	Rockefeller Foundation
	American Cancer Society
	American Heart Association
	American Diabetes Foundation
STATE	
Public	State department of health
	Department of family and social services
	State universities
Private/voluntary	March of Dimes
	State hospital association
	State cancer society
	State heart association
	State nurses association
	Corporations
LOCAL	
Public	Health department
Private/voluntary	Sigma Theta Tau chapters
	Regional nursing research societies
	March of Dimes
	Business and industry

SUGGESTIONS FOR PARTICIPATION IN RESEARCH

Practicing nurses can participate in each stage of the research process. They are in key positions to identify clinical problems to be researched. Nurses can take anecdotal notes about clinical situations that will help in identifying key variables for study. They also can read research on the topic of concern and discuss observations with other nursing colleagues, including researchers. Frequently, nurse researchers work in universities and are more than willing to collaborate in joint research efforts. Practicing community health nurses can assist researchers in securing institutional approval to conduct research and in facilitating access to research participants. They also may be involved in data collection, whether for pilot studies, replication studies, or original research. The nurse may be a participant in research by answering questionnaires and participating in interviews or by being observed in practice.

Community health nurses can provide valuable insights into study findings, often explaining relationships, or a lack thereof, to researchers. They can apply relevant research findings in practice. They also can explain or report on research findings to community members, administrators, policy makers, and others, thus initiating action for social change.

Community health nurses work with community members in improving their health. They can help seek and identify scientifically oriented solutions to health and nursing problems; thus, they are in a key position to develop knowledge that can be used in practice.

 ## Clinical Application

Selected examples of research studies are presented here because they are generated by community health nursing practice, involve a community health nurse as an investigator, or have implications for the use of research findings in community health nursing practice and policy change.

Case 1: AIDS Prevention in Inner-City Black Female Adolescents

AIDS disproportionately affects inner-city black women of childbearing age; therefore it is imperative to design interventions to reduce the risks. Nurse researchers tested the value of culturally sensitive AIDS risk reduction interventions for inner-city black adolescent women (Jemmott and Jemmott, 1992). Before the intervention, individual and focus group interviews were conducted with adolescents from the community to determine a culturally appropriate way

to present the AIDS program to the target population.

During implementation, the participants received the intervention in small groups of adolescents led by a specially trained black female health educator who was a local resident. The intervention increased their intention to use condoms among the participants. Findings were consistent with other studies that suggested that knowledge alone was not sufficient to change risky behavior. "Tailoring advice to the culture of the target community is essential to the success of risk-reduction interventions for ethnic minority women" (Jemmott and Jemmott, 1992, p. 275).

Case 2: Updating Quality-of-Life Assessments for Elderly People

Most of the instruments for quality-of-life assessment of elderly people were originally developed for use with chronically ill and disabled populations; they ob-

Clinical Application—cont'd

jectively measured functioning in activities of daily living. Now, since more than half of elderly people are living with spouses in independent households and subjectively rate their health as good, the need arose for a more encompassing measure of quality of life for elderly persons in the community.

To address this need, nurse researchers designed and tested a Life Situation Survey to measure subjectively perceived quality of life (Rickelman et al., 1994). Research findings indicated a strong level of attachment to a special person, primarily a spouse. This attachment was significantly and positively correlated with perceived quality of life and self-rated health. Information about these relationships can be explored by nurses as they interact with elderly people in community settings.

Case 3: Sociodemographic Barriers to Prenatal Care

A study to determine the effect of sociodemographic factors on quality of prenatal care revealed the discrepancies in use and quality of care for many women (Hansell, 1991). Research findings indicated that the groups receiving the most inadequate care were teenagers, minorities, less educated persons, single persons, and poor people.

Attitudinal barriers were a major factor influencing use of services. Disadvantaged women had experienced low quality of health services. Subsequently, they thought that the benefits of prenatal care were not worth it when weighed against the costs of child care, transportation, and lost wages. Community health nurses can apply findings from this study in their practice and examine mechanisms to reduce the barriers to use of prenatal care for high-risk women.

Case 4: Health-Promoting Behaviors Among African-American Women

High rates of morbidity and mortality exist among minority populations. Information about their health care beliefs and practices are therefore important in developing, implementing, and evaluating culturally competent health-promoting interventions. A study was conducted to describe health-promoting life-style behaviors among African-American women.

The study also compared findings with published reports on the Health-Promoting Lifestyle Profile, a tool that assesses the likelihood of engaging in health-promoting behaviors. The authors concluded that the tool may have "a middle class bias that is inappropriate for some people, such as those who live in unsafe neighborhoods and fear crime" (Ahljevych and Bernhard, 1994, p. 89).

The tool measures behaviors over which people have control. Many women who participated in the study lacked control over living arrangements, adequate resources for food purchases, or a safe place to exercise. Therefore, it was concluded that their low scores on the profile should not be interpreted as a lack of interest in promoting healthy life-styles. Implications for nursing research include developing culturally sensitive instruments to measure health-promoting behaviors and working with communities to create environments conducive to health promotion.

Case 5: Interventions to Encourage Health Promotion in Elderly People

This example illustrates how findings from a nursing research study employing quantitative methods may be used to recommend a follow-up study using qualitative methods. Despite the recommendation that elderly people receive an annual influenza vaccine, the vaccination rate remains at 20% to 30%. A study of public health nursing interventions to encourage annual vaccination against influenza among persons 65 years of age and older was designed (Black et al., 1993). Public health clients were randomly assigned to either a control group or a study group that promoted the influenza vaccine during a home visit.

Beliefs regarding immunization, rather than the presence of chronic health conditions, were found to be the strongest reason for not receiving the vaccine, thus refuting previous studies. Recommendations for further study included assessing beliefs constituting barriers to vaccine acceptance. The researchers suggested that a study using "qualitative methods may contribute to our understanding of older clients' perceptions and willingness to participate in preventive self-care", such as influenza immunization (Black et al., 1994, p. 1753).

Case 6: Perceptions of Long-Term Care Needs Among Elderly People

A nursing research study that used qualitative methodology examined the perceptions of elderly people at risk for nursing home admission. The purpose of the study was to learn this population's perceptions regarding their needs for community-based long-term care (Krothe, 1992). This information is essential for informed and responsive policy and program development that is sensitive to clients' needs and for cost-effective alternatives to institutionalization. Findings from the study indicated that the concept of control over decision making related to one's life is predominant in elderly people's desire and ability to stay at home. Policy implications to create environments that promote self-reliance in elderly people were suggested from the research findings. The implications included policy changes for community-based long-term care, family members, formal and informal care providers, and nursing homes.

Key Concepts

- Although research for community health nursing practice has developed over the years, community health nurses need to increase their scientific research base.
- Community health nursing, primary health care, and health promotion are complementary. Research conducted by community health nurses can make a significant contribution to nursing practice and also to primary health care.
- The research process is a problem-solving process. It involves assessment, planning, implementation, evaluation, and action.
- Significant questions for research can be generated from community health nursing practice and linked with the key concepts of primary health care.
- Community participation is a key concept of primary health care and is concerned with the level of citizen involvement in health decision making.
- Potential questions to be answered by research address the basic concepts of primary health care and health promotion.
- The ethical issues in research need thoughtful attention by the nurse researcher.
- The issue of who employs the researcher and potential uncertainties about the authority structure are often major sources of concern for the nurse researcher.
- Federal money for research continues to be competitive. Researchers and others need to explore alternative funding sources and use creative financing options.
- Clinical applications of selected community health nursing studies are suggested to improve services and promote policy change.

Critical Thinking Activities

1. Read the newspaper, and identify one priority problem that has relevance to community health nursing practice that could be researched in the community.
2. From your community health nursing experiences, specify a research question that you could relate to one of the concepts of primary health care.
3. Identify a research study in the literature relevant to community health nursing, and identify the strengths and limitations of the research.
4. Talk with a community member, a community health nurse, a researcher, and an administrator who have been involved in research. Ask them about their roles and functions in research. What were the sources of role strain?
5. Identify from the literature three funding sources for research in community health nursing.
6. From the literature, identify research findings, one in a research study that uses quantitative methods and one that uses qualitative methods, that can be applied in community health nursing practice.
7. Identify a researchable topic based on your community health nursing practice that has implications for health care reform.
8. Communicate to a policy maker at the local, state, or national level the findings of a nursing research study that supports community-based care.

Bibliography

Ahljevych K, Bernhard L: Health-promoting behaviors of African American women, *Nurs Res* 43(2):86-89, 1994.

Black ME, Ploeg J, Walter SD, Hutchinson BG, Scott EAF, Chambers LW: The impact of a public health nurse intervention on influenza vaccine acceptance, *Am J Public Health* 83(12):1751-1753, 1993.

Brink PJ, Wood MJ: *Basic steps in planning nursing research: from question to proposal,* Boston, 1994, Jones & Bartlett.

Brockopp DY, Hastings-Tolsma MT: *Fundamentals of nursing research,* Boston, 1994, Jones & Bartlett.

Buhler-Wilkerson K: Bringing care to the people: Lillian Wald's legacy to public health nursing, *Am J Public Health* 83(12):1778-1786, 1993.

Flynn BC, Rider M, Ray DW: Healthy cities: the Indiana model of community development in public health, *Health Educ Q* 18(3):331-347, 1991.

Hansell MJ: Sociodemographic factors and the quality of prenatal care, *Am J Public Health* 81(8):1023-1028, 1991.

Healthy People 2000: national health promotion and disease prevention objectives, Washington, DC, 1991, USDHHS, Public Health Service.

Jemmott LS, Jemmott JB: Increasing condom-use intentions among sexually active black adolescent women, *Nurs Res* 41(5):273-277, 1992.

Krothe JS: *Constructions of elderly people's perceived needs for community based–long term care,* doctoral dissertation, Bloomington, 1992, Indiana University.

Long KA, Boik RJ: Predicting alcohol use in rural children: a longitudinal study, *Nurs Res* 42(2):79-85, 1993.

Munhall PL, Boyd CO: *Nursing Research: a qualitative perspective,* New York, 1993, National League for Nursing.

National Science Foundation: NSF announcements for December, NSF bulletin, Washington, DC, 1979, The Foundation.

Ottawa Charter for Health Promotion, Copenhagen, 1986, World Health Organization.

Polit DF, Hungler, BP: *Essentials of nursing research: methods, appraisal, and utilization,* Philadelphia, 1993, JB Lippincott.

Rickelman BL, Gallman L, Parra H: Attachment and quality of life in older, community-residing men, *Nurs Res* 43(2);68-72, 1994.

Sarter B, editor: *Paths to knowledge: innovative research methods for nursing,* New York, 1988, National League for Nursing.

Tornquist EM, Funk SG: How to write a research grant proposal, *Image J Nurs Scholarship* 22:44-51, 1990.

Tornquist EM, Funk SG, Champagne MT: Writing research reports for clinical audiences, *West J Nurs Res* 11:576-582, 1989.

World Health Organization, UNICEF: *Primary health care: a joint report,* Geneva, 1978, World Health Organization.

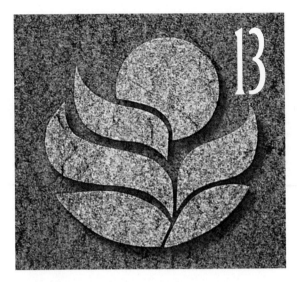

13

Educational Theories, Models, and Principles Applied to Community Health Nursing

Jeanette Lancaster ◆ Lisa Onega ◆ Douglas Forness

Jeanette Lancaster ◆ Lisa Onega ◆ Douglas Forness

Key Terms

affective domain
behavioral theory
cognitive domain
cognitive theory
critical theory
developmental theory
health belief model
health promotion model
humanist theory
long-term evaluation
PRECEDE-PROCEED model
psychomotor domain
short-term evaluation
social learning theory

Objectives ▼

After reading this chapter, the student should be able to do the following:

◆ Discuss six educational theories as they relate to community health nurse educators.
◆ Describe three models for effective health education.
◆ Discuss three categories of educational principles.
◆ Identify and describe the five steps of the educational process.
◆ Describe the importance of evaluating the educational product.

Outline ▼

Health education is a vital part of community health nursing. The promotion, maintenance, and restoration of health requires that community health clients receive a practical understanding of health-related information.

Community health clients include individuals, families, and communities. An individual is any person, regardless of age, gender, or other characteristic. Families are a group of individuals linked by ancestry, marriage, or household and may consist of nuclear, extended, biological, adoptive, or other alternative makeup. A community may be a small group, support system, club, church, school, neighborhood, or loosely tied and widely scattered group with a common interest or cause.

Because community health nurses see clients with varying needs and abilities in a variety of settings, they are in key positions to deliver health education. The information that the community health nurse provides enables clients to make knowledgeable decisions, cope more effectively with alterations in their health and life-styles, and assume greater personal responsibility for their health (Graham, 1992).

In an era of growing health costs and increasing collaboration between health service providers and consumers, clients are increasingly encouraged to share responsibility for their own health maintenance. Community health nurse educators empower consumers by educating them about ways to manage their own health processes more effectively (Clarke et al., 1993). As lifespan increases, people are more likely to experience the chronic illnesses related to aging that require complex changes in diet, exercise, life-style, and medical treatments. Health education becomes crucial to health care because of such social changes (Annand, 1993). Also, attainment of the objectives of *Healthy People 2000* will rely heavily on community-based programs to promote healthy habits and life-styles.

As discussed in Chapter 3, the goal of *Healthy People 2000* is to set forth a national strategy for improving national health. *Healthy People 2000* describes objectives that, if attained, will prevent major chronic illness, injuries, and infectious diseases. Education is a primary strategy in assisting people to change their habits. Education is therefore provided in a wide variety of community health settings, including schools, homes, the workplace and ambulatory and inpatient health care facilities.

While the accomplishment of a number of the objectives of *Healthy People 2000* relies on educational strategies, several objectives specifically address health education. These are listed in the box above.

The ability to apply learning theories in a variety of educational settings is essential to guide the thinking, decision making, and practice of community health nurses. To promote the health of clients, it is necessary to teach health concepts and self-care skills in understandable ways.

Healthy People 2000 Educational Objectives

- Increase to at least 75% the proportion of people aged 10 years or older who have discussed issues related to nutrition, physical activity, sexual behavior, tobacco, alcohol, other drugs, or safety with family members on at least one occasion during the preceding month.
- Increase to at least 50% the proportion of counties that have established culturally and linguistically appropriate community health promotion programs for racial and ethnic minority populations.
- Increase to at least 90% the proportion of hospitals, health maintenance organizations, and large group practices that provide client education programs, and to at least 90% the proportion of community hospitals that offer community health promotion programs addressing the priority health needs of their communities.
- Increase to at least 75% the proportion of local television affiliates in the top 20 television markets that have become partners with one or more community organizations around one of the health problems addressed by the *Healthy People 2000* objectives.

From *Healthy People 2000: national health promotion and disease prevention objectives*, Washington, DC, 1991, USDHHS, Public Health Service.

Learning is defined in a variety of ways. Most definitions of the learning process include a measurable change in behavior that persists over time. Newly learned knowledge and behaviors are practiced and thus are repeatedly reinforced (Padilla and Bulcavage, 1991). Although many theories and principles related to learning are applicable to community health nursing, only samples of the most useful and readily adaptable ones are included here. A solid theoretical foundation of health education enables the community health nurse to educate clients successfully. (See Figure 13-1 for the sequence of actions that a community health nurse follows when developing an educational program.)

GENERAL EDUCATIONAL THEORIES

Educational theories help community health nurses understand how people learn and how to design and implement client education. Table 13-1 provides an overview of six major educational theories useful in community health nursing. It is important to understand each of these educational theories and be able to choose and then apply the most appropriate theory to a wide variety of health education situations. Often it is necessary to combine a number of these perspectives in the education process.

Behavioral Theory

Behavioral theory approaches the study of learning by concentrating on behaviors that can be observed and measured. The goal of behavioral ap-

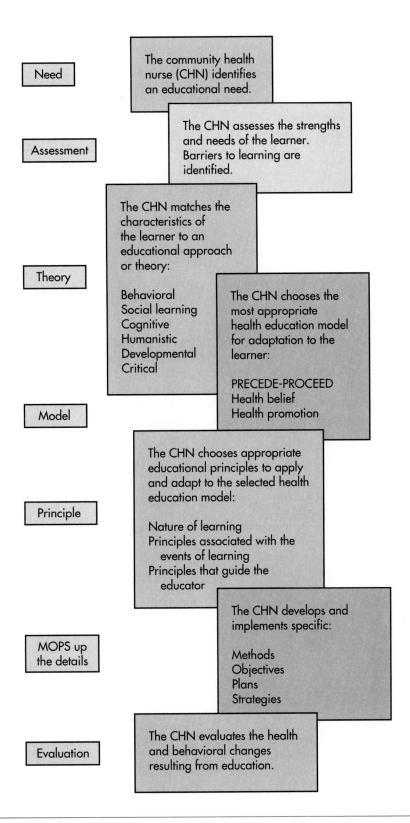

FIGURE 13-1

The sequence of actions that a community health nurse follows when developing an education program.

Table 13-1   Overview of Six General Educational Theories

Theory	Focus	Method
Behavioral	Change behavior	Reinforcement/punishment
Social Learning	Change expectations and beliefs	Provide information
Cognitive	Change thought patterns	Variety of sensory input and repetition
Humanist	Use feelings and relationships	Self-determination of learners to do what is best for themselves
Developmental	Consider human developmental stage	Provide opportunities matching readiness to learn
Critical	Increase depth of knowledge	Ongoing dialogue and open inquiry

Data from Driscoll MP: *Psychology of learning for instruction*, Boston, 1994, Allyn & Bacon; and Edwards L: In Edelman CL, Mandle CL, editors: *Health promotion throughout the lifespan*, St Louis, 1990, Mosby.

proaches to learning is behavioral change. A *target behavior*, which the educator seeks to either increase or decrease, is identified. To increase a behavior, one identifies and consistently uses a *reinforcer* to modify the target behavior. To decrease a behavior, one identifies and consistently uses the *withdrawal of a reinforcer* or a *punishment* to modify the target behavior (Dembo, 1994; Dignam, 1992; Driscoll, 1994).

The behavioral approach is useful when the educator has full control over the reward/consequences environment, that is, the feedback system. This approach is also useful when the learner has cognitive limitations because the behavioral approach requires only the most rudimentary use of cognition.

For example, a community health nurse working in a school system might want to decrease the number of adolescent deaths associated with alcohol use. The nurse identifies the target behavior as use of a designated driver. The nurse works to increase the use of designated drivers for transporting students from school-related functions. Therefore, after every school-related sporting or social event, four trained adults sit at the exit doors, evaluate the sobriety of designated drivers, and assign designated drivers to cars. Designated drivers each receive $10 for gasoline from raised funds, have their names printed in the weekly school newspaper, and become eligible for a weekly prize drawing of $20.

Social Learning Theory

Social learning theory builds on the principles of behavioral theorists. They believe that behavior is a function of an individual's *expectations* about the *value of an outcome* (Do I want the outcome?) or *self-efficacy* (Can I achieve the outcome?). If clients believe that an outcome is desired and attainable, they are more likely to change their behavior to achieve that goal. Thus, educators may use this theory to change behaviors by enabling clients to either change their expectations about the value of a certain outcome or their ability to achieve the desired outcome or both (Blair,

1993; Dembo, 1994; Padilla and Bulcavage, 1991).

For example, if the community health nurse wants to help a group of obese women lose weight, the nurse instructs the women to eat less, select healthful foods, and exercise more. Through the presentation of scientific data describing balanced eating and the positive effects of exercise, the nurse helps the women develop the expectation that decreased food intake and increased exercise will result in weight loss. Thus, through case study presentations and before-and-after photos, the nurse helps the women change their expectations about their power to achieve the goal of weight loss. Without the belief in their power to change, the women may be unable to remain motivated to change their target behaviors.

Cognitive Theory

Cognitive theory maintains that by changing *thought patterns* and *providing information*, learners' behavior will change. It posits that people's thought patterns undergo constant change as they interact with their environment. Thus the educator seeks to provide information in a variety of ways that will change clients' thought patterns and ultimately will be followed by changes in behavior (Dembo, 1994; Dignam, 1992; Driscoll, 1994).

For example, if a woman does not do monthly breast self-examinations (BSEs), the nurse instructs the client to begin doing so. The nurse seeks to change the woman's thought patterns by providing information about BSE in a variety of ways. The nurse verbally teaches the client about the procedure and reasons for BSE. The nurse next shows the woman a video about BSE. The nurse then observes as the client practices BSE on a breast model. Finally, the nurse gives the woman a handout with the procedure on it. The nurse instructs the client to hang the handout next to the bathroom mirror to remind her to do monthly BSEs. Thus, by using a variety of environmental cues and sensory input, the client's thought patterns can be changed, thereby influencing her behavior related to BSE.

Humanist Theory

Humanist theory describes the influence that *feelings, emotions,* and *personal relationships* have on behavior. These theorists believe that learners should be encouraged to examine their feelings and engage in various forms of *self-expression.* In addition, humanists think that people need to be aware of and able to clarify their values. If people are given *free choice,* they will do what is best for themselves. Humanists encourage health educators not to be overly controlling and restrictive with learners, but rather to help them grow and develop according to their natural inclinations (Dembo, 1994; Dignam, 1992).

For example, if a retirement community wants to develop a health promotion program, it might encourage the nurse to schedule meetings with members. At the meetings, the nurse facilitates group discussion about the goals and strategies for the program and provides a variety of handouts related to health promotion. Finally, the nurse answers questions and offers encouragement to the group members as they develop their own health promotion program.

Developmental Theory

Developmental theory maintains that learning occurs in concert with *developmental stages.* Each stage is a major transformation from the previous one, and learning occurs quite differently in each developmental period. *Readiness to learn* depends on the individual's developmental stage (Hancock and Mandle, 1990).

For example, to help a family with a toddler prevent accidents in the home, the nurse would educate parents about safety practices. The nurse would also teach the parents how to educate the toddler simply and clearly about safety according to the toddler's developmental stage and readiness to understand concepts and behavioral patterns. The nurse recognizes that the parents' and the toddler's levels of readiness to learn are quite different. Since the toddler cannot reach the stove top, teaching about the dangers of a hot stove at this stage of physical development is unnecessary. However, the toddler is at risk for accidental poisoning. Although the parents may teach the toddler not to open bottles and jars without their help, all poisons must be removed from the toddler's possible reach as a necessary precaution. The risk of poison ingestion is incomprehensible to the toddler because of the stage of both language and cognitive development.

Critical Theory

Critical theory approaches learning as an *ongoing dialogue.* An individual holds a belief about a health matter. The educator attempts to change this belief by *questioning* the learner. As the learner answers the questions, the learner's beliefs begin to change, new questions arise, and the learner then asks the educator questions. The educator responds to these questions. This process of *discourse* ultimately changes thinking and behavior (Dignam, 1992; Welton, 1993).

For example, the nurse would like a newly diagnosed group of diabetic clients to assume responsibility for the management of their diabetes. The nurse asks the clients what they know about diabetes. The clients demonstrate that they can check their own blood sugar and prepare their own insulin injections. However, on further questioning, it is discovered that the clients are not familiar with the long-term complications of diabetes. The nurse then educates them. As a result, the clients begin to go to an ophthalmologist every year and check their feet daily for alterations in skin color or integrity.

HEALTH EDUCATION MODELS

Conceptual models organize global ideas and simplify complete systems into succinct formats. Thus, conceptual models provide meaningful descriptions to guide the thinking, observations, and practice of educators (Driscoll, 1994; Edwards, 1990). Three health education models are described here:
1. PRECEDE-PROCEED
2. Health belief
3. Health promotion

These three models are directly applicable to the community health role and provide a practical way of viewing the process of health education.

 PRECEDE-PROCEED are Acronyms

PRECEDE IS AN ACRONYM FOR:

P redisposing,
R einforcing, and
E nabling
C auses in
E ducational
D iagnosis and
E valuation

PROCEED IS AN ACRONYM FOR:

P olicy,
R egulatory, and
O rganizational
C onstructs in
E ducational and
E nvironmental
D evelopment

From Green LW, Kreuter MW: *J Health Educ* 23(3):140-147, 1992.

Table 13-2 The Nine Phases of the PRECEDE-PROCEED Model

Phase	Title	Description
1	Social diagnosis	The social concerns of the community are identified.
2	Epidemiological diagnosis	Epidemiological data are used to suggest health problems.
3	Behavioral and environmental diagnosis	Behavioral and environmental risk factors that seem to affect health are identified.
4	Educational and organizational diagnosis	Predisposing, reinforcing, and enabling factors are identified.
5	Administrative and policy diagnosis	Planning related to health education and policy regulations occurs.
6	Implementation	The health education program is implemented.
7	Process evaluation	The education process is evaluated in an ongoing fashion.
8	Impact evaluation	The immediate effects or objectives of the educational program are evaluated.
9	Outcome evaluation	The short-term and long-term effects of the educational program are evaluated.

Data from Green LW, Kreuter MW: J *Health Educ* 23(3):140-147, 1992; Green LW, Ottoson JM: *Community health*, ed 7, St Louis, 1994, Mosby; and Hawe P, Degeling D, Hall J: *Evaluating health promotion: a health worker's guide*, Philadelphia, 1990, MacLennan & Petty.

PRECEDE-PROCEED Model

The **PRECEDE-PROCEED model** focuses primarily on planning and evaluating community health education programs. The PRECEDE-PROCEED acronym is shown in the box on p. 251, and the nine phases of the model are outlined in Table 13-2.

One strength of the PRECEDE-PROCEED model is that it consistently involves the client in a problem-solving approach to provide health education for an identified area of need. The PRECEDE-PROCEED model focuses on helping communities change their behaviors. It begins by assessing the environment in which the group lives and considering the social factors that influence health behaviors. Next, the model examines both the internal and the environmental factors of the group that predispose it (PRECEDE) to certain behaviors or health problems. The model then calls for the identification of factors that will help the group in adopting healthy actions. Priorities are set. The program is developed, implemented, and finally evaluated (PROCEED). The PRECEDE-PROCEED model is easy to use; its steps are a checklist for ensuring that all stages of the problem-solving process are followed (Edwards, 1990; Green and Kreuter, 1992; Padilla and Bulcavage, 1991).

Health Belief Model

The **health belief model** was developed to provide a framework for understanding why some people take specific actions to avoid illness, whereas others fail to protect themselves. When the model was developed, both the public and the private health sectors were concerned that people were reluctant to be screened for tuberculosis, to have Pap smears to detect cervical cancer, to be immunized, or to take other preventive measures that were either free or available at nominal cost. The model was designed to predict which people would and would not use preventive measures and to suggest interventions that might reduce client reluctance to assess health care (Padilla and Bulcavage, 1991; Salazar, 1991). The box on p. 253 (top) outlines the three major components of the health belief model: individual perceptions, modifying factors, and variables affecting the likelihood of action. In addition, cues to action such as mass media campaigns, advice from others, reminder postcards from health care providers, illnesses of family members or friends, and newspaper or magazine articles may help motivate clients to take action (Salazar, 1991).

The health belief model is beneficial in assessing health protection or disease prevention behaviors. It is also useful in organizing information about clients' views of their state of health and what factors may influence them to change their behavior. The health belief model, when used appropriately, provides organized assessment data about clients' abilities and motivation to change their health status. Health education programs can then be developed to better fit the needs of clients (Salazar, 1991).

Health Promotion Model

The **health promotion model** was developed as a complement to other health-protecting models such as the health belief model. The health promotion model explains the likelihood that healthy life-style patterns or health-promoting behaviors will occur (Palank, 1991; Simmons, 1990). The box on p. 253 (bottom) outlines the three major categories of determinants of health-promoting behavior: cognitive-perceptual factors, modifying factors, and variables affecting the like-

The Three Major Components of the Health Belief Model

INDIVIDUAL PERCEPTIONS

Person's *beliefs* about his or her own susceptibility to disease

PLUS
The *seriousness* with which he or she views the disease

EQUALS
The *perceived threat* of an illness for each person

MODIFYING FACTORS

Demographic Variables

Age
Gender
Race
Ethnicity

Sociopsychological Variables

Personality
Social class
Peer pressure

Structural Variables

Knowledge about the disease
Prior contact with the disease

VARIABLES AFFECTING THE LIKELIHOOD OF INITIATING ACTIONS

Person's *perceived benefits* of action

MINUS
His or her *perceived barriers* to accomplishing action

EQUALS
The *likelihood* that person will take action to change his or her behaviors

From Salazar MK: *AAOHN J*, 39(3):128-135, 1991.

 Three Categories of Determinants of Health-Promoting Behavior

COGNITIVE-PERCEPTUAL FACTORS

Definition of health
Importance of health
Perceived health *status*
Perceived *control* of health
Perceived *self-efficacy*
Perceived *benefits* of health-promoting behavior
Perceived *barriers* to health-promoting behavior

MODIFYING FACTORS

Demographic Factors

Age
Gender
Race
Ethnicity
Education
Income

Biological Characteristics

Body weight
Body fat
Height

Interpersonal Influences

Expectations of significant others
Family patterns of health care
Interactions with health professionals

Situational (Environmental) Factor

Access to care

Behavioral Factors

Cognitive and psychomotor skills necessary to carry out healthy behaviors

VARIABLES AFFECTING THE LIKELIHOOD OF INITIATING ACTIONS

Depend on internal and external cues:
 The desire to feel well
 Individualized health teaching
 Mass media health promotion campaigns

Data from Palank CL: *Nurs Clin North* 26(4):815-832, 1991; and Simmons SJ: *J Adv Nurs* 15(10):1162-1166, 1990.

lihood of action. Although these three categories are similar to the three factors of the health belief model, the health promotion model expands and modifies them.

This model, as with the health belief model, is useful to the community health nurse as a framework for client assessment. However, the health promotion model expands the principles of the health belief model and posits that individuals are likely to change their behavior to feel better physically, psychologically, socially, and spiritually.

Community Health Nurses' Application of Health Education Models

It is up to the community health nurse to select the most appropriate model for educational programs. For example, when providing educational programs to communities, the nurse may use the PRECEDE-PROCEED model to organize the teaching program. However, when delivering education to individuals or families, the nurse may use the health belief model or the health promotion model to identify the specific beliefs, behaviors, or cultural factors that must be modified to change behavior.

The health belief model is particularly useful in assessing the likelihood that clients will change their health behaviors and in developing concrete plans aimed at changing health beliefs. The health promotion model borrows concepts from general education theories and other health education models. It provides a broad base for assessing health perceptions and attempting to help clients modify their health behaviors by changing their perceptions of the factors affecting health. Many other health education models may also be used by the community health nurse to plan educational interventions.

EDUCATIONAL PRINCIPLES

A variety of educational principles can be used to guide the selection of health information for individuals, families, and communities. Three of the most useful categories of educational principles include those associated with (1) the nature of learning, (2) the events of instruction, and (3) guidelines for the educator.

The Nature of Learning

One way to learn about the nature of learning is to examine the cognitive, affective, and psychomotor domains of learning (Dembo, 1994). Each domain has specific behavioral components that form a hierarchy of steps or levels. Each level builds on the previous one. Understanding these three learning domains is crucial in providing effective health education.

The **cognitive domain** concerns memory, recognition, understanding, and application and is divided into a hierarchical classification of behaviors. Learners master each level of cognition in order of difficulty (Dembo, 1994). For health education to be effective, the instructor must first assess the cognitive abilities of the learner so that the instructor's expectations and plans are directed toward the correct level. Teaching above or below the client's level of understanding may lead to frustration and discouragement.

The **affective domain** describes changes in attitudes and the development of values. In affective learning, nurses consider and attempt to influence what clients, families, and communities think, value, and feel. Since the values and attitudes of nurses may differ from those of their clients, it is important to listen carefully to detect clues to feelings that may influence learning. As with cognitive learning, affective learning comprises a series of steps (Dembo, 1994). Steps in the affective domain as compared with the cognitive domain are listed in Table 13-3. It is difficult to change deep-seated qualities such as values, attitudes, beliefs, and interests. To make such changes, people need support and encouragement from those around them to reinforce new behaviors.

The **psychomotor domain** includes the performance of skills that require some degree of neuromuscular coordination. Community health clients are taught a variety of psychomotor skills, including giving injections, taking blood pressure, measuring blood sugar, bathing infants, changing dressings, and walking with crutches. The levels of psychomotor learning from the simplest to the most complex level of observable movements are outlined in the box on p. 255.

Three conditions must be met before psychomotor learning occurs (Dembo, 1994):

1. The learner must have the *necessary ability*. For example, the nurse may find that a client with Alzheimer's disease may only be capable of fol-

Table 13-3   Steps in the Cognitive Domain as Compared With the Affective Domain

	Cognitive domain	Affective domain
Knowledge	Requires *recall* of information	Learner *receives* the information.
Comprehension	*Combines* recall with understanding	Learner *responds* to what is being taught.
Application	Takes new information and *uses it in a different way*	Learner *values* the information.
Analysis	Breaks down communication into constituent parts to understand the parts and their *relationships*	Learner *makes sense* of the information.
Synthesis	Builds on the previous four levels by putting the parts back together into a *unified whole*	Learner *organizes* the information.
Evaluation	*Judges* the value of what has been learned	Learner *adopts* behaviors consistent with the new value system.

From Dembo MH: *Applying educational psychology*, ed 5, New York, 1994, Longman.

Levels of Psychomotor Learning

REFLEX MOVEMENTS

Occur in response to a stimulus without conscious awareness

BASIC MOVEMENTS

Develop from a combination of reflex movements

PERCEPTUAL ABILITIES

Transfer visual stimuli into appropriate movements

PHYSICAL ABILITIES

Combine basic body movements by incorporating endurance, strength, flexibility, and agility

SKILLED MOVEMENTS

Are indicative of a degree of proficiency

NONDISCURSIVE COMMUNICATION

Complex movements are used to communicate feelings, needs, or interests to others

From Dembo MH: *Applying educational psychology*, ed 5, New York, 1994, Longman.

lowing instructions of one or two steps. Therefore the nurse must adapt the education plan to fit the client's abilities.

2. The learner must have a *sensory image* of how to carry out the skill. For instance, when educating a group of pregnant women about techniques to manage labor, the nurse asks the clients to visualize themselves in calm control of their delivery.

3. The learner must have *opportunities to practice* the new skills being learned. Practice sessions should be provided during the program because many clients will not have the facilities, motivation, or time to practice what they have learned at home.

To facilitate skill learning, the educator should show the learner the skill either in person, on a video, or with pictures. Then the educator should allow the learner to practice and immediately correct any errors in performing the skill.

In assessing a client's ability to learn a skill, the educator should evaluate physical, intellectual, and emotional ability. For example, a tremulous person with poor eyesight may be incapable of learning insulin self-injection. Similarly, some clients do not have the intellectual ability to learn the steps that make up a complex procedure. The community health nurse should teach at the level of the learner's ability.

The Events of Instruction

To educate others effectively, the nurse needs to understand the basic sequence of instruction. When nurses consider the following nine steps of instructing others, they can systematically plan health education

so that learners gain as much as possible from the instruction (Driscoll, 1994).

1. *Gaining attention.* Before learning can take place, the educator must gain the learner's attention. One way to do this is by convincing the learner that the information about to be presented is important and beneficial to the learner.

2. *Informing the learner of the objectives of instruction.* Before teaching begins, the major goals and objectives of instruction should be outlined so that learners develop expectations about what they are supposed to learn.

3. *Stimulating recall of prior learning.* The educator should have learners recall previous knowledge related to the topic of interest. This assists learners in linking new knowledge with prior knowledge.

4. *Presenting the stimulus.* The essential elements of a topic should be presented in as clear, organized, and simple a manner as possible. The material should be presented in a way that is congruent with the learner's strengths, needs, and limitations.

5. *Providing learning guidance.* For long-lasting behavioral changes to occur, the learner must store information in long-term memory. With guidance from the educator, the learner can transform general information that has been presented into meaningful information that the learner can recall.

6. *Eliciting performance.* Learners should be encouraged to demonstrate what they have learned. Educators should expect that during the educational process learners will need to correct errors and improve skills.

7. *Providing feedback.* Educators should provide feedback to learners to assist them in improving their knowledge and skills. Learners can then modify their thinking patterns and behaviors based on this feedback.

8. *Assessing performance.* Learning should be evaluated. Knowledge and skills should be formally assessed with the expectation that new information has been understood.

9. *Enhancing retention and transfer of knowledge.* Once a baseline level of knowledge and skills has been attained, educators should assist learners in applying this information to new situations.

By using these instructional principles, nurses may help clients to maximize learning experiences. If steps of this process are omitted, superficial and fragmented learning may occur.

The Effective Educator

Community health nurse educators must be effective teachers. Six basic principles that guide the effective educator are listed in the box on p. 256 (top, left) and discussed next.

Sending a Clear Message

Regardless of the importance of the content or the interest level of the learner, if the material is not pre-

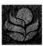

Six Principles that Guide the Educator

MESSAGE
Sending a clear message to the learner

FORMAT
Selecting the most appropriate learning format

ENVIRONMENT
Creating the best possible learning environment

EXPERIENCE
Organizing positive and meaningful learning experiences

PARTICIPATION
Engaging the learner in participatory learning

EVALUATION
Evaluating and giving objective feedback to the learner

From Knowles M: *The adult learner: a neglected species*, ed 4, Houston, 1990, Gulf.

Communication Guidelines for Educational Interactions

- Begin strongly—people remember the first point.
- Use a clear, direct, and succinct style—this helps the learner to remain focused.
- Use the active voice—for example, the educator may say, "We will discuss relaxation techniques," instead of "Relaxation techniques will be discussed."
- Accentuate the positive—for example, the educator may say, "The majority of individuals are able to lose weight with a well-balanced diet and exercise," instead of "A few people have not been able to lose weight with a well-balanced diet and exercise."
- Use vivid communication, not statistics or jargon—specific case histories are often more meaningful than general, non-specific terms or dry statistics.
- Refer to trustworthy sources—for example, "the surgeon general" is a more credible source than "some people."
- Base strategies on a knowledge of the audience—be aware of the perceptions and perspectives of the audience.
- Make points explicitly—be direct, and give clear instructions.
- End strongly—the last point made is likely to be remembered.

Modified from Damrosch S: *Nurs Clin North Am* 26(4):833-843, 1991.

sented in a clear and organized manner, the learner will not receive or retain an optimum level of information. At various stages in the educational process, the educator must reassess learner readiness and be aware of possible barriers to effective communication (Hamachek, 1990). Emotional stress and physical illness are only two factors that may limit the amount of information a learner is able to absorb. The nurse educator must be aware of various factors affecting the learner and recognize that the needs and barriers influencing the learner's receptivity may vary from session to session. Educational strategies and activities can be developed and adjusted to fit the dynamic needs of the learner.

The educator is responsible for providing information that is understandable. Medical jargon and technical terms may interfere with the clarity of the intended message (Damrosch, 1991). For example, in helping clients understand diet control for hypertension, the nurse might use the phrase "high blood pressure" rather than the term "hypertension" to tailor the message to the learner's ability to understand. (See the box above, right, for communication guidelines in educational interactions.)

Selecting the Learning Format

The educator must decide how to teach. The educator selects an appropriate learning format, or strategy, for implementing the learning program. A format should be chosen that matches the goals and objectives of the program and should be adapted to meet the learning needs of the client. In addition, teaching tools such as printed materials or audiovisual aids that will enhance learning should be selected (MacDonald, 1991). Three examples of learning formats are outlined in the box on p. 257 (top, left).

Research Brief

Estey A, Musseau Al, Keehn L: Comprehension levels of patients reading health information, *Patient Educ Counseling* 18:165-169, 1991.

Printed educational materials are among the most convenient and economical methods of health education. Estey, Musseau, and Keehn evaluated reading materials developed at both the fifth- and the ninth-grade levels with general medical and surgical patients. They used the Wide Range Achievement Test–Revised (WRAT-R) to assess the reading levels of patients and the Cloze test to determine the reader's level of comprehension. They found that more subjects were able to understand the materials written at the fifth-grade reading level than those written at the ninth-grade level.

Selecting the Learning Environment

Educational programs quickly lose their effectiveness if the environment is not conducive to learning. The nurse can begin to establish an appropriate learning climate for an educational event when announcements of the program are made. The tone and appearance of letters, flyers, and media messages announcing the program draw a mental picture for participants of what the activity will be like. By carefully considering program objectives and information about the culture, beliefs, and educational level of learners, the nurse can develop preparatory materials

Examples of Learning Formats

1. The client is a large class of university students studying communicable diseases. The selected format is a lecture followed by a question-and-answer period.
2. The client is a group from a shelter for victims of domestic violence. The chosen format is an informal, small-group, open discussion following a short poster presentation.
3. The client is a family with a newly diagnosed, insulin-dependent, diabetic, 6-year-old child. The objectives are different for each family member. Therefore the format must be adapted to each member as well. The child requires materials appropriate to his or her developmental stage. The objectives for the child are to overcome fear of injections and to begin to deal with possible life-style changes. The material will be presented in the form of a picture book and storytelling that provides a realistic yet nonthreatening look at both the illness and the treatment. The objectives for the parents are to understand both the short- and the long-term ramifications of their child's disease and to learn the specific skills needed to manage the illness at home.
   a. Informational handouts will be gathered, and several medical journal articles will be copied and given to the parents to read.
   b. Insulin injection demonstrations and practice sessions will be provided.
   c. The nurse will provide the phone number of the clinic for follow-up questions, as well as phone numbers of several diabetes associations.
   d. The family members will be introduced to the local chapter of a support group appropriate to their specific needs. This support group will help them process their fears and concerns.

Environmental Realms

THE PHYSICAL REALM

This realm includes setting up the program and positioning the presenter and the clients in physical relation to one another. It also includes lighting and temperature of the room, volume of amplification equipment, furniture, and bathroom facilities. The more subtle effects of environment are those that create a stimulating setting, allow for few external distractions, and assist the learner in concentration and attention.

THE INTERPERSONAL REALM

This realm consists of human relationships and should be therapeutic, supportive, and conducive to producing quality educational interactions. The interpersonal dynamic should be one in which learners experience a clear sense that the educator cares about their progress and needs. Learners also can contribute to the interpersonal environment by showing interest in the subject and remaining responsive both to peer and to group interactions.

THE ORGANIZATIONAL REALM

This realm entails the administrative aspects of the educational program. Beginning with scheduling, announcements, and other preparations, this is the realm that makes the components of the program merge into an effective learning session. Arrangements for parking, delivery of audiovisual materials, ensuring readability of printed or projected materials, and responsiveness to ongoing learner needs and requests are a few examples of organizational aspects of environment.

From Knowles M: *The adult learner: a neglected species,* ed 4, Houston, 1990, Gulf.

---

that appeal to the target population (Knowles, 1990). During the program, it is important to create a positive, supportive, and pleasant atmosphere for the client so that learning can be maximized. Three environmental realms that should be considered are described in the box above, right.

Organizing Learning Experiences

Regardless of the educator's level of knowledge or the quality of the interpersonal relationship that the educator has developed with the learner, sound organization of the material is essential for learning to occur. Materials should be presented in a logical and integrated manner, from simple foundational concepts to more complex ideas. These should represent building blocks in a well-designed structure with a clear and unambiguous blueprint. The educator should reduce difficult or confusing concepts to their component parts and show the learner how to reassemble them one at a time. The pace of the presentation should match the ability of the learner and leave adequate pause for the learner to absorb the material.

The principles of continuity, sequence, and integration are important aids in the organization of educational programs. A lack of *continuity* causes a break in the flow of logical thought and may confuse the learner. One valuable technique that helps maintain continuity for the learner is repeated emphasis of essential points.

Sequencing means that each learning experience builds on the previous one and requires a higher level of functioning. Learning activities should be sequenced so that participants start with simple, easy-to-master exercises or materials and progress to more complex ones requiring greater skill, coordination, or understanding.

Integration of various aspects of the material demonstrates how each component fits into the whole. Without integration, the learner is left with a puzzle of disjointed facts or concepts that is difficult to assimilate in a productive way (Knowles, 1990).

Encouraging Participatory Learning

People learn better when they are actively involved in the learning process. Participation increases motivation, flexibility, and learning rate. Participatory learning is not limited to the psychomotor domain. The cognitive and affective domains also call for a teaching strategy in which the instructor enlists the active involvement of the learner. Verbal response or feedback, as long as it engages the learner, is participatory. Merely sitting and listening is not as effective as is discussion, even when the presentation is stimulating, interesting, and dynamic. Role play, acting out an experience, storytelling, "hands-on" training, and similar activities are good examples of participatory learning. Immediate feedback, an important advantage of participatory learning, ensures that errors are corrected before problematic habits or misconceptions develop. Computer-assisted learning provides immediate feedback to learners (Knowles, 1990).

The educator can structure learning activities and the environment to facilitate participatory learning. Using proper teaching materials, learners can be provided with adequate prompting and modeling to ensure their ability to practice and to demonstrate mastery of the material. By using the principle of participatory learning, the material becomes more accessible and meaningful to learners and is more likely to be retained and used in the future (Knowles, 1990).

Providing Evaluation and Feedback

It is essential to evaluate learning and provide constructive and helpful feedback to the learner throughout the educational process to avoid discouraging or offending the learner. Through clear and behaviorally focused feedback, clients can monitor their progress, level of knowledge, and learning needs. The educator may use tools such as quizzes, tests, completed study sheets, observation of skills, small-group tasks, and competency rating scales to evaluate learning outcomes. Not only should learners receive feedback, but the educator should also elicit feedback from learners throughout the educational process. Based on the feedback that the educator receives from learners, modifications in the implementation and presentation of the educational program can be made (Knowles, 1990).

THE EDUCATIONAL PROCESS

In addition to understanding the nature of learning, the events of instruction, and strategies for effective education, knowledge of the educational process is essential for the community health nurse. Interestingly, the educational and nursing processes are similar, and both are used at the individual, family, and community levels (Bigbee and Jansa, 1991). (See Table 13-4 for a comparison of the two processes.) Each step of the educational process is outlined in this section.

Identify Educational Needs

Community health nurses learn about the health education needs of their clients by performing a systematic and thorough client needs assessment. The steps of a needs assessment are listed in the box below. Once needs have been identified, they are prioritized so that the most critical educational needs are met first (Strodtman, 1984).

A variety of factors influence clients' learning needs and their ability to learn. Demographic, physical, geographical, economic, psychological, social, and spiritual characteristics of learners should be considered when identifying learning needs.

The educator must also understand how the learner's existing knowledge, skills, and motivation influence learning. Resources for and barriers to learning should be identified. Resources include printed materials, equipment, agencies, and other individuals. Barriers include lack of time, money, space, energy, confidence, and organizational support (Edwards, 1990). Communication barriers may result from cultural and language differences between the nurse and the client or from printed materials that are inappropriate to the client's reading level. Such adverse influences on the learning process can be minimized with a vigilant awareness of both initial and newly developing barriers during the educational process (Volker, 1991).

Establish Educational Goals and Objectives

Once learner needs are determined, goals and objectives to guide the educational program must be identified. Goals are broad, long-term expected outcomes such as, "Mr. Williams will become independently proficient in the care of his ostomy bag within 3

Table 13-4   A Comparison of the Nursing and Educational Processes

Nursing process	Educational process
Assessment	Identify educational needs
Diagnosis	Establish educational goals and objectives
Planning	Select appropriate educational methods
Implementation	Implement the educational plan
Evaluation	Evaluation of process and product

Data from Edwards L: In Edelman CL, Mandle CL, editors: *Health promotion throughout the lifespan*, St Louis, 1990, Mosby; Hawe P, Degeling D, Hall J: *Evaluating health promotion: a health worker's guide*, Philadelphia, 1990, MacLennan & Petty; and Strodtman LK: *Patient Educ Counseling* 5(4):189-200, 1984.

   The Steps of a Needs Assessment

1. Identify what the client wants to know.
2. Determine how the client wants to learn.
3. Discern what will enhance the client's ability and motivation to learn.
4. Collect data systematically from the client, family, and other sources to assess learning needs, readiness to learn, and situational and psychosocial factors influencing learning.
5. Analyze assessment data to identify cognitive, psychomotor, and affective learning needs.
6. Encourage client participation in the process.
7. Assist the client in prioritizing learning needs.

From Volker DL: *Oncol Nurs Forum* 18(1):119-123, 1991.

months." Goals of the program should directly address the client's overall learning needs.

Objectives are specific, short-term criteria that need to be met as steps toward achieving the long-term goal such as, "Mr. Williams will properly reattach his own ostomy bag, after the nurse has cleaned the site five consecutive times within 2 weeks." Objectives are written statements of an intended outcome or expected change in behavior and should define the minimum degree of knowledge or ability needed by a client (Green and Ottoson, 1994; Hawe et al., 1990; Strodtman, 1984). Objectives must be stated clearly, and expected outcomes must be defined in measurable terms. The four parts of an objective may be developed by answering the questions outlined in Table 13-5.

Select Appropriate Educational Methods

Methods should be chosen to facilitate the efficient and successful accomplishment of program goals and objectives. The methods should also be appropriately matched to the client's strengths and needs. Caution should be used to avoid complex methodological designs. The educator should choose the simplest, clearest, and most succinct manner of presentation. The educator should be proficient in using a broad array of tools designed to convey information (Knowles, 1990). A few examples of strategies that may be used to enhance learning are listed in the box above.

When nurses select educational methods, they should consider developmental disabilities, age, educational level, knowledge of the subject, and size of the group. Matching the media and other tools the needs of the learner is an important skill for educators to develop.

For example, clients with a visual impairment may need more verbal description. Clients with hearing

Strategies to Enhance Learning

Printed materials
Audiovisual materials
Computer-assisted learning
Demonstrations
Guest speakers
Role play
Field trips
Peer presentations
Peer counseling and tutoring

impairments may need increased visual description. Speakers who can use sign language may be necessary. Also, limitations in attention and concentration require creative methods and tools for keeping the learner focused. Such methods and tools include frequent breaks; austere, nondistractive surroundings; small-group interactions that keep the learner involved and interested; and the use of "hands-on" equipment such as mannequins, models, and other materials the learner can physically manipulate. Comprehension and retention are related to the depth or intensity of the learner's involvement. The educator tries to involve the learner appropriately and creatively in a variety of ways and as actively as possible.

Implement the Educational Plan

Once educational methods have been selected, they should be implemented through management of the educational process. Implementation entails (1) control over starting, sustaining, and stopping each method and strategy in the most effective and appropriate time and manner; (2) the coordination and control of environmental factors, the flow of presenta-

Table 13-5 The Four Parts of an Objective

Question	Example
	String all "a" phrases together as one sentence for one example. String all "b" and "c" phrases together in like manner.
Who is to exhibit the behavior?	a. Each member of the Jones family b. Ms. Smith c. Eighty percent of the target population
What behavior is expected?	a. will give an insulin injection to Billy b. will perform a blood sugar test on herself c. will take their children to receive immunizations
Conditions and qualifiers of behavior.	a. with accuracy regarding dosage b. with accuracy regarding the blood sugar reading c. within 1 month of the immunization due date
Standards of behavior or performance.	a. 100% of the time for ten consecutive trials. b. within 10 points of the educator's reading for ten consecutive trials. c. for 100% of standard childhood disease immunizations.

From Green LW, Ottoson JM: *Community health*, ed 7, St Louis, 1994, Mosby; and Hawe P, Degeling D, Hall J: *Evaluating health promotion: a health worker's guide*, Philadelphia, 1990, MacLennan & Petty.

tion, and other contributory facets of the program; and (3) keeping the materials logically related to the core theme and overall program goals.

The educator must be flexible. He or she must modify educational methods and strategies to meet unexpected challenges that may confront both the educator and the learner. External influences such as time limitations, expense, administrative and political factors, and learner needs require an ongoing evaluation of their impact on the educational program (Knowles, 1990; Strodtman, 1984). Thus, implementation is a dynamic element in the educational process.

Evaluate the Educational Process

Evaluation is as important in the educational process as it is in the nursing process. Evaluation provides a systematic and logical method for making decisions to improve the educational program. Educational evaluation involves three areas (Hawe et al., 1990):
1. Educator evaluation
2. Process evaluation
3. Product evaluation

Both educator and process evaluation are described in this section. Product evaluation is described in the next section.

Educator Evaluation

Feedback to the educator allows for modifications in the teaching process and enables the nurse to better meet the learner's needs. The learner's evaluation of the educator occurs continuously throughout the educational program. The educator may receive feedback from the learner in written form, such as an evaluation sheet. The educator may also receive feedback verbally or nonverbally, as in return demonstrations and by facial expressions (Knowles, 1990).

The educator should assume that inadequate learner responses reflect an inadequate program, not an inadequate learner. If evaluation reveals that the learning objectives are not being met, the nurse must determine why the instruction is not effective. It is then the educator's responsibility to present the material creatively and meaningfully in new ways that will increase learner retention and the learner's ability to apply the new knowledge (Hawe et al., 1990; Knowles, 1990). Ultimately, the educator must assume responsibility for the success or failure of the educational process and the development of learner knowledge, skills, and abilities.

Process Evaluation

Process evaluation examines the dynamic components of the educational program. It follows and assesses the movements and management of information transfer and attempts to keep the objectives on track. Process evaluation is necessary *throughout* the educational program to determine whether goals and objectives are being met and the time required for

their accomplishment. Ongoing evaluation also allows the teacher to correct misinformation, misinterpretation, or confusion.

Goals and objectives also should be periodically reconsidered. The nurse must ask if the desired health behavior change is really necessary. Such a question inevitably leads back to the original learning objectives and encourages the nurse to rethink the practicality and merit of each of the objectives. Finally, factors that influence learner readiness and motivation should be reassessed if teaching seems to be ineffective. Process evaluation uses information gathered from the educator as well as from learner evaluations and assesses the dynamics of their interactions (Hawe et al., 1990; Knowes, 1990).

THE EDUCATIONAL PRODUCT

The educational product is the outcome of the educational process. The product is measured both qualitatively and quantitatively. For instance, a qualitative assessment should answer the question, "How well does the learner appear to understand the content?" A quantitative assessment should answer the question, "How much of the content does the learner retain?" Thus the quality of the product is measured by improvement and increase, or the lack thereof, of the learner's knowledge, skill, and abilities related to the content of the educational program.

In community health nursing the educational product is assessed as a measurable change in the health or behavior of the client. Evaluation of the educational product can be divided into three components:
1. Evaluation of health and behavioral changes
2. Short-term evaluation
3. Long-term evaluation

Did You Know?

Whichever methods of evaluation the nurse uses to determine teaching and program effectiveness, a helpful concept to keep in mind is that of the curve of normal distribution. In any group of learners, about 2% will be extremely negative, and 2% will be extrememly positive in their evaluation of the program. Another 14% will be fairly negative, and 14% will be quite enthusiastic. The majority of participants (68%) will be somewhat neutral in their responses. Therefore, even though the nurse should consider the extremely negative responses, alarm or discouragement should not appear until the proportion of extremely negative responses rises above 16%.

From Knowles MS: *The modern practice of adult educatoin: from pedagogy to andragogy,* ed 4, Chicago, 1980, Follett.

Evaluation of Health and Behavioral Changes

A variety of approaches, methods, and tools can be used to evaluate health and behavioral change. These include questionnaires, surveys, skills demonstrations, testing, subjective client feedback, and direct observation of improvements in client mastery of materials. Qualitative or quantitative strategies may be used, depending on the nature of the expected educational outcome. Evaluation of outcomes measured includes changes in knowledge, skills, abilities, attitudes, behavior, health status, and quality of life (Hawe et al., 1990).

Approaches to evaluating health education effects will vary, depending on the situation. For example, when considering a client's ability to perform a psychomotor skill, such as changing a dressing, viewing the actual performance of the skill is the most appropriate means of evaluation. A second, more complex example is the nurse's completion of the implementation phase of a family education program. The nurse might use a specific tool, such as the Family Assessment Device, a self-report instrument designed specifically to evaluate the effects of clinical interventions for families, to measure learning. The family functioning components that the Family Assessment Device measures are problem solving, communication, roles, affective responsiveness, affective involvement, behavior control, and general functioning (Reeber, 1992). This type of evaluation tool is necessary to measure a wide array of variables; when working with families, educational outcomes may sometimes be manifested in unexpected ways.

If evaluation of the educational product shows positive changes in health status and health-related behaviors, the educator can expect good results in similar health educational programs. If evaluation of the educational product shows that either no changes or negative changes in health status and health-related behaviors resulted, then various components of the educational process can be examined and modified to produce better results in the future (Redman, 1993).

Short-Term Evaluation

It is important to evaluate short-term health and behavioral effects of health education programs and determine if they are really caused by the educational program. Short-term objectives are often easy to evaluate (Edwards, 1990; Green and Ottoson, 1994; Hawe et al., 1990). For example, a **short-term evaluation** of whether or not a client can perform a return demonstration of breast self-examination requires minimal energy, expense, or time; skill mastery can be determined within a matter of minutes. If the short-term objective is not met, the nurse determines why and identifies possible solutions so that successful learning can occur. If the short-term objective is met, the nurse can then focus on the long-term evaluation designed to assess the lasting effects of the education program, in this case, that of ongoing monthly breast self-examinations performed by the learner independently and at home.

Long-Term Evaluation

The ultimate goal of health education is to help clients make lasting behavioral changes that will improve their overall health status. Long-term follow-up with clients is a challenging task. Even though clients make positive behavioral changes and their health status improves, they often no longer use the health care services of the nurse (Redman, 1993). Some of the other reasons long-term evaluation can be challenging are listed in the box below.

Long-term evaluation is geared toward following and assessing the status of an individual client, family, or community over time. The tools of evaluation are designed to assess whether or not specific goals and objectives were met. Also, the extent and direction of changes in health status and health behaviors that the client has experienced are monitored (Redman, 1993).

For community health nurse educators, the goal of long-term evaluation is to analyze the effectiveness of the education program, not the specific health status of the individual client. Nurses track the client's (who may be an entire community) performance of objectives over time. They do not track the community members themselves. Thus, in a changing population, long-term evaluation of the results of an education program is still possible. The percentage of objectives and goals met by a sampling of the target population gives valid statistics for program assessment,

 Why Long-Term Evaluation is Challenging

COOPERATION

Clients may not comply with return appointments or calls.
May show a lack of interest in their own health care.
Clients may think it is too time-consuming or expensive to follow up.

TIME

Follow-up requires making phone calls, evaluating clients, and reviewing and analyzing the results of the evaluation.

ENERGY

Follow-up requires the educator to keep track of clients and to relocate those who have moved.
The nurse must obtain the cooperation of clients.
The nurse must balance long-term evaluation responsibilities with other demands.

EXPENSE

Travel, phone calls, mail, and staff time are all expenses related to long-term evaluation follow-up.

even though the individual population may have experienced a complete turnover.

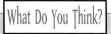

What Do You Think?

Community health nurse educators should be involved in health education related to sexual education for adolescents because information about abortion, abstinence, birth control, peer pressure, rape, and sexually transmitted diseases is important for this age group.

For example, a community health nurse notes that according to annual health department data, 60% of all pregnant women in the nurse's catchment area received some prenatal care. Wanting to increase this percentage to 100%, the nurse tries an educational intervention in which radio and television stations make public service announcements about the importance and availability of prenatal services.

After 1 year, the nurse discovers that 80% of all pregnant women now receive prenatal care. The nurse continues to use public service announcements the following year because good results are evident. The long-term goal is to reach 100% compliance with the education program. Therefore the community health nurse also enlists volunteers to put informational posters in shopping malls, grocery stores, public transportation stops, laundries, and on public transportation vehicles. The second year after implementing interventions, again using the statistics from the health department, the nurse finds that 95% of all pregnant women in the target area now receive prenatal care. The nurse can thus evaluate a community educational program over time and increase the rate, range, and consistency of progress made toward meeting the goals of the project.

Clinical Application

In this section the educational concepts that have been highlighted in this chapter are applied to a clinical situation. (Refer to Figure 13-1, which shows the sequence of actions that a community health nurse follows when developing an educational program.)

Identifying an Educational Need

During an initial survey of a community, the nurse finds in local school records that an unusually large percentage of elementary school children are not receiving standard immunizations for communicable childhood diseases. The nurse identifies education about immunizations as a need in the community.

Assessing Strengths, Needs, and Barriers

The nurse then performs an assessment, which shows that the majority of the parents are of a certain ethnic group, are single, work full time, and are of a lower socioeconomic status. The nurse designs a simple verbal questionnaire that includes questions about attitudes and beliefs related to immunizations and assigns several pollsters to speak with a sampling of the parents. The following barriers to learning are identified:

1. Lack of awareness about the need for and the benefits of immunization
2. Belief that immunizations can be harmful to children
3. Belief that immunizations are expensive
4. Inability to get time off from work to have children immunized

The nurse next develops a strengths-and-needs list from the information gathered in the survey. Strengths that the nurse finds in the community members are their desire to be good parents and their involvement in the parent/teacher organization. The survey also demonstrates that the average education of the parents is at a tenth-grade level, another strength. The nurse identifies the following as client needs: knowledge about the existence and benefits of immunization, valid information about the risks of immunization, knowledge that immunizations are free, and information about the availability and accessibility of immunizations through the school system. Parents also need to know that the community has a mobile immunization unit. It operates in the evenings for families with infants and preschoolers and who do not have transportation available to them.

Choosing an Educational Theory

The nurse next matches the characteristics of the learner to an educational theory. In this case, the community health nurse educator chooses to combine and apply three theories to the educational situation. The social learning theory is chosen because of the desire to influence the parents' beliefs and expectations. The cognitive theory is chosen because the nurse believes that the parents will respond to a variety of information. The humanistic theory is selected because the client is a close-knit, supportive community and is strongly devoted to its children.

Choosing A Health Educational Model

The nurse educator selects a health education model for adaptation to the learner. The health belief model is chosen because of the need to change many of the parents' beliefs about immunizations. Based on the principles of this model, the nurse expects that the

Clinical Application—cont'd

behaviors of the parents will change once their beliefs change.

Choosing Educational Principles

The nurse considers educational principles and determines that the educational format should be that of a "town meeting." The most convenient environment conducive to the concentration and comfort of the group is the local high-school theater. To complete the design of the format, the nurse plans an informal lecture about immunizations. A local family physician, who grew up in the neighborhood and has family still living in the community, will give the lecture. After the talk, parents will be invited to ask questions and discuss issues. The program will conclude by encouraging parents to enjoy snacks and socialize with each other. Small discussion groups will be encouraged to develop into community action groups of those who think that immunizations are important.

MOPping up the Details

The community health nurse also organizes other educational methods, objectives, plans, and strategies (MOPS). For example, the nurse may ask interested parents to volunteer in the arrangement of further meetings.

Once the previously listed plans and strategies have been developed, the nurse then implements them. First, the nurse arranges a meeting with as many of the target group as possible through the local parent/teacher organization. The meeting is widely advertised through direct mailing to the target group and through notices that the children take home with their report cards. Public service announcements on the local television news and radio broadcasts are made. Carpools and shuttle vans are arranged for those who call for assistance with transportation. The date and time of the program are made as convenient as possible.

Evaluating the Educational Program

Soon after the strategies for these objectives have been implemented, the community health nurse educator develops an evaluation program for 3 months, 6 months, 9 months, and 1 year after the initiation of the educational program to evaluate the success of the program. The central criterion for the determination of success is the number of children receiving immunizations. Thus, even as the specific individuals change over time, the program evaluation process can be applied far into the future without the need for fundamental revision.

Key Concepts

- Health education is a vital component of community health nursing because the promotion, maintenance, and restoration of health rely on client's understanding of health care requirements.
- Six important general educational theories used to guide the practice of the community health nurse educator are behavioral, social learning, cognitive, humanist, developmental, and critical theories.
- Three current and useful models for organizing health education are the PRECEDE-PROCEED, health belief, and health promotion models.
- Three domains of learning are cognitive, affective, and psychomotor. Depending on the needs of the learner, one or more of these domains may be important for the community health nurse educator to consider as learning programs are developed.

- Nine principles associated with instruction are gaining attention, informing the learner of the objectives of instruction, stimulating recall of prior learning, presenting the stimulus, providing learning guidance, eliciting performance, providing feedback, assessing performance, and enhancing retention and transfer of knowledge.
- Principles that guide the effective educator include message, format, environment, experience, participation, and evaluation.
- The five phases of the educational process are to identify educational needs, establish educational goals and objectives, select appropriate educational methods, implement the educational plan, and evaluate the educational process and product.
- Evaluation of the product includes the measurement of short-term and long-term goals and objectives related to improving health and promoting behavioral changes.

Critical Thinking Activities

1. Review the general theories of learning summarized in the chapter, and decide which one would most effectively fit the learning needs of an individual who has been recently diagnosed with lung cancer, a family caring for an individual with Alzheimer's disease, and a community in which adolescent cigarette smoking is on the rise.

2. Recall an educational interaction with a client that did not seem to go well. Identify what might have been the problem, based on educational principles. Develop a plan for ways in which the interaction could have been improved, again based on educational principles.

3. Recall a learning experience in which either the message, format, environment, experience, participation, or evaluation were problematic. Then, develop a plan for how the problem could have been overcome and turned from a negative or neutral learning situation into a positive one.

4. Review the phases of the educational process, and apply this process to an individual with hypertension, a family with a child who has attention deficit disorder, and a community in which tuberculosis is on the rise.

Bibliography

Annand F: A challenge for the 1990s: patient education, *Today's OR Nurse* 15(1)31-35, 1993.

Bigbee JL, Jansa N: Strategies for promoting health protection, *Nurs Clin North Am* 26(4):895-912, 1991.

Blair JE: Social learning theory: strategies for health promotion, *AAOHN J* 41(5):245-249, 1993.

Clarke HF Beddome G, Whyte NB: Public health nurses' vision of their future reflects changing paradigms, *Image J Nurs Scholarship* 25(4):305-310, 1993.

Damrosch S: General strategies for motivating people to change their behavior, *Nurs Clin North Am* 26(4):833-843, 1991.

Dembo MH: *Applying educational psychology,* ed 5, New York, 1994, Longman.

Dignam D: Cinderella and the four learning theories, *Nurs Praxis NZ* 7(3):17-20, 1992.

Driscoll MP: *Psychology of learning for instruction,* Boston, 1994, Allyn & Bacon.

Edwards L: Health education. In Edelman CL, Mandle CL, editors: *Health promotion throughout the lifespan,* St Louis, 1990, Mosby.

Estey A, Musseau A, Keehn L: Comprehension levels of patients reading health information, *Patient Educ Counseling* 18:165-169, 1991.

Graham KY: Health care reform and public health nursing, *Public Health Nurs* 9(2):73, 1992.

Green LW, Kreuter MW: CDC's planned approach to community health as an application or PRECEDE and an inspiration for PROCEED, *J Health Educ* 23(3):140-147, 1992.

Green, LW, Ottoson JM: *Community health,* ed 7, St Louis, 1994, Mosby.

Hamachek D: *Psychology in teaching, learning, and growth,* ed 4, Boston, 1990, Allyn & Bacon.

Hancock LA, Mandle CL: Overview of growth and developmental framework. In Edelman CL, Mandle CL, editors: *Health promotion throughout the lifespan,* St Louis, 1990, Mosby.

Hawe P, Degeling D, Hall J: *Evaluating health promotion: a health worker's guide,* Philadelphia, 1990, MacLennan & Petty.

Knowles M: *The adult learner: a neglected species,* ed 4, Houston, 1990, Gulf.

Knowles MS: *The modern practice of adult education: from pedagogy to andragogy,* ed 4, Chicago, 1980, Follett.

MacDonald RE: *A handbook of basic skills and strategies for beginning teachers: facing the challenge of teaching in today's schools,* Chico, Calif, 1991, Longman.

Padilla GV, Bulcavage LM: Theories used in patient/health education, *Semin Oncol Nurs* 7(2):87-96, 1991.

Palank CL: Determinants of health-promotive behavior: a review of current research, *Nurs Clin North Am* 26(4):815-832, 1991.

Redman BK: Patient education at 25 years: where we have been and where we are going, *J Adv Nurs* 18(5):725-730, 1993.

Reeber BJ: Evaluating the effects of a family education intervention, *Rehabil Nurs,* 17(6):332-336, 1992.

Salazar MK: Comparison of four behavioral theories, *AAOHN J* 39(3):128-135, 1991.

Simmons SJ: The Health-Promoting Self-Care System Model: directions for nursing research and practice, *J Adv Nurs* 15(10):1162-1166, 1990.

Strodtman LK: A decision-making process for planning patient education, *Patient Educ Counseling* 5(4):189-200, 1984.

Volker DL: Patient education: needs assessment and resource identification, *Oncol Nurs Forum* 18(1):119-123, 1991.

Welton MR: The contribution of critical theory to our understanding of adult learning. In Merriam SB, editor: *An update on adult learning theory,* San Francisco, 1993, Jossey-Bass.

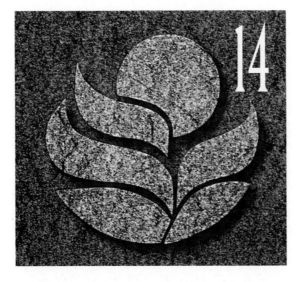

14

Community Health Promotion: A Multilevel Framework for Practice

Pamela A. Kulbok ◆ Shirley C. Laffrey ◆ Jean Goeppinger

Objectives

After reading this chapter, the student should be able to do the following:

◆ Compare and contrast definitions of health.
◆ Describe the influence of his or her definition of health on nursing practice.
◆ Contrast the health paradigm and the pathogenic paradigm as the basis for health promotion and illness prevention interventions.
◆ Discuss the interrelationship of individual, family, aggregate, and community as the target of health promotion strategies.
◆ Describe and use methods of assessing the health risks of individuals, families, aggregates, and community groups.
◆ Discuss multilevel approaches to promote health, prevent illness and reduce risk in individuals, families, aggregates, and community groups.
◆ State the reasons why community health nursing roles are essential to health promotion and illness prevention.

Outline

Life-style is the most critical modifiable factor influencing the health of Americans today. There has been sustained interest in healthy life-styles since the rise of the self-care movement of the 1960s. Many Americans exercise regularly, maintain their weight at recommended levels, and deliberately attempt to manage their stress. Some drive at reduced speeds, drink fewer alcoholic beverages than in the past, and smoke less or not at all. Others jog or walk on country lanes and in city parks, participate in structured physical fitness programs, and engage in a variety of relaxation techniques at home and at work. Similarly, evidence indicates a growing interest among nurses in the promotion of health through healthy life-styles. This has been demonstrated in the work of such researchers as Kulbok and Baldwin (1992), Laffrey et al. (1986), Pender (1987), and Woods (1989).

Community health nursing is based on a synthesis of public health and nursing knowledge. Three concepts—health, health promotion, and community—provide the major cornerstones for a multilevel framework for community health nursing practice. These concepts and the particular way they are linked together determine the direction and methods for community health nursing practice. This chapter focuses on the historical roots and definitions of the three concepts and a discussion of the community frameworks used by community health nurses to guide their practice, education, and research. We discuss and emphasize that the manner in which health, health promotion, and community are related is an important factor in the nurse's orientation to practice.

HEALTH AND HEALTH PROMOTION
Historical Perspectives

Health is the pivotal term in a framework for community health nursing practice. Beginning with Nightingale's efforts to discover and use the laws to serve humanity and moving to a contemporary view of nursing's central concern—the meaning attached to life and health (Fitzpatrick, 1989)—community health nursing is concerned with promoting the health of populations and of the total community. The concept of health shapes the process of community health nursing from assessment of the health-related needs of individuals, families, aggregates, and communities to evaluation of behavioral outcomes. Although health ranks among nursing's essential concepts—person, health, environment, and nursing—it is the least well understood and the most elusive of the four concepts.

Descriptions of the nature of health evolved through philosophical and scientific inquiry. The ancient Greek view of health was that the totality of environmental forces, including living habits, climate, and quality of air, water, and food, influences the condition of human well-being. Just as this holistic view of health very likely began before recorded history, the concept of

people helping themselves in health matters is not new. References to self-care in classical literature include mythical and religious elements, as well as pragmatic components. For instance, in Greek literature the goddess Hygeia represented the belief that humans could remain healthy if they lived rationally. Certain activities of daily living, such as exercise, were considered essential to the maintenance of health. Similarly, in biblical times, various food laws were instituted that promoted health. (See box on p. 267 for the development of the concept of health over time.)

Scientific medicine emerged slowly during the sixteenth to the nineteenth centuries. Formidable resistance to scientific discoveries, such as the germ theory of disease and the principle of antisepsis, impeded the translation of new medical science into medical practice. However, in the twentieth century, medical science grew in power, and the dramatic pace of scientific progress was characterized as a revolution (Somers and Somers, 1961). With the development of scientific and biological orientation toward disease, self-care was steadily deemphasized in favor of professional care.

The holistic view of health was formally introduced by the South African philosopher Jan Christian Smuts in 1926 as an antidote to the prevailing reductionistic view of medical science. It was a way of comprehending whole organisms and systems as entities greater than and different from the sum of their parts (Smuts, 1926). Smuts' holistic perspective of health was overshadowed by the scientific view of disease as a deviation from the biochemical norm. A focus on treatment and cure, with its dependence on health professionals, continued to overshadow self-care, health promotion, and illness prevention. Despite a growing emphasis on self-care, the biomedical emphasis continues to this day.

During the past three decades, the idea of *self-care* as derived from a positive idea of health has reemerged. In some cases, self-care competes with professional care. For example, some proponents of self-care emphasize lay diagnosis and self-treatment, as opposed to professional diagnosis and collaborative management. Other, more conservative versions of self-care focus on teaching people how to work with their health care providers. In either case, the professional health care system is dramatically affected, and professional roles are being renegotiated with an emphasis on collaboration between consumers and providers.

The revitalization of self-care in the United States may represent a cyclical recurrence of the more general self-help theme. Americans on the frontier did not have the benefit of expert advice and often lived far from professional medical help. In the true spirit of Jacksonian democracy, they not only depended on themselves, but often scorned advice from outsiders. In health matters, as in other areas, the older, wiser, and more experienced family members were the experts. They may have consulted the medical encyclopedia on the parlor bookshelf or used folk remedies.

In either case, self-care retained its original religious links. Early popular self-care books, such as the *Primitive Physic* by John Wesley (1747), were recommended regularly at prairie revivals.

The reemergence of the self-care movement also was accelerated by the political climate of the 1960s and 1970s. Authority, in general, was challenged. Racial minorities began to demand their rights in the 1960s; women and elderly persons began to make their demands public in the 1970s. A challenge to the professional health care system, which many believe exemplifies elite rather than democratic control, is illustrated clearly in the ideology of self-care. Illich, for example, wrote, "The medical establishment has become a major threat to health. The disabling impact of professional control over medicine has reached the proportions of an epidemic" (1976, p. 3). Illich chastised U.S. health professionals and society for robbing individuals of their self-care skills. He warned that politicians and legislators may promote self-care because of their interest in cost containment rather than a genuine belief in individuals' abilities to preserve health.

The viewpoint that the individual is in a position to produce health is shared by many health professionals. Fuchs (1974), in his study *Who Shall Live,* suggested that the "greatest potential for improving health lies in what we do and don't do for and to ourselves." Other self-care advocates believe that modern medicine has been given too much credit for improvements in health. Wildavsky (1977) asserted that the medical system affects only 10% of the variability in health indicators such as infant mortality, disability

Health Perspectives Over Time

Ancient Greek View
  Health was the totality of environmental forces influencing human well-being.
  Ways of living were essential to maintain health.
1700s to 1800s
  Scientific discoveries were opposed, such as the germ theory of disease and the principle of antisepsis.
  Translation of new medical science into medical practice was impeded.
Early to middle 1900s
  Holistic view of health was reintroduced as an antidote to the medical science model.
  Scientific and biologic view of disease dominated.
  Self-care was deemphasized.
Late 1900s
  Reemergence of the ideal of self-care was accelerated by the climate of political activism.
  Increased recognition that people produce health by what they do and don't do for themselves.
  Collaboration between consumers and providers and renegotiation of professional roles in health care.

days, and adult mortality. He attributed the remaining 90% to factors over which physicians lack control, "from individual lifestyle (smoking, exercise, worry), to social conditions (income, eating habits, physiological inheritance), to the physical environment (air and water quality)" (p. 105).

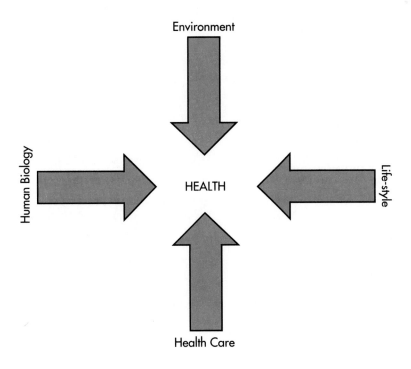

FIGURE 14-1

Determinants of health. (Modified from LaLonde M: *A new perspective on the health of Canadians,* Ottawa, 1974, Government of Canada.)

In the political arena, these conclusions were supported first by LaLonde in *A New Perspective on the Health of Canadians* (1974). As the Canadian Minister of National Health and Welfare, LaLonde urged a more comprehensive approach to health care. He identified four major determinants of health: human biology, environment, life-style, and health care (Figure 14-1). LaLonde's ideas were echoed by policy makers in the United States. The *Forward Plan for Health, FY 1978-82* acknowledged that ". . . the best hope of achieving any significant extension of life expectancy lies in the area of . . . prevention . . . the greatest benefits are likely to accrue from efforts to improve the health habits of all Americans and the environment in which they live and work" (U.S. Department of Health, Education and Welfare, 1976, p. 69). (The box at right lists some landmark initiatives in health promotion and disease prevention.)

The U.S. Public Health Service first established national objectives involving disease prevention, health protection, and health promotion strategies in the surgeon general's report *Healthy People* (U.S. Department of Health, Education and Welfare, 1979). Disease prevention strategies focused on priority services such as family planning, immunizations, and high blood pressure control, delivered in public and private clinical settings. Health protection strategies are directed to environmental or regulatory measures designed to "significantly improve health and the quality of life for this and future generations of Americans . . ." (p. 101), including occupational safety and health and accidental injury control. Health promotion strategies are designed to achieve well-being through community and individual life-style change measures. Health promotion is described as beginning with people who are basically healthy and who are seeking to enhance their life-styles. The surgeon general's report (1979) also described inherited biological factors, the environment, and behavioral factors as the three categories of risks to health. These are identical to LaLonde's first three major determinants of health.

Although a national initiative for health promotion was slowly gaining momentum in the United States, disease prevention continued to be the main focus for intervention. In 1990 a shift was evident in the new report on national health objectives, *Healthy People 2000* (1991). The 1991 report described the same three strategies for health as the 1979 report. However, in *Healthy People 2000* the three terms were reordered. The emphasis was placed on health promotion *first*, then health protection, and finally, preventive services (Kulbok and Baldwin, 1992). The objectives listed in *Healthy People 2000* address the determinants of health status as originally described by LaLonde: human biology, environment, life-style, and health care. All four determinants are essential for community health nursing practice.

The politics of the existing illness care system poses a major difficulty for promoting holistic health. The health care industry is a big business, with a vested in-

Landmark Health Promotion/Disease Prevention Initiatives*

1974 LaLonde's *New Perspectives on the Health of Canadians*
1976 *Forward Plan for Health*, FY 1978-82
1979 The surgeon general's report *Healthy People*
1989 *Guide to Clinical Preventive Services*
1990 *Healthy People: 2000*
1991 Nursing's Agenda for Health Care Reform
1994 Put Prevention into Practice (PPIP) program

---

*1974, Canada; 1976 to 1994 entries, United States.

terest in keeping the biomedical model in place. Nursing's Agenda for Health Care Reform (American Nurses Association [ANA], 1991) challenges the utility of the medical care system. Under the joint leadership of the ANA and the National League for Nursing (NLN), more than 60 nursing and allied health care organizations, representing 1 million nurses, health professionals, and consumers, have endorsed a landmark reform agenda for a true "health" care system (Reifsnider, 1992). Historically, community health nurses have been leaders in providing primary health care (Stanhope, 1995) and enhancing wellness in populations (Fry, 1983). Their rich experience positions community health nurses to assume leadership in "health" care reform endeavors.

What Do You Think?

The politics of the existing illness care system is a major obstacle to holistic health promotion. The health care industry is a big business, with a vested interest in keeping the biomedical model in place.

Definitions of Health

The World Health Organization (WHO, 1958) reflected a holistic perspective in its classic definition of multidimensional **health** as a state of complete physical, mental, and social well-being and not merely the absence of disease and infirmity. This definition was considered both visionary and idealistic. However, the WHO perspective did have problems with definition and measurement (Ahmed et al., 1979; Kulbok, 1983).

In 1975, Terris noted that the WHO definition of health was considered by epidemiologists to be "vague and imprecise with a Utopian aura" (p. 1037). Terris therefore expanded the WHO definition: "Health is a state of physical, mental and social well-being and the ability to function and not merely the absence of illness and infirmity" (p. 1038). In adding "ability to function" and deleting the word "complete" from the WHO definition, the WHO definition was placed in a more realistic context, providing an important and useful framework for health promotion practice, education, and research.

Smith (1981) maintained that nursing's idea of health directs the nature of our practice, education, and research. She further clarified the idea of health by observing that, in existing literature, health was consistently described as a comparative concept, allowing for "more" or "less," or gradations, along a health-illness continuum. Smith proposed four models of health, ordered from narrow and concrete to broad and abstract: (1) clinical health, or the absence of disease; (2) role performance health, or the ability to perform one's social roles satisfactorily; (3) adaptive health, or flexible adaptation to the environment; and (4) eudaemonistic health, or self-actualization and the attainment of one's greatest human potential.

It is important for community health nurses to examine their personal conception of health and recognize how their definition of health and their nursing care are directed by their health conception. A nurse who defines health as the absence of disease is likely to focus primarily on physical and biological signs and symptoms of disease with minimal attention to the quality of social roles and evidence of subjective well-being. A nurse who broadly defines health as self-actualization is more likely to consider indicators of physical health, social health, and the potential for maximum well-being when planning nursing care.

Many unanswered questions surround the nature of health. Are health and illness two distinct states, or are they opposite ends of a single continuum? If health is accepted as a multidimensional concept, is one health dimension dominant? Does the presence of "more" mental or social health compensate for "less" physical health or the inability to function? In Smith's (1981) categories of health, eudaemonistic health or well-being subsumes the adaptive, role performance, and clinical models of health. This implies the dominance of self-actualization or well-being over biological health and social function. Does this mean that the greatest capacity for health exists in the human potential for self-actualization, regardless of whether one is ill or is able to function within one's socially and personally defined roles? Community health nurses have contributed to this ongoing discussion of the nature of health in individuals and communities by emphasizing positive health and health promotion, while acknowledging the importance of illness and disease.

Definitions of Health Promotion

Health promotion is an accepted aim of community health nursing practice, although it is rarely defined and is not consistently differentiated from disease prevention or health maintenance (Brubaker, 1983). It has even been observed that health promotion and

disease prevention are "two sides of one coin" (Breslow, 1990).

Leavell and Clark (1965) strongly influenced the evolution of health promotion and disease prevention strategies. They presented classic definitions of primary, secondary, and tertiary levels of prevention that were rooted in the biomedical model of health and epidemiology. The application of any preventive measure, according to Leavell and Clark, corresponds to the natural history of any human disease. Primary preventive measures are directed toward "well" individuals in the prepathogenesis period to promote their health and to provide specific protection from disease. Secondary and tertiary preventive measures are applied to diagnose or to treat individuals in the period of disease pathogenesis (Figure 14-2).

Even though primary, secondary, and tertiary levels of prevention had their origins in the medical model, Leavell and Clark moved beyond the medical model. They conceptualized primary prevention as two distinct components: health promotion and specific protection. Health promotion focuses on general positive measures such as education for healthy living and promotion of favorable environmental conditions. According to Leavell and Clark, health promotion includes periodic selective examinations such as routine well-child evaluation for developmental assessment and health education. The other aspect of primary prevention, specific protection, includes measures to reduce the threat of specific diseases. Among these measures are immunizations, hygiene, and the elimination of hazards in one's workplace (Kulbok and Baldwin, 1992).

When health promotion and specific protection are described as subconcepts of primary "prevention," they appear to stem from a definition of health as the absence of disease. However, differences in health promotion and specific protection strategies suggest they are not the same. Some terms used to describe health promotion are linked to a positive view of health, including health behavior, health-enhancing behavior, health habits, health practices, healthy life-style, and self-care behavior. Other terms are linked to a negative view of health as the absence of disease and include preventive health behavior, disease or illness prevention, health-protecting behavior, health-negating behavior, and risk reduction (Kulbok and Baldwin, 1992). The confusion in terminology is increased when actions to promote health, protect health, and prevent disease are used interchangeably as indicators of preventive behavior (Coburn and Pope, 1974; Green, 1969; Kulbok, 1983; Langlie, 1977).

Kasl and Cobb (1966) presented a set of definitions to distinguish health behavior from illness and sick role behavior. **Health behavior** was defined as any action to prevent or detect disease in the asymptomatic stage undertaken by a person who believes himself or herself to be healthy. This definition represented a beginning focus on prevention and detection but, because it was restricted to actions to prevent or detect

The Natural History of Any Disease of Man

Prepathogenesis period			Period of pathogenesis	
Health promotion	**Specific protection**	**Early diagnosis and prompt treatment**	**Disability limitation**	**Rehabilitation**
Health education	Use of specific immunizations	Case-finding measures, individual and mass	Adequate treatment to arrest the disease process and to prevent further complications and sequelae	Provision of hospital and community facilities for retraining and education for maximum use of remaining capacities
Good standard of nutrition adjusted to developmental phases of life	Attention to personal hygiene	Screening surveys		
	Use of environmental sanitation	Selective examinations		Education of the public and industry to utilize the rehabilitated
Attention to personality development	Protection against occupational hazards	Objectives: To cure and prevent disease processes	Provision of facilities to limit disability and to prevent death	
Provision of adequate housing, recreation, and agreeable working conditions	Protection from accidents	To prevent the spread of communicable diseases		As full employment as possible
	Use of specific nutrients	To prevent complications and sequelae		Selective placement
Marriage counseling and sex education	Protection from carcinogens	To shorten period of disability		Work therapy in hospitals
Genetics	Avoidance of all allergens			Use of sheltered colony
Periodic selective examinations				
Primary prevention		**Secondary prevention**		**Tertiary prevention**
Levels of application of preventive measures				

FIGURE 14-2

Levels of application of preventive measures in the natural history of disease. (From Leavell HR, Clark EG: *Preventive medicine for the doctor in his community: an epidemiological approach,* New York, 1965, McGraw-Hill.)

illness or disease, did not include health maintenance, health promotion, or wellness behaviors. *Illness behavior* was defined as any action undertaken by a person who thinks he or she may have a symptom of illness. *Sick role behavior* was defined as any activity undertaken to facilitate recovery from illness (Kasl and Cobb, 1966).

An equally important definition (Harris and Guten, 1979) described self-reported behaviors used by adults to protect their health. *Health protective behavior* (HPB) was defined as all behaviors that individuals perform to protect their health, regardless of their actual or perceived health status and regardless of whether the behavior is proved effective. Thus, HPB moved beyond the realm of medically prescribed behaviors (i.e., those behaviors that the medical community accepts as effective). Harris and Guten's research was important because it assisted health professionals and the public to conceptualize health behavior as self-defined behaviors performed to protect against disease and to promote a higher level of health.

Community health nurses have attempted to clarify health promotion and disease and illness prevention definitions because of their goal of a healthy population and a healthy community. Kulbok (1985) built on Harris and Guten's (1979) definitions and presented the term *preventive health behavior* to describe behaviors that promote health and prevent disease.

Kulbok (1983, 1985) proposed a Resource Model of Health Behavior, in which social and health resources were viewed as correlates of health behaviors. In a study to test this model, Kulbok (1983) found that (1) health behavior is multidimensional, and several unrelated categories of health behavior consist of checkups, dental care behaviors, physical fitness activities, consumption of harmful substances, and health-protecting actions such as seat belt use; and (2) different health and social resources are associated with the performance of different health behaviors. Strategies to promote well-being often focus on assisting clients to practice new, healthy behaviors or to change unhealthy behaviors. Successful intervention is more likely when nurses understand how individuals' social and health resources are related to their health behaviors and how personal and community resources may affect behavior choices.

Laffrey (1985, 1986, 1990) differentiated between health promotion and illness or disease prevention. **Health promotion behavior** was defined as behavior directed toward achieving a greater level of health and well-being. **Illness prevention,** or **disease prevention,** was defined as behavior directed toward reducing the threat of illness, disease, or complications. A third definition proposed by Laffrey (1990) was **health maintenance behavior,** directed toward keeping a current state of health and well-being. These definitions require that one assess not only the behavior, but also the basis on which one makes a choice to perform a given behavior. In a study of community-residing men and women with and without chronic diseases, Laffrey (1990) asked subjects to identify their five most important health behaviors. For each behavior reported, subjects were asked the major reason why they usually performed that behavior. Responses indicated that behaviors were performed for each of the three reasons. For example, one individual reported that he exercises because he has several risk factors for coronary artery disease. Exercise, for him, is an illness-preventing behavior. Another person reported that he exercises because regular, vigorous exercise makes him feel more energetic and he functions at a higher level than he did when he was more sedentary. For this individual, exercise is a health promotion behavior. Yet a third individual reported exercising regularly to maintain her weight at a good level. For this individual, exercising is a health maintenance behavior.

Pender (1987) also differentiated between health-protecting and health-promoting behaviors. Health protection refers to behaviors that decrease one's probability of becoming ill, whereas health promotion refers to behaviors that increase well-being of either an individual or a group. Although health protection and health promotion are complementary, health promotion is a broader concept that encompasses both individuals and groups.

The WHO described health promotion as ". . . the process of enabling people to increase control over, and improve their health" (1984, p. 3). Health promotion combines both individual and community level strategies, including communication, education, legislation, organizational change, and community development. From the WHO perspective, health is more than the absence of disease, it is a resource for daily living. For individuals or communities to realize physical, mental, and social well-being, they must become aware of, and learn to use, the social and personal resources available within their environment. Kulbok's (1985) model of health resources, Laffrey's (1990) health behavior choices, and Pender's (1987) definition of health promotion are congruent with the WHO process of health promotion. Health promotion and self-care are consistent with the goals of community health nursing.

Kulbok et al. (1991) studied a group of 16 health promotion experts and found differences between the terms *health promotion* and *health promotion behavior*. The group defined health promotion as activities undertaken by health professionals to promote health in their clients. Examples of these activities are health education and counseling. Health promotion behavior, on the other hand, was defined as behavior that an individual performs to promote his or her own health and well-being.

The increase in terms used to describe health behavior may be viewed as part of the movement to de-fine health from a positive perspective (Pender, 1987). However, Reynolds (1988) cautions that although nurses increasingly view health holistically, the biomedical model continues to predominate and has a great impact on the way nurses think about, and practice, nursing.

Definitions of Self-Care

The term *self-care* has been very influential in nursing's approach to health promotion. Orem (1995) has developed a nursing framework in which **self-care** is used to describe activities individuals initiate and perform on their own behalf to maintain life, health, and well-being. According to Orem, individuals are not always able to be completely self-sufficient in their self-care. Consequently, although self-care is a lay responsibility, professional care may be required to enhance an individual's capability for self-care. Within this framework, nursing care depends on the capability of individuals and can range from total care to partial care to education and support of individuals to assist them increase their self-care capability. Orem's self-care focus is on the individual. However, her conceptualization of self-care includes a full range of activities that individuals can do for themselves in a variety of health and illness matters. These activities complement professional health care services.

A broader description of self-care was presented by Goeppinger (1982), who noted that self-care activities may be carried out by the individual, the community, or the society and are based on scientific, religious, philosophical, and cultural influences. Health care provided by community health nurses and other primary care workers may be directed toward the individual by changing health beliefs and behaviors. From a public health and political perspective, it is important that self-care also emphasize community responsibility and social change. For example, the WHO definition of health promotion noted earlier included one's use of personal and social resources within the environment to promote health and well-being. However, an important precursor to the use of resources by the population is to develop adequate resources within the environment to enhance the health of the population. In the following discussion, we consider disease prevention, risk appraisal, and reduction in the light of the broad perspective of health promotion and self-care.

Disease Prevention, Risk Appraisal, and Risk Reduction

The disease prevention strategy of risk appraisal and risk reduction is a quantitative approach health professionals can use to help individuals and groups maximize their self-care activities. It compares information supplied by individuals about their health-related practices, health habits, demographic characteristics, and personal and family medical history with data

Three Most Common Health Risk Appraisal Approaches

1. Health hazard appraisal and its many versions
2. Clinical guidelines and recommendations for preventive services
3. Wellness appraisals or inventories

from epidemiological studies and vital statistics. It uses these comparisons as the basis to predict individuals' risks of morbidity and mortality and to determine recommendations to reduce risks and promote healthful behavior. The goal of **risk appraisal** and **risk reduction** is to prevent disease or detect disease in its earliest stages. The knowledge base for risk appraisal and risk reduction is the scientific evidence regarding the relation between risk factors and mortality and the effectiveness of planned interventions in reducing both mortality and risks of mortality.

Since the early 1970s, risk appraisal and reduction have gained popularity among health professionals. This trend has been influenced by three factors: (1) the renewed emphasis on health promotion and disease prevention, (2) epidemiological studies that have provided an empirical data base for making predictions from risk appraisal methods, and (3) a proliferation of risk appraisal tools for use in clinical practice. The health insurance industry has recognized the potential of risk reduction for cost containment and has promoted the approach in occupational and health care settings.

In health risk appraisal, data about health risks experienced by an individual or group are collected and analyzed, and a health risk profile is generated. Health risk appraisal may be done at both individual and community levels. A clinical approach is typically used to identify the presence or absence of risks at the individual level, and an epidemiological approach is frequently used to identify risks at the community level. Both of these approaches are important to community health nurses. In this section, we discuss methods of individual and community health risk appraisal. Later in the chapter, some influential community and epidemiological studies are reviewed.

The box above lists the three most common types of individual health risk appraisal approaches. Each type of risk appraisal is complex, and only the basic concepts and selected procedures are described in this chapter. More complete explanations can be found in the references cited at the end of the chapter. An example of a risk appraisal tool and clinical preventive services guidelines are shown in Appendix A.2.

Health Hazard Appraisal

Robbins and Hall (1970) were among the earliest proponents of individual health-risk appraisal. Unlike physicians in conventional clinical practice, they wanted to approach an individual's health from the perspective of what was likely to occur, rather than what had already occurred. They recognized that most chronic diseases have a predictable sequence and that the characteristic precursors of many diseases can be monitored and controlled. Robbins and Hall put the concept of prospective medicine into practice by developing a method to profile risk called the health hazard appraisal. The objectives of the health hazard appraisal are to (1) assess the total risks to a client's health based on knowledge of the client, the natural history of certain diseases, and the major causes of mortality for aggregates of the client's age, sex, race, and family history; (2) initiate life-style changes in the client to avoid disease precursors or to minimize their pathogenic influence; and (3) institute medical treatment and life-style changes as early in the course of disease as possible.

To accomplish these objectives, data are collected by a self-administered questionnaire, basic laboratory tests, and clinical examination. The questionnaire elicits information about personal characteristics and behaviors known to predict health status. These personal data are compared with data compiled from the 10 major causes of death of an aggregate of the same age, sex, and race as the client. Based on the comparison of data, the client's appraisal age and achievable age are calculated. The appraisal age is the health age of the average person in the client's racial, sex, and age aggregate with a similar risk profile. For example, a 20-year-old white woman might have an appraisal age of 15 if she has good health habits and no family history of chronic disease. Another 20-year-old white woman might have an appraisal age of 26 if she smokes, fails to wear a seat belt while driving, does not perform regular breast self-examinations, and has a family history of hypertension. *Achievable age* refers to the health age the client could achieve by modifying health hazards. The second woman's achievable age could be lowered considerably if she were to modify her behavior.

Risk appraisal instruments are convenient tools that can be used to determine individual health risks. Existing instruments vary in their intent and methods. Some are medically focused; others include risks related to mental, social, and environmental health; and still others include risk assessments and wellness appraisals.

One of the most comprehensive health risk appraisals is the Healthier People Questionnaire developed by the Carter Center of Emory University and the Centers for Disease Control (CDC). The Healthier People Project was initiated in 1986 after a decade of development work by the CDC and a network of state health departments and collaborating universities and after completion of the Risk Factor Update Project (Breslow et al., 1985).

Healthier People is a comprehensive program for health risk appraisal and reduction available to the public. The program includes a computer-scored Healthier People Questionnaire and materials to facilitate easy use. The user materials include (1) instructions on how to administer the questionnaire and use the software, (2) guidance in planning and implementing a comprehensive health promotion program, (3) procedures for modifying the software for special population groups, (4) epidemiological data and mortality tables used to support Healthier People, and (5) software design information for programmers. The most recent version of Healthier People is Version 4.0, published in 1991 by the Carter Center of Emory University. Current program information can be obtained from Risk Assessment Systems, Inc.,* who purchased the marketing and development rights to the Healthier People Program in 1994.

The Lifestyle Assessment Questionnaire (LAQ) (National Wellness Institute, 1989) includes the health risk appraisal questionnaire from the Healthier People Program, a wellness inventory, and a "topics for personal growth" section. Only data from the health risk appraisal portion, however, are compared with mortality data. Users are provided with a *Personal Wellness Report,* which includes summaries of the results from the wellness inventory, a health risk appraisal, a personal growth section, and a sample action plan for behavior change to increase wellness. In addition to the comprehensive LAQ, the Wellness Institute† offers age-specific risk appraisals and wellness inventories.

Clinical Preventive Services Guidelines

Gradual acceptance of the scientific evidence of the benefits associated with key preventive measures led to the development of clinical practice guidelines in the late 1970s. The lifetime health-monitoring program was proposed by Breslow and Somers in the United States in 1977, and comparable recommendations were set forth by the Canadian Task Force on Periodic Health Examination in 1979. As with the health hazard appraisal, these guidelines use clinical and epidemiological data to identify specific needs for health care. However, they do more than assess individual health risks. For example, the lifetime health-monitoring program provides a detailed list of recommendations for preventive measures appropriate for each of 10 different age groups.

In 1989 the U.S. Public Services Task Force published the *Guide to Clinical Preventive Services,* which was based on its review of the scientific evidence on 169 clinical preventive services for 60 target conditions. These guidelines were the work of a 20-member expert panel, including one nursing representative, Dr. Carolyn Williams. The *Guide,* developed for primary care clinicians, included information about the appropriate content of periodic health examinations (Griffith and Diguiseppi, 1994). Clinical preventive services refer to disease prevention and health promotion services delivered to individuals in health care settings,

including immunizations (e.g., influenza, pneumococcus, and childhood vaccines), screening (e.g., blood pressure measurement, Papanicolaou smear, mammogram), counseling (e.g., smoking cessation, diet, and exercise guidance), and chemoprophylactic regimens (e.g., hormone replacement and aspirin). Many of these preventive measures are routine nursing interventions.

In 1990 the U.S. Preventive Services Task Force was reconstituted and charged to update these scientific assessments of preventive services. The current task force is appointed to examine additional clinical preventive services and to reevaluate existing preventive interventions for which new scientific evidence exists. The second edition of the *Guide* was published in late 1995.

These clinical preventive services guidelines are designed to tell primary care clinicians "what to do" in the delivery of preventive services to individuals. However, to ensure implementation of the guidelines, the Public Health Service of the DHHS, provider organizations, and major health-related groups collaborated to develop a program entitled "Put Prevention into Practice" (PPIP). The PPIP program uses a kit of materials designed to improve delivery of preventive services. The *Put Prevention Into Practice Education and Action Kit* includes materials for the provider, the office/clinic staff and systems, and the health care consumer. The health care consumer materials include the Child Health Guide and the Adult Personal Health Guide; these guides are passport-size, consumer-held minirecords. A Spanish version is also available (Griffith and Diguiseppi, 1994). The PPIP program is designed to influence the health promotion and disease prevention practices of health care professionals and consumers. PPIP materials are available through the U.S. Government Printing Office.

Wellness Inventories

The various wellness inventories are slightly different from most health risk appraisal instruments and guidelines for preventive services, since they tend to define health risks more broadly and emphasize empowerment of individuals to achieve health. Wellness appraisals also lead to disease prevention, but do so by advocating health enhancement or promotion. Typical wellness instruments include inventories related to self-responsibility, nutritional awareness, physical fitness, stress management, and environmental sensitivity (Ardell, 1977). Travis' Wellness Self-Evaluation (1977) includes a Life Change Index, Eating Habits Survey, Wellness Inventory Symptom Checklist, Medical History, Purpose in Life Test, Stress Assessments, and Creativity Index. The Wellness Inventory of the LAQ (National Wellness Institute, 1989) covers six dimensions: physical, social, emotional, intellectual, occupational, and spiritual. These wellness appraisal instruments are broader in scope than the health hazard appraisal in that they address health-promoting aspects of life-style, whereas health hazard appraisals as-

*5846 Distribution Dr., Memphis, TN 38141, (901) 795-1700.
†1045 Clark St, Suite 210, PO Box 827, Stevens Point, WI 54481-0827, (715) 342-2969.

sess only the health behaviors that have clearly documented relationships to specific diseases.

Advantages and Disadvantages

Because risk appraisal instruments include recommendations for preventive actions, they may support the individual's self-care behaviors. Further, the recommendations may provide support and direction to nurses in their counseling and educational activities with these clients. Studies of health risk appraisals in clinical settings indicate that clients who complete the instruments generally are more aware of their health risks (Avis et al., 1989; Bartlett et al., 1983; Schultz, 1984), are more willing to discuss their health behaviors (Skinner et al., 1985), and in some cases, initiate recommended changes (Bartlett et al., 1983; Schultz, 1984). Risk appraisals also may be useful for measuring the effectiveness of planned interventions for risk reduction. Completed by individuals and groups at different time periods, they provide feedback about how behavioral changes have influenced health risks and life expectancy.

Despite these advantages, it is important to be aware of the limitations of risk appraisal instruments. Some of these limitations are inherent in the tools themselves, whereas others relate more to problems in usage (Kirscht, 1989). Actual tool limitations include (1) questionable validity and reliability of the instruments, (2) the inconsistency with which different appraisal instruments measure and analyze health characteristics, and (3) an overemphasis on life-style factors and lack of attention to other important risks, such as environmental hazards and inadequate health care (Meeker, 1988; Smith et al., 1987, 1989). For example, an instrument may be weak in measuring particular risks such as smoking, alcohol consumption, or violent behavior (Killeen, 1989). When selecting a risk appraisal instrument, it is important to assess the overall strengths and limitations of the tool, as well as its advantages and disadvantages for specific populations.

The best results can often be obtained by using health risk appraisals in conjunction with clinical observation and assessment. Although an educational message may have a great impact on some individuals, others may deny the message or avoid its implications (Becker and Janz, 1987). Even when individuals are motivated by health appraisal feedback, they may not have the behavioral skills necessary to initiate and sustain changes in life-style. This is especially true regarding those behaviors that are difficult to change, such as smoking habits.

Another limitation of health risk appraisals is that they are probably more suitable for use with middle-age people than for those younger than 35 or older than 65 (Doerr and Hutchins, 1981). Health risk appraisals provide little incentive to the very young to change poor health habits because the effects of life-style on illness are usually not detected until middle to late adulthood. Furthermore, health risk appraisals are not good predictors of illness for persons over 65 years of age. In addition, because they were developed and tested with white, middle-class populations, existing appraisals are probably not useful with blue-collar workers (Shy et al., 1985). Their use with minorities is further compromised by the inadequacy of epidemiological data on risk factors, such as the lack of available and accessible health services, especially for those who are poor. An individual's ability to change lifestyle is limited by the realities of living in a system that may restrict participation in decision making and restrict economic and educational opportunities or is limited by living in an environment where external threats to health, such as violence, are common (Rowley, 1985).

COMMUNITY
Historical Perspectives

After health and health promotion, the third major concept in a framework for community health nursing is **community.** The emphasis on community versus the individual as the focus of practice is not new but is receiving greater attention since the mid-1970s. McKinley and McKinley (1977) attributed declining mortality and morbidity rates to better standards of living, including the environmental factors of living conditions and sanitation, as well as better nutrition. In a much publicized report, the Institute of Medicine's Committee for the Study of the Future of Public Health also emphasized the concept of community in their statement that "the primary mission of public health is to assure conditions in which people can be healthy by generating organized community effort to . . . prevent disease and promote health (Institute of Medicine [IOM], 1988, p. 7).

> ### Did You Know?
>
> The Institute of Medicine's Committee for the Study of the Future of Public Health stressed the importance of community by asserting that the mission of public health is "to assure conditions in which people can be healthy by generating organized community effort . . . to prevent disease and promote health."

The environmental and community emphases for health are even more clear in the national health promotion and disease prevention objectives outlined in *Healthy People 2000* (1991) than they were in the 1979 surgeon general's report. Two categories of national health goals reflect the importance of environment and community. One category, health promotion, is described as "personal health choices within a social context" (p. 6) and includes educational and community-based programs that address life-style. The other category, health protection, is defined as "environmental or regulatory measures that confer protection on large population groups" (p. 6). The year 2000 objectives emphasize the necessity of community-wide strategies rather than relying on individually oriented strategies if nursing is to achieve the goals set forth by the year 2000.

In 1991 the American Public Health Association (APHA) published *Healthy Communities 2000: Model Standards for Community Attainment of the Year 2000 National Health Objectives.* These model standards can be used by local communities to accomplish the following: translate national health objectives into community planning tailored to meet local needs; establish community-specific, measurable health objectives; encourage communication and coordination of community efforts; encourage a sharing of responsibilities among community groups; determine priorities based on existing local patterns, health needs and resources; and assist communities to justify needed programs and budgets to legislative bodies.

All the national objectives in *Healthy People 2000* are included in the model standards of *Healthy Communities 2000,* and a practical outline is provided for each objective that communities can tailor to their own local needs and their own health situations. Directors and supervisors of health departments work with these model standards to tailor programs to their own communities. Community health nurses participate in this process through community assessments, community development activities, and identification of key persons in the community with whom to build partnerships for health programs that can benefit the population. These model standards therefore provide an important link between the concepts of health promotion and disease prevention and community-wide health planning and programs.

Although the model standards provide an excellent opportunity for community health nurses to participate in community-wide health care, nurses generally have not been as involved in the process. Edwards and Dees (1990) argued that the contribution of community health nursing to problems of the environment lies in our ability to integrate concepts of health and disease, individual and aggregate, public health and nursing, and health promotion and disease prevention. This integration is reflected in the relationship between the personal and environmental forces that affect health. One makes choices about various health practices, but the degree of freedom in one's personal choices is affected greatly by others in one's peer group, one's family, options available within the immediate environment, and the norms and values within the environment. It would be naive to think that lasting individual behavior change can take place by intervening with the person without also assessing and intervening at the level of the immediate and surrounding environment.

Models and Frameworks

The theoretical frameworks developed within nursing primarily are oriented to individuals. An assumption exists in the nursing profession that simply changing the word "man" or "human being" to "aggregate" or "community" is sufficient (Hanchett, 1988). In community health nursing practice, nurses soon become aware that the community is more than the sum of the individuals, families, and aggregates within it, and that for any real change to occur, the larger community must be considered.

Despite this community-oriented ideal, community health nursing practice continues to focus on ill and disadvantaged individuals in various community settings. The concept of the community as client has not been easily integrated into practice. Consequently, nursing practice directed *to* the community has been neglected in favor of providing care to individuals *in* the community. There has been much discussion about how community is conceptualized; is the community the setting for practice, or is it the client for practice? Another way of asking this question is whether the community provides the environment or the context for individual and family clients, or whether the community itself is the object of nursing care in its own right.

Chopoorian (1986) argues that a lack of consciousness of community may "contribute to the peripheral role of nurses in the larger arena of social, economic, and political affairs" (p. 42). Community health nurses have great potential for strengthening their position with the community. Chopoorian urges that nurses look not at the profession or to individual clients as the object of reform or revision, but rather at the larger community. She suggests that environment be reconceptualized as social, economic, and political structures; as human social relations; and as everyday life. Such a dynamic perspective would lead to greater involvement by community health nurses in the process of community life.

Several authors have described community from a systems perspective (Blum, 1981; Hanchett, 1979, 1988; Minkler, 1990). Within a *systems perspective,* human beings are viewed within a hierarchy of natural systems, and health is viewed as a function of the harmony of the interrelationships among various levels of the hierarchy. Each movement in one level of the hierarchy has a corresponding movement in all the levels. If individual, family, aggregate, community, and society are seen as different levels of the systems' hierarchy, any change in one level has a corresponding change in all the other levels.

Hanchett (1979, 1988) defines community within a systems perspective, noting that people in relation to one another, to their geographical location, and to available services and resources are the essential aspects of the community system with which the community health nurse must be concerned. Hanchett notes the importance of considering the whole community as more than and different from the sum of its people and their interrelations. She moves beyond definitions of a community as structure or process to one that incorporates a wholeness of energy. Hanchett asks about a community, "Do you feel energized or devitalized by being there? What is the level of fear, hope, spontaneity, joy, or of sadness there? Is it a young, vibrant, growing community, or is it a community that is mature, calm, and knowledgeable about itself and its directions? Is it aging? If so, is it aging well or decaying?" (1979, p. 26). Hanchett notes that "community health is a function of the energy, the individuality, and the relationships of the community as a whole, and of the individuals and groups within the community" (p. 34).

Minkler (1990) describes two basic perspectives about the nature of community. One is an ecological system perspective, which includes population characteristics, physical environment, social organization, and technology. The other is a more dynamic social systems view of social, economic, and political interactions within the community and between the community and outside entities.

Anderson et al. developed a community-as-client model (1995) that included eight major community subsystems: housing, education, fire and safety, politics and government, health, communication, economics, and recreation. The basic structure or core of the community, according to these authors, is its people, their values, beliefs, culture, religion, laws, and mores. Within a community system, the people interact dynamically with the other subsystems. A community health assessment must therefore incorporate information about the subsystems and the pattern of interactions among the subsystems and of the total community with the systems external to it. In this regard, the community-as-client model is congruent with Hanchett's definition.

Salmon and White (1982) developed a systems model to guide community health practice. Their model is based on a definition of public health as the "effort organized by society to protect, promote, and restore people's health." Priorities for community health nursing practice are derived from multiple determinants of health (human-biologic, environmental, social, and medical-technological-organizational). Salmon and White proposed that community health nursing encompasses prevention, protection, and promotion strategies. Their model includes multiple health determinants and is congruent with the Canadian Framework for Health (LaLonde, 1974) and with the IOM determinants of health (IOM, 1988).

The two models just described are based on a systems view of community and on an assumption that a healthy community is facilitated by assessing the various components of the system. Interventions are planned at the system level by participating with relevant components or subsystems. Although these models provide guidance for assessing community and ag-

gregate systems, less guidance is provided for interventions. Furthermore, because the ultimate goal of community health nursing within these models is stability and equilibrium, to be achieved by protection of the community from specific disease risks, less attention is focused on factors that would promote an optimally healthy community. Nevertheless, the major community-wide studies have drawn on concepts such as those presented in these models. These community and epidemiological studies are described next.

Community Studies

Two of the most influential community-wide studies of health risks are the Framingham Heart Study, initiated in 1949, and the Human Population Laboratory's longitudinal survey in Alameda County, Calif, initiated in the early 1970s. Both studies support the hypothesis that selected risk factors are directly related to morbidity and mortality.

In the Framingham Heart Study, 5209 adult residents of a small town in Massachusetts agreed to be followed over their life spans to help researchers identify factors contributing to the development of coronary heart disease and high blood pressure. The subjects received periodic health and life-style assessments, and morbidity and mortality statistics were collected. The longitudinal study was successful in meeting its objectives. Heart disease was found to be more prevalent among smokers and among those with elevated blood pressure, cholesterol levels, or low levels of exercise. Obesity also was identified as a contributor to high blood pressure and elevated cholesterol levels and thus to heart disease (Haynes et al., 1980).

The Alameda County Study was designed to follow a probability sample of 6928 individuals over a 4-year period (Breslow, 1972). Social and behavioral factors were studied in relation to mortality. The health behaviors studied included eating three meals daily at regular intervals, eating breakfast, sleeping 7 to 8 hours a night, using alcohol moderately, exercising regularly, not smoking, and maintaining a desirable height-to-weight ratio (Belloc, 1973). Cigarette smoking, alcohol consumption, physical exercise, hours of sleep, and weight in relation to height were found to be related to mortality (Berkman and Breslow, 1983; Cohn et al., 1988; Kaplan and Camacho, 1983; Wiley and Camacho, 1980; Wingard et al., 1982). Social factors were identified as being important influences on health.

Renne (1974) found that the strength of social networks (e.g., marriage, contact with close friends and relatives, church membership, ties with formal and informal groups) was inversely related to mortality. These findings were initially received with great controversy. However, they led to the inclusion of social and environmental variables, as well as personal behaviors, in health risk appraisals. Subsequent studies have verified the early findings (Kotler and Wingard, 1989).

Findings from large-scale surveys such as the Framingham and Alameda County studies prompted a number of **multilevel intervention** programs based on a public health model. Projects developed to promote community-based, risk reduction interventions were the Stanford Heart Disease Prevention Program (Farquhar et al., 1990), the North Karelia Study (Puska et al., 1983), the Pawtucket Study (Lasaster et al., 1984), and the Minnesota Heart Health Program (Luepker et al., 1994; Perry et al., 1992).

The findings of the initial Stanford Three-City Program were encouraging (Maccoby et al., 1977). A mass media campaign was provided alone in one community and in conjunction with face-to-face instruction in two other communities. Reductions in cigarette smoking, blood pressure, and serum cholesterol were greater in the two communities that received the combined program than in the community that received only the mass media campaign.

Subsequently, the Stanford Five-City Project was initiated (Farquhar et al., 1985). Two treatment cities received a low-cost, comprehensive intervention program based on principles from social learning theory (Perry et al., 1990), communication–behavior change theory, community organization, and social marketing. Once again, improvements in serum cholesterol, blood pressure, smoking rate, and resting pulse were observed in these cities after the program (Farquhar et al., 1990; Winkleby, 1994; Winkleby et al., 1994).

Positive changes likewise were found in the North Karelia Study (Puska et al., 1983). Citizens of North Karelia, a rural area in Finland, were selected for this program because they had extraordinarily high mortality from cardiovascular disease in the early 1970s. More than half of the North Karelia men smoked, consumed large amounts of animal fats, and had elevated serum cholesterol levels. In addition, many had untreated hypertension. The government initiated the intervention program at both an individual and a community level to assist the population to modify their high-risk behaviors.

The North Karelia Project involved extensive retraining of health professionals, reorganization of public health services, production of low-fat and low-salt dairy products and meat, and development of community health education programs. Follow-up studies demonstrated that the prevalence of the three major risk factors for cardiovascular disease decreased much more in North Karelia than in a comparison county (Puska et al., 1983).

The Pawtucket Study is an ongoing intervention project in a Rhode Island community that traditionally has had very high rates of cardiovascular disease. As in North Karelia, the interventions in Pawtucket are directed toward both individuals and the community. The news media, churches, social groups, and business community were employed to provide the community with an education intervention. The food industry offered "Heart Healthy" food items and menus, and extensive campaigns were launched to inform citizens about their cholesterol levels and other cardiovascular risk factors (Lefebvre et al., 1986). Although morbidity and mortality data have not yet been published (Winkleby, 1994), positive changes in cardiovascular risks have been documented for both the city that received the intervention and for a comparison city, indicating that health awareness, knowledge, and behavior are improving among the general public. This is likely a result of a mass media concern with health (Niknian et al., 1991).

The Minnesota Heart Health Program (Luepker et al., 1994) was initiated in 1980 with 400,000 persons in six Midwest communities. Three communities received the program, and three communities served as controls. Risk factor improvements were seen in all six communities, and only modest, nonstatistically significant differences were found between the treatment and control cities (Luepker et al., 1994). The favorable health risk changes were found across all age and education groups and for both the men and women. Winkleby (1994) notes that these findings reflect the effect of a strong contemporary health promotion movement. Future programs must build around public policy initiatives, combined with health education strategies for the community at large as well as smaller interventions directed to specific high-risk populations (Luepker et al., 1994).

These programs, among others, have provided the beginning of a scientific knowledge base for the implementation of risk appraisal and risk reduction programs. However, information on the relative effectiveness of specific interventions in reducing risk still remains limited (Frank et al., 1993; Luepker et al., 1994; Schoenbach et al., 1987).

From the programs described, multiple levels of intervention will be necessary if community health nurses are to reach the community in a meaningful way. Community health nurses have traditionally had a close relationship with individuals, families, high-risk groups, and organizations such as schools and workplaces. Therefore, they are well positioned to make meaningful contributions to risk reduction, disease and illness prevention, and health promotion. This can be accomplished by participating in large community projects, such as the ones described here. Just as important is that community health nurses develop and document health programs and improvements targeted to the specific high-risk populations with whom they interact on a day-to-day basis.

Community Health Nursing Applications

About 20 years ago, Milio (1976) offered a set of propositions for improving health behavior by considering personal choices in the context of available societal resources. These propositions constitute a fitting model for health promotion that articulates the combined importance of personal and societal resources as

Milio's Propositions for Improving Health Behavior

1. Health status of populations is a function of the lack or excess of health-sustaining resources.
2. Behavior patterns of populations are related to habits of choice from actual or perceived limited resources and related attitudes.
3. Organizational decisions determine the range of personal resources available.
4. Individual health-related decisions are influenced by efforts to maximize valued resources in both the personal and the societal domains.
5. Social change reflects a change in population behavior patterns.
6. Health education impacts behavior patterns minimally without new health-promoting options for investing personal resources.

Modified from Milio N: Am J *Public Health* 66(5):435-439, 1976.

community health nursing moves toward the year 2000 (see box above).

Stevens (1989) advocated critical social theory as a useful method of "consciousness raising" with community residents. As citizens "dialogue with each other and reflect critically upon their own situations with respect to oppressive environmental conditions, they begin to take collective action based on their common interests, risks they are willing to undergo, consequences they can expect, and knowledge of the circumstances of their own lives" (p. 4).

Within this approach, the nursing process can be used to assess the community's health by various means, such as assessing the number and adequacy of health facilities, surveying community population samples and key persons in the community for their perception of needs, and reviewing written information and census data about the community (Laffrey et al., 1989). Planning for health care is based on the assessment and prioritization of needs. Community-oriented interventions can take many forms and often provide multiple approaches to address identified needs. Evaluation allows a reassessment of the process as well as the resolution of the identified health need.

Chapter 15 describes levels of partnership with the community. In a *passive* partnership, community health nurses are involved with implementing change as determined and directed by professional leaders for the benefit of the community. As the partnership becomes more active, community residents become increasingly more involved in assessing, planning, implementing, and evaluating community change. In an *active* partnership, health needs are determined by both professionals and community residents. Planning groups include providers and consumers who represent as many different facets of the community as possible.

The approaches proposed by Milio (1976) and Stevens (1989) reflect an active partnership between community residents and health professionals. The aim of community health nursing within this approach is to facilitate community residents' ability to increase their awareness of their own health situations and to become empowered to determine what they want for themselves, their families, and their community.

The presence and availability of health-related resources and community residents' attitudes toward these resources would be assessed within this approach. The community health nurse would then assess health behaviors in relation to the resources and opportunities that community residents see within their environment. The community health nursing assessment would be conducted in such a way that the residents would become aware of their resources or lack of resources and would participate in planning for their own health-related needs and activities. The residents would make the major decisions about how to develop and make available the resources they require to meet their health needs. Thus, health-related actions can be realistically based on clients' particular life situations.

Stoner et al. (1992) made use of the principles advocated by Milio (1976) and Stevens (1989) in a community analysis with an emphasis on health, as perceived by the population, rather than health problems. Flick et al. (1994) described another community project that used these principles. A partnership was developed by community health nurses with a local neighborhood to enhance its capacity to improve its own health. This project, conducted over 7 years, was

Research Brief

Flick LH, Reese CG, Rogers G, Sonn J: Building community for health: lessons from a seven-year-old neighborhood/university partnership, *Health Educ Q* 21(3):369-380, 1994.

Two case studies of community conflict situations that occurred in the process of community empowerment were analyzed. A partnership was formed between a community health nursing graduate program and a racially diverse neighborhood in a large Midwestern city. The twofold aim of the partnership was to enhance the community's capacity to promote its health and to teach community organizing for health promotion to community health nurses.

The community and professional partnership was based on concepts of multidimensional health, reciprocity, trust, social justice, and education as a liberating process. Community conflicts served as both incentives and obstacles in the process of community activation and organization. Improved conflict identification and conflict management skills were required by both community and professional participants. The authors determined that conflict management theory is essential when an empowerment education model is implemented in a diverse, integrated community.

based on a community-organizing model in which community mobilization occurs through community participation and control, with health professionals serving as a resource to the community.

Community health nurses have a great opportunity to work in multidisciplinary teams in public health and community-based settings to conduct assessments, develop strategies with the community and its populations, and facilitate the empowerment of community residents to increase their own awareness of their current health situations. As community groups are able to see their own health choices in light of environmental constraints and resources, they become empowered to make meaningful decisions about their own health at an individual level, at the level of their families, and also collectively, within neighborhoods or groups and at the larger community level. As the year 2000 approaches, it is increasingly important that community health nurses incorporate these strategies into their practice. Therefore, nursing concerns seen from a community health nursing perspective require a framework that can take into account aspects of health promotion, disease and illness prevention, and illness care of individuals, families, aggregates, and the total community.

The two concepts of health and community are inextricably linked. As described throughout this chapter, it is difficult to talk of one without including the other. However, it is also important that community health nurses examine their definitions and beliefs about each concept as the basis for developing models to guide practice. Moe (1977) defines community as "people and the relationships that emerge among them as they develop and use in common some agencies and institutions and a physical environment." If this definition is accepted, it is imperative that community health nursing activity consider the people, the community, and the pattern of the interrelationships among them.

The essence of the community health nursing perspective is the ability to see the totality of community while addressing its component parts and, at the same time, see the totality of health promotion while addressing its component parts: health protection, illness and disease prevention, and illness care. It is the dynamic relationship among all these levels that distinguishes community health nursing from nursing in more circumscribed settings, such as hospitals and clinics.

SHIFTING EMPHASIS FROM ILLNESS TO WELLNESS

An understanding of the need to shift the emphasis from illness to wellness is gradually increasing among professional nurses. In community health nursing practice, it is clear that although illness and disease affect the health of individuals, families, and communities, so do many other factors. The biomedical model of health, defined as absence of disease, cannot explain why some individuals exposed to recognized illness-producing stressors do not become ill, whereas

other individuals who appear to be in the most health-conducive circumstances become ill. Community health nurses recognize and work to enhance a health potential within clients, whether the client is an individual, a family, an aggregate, or the total community. This health potential is greater than a mere absence of illness or disease, but it would not be detected if one were operating from the biomedical model alone.

A growing population of vulnerable persons in our society necessitates that community health nurses define health in more optimistic terms than allowed within the biomedical model. Because a large proportion of those over age 65 have at least one diagnosed chronic disease, defined health as absence of disease severely limits the health promotion aspect of nursing care of older adults since, by that definition, these individuals can never be healthy. Similarly, in other culturally diverse, high-risk, and vulnerable populations, the meaning and lived experience of health are not adequately reflected by the clinical or biomedical model of health as absence of disease. The role performance, adaptive, and eudaemonistic models of health probably are more meaningful to these individuals. The goal of health care must be directed toward optimizing health within these models rather than focusing solely on disease care.

Laffrey et al. (1986) proposed two paradigms from which the concepts person, health, environment, and nursing could be viewed. The most prominent is the *pathogenic,* or *disease, paradigm,* in which health is viewed as the absence of disease. The pathogenic paradigm assumes a narrow view of human beings and human behavior. The second paradigm is the *health paradigm,* in which "health is a fluid, flexible process, a subjective phenomenon of each human being" (p. 97). The health paradigm is based on a holistic view of human beings and their life situations and is consistent with high-level wellness as defined by Dunn (1973).

Laffrey et al. (1986) suggest that both paradigms can be useful for advancing the specific aims and processes of community health nursing. The pathogenic approach directs nursing toward disease prevention, risk reduction, prompt treatment, and rehabilitation. The health approach directs community nursing practice toward promotion of greater levels of positive health. If health is defined broadly as the totality of the life process, in mutual and simultaneous interaction with the environment, disease and illness can be seen as potential manifestations of that interaction. Therefore, the health paradigm cannot exclude any part of the life process and, as such, subsumes disease treatment and disease prevention (Laffrey et al., 1986).

A danger of "victim blaming" is inherent in the emphasis on individual responsibility for health behavior for either disease prevention or health promotion. Downie et al. (1990) have cautioned against this approach, arguing that it is not realistic to emphasize individual responsibility for health while excluding community responsibility. Likewise, conceptualizing health as the sole responsibility of the community in a "top down" manner is patronizing and serves to keep people in a victim position. Downie et al. advocate a "new sense of community responsibility or citizenship" (1990, p. 171), combining empowerment of individuals to be autonomous, knowledgeable, and self-determining in matters of their own health with the activity of the larger community to provide leadership and professional assistance for community development—to work with and through the community to promote health. "Health and well-being are, in the end, a set of relationships among citizens" (p. 170).

Confusion will continue to exist during this evolutionary period. Although a broader conception of health is becoming more generally accepted, indicators of health promotion continue to be derived from the biomedical model. Downie et al. (1990) provide a compelling argument for the dangers inherent in simply adding health promotion to the biomedical model. This medicalization of health promotion has led to a "new generation of experts dominating the media with the high-pressure selling of positive health" (p. 168). Tillich (1961) argued that health care workers are overprofessionalized, giving the impression that ordinary people are not able to manage their own health but that expert professionals can do so with medical technology and pills.

To simply incorporate health promotion into the present models of health care may therefore violate the very premises on which community health nursing is based. The WHO (1984) supports an approach that considers both the community and the individuals within the community in their emphasis on full (public) participation in health-promoting activities.

A MODEL OF COMMUNITY HEALTH PROMOTION

A model of community health promotion was developed by Laffrey and Kulbok (1995) to guide community health nursing practice. This model, shown in Figure 14-3, is based on two complementary paradigms for nursing, the health paradigm and the pathogenic (disease) paradigm as described by Laffrey et al. (1986). The health paradigm is focused on promoting health as a dynamic, creative, and positive quality of life. The goal of positive health involves the promotion of physical, mental, emotional, spiritual, functional, and social well-being. The pathogenic paradigm includes both the care and the prevention of illness, disease, and disability and focuses on reducing known risks and threats to health and preventing disease. Although existing clinical strategies may be similar within the two paradigms, the ultimate goal of each paradigm contains fundamental differences. These differences are seen in the specific purpose of the nursing care and whether it is directed to the individual, family, aggregate, or community.

Laffrey and Kulbok's model includes two major dimensions: client system and focus of care. *Client system* refers to the level of client toward which community

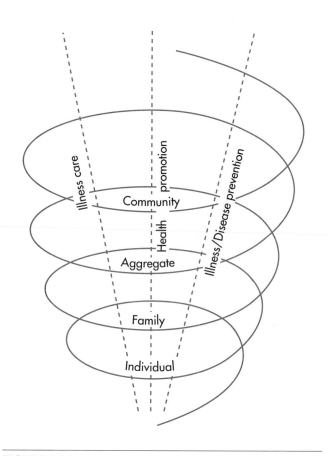

FIGURE 14-3

A model of community health promotion. (Laffrey SC, Kulbok PA: A *integrative model for community nursing*, 1995 [under review].)

health nursing is targeted. Client system is conceptualized from its narrow, most delimited target, the individual, in which the environment is principally the family and extends to the population group and community as these affect the individual. The client system can also be the family, population group or aggregate, the total community, or the society at large.

The *focus of care* within the model is illness care, illness or disease prevention, or health promotion. Each focus is appropriate for some aspects of community health nursing care. Even more important is the awareness that ultimately the goal is a healthier community, achieved through health promotion interventions. The model reflects the continuity and expansiveness of the client system and the focus of care. The core of the model, depicted by its central axis, is health promotion. At its narrowest focus, illness care is provided to individuals. At the model's broadest level of care, the community health nurse works with community leaders to plan for community facilities for the purpose of promoting optimal health of its citizens.

Community health nursing care, within this model, must extend beyond resolving a specific illness to preventing the illness and promoting optimal health for the individual, the family, the aggregate, and the total community. All levels are important to the health of the community and its populations.

Table 14-1   Community Health Levels of Care: Malnutrition/Failure to Thrive

Focus of care	Client system			
	Individual	**Family**	**Aggregate**	**Community**
Illness care	Weigh and measure child. Monitor child's symptoms. Teach mother basic nutrition and child care for failure-to-thrive child.	Teach signs/symptoms of malnutrition to high-risk family members. Refer family for care for nutrition-related problems.	Assess prevalence of failure-to-thrive children in community. Teach classes about emergency food sources and referral sources for aggregate of failure-to-thrive children.	Assess community for accessibility and adequacy of care providers to treat malnutrition and failure to thrive in community.
Illness/disease prevention	Teach mother well-balanced nutrition and child care to prevent recurrence of malnutrition and failure to thrive.	Teach nutrition to high-risk family members to prevent nutrition-related problems.	Assess community for prevalence of children at risk of malnutrition. Develop classes about reducing risks of malnutrition in aggregate of high-risk children.	Participate in providing community-wide multimedia education for reduction of malnutrition. Lobby for legislation to promote resources to ensure adequate nutrition to community.
Health promotion	Support individual efforts to adopt health promotion life-style, including healthy nutrition.	Plan with family to adopt healthy life-style and incorporate healthy foods into daily eating patterns.	Educate school personnel regarding healthy school lunches for aggregate of school-children.	Work with community leaders and citizens to establish nutrition education programs in community.

Clinical Application

One example of community health nursing care that reflects the four client systems and multiple foci of care is shown in Table 14-1. The health problem that comes to the community health nurse's attention in this example is a young child with a diagnosis of failure to thrive.

Illness Care

The community health nurse initiates care at the individual level with a goal of resolving the failure to thrive. The individual child's health is assessed and monitored, and the mother is taught principles of nutrition, feeding, and care of the ill child. At the family-as-client level, the community health nurse would assess the presence of malnutrition within the family and refer other family members for care as needed. Another family intervention might be referring the family for counseling to relieve the stress related to the child's illness. At the aggregate-as-client level, the community health nurse would assess the community for the prevalence of failure-to-thrive children. Another aggregate intervention would be to teach classes to raise the awareness of the community members about the prevalence of this condition and to educate groups of people about referral

sources and emergency food for failure-to-thrive children. At the community-as-client level, the community health nurse might become involved with other community leaders and citizens to assess the prevalence of malnutrition and nutrition-related illnesses in the community.

Illness/Disease Prevention

At the individual-as-client level, well-balanced nutrition and child care might be taught to mothers to prevent a recurrence of malnutrition and failure to thrive in the child. Recommendations from the *Guide to Clinical Preventive Services* provide direction for age-specific periodic health examination, screening, and counseling interventions. In addition, the nurse could select an appropriate health risk appraisal tool for use in conjunction with clinical observation and assessment. The high-risk family would be taught nutrition principles and assisted to incorporate healthy food into their diets to prevent nutrition-related problems. An aggregate-as-client perspective would include assessing the community for aggregates at risk for malnutrition (e.g., schoolchildren, poor persons, the elderly, homeless persons), analyzing baseline health risk data, and working with others to in-

Continued.

Clinical Application—cont'd

stitute programs to reduce their risk, thereby preventing malnutrition. Community-wide multimedia education for reduction of risk factors for malnutrition and lobbying for legislation to promote resources for adequate nutrition within the community are examples of a community-as-client approach.

Health Promotion

At the individual-as-client level, the community health nurse would focus on empowering the individual to adopt healthy life-style as appropriate to his or her age, culture, and resources. For young children, this may include working with the parent as the primary caregiver to support him or her in providing health-enhancing care to the child. Within a family-as-client perspective, the approach would include the entire family and could include planning with the family on how to adopt healthy activities into their life-style. These activities could range from well-balanced nutrition to planning for enjoyable relaxation activities for the family. The use of a wellness inventory would assist the nurse in designing an intervention and would increase the family's awareness of a wide range of personal self-care behaviors. At the aggre-

gate-as-client level, the community health nurse might provide education to school personnel regarding healthy lunches for the aggregate of students or teachers. Regardless of the level of health need or client system at which care begins, the ultimate goal of the community health nurse is health promotion of the total community and all its constituents. Participating with community leaders and citizens to establish nutrition education or preparation for parenthood classes throughout the community are examples of a community-as-client approach.

Although an important starting point may be the care of the failure-to-thrive child, the community health nurse recognizes that solving the immediate problem is not sufficient. The child's health problem is viewed within a broader context of an optimally healthy child, family, aggregate of children, and community. This approach necessitates that the nursing intervention not be limited to solving the immediate problem of weight gain, but rather that care be oriented toward interventions that promote optimal health for the child, family, aggregate of high-risk children, and the total community.

Key Concepts

- ◆ Community health nursing is concerned with promoting the health of populations and of the total community. The concept of health shapes the process of community health nursing from assessment of health-related needs of individuals, families, aggregates, and communities to evaluation of behavioral outcomes.
- ◆ The greatest benefits in public health are likely to accrue from efforts to improve individual life-style, social conditions, and the physical environment.
- ◆ Community health nurses have a history of commitment to primary health care and to enhancing levels of wellness in populations. Rich opportunities to guide "health" care reform endeavors await future community health nursing leaders.
- ◆ It is important for community health nurses to examine their personal definition of health and to recognize how nursing care is directed by this health definition. A nurse who defines health broadly as self-actualization is more likely to consider multiple indicators of physical health, social health, the ability to adapt to the changing environment, and potential for

maximum well-being when planning nursing care.
- ◆ The goal of risk appraisal and reduction is the prevention or early detection of disease. The knowledge base for this approach is the scientific evidence regarding the relation between risk factors and mortality and the effectiveness of planned interventions in reducing both risks and mortality.
- ◆ Health hazard appraisal is used to assess the total risks to an individual's health, to initiate disease-preventing life-style changes, and to institute treatment and life-style changes as early in the course of disease as possible.
- ◆ Clinical preventive guidelines use clinical and epidemiological data to identify specific individual health risks, and they provide a detailed list of recommendations for preventive measures appropriate to different age groups.
- ◆ Wellness inventories define health risks broadly and emphasize empowerment of individuals to achieve health.
- ◆ Clinical observation, assessment, and nursing interventions used in conjunction with health risk appraisals are essential to obtain the best

Key Concepts—cont'd

results. Although educational messages have an impact on some individuals, others may deny the implications. Even when individuals are motivated by health appraisal feedback, they may not have the behavioral skills necessary to initiate and sustain changes in lifestyle.

◆ The Stanford Heart Disease Prevention Program, the North Karelia Study, the Pawtucket Study, and the Minnesota Heart Health Program provided a beginning scientific knowledge base for the implementation of risk appraisal and risk reduction programs.

◆ Community health nursing care must extend beyond resolving a specific illness to preventing the illness and promoting optimal health for the individual, the family, the aggregate, and the total community. All these levels are important to the health of the community and its populations.

Critical Thinking Activities

1. State your personal definition of health, and interview a nurse, client, and physician about their definitions of health. Discuss the range of definitions using Smith's four models of health as a frame of reference.

2. Compare and contrast definitions of health promotion and disease prevention. Propose a rationale for the statement that health promotion and disease prevention are "two sides of one coin." Can the same strategies, such as a physical fitness or stress management program, be defined as health promoting and disease preventing?

3. Develop a community health nursing plan in relation to adolescent substance abuse using Milio's propositions as a frame of reference.

4. What are the critical elements or characteristics of the concept of community as applied in community health nursing practice? Define community health promotion, and provide examples of health status indicators for a specified community.

5. Discuss community health nursing practice using the framework of individual-family-aggregate-community as the client system and illness care, illness/disease prevention, and health promotion as the focus of care. Analyze the role of partnership with the community in various practice settings, such as school health, public health, and home health.

6. Describe community health levels of care, including the client system and the focus of care: (a) for teenage pregnancy, beginning with health promotion at the individual level, and (b) for breast cancer, starting from the level of community illness/disease prevention.

Bibliography

Ahmed PI, Kolker A, Coelho GV: Toward a new definition of health: an overview. In Ahmed PI, Coelho GV, editors: *Toward a new definition of health: psycho-social dimensions*, New York, 1979, Plenum.

American Nurses Association: *Nursing's agenda for health care reform*, supplement to *Am Nurse*, Washington, DC, 1991, The Association.

American Public Health Association: *Healthy Communities 2000: model standards for community attainment of the year 2000 national health objectives*, ed 3, Washington, DC, 1991, The Association.

Anderson E, McFarlane J: *Community-as-client: application of the nursing process*, Philadelphia, 1988, Lippincott.

Anderson E, McFarlane J, Helton A: Community-as-client: a model for practice, *Nurs Outlook* 34(5):220-224, 1986.

Ardell DB: *High level wellness: an alternative to doctors, drugs, and disease*, Emmaus, Pa, 1977, Rodale.

Avis NE, Smith KW, McKinlay JB: Accuracy of perceptions of heart attack risk: what influences perceptions and can they be changed? *Am J Public Health* 79(12):1608, 1989.

Bartlett EE, Pegues HU, Shaffer CR, Crump W: Health hazard appraisal in a family practice center: an exploratory study, *J Community Health* 9(2):135, 1983.

Becker MH, Janz NK: Behavioral science perspectives on health hazard/health risk appraisal, *Health Services Res* 22(4):537, 1987.

Belloc NB: Relationship of health practices and mortality, *Prev Med* 2(1):67, 1973.

Berkman LF, Breslow L: *Health and ways of living, the Alameda County Study*, New York, 1983, Oxford University Press.

Blum HL: *Planning for health*, ed 2, New York, 1981, Human Sciences.

Breslow L: A quantitative approach to the World Health Organization's definition of health: physical, mental, and social well-being, *Int J Epidemiol* 1(4):347, 1972.

Breslow L: A health promotion primer for the 1990's, *Health Affairs* 9(2):6-21, 1990.

Breslow L, Somers AR: The lifetime health-monitoring program: a practical approach to preventive medicine, *N Engl J Med* 296(11):601, 1977.

Breslow L, Fielding J, Afifi AA, et al: *Risk Factor Update Project: final report*, Atlanta, 1985, US Department of Health and Human Services.

Brubaker BH: Health promotion: a linguistic analysis, *Adv Nurs Sci* 5(3):1-14, 1983.

Chopoorian TL: Reconceptualizing the environment. In Moccia P, editor: *New approaches to theory development*, Pub No 15-1992, New York, 1986, National League for Nursing.

Coburn D, Pope CR: Socioeconomic status and preventive health behavior, *J Health Soc Behav* 15:67-78, 1974.

Cohn BA, Kaplan GA, Cohen RD: Did early detection and treatment contribute to the decline in ischemic heart disease mortality? Prospective evidence from the Alameda County Study, *Am J Epidemiol* 127(6):1143, 1988.

Doerr BT, Hutchins EB: Health risk appraisal: process, problems, and prospects for nursing practice and research, *Nurs Res* 30(5):299, 1981.

Downie RS, Fyfe C, Tannahill A: *Health promotion models and values,* New York, 1990, Oxford University Press.

Dunn HL: *High-level wellness,* Arlington, Va, 1973, Beatty.

Edwards LH, Dees RL: Environmental health: the effects of life-style on the world around us. In Wold SJ, editor: *Community health nursing: issues and topics,* East Norwalk, Conn, 1990, Appleton & Lange.

Farquhar JW, Fortmann SP, Flora JA, et al: Stanford Five-City Project: design and methods, *Am J Epidemiol* 122(2):323, 1985.

Farquhar JW, Fortmann SP, Flora JA, et al: Effects of community-wide education on cardiovascular disease risk factors: the Stanford five-city project, *JAMA* 264:359-365, 1990.

Fitzpatrick J: A life perspective rhythm model. In Fitzpatrick J, Whall AL, editors: *Conceptual models of nursing: analysis and application,* ed 2, East Norwalk, Conn, 1989, Appleton & Lange.

Flick LH, Reese CG, Rogers G, Sonn J: Building community for health: lessons from a seven-year-old neighborhood/university partnership, *Health Educ Q* 21(3):369-380, 1994.

Frank E, Winkleby M, Fortmann SP, Farquhar JW: Cardiovascular disease risk factors: improvements in knowledge and behavior in the 1980's, *Am J Public Health* 83(4):590-593, 1993.

Fry ST: Dilemma in community health ethics, *Nurs Outlook* 31:176-179, 1983.

Fuchs V: *Who shall live,* New York, 1974, Basic Books.

Goeppinger J: Changing health behaviors and outcomes through self-care. In Lancaster J, Lancaster W, editors: *Concepts for advanced nursing practice: the nurse as a change agent,* St Louis, 1982, Mosby.

Green LW: *Status inconsistency, reference group theory, and preventive health behavior,* doctoral dissertation, University of California, Ann Arbor, Mich, 1969, University Microfilms.

Griffith HM, Diguiseppi C: Guidelines for clinical preventive services: essential for nurse practitioners in practice, education, and research, *Nurse Pract* 19(9):25-35, 1994.

Hanchett ES: *Community health assessment: a conceptual tool kit,* New York, 1979, Wiley.

Hanchett ES: *Nursing frameworks and community as client: bridging the gap,* East Norwalk, Conn, 1988, Appleton & Lange.

Harris DM, Guten S: Health protective behavior: an exploratory study, *J Health Soc Behav* 20:17-29, 1979.

Haynes SG, Feinlieb M, Kannel WB: The relationship of psychosocial factors to coronary heart disease in the Framingham Study III: eight year incidence of coronary heart disease, *Am J Epidemiol* 111:37, 1980.

Healthy People 2000: national health promotion and disease prevention objectives, Washington, DC, 1992, USDHHS, Public Health Service.

Illich I: *Medical nemesis: the expropriation of health,* New York, 1976, Random House.

Institute of Medicine: *The future of public health,* Washington, DC, 1988, National Academy Press.

Kaplan GA, Camacho T: Perceived health and mortality: a nine year follow-up of the Human Population Laboratory chart, *Am J Epidemiol* 117(3):292, 1983.

Kasl SV, Cobb S: Health behavior, illness behavior and sick-role behavior, *Arch Environ Health* 12:246-266, 1966.

Killeen ML: What is the health risk appraisal telling us? *West J Nurs Res* 11(5):614, 1989.

Kirscht JP: Process and measurement issues in health risk appraisal, *Am J Public Health* 79(12):1598, 1989 (editorial).

Kotler P, Wingard DL: The effect of occupational, marital and parental role on mortality: the Alameda County Study, *Am J Public Health* 79(5):607, 1989.

Kulbok PA: A concept analysis of preventive health behavior. In Chinn PL, editor: *Advances in nursing theory development,* Rockville, Md, 1983, Aspen.

Kulbok PA: Social resources, health resources, and preventive health behavior: patterns and predictors, *Public Health Nurs* 2(2):67-81, 1985.

Kulbok PA, Baldwin JH: From preventive health behavior to health promotion: advancing a positive construct of health, *Adv Nurs Sci* 14(4):50-64, 1992.

Kulbok PA, Baldwin JH, Duffy R: *Content validity: developing an inventory of multidimensional behavior for health promotion.* Unpublished paper presented at the American Public Health Association Annual Meeting, Washington, DC, 1991.

Laffrey SC: Health behavior choice as related to self-actualization and health conception, *West J Nurs Res* 7(3):279-300, 1985.

Laffrey SC: Development of a health conception scale, *Res Nurs Health* 9:107-113, 1986.

Laffrey SC: An exploration of adult health behaviors, *West J Nurs Res* 12(4):434-447, 1990.

Laffrey SC, Dickinson D: *How community health nurses view their roles,* 1994 (submitted for publication).

Laffrey SC, Kulbok PA: *An integrative model for community nursing,* 1995 (under review).

Laffrey SC, Loveland-Cherry CJ, Winkler SJ: Health behavior: evolution of two paradigms, *Public Health Nurs* 3(2):92-100, 1986.

Laffrey SC, Meleis AI, Lipson JG, Solomon M, Omidian PA: Assessing Arab-American health care needs, *Soc Sci Med* 29(7):877-883, 1989.

LaLonde M: *A new perspective on the health of Canadians,* Ottawa, 1974, Government of Canada.

Langlie JK: Social networks, health beliefs and preventive health behavior, *J Health Soc Behav* 18:244-260, 1977.

Lasater T, et al: Lay volunteer delivery of a community-based cardiovascular risk factor change program: the Pawtucket Experiment. In Matarazzo JD, Weiss SM, Herd JA, Miller NE, Weiss SM, editors: *Behavioral health: a handbook of health enhancement and disease prevention,* Silver Spring, Md, 1984, Wiley.

Leavell HR, Clark EG: *Preventive medicine for the doctor in his community: an epidemiological approach,* ed 3, New York, 1965, McGraw-Hill.

Lefebvre RC, et al: Community intervention to lower blood cholesterol: the "know your cholesterol" campaign in Pawtucket, Rhode Island, *Health Educ Q* 13(2):117, 1986.

Luepker RV, Murray DM, Jacobs DR, et al: Community education for cardiovascular disease prevention: risk factor changes in the Minnesota Heart Health Program, *Am J Public Health* 84(9):1383-1392, 1994.

Maccoby N, Farquhar JW, Wood PD, Alexander J: Reducing the risk of cardiovascular disease: effects of a community-based campaign on knowledge and behavior, *J Community Health* 3(2):100, 1977.

McKinlay JB, McKinlay SM: The questionable contribution of medical measures to the decline of mortality in the United States in the twentieth century, *Milbank Q* 55(3):405, 1977.

Meeker WC: A review of the validity and efficacy of the health risk appraisal instrument, *J Manipulative Physiol Ther* 11(2):108, 1988.

Milio N: A framework for prevention: changing health-damaging to health-generating life patterns, *Am J Public Health* 66(5):435-439, 1976.

Minkler M: Improving health through community organization. In Glanz K, Lewis FM, Rimer BK, editors: *Health behavior and health education: theory, research, and practice,* San Francisco, 1990, Jossey-Bass.

Moe EV: Nature of today's community. In Reinhardt AM, Quinn MD, editors: *Current practice in community health nursing,* St Louis, 1977, Mosby.

National Wellness Institute: *Lifestyle Assessment Questionnaire,* Stevens Point, Wis, 1989, The Institute.

Niknian M, Lefebvre RC, Carlton RA: Are people more health conscious? A longitudinal study of one community, *Am J Public Health* 8(2):205-207, 1991.

Orem D: *Nursing: concepts of practice*, ed 5, St Louis, 1995, Mosby.

Pender N: *Health promotion in nursing practice*, ed 2, East Norwalk, Conn, 1987, Appleton & Lange.

Perry CL, Baranowski T, Parcel GS: How individuals, environments, and health behavior interact: social learning theory. In Glanz K, Lewis FM, Rimer BK, editors: *Health behavior and health education: theory, research, and practice*, San Francisco, 1990, Jossey-Bass.

Perry CL, Kelder SH, Murray DM, Knut-Inge K: Community-wide smoking prevention: long-term outcomes of the Minnesota Heart Health Program and the Class of 1989 Study, *Am J Public Health* 82(9):1210-1216, 1992.

Puska P, et al: Change in risk factors for coronary heart disease during 10 years of a community intervention programme (North Karelia Project), *Br Med J* 287(6408):1840, 1983.

Reifsnider E: Restructuring the American health care system: an analysis of nursing's agenda for health care reform, *Nurse Pract* 17(5):65-75, 1992.

Renne KS: Measurement of social health in a general population survey, *Soc Sci Res* 3:25, 1974.

Reynolds CL: The measurement of health in nursing research, *Adv Nurs Sci* 10:23-31, 1988.

Robbins LC, Hall JN: *How to practice prospective medicine*, Indianapolis, 1970, Methodist Hospital of Indiana.

Rowley DL: Are current health risk appraisals suitable for black women? In *Proceedings of the 21st Annual Meeting of the Society of Prospective Medicine*, Bethesda, Md, 1985, Society of Prospective Medicine.

Salmon M, White M: Construct for public health nursing, *Nurs Outlook* 30(9):527-530, 1982.

Schoenbach VJ, Wagner EH, Beery WL: Health risk appraisal: review of the evidence for effectiveness, *Health Services Res* 22(4):553, 1987.

Schultz CM: Lifestyle assessment: a tool for practice, *Nurs Clin North Am* 19(2):271, 1984.

Shy CM, et al: Project to modify the CDC Health Risk Appraisal for blue collar workers. In *Proceedings of the 21st Annual Meeting of the Society of Prospective Medicine*, Bethesda, Md, 1985, Society of Prospective Medicine.

Skinner HA, Allen BA, McIntosh MC, Palmer WH: Lifestyle assessment: just asking makes a difference, *Br Med J* 290:214, 1985.

Smith JA: The idea of health: a philosophical inquiry, *Adv Nurs Sci* 3(3):43-50, 1981.

Smith KW, McKinlay SM, McKinlay JB: The reliability of health risk appraisals: a field trial of four instruments, *Am J Public Health* 79(12):1603, 1989.

Smith KW, McKinlay SM, Thorington BD: The validity of health risk appraisal instruments for assessing coronary heart disease risk, *Am J Public Health* 77(4):419, 1987.

Smuts JC: *Holism and evolution*, New York, 1926, Macmillan.

Somers HM, Somers AR: *Doctors, patients and health insurance: the organization and financing of medical care*, Washington, DC, 1961, The Brookings Institute.

Stanhope MK: Primary health care pratice: is nursing part of the solution or the problem? *Family Community Health* 18(1):49-68, 1995.

Stevens PE: A critical social re-conceptualization of environment in nursing: implications for methodology, *Adv Nurs Sci* 11(4):56-68, 1989.

Stoner MH, Magilvy JK, Schultz PR: Community analysis in community health nursing practice: the GENESIS model, *Pub Health Nurs* 9(4):223-227, 1992.

Terris M: Approaches to an epidemiology of health, *Am J Public Health* 65(10):1037-1045, 1975.

Tillich P: The meaning of health perspective, *Biol Med*, 1961, pp 92-100.

Travis JW: *Wellness workbook for health professionals*, Mill Valley, Calif, 1977, Wellness Resource Center.

US Department of Health, Education and Welfare: *Forward plan for health, FY 1978-82*, DHEW PHS Pub No (OS) 76-50046, Washington, DC, 1976, US Government Printing Office.

US Department of Health, Education and Welfare: *Healthy People: the surgeon general's report on health promotion and disease prevention*, DHEW Pub No 79-55071, Washington, DC, 1979, US Government Printing Office.

US Preventive Services Task Force: *A guide to clinical preventive services: an assessment of the effectiveness of 169 interventions*, Baltimore, Md, 1989, Williams & Wilkins.

Wesley J: *Primitive physic: or an easy and natural method for curing most diseases*, London, 1747, T Trye.

Wildavsky A: Doing better and feeling worse: the political pathology of health policy, *Daedalus* 106:105, 1977.

Wiley JA, Camacho TC: Life-style and future health: evidence from the Alameda County Study, *Prev Med* 9(3):371, 1980.

Wingard DL, Berkman LF, Brand RJ: A multivariate analysis of health-related practices: a nine-year mortality follow-up of the Alameda County Study, *Am J Epidemiol* 116(5):765, 1982.

Winkleby MA: The future of community-based cardiovascular disease intervention studies, *AJBH* 84(5):1369-1372, 1994.

Winkleby MA, Flora JA, Kraemer HC: A community-based heart disease intervention: predictors of change, *Am J Public Health* 84(5):767-772, 1994.

Woods N: Conceptualization of self-care: toward health oriented models, *Adv Nurs Sci* 12(1):1, 1989.

World Health Organization: *The first ten years of the World Health Organization*, New York, 1958, WHO.

World Health Organizations: *Health promotion: a discussion document on the concept and principles*, Copenhagen, 1984, WHO Regional Office for Europe.

Part Four Issues and Approaches in Aggregate Health Care

The primary orientation of health care delivery has been toward care and cure of the individual. There is increasing evidence that life-style and personal health habits influence the health of individuals, families, groups, and communities.

Although it is necessary to identify health-risk factors among individuals and groups in the community, it is of paramount importance that community health nurses learn to identify and work with health problems of the total community. This is often referred to as an aggregate approach to health care delivery. Healthy communities provide greater resources for growth and nurturing of individuals and families than do their unhealthy counterparts.

Certainly, community health nurses use a public health approach to work with individuals and families in promoting health, intervening in disease onset or progression, and assisting with rehabilitation. Likewise, nurses often find that strategies used to introduce health behaviors directed at illness prevention and life-style changes are applicable to groups in the community and to the community at large. Group concepts promoting health behaviors through groups, identifying community groups and their contributions to community life, and assisting groups to work toward community health goals are essential to community health nursing practices.

Healthy communities/healthy cities is an organized approach to helping communities organize and move to provide environments for healthful living for their populations. In this approach health is defined to encompass the physical and mental health of individuals and families plus the social, political, economic, educational, cultural, and environmental milieus of the total community.

The nurse will be able to assist communities in attaining their health goals by understanding the organization of communities, the effects of rural versus urban settings on health issues, how and why programs are managed, and how to evaluate programs for quality and effectiveness. A community assessment provides the basis for helping communities establish their goals. The use of a nurse-managed clinic is one approach community health nurses have found to be successful in meeting the needs of aggregates, or vulnerable at-risk populations, whose needs must be considered when trying to improve the health of a community. Case management is an approach that has been used by community health nurses since its inception to match the most appropriate services and health care delivery interventions to population needs.

While all communities strive to protect their populations and provide a safe living environment, natural and person-made disasters may occur; community health nurses can play a significant role in helping a community through such a crisis. The chapters in this section of the text assist the community health nurse in learning how to work with aggregates and how to develop healthy communities. ▼

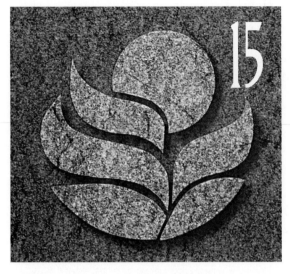

15

Community as Client: Using the Nursing Process to Promote Health

George F. Shuster ◆ Jean Goeppinger

Objectives ▼

After reading this chapter, the student should be able to do the following:

◆ Decide whether nursing practice is community oriented.
◆ Illustrate selected concepts basic to community-oriented nursing practice—community, community client, community health, and partnership for health.
◆ Understand the relevance of the nursing process to community-oriented nursing practice.
◆ Decide which methods of assessment, intervention, and evaluation are most appropriate in selected situations.
◆ Develop a community-oriented nursing care plan.

Outline ▼

Although nurses traditionally have viewed the community as a client (Schultz, 1987), many community health nurses consider it their most important client (Ervin and Kuehnert, 1993; Kuehnert, 1991), and more recently, their partner (Anderson and McFarlane, 1995). This chapter clarifies community concepts and provides guidelines for nursing practice with the community client, emphasizing the use of the nursing process to promote community health.

COMMUNITY DEFINED

The concept of community varies widely. Dever (1991, p. 45) defines it as "the entire fabric of society and its institutions." Hanchett (1990), like Dever, views the community as a whole. The Expert Committee Report on community health nursing of the World Health Organization (1974, p. 7) includes this definition: "A community is a social group determined by geographic boundaries and/or common values and interests. Its members know and interact with one another. It functions within a particular social structure and exhibits and creates norms, values and social institutions."

Still other theorists and writers present **typologies** (which involves classification of communities by category) rather than single definitions. One such typology of community was described by Blum in the 1974 edition of his classic text, *Planning for Health.* The categories or types of communities include communities defined by geopolitical boundaries, their interactions (such as between schools, social services, and governmental agencies), and problem-solving dimensions (see box below).

Blum's work (1974) shows the complexity of contemporary society. Nurses working in communities quickly learn society actually consists of many different kinds of communities; some of the communities listed in the box are communities of place because interactions occur within a specific geographic area.

Neighborhood and face-to-face communities are two examples of this type of community. Other communities, such as communities of special interest or resource communities, are spread out across widely scattered geographic areas. They are brought together by common concerns and interests that can be long term or temporary in nature. Yet another type of community is illustrated by a community of problem ecology, which is created when environmental problems like water pollution affect a widespread area. For instance a problem such as water pollution can bring people together from areas that would not normally share a common interest. Nurses also may work in partnership with communities of political jurisdiction, such as school districts, townships, or counties. Because the nature of each type of community varies, nurses planning interventions with communities must take into consideration the characteristics of that specific community. Each community is unique, and its unique characteristics will influence the nature of the partnership.

In most definitions, the concept of community includes three dimensions: people, place, and function. The people are the community residents. *Place* refers both to geographical and time dimensions, and *function* refers to the aims and activities of the community. Community-oriented nurses regularly need to examine how the personal, geographical, and functional dimensions of community shape their nursing practice. They are able to use both a conceptual definition of "community" and a set of indicators for the concept of "community" in their practice.

In this chapter we use the following definition: **Community** is a locality-based entity, composed of systems of formal organizations reflecting societal institutions, informal groups, and **aggregates.** These components are *interdependent* and their function is to meet a wide variety of collective needs (Bogan et al., 1992). This definition includes personal, geographical, and functional dimensions and recognizes interdependence, or interaction, among the systems within a community. Indicators of the dimensions of this definition are listed in Table 15-1.

THE COMMUNITY AS CLIENT

The uniqueness of community health nursing customarily has been attributed to its **practice setting.** The idea of health-related care being provided within the community is not new. Indeed, at the turn of the century most persons stayed at home during illnesses. Consequently, the practice environment for all nurses was the home rather than the hospital.

Types of Communities

Face-to-face community
Neighborhood
Community of identifiable need
Community of problem ecology
Community of concern
Community of special interest
Community of viability
Community of action capability
Community of political jurisdiction
Resource community
Community of solution

From Blum HL: *Planning for health,* New York, 1974, Human Sciences Press.

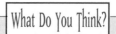

What Do You Think?

It is impossible to provide nursing care to a community. The nurse's only client is the individual.

Table 15-1   The Concept of Comunity Specified

Dimensions	Indicators
Space and time	Geopolitical boundaries Local or folk name for area Size in square miles, acres, blocks, or census tracts Transportation avenues, such as rivers, highways, railroads, and sidewalks History Physical environment, such as land-use patterns and condition of housing
People or person	Number and density of population Demographic structure of population, such as age, sex, socioeconomic, and racial distributions; rural and urban character and dependency ratio Informal groups, such as block clubs, service clubs, and friendship networks Formal groups, such as schools, churches, businesses, industries, governmental bodies, unions, and health and welfare agencies Linking structures (intercommunity and intracommunity contacts among organizations)
Function	Production, distribution, and consumption of goods and services Socialization of new numbers Maintenance of social control Adapting to ongoing and expected change Provision of mutual aid

As the range of community-based nursing services expanded, many different kinds of agencies were established, and their services often overlapped. For instance, both privately established voluntary agencies and official local health agencies worked to control tuberculosis. These nurses were called community health nurses, public health nurses, or visiting nurses. Nurses from both types of agencies practiced in clients' homes and not in the hospital. Early community health nursing textbooks included lengthy descriptions of the home environment and tools for assessing the extent to which that environment promoted the health of family members. Health education about the domestic environment was frequently a major part of home nursing care.

By the 1950s, visiting nurse associations, health departments, schools, prisons, industries, and neighborhood health centers, as well as homes, had all become areas of practice for community nurses. Many of the new community nurses did not consider the environments in which they practiced. Although their practices took place within the community, they focused on the individual patient or family seeking care. The care provided was not community oriented; rather, it was oriented towards the individual or family who lived—and was ill—in the community. This commitment to direct "hands-on" clinical nursing care delivered to individuals or families in community settings has been and remains a more popular conception of community nursing practice than the idea of the whole community as the target of nursing practice. This remains true despite the American Nurses Association's (ANA) statement in *Standards of Community Health Nursing Practice* which says: "while community health nursing practice includes nursing directed to individuals, families, and groups, the dominant responsibility is to the population as a whole" (ANA, 1986, p. 2). When the location of the practice is in the community and the focus of the practice is the individual or family, then the client remains the individual or family—not the whole community.

Therefore, the community is considered the client only when the nursing focus is on the collective or common good instead of individual health. Community-oriented practice seeks healthful change for the whole community's benefit (Wallerstein, 1992). Although the units of service may be individuals, families or other interacting groups, aggregates, institutions, and communities, the resulting changes are intended to affect the whole community—not just the individual, family, or specific aggregate. For example, an occupational health nurse's target might be preventing illness and injury and maintaining or promoting the health of an entire company work force. Because of this focus, the nurse not only would help the individual disabled worker seeking service to achieve independence in activities of daily living, but also would become involved with promoting vocational rehabilitation and seeking reasonable employment policies for all disabled workers.

Community as Client and Nursing Practice

Population-based care is experiencing a rebirth, and the community as client is relevant to nursing practice for several reasons. The concept of community as client makes direct clinical care an aspect of community health practice. For instance, sometimes direct nursing care is provided to individuals and family members because their health needs represent common community-related problems rather than problems that are unique to their situations. Changes in their health will affect the health of their communities (Coelho et al., 1993). In such cases, decisions are made at the individual level because the individual's health is related to the health of the population as a whole and because the individual has an effect on community health. Improved health of the community remains the overall goal of nursing intervention. Interventions to stop spouse and elder abuse are two examples of nursing interventions undertaken primarily because of the effects of abuse upon society and therefore upon the population as a whole.

The concept of community as client also highlights the complexity of the change process (Kenney, 1992). Change for the benefit of the community as client often must occur at several levels, ranging from the individual to the societal. As Ryan (1976) points out, the "victim" cannot always be blamed and expected to correct the deficit without concurrent changes in the helping professions and public policy. For instance, lifestyle-induced health problems, such as smoking, overeating, and speeding, cannot be solved simply by asking individuals to choose health-promoting habits. Society also must provide healthy choices. Most individuals cannot change their habits alone; they require the support of family members, friends, community health care systems, and relevant social policies.

A commitment to the health of the community client requires a process of change at each of these levels. Both collaborative practice models involving the community and nurses in joint decision making and specific nursing roles are required for each of the units of service (Oppewal, 1992). One nursing role emphasizes individual and direct personal care skills. Another nursing role focuses on the family as the unit of service. A third nursing role focuses on the community as a unit of service, especially constituent community groups (Chalmers and Kristajanson, 1990; Russell, 1992).

Viewing the community as client and thus as the target of service means embracing two key concepts: community health and partnership for community health. Together these form not only the goal but also the means of community-oriented practice.

GOALS AND MEANS OF COMMUNITY-ORIENTED PRACTICE

In community-oriented practice the nurse and community seek healthful change together (Braddy et al., 1992; Lexau et al., 1993). Their common goal of community health involves an ongoing series of health-promoting changes rather than a fixed state. The most effective means of achieving healthy changes in the community is through this same partnership. Specific examples of partnership between the nurse and the community (Jefferson County) are provided throughout this chapter.

Community Health

Like the concept of community, community health has three common characteristics, or dimensions: status, structure, and process. Each dimension has a unique effect on community health as the goal of community-oriented practice.

Status

Community health in terms of status or outcome is the most well-known and accepted approach; it in-

Consensus Set of Indicators* for Assessing Community Health Status

INDICATORS OF HEALTH STATUS OUTCOME

1. Race/ethnicity-specific infant mortality, as measured by the rate (per 1000 live births) of deaths among infants <1 year of age

Death rates (per 100,000 population)† for:

2. Motor vehicle crashes
3. Work-related injury
4. Suicide
5. Lung cancer
6. Breast cancer
7. Cardiovascular disease
8. Homicide
9. All causes

Reported incidence (per 100,000 population) of:

10. Acquired immunodeficiency syndrome
11. Measles
12. Tuberculosis
13. Primary and secondary syphilis

INDICATORS OF RISK FACTORS

14. Incidence of low birth weight, as measured by percentage of total number of live-born infants weighing <2500 g at birth
15. Births to adolescents (females aged 10 to 17 years) as a percentage of total live births
16. Prenatal care, as measured by percentage of mothers delivering live infants who did not receive prenatal care during first trimester
17. Childhood poverty, as measured by the proportion of children <15 years of age living in families at or below the poverty level
18. Proportion of persons living in counties exceeding U.S. Environmental Protection Agency standards for air quality during previous year

From *Morbidity and Mortality Weekly Report* 40(27):449-451, 1991.
*Position or number of the indicator does not imply priority.
†Age-adjusted to the 1940 standard population.

volves biological, emotional, and social components. The physical component of community health frequently is measured by traditional morbidity and mortality rates, life expectancy indices, and risk factor profiles. The question of exactly which risk factors are most important has been a matter of ongoing controversy. In an effort to help resolve this question, *Morbidity and Mortality Weekly Report* recently published the work of a consensus committee involving representatives from a number of community-health-related organizations. This committee identified by consensus 18 community health status indicators (see box above).

The emotional component of health status can be measured by consumer satisfaction and mental health indices. Crime rates and functional levels reflect the social component of community health. Other status measures, such as worker absenteeism and infant mortality rates, reflect the effects of all three components.

Table 15-2   Eight Essential Conditions of Community Competence

Condition	Definition
Commitment	The affective and cognitive attachment to a community "that is worthy of substantial effort to sustain and enhance" (Cottrell, 1976, p. 198)
Self-other awareness and clarity of situational definitions	The lucid and realistic perception of one's own and the other's community components, identities, and positions on issues
Articulateness	The technical aspects of formulating and stating one's views in relation to the other's views
Effective communication	The accurate transmission of information, based on the development of common meaning among the communicators
Conflict containment and accommodation	The inventive and effective assimilation and management of true, or realistically, perceived differences
Participation	Active, community-oriented involvement
Management of relations with larger society	Adeptness at recognizing, obtaining, and using external resources and supports and, when necessary, stimulating the creation and use of alternative or supplementary resources
Machinery for facilitating participant interaction and decision-making	Flexible and responsible procedures, formal and informal, facilitates interaction and decision-making

From Goeppinger J, Lassiter PG, Wilcox B: *Nurs Outlook* 30(8):464-467, 1982.

Structure

Community health as viewed from a structural perspective usually comprises community health services and resources, as well as attributes of the community structure itself. Indicators used to measure community health services and resources include utilization patterns, treatment data from various health institutions, and provider/patient ratios. These data provide information, such as the number of available hospital beds or the number of emergency room visits to a particular facility. The problems with using these measures are serious. For instance, inequities in access to care and quality of care are well known (Selby-Harrington and Riportella-Muller, 1993). Less well known, but equally problematic, is the erroneous assumption of a direct causal relationship between the provision of health care and improved health (Ugarte et al., 1992). Such problems necessitate cautious use of health services and resources as measures of community health.

Attributes of the community structure are commonly identified as social indicators, or correlates, of health. Measures of community structure include demographic characteristics, such as socioeconomic and racial distributions, and educational levels. Their relationships to health status have been thoroughly documented. For instance, health status is inversely related to age and directly related to socioeconomic level (Dever, 1991).

Process

The view of community health as the process of effective community functioning of problem solving is well

established. However, it is especially appropriate to community-oriented nursing because it directs the study of community health to the "promotion of effective community action" or "wellness" (Goodman et al., 1993), which is an important aim of community-oriented nurses. Chalmers and Kristajanson (1990) have recently presented a model of community level practice that reflects the process dimension. They call it the Health Promotion Model and describe it as "a mediating, enabling, and advocacy strategy that aims to develop community systems and make health a politically accountable issue."

The concept of community competence, defined originally in a classic work by Cottrell (1976), provides a basic understanding of the process dimension of community health. **Community competence** is a process whereby the components of a community—organizations, groups, and aggregates—"are able to collaborate effectively in identifying the problems and needs of the community; can achieve a working consensus on goals and priorities; can agree on ways and means to implement the agreed-on goals; and can collaborate effectively in the required actions" (Cottrell, 1976, p. 197). Cottrell (1976) also proposed eight essential conditions of competence. The conditions are listed and defined in Table 15-2.

The term **community health** as used in this chapter is the meeting of collective needs by identifying problems and managing interactions within the community itself and between the community and the larger society (Braddy et al., 1992; Hoover and Schwartz, 1992). This definition emphasizes the process dimension but also includes the dimensions of

Table 15-3   The Concept of Community
             Health Specified

Dimension	Indicators
Status	Vital statistics—live births, neonatal deaths, infant deaths, maternal deaths
	Incidence and prevalence of leading causes of mortality and morbidity
	Health risk profiles of selected aggregates
	Functional ability levels
Structure	Health facilities, such as hospitals, nursing homes, industrial and school health services, health departments, voluntary health associations, categorical grant programs, and prepaid health plans
	Health-related planning groups
	Health manpower, such as physicians, dentists, nurses, environmental sanitarians, social workers, and others
	Health resource utilization patterns, such as bed occupancy days and patient/provider visits
Process	Commitment
	Self-other awareness and clarity of situational definitions
	Articulateness
	Effective communication
	Conflict containment and accommodation.
	Participation
	Management of relationships with the larger society
	Machinery for facilitating participant interaction and decision-making

status and structure. Indicators for all three dimensions are listed in Table 15-3.

The use of status, structure, and process dimensions to define community health, as illustrated in Table 15-3, is an effort to develop a broad definition of community health involving indicators that are often not included when discussions focus only on risk factors as the basis for community health. Indeed the meaning of the term "risk" has evolved over the past 30 years until it is used in several different, sometimes confusing contexts (Hayes, 1992). Nevertheless, epidemiological data related to health risks of aggregates and communities, commonly expressed as rates and confidence intervals, are vital indicators of health status. Dever (1991) provides a good discussion of risk factors, health status indicators and indexes in relation to risk factors, whereas Muecke (1984) presents a community health nursing approach describing health risks as factors identified with either the defined community or its related environmental characteristics. Data about the structure of the community and its processes provide different information that is complementary to the health risk data and therefore necessary for the development of a clear understanding of the community.

Strategies to Improve Community Health

One important guideline that is available for nurses working to improve the health of the community is *Healthy People 2000,* a publication that offers a vision of the future for public health and specific objectives to help attain that vision (Healthy People 2000, 1991).

Healthy People 2000 has stimulated a number of joint efforts to develop strategies for achieving its goals. These efforts have involved such organizations as the Centers for Disease Control and Prevention (CDC), American Public Health Association (APHA), Association of State and Territorial Health Officials (ASTHO), and National Association of County Health Officials (NACHO). The results of these efforts are a number of publications and guidelines that provide detailed strategies for achieving the objectives in *Healthy People 2000.* These publications include *Healthy Communities 2000: Model Standards, Assessment Protocol for Excellence in Public Health (APEXPH),* and *Planned Approach To Community Health (PATCH).* Each of these three approaches offers step-by-step guidelines for community interventions. *Healthy Communities 2000: Model Standards,* for example, is a guidebook using an 11-step process written to help plan community public health services. It emphasizes health outcomes, a community focus, and a government presence at the local level that is often in the form of a local public health agency.

Did You Know?

The development of the concept of healthy communities/healthy cities has revitalized nursing's interest in developing partnerships with communities to provide a healthy environment for citizens.

APEXPH and *PATCH* are two planning tools that can be used to help implement the *Healthy Communities 2000: Model Standards. APEXPH* is a process emphasizing local level activity and focuses on improving the public health of communities by increasing the capacity of the local health care agencies to provide core functions, such as assessment and policy development. *PATCH* materials focus more on the prevention of identified chronic disease and health promotion programs and their associated planning and implementation processes (APHA, 1994; APHA Model Standards, 1993). Readers interested in contacting these organizations can refer to the box on p. 295.

The World Health Organization's (WHO) Healthy Cities initiative offers yet another approach to community-oriented health promotion. First initiated in Europe during the middle 1980s, Healthy Cities has

Information You Can Use

become a movement on a global scale with hundreds of Healthy Cities' initiatives (Tsouros, 1990). Healthy Cities' initiatives are based on recognition that the health of the community is affected by political, economic, environmental, and social factors. The Healthy Cities' approach emphasizes community development through broad-based local citizen involvement to address local problems (Flynn et al., 1992). Healthy Cities initiatives focus on social change, including developing supportive environments, developing personal skills, reorienting health care services, health policy, and community action (Flynn, 1992).

Several different community-oriented health promotion approaches have been noted here but regardless of what approach is taken, specific strategies to improve community health often depend on whether the status, structure, or process dimension of community health is being emphasized (Kulbok and Baldwin, 1992; Shea, 1992). If the emphasis is on the status dimension, the most appropriate strategy is usually at the level of primary prevention because the objective is either to prevent a disease or treat it in its presymptomatic stages (Fries et al., 1992). Immunization programs are an example of a primary level nursing intervention that would be reflected in morbidity and mortality measures.

Nursing intervention strategies focused on the structural dimension are directed to either health services or demographic characteristics. Intervention aimed at altering health services might include program planning. Interventions aimed at affecting demographic characteristics might include community development (Kreuter, 1992).

When the emphasis is on the process dimension, the most appropriate strategy is usually health promotion. For example, if family-life education is lacking in a community because of ineffective communication among families, children, school board members, reli-

gious leaders, and health professionals, then the most effective strategy may be to open discussion among these groups and assist community members to develop education programs.

Community Partnerships

Community partnership is crucial because community members and professionals who are active participants in a collaborative decision-making process have a vested interest in the success of efforts to improve the health of their community (Rienzo and Button, 1993). Consequently, successful strategies for improving community health must include community partnership as the basic means, or key, for improvement (Orenstein et al., 1992). Community partnership is a basic tenet of such community-oriented approaches as Healthy Cities.

Most changes must aim at improving community health through active partnerships between community residents and health workers from a variety of disciplines (Dahl et al., 1993). Unfortunately, community residents often are viewed only as data sources and recipients of intervention. This form of partnership is called *passive participation* (Feuerstein, 1980). In contrast is the type of lay-professional partnership used here. This approach specifically emphasizes *active participation*. Here, power is shared among lay and professional persons throughout the assessment, planning, implementation, and evaluation process.

In the past, nurses have not been influential in initiating community changes, although they generally have been actively involved in the implementation phase. Intervention by the nurse for the community's benefit, or passive participation, has been a common practice mode (Lassiter, 1992). Passive participation contrasts with the partnership approach proposed below in which all involved are assessing, planning, and implementing needed community changes (Chapman and Jurs, 1993).

Partnership often is equated with participation and involvement of the community or its representatives in healthful change (Eng et al., 1992). **Partnership** is defined here as the informed, flexible, and negotiated distribution (and redistribution) of power among all participants in the processes of change for improved community health. The three main characteristics of partnership are denoted by the adjectives *informed, flexible,* and *negotiated.*

First, partnership is informed. Lay and professional partners must be aware of their own and other's perceptions, rights, and responsibilities. Second, partnership is flexible. Lay and professional partners must recognize the unique and similar contributions each can make to a given situation. For example, professionals often contribute substantive expertise that laypersons lack. On the other hand, laypersons' definitions of community health problems are often more accurate than those of professionals. And third, because contributions vary and each situation is different, the distribution of power must be negotiated at every stage of the change process.

Partnership, as defined here, is a concept that is as essential for community health nurses to know and use as are the concepts of community, community as client, and community health. Experienced community health nurses know partnership is important because health is not given, but rather it is generated through new and increasingly effective forms of lay-professional collaboration. For example, maternal-child health in both developed and developing countries is affected more by wise grocery shopping and menu planning or improvements in home gardening than by the ingestion of vitamin and mineral supplements (Combs-Orme et al., 1985). Changes in grocery shopping and gardening practices require active participation of both lay and professional people. Partnership in identifying problems and setting goals is especially important because it elicits the commitment essential to successful change.

The significance and effectiveness of partnership in improving community health is supported by a growing body of literature (Eng and Young, 1992; Eng and Hatch, 1991; Watkins et al., 1991). Classic studies document the utility of partnership models involving Latina opinion leaders (Lorig and Walters, 1980-1981), health facilitators (Salber, 1981), lay advisors (Salber, 1979), and health guides (Warnecke et al., 1976). The roles of these partners-in-health have included sympathetic listening, offering advice, making referrals, and instituting programs. More recently the effectiveness of partnership models between nurses and communities has been demonstrated in arthritis self-care (Goeppinger et al., 1989; Lorig et al., 1989), rural minority health (Sutherland et al., 1989) migrant health (Smith and Gentry, 1987), child health (Armstrong-Ester et al., 1987), and care of the elderly (Jamieson, 1990). Recent work by Swannel and co-workers (1992) has demonstrated the continuing utility of partnership models in improved health in other countries. In international health, partnership models generally are viewed as empowering people, through their lay leaders, to control their own health destinies and lives. In the United States partnership models have involved churches (King et al., 1993) and informal community leaders.

Despite supportive data, professional health workers often have challenged the notion of partnership. Unfortunately, passive compliance is more frequently sought than the true collaboration inherent in a partnership. Also, questions frequently are raised about the ability of health care consumers to determine health needs accurately and to evaluate professional practice.

◆ Community-Focused Nursing Process

Most nurses are familiar with the nursing process as it applies to individually focused nursing care. Using it to promote community health makes this same nursing process community focused. The phases of the nursing process that directly involve the community as client begin with establishment of the contract/partnership and include assessment, diagnosis, planning, implementation, and evaluation. Figure 15-1 provides an overview of the nursing process with the community as client.

Application of the nursing process to the community as client is illustrated in the following sections with a case study taken from the practice of a community health nurse. For clarity, infant malnutrition is the only community health problem used to illustrate application of the nursing process. In reality, several different community-health problems were identified by the partnership. Their relative importance was determined, and infant malnutrition was designated the most important problem from among all of the identified problems before continuing with intervention.

ASSESSING COMMUNITY HEALTH

Assessing community health requires gathering relevant existing data, generating missing data, and interpreting the data base. Gathering the data and its initial interpretation are the first steps in the assessment phase of the nursing process.

Data Collection and Interpretation

The primary goal of **data collection** is to acquire usable information about the community and its health. The systematic collection of data about community health necessitates gathering or compiling existing data and generating missing data. These data are then interpreted, and community health problems and capabilities are identified.

Data Gathering

Data gathering is the process of obtaining existing, readily available data. These data usually describe the demography of a community: age, sex, socioeconomic, and racial distributions; vital statistics, including selected mortality and morbidity data; community institutions, including health care organizations and the services they provide; and health manpower characteristics. Often these data have been collected by others via structured interviews, questionnaires, or surveys and are available in published reports (Stoner et al., 1992).

Data Generation

Data generation is the process of developing data that do not already exist through interaction with community members or groups. This type of information is less easily acquired and is generally not statistical in nature. Data that frequently must be generated include information about a community's knowledge and beliefs, values and sentiments, goals and per-

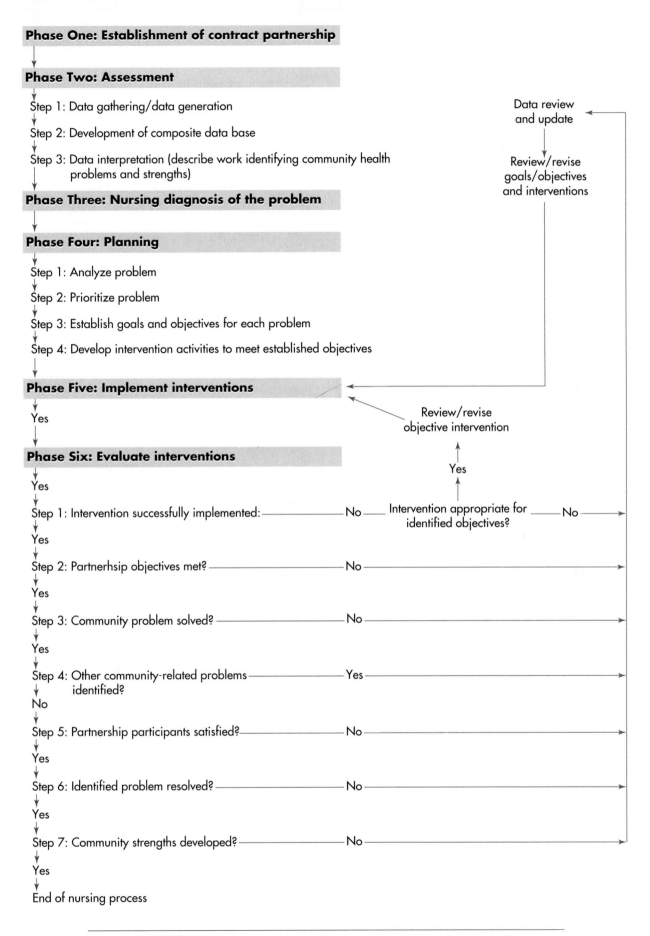

Phase One: Establishment of contract partnership

Phase Two: Assessment

Step 1: Data gathering/data generation

Step 2: Development of composite data base

Step 3: Data interpretation (describe work identifying community health problems and strengths)

Phase Three: Nursing diagnosis of the problem

Phase Four: Planning

Step 1: Analyze problem

Step 2: Prioritize problem

Step 3: Establish goals and objectives for each problem

Step 4: Develop intervention activities to meet established objectives

Phase Five: Implement interventions

Yes

Phase Six: Evaluate interventions

Yes

Yes

Step 1: Intervention successfully implemented: ————— No —— Intervention appropriate for ———— No ———→
identified objectives?

Yes

Step 2: Partnerhsip objectives met? ————————— No ————————————————————→

Yes

Step 3: Community problem solved? ——————— No ————————————————————→

Yes

Step 4: Other community-related problems ———— Yes ————————————————————→
identified?

No

Step 5: Partnership participants satisfied? ———— No ————————————————————→

Yes

Step 6: Identified problem resolved? ————— No ————————————————————→

Yes

Step 7: Community strengths developed? ———— No ————————————————————→

Yes

End of nursing process

Data review
and update

Review/revise
goals/objectives
and interventions

Review/revise
objective intervention

Yes

Yes

FIGURE 15-1

Flow chart illustrating the nursing process with the community client.

ceived needs, norms, problem-solving processes, and power, leadership, and influence structures. These data are more apt to be collected via interviews and observation and to be qualitative.

Composite Data Base

A *composite data base* is created by combining the gathered and generated data. Data interpretation seeks to attribute meaning to the data. First, data are analyzed and synthesized and themes are noted (Hettinger and Brazile, 1992). Community health problems, or needs for action, and community health strengths, or capabilities, are determined. Next, the resources available to meet the needs are identified. Problems are indicated by differences between the nurse's and community's goals for community health and the themes or findings from the data analysis. Strengths, on the other hand, are suggested by similarities between the nurse's and community's concepts of community health and available data. The nurse and community, working in a partnership, identify problems. Next, the resources available to meet the needs are identified. Active community participation is critical for the data interpretation process, particularly in identifying problems.

The Program Planning Model, initially proposed by Delbecq and Van de Ven (1971), is a widely accepted technique for encouraging lay participation in problem identification. The model illustrates active community participation in problem identification and program planning. It maximizes the contributions of various groups with diverse interests and expertise. This model depends heavily on **nominal groups,** "groups in which individuals work in the presence of one another but do not interact" (Delbecq and Van de Ven, 1971, p. 467), the separation of individual from collective problems, and a round-robin procedure for listing problems without concurrently evaluating or elaborating on them. This model is popularly known as the *nominal group process.*

Other consensus methods, such as the Delphi technique, also are used to define the extent of agreement among content experts, policymakers, and community members about the presence and importance of certain health problems. Experience shows that consensus methods will produce useful and credible results if the following conditions are met: problems are carefully selected; participants in the process are deliberately selected and closely monitored; justifiable and reasonable levels of consensus are expected; and the findings are used as guides to decisions.

Data Collection Methods

A variety of methods to collect data is essential. Methods that encourage the nurse to consider the community's perception of its health problems and capabilities are as important as those methods structured to yield knowledge the nurse considers essential.

Five useful methods of collecting data are informant interviews, participant observation, windshield surveys, secondary analysis of existing data, and surveys. These methods can be clustered into two distinct but complementary categories: methods that rely on what is directly observed by the data collector and methods that rely on what is reported to the data collector. Both categories of data collection are described in more detail in the next two sections.

Collection of Direct Data

Informant interviews, participant observation, and windshield surveys are three methods of directly collecting data. All three methods require sensitivity, openness, curiosity, and the ability to listen, taste, touch, smell, and see life as it is lived in a community. **Informant interviews,** which consist of directed conversation with selected members of a community about community members or groups and events, are basic to effective data collection. Also basic is **participant observation,** the deliberate sharing, in so far as circumstances permit, in the life of a community. Informant interviews and participant observation are particularly suitable techniques for generating information about community beliefs, norms, values, power and influence structures, and problem-solving processes (Rivo et al., 1992). Such data can seldom be reported in numbers, so often they are not collected. Even worse, conclusions that are intuitive and unverified—are sometimes substituted for this type of data. Conclusions from direct data collection methods should be validated by those people providing information.

In the example of the community with the infant malnutrition problem, informant interviewing with social workers and religious leaders provided data indicating a community with well-defined clusters of persons with low incomes, concerns about adolescent pregnancy, and worries about the health of its babies. This data, which reflected the concerns and worries of the Jefferson County community, would have been difficult to acquire without personal interviews.

Windshield surveys are the motorized equivalent of simple observation. The nurse, driving a car or riding public transportation, can observe many dimensions of a community's life and environment through the windshield. Common characteristics of people on the street, neighborhood gathering places, the rhythm of community life, housing quality, and geographic boundaries can be observed readily. Again, using the infant malnutrition example, the windshield survey suggested the community had a significant unemployed population because adults were observed "hanging out" at country crossroads during the daytime. An example of a windshield survey can be found in Appendix C.1.

Collection of Reported Data

Secondary analysis and surveys are two methods of collecting reported data. In **secondary analysis,** the community health nurse uses previously gathered data, such as minutes from community meetings. This type of analysis is extremely valuable because it is efficient and economical. Many sources of data are readily available and useful for secondary analysis including public documents, health surveys, minutes from meetings, statistical data, and health records (Kieffer et al., 1992). In the Jefferson County infant malnutrition example, birth records noting low birth weights and health department clinic records of low-weight-for-height children provided information that reflected a higher-than-average rate of infant malnutrition.

Surveys report data from a sample of persons. They are equally useful but somewhat less efficient and economical than observational methods and secondary analyses because they require time-consuming and costly data collection (Guendelman and Silberg, 1993). Thus the survey method is not often used by the community health nurse. However, surveys are necessary for identifying certain community problems (Brownson et al., 1992). For example, a lack of accessible personal health services cannot be documented readily and reliably in any other fashion.

Because no data collection method is without bias, it is best to use several methods with different strengths and weaknesses. This is called **triangulation.** Using multiple complementary methods is essential to and consistent with community health nursing practices. Readers interested in further information about survey and secondary analysis methods should refer to *The Practice of Social Research* (Babbie, 1989). Readers interested in additional information about observational methods should refer to *The Practice of Nursing Research* (Burns and Grove, 1993).

Assessment Guides

Nursing assessment of community health—data collection and interpretation—must be focused. Focus, or perspective, can be provided by detailed assessment guides, which are built on a conceptual framework of definitions of community and community health.

Concepts that are measurable in behavioral or observable terms can serve as assessment guides. The concepts of community and community health have already been defined in such terms. The concept of community has been specified (see Table 15-1). The definition previously given includes three dimensions: people or person, place and time, and function. Each of these dimensions is specified by several indicators. For example, the geographical dimension is represented by indicators, such as size in square miles and political boundaries.

The specification of community health—its status, structure, and process dimensions—are presented in Table 15-3. In the infant malnutrition example, status dimension data were gathered from morbidity/mortality data; structural dimension data were gathered from vital statistics and from informant interviews with social workers; and process dimension

data were gathered from informant interviews with community religious leaders. In this way the concepts of community and community health provide the framework for the Assessment Guide in Appendix C.1. Together, the concepts and Assessment Guide constitute the Community Health Assessment Model, the basis of the *Community-Oriented Health Record* (COHR) (see Appendix C.1). Data, problems, and capabilities are all organized by using the Community Health Assessment Model.

The Community-as-Partner Model is another example of an assessment guide developed to illustrate the bringing together of nursing philosophy and public health to show that nurses can work with communities as partners (Anderson and McFarlane, 1995). This model illustrates how communities change and grow best by full involvement and self-empowerment. The heart of this model is an assessment wheel that illustrates that the people actually are the community. Surrounding the people, and integral to the community, are eight identified subsystems: housing, education, fire and safety, politics and government, health, communication, economics, and recreation. These subsystems both affect and are affected by the people who make up the community. This model and additional information to understand it can be found in Appendix H.1.

Assessment Issues

Gaining entry or acceptance into the community is perhaps the biggest challenge in assessment. The community health nurse is usually an outsider and often represents an established health care system that is neither known nor trusted by community members who may therefore react with indifference or even active hostility to the nurse. In addition, community health nurses may feel insecure about their skills as a community worker, and the community may refuse to acknowledge its need for those skills. Because the nurse's success largely depends on the way he or she is viewed, entry into the community is critical. Often the nurse can gain entry by participating in community events, looking and listening attentively, visiting people in formal leadership positions, employing an assessment guide, and using a peer group for support.

Once the nurse gains entry at an initial level, **role negotiation** often becomes an issue. The concept of role involves the values, behaviors, or goals that govern an individual's interactions with others. The nurse must decide how long to separate the roles of data collector and intervenor. Effective implementation of the nursing process requires initial collection of an adequate data base. The danger of premature response to health needs and social injustice is great. Nurses can facilitate role negotiation by a thoughtful and consistent presentation of the reasons for their presence in the community and by sincere demonstrations of their commitment to the community. Keeping appointments, clarifying community members' perceptions of health needs, and respecting an individual's right to choose whether he or she will work with the nurse are often useful techniques.

Maintaining *confidentiality* is also important. Nurses must scrupulously protect the identity of community members who provide sensitive or controversial data. In some cases the nurse may consider withholding data; in other situations she may be legally required to disclose data. For example, nurses are required by law to report child abuse.

Of a less personal nature is the issue of small-area analysis. Dever (1991) presents a more in-depth discussion about potential problems of small-area analysis although the issue raised here concerns the inappropriateness of reaching conclusions based on data gathered from small areas. For example, calculation of mortality rates in a rural county when the denominator is as small as 5000 may be skewed. This issue frequently compromises the validity of many identified health problems. It also reinforces the usefulness of triangulation, because if similar health problems are identified using several assessment methods, the nurse can be more confident of their validity.

Remember, a community assessment will identify multiple community health problems. Each one of these problems must be analyzed and assigned a priority score to determine which are the most serious problems. In the next sections, the infant malnutrition example is used to illustrate how an identified problem generates a community-based nursing diagnosis, which is analyzed and assigned a priority score.

COMMUNITY-ORIENTED NURSING DIAGNOSIS

The assessment activities and the creation of a composite data base will result in the identification of community health problems. Each problem needs to be identified clearly and stated as a community health diagnosis. The statement of the problem in a community health diagnosis format is the third phase of the community as client process. The development of the community health diagnosis in this phase of the process helps to clarify the problem and is an important precursor to planning. In the planning phase, where each community nursing diagnosis is analyzed, priorities are established and community-focused interventions are identified. Community nursing diagnoses clarify the recipient of care (the community as opposed to an individual) they provide a statement identifying problems faced by the recipient, and they identify factors contributing to the problem.

Although the North American Nursing Diagnosis Association (NANDA) is a familiar nursing diagnosis *taxonomy* for most students, NANDA's focus has been at the individual rather than the community level of diagnosis. Nor is NANDA the only accepted system of nursing diagnosis; for example, home health nurses are familiar with the OMAHA system of nurs-

ing diagnosis. In this chapter we use a modification of a nursing diagnosis format proposed by Muecke (1984) and consisting of three parts:
1. Risk of _____
2. Among _____
3. Related to _____

"Risk of" identifies a specific problem or health risk faced by the community. "Among" identifies the specific community client the nurse will be working with in relation to the identified problem or risk. (See the box, Types of Communities, on p. 290). "Related to" describes characteristics of the community and its environment that were identified in the composite database of the assessment phase. Each community has its own unique characteristics. Some of these characteristics are strengths that the community nurse can build upon, but other characteristics contribute to the problem identified in the community health diagnosis. The characteristics that are contributing factors related to the identified problem are listed after the "related to" statement as the third part of the community health diagnosis.

The example being used for illustration in this chapter is infant malnutrition. Based on assessment data the community diagnosis for infant malnutrition using this format would be the following:
1. Risk of infant malnutrition
2. Among families in Jefferson County
3. Related to: lack of consistent developmental screening; no outreach program to identify at-risk infants; families lack of knowledge about WIC; confusion among community families about WIC program enrollment criteria; community families' lack of infant-related nutritional knowledge.

Frequently, a number of community health diagnoses will be made based upon the different problems identified during the assessment data. In the next phase, "Planning for Community Health," weights and priorities are established among the problems identified in the assessment phase, and the problems have now been stated in a community health nursing diagnosis format.

PLANNING FOR COMMUNITY HEALTH

The planning phase includes analyzing the community health problems identified in the community nursing diagnoses and establishing priorities among them, establishing goals and objectives, and identifying intervention activities that will accomplish the objectives.

Problem Analysis

Problem analysis seeks to clarify the nature of the problem. The nurse identifies the origins and impact of the problem, the points at which intervention might be undertaken, and the parties that have an interest in the problem and its solution. Analysis often

Table 15-4 Problem Analysis

Name of community: Jefferson County

Problem statement: Infant malnutrition in Jefferson County

Problem correlates (precursors and consequences)	Relationship of correlates to problems	Data supportive to relationships (refer to appropriate sections of data base and relevant research findings in current literature)
1. Inadequate diet	Diets lacking in required nutrients contribute to malnutrition.	All county infants and their mothers seen by PHNs in 1993 referred to nutritionist because of poor diets.
2. Community norms	Bottle fed babies less apt to receive adequate amounts of safe milk containing necessary nutrients.	Area general practitioners and nurses agree that 90% of mothers in county bottle-feed.
3. Poverty	Infant formulas are expensive.	60% of new mothers in county are receiving welfare.
4. Disturbed mother-child relationship	Poor mother-child relationship may result in infant's failure to thrive.	Data from nursing charts of 43 mothers with infants diagnosed as "failure to thrive."
5. Teenage pregnancy	Teenage mothers most apt to have inadequate diets prenatally, to bottle feed, to be poor, and to lack parenting skills.	70% of births in 1994 were to women 19 years of age or younger.

requires the development of a problem matrix, in which the direct and indirect precursors and consequences are identified and interrelationships among the problems, precursors, and consequences are mapped. The matrix is important because the nurse can anticipate that several of the same precursors and consequences underlie many of the problems. The problem of highest priority may be among the common precursors and consequences.

Problem analysis should be undertaken for each identified problem. It often requires organizing a special group composed of the nurse, persons whose areas of expertise relate to the problem, persons whose organizations are capable of intervening, and representatives of the community experiencing the problem. Both content and process specialists must participate. Together they can identify the problem correlates and explain the relationships between each correlate and the problem.

This process is seen in the following example of problem analysis (see Table 15-4). Problem correlates (precursors and consequences) of infant malnutrition are listed in the first column. Correlates are from all facets of community life. Social or environmental correlates are as appropriate as those oriented to the individual. For example, teenage pregnancy is a social correlate of infant malnutrition, and high unemployment is an environmental correlate. In the second column the relationships between each correlate and the problem are noted. The third column contains data from the community and the literature that support the relationship, using the suspected infant malnutri-

tion example and a few of its correlates. Infant malnutrition is thought to be correlated with inadequate diet, community norms, poverty, disturbed mother-child relationship, and teenage pregnancy.

Problem Prioritization

Infant malnutrition represents only one of several community health problems identified by the community assessment. In reality, several community-health problems besides infant malnutrition were identified. They included a mortality rate from cardiovascular disease that was higher than the national norm and, as expressed by many residents, a desire to quit smoking.

Each problem identified as part of the assessment process must be put through a ranking process to determine its relative importance. This ranking process, in which problems are evaluated and priorities established according to predetermined criteria, is termed **problem prioritization.** It takes into consideration the contributions of community members, substantive experts, and administrators and resource controllers (Damazzo and Hanson, 1992).

Problem Prioritization Criteria

Criteria that have been helpful in ranking identified problems include: (1) community awareness of the problem; (2) community motivation to resolve or better manage the problem; (3) the nurse's ability to influence problem solution; (4) availability of expertise relevant to problem solution; (5) severity of conse-

Table 15-5   Problem Prioritization

Criteria	Criteria weights (1-10)	Problem	Rating (1-10)	Rationale for rating teachers	Problem significance (weight × rate)
1. Community awareness of the problem	5	Infant malnutrition in Jefferson County	10	Health service providers, teachers, and a variety of parents have mentioned problem.	50
2. Community motivation to resolve the problem	10		3	Most feel this problem is irresolvable because majority of those affected are indigent.	30
3. Nurse's ability to influence problem resolution	5		8	Nurse skilled at consciousness raising and mobilizing support.	40
4. Ready availability of expertise relevant to problem resolution	7		10	WIC program, nutritionists available. County extension agent interested.	70
5. Severity of consequences if problem is left unresolved	8		5	Effects of marginal malnutrition not too well documented.	40
6. Quickness with which problem resolution can be achieved	3		3	Time to mobilize rural community with no history of social action lengthy.	9
					Total: 239

quences if the problem is unresolved; and (6) speed with which resolution can be achieved. Using the example of infant malnutrition again, these six criteria are listed in the first column of Table 15-5.

Given an acceptable and comprehensive set of criteria and a list of community health problems, the process of assigning priorities is rather simple. Each problem is considered independently, and an overall priority score is calculated. This calculation involves two separate but related weighted factors: the first factor involves criteria related to the identified problem itself and the second factor involves these same criteria, but the second factor is weighted based on the partnership's ability to influence each of the criteria in factor one.

Each of the six criteria listed in Table 15-5 is considered separately and independently and then assigned a criterion weight. The criteria are weighted on a scale ranging from a low score of one to a high score of ten. Listed in the second column of Table 15-5, these criteria are weighted jointly by the members of the partnership based on the perceived importance of each criterion to the identified community health problem. For instance, when members of the partnership assigned a weight to the first criterion listed in Table 15-5, they had to ask each other: "How important is community awareness of infant malnutrition in Jefferson County for problem resolution?"

Then the second factor, the importance of each criterion relative to the problem, also must be considered and rated relative to the partnership's ability to resolve the problem. In deciding the rating to be assigned, the members of the partnership answer questions related to their ability to influence and/or change the situation relative to the criterion. In the infant malnutrition example, they asked each other to identify the extent of the community's awareness of the problem. After members have discussed questions about the criterion's significance and have agreed on its rating, the score is recorded. In differentiating between the ideas of criteria weight and problem rating, it may be helpful to remember that a criterion could be extremely important in considering priorities, but rate low for a particular problem because the members of the community partnership feel it would be difficult to influence or change things relative to that particular criterion. One example of the difference between the perceptions of the nurse and community members is smoking in public buildings; the community nurse might identify smoking as a public health problem but community members might view smoking as an issue of individual choice and personal freedom.

This process is repeated separately for each identified problem and a significance score is determined; then the significance scores for all the problems are compared. Priorities among the identified problems

Table 15-6   Goals and Objectives

Name of community: Jefferson County

Problem/concern: Infant malnutrition

Goal statement: To reduce the incidence and prevalence of infant malnutrition

Present date	Objectives (number and statement)	Completion date
1-94	No. 1 80% of infants seen by health department, neighborhood health center, and private physicians will have their developmental levels assessed.	8-94
1-94	No. 2 WIC program eligibility will be determined for 80% of infants, seen by health department, neighborhood health center, and private physicians.	5-94
1-94	No. 3 An outreach program will be implemented to identify at-risk infants not now known to health care providers.	8-94
1-94	No. 4 WIC program eligibility will be determined for 25% of at-risk infants.	1-95
1-94	No. 5 75% of all infants eligible for WIC food supplements will be enrolled in the program.	12-94
1-94	No. 6 50% of the mothers of infants enrolled in WIC will demonstrate three ways of incorporating WIC supplements into their infants' diets.	10-95

are established. The problems with the highest priority scores are the ones selected as the focus for intervention.

Establishing a priority score for each identified problem can appear complicated; however, it helps to recall that the criteria were established and weighted by participants in the community partnership before prioritization began. Also, the rationale for rating as well as each problem rating score is established via the participation of all members in the community partnership. Although the numerical scores are subjective, the active involvement of the nurse and various community representatives, along with the use of triangulation, helps ensure that the data used to establish the rationale are relevant and accurate. Community participation also helps ensure that the significance score established for each problem reflects its importance relative to other community health problems.

The process of establishing a total significance score for the problem of suspected infant malnutrition is called problem prioritization and is depicted in Table 15-5 where criterion two, community motivation to resolve the problem, is used as an example. Community motivation to resolve the problem was the criterion weighted as most important to problem resolution as indicated by the criterion weight of 10. Yet most community residents believed the problem was irremediable because of the poverty of those affected and because partnership members did not believe they could effectively influence poverty, so they rated their ability to intervene low as indicated by the rating of 3. As a result the relative significance of this criterion when applied to the problem of infant malnutrition was low in comparison to the other criteria. This is indicated by the score of 30.

A similar process with the remaining five criteria listed in Table 15-5, yielded a total significance score of 239 for the suspected infant malnutrition problem. Assuming 239 is the highest significance score among the several identified community health problems, infant malnutrition is justified as the priority problem for intervention.

Establishing Goals and Objectives

Once high-priority problems are identified, relevant goals and objectives are developed. **Goals** are generally broad statements of desired outcomes. **Objectives** are the precise statements of the desired outcomes.

An example of one of the goals and the specific objectives associated with it for the infant malnutrition problem is depicted in Table 15-6. The goal presented is to reduce the incidence and prevalence of infant malnutrition. *The objectives must be precise, behaviorally stated, incremental, and measurable.* In this example the specific objectives pertain to assessing infant developmental levels, determining Women, Infants and Children Program (WIC) eligibility, implementing an outreach program, enrolling infants in the WIC program, and incorporating supplemental foods into existing diets.

As noted earlier, establishing these goals and objectives involves collaboration between the nurse and representatives of the community groups affected by both the problem and the proposed intervention. This often requires considerable negotiation among all participants in the planning process. One important advantage offered by the continuous active involvement of people affected by the outcomes is that they have a vested interest in those outcomes and therefore are

Table 15-7   Plan: Intervention Activities to Assess Infants' Developmental Levels

Name of community: Jefferson County

Objective number 1   80% of infants seen by health department, neighborhood health center, and private physicians will have
and statement.   their development levels assessed.

Date	Intervenor activities/means	Value to achieving objective (1-10)	Activity/means selected for implementation*	Probability of implementing activity (1-10)	Activity significance (value × probability)
1-94	1. WIC program supplies personnel to assess infant developmental levels.	1	Insufficient personnel and time. Existing community resources (potential) ignored.	10	10
1-94	2. WIC program provides in-service education to staff an assessment of infant development.	5	Antipathy between WIC personnel and other health workers high. Need for education must be assessed first and enthusiasm for objectives created.	5	25
1-94	3. CN provides in-service education to staff an assessment of infant development.	3	CN cannot do it alone!	10	30
1-94	4.* CN assists WIC personnel to identify in-service educational needs of area health care providers about assessment of infant development.	8	Most likely to build on existing community strengths. CN skilled in needs assessment and interpersonal techniques needed to decrease antipathy.	8	64
1-94	5.* CN assists WIC personnel to identify driving and restraining forces relative to implementation of objective.	10	Without this, change effort likely to fail.	8	80

*See the text below.

supportive of and committed to the success of the intervention. Once goals and objectives are established, intervention activities to accomplish the objectives can be identified.

Identifying Intervention Activities

Intervention activities, the means by which objectives are met, are the strategies that achieve the objectives, the ways change will be affected, and the ways the problem cycle will be interrupted. Because alternative intervention activities do exist, they must be identified and evaluated. Sketching out possible interventions and selecting the best set of activities to achieve the goal of documenting and reducing infant malnutrition are depicted in Tables 15-7 and 15-8.

To achieve the objective related to assessment of infant developmental levels (see Table 15-6, objective 1), five intervenor activities are listed in the second column of Table 15-7. Each is relevant to the first objective: 80% of infants seen by the health department, neighborhood health center, and private physicians will have their developmental levels assessed. The first two activities involve WIC program personnel as the principal change agents. The last three involve the community nurse (CN), WIC program personnel, and

the staff of the health department, neighborhood health center, and private physicians' offices as the change partners.

The probable effectiveness for each of the activities is considered in the third and fifth columns. The **value,*** or the likelihood that the activity will foster achievement of the objective and eventful resolution of the problem, is noted in the third column. Clearly it is more valuable in the long-term to educate others in how to assess infant development (activity four) than to do it for them (activity one). It is also valuable to analyze the change process necessary to accomplish the objective (activity 5). Consequently, activities four and five have higher value scores than activity one, in which the professional staff alone carries out the intervention.

On the other hand, the **probability,*** or the likelihood that the means can be implemented, is highest when only the community nurse is involved, because the nurse has more control over her own behavior than over the behavior of others. Therefore activities one and three have higher probabilities than activi-

---

*The value and probability scores of intervenor activities may range from 1 (low) to 10 (high). The range of 1 to 10 was arbitrarily determined.

Table 15-8   Plan: Intervention Activities to Implement an Outreach Program

Name of community: Jefferson County

Objective number 3   An outreach program is implemented to identify at-risk infants not now known to health care providers and statement.

Date	Intervenor activities/means	Value to achieving objective (1-10)	Activity/means selected for implementation*	Probability of implementing activity (1-10)	Activity significance (value × probability)
1-94	1.* CN identifies and trains lay advisors in community as case finders.	8	Lay leaders already known, proven to be effective change agents; can't however, be paid.	6	48
1-94	2.* Local hospital administrators alter job descriptions of nurses in maternity and pediatrics to include case finding and referral.	8	All babies in Jefferson County born in hospital since 1994. Administrator interested in community. Administration powerful and can alter nurses' job descriptions.	5	40
1-94	3. CN encourages public health nurses to do better job of case finding.	8	Public health nurses have historic role in case finding. CN not well known by PHNs. PHNs reported to be overworked.	2	16
1-94	4. WIC personnel devote 1 evening/week to case finding.	1	One nurse (nonresident) eager to do this. Doesn't develop existing community resources.	10	10

*See the text below.

ties two, four, and five, as recorded in the fifth column. Conditions explaining the numerical scores are noted briefly in the fourth column. A total score is computed by multiplying the value of the activity by the probability. These scores are listed in the last column. The activities with the highest total scores become the priority intervention activities because it is important to be able to both affect the objective (value) and carry out the means (probability). In this case, activities four and five, with total scores of 64 and 80 respectively, would be selected.

Although the numbers assigned by the nurse to both value and probability are based on subjective judgment, their products are quite useful. When the scores in the two columns are multiplied together, the resulting totals establish a relative basis for judging which of the potential intervenor activities will be most effective in meeting the objectives.

A second example of plan development is depicted in Table 15-8. The activities relate to objective three of the goals and objectives (see Table 15-6) in the implementation of an outreach program and involve using lay advisors, hospital nurses, public health nurses, and WIC program personnel. Activities one and two, with total scores of 48 and 40 respectively, were selected. Activity one builds on existing informal community leaders and activity two addresses needed changes in the formal health care delivery system.

IMPLEMENTATION FOR COMMUNITY HEALTH

Implementation, the fourth phase of the nursing process, comprises the work/activities aimed at achieving the goals and objectives. Implementation efforts may be made by the person or group who established the goals and objectives, or they may be shared with or even delegated to others. The issue of centralizing implementation efforts is important, and the community health nurse's position on this issue can be influenced by a variety of factors.

Factors Influencing Implementation

Implementation is shaped by the nurse's chosen roles, the type of health problem selected as the focus for intervention, the community's readiness to participate in problem resolution, and characteristics of the social change process. The nurse participating in community-oriented intervention commands knowledge and skills not possessed by the other intervenors. The question is how the nurse uses the position, knowledge, and skills.

Nurse's Role

Nurses can act as content experts, helping communities to select and attain task-related goals. In the example of infant malnutrition, the nurse used epidemiological skills to determine the incidence and prevalence of malnutrition. The nurse also served as a process expert by increasing the community's own capabilities in documenting the problem rather than by only contributing substantive expertise.

Content-dominated roles often are considered *change agent* roles, whereas process roles are termed *change partner* roles. Change agent roles emphasize gathering and analyzing facts and implementing programs, whereas change partner roles include those of enabler-catalyst, teacher of problem-solving skills, and activist advocate (Eng and Young, 1992; Fulmer et al., 1992; Rothman, 1974).

The Problem

The role the nurse chooses depends on the nature of the health problem and the community's decision-making ability and on professional and personal preferences. Some health problems clearly necessitate certain intervention roles. If a community lacks democratic problem-solving abilities, the nurse may select teacher, facilitator, and advocate roles. Problem-solving skills must be explained and modeled. A problem with ascertaining the status of community health, on the other hand, frequently requires fact-gatherer and analyst roles. Some problems, such as the example of infant malnutrition, require multiple roles. In that case, managing conflict among the involved health care providers demanded process skills. Collecting and interpreting the data necessary to document the problem required both interpersonal and analytical skills.

The community's history of participation in decision making is a critical factor. In a community skilled in identifying and successfully managing its problems, the nurse may serve appropriately as technical expert or advisor. Quite different roles may be required if the community lacks problem-solving skills or has a history of unsuccessful change efforts. The nurse may have to focus on developing problem-solving capabilities or achieving one successful change so that the community becomes empowered to assume responsibility for promoting change on its own behalf.

Social Change Process

The nurse's role also depends on the social change process. Not all communities are receptive to *innovation*. Receptivity to change is often inversely related to the extent to which a community adheres to traditional norms. Innovation is often directly related to high socioeconomic status, a perceived need for change, the presence of liberal, scientific, and democratic values, and a high level of social participation by community residents (Rogers 1995). The innovation itself affects its acceptance. Innovations with the highest adoption rates are perceived as more advantageous than the other alternatives, compatible with existing values, amenable to a limited trial, easily explained or demonstrated, geographically accessible, and simple (Rogers 1995). For example, community residents might go to an immunization clinic rather than a private physician if the clinic is nearby and less expensive and if the physician is not always available when needed.

Innovations also are accepted more readily when the innovation is disseminated in ways compatible with the community's norms, values, and customs and when information is relayed through the appropriate communication mode (mass media for early adopters and face-to-face for late adopters). Other factors that positively influence acceptance include the support of other communities for the change efforts, identification and use of opinion leaders, and clear, unambiguous communication about the innovation (Rogers, 1995).

Many complex and varied factors combine to shape implementation and its effects on the change process. Therefore, the community health nurse must be adaptable. The roles required to initiate change may differ from those used to maintain or stabilize it. Also, the roles required to initiate, maintain, and stabilize change may vary from community to community and from one intervention to another within the same community. Thus the nurse must be skilled in a variety of implementation mechanisms.

Implementation Mechanisms

Implementation mechanisms are the vehicles, or modes, by which innovations are transferred from the planners to the units of service. The community health nurse alone is never considered an implementation mechanism, for change on behalf of the community client requires multiple implementation mechanisms. The nurse must identify and appropriately use all of them. Some important implementation mechanisms, or aids, include small interacting groups, lay advisors, the mass media, and health policy.

Small Interacting Groups

Small interacting groups, formal and informal, are essential implementation mechanisms. Many of the groups in the community—families, legislative bodies, health-care recipients, and service providers—are fully considered elsewhere in the text. Some of the informal groups, such as neighborhoods and social action groups, also have been discussed. The common tie among these diverse groups is their location between the community and individual levels. Because of their intermediate position, they can and do act both to support and to constrain change efforts at the community and individual levels. They are potentially powerful precisely because they are mediating structures.

Consequently, the community health nurse needs to ascertain which groups view the proposed change as beneficial and which do not. New small groups may need to be formed to facilitate the change. Accommo-

Table 15-9   Progress Notes

Name of community: Jefferson County

Goal: To reduce the incidence and prevalence of infant malnutrition

Date	Narrative, Assessment, Plan (NAP)	Budget, time
	(Record both objective and subjective data. Interpret these data in terms of whether the objectives were achieved and whether the intervenor activities used were effective. The plan is dependent on the assessment and may include both new or revised objectives and activities.)	
2-14-94	Objective 1, Means 4	
	Narrative: Meeting to develop needs assessment was attended by CN, two WIC personnel, and physicians from health department, neighborhood health center, and local medical society. Consensus rapidly achieved among five of six participants that goal, objectives, and means (especially Objective 1, Means 4) were appropriate. Physician representing medical society consistently objected, stating vehemently that private sector had long provided adequate medical care for area youngsters. Physician would not recommend that medical society support the effort. CN afraid that this would jeopardize entire effort. Eventually, however, physician left and plans were made to develop and conduct needs assessment, and to continue seeking medical society's help.	
	Agenda: CN to develop needs assessment tool with WIC personnel and health systems agency planner. Physicians to develop list of providers to be contacted. Neighborhood health center physician to get a place on medical society agenda and attempt to clarify our plans. WIC personnel to contact nonphysician health workers to introduce plan and develop provider list.	
	Assessment: Plans made to proceed with needs assessment and partner support essential to accomplishment of objective. Group process problematic, and CN ineffective because of discomfort with conflict between physician and WIC staff member.	$200, 2 hours meeting and 2 hours preparation time
	Plans: Meeting scheduled for 2-28-94 to deal with agreed-on agenda.	
	Before 2-28 meeting, CN will discuss ways to better handle conflict with consultation group, collaborate in drafting needs assessment, and telephone others to determine their progress.	
	J. Goeppinger, RN, CN	

dations may be necessary in the innovation or in the dissemination process to increase acceptance. Initially the innovation may have to be directed to groups with a majority of early adopters (those with broad perspectives and abilities to adopt new ideas from mass media information sources) and to groups whose goals parallel those of the intervention plan (Rothman, 1974). Using a small group to initiate community-oriented change is illustrated in the Progress Notes (see Table 15-9).

Lay Advisors

Lay advisors are individuals who are influential in approving or vetoing new ideas and from whom others seek advice and information about new ideas (Rothman, 1974). They often perform a similar function to that of early adopters. Lay advisors, or opinion leaders, are characterized by conformity to community norms, heavy involvement in formal social groups, specific areas of expertise, and a slightly higher social status than their followers (Rogers, 1995).

Mass Media

Both small interacting groups and lay advisors are particularly useful in instituting change among late adopters. But groups dominated by early adopters and lay advisors can be reached through the mass media. **Mass media,** like newspapers, television, and radio, represent an impersonal and formal type of communication and are useful in providing information quickly to large numbers of people. Using the mass media is efficient because the proportion of resources expended to population covered is low and populations can be targeted. For example, information about teenage pregnancy can be efficiently disseminated through rock music stations.

In addition to being efficient, the mass media are effective aids in intervention. The Stanford Five-City-Project used mass media as a major portion of the project's education intervention, and recent risk factor scores for cardiovascular disease have improved as a result (Winkleby et al., 1994). A small (N100) pilot study conducted in North Carolina also found that mailed pamphlets were as effective as telephone calls and home visits in increasing the use of selected health services (Selby et al., 1990). Similarly, community residents in upstate New York were mobilized successfully for a community-based health intervention using bulk-mailed "Help Yourself to Health" flyers (Hanson, 1988-1989).

Health Policy

Health policy also can play a critical part in the adoption of healthful community-oriented change (Dever, 1991). The major intent of public policy in the health field is to address collective human needs, and it frequently serves to constrain individual choice for the public good. For instance, drivers have been urged for several years to wear automobile seat belts. However, the incidence of automobile fatalities was not reduced until drivers were required to observe lowered speed limits and, in some states, to wear seat belts and use special restraining seats for children. Obviously health policy can facilitate interventions that promote community health.

If public policy that will encourage or even simply allow health-generating choices is to be enacted, the community health nurse must actively lobby for it. The nurse also must use small groups, lay advisors, and the mass media as aids to implementation. Working with naturally occurring small groups like the family and with lay advisors is familiar to most community health nurses. Working with legislators and the mass media is less familiar. Yet all resources must be used to achieve healthful change in the community client.

No matter what mechanisms are used, all implementation efforts must be documented. Evaluation, the sixth phase of this process, is also important to determine and improve the effectiveness of community-oriented nursing practice and thereby increase our knowledge base and improve our success in competing for funds.

EVALUATING THE INTERVENTION FOR COMMUNITY HEALTH

Simply defined, **evaluation** is the appraisal of the effects of some organized activity or program. An example of evaluation research is provided in the Research Brief at right. Evaluation may involve the design and conduct of evaluation research, in which social science research methods are used to determine program effectiveness, efficiency, adequacy, appropriateness, and unintended consequences (Harris, 1992: Kaluzny et al., 1992). Evaluation also may involve the more elementary process of assessing progress by contrasting the objectives and the results. (Green and Kreuter, 1992) This section deals with the basic approach of contrasting objectives and results (Bennett, 1993; Cook et al., 1992; Steckler et al., 1992; Wiesbred et al., 1992).

Evaluation begins in the planning phase, when goals and measurable objectives are established and

Research Brief

Bennett EJ: Health needs assessment of a rural county: impact evaluation of a student project, *Fam Community Health* 16(1):28-35, 1993.

A comprehensive needs assessment to identify the perceived health needs of a rural Arizona county was done by the Arizona State University College of Nursing. The project's goal was to involve the community in the assessment phase by using three specific target population groups identified by key informants: residents over 65; women with infants under 12 months; and children under 18. Data were collected from a large convenience sample recruited from each of the three groups. This article described the impact of the assessment 1 year later on community participation in health and human services planning, as well as community agencies' use of the survey data related to the delivery of their services.

Survey results have been used by state agencies for planning, and by the local hospital, as well as the Head Start program in transportation planning and development. Nursing students participated in this research over the course of a year. The study suggests that projects such as this can have a significant impact upon the community while providing students with an opportunity to be involved in community health nursing research.

goal-attaining activities are identified. After implementing the intervention, only the accomplishment of objectives and the effects of intervention activities have to be assessed. The Progress Notes direct the nurse to perform such appraisals concurrently with implementation. In assessing the data recorded there, the nurse is requested to evaluate whether the objectives were achieved and whether the intervention activities used were effective. The nurse also must decide whether the costs in money and time were commensurate with the benefits. This process is depicted in the progress notes (see Table 15-9). Here the nurse has noted progress toward the needs assessment and difficulties encountered in handling conflict among the group members.

Such an evaluation process is oriented to community health because the intervention goals and objectives are derived from the nurse's and the community's conceptions of health. Simplistic as it appears, it is not without problems. The lack of a control community or even adequate baseline information casts doubts about attributing success, or failure, to the intervention (Wickizer et al., 1993). Nursing interventions also may have such diffuse and therefore weak effects that our crude measures do not discern them. Models for the practitioner to use in determining cost-benefit and cost-effectiveness figures are complicated and therefore, not commonplace. And finally, the lay

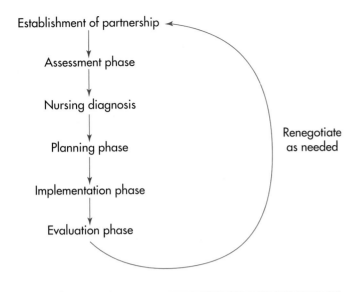

FIGURE 15-2
Flow chart illustrating the circular nature of nursing process with the community client.

role in evaluation has never been fully accepted. Professionals have adopted partnership in assessment and implementation more readily than in evaluation. The issue of who has the power to define, judge, and institute change in professional activities is by no means resolved. With evaluation the entire process is open to renegotiation to achieve community health (Figure 15-2).

PERSONAL SAFETY IN COMMUNITY PRACTICE

Personal safety is a prerequisite for effective community nursing practice and it should be a consideration throughout the process. An awareness of the community and common sense are the two best guidelines for judgment. For example, common sense suggests not leaving anything valuable on a car seat or leaving your car unlocked. Similar guidelines apply to the use of public transportation. Calling ahead to schedule meetings will help prevent delays or confusion, and it gives the CN an opportunity to lay the groundwork for the meeting. If there is no telephone or no access to a neighbor's telephone, plan to establish a time for any future meetings during the initial visit. Regardless of whether there has been telephone contact, there are very rare situations when a meeting may be postponed because the CN arrives at a location where people are unexpectedly loitering by the entrance and the CN has concerns about personal safety.

For nurses who are either just beginning their careers in community health or who are just starting a new position, there are three clear sources of information that will help answer any questions about personal safety. The first source is other nurses, social workers, or health care providers who are familiar with the dynamics of a given community; they can provide valuable insights into when to visit, how to get there and what to expect because they function in the community themselves. However, the best sources of information about the community are the community members themselves and one benefit of developing an active partnership with community members is their willingness to share their insight about day to day community life. The third source is your own observations. Knowledge gained during the data collection phase of the process should provide a solid basis for an awareness of day-to-day community activity. Nurses with experience practicing in the community generally agree, "If you feel uncomfortable in a situation, leave—trust your feelings."

 ## Clinical Application

A clinical application is presented here in a phase-by-phase summary format for further clarification of how the nursing process can be used to promote community health. In this clinical application the flow chart in Figure 15-1 provides an overview of the entire process. Therefore, throughout this example reference will be made back to Figure 15-1.

Cigarette smoking is used here as an example of applying the nursing process to the community client. Cigarette smoking is only one of several community-health-related problems identified during the assessment phase. However, for clarity it will be the only problem used here.

Recall from the infant malnutrition example earlier in the chapter that the phases of this process include: establishment of the contract/partnership, assessment, nursing diagnosis, planning, implementing interventions, and evaluating interventions.

Establishing the contract/partnership for community health is the first phase of the nursing process. In the example, community interest in the question of cigarette smoking in Jefferson County was stimulated by community-wide discussion of a proposed local ordinance limiting smoking in public buildings. Many questions about cigarette smoking were raised by this discussion and debate. Some members of the community decided to pursue this question further, and their decision resulted in the formation of a partnership. This partnership included the community health nurse, community members who supported the local chapter of the American Lung Association (ALA), and the ALA regional director.

Continued.

Clinical Application—cont'd

Assessing Community Health

Assessing community health is the second phase of this process. In Figure 15-1, Assessment, Step 1 involves both data gathering and data generation, using the COHR. Table 15-3 specifies different types of status, structure, and process indicators of community health that can be used for assessment. One example of status data gathered for this community health assessment is a recently commissioned district-wide health study that provided vital statistics, such as mortality and morbidity data for Jefferson County. On the other hand, one example of data generation involved talking with local church leaders, health workers, and other interested lay people about perceived community health needs. These interviews provided important information about the structural and process dimensions of this community's health. Data that are gathered and data that are generated about a community health status are combined during the development of a composite data base (Figure 15-1, Assessment, Step 2).

Data interpretation (Assessment, Step 3) requires examination of the composite data base in order to identify problems. Here the identified community health problems included concerns about drugs in the community, a highly perceived prevalence of smokers in the community, and an increased need for low-income housing. Community strengths also were identified and included such things as the presence of an established community church coalition interested in promoting community health. Once community health problems and community strengths are identified the third phase involves the nursing diagnosis.

Nursing Diagnosis for Community Health

In this clinical application the nursing diagnosis is:
1. Risk of increased incidence of respiratory diseases associated with a high prevalence of cigarette smoking
2. Among families in Jefferson County
3. Related to known relationship between smoking and increased prevalence of respiratory infections; cigarette smoking portrayed to young women by tobacco advertising as a means of self-expression; smokers believe that "only a few a day" is not really smoking, and therefore it will not cause any harm; smokers lack of knowledge about the effects of second-hand smoke on other family members.

Planning for Community Health

Problem Analysis (Figure 15-1, Planning, Step 1)
The first planning step is to analyze each of the identified problems. Analysis is necessary to understand the nature of the identified problem.

Problem Prioritization (Figure 15-1, Planning, Step 2)
Because community resources are limited and the community health assessment usually identifies more than one problem, some means of comparison is needed in order to decide where to start and which identified problem is most significant to the members of the community partnership. In this example, six preselected criteria are used and are listed here as: community awareness of the problem, community motivation to resolve the problem, nurse's ability to influence problem resolution, the ready availability of expertise relevant to problem resolution, the severity of consequences if the problem is left unresolved, and the quickness with which the problem resolution can be achieved. These six criteria are the same criteria as those listed in Table 15-5, and they were selected as a framework for analysis before completion of the community assessment.

When these criteria were applied to the problem of increased incidence of respiratory diseases associated with a high prevalence of smoking in Jefferson County, criteria weights were established by the community partnership participants. This meant examining how important each criterion was relative to any plan of action for resolving the particular community health problem being evaluated (that is, the increased incidence of respiratory diseases caused by a high prevalence of smoking). Determining a problem rating score requires community partnership participants to ask themselves questions about their ability to affect the current situation in their community regarding the specific criterion under consideration. In this clinical application, community motivation to resolve the problem was considered the most important criterion because any community-based effort to reduce smoking would require a great deal of motivation by both the community at-large and individual smokers interested in quitting. Therefore, it received the highest assigned significance score among the six criteria scores that were assigned.

Establish Goals and Objectives (Figure 15-1, Planning, Step 3)
The high prevalence of smoking-related respiratory diseases was identified as the priority problem when compared to other problems identified in the community assessment. Consequently, the next step involved establishing broad goals and specific objectives, that is precise statements of desired outcomes. The goal statement comes from the Nursing Diagnosis and is identified here as "Reduce the incidence and prevalence of smoking-related respiratory diseases by reducing the prevalence of cigarette smoking." The number of specific objectives associated with each broad goal will vary from problem to problem. One specific objective identified as part of this clinical application was "Volunteers will be instructed about enrolling people interested in smoking cessation."

Intervention activities provide specific ways to meet each of the objectives established by the community partnership to help address the problem of

Clinical Application—cont'd

the high prevalence of cigarette smoking. Each identified objective always requires a plan. Only the plan for one objective, "Volunteers will be instructed about enrolling people interested in smoking cessation," is presented here.

Develop Intervention Activities (Figure 15-1, Planning, Step 4)

A number of specific intervenor activities were developed for the objective "Volunteers will be instructed about enrolling people interested in smoking cessation." They included: (1) the provision of volunteers by a community health-promotion coalition to enroll participants; (2) the provision of volunteers and staff to assemble self-help information packets for volunteer distribution; and (3) the writing of step-by-step written directions for community volunteers. An estimated value of each intervenor activity for the identified objective must be identified, as should the anticipated relative probability of implementing each intervenor activity vis-à-vis successful implementation of the identified objective. A total for each intervenor activity is obtained by multiplying these two numbers. For example, the first intervenor activity noted above is to identify volunteers from community organizations to support the program. It was given a value of 10 on a 1 to 10 scale because without identification and recruiting of volunteers from community organizations the goal will not be met. So this intervenor ac-

tivity is critical. However, the nurse can expect some organizations to decline participation and others to withdraw as the process of implementation takes place. The probability assigned is 7, therefore, rather than 10. And the total score would be $10 \times 7 = 70$. A similar process was repeated for each of the other two intervenor activities listed above.

Implementing the Plan for Community Health

The process of implementing the plan itself takes place over time (Figure 15-1, Implement Interventions). It is guided by the results of the planning phase, using the different intervention activities identified as guidelines for reaching each specific objective. The three intervenor activities noted above took 6 months to implement.

Evaluating the Intervention for Community Health

Evaluation of the community health intervention starts while planning is taking place (see Figure 15-1, Evaluate Interventions, Steps 1-7). It is an ongoing part of implementation of each selected intervenor activity, and it also may include retrospective evaluation to assess how successfully each specific objective was completed. Because this assessment is an ongoing process, intervenor activities that are ineffective can be modified or changed. Objectives may be added. This might happen if the intervenor activities were ineffective or unworkable.

Key Concepts

◆ Most definitions of community include three dimensions: (1) networks of interpersonal relationships that provide friendship and support to members; (2) residence in a common locality; and (3) "solidarity, sentiments, and activities."

◆ A community is defined as a locality-based entity, composed of systems of formal organizations reflecting societal institutions, informal groups, and aggregates that are interdependent and whose function or expressed intent is to meet a wide variety of collective needs.

◆ A community practice setting is insufficient reason for saying practice is oriented toward the community client. When the location of the practice is in the community but the focus of the practice is the individual or family, then the nursing client remains the individual or family—not the whole community.

◆ Community-oriented practice is targeted to the community, the population group in which healthful change is sought.

◆ Community health as used in this chapter is defined as the meeting of collective needs through identifying problems and managing interactions within the community itself and between the community and the larger society.

◆ Most changes aimed at improving community health involve, of necessity, partnerships among community residents and health workers from a variety of disciplines.

◆ Assessing community health requires gathering existing data, generating missing data, and interpreting the data base.

◆ Five methods of collecting data useful to the community health nurse are informant interviews, participant observation, secondary analysis of existing data, surveys, and windshield surveys.

Continued.

Key Concepts—cont'd

♦ Gaining entry or acceptance into the community is perhaps the biggest challenge in assessment. The community health nurse is usually an outsider and often represents an established health care system that is neither known nor trusted by community members, who may react with indifference or even active hostility.

♦ The planning phase includes analyzing and establishing priorities among community health problems already identified, establishing goals and objectives, and identifying intervention activities that will accomplish the objectives.

♦ Once high-priority problems are identified, broad relevant goals and objectives are developed.

♦ The goal, generally a broad statement of desired outcome, and objectives, the precise statements of the desired outcome, are carefully selected.

♦ Intervention activities, the means by which objectives are met, are the strategies that clarify what must be done to achieve the objectives, the ways change will be affected, and the way the problem will be interrupted.

♦ Implementation, the third phase of the nursing process, is transforming a plan for improved community health into achievement of goals and objectives.

♦ Simply defined, evaluation is the appraisal of the effects of some organized activity or program.

Critical Thinking Activities

1. Observe an occupational health nurse, community health nurse, school nurse, family nurse practitioner, or emergency room nurse for several hours. Determine which of the nurse's activities are community-oriented and state the reasons for your judgment.

2. Using your own community as a frame of reference, develop examples illustrating the concepts of community, community client, community health, and partnership for health.

3. Read your local newspaper and identify articles illustrating the concepts of community, community client, community health, and partnership for health.

4. Using any two of the conditions of community competence given in the chapter, briefly analyze your own community. Give examples of each condition.

Bibliography

American Nurses Association Task Force to Revise Community Health Standards: *Standards of community health practice*, Washington, DC, 1986, American Nurses Association.

Anderson ET, McFarlane J: *Community-as-partner: theory and practice in nursing*, Philadelphia, Lippincott, 1995.

Anonymous: Consensus set of health status indicators for the general assessment of community health status—United States, *Morb Mortal Wkly Rep* 40(27):449-451, 1991.

APHA: *Community strategies for health: fitting in the pieces*, Washington, DC, 1994, American Public Health Association.

APHA Model Standards: *The guide to implementing model standards: eleven steps toward a healthy community*, Washington, DC, 1993, American Public Health Association.

Armstrong-Esther CA, Lacey B, Sandilands R, Browne KD: Partnership in care, *J Adv Nurs* 12:735-741, 1987.

Babbie E: *The practice of social research*, ed 5, Belmont, Calif, 1989, Wadsworth Publishing.

Bennett EJ: Health needs assessment of a rural county: impact evaluation of a student project, *Fam Community Health* 16(1):28-35, 1993.

Blum HL: *Planning for health*, New York, 1974, Human Sciences Press.

Bogan G, Omar A, Knobloch RS, Liburd LC, O'Rourke TW: Organizing an urban African-American community for health promotion: lessons from Chicago, *J Health Educ* 23(3):157-159, 1992.

Bowling A: Health care research: measuring health status, *Nurs Pract* 4(4);2-8, 1991.

Braddy BA, Orenstein D, Brownstein JN, Cook TJ: PATCH: an example of community empowerment for health, *J Health Educ* 23(3):179-182, 1992.

Brownson RC, Smith CA, Jorge NE, Deprima LT, Dean CG, Cates RW: The role of data-driven planning and coalition development preventing cardiovascular disease, *Public Health Rep* 107(1):32-37, 1992.

Burns N, Grove SK: *The practice of nursing research*, ed 2, Philadelphia, 1993, WB Saunders.

Chalmers K, Kristajanson L: *The theoretical basis for nursing at the community level: models for community health practice.* Paper presented at the 118th annual meeting of the American Public Health Association, New York, 1990.

Chapman L, Jurs J: Conducting community health planning through a hospital sponsored coalition, *J Health Educ* 24(2):119-120, 1993.

Coelho RJ, Kelley PS, Deatsman-Kelly C: An experimental investigation of an innovative community treatment model for persons with a dual diagnosis (DD/MI), *J Rehabil* 59(2):37-42, 1993.

Combs-Orme T, Reis J, Ward LO: Effectiveness of home visits by public health nurses in maternal and child health: an empirical view, *Public Health Rep* 100:490-499, 1985.

Cook TJ, Schmid TL, Braddy BA, Orenstein D: Evaluating community-based program impacts, *J Health Educ* 23(3):183-186, 1992.

Cottrell LS: The competent community. In Kaplan BH, Wilson RN, Leighton AH, editors: *Further explorations in social psychiatry*, New York, 1976, Basic Books.

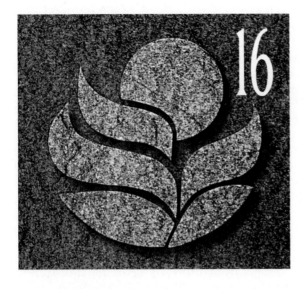

16 Community Health Nursing in Rural Environments

Angeline Bushy

Objectives

After reading this chapter, the student should be able to do the following:

◆ Compare and contrast definitions of rural as opposed to urban.
◆ Describe residency as a continuum, ranging from farm residency to core inner city.
◆ Compare and contrast the health status of rural and urban populations on select health measures.
◆ Discuss barriers to care in health professional shortage areas and for underserved populations.
◆ Review issues related to delivery of services for rural underserved populations.
◆ Describe characteristics of rural and small-town residency.
◆ Examine the role and scope of community health nursing practice in rural and underserved areas.
◆ Highlight two professional-client-community partnership models that are effective in providing a continuum of care to residents living in an environment with sparse resources.

Outline

Universal access to health care has become a national priority, especially in regions with insufficient numbers of all types of health care providers. Recruiting and retaining qualified health professionals in underserved communities, particularly the inner city and rural areas of the United States, is difficult. Until recently, however, limited research has been undertaken on the special challenges, problems and opportunities of nursing practice, especially community health nursing (CHN) in rural settings.

This chapter discusses the issues surrounding health care delivery in rural environments and presents the definitions and perceptions of the term rural, the lifestyle and health status of rural populations, barriers to obtaining a continuum of health care services, nursing practice issues, and strategies to deliver more effective community-based services to clients who live in more isolated environments with sparse resources. The chapter acquaints readers with rural nursing practices and can be used by students, nurses who practice in rural health departments, and those who work in agencies located in an urban area that offer outreach services to rural populations in their catchment area.

HISTORICAL OVERVIEW

Formal rural community health nursing originated with the Red Cross Rural Nursing Service. Before that agency came into existence, care of the sick in a small community was provided by informal social support systems. Generally, this task was assigned to healing women who lived within the geographical area if self-care and family care did not prove effective to bring about healing. Historically, the health needs of rural Americans have been numerous—not necessarily unique—but nevertheless different from those of urban populations. Consistent problems of maldistribution of health professionals, poverty, limited access to services, ignorance, and social neglect have plagued many rural communities for generations. Over the years, the history of the Red Cross Rural Nursing Services shows a consistent movement away from its initial rural focus, as demonstrated by its frequent name changes. Unfortunately, as with the Rural Red Cross Service, concern for rural health often is a passing fad that is preempted by other areas of greater need (Bigbee and Crowder, 1985). Hopefully, this will not be the case with health care reform in its efforts to assure universal access to care for rural and urban residents.

DEFINITION OF TERMS
Rurality: A Subjective Concept

Everyone has an idea as to what constitutes "rural" versus urban. Rural can be defined in terms of the geographic location and population density, or it may be described in terms of the distance from (i.e., 20 miles) or the time (i.e., 30 minutes) needed to commute to an urban center. Other definitions equate rural with farm residency and urban with nonfarm residency. Some consider "rural" to be a state of mind. For the more affluent, rural may bring to mind a recreational, retirement, or resort community located in the mountains or in lake country where one can relax and participate in outdoor activities, such as skiing, fishing, hiking, or hunting. For the less affluent, the term can impose grim scenes. For example, some people may think of an impoverished Indian reservation that is comparable to a third-world country, or it may bring to mind images of a migrant labor camp with several families living in a one-room shanty with no access to safe drinking water or adequate sanitation.

It is difficult to describe a "typical rural town" because of the wide population and geographic diversity. For example, rural towns in Florida, Oregon, Alaska, Hawaii, and Idaho are different from each other, and quite different from those in Vermont, Texas, Tennessee, Alabama, or California. Furthermore, there can be vast differences among rural areas within one state. The descriptions and definitions for rural are more subjective and relative in nature than for urban.

For instance, "small" communities with populations of more than 20,000 have some features that one may expect to find in a city. Then again, residents who live in a community having a population of less than 2000 may perceive a community with a population of 5000 to 10,000 to be a city. As for communities that seem geographically remote on a map, the residents who live there may not feel isolated. Those residents believe they are within easy reach of services through telecommunication and dependable transportation, albeit extensive shopping amenities may be 50 to 100 miles from the family home or obstetric care may be 150 miles away or nursing services in the district health department in an adjacent county may be 75 or more miles away.

Rural versus Urban: A Continuum

Frequently used definitions to describe **rural** versus **urban** are provided by several federal agencies, as shown in the box on p. 317 (Braden and Beauregard, 1994; Bureau of the Census, 1991; USBHP, 1990; USOTA, 1990). These definitions, often dichotomous in nature, fail to take into account the relative nature of ruralness. Rural-urban residency, realistically, is a continuum ranging from living on a remote farm, to a village or small town, to a larger town or city, to a large metropolitan area with a **"core inner city"** (Hewitt, 1989; Lee, 1991) (see Figure 16-1).

As beliefs and values change over time, urban/rural differences may narrow in some aspects and enlarge in others. Depending on the definition that is used, the actual rural population may vary slightly. Generally speaking, about 25% of all U.S. residents live in rural settings. For this chapter, rural refers to areas having fewer than 99 persons per square mile and communities having 20,000 or fewer inhabitants.

Terms and Definitions

TERM	DEFINITIONS
Frontier	Fewer than six persons per square mile
Rural	Community with less than 2500 residents
	Less than 99 persons per square mile*
	Community with less than 20,000 residents*
Farm Residency	Residence outside the city limits; involvement in agriculture industry
Nonfarm Residency	Residence within the city limits
Urban	Community with more than 2500 residents
	More than 99 persons per square mile
Suburban	Areas outlying highly populated cities
Standard Metropolitan Statistical Area (SMSA)	County with a central city of at least 50,000 residents
Nonmetropolitan Statistical Area (non-SMSA)	Counties that do not meet SMSA Criteria
Core Metropolitan	Densely populated counties with more than 1 million residents
Other Metropolitan	Fringe counties of Core Metropolitan; all other Metropolitan
Urban Nonmetropolitan	Cities with a population of at least 20,000 but less than 50,000

*Definition of rural as used in this chapter.

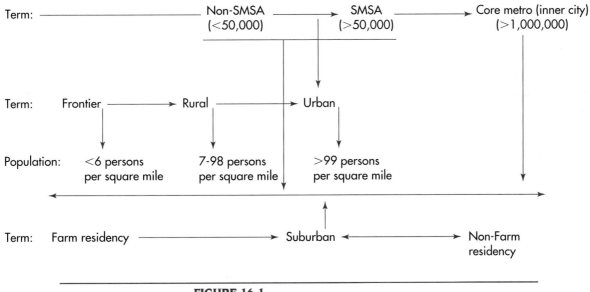

FIGURE 16-1

The continuum of rural-urban residency.

CURRENT PERSPECTIVES

Population Characteristics

Adding to the confusion about the notion of rural as opposed to urban residency are the special needs of the numerous underrepresented groups (minorities, subgroups) who reside across the 50 states. In general, there is a higher proportion of Caucasians in rural areas (about 82%) than in core metropolitan areas (about 62%). There are, however, regional variations, and some rural counties have significant numbers of minorities. Of the total rural population, nearly 4 million are African-American, almost 2 million are Native American, 34 million are Asian-Pacific Islanders and 75 million are of other races (Bureau of the Census, 1992; NRHA, 1994). Little is documented on the needs and health status of special rural populations. Anthropologists are quick to report that, within a group, there often exists a wide range of life-styles. Consequently, even in the smallest or most remote town or village, a subgroup may behave differently

Table 16-1 Selected Population Characteristics by Place of Residence in regard to Age, Marital Status, Education Level, Poverty Rate (Percentage of population)

Demo factor	Core metro	Other metro	Urban nonmetro	Rural
Age				
6-17 yrs	15.2	17.3	—	20
25-54 yrs	43.3	42	40.8	38.3
65+ yrs	12	—	10	17.3
Marital Status (over 17)				
Never married	26.5	21	19.3	16.5
Were married	52.7	60.5	61	64.6
Education				
12 yrs	25	25	40	36
12+ yrs	40	40	30	24
Poverty Rate				
Below indices	19	15	22	26

and have different values regarding health, illness, and patterns of accessing health care. Their lifestyle too may be associated with health problems that are different from the predominant cultural group within a given community. Background information on those particular populations can be found in other chapters of this text.

Table 16-1 presents demographic data comparing the rural and urban population. Demographically, rural communities are described as "bipolar" in age distribution because they have a higher than average number of younger and older residents. In other words, one finds a higher proportion of persons between 6 and 17 years of age and over 65 years of age living in rural compared to urban areas. Persons 18 years of age and over living in rural areas are more likely to be, or to have been, married than adults in the three urban categories. As a group, rural people also are more likely to be widowed. As for level of education, adults in rural areas have fewer years of formal schooling than do urban adults.

Rural families tend to be poorer than their urban counterparts. Comparing annual incomes with the standardized index established by the Bureau of Census, more than one-fourth of rural Americans live in or near poverty and nearly 40% of all rural children are impoverished (Children's Defense Fund, 1991; Rowland and Lyons, 1989). Compared with those in metropolitan settings, a substantially smaller percentage of families living in rural and nonmetropolitan areas are at the high end of the income scale. Level of income is a critical factor in whether or not a family has health insurance or qualifies for public insurance. Hence, rural families are less likely to have private insurance and more likely to have public insurance or to be uninsured.

The working poor, of which there is a high number in rural areas, are particularly at risk for being underinsured or uninsured (NRHA, 1994). In working poor families one or more of the adults is employed but still cannot afford private health insurance. Furthermore, their annual income is such that it disqualifies the family from obtaining public insurance. A number of reasons are cited for this phenomenon occurring more often in rural settings. For instance, a large number of individuals are self-employed in a family business, such as ranching or farming, or they work in small enterprises, such as a service station, restaurant, or grocery store. Or, an individual may be employed in part-time or seasonal occupations, such as farm laborer and construction in which health insurance often is not an employee benefit. In other situations, a family member may have a preexisting health condition that makes the cost of insurance prohibitive, if it is even available to them.

A few rural families "fall through the cracks" and are unable to access any type of public assistance because of other deterrents. For example, language barriers, being physically compromised, the geographic location of an agency, lack of transportation, or having the status of "undocumented" worker. Insurance, or the lack of it, has serious implications for the overall health status of rural residents and the community health nurses who provide services to them.

Health Status of Rural Residents

Even though rural communities constitute about one-fourth of the total population, we do not fully understand the health problems or the health behaviors of those residents. This section summarizes the overall health status for rural adults and children. The health status measures that are addressed herein are perceived health status, diagnosed chronic conditions, physical limitations, frequency of seeking medical treatment, usual source of care, maternal-infant health, children's health, mental health, minorities' health, and environmental and occupational health risks (Braden and Beauregard, 1994; Gesler and Ricketts, 1992; Wakefield, 1990).

Perceived Health Status

In general, rural populations have a poorer perception of their overall health and functional status than their urban counterparts. Specifically, rural residents over the age of 18 assess their health status less favorably than urban residents. Studies show that rural adults are less likely to engage in preventive behavior, which increases their exposure to risk. Specifically they are less likely to wear seat belts, have regular blood pressure checks, have pap smears, and complete self-breast examinations. Ultimately, failure to participate in these life-style behaviors affects overall health status of rural residents, their level of function, physical limitations, degree of mobility, and level of self-care activities (Sullivan et al., 1993; Weinert and Long, 1993).

Chronic Illness

Compared with their urban counterparts, rural adults are more likely to have one or more of the following chronic conditions: hypertension, arthritis/rheumatism, diabetes, cardiovascular disease, or cancer. Nearly half of all rural adults have been diagnosed with at least one of these chronic conditions compared to about a quarter of nonrural adults. More specifically, the prevalence rate of diagnosed diabetes in rural adults is about 7 out of 100 as opposed to 5 out of 100 in nonrural environments. As for cancer, more rural adults have this diagnosis (almost 7%) compared to urban adults (about 5%).

A higher percentage of rural adults receive medical treatment for both life-threatening illness and degenerative or chronic conditions than do urban adults. Life-threatening conditions include malignant neoplasms, heart disease, cardiovascular problems, and liver disorders. Degenerative or chronic diseases include diabetes, kidney disease, arthritis and rheumatism, and chronic diseases of the blood, nervous, respiratory and digestive system. In essence, chronic health conditions, coupled with their poor health status, limit the physical activities of a larger proportion of rural residents compared with their urban counterparts (Dickey and Kamerow, 1992; Frame, 1992; Geller et al., 1990; Goeppinger, 1993; McManus et al., 1990).

Physical Limitations

Limitations in mobility and self-care are strong indicators of an individual's overall health status. Specifically assessed measures on a national health survey included (1) walking one block, (2) walking uphill or climbing stairs, (3) bending, lifting, stooping, and (4) feeding, dressing, bathing, or toileting. More rural adults (9%) experience at least three of these limitations compared with metropolitan adults (6%) who were limited to that degree. The increased prevalence of poor health status and impaired function is not necessarily due to the increased number of older adults found in rural areas. Similar patterns are evident in adults ages 18 to 64. Rural adults under age 65 are more likely than urban to assess their health status as fair to poor and a greater percentage have been diagnosed with a chronic health condition.

Based on data from national health surveys, the overall health status of rural adults leaves much to be desired. This is attributed to a number of factors, including impaired access to health care providers and services coupled with other rural factors. Hence, community health nurses in rural practice settings play an important role in providing a continuum of care to clients living in these underserved areas, for instance, by teaching rural clients how to prevent accidents, engage in more healthful life-style behaviors, and reduce the risk of chronic health problems. Once diagnosed with a long-term problem, community health nurses can help clients in rural environments manage chronic conditions to maintain an optimal level of health and function.

Utilization Patterns of Health Services

In measuring the utilization of health care services, more than three-fourths of adults in rural areas received medical care on at least one occasion during that year. Table 16-2 summarizes the frequency of visits to ambulatory care settings by rural and metro residents (Braden and Beauregard, 1994). Despite their overall poorer health status and higher incidence of chronic health conditions, rural adults seek medical care less often than urban adults. In part this discrepancy can be attributed to scarce resources and lack of providers in rural areas. Other reasons for this phenomenon are discussed in a subsequent part of this chapter focusing on barriers to accessing health care.

Availability and Access of Health Care

The ability of a person to identify a "usual" source of care has been viewed as a favorable indicator of access to health care and a person's overall health status. In

Table 16-2 Annual Number of Visits Per Person to an Ambulatory Care Setting by Place of Residence

Uninsured/Public Coverage

Rural/Nonmetro	7.5 visits
All metro	7.5 visits

Private Insurance

Rural/Nonmetro	6.3 visits
All metro	7.4 visits

Number of Visits by Place of Residence

Rural	9.5 visits
Urban nonmetropolitan	10.4 visits
Core metropolitan	12.1 visits
Other metropolitan	10.9 visits

Table 16-3 Residency and Rate of Infant Mortality and Low Birth Weight (per 1000 population)

	National average	Non-HPSA	HPSA
Infant mortality	10.4	9.1	12.6
Low birth weight	6.8	5.8	8.3

essence, a person who has a usual source of care is more likely to seek care when ill and is more compliant with prescribed regimens. Having the same provider of care can enhance continuity of care, as well as a client's perceived perception of the quality of that care. Rural adults (85%) are more likely than urban (78%) to identify a particular medical provider as their usual source of care. As for the type of provider who delivers the care, general practitioners usually are seen by rural adults, whereas urban adults are more likely to seek care from a specialist.

Another measure of access to care is traveling time and/or distance to ambulatory care services. Rural persons who seek ambulatory care are more likely to travel more than 30 minutes to reach their usual source of care. Extended commuting time also may be a factor for residents in highly populated urban areas and those who must rely on public transportation. Upon arriving at the clinic or doctor's office, however, no differences have been found in the waiting time to see the provider between rural and urban residents.

Measure of usual place and usual provider, in and of itself, suggests that rural residents are at least as well off as urban residents in regard to access to care. Caution must be used when making this generalization, though, since 1 out of 17 rural counties is reported to have no physicians. Among rural respondents on national surveys the ability to identify a usual site of care or a particular provider often stems from a community or county having only one, perhaps two, health care providers. The limited number of health care facilities is reinforced by the finding that nearly all rural residents (95%) who seek health care use ambulatory services that are provided in a doctor's office as opposed to a clinic, community health center, hospital outpatient department, or emergency room (NRHA, 1993; University of Iowa, 1993a, 1993b; USBHP, 1990; USGAO, 1991).

It is not unusual for rural professionals to live and practice in a particular community for decades. Moreover, in a **Health Professional Shortage Area**

(HPSA) a doctor, a nurse practitioner, or community health nurse often provides services to residents who live in several counties. In the case of community health nursing, one or two nurses in a county health department usually offer a full range of services for all residents in a catchment area, which may span more than a hundred miles from one end of a county to the other. Consequently, rural physicians and nurses frequently report, "I provide care to individuals and families with all kinds of conditions, in all stages of life, and across several generations." In turn, it should not come as a surprise that rural respondents who participate in national surveys are able to identify a usual source and usual provider of health care.

Maternal-Infant Health

There are conflicting reports in the literature regarding pregnancy outcomes in rural areas. Overall, rural populations have higher infant and maternal morbidity rates, especially counties designated as HPSAs (Table 16-3). Here, one also finds fewer specialists, such as pediatricians, obstetricians, and gynecologists to provide care to at-risk populations.

It is important to emphasize, there are extreme variations in pregnancy outcomes from one part of the country to another, even within states. For instance, in several counties located in the north central and intermountain states, the pregnancy outcome is among the finest in the United States. However, in several other counties within those same states, the pregnancy outcome is among the worst. Particularly at risk are women who live on or near Indian reservations, are migrant workers, and are of African-American origins and live in rural counties of states located in the deep south (Bronstein and Morrisey, 1991; Henshaw and VanVort, 1991; Nesbitt et al., 1990).

Most nurses understand the effects of socioeconomic factors on pregnancy outcomes, such as income level (poverty), education levels, age, employment/unemployment patterns, and use of prenatal services. There are other less well-known determinants, such as environmental hazards, occupational risks, and the cultural meaning placed on childbearing and child rearing practices by a community. The effects of these multifaceted factors vary, and because of space limitations, they will not be examined in depth in this chapter.

Children's Health

Reports on the health status of rural children show regional variations and conflicting data. Comparing rural with urban children under 6 years of age on the measures of access to providers and utilization of services reveals the following findings. Urban children are less likely to have a usual provider but are more likely to see a pediatrician when they are ill. Similar to rural adults, their children also are more likely to have care from a general practitioner who is identified as their usual care giver.

School nurses are an important factor in the overall health status of children in the United States. The availability of school nurses in rural communities also varies from region to region. More specifically, in frontier and rural areas of the United States, school nurses usually are scarce. In part this deficit can be attributed to limited resources associated with low tax revenues and shortages of health personnel in those counties. In other words, there are fewer tax payers living in those large geographical areas. Some frontier areas have fewer than four persons per square mile and a few have less than two persons per square mile.

Consequently, rural county commissioners like their urban counterparts are forced to prioritize the allocation of scarce resources among such services as maintaining public utilities, roads, bridges, schools, supporting a financially suffering county hospital, hiring a county health nurse, and offering school health services. In rural communities there are fewer resources to begin with. Yet, certain public services must still be provided to local residents.

Obviously, creativity is required by both community residents and local health care providers to resolve health care and school nursing needs. Partnership arrangements, for example, have been negotiated by two or more counties that agree to share the cost of a "district" health nurse. Other county commissioners have forged partnerships with an agency in an urban setting and contracted for specific health care services. In both of these situations, it is not unusual for the community health nurse to provide services to all children attending schools in the participating counties. In some frontier states, schools may be situated more than 100 miles apart and as many miles or more from the district health office. Because of the number of schools and distances between them, the county nurse may only be able to visit each school once, maybe twice, in a school term. Usually the nurse's visit is to update preschool immunizations and, perhaps, to teach maturation classes to students in the upper grades.

The health status of rural women, infants, and children is less than optimal. In part this can be attributed to inadequate preventative, primary, and emergency services to meet their particular health care needs. On the one hand, scarce resources can pose a challenge to a community health nurse who provides care to rural residents, especially those in underserved areas. On the other, resource deficits encourage creativity and innovation, an espoused characteristic of community health nursing in general, and of rural nurses in particular (ANA, 1991; Children's Defense Fund, 1991;

Greydanus, 1992; Kirby, 1990; Monheit and Cunningham, 1992; Perloff, 1992; Washington State Nursing Network, 1992).

Mental Health

As with other dimensions on the health of rural populations, the facts about their mental health status also are ambiguous and conflicting. We do know that stress, stress-related conditions, and mental illness are prevalent among populations when severe economic difficulties persist. The depressed agriculture, lumber, and mining industries during the 1980s resulted in numerous job losses in rural communities; hence, the term "farm stress." Economic recession also is a contributing factor to a family not having insurance or being underinsured. Interestingly, even if mental health services are available and accessible, rural residents delay seeking care when they have an emotional problem until there is an emergency or a crisis (Abraham et al., 1994). This phenomenon is reflected in the lower number of annual visits to mental health services by rural residents, as is the case for those with chronic health problems.

Mental health professionals who provide services to this target population report a persistent, endemic level of depression among rural residents. They speculate this condition is associated with the high rate of poverty, geographic isolation, and insufficient numbers of mental health services. Depression also may be a contributing factor to the escalating incidence of accidents and suicides, especially among rural male adolescents and young men. The incidents have increased dramatically over the last decade and continue to rise in this group, to the point of being epidemic in some small communities (Dunbar, 1992; Human and Wasem, 1991; Murray and Keller, 1991; NCHADI, 1991; USGAO, 1990; Wagenfeld and Wagenfeld, 1990).

Reports on the incidence in rural populations of domestic violence, alcohol and chemical substance use/abuse also are conflicting. These behaviors are less likely to be reported in areas where residents are related or personally acquainted. After a period of time, in small, tight-knit communities destructive coping behaviors often come to be accepted as, "business as usual, and nothing out of the ordinary in that family." Family problems also may be ignored if formal social services and public health services are sparse or nonexistent and if the community does not trust the professionals who provide services within a local agency. In underserved rural areas there are gaps in the continuum of mental health services which, ideally, should include preventive education, anticipatory guidance, early intervention programs, crises and acute care services, and follow-up care. As with other aspects of health care, community health nurses in rural areas play an important role in community education, case finding, advocacy, and case management of client systems experiencing emotional problems and chronic mental health problems.

Table 16-4   Special Rural Populations' Health Care Needs and Required Nursing Skills

Population/Community	Needs/Skills
Farming/ranching	Advanced life support for cardiac emergencies Emergency care for accident/trauma victims Environmental hazards Perinatal-health care Farmer's lung Dermatitis Farm stress/depression
Native Americans	Diabetes Alcohol/substance abuse Cirrhosis of the liver Vehicular accidents Hypothermic injuries Trauma-related injuries Tuberculosis Sudden infant death syndrome (SIDS) Perinatal health care
African Americans	Hypertension Cardiovascular disease Sickle cell anemia Perinatal health care
Migrant farm workers	Field sanitation Safe drinking water Exposures to pesticides, herbicides Infectious diseases (e.g., hepatitis, typhoid)
Native Alaskans	Exposures to petroleum by-products Toxic residue contaminated seafood Diabetes Alcohol/substance abuse Cirrhosis of the liver Vehicular accidents Hypothermic injuries Trauma-related injuries Tuberculosis Sudden infant death syndrome (SIDS) Perinatal health care
Miners (coal)	OSHA Standards Respiratory diseases (black lung, COPD) Air/Water quality standards Substance abuse Depression Trauma care

Minorities' Health

As mentioned previously, there are a significant number of at risk minority groups in rural America who have some rather unique concerns, in particular, children, the elderly, American Indians, Native Alaskans, Native Hawaiians, migrant workers, African-Americans, and the homeless (NRHA, 1994; USDHHS, 1989) (see Table 16-4). The rural homeless, for instance, may be seasonal farm workers or families from within a community who had their farm foreclosed. Sometimes the family may be allowed, according to the law, to continue living in the house on the farm that once was theirs. The family no longer has a means of livelihood and often remains hidden in the community with insufficient income to purchase food or other necessary services. The particular health problems of these at-risk groups are discussed in other chapters of this text. Community health nurses should be aware, however, that at-risk and underrepresented groups may experience some unique concerns related to the rural lifestyle, isolation, and sparse resources.

Environmental and Occupational Health Risks

A community's primary industry also is an influencing factor in the local lifestyle, the health status of its residents, and the number and types of health care services it may need. For instance, three high risk industries identified by OSHA that are found in predominantly rural environments are lumbering/forestry, mining, and agriculture. Associated health risks of those industries are machinery and vehicular accidents, trauma, select types of cancer, and respiratory disease stemming from repeated exposure to toxins, pesticides and herbicides (Geller et al., 1990; National Safety Council, 1990-1993; Wakefield, 1990).

More specifically, agriculture-type businesses, such as farming and ranching, often are owned and operated by a family. Small enterprises do not fall under OSHA guidelines; hence, safety standards are not enforceable on most farms and ranches. Moreover, small businesses, such as farming, are not covered under workman's compensation insurance. Additional concerns arise because family members participate in the farm/ranch work. This means that some adults and children may operate dangerous farm machinery with minimal operating instructions on the hazards and safety precautions. Consequently, agriculture-related accidents result in a significant number of deaths and long-term injuries, particularly among children and women, but also among males. The morbidity and mortality rates associated with agriculture vary from state to state. The rising incidence of these injuries and deaths, however, has become a national concern (USOTA, 1990). To this end, community health nurses in rural settings can help address this problem by including farm safety content in school education programs and in public presentations to church and civic groups.

In summary, it is risky to generalize about the health status of rural Americans because of their di-

Characteristics of Rural Life

More space; greater distances between residents/services
Cyclic/seasonal work and leisure activities
Informal social/professional interactions
Access to extended kinship systems
Residents are related or acquainted
Lack of anonymity
Small enterprises (family); fewer large industries
Economic orientation to land and nature (e.g., agriculture,
   mining, lumbering, fishing)
High-risk occupations more prevalent
Town is center of trade
Churches and schools are socialization centers
Preference for interacting with localities (insiders)
Mistrust of newcomers to the community (outsiders)

Barriers to Health Care

Great distances to obtain services
Lack of personal transportation
Unavailable public transportation
Lack of telephone services
Unavailable outreach services
Inequitable reimbursement policies for providers
Unpredictable weather conditions
Inability to pay for care
Lack of "know how" to procure entitlements/services
Providers' attitudes and knowledge levels about rural
   populations

versity coupled with conflicting definitions as to what differentiates rural from urban residences. There are a significant number of vulnerable individuals and families living in rural communities across the 50 states, but little is known about many of them. This void is a potential research area for community health nurses who practice in rural environments across America.

RURAL HEALTH CARE DELIVERY ISSUES AND BARRIERS TO CARE

Even though each rural community is unique, the experience of living in a rural area has several common characteristics (Ludloff and Swanson, 1990) (see box above, left). Concomitantly, barriers to health care may be associated with these characteristics, that is to say, whether or not services and professionals are available, affordable, accessible, or acceptable to rural consumers.

Availability implies the existence of health services, as well as the necessary personnel to provide essential services. Sparseness of population limits the number and array of health care services in a given geographical region. Hence, the cost of providing special services to a few people often is prohibitive, particularly in frontier states where there are insufficient numbers of physicians, nurses, and other types of health providers. Consequently, where services and personnel are scarce they must be allocated prudently. *Accessibility* implies that a person has logistical access to, as well as the ability to purchase, needed services. *Affordability* is associated with both availability and accessibility of care. It infers that services are of "reasonable cost" and that a family has sufficient resources to purchase them when they are needed. *Acceptability* of care means that a particular service is appropriate and offered in a manner that is congruent with the values of a target population. This can be hampered by both the client's cultural preference and the urban orienta-

tion of health professions (Conway-Welch, 1991; Gesler and Ricketts, 1992; NACHC, 1992; Summer, 1991) (see box above, right).

A few comments are in order regarding providers' attitudes, insights and knowledge about rural populations. A demeaning attitude, lack of accurate knowledge about rural populations, or insensitivity about the rural life-style on the part of a community health nurse can perpetuate difficulties in relating to those clients. Moreover, insensitivity perpetuates mistrust, resulting in rural clients perceiving professionals as "outsiders to our community." Conversely, some professionals in rural practice express feelings of "professional isolation and community nonacceptance." To resolve these conflicting views, it behooves nursing faculty to expose students to the rural environment. Clinical experiences should include opportunities to provide care to clients in their natural setting (i.e., rural) in order to gain accurate insight about that particular community.

To design community-based programs that are available, accessible, affordable, and appropriate, community health nurses must design strategies and implement interventions that mesh with a client's belief system. This infers that a family and a community are actively involved in planning and delivering care for a member who needs it. Community health nurses must have an accurate perspective from rural clients. Although the importance of forming partnerships and assuring mutual exchange seems obvious, to date most of the research about rural communities has been for policy or reimbursement purposes. There is minimal empirical data about rural family systems in terms of their health beliefs, values, perceptions of illness, health care seeking behaviors, and what constitutes appropriate care. Hence, nurses must assume a more active role in implementing research on the community nursing needs of rural populations, in order to expand our profession's theoretical base and subsequently implement empirically based clinical interventions.

Characteristics of Nursing Practice in Rural Environments

Variety/diversity in clinical experiences
Broader/expanding scope of practice
Generalist skills
Flexibility/creativity in delivering care
Sparse resources (materials, professionals, equipment, fiscal)
Professional/personal isolation
Greater independence
More autonomy
Role overlap with other disciplines
Slower paced
Lack of anonymity
Increased opportunity for informal interactions with patients/
  co-workers
Opportunity for client follow-up upon discharge in informal
  community settings
Discharge planning allows for integration of formal with informal
  resources
Care for clients across the lifespan
Exposed to clients with a full range of conditions/diagnoses
Status in the community; viewed as an occupation of prestige
Viewed as a professional "role model"
Opportunity for community involvement and informal health
  education

NURSING CARE IN RURAL ENVIRONMENTS

Rural Nursing Theory, Research, and Practice

There is a growing body of literature on nursing practice in small towns and rural environments and several themes have emerged (see box above). As with everything in life, each of these dimensions can be viewed as an opportunity or a challenge by a nurse who practices here.

Researchers from the University of Montana contend that existing theories do not fully explain rural nursing practice (Long and Weinert, 1989; Weinert and Long, 1990; 1991; 1993). They examined the four concepts pertinent to a nursing theory (health; person; environment; nursing/caring) and described relational statements that are relevant to clients and nurses in rural environments. Since the focus of their research was Anglo-Americans living in the Rocky Mountain area, care must be taken about generalizing those findings to other geographical regions and minorities. In essence, they propose that rural residents often judge their health by their ability to work. They consider themselves healthy, even though they may suffer from several chronic illnesses, so long as they are able to continue working. For them, being healthy is the ability to be productive. Chronically ill people emphasize emotional and spiritual well-being rather than physical wellness.

Distance, isolation, and sparse resources are inherent in rural life and are reflected in residents' independent and innovative coping strategies. Self-

Long K, Weinert C: Rural nursing: developing a theory base. *Sch Inq Nurs Pract* 3:113-127, 1989.
Weinert C, Long K: Rural families and health care: refining the knowledge base, *J Marriage Fam Rev* 15(1, 2):57-76, 1990.

The following theoretical concepts and dimensions of rural nursing were proposed by Long and Weinert at Montana State University:

Health Defined by rural residents as the ability to work. Work and health beliefs are closely related for rural Montana sample.

Environment Distance and isolation are particularly important for rural dwellers. Those who live long distances neither perceive themselves as isolated nor do they perceive health care services as inaccessible.

Nursing Lack of anonymity, outsider/insider, old-timer/newcomer. Lack of anonymity is a common theme among rural nurses who report knowing most people whom they care for, not only in the nurse-client relationship but in a variety of social roles, such as family member, friend, or neighbor. Acceptance as a health care provider in the community is closely linked to the outsider/insider–newcomer/oldtimer phenomenon. Gaining trust and acceptance of local people is identified as a unique challenge that must be successfully negotiated by nurses before they can begin to function as effective health care providers.

Person Self-reliance and independence in relation to health care are strong characteristics of rural individuals. They prefer to have people they know care for them (informal services) as opposed to that provided by an outsider in a formal agency.

reliance and independence are demonstrated through their self-care practices and preference for family and community support. Community networks provide support but still allow for each person's and family's independence. Ruralites prefer and usually seek help through their informal networks, such as neighbors, extended family, church, and civic clubs, rather than seeking a professional's care in the formal system of health care, including services such as those provided by a mental health clinic, social service agency, or health department.

The work and home roles for professional nursing practice in rural areas may not be distinct. In many instances a nurse may have more than one work role in the community, such as a nurse who is also a Sears' catalogue store owner, or a nurse who works at the local hospital or doctor's office and also is actively involved in the management of a family farm. For nurses, this means that many, if not all, patients are personally known as neighbors, friends of an immediate family member, or perhaps part of one's extended family. Associated with the social informality, there is a corresponding lack of anonymity in a small town. Some rural nurses say, "I never really feel like I am off duty because everybody in the county knows me through my work." In part this can be attributed to nurses being highly regarded by the community and viewed by local people as an "expert" on health and illness. It is not unusual for residents to informally seek a nurse's advice, that is "to be checked out," before seeking the services of a doctor for a health problem. Moreover, health-related questions are asked by residents when they encounter the nurse (who may be a family neighbor, a friend, or a relative) in a grocery store, service station, basketball game, or at church functions.

Nurses in rural practice must make decisions about individuals of all ages, with a variety of health conditions. They are expected to assume multiple roles stemming from the range of services that must be provided in a rural health care facility. At various times, a nurse may assume several roles because of the low numbers of nursing and other health professionals within the facility. Stemming from rural residents' expectations of the health care delivery system, the skills needed by nurses in rural practice include technical and clinical competency, adaptability, flexibility, refined assessment skills, organizational abilities, independence, open attitude about continuing education, sound decision-making skills, leadership ability, self-confidence, skills in handling emergencies, teaching, and public relations. Nurse administrators also are expected to be a "jack-of-all-trades" (generalists) and to demonstrate competence in several clinical specialties in addition to managing and organizing staff within the facility for which they are responsible (DeLao, 1992; Jamie, 1992; Moser, 1992; Moulton, 1992).

There are challenges, opportunities, and rewards in rural community nursing practice. The manner in which each factor is perceived depends on individual preferences and the situation in a given community. Frequently cited challenges of rural practice include limited educational opportunities, professional isolation, lack of other kinds of health personnel/professionals with whom one can interact, heavy work loads, the ability to function well in several clinical areas, lack of anonymity, and, for some, a restricted social life.

There are equally as many, if not more, opportunities and rewards in rural nursing practice. Those most commonly cited include close relationships with clients and co-workers, diverse clinical experiences that evolve from caring for patients of all ages who have a variety of health problems, caring for patients and client systems for long periods of time (in some cases, across several generations), opportunities for professional development, and greater autonomy. Many appreciate the solitude and quality of life afforded in a rural community—personally, as well as for their family. Others thrive on the outdoor recreational activities. And still others thoroughly enjoy the informal, face-to-face interactions coupled with the public recognition and status associated with living and working as a nurse in a small community.

Community Health Nursing in Rural Environments

Although most of the publications about rural health care and nursing focus on hospital practice, much of that information is applicable to community-based agencies and community health nursing as well (Davis, 1991; Davis and Droes, 1993; Hamel-Bissel, 1992; Washington State Nursing Network, 1993). The work-related stressors of community health nursing have received some attention in the literature. Case (1991) focused on stressful experiences of nurses working in rural Oklahoma Health Departments (see box below). Similar stressors are cited by nurses who work in urban agencies. However, the rural informants elaborated with anecdotal reports describing the stressors associated with geographic distance, isolation, sparse resources, and other environmental factors that characterize ruralness.

Community health nursing in rural practice settings is characterized by physical isolation that may lend itself to any one of the following: professional isolation; scarce financial, human, and health care resources; and a scope of practice that is broad in nature. As a result of personal familiarity with local residents, a community health nurse often possesses in-depth knowledge of clients and their family systems. Along with the acknowledged benefits, informal (face-to-face) interactions can significantly reduce a nurse's anonymity in the community and at times be a barrier to completing objective assessment on a client. Like urban practice, rural community health nursing takes place in a variety of locations, including the home, clinics, school, occupational settings, correctional facilities, and at community events, such as the county

 Work Stressors of Community Health Nurses in Rural Practice

Political/bureaucratic problems
Understaffing; overworked
Intraprofessional/interpersonal conflicts
Difficult/unpleasant nurse-patient encounters
Unsatisfactory work environment
Relatives refuse to deliver needed care to client
Patients who are hostile, apathetic, dependent, low intelligence
Inadequate communication
Fear for personal safety
Difficulty locating patients for care and/or follow-up
"Falling through the cracks"

From Case T: In Bushy A, editor: *Rural nursing*, vol II, Newbury Park, Calif, 1991, Sage Publications.

fair, rodeos, civic and church-sponsored functions, and school athletic events.

Future Research Needs

Since there only are a few empirical studies on rural nursing practice, with much of it consisting of anecdotal reports by nurses, the research needs are endless. There are several specific areas that are of particular importance to community health nursing practice in rural environments.

First, most nurses indicate that they enjoy practicing in rural areas and are extremely proud of what they do. They believe, however, their work deserves more recognition by professional nursing organizations. Furthermore, the retention rate of nurses in some practice settings is quite poor. The perspective of nurses who are dissatisfied with rural nursing is necessary to have a more complete picture of the rural experience, especially from community health nurses. This data could be useful to a variety of people: other nurses who are considering rural practice; nurse managers in need of better screening tools to assess fit of nurse-person-environment when interviewing applicants; planners of continuing nursing education programs; and faculty who teach community health to undergraduate and graduate students.

Second, more information is needed about the stressors and rewards of rural practice. This data could be used to develop stress management techniques by community health nurses and their supervisors to retain nurses and to improve the quality of their workplace environment.

Third, with the increasing numbers of rural residents in all regions of the United States, empirical data are needed on the particular community nursing needs of rural-client systems, especially underrepresented groups, minorities, and other at-risk populations that vary by region and state.

Finally, since most of the reported research studies on rural nursing have been undertaken with Anglo-Americans living in the intermountain and midwest regions, data is needed from residents in other areas, especially the states east of the Mississippi River.

Preparing Nurses for Rural Practice Settings

Nurses in rural practice must have broad knowledge about nursing theory. Health promotion, primary prevention, rehabilitation, obstetrics, medical-surgical, pediatrics, competency in planning and implementing community assessments, and an awareness and understanding of the particular health concerns in a specific state are important in this practice environment. A community's demographic profile and its principal industry can present a snapshot of some of its social, political, and health risks. From this kind of information, a community health nurse can anticipate the particular skills that will be needed to care for clients in a catchment area.

Stemming from their knowledge of resources and their ability to coordinate formal and informal services, community health nurses have and will continue to play an important role in offering a continuum of services for rural clients, in spite of sparse resources and fragmentation in the health care delivery system. Preparing nurses to practice in rural environments mandates creative and innovative nursing educational opportunities on the part of nursing educators. Collaboration and partnerships must be established between educators, rural community health nurses, and administrators of health care facilities in rural settings. In order to meet the demands and expectations of practice in that setting, nursing faculty must expose students to the rural environment, facilitate the development of generalists skills, and enhance their ability to function in several roles.

What Do You Think?
Within the nursing profession, there is a disagreement as to whether or not rural nursing is a specialty practice.

FUTURE PERSPECTIVES

Those concerned with rural health, including residents of rural communities, their elected representatives, and the administrators of public and private health care agencies, should be aware of the problems inherent in providing a continuum of care to underserved populations. Typically, media accounts focus exclusively on rural hospitals and the lack of primary care providers. Those reports, generally neglect the public and community health perspective when discussing the continuum of health care in rural environments (Gahr, 1993; NRHA, 1993; RWJF, 1993). Case management and community-oriented primary care (COPC), however, have proven to be effective models in helping to address some of those deficits.

Scarce Resources and a Comprehensive Health Care Continuum

Our current health care system is fragmented, thereby creating even greater difficulty in providing a comprehensive continuum of care to populations living in areas having scarce resources, such as money, personnel, equipment, and ancillary services. In rural communities, the most critically needed services usually are preventive services, such as health screening clinics, nutrition counseling, and wellness education.

Community health nursing needs vary by community. However, there is a prevailing plea in most rural areas, especially those designated as shortage areas for school nurses, family planning services, prenatal care, care for individuals with AIDS and their families, emergency care services, services for children with special needs, including those who are physically and mentally challenged, mental health services, and community-based programs for the elderly. Especially needed are services for the frail elderly and those with Alzheimer's disease, such as adult day care, hospice, respite care, homemaker services, and meal deliveries to help the elderly who remain at home in small-town America.

Providing a continuum of care has been hindered by closures of small hospitals. More than 160 rural hospitals have closed since 1980. Of the remaining 2700 rural hospitals, 600 report financial problems that could lead to closure. A shortage or the absence of even one provider, most often a physician or nurse, could mean that a small hospital must close its doors. This phenomenon has a ripple effect on the health of local residents, other health care services, and the economic development efforts in many small communities (Nadel, 1991).

The short supply and increasing demand for primary care providers in general, and community health nurses in particular, will continue for some time. To help solve this problem, elected officials and policy developers are looking at nurses to provide vital services in underserved areas. To respond to this opportunity, creativity is needed on the part of nursing to ensure delivery of appropriate and acceptable services to at-risk and vulnerable populations who live in rural and underserved regions. Nurses must be sensitive to the health beliefs of clients, then plan and provide nursing interventions that mesh with communities' cultural values and preferences (Aitken et al., 1990; ANA, 1991; Fenton et al., 1991).

"Year 2000" National Health Objectives Related to Rural Health

Since the demographic profile varies from community to community, each state has variations in the health status of its population. *Healthy People 2000* has important implications for community health nurses in that a significant number of at-risk populations cited in that policy-guiding document reside in rural areas across the 50 states (Healthy People 2000, 1991). Consequently, priority objectives vary, depending on population mix, health risks, and health status of residents in the state.

At the local level, communities have been encouraged to use *Healthy People 2000* as a guide for action and each should identify objectives and establish meaningful goals based on its situation. *Healthy Communities 2000: Model Standards* (APHA, 1991) was designed to assist local officials in tailoring the objectives to their community's needs. This document encourages the establishment of professional-community partnerships. Translating national objectives into achievable community health targets requires integration of the following components to ensure that services will be acceptable and appropriate for rural clients:

- Health statistics must be meaningful, understandable, and include appropriate process objectives that can be measured readily.
- Strategies must be designed that involve the public, private, and voluntary sectors of the community to achieve agreed-upon local objectives.
- Coordinated efforts are needed to ensure that the community works together to achieve the goals.

Consider, for example, these components in developing a health plan for a rural county having a large population of lower than average age. *Healthy People 2000* objectives for the county would target women of childbearing age, children, and adolescents. Priority objectives should include offering accessible prenatal care programs, improving immunization levels, providing preventive dental care instructions, implementing vehicular accident prevention and firearm safety programs, as well as educating teachers and health professionals for early identification of cases of domestic violence. Or, consider a rural county that has a higher number of individuals over age 65 than the national average. Priority objectives in the health plan would target the health risks and problems of the elderly in that community. Specific objectives might include development of health promoting programs to prevent chronic health problems and establishing community-based programs to meet the needs of those having chronic illness, specifically cardiovascular disease, diabetes, hypertension, and accident-related disabilities.

When implementing community-focused health plans that flow from *Healthy Community: 2000*, consideration always must be given to rural factors, such as sparse population, geographic remoteness, scarce resources, personnel shortages, and physical, emotional and social isolation. In addition to being actively involved in empowering the community and planning and delivering care, nurses play an important role in representing their community's perspective to local, state, regional, and national health planners and to their elected officials.

BUILDING PROFESSIONAL-COMMUNITY-CLIENT PARTNERSHIPS IN RURAL SETTINGS

The agenda for health care reform emphasizes providing universal access and a continuum of care for all U.S. citizens, especially vulnerable and underserved populations. The Federal Office of Rural Health Policy emphasizes that community-based programming, which actively involves the state and local element, is an essential element for any kind of reform to be successful, especially in rural areas. In other words, professional-client-community partnerships are critical elements for reform to be meaningful at the local level. Two models have been found to be particularly useful in rural environments: case management and community-oriented primary care (COPC).

Community-Oriented Primary Care (COPC)—A Partnership Process

Define and characterize the community.
Identify the community's health problems.
Develop or modify health care services in response to the community's identified needs.
Monitor and evaluate program process and patient outcomes.

Case Management in Rural Settings

Case management is a client-professional partnership that can be an effective strategy for arranging a continuum of care for rural clients (Parker et al., 1991), with the case manager tailoring and blending formal and informal resources. Collaborative efforts between a client and case manager allow clients to participate in their plan of care in an acceptable and appropriate way, especially when local resources are few and far between.

Community-Oriented Primary Care in Rural Settings

Community-oriented primary care is an effective model for delivering available, accessible, and acceptable services to vulnerable populations living in underserved areas. This model emphasizes flexibility, grass-root involvement, and professional-community partnerships. It blends primary care, public health, and prevention services, which are offered in a familiar and accessible setting. The COPC model is interdisciplinary in nature, uses a problem-oriented approach, and mandates community involvement in all phases of the process (see box above, left).

Building professional-community partnerships is an ongoing process. At various times, community health nurses, other health professionals, and community leaders must assume the role(s) of advocate, change agent, educator, expert, and/or group facilitator to gain both active and passive support from the community. Partnerships involve "give and take" by all the participants in the negotiations in order to reach consensus. Essentially, the process begins with professionals gaining entrance into a community, establishing rapport and trust with localities, then working together to empower the community to resolve mutually defined problems and goals. As mentioned earlier, *Healthy Communities: 2000* is an excellent guide for developing and defining those goals. Stemming from churches' and schools' central importance in a rural community, leaders from those institutions can be key players in building provider-community partnerships. Remember, the organizational phase precedes all others. Those efforts lay the foundation for all other activities related to planning, implementing, and evaluating community-based services.

Building Professional-Community-Client Partnerships

Gain the local perspective.
Assess the degree of public awareness and support for the cause.
Identify special-interest groups.
List existing services to avoid duplication of programs.
Note real and potential barriers to existing resources/services.
Generate a list of potential community volunteers and professionals who are willing to assist with the project.
Create awareness among target groups of a particular program (e.g., individuals, families, senior centers, church and recreation groups, health care professionals, law enforcement personnel, and other religious, service, and civic clubs).
Identify potential funding sources to implement the program.
Establish the community's health care priority list and involve large numbers of community members in considering and selecting their health care options.
Incorporate business principles in marketing the program.
Measure the health system's local economic impact.
Educate residents to the important role the local health care system plays in the economic infrastructure of the community and the consequences of a system failure.
Develop [new] local leadership and support for the community's health system through training and providing experience in decision making.

As with case management for a client, professional-community partnerships allow for more effective identification of existing informal social support systems that are accepted by rural residents. The goal is to integrate community preferences with new, or existing, formal services. Encourage public input early in the planning process. Public input must continue throughout the process to allow the community to feel it has "ownership in the project," as opposed to residents viewing it as "an outsider bringing another bureaucratic program into town." The box above, right, highlights strategies that community health nurses can use to enhance the building of professional-community partnerships in rural environments.

Partnership models, such as case management and COPC, have proven to be highly effective in areas with scarce resources and insufficient numbers of health care providers. Individuals and communities who are informed and active participants in planning their health care are more likely to develop consensus about the most appropriate solution for local problems. Subsequently, they are more likely to use and support that system after it is implemented. Partnership models enhance the ability of rural communities to do what they historically have done well. That is, assume responsibility for the services and institutions that serve its residents. Knowledge about partnership models and the skills to effectively implement them is useful for community health nurses who coordinate services that are accessible, available, and acceptable for rural populations in their catchment area.

Clinical Application

Ethyl, a 73-year-old widow, was diagnosed more than 10 years ago with progressive Parkinson's disease. Her husband of more than 40 years suddenly died 3 years ago following a serious stroke. She has two married daughters; one lives in California, and one lives in Illinois. The South Dakota town in which she and her husband lived all of their lives has a steadily decreasing population, with a current population of less than 1200 residents. Two years ago the only doctor who had been there for more than 40 years had a fatal heart attack; now the residents must drive 100 miles to Rapid City for their health care.

Her older widowed sister, Suzanna (age 75) also lives in town. This past year their brother, Bill (age 71), entered the County Nursing Home located in a town 20 miles away. Despite her physical rigidity and ataxia, Ethyl manages to live alone in her two-bedroom home with her dog and cat. Ethyl insists that she will not relinquish her private, independent lifestyle as her brother Bill has. Yet, within this past year she was hospitalized three times at the medical center in Rapid City. She says the reasons for being hospitalized were "for a bad chest cold, a bladder infection, and after a neighbor found me laying unconscious in the garden." Her doctor says this episode was related to "a heart problem."

Following discharge for the first hospitalization a home health nurse, Liz, was assigned as her case manager. Now, Ethyl refers to her as "my nurse." Liz's office is based at the County Senior Center, near the nursing home where Bill is now a resident. He, too, is one of the clients that Liz checks on weekly. Liz provides outreach services to all the residents in the county who are referred by a Rapid City home health agency. As a case manager, she works closely with the hospital's discharge planners to arrange a continuum of care for clients in the two-county area. Her activities include coordinating formal with informal services for clients, including nutrition, hydration, pharmacologic, personal care, homemaker, and routine activities, such as writing checks, home maintenance, and emergency back-up services.

As for Ethyl, formal services were integrated with her preferences of informal supports. Specifically she gets a daily hot meal from Meals-on-Wheels. The food is prepared at the County Senior Center and extra meals are brought on Friday for the weekend. The individual who delivers the meals has been educated to notice if the recipient exhibits any unusual behaviors or if there is need for professional assistance. If so, the driver calls, via cellular phone, either Liz or the county Coordinating Assessment and Monitoring (CAM) Agency, which is located in the hospital emergency room (ER) at Rapid City. Upon receiving such a call the ER staff may decide to dispatch emergency care via helicopter to the scene.

The County Senior Center also provides van services to small towns in the county to transport elderly residents to Rapid City for weekly shopping and visits to the doctor. Until recently Ethyl used this mode of public transportation. The service is convenient. The van stops in front of her house at 7:30 AM but often does not return until after 8:00 PM. Recently, she became too unsteady to use this service. Liz also worked with the Women's Circle in Ethyl's church to coordinate regular visits by members to "check on Ethyl," deliver groceries, "take in frozen meals" to augment Meals-on Wheels, and take her to the doctor for her appointments.

When Ethyl was found in the yard, it took a neighbor and Suzanna a half day to convince her to go to the doctor. Following that hospitalization, Communi-Call (a remote communication system) was placed in her home so Ethyl can call CAM for assistance when she does not feel "up to par." Her cardiac status is monitored remotely in the hospital's ER by LifeLine. This technology helps to detect changes earlier without traveling to see the doctor. Hopefully, it will help to avoid another emergency. To ensure continuity of care between the nurse's twice-weekly home visit, homemaking services have been coordinated on Thursday mornings. A personal attendant assists Ethyl three times a week with hygiene activities. These in-home services are provided by two local women who also work part-time for the home health agency.

In the winter, when the county roads are not plowed, professional services can be interrupted and a client may be without help for a week or more. At these times Suzanna and a neighbor check on Ethyl by telephone. As part of a group volunteer project, the local boy scout troop assists in snow removal and lawn care.

Arranging for home and plumbing repairs is more difficult for the case manager, with delays of 2 weeks or longer. When a water line ruptured, neighbors brought bottled water to Ethyl's home while she was waiting for the repair part to arrive. The local VFW Club purchased a hydraulic chair lift for her use and two members volunteered to place safety rails in her remodeled bathroom. Even though she is on a fixed income below the poverty level, she has been able to heat her home through the Fuel Assistance Program. In spite of her disabilities, Ethyl says she is extremely satisfied with how she is managing. She thanks her nurse Liz, and God, for the time she can spend at home near her friends, neighbors, and relatives.

Ethyl's case illustrates how formal and informal services can be integrated by a community health nurse. This plan of care offers the client a quality of life that she prefers, ensures that her living arrangement is physically safe, and her care is medically appropriate. With the expertise and personal touch of a home health nurse, a comprehensive array of formal and informal services was coordinated for a physically impaired, elderly woman. Certainly, Ethyl had input into her plan of care. Without collaboration and mutual goal setting, she probably would have been hospitalized far more frequently or perhaps even placed in a long-term care facility.

Key Concepts

- There is great diversity in rural environments across the 50 states.
- There are variations in the health status of rural populations, depending upon genetic, social, environmental, economic, and political factors.
- There is a higher incidence of working poor in rural America than in more populated areas.
- Rural adults, age 18 and over, are in poorer health than their urban counterparts; nearly 50% have been diagnosed with at least one major chronic condition. Yet, they average one less physician visit each year than healthier urban counterparts.
- About 26% of rural families are below the poverty level; more than 40% of all rural children under age 18 live in poverty.

- General practitioners are the usual providers of care for rural adults and children.
- Rural residents often must travel for more than 30 minutes to access a health care provider.
- Nurses must take into consideration the belief systems and life-styles of a rural population when planning, implementing, and evaluating community-based services.
- Barriers to rural health care include the availability, affordability, accessibility, and acceptability of services.
- Partnership models, in particular case management and community-oriented primary care (COPC) are effective models to provide a comprehensive continuum of care in environments with scarce resources.

Critical Thinking Activities

1. Compare and contrast the terms urban, suburban, rural, frontier, farm, nonfarm residency, metropolitan, and nonmetropolitan.
2. Describe residency as a continuum, ranging from farm residency to core metropolitan.
3. Discuss economic, social, and cultural factors that impact rural life-style and the health care seeking behaviors of residents who live there.
4. Identify barriers that impact accessibility, affordability, availability, and acceptability of services in the health care delivery system.
5. Summarize key nursing concepts as these fit with practice in rural environments.
6. Examine the characteristics of rural community nursing practice and how this differs from practice in more populated settings.
7. Identify challenges, opportunities and benefits of living and practicing as a community health nurse in the rural environment.
8. Debate case management and community-oriented primary care as partnership models that can help community health nurses enhance the continuum of care for clients living in an environment with sparse resources.

Bibliography

Abraham I, Buckwalter K, Neese K, Fox J: Mental health of rural elderly, *Issues Ment Health Nurs* 15(3):203-213, 1994.

Aitken T, VanArsdale S, Barry L: Strategies for practice as a clinical nurse specialist in a small setting, *Clinical Nurse Specialist* 4(1):28-32, 1990.

American Nurses Association (ANA) Council of Community Health Nurses: *Community-based nursing services: innovative models,* Washington, DC, 1991, ANA Council of Community Health Nurses, (Pub No CH13:1-91).

American Public Health Association (APHA): *Healthy Communities 2000: Model Standards,* Washington, DC, 1991, APHA.

Bigbee J, Crowder E: The Red Cross Rural Nursing Service: an innovation of public health nursing delivery, *Public Health Nurs* 2(2):109-121, 1985.

Braden J, Beauregard K: *National medical expenditure survey—health status and access to care of rural and urban populations,* Research Findings 18, Rockville, Md, Agency for Health Care Policy and Research, 1994, Public Health Service, (Pub No 94-0031).

Bronstein J, Morrisey M: Bypassing rural hospitals for obstetrics service care, *J Health Polit Policy Law* 16:87-118, 1991.

Bureau of the Census: *Residents of farms and rural areas: 1990,* Washington, DC, 1991, US Department of Commerce, (Current Population Reports, Series P-20, No 446).

Bureau of the Census: *Statistical abstract of the United States: 1990, national general population characteristics,* Hyattsville, Md, 1992, Bureau of the Census.

Case T: Work stresses of community health nurses in Oklahoma. In Bushy A, editor: *Rural nursing,* vol II, Newbury Park, Calif, 1991, Sage Publications.

Children's Defense Fund: *Falling by the wayside: children in rural America,* Washington, DC, 1991, Children's Defense Fund.

Conway-Welch C: Issues surrounding the distribution and utilization of nurse nonphysician providers in rural America, *J Rural Health* 7(suppl):388-401, 1991.

Davis D: *A study of rural nursing: domains of practice—a characteristic of excellence,* Reno, Nev, 1991, University of Nevada (unpublished thesis).

Davis D, Droes N: Community health nursing in rural and frontier counties, *Nurs Clin North Am* 28(1):159-169, 1993.

DeLao R: A day in the life of a rural community health nurse: tales from the trenches, *Caring* 11(2):10-12, 1992.

Dickey L, Kamerow D: *How to put "prevention" into practice.* Presentation at the 1992 National Rural Heath Conference, Washington, DC, May, 1992.

Dunbar E: Rural mental health administration. In Austin M, Hersey W, editors: *Handbook of mental health administration: the middle management perspective,* San Francisco, 1992, Jossey-Bass.

Fenton M, Rounds L, Anderson E: Combining the role of the nurse practitioner and the community health nurse: an educational model for implementing community-based primary care, *J Am Acad Nurs Pract* 3(3):99-105, 1991.

Frame P: Health maintenance in clinical practice: strategies and barriers, *Am Fam Physician* 43(3):1192-1200, 1992.

Gahr W: *Rural America: blueprint for tomorrow,* Newbury Park, Calif, 1993, Sage Publications.

Geller J, Ludtke R, Stratton T: Nonfatal farm injuries in North Dakota: a sociological analysis, *J Rural Health* 6(2):185-195, 1990.

Gesler W, Ricketts T: *Health in rural North America: the geography of health care services and delivery,* New Brunswick, NJ, 1992, Rutgers University Press.

Goeppinger J: Health promotion for rural populations: partnership interventions, *Fam Community Health* 16(1):1-9, 1993.

Greydanus D: *Adolescent care: common problems and concerns.* Presented at the National Rural Health Association 15th Annual Conference on Rural Health, Washington, DC, May, 1992.

Hamel-Bissel B: On fear and courage: a first encounter with AIDS in rural Vermont. In Winsted-Fry P, editor: *Rural health nursing: stories of creativity, commitment and connectedness,* New York, 1992, NLN Publications, (Pub No 21-2408).

Healthy People 2000: national health promotion and disease prevention objectives, Washington, DC, 1991, USDHHS, Public Health Service.

Henshaw S, VanVort J: The accessibility of abortion services in the United States, *Fam Plann Perspect* 23:245-263, 1991.

Hewitt M: *Defining "rural" areas: impact on healthcare policy and research,* Washington, DC, 1989, US Government Printing Office.

Human J, Wasem K: Rural mental health in America, *Am Psychologist* 46(3):232-239, 1991.

Jamie D: Managing at-risk situations: tales from the trenches, *Caring* 11(2):14-15, 1992.

Kirby D: School and community relationships, *J Sch Health* 60(4):170-178, 1990.

Lee H: Definitions of rural: a review of the literature. In Bushy A, editor: *Rural Nursing,* vol I, Newbury Park, Calif, 1991, Sage Publications.

Long K, Weinert C: Rural nursing: developing a theory base, *Sch Inq Nurs Pract* 3:113-127, 1989.

Ludloff A, Swanson L: *America's rural communities,* Boulder, Colo, 1990, Westview Press.

McManus M, Newacheck P, Greany A: Young adults with special health care needs: prevalence, severity and access to health services, *Pediatrics* 86:674-682, 1990.

Monheit A, Cunningham P: Children without insurance, *Future Child* 2(2):154-183, 1992.

Moser E: The special needs of rural clients: tales from the trenches, *Caring* 11(2):18-20, 1992.

Murray J, Keller P: Psychology in rural America: current status and future directions, *Am Psychologist* 46(3):220-231, 1991.

Moulton K: The frontier home care nurse: tales from the trenches, *Caring* 11(2):16-17, 1992.

Nadel M: *Rural hospitals: closures and issues of access.* Testimony of US General Accounting Office before US House of Representatives Task Force on Rural Elderly. Select Committee on Aging, Sept 4, 1991.

National Association of Community Health Centers (NACHC): *National health reform and access to health care,* Academy, DC, 1992, NACHC.

National Clearing House for Alcohol and Drug Information (NCHADI): *The rural communities prevention resource guide,* Rockville, Md, 1991, NCHADI.

National Rural Health Association (NRHA): *Study of models to meet rural health needs through mobilization of health professionals, education, and services resources,* Kansas City, Mo, 1993, NRHA.

National Rural Health Association (NRHA): *A shared vision: building bridges for rural health access.* Conference Proceedings of National Rural Minorities, Kansas City, Mo, 1994, NRHA.

National Safety Council: *Accident Facts,* (yearly editions), Chicago, Ill, 1990-1993, National Safety Council.

Nesbitt T, Conne F, Hart T, Rosenblatt R: Access to obstetrical care in rural areas: effect on birth outcomes, *Am J Public Health* 80:814-818, 1990.

Parker M, Quinn J, Viehl M, McKinley A, Polich C, Detzner D, Hartwell S, Korn K: Case management in rural areas: definitions, clients, financing, staffing and service delivery issues. In Bushy A, editor: *Rural nursing,* Vol II, Newbury Park, Calif, 1991, Sage Publications.

Perloff J: Health care resources for children and pregnant women, *Futur Child* 2(2):78-93, 1992.

Robert Wood Johnson Foundation (RWJF): *Rural health challenges in the 1990s: strategies from the hospital-based rural health care programs.* Princeton, NJ, 1993, RWJF.

Rowland D, Lyons B: Triple jeopardy: rural, poor and uninsured, *Health Serv Res* 23(6):975-1004, 1989.

Sullivan T, Weinert C, Fulton R: Living with cancer: self-identified needs of rural dwellers, *Fam Community Health* 16(1):41-49, 1993.

Summer L: *Limited access: health care for the rural poor,* Washington, DC, 1991, Center on Budget and Policy Priorities.

University of Iowa: *Conference proceedings—implementing health care reform in rural America: state and community roles,* Des Moines, Ia, 1993a, University of Iowa.

University of Iowa: *Federal and state rural health care reform legislation: a compendium prepared for health care reform conference,* Des Moines, Ia, 1993b, University of Iowa.

US Bureau of Health Professions (USBHP): *Seventh report to the president and congress on the status of health personnel in the US,* Washington, DC, 1990, USBPH, (DHHS Pub No HRS-OD-90-3).

US Department of Health and Human Services (USDHHS): *Indian health services: trends in Indian health,* Washington, DC, 1989, Indian Health Service.

US General Accounting Office (USGAO): *Report to congressional requesters: rural drug abuse: prevalence, relation to crime and programs,* Washington, DC, 1990, USGAO, (GAO/PEMD-90-24, B-240854).

US General Accounting Office (USGAO): *Physician supply from the National Health Service,* Washington, DC, 1991, USGAO, (# GAO/HRD 90-128).

US Office of Technology Assessment (USOTA): *Health care in rural America,* Washington, DC, Sept, 1990, Government Printing Office, (QTA-H-434).

Wagenfeld M, Wagenfeld J: Mental health and rural America: a decade review, *J Rural Health* 7(6):707-722, 1990.

Wakefield M: Health care in rural America: a view from the nations capitol, *Nurs Econ* 8(2):83-89, 1990.

Washington State Nursing Network—Celebration of Public Health Nurse Committee: *Opening doors: stories of public health nursing,* Olympia, Wa, 1992, Washington State Department of Health.

Weinert C, Long K: Rural families and health care: refining the knowledge base, *J Marriage Fam Rev* 15(1, 2):57-76, 1990.

Weinert C, Long K: The theory and research base for rural nursing practice. In Bushy A, editor: *Rural nursing,* vol II, Newbury Park, Calif, 1991, Sage Publications.

Weinert C, Long K: Support systems for the spouses of chronically ill persons in rural areas, *Family Community Health* 16(1):46-54, 1993.

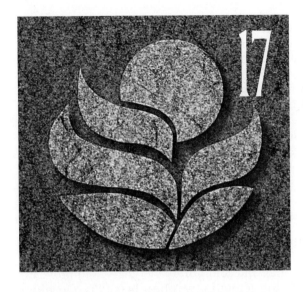

17 Health Promotion Through Healthy Cities

Beverly C. Flynn ◆ Louise I. Dennis

Objectives ▼

After reading this chapter, the student should be able to do the following:

◆ Trace the Healthy Cities Movement.
◆ Describe the relationship between primary health care, health promotion, and the Healthy Cities Movement.
◆ Describe the steps in the CITYNET-Healthy Cities process.
◆ Discuss application of the CITYNET-Healthy Cities process in health promotion.
◆ Provide examples of the implications for community health nursing in a Healthy City.
◆ Analyze the impact of the CITYNET-Healthy Cities process in health promotion at the community level.

Key Terms ▼

appropriate technology
CITYNET process
community participation
equity
health promotion
Healthy Cities
healthy public policy
international cooperation
multisectoral cooperation
primary health care

Outline ▼

The Healthy Cities Movement is mobilizing local governments, professionals, citizens, and private and voluntary organizations to put health promotion on the political agenda of cities. This is accomplished through application of the World Health Organization's (*Primary Health Care*, 1978) goal of health for all by the year 2000, the strategy of primary care, and the principles of health promotion outlined in the *Ottawa Charter for Health Promotion* (1986). Cities are challenged (1) to develop projects that reduce inequalities in health status and access to services, (2) to develop healthy public policies at the local level, (3) to create physical and social environments that support health, strengthen community action for health, help people develop new skills for health, and (4) to reorient health services consistent with the strategy of primary health care and the principles of health promotion (Tsouros, 1990).

HISTORY OF THE HEALTHY CITIES MOVEMENT

Although the Healthy Cities movement has been labeled "the new public health" (Ashton and Seymour, 1988), others would say the concept of a healthy city is not new (Hancock, 1993). It is based on the belief that the health of the community is largely influenced by the environment in which people live and that health problems have multiple causes—social, economic, political, environmental, and behavioral. Healthy Cities is consistent with the definition of health promotion that promotes change in the broader environment to support health (*Ottawa Charter for Health Promotion*, 1986).

Healthy Cities is based on the recognition that about half of the world's population lives in urban areas, where the human and health-related problems are most complex and are coupled with increasingly fragmented policy and scarce resources. A key strategy of Healthy Cities is to mobilize the community by developing public, private, and not-for-profit partnerships to address the complex health and environmental problems in the city. The Healthy Cities process involves specific steps to conduct community assessments; establish priorities, goals, and city-wide action plans; secure resources; establish steering groups to carry out the action; monitor and evaluate progress; and review and adjust policies (Tsouros, 1990). The Healthy Cities process has been applied to rural and metropolitan areas (Flynn, 1992). Healthy Cities engages local residents for action in health and is based on the premise that when people have the opportunity to work out their own locally defined health problems they will find sustainable solutions to those problems (Flynn, 1994).

The Healthy Cities movement began in 1984 in Canada, and in 1986 the WHO Regional Office for Europe initiated the WHO Healthy Cities Project. It now has become an international movement involving about one thousand cities. Although eleven cities were selected to participate in the WHO Healthy Cities project in the early years, the current phase includes 35 participating cities. In addition, there are 23 national networks and over 650 participating cities and towns throughout Europe. National networks also have developed in Canada, the United States, Australia, Iran, and Egypt to name a few. Regional networks are developing in Francophone Africa, Southeast Asia, and the Western Pacific.

DEFINITION OF TERMS

Healthy Cities is an international movement of cities focused on mobilizing local resources and political, professional, and community members to improve the health of the community. A healthy city is one whose priority is to improve its environment and expand its resources so that community members can support each other in achieving their highest potential.

Guiding the Healthy Cities movement are the principles of health for all (*Primary Health Care*, 1978) and the *Ottawa Charter for Health Promotion* (1986). The principles of health for all include equity, health promotion, community participation, multisectoral cooperation, appropriate technology, primary health care, and international cooperation. **Equity** implies providing accessible services in order to promote the health of populations most at risk to health problems, for example, the poor, youth, elderly, minorities, the homeless, and refugees. **Health promotion** and disease prevention are focused on providing community members with a positive sense of health that enables physical, mental, and emotional capacities. In order to achieve health for all, individuals within communities must become involved in health promotion. The key to obtaining health for all is through **community participation,** whereby well-informed and motivated community members participate in planning, implementing, and evaluating health programs. In addition, achieving health for all requires **multisectoral cooperation.** This refers to coordinated action by all parts of a community, from local government officials to grass-roots community members. **Appropriate technology** refers to affordable social, biomedical, and health services that are relevant and acceptable to individuals' health, needs, and concerns.

Primary health care is the focus of health care system reform. It means meeting the basic health needs of a community by providing readily accessible health services. Since health problems transcend international borders, **international cooperation** is needed to ensure that the goal of health for all by the year 2000 is reached.

Health promotion had become a key strategy for the goal of health for all by the time the *Ottawa Charter for Health Promotion* was adopted in 1986. This charter provided a clear definition of health promotion and the framework for the Healthy Cities movement (Ashton, 1992; *Twenty Steps for Developing a Healthy Cities Project*, 1992). Health promotion was officially defined as the "process of enabling people to take control over and to improve their health" (*Ottawa Charter for Health Promotion*, 1986, p. 1). This is accomplished through enabling community members to increase control over and assume more responsibility for health, mediating between public, private, voluntary, and community sectors; and advocating on behalf of people powerless to make the necessary changes to promote health.

Five elements make up the strategic framework provided by the Charter and are listed in order of priority for health promotion action. The elements include building healthy public policy, creating supportive environments, strengthening community action, developing personal skills, and reorienting health services. **Healthy public policy** refers to public policy for health that is based on an ecological perspective and multisectoral and participatory strategies (Pederson et al., 1988). Healthy public policy is future oriented and deals with local health problems, as well as global health issues. In contrast, medical policy is mainly concerned with the existing medical care system and use of technology and biomedical science to treat disease. Creating supportive environments refers to physical, political, economic, and social systems that will support the community's health. Strengthening community action refers to promoting the community's capacity, ability, and opportunity to take appropriate action to protect and improve the health of the community. Developing personal skills is helping people develop the life-style skills they need to be healthy. Reorienting health services refers to changing the focus of health services toward primary health care, health promotion, disease prevention, and community-based care.

The CITYNET-Healthy Cities process is an adaptation of the European and Canadian models of Healthy Cities in the United States. The nine-step **CITYNET process** includes the following: building the partnership for health, obtaining community commitment, developing the Healthy City Committee, developing leadership in Healthy Cities, assessing the community, community-wide planning for health, community ac-

tion for health, providing data-based information to policy makers, and monitoring and evaluating Healthy City initiatives (Rider et al., 1993).

MODELS OF COMMUNITY PRACTICE

The assumptions that professionals have about communities shape the implementation of the Healthy Cities process. Rothman and Tropman (1987) propose three distinct models of community practice: locality development, social planning, and social action. Locality development is a process-oriented model that emphasizes consensus, cooperation, and building group identity and a sense of community. Social planning stresses rational-empirical problem solving, usually by outside professional experts. The authors note that social planning does not focus on building community capacity or fostering fundamental social change. Social action, on the other hand, aims to increase the problem-solving ability of the community along with concrete actions to correct the imbalance of power and privilege of an oppressed or disadvantaged group in the community (Minkler, 1990). Although it is argued that these models of community practice are not mutually exclusive, efforts generally can be categorized within one model.

Arnstein (1969) depicted a ladder of citizen participation with the lower levels of participation as manipulation, therapy, and informing. The higher levels of participation include partnership, delegated power, and citizen control.

These models of community practice can be summarized as top-down and bottom-up approaches. In a top-down approach, experts and health professionals take the lead in identifying community health problems and implementing programs with little input from the individuals for whom these programs are being planned. A bottom-up approach utilizes broad-based community problem solving that includes health professionals, local officials, service providers, and other community members, including those at risk for health problems.

Rothman and Tropman's (1987) locality development and social action are examples of a bottom-up approach in which community participation is evident in all stages of community health planning and practice. Social planning portrays a top-down approach where rational-empirical problem solving usually is conducted by outside experts.

Arnstein's (1969) lower levels of the ladder—manipulation, therapy, and informing—can be equated with a top-down approach in which community practice and action are planned by professionals and experts. The higher levels of the ladder—partnership, delegated power, and citizen control—represent a bottom-up approach, reflecting a multisectoral approach with community participation.

Healthy Cities emphasizes a bottom-up approach with multisectoral planning and action for health. The

---

Did You Know?

Implementing the steps of the CITYNET-Healthy Cities process will enable nurses to gain an understanding of the linkages between health, community, and the policy process. Benefits to the community include increased access to services and improved health status, thus promoting equity in health.

| What Do You Think? |

Community participation in health decisions is more effective in promoting healthy public policy than decision-making by outside professional experts.

CITYNET-Healthy Cities process aims at partnerships within the community and focuses on community leadership development for health that is consistent with Rothman and Tropman's (1987) locality development model.

HEALTHY CITIES TODAY

Because cities in Europe and Canada have the longest history in the Healthy Cities movement, examples of Healthy Cities' initiatives from these regions of the world are highlighted below. These examples suggest that different models of community practice are being implemented in the Healthy Cities movement. The locality development and social planning models are utilized most frequently.

Europe

The largest Healthy City in the European Healthy Cities project is St. Petersburg, Russia. In 1992, government officials, health professionals, and consultants from the WHO European Region Healthy Cities Project met to identify the major health problems in St. Petersburg. They decided to begin their health initiative by focusing on programs to decrease the city's high maternal and infant mortality rates. Four projects were developed. These included a Family Planning Center, Teen Center, Maternity Home with rooming in and breast feeding (Baby Friendly Campaign), and Rehabilitation Center for socially disadvantaged pregnant women (Flynn and Dennis, 1993). A Consensus Conference was held late in 1992 with international consultants to address how to improve the four projects. The local individuals who attended the conference were largely health professionals, including physicians, nurses, and midwives. This was the first time many of these professionals met together in an interdisciplinary approach to address health problems.

Horsens Healthy City (Denmark) identified six steps necessary to transform a health promotion idea into action (Bragh-Matzon, 1992). These six steps follow:
1. Political commitment and legitimacy
2. Building a small catalyst unit to secure the transformation process
3. Building an infrastructure to secure involvement and legitimization from essential powers in city life
4. Information, communication, visibility, and public debates on health issues
5. Combining short-term action and long-term planning
6. Promoting and securing the process over time.

The first step involved obtaining a commitment from the City Council to support the health-for-all strategy through the Healthy City model. In the second step, the catalyst unit was a small team that bridged the existing government and health structures with the multiple powers and resources within in the city. The team included highly experienced professional community members from different disciplines. Nonprofessional community members, or "grass-roots" people, were not directly involved on this team. However, their input was sought by professional team members. It was not until the third step that direct community participation occurred. Ordinary citizens were included on a steering committee that became the Health Committee for the city. The function of the Health Committee was to oversee projects and communicate with appropriate individuals and agencies in the city, thereby creating more effective links among politicians, health professionals, and citizens.

Horsens' first health initiative involved conducting a Health Survey to obtain a health profile for the city. This resulted in the "Torsted West Project." The goal of this project was to plan a new residential area along ecological principles. This was accomplished through the six steps. Consultants from other Healthy Cities were involved in providing their expertise to the project (Draper et al., 1992).

Munich Healthy City (Germany) initiated a hospital nutrition project. Input from consultants was sought once the problem was identified by concerned community members (Draper et al., 1992). A concerned group of parents initiated the project. The Parents' Board for Chronically Ill Children was developed. They wrote a proposal on the food needs of hospitalized children to increase community awareness of this problem. They noticed that only medical aspects of diets (i.e., diabetic diets) were being considered during children's hospitalizations rather than providing overall healthy nutrition. The Parents' Board initiated networking with appropriate professionals within the hospital to consider the importance of healthy and child-focused menus. Collaboration with nurses, doctors, hospital cooks, dietitians, hospital administration, the city health department, and young patients and their families resulted in improved meals for hospitalized children. This initiative also resulted in improving the provision of healthy food in nurseries and schools.

Multi-City Action Plans—Linking of Cities

Multi-City Action Plans (MCAP) provide platforms for international cooperation in health planning and sharing of professional experts. Groups of Healthy

Cities in Europe work together to address common health concerns. This enables smaller cities and cities new in the Healthy Cities movement to work together on common health problems, thereby expanding the number of partners and resources available to deal with problems. The goal of the MCAPs is to jointly develop, implement, and disseminate innovative models of health promotion. To achieve this goal, a business partnership is developed between cities involved in the European Healthy Cities movement. These cities are committed to working together on one common health problem for at least 2 years. The result is "open market events" that provide forums to present models of successful health promotion projects, exchange information, and monitor progress (Tsouros, 1990).

Examples of health concerns that MCAPs address include AIDS, alcohol, environment and health, diabetes, disability, health-promoting hospitals, nutrition, sports, tobacco-free cities, unemployment, and women's health (World Health Organization, 1994). Specific MCAPs on AIDS activities include surveying user views on existing services and opinions on needed services; encouraging participation of gay/lesbian and other community-based organizations in the HIV/AIDS work and policy development; exchanging educational material and expertise on prevention methods; and developing a guide on services available to travellers with HIV/AIDS. In addition, an MCAP on AIDS newsletter is published and distributed to member cities as a method of communicating and networking.

United States

Healthy Cities in the United States has the longest history in Indiana and California. Healthy Cities Indiana began as a pilot program in 1988 with a grant from the W. K. Kellogg foundation as a collaborative effort between Indiana University School of Nursing, Indiana Public Health Association, and six Indiana cities. Based on the success of this project, the W.K. Kellogg Foundation funded the dissemination phase called CITYNET-Healthy Cities, in cooperation with the National League of Cities through their network of 19,000 local officials (Flynn et al., 1991). The CITYNET process begins with building a partnership and establishing city leaders' commitment to the Healthy City process. Once the commitment is obtained, a Healthy City Committee is established that includes multisectoral representation of the community, as well as citizen participation. Broad multisectoral involvement and citizen participation occur in all the remaining stages of the CITYNET process (leadership development, community assessment, community-wide planning for health, community action, providing data-based information to policy makers, and monitoring and evaluation). CITYNET-Healthy Cities aims at partnerships within the community that require

health professionals to recognize that because of the city's complex nature, community problems cannot be medicalized. "Professionalizing" community problems is working at the lowest level of participation—that of providing therapy or treatment rather than community partnership (Arnstein, 1969).

Six cities were initially involved in Healthy Cities Indiana. Actions of these cities focused on problems of diverse populations. For example, actions have been directed to local priorities that include problems of children, teen parents, the homeless, access to health care, crime and violence, and the elderly. Action also has been taken on the broader environmental policy issues, including management of solid waste and promotion of air quality. For each of these projects, the CITYNET-Healthy Cities process was followed, thereby providing a broad base of community participation at all stages of community planning.

Research Brief

Flynn B, Ray D, Rider M: Empowering communities: action research through Healthy Cities, *Health Educ Q* 21(3):394-405, 1994.

The Healthy Cities process uses action research to empower communities to take action for health. Five concepts that link community empowerment and action research are focus on community, citizen participation, information and problem solving, sharing of power, and quality of life. Two case studies from Healthy Cities Indiana (a pilot program of CITYNET-Healthy Cities) provide illustrations of these concepts. The dynamics of community participation in action research and the successes and barriers to community participation are presented. Outcomes found to empower the community are the extent to which Healthy City projects are initiated, their progress monitored, continued action in health supported, resources obtained, and policies promoted that contribute to equity in health.

During the assessment of their community, the New Castle Healthy City (Indiana) Committee questioned their community's high death rates caused by cancer, chronic obstructive pulmonary disease, and heart disease. The committee asked the following questions: Why were these rates higher than the state and nation? What were the life-style choices of community people? What in the environment supported or inhibited healthy choices? They decided to work with CITYNET staff and constructed a survey to obtain baseline data on health behaviors in the community. CITYNET staff trained local volunteers in survey data collection. One thousand surveys were distributed door-to-door using a system to ensure appropriate geographic coverage in the community. They obtained a 50% response rate that demonstrated the community's interest in health concerns. The committee used the national health objectives to compare their findings (Healthy People 2000, 1991). They found high levels of unhealthy behaviors, such as higher cigarette smoking behavior and inadequate exercise than suggested in the national objectives. They used the survey results to target their Healthy Cities initiatives. The data were used to testify before the County Commissioners on the need for health education and to support the employment of a health educator in the local health department. The cigarette smoking results were used by the committee to testify before the city council in support of an ordinance banning smoking in city buildings. During the last several years, the committee also has sponsored health awareness programs in the community. The 1994 program included a family fitness walk, safety checks of bicycles, and presentations on healthy food preparation emphasizing reduced fat and salt in meals. The committee obtained broad community support and cooperation not only in defining their local problems but also in setting priorities and implementing their initiatives. Their interventions integrated individual life-style change and policy change aimed at promoting supportive environments for health. Plans are underway to repeat the survey in order to evaluate progress of their Healthy Cities initiatives in reaching the year 2000 health objectives.

The California Healthy Cities project has grown from six initial cities to about 30 and is administered throughout the state department of health and social services. It is built on the premise of shared responsibility among community members, local officials, and the private sector. Community participation is the cornerstone of the projects while the mission is to reduce inequities in health status that exist between diverse populations in cities.

An example of one of the first California Healthy Cities is the Bell Healthy City project. Bell's residents are largely ethnic minorities with an average income of $10,000 per year (Hafey et al., 1992). The City Council voiced concern over the plight of the city and launched a series of Town Hall meetings to learn how to improve the city's quality of life. Community participation was encouraged. A number of goals were set to improve the quality of life in Bell, including developing recreational alternatives for all age groups; educating the community about graffiti, drug abuse, and vandalism; and providing the community with activities that foster a sense of community pride. Many of these goals currently are being implemented.

Canada

Toronto, Ontario was one of the first cities to become involved in the Healthy Cities movement in North

America. The movement began with a strategic planning committee to develop an overall strategy (Hancock, 1992). The committee conducted vision workshops in the community and a comprehensive environmental scan to help identify health needs in Toronto. The outcome was a final report outlining major issues with a strategic mission, priorities, and recommendations for action.

The Toronto Healthy City is involved in a number of projects. One of them is called Healthiest Babies Possible. This is an intensive antenatal education and nutritional supplement program for pregnant women who are identified by health and social agencies as high risk. The program includes intensive contact and follow-up of women along with food supplements. It has been successful in decreasing the incidence of low-birth-weight infants.

Another project known as Parents Helping Parents identifies children at high risk for neglect or abuse. Parents of these children are linked with specially trained health workers from similar sociocultural backgrounds to help them cope with problems of parenting and learn new and more effective parenting skills. Community participation is especially evident in this program in which community members, frequently from disadvantaged communities, are trained as health workers. The health workers are provided with new skills, a useful role in their communities, and a sense of self-esteem.

Halton Ontario Healthy City Project focused on healthy eating. Through cooperation of community volunteers, community groups, the District Health Council, and the Halton Regional Health Department, Community Kitchens were established (Healthy Lifestyles Take Hold in Halton, 1994). Through pooling of resources (recipes, knowledge, and time) each member of the Community Kitchen was able to take home a variety of prepared meals, thereby reducing food costs. Classes on nutrition, food preparation, and shopping skills were offered to all participants. The spirit of this project spread to the local Salvation Army where ready-to-serve meals for the homeless were made available. In addition, the Girl Scouts Association became involved in Community Kitchens, resulting in a Brownie nutrition badge for girls working at the Kitchens.

FUTURE OF THE HEALTHY CITIES MOVEMENT

Facilitators

The continuance of the Healthy Cities movement is contingent upon a number of factors that can facilitate the process. The facilitators of the Healthy Cities movement have been identified as follows:

1. Overt and covert political support of the official power structure
2. Participation by smaller cities

3. Broad-based representation on Healthy City committees
4. Committee action that includes affirming values and envisioning common goals, resolving conflict, implementing projects, developing long-term plans that build healthy public policy, and building support for long-term actions
5. Technical support
6. Positive media response (Flynn et al., 1991).

Official political support has been found to be of major importance in facilitating the Healthy City committee. In addition, the level of political commitment can determine action taken by the committee. The size of the city affects the pace at which a Healthy City project is developed and implemented, with smaller cities typically moving faster. Healthy City committees that have been able to obtain broad-based representation are better able to identify community problems, develop and implement appropriate solutions to the problems, and build consensus in the community for support of the solutions. When Healthy City committee action is successful, this empowers the committee to continue to take additional health promotion action. Technical assistance to research problems and solutions, as well as to evaluate existing programs, facilitates the process. Finally, support of the media at the local level can facilitate a positive image of the work conducted by the Healthy City committee (Flynn et al., 1991).

Barriers

Although the barriers to the Healthy City process can be viewed as the opposite of the facilitators, three major barriers are noteworthy. The first is lack of political support. Without support of local political officials, good ideas for health promotion action may not be realized and may not lead to new health-related policies. The second barrier is lack of broad-based representation on the Healthy City committee. This may lead to action that reflects the needs of a select group within the community rather than comprehensive community health action. In addition, lack of broad-based representation frequently leads to a "top-down"

approach in which programs are planned by a few people with little community participation. The outcome of this approach is not likely to change the community's health. A third barrier is a city's size. Larger cities are more complex, making communication across various sectors of the city more difficult and time consuming (see Table 17-1).

Healthy Public Policy

Healthy public policy is defined as health policies developed through a multisectoral and collaborative process with participation from community members that will be most affected by the policy (Pederson et al., 1988). Healthy public policy supports health in a broad ecological sense that includes environmental, physical, social, and mental well-being. It transcends traditional departmental and governmental boundaries to include dialogue between policy makers and the "public." The health effects of all public decisions are considered. In this sense, healthy public policy proposes a new way of thinking about health and government policy and links policymakers, professionals, and common citizens through a concern for health. Examples of healthy public policies are seat-belt legislation, no-smoking policies in public buildings, motorcycle-helmet laws, and immunization policies for school-age children. Healthy public policies create supportive environments for health by "making the healthy choices the easy choices" for people to make (Ashton, 1987).

The Healthy Cities movement supports the promotion of healthy public policy at the local level through multisectoral action and community participation. As the Healthy Cities movement spreads worldwide, healthy public policies may become the norm for providing healthier environments in which to live.

IMPLICATIONS FOR COMMUNITY HEALTH NURSING

Community health nurses can use *The CITYNET Manual* developed by CITYNET-Healthy Cities staff to help

Table 17-1 Facilitators and Barriers of the Healthy Cities Movement

Facilitators	Barriers
Overt and covert political support	Lack of support by local officials
Smaller cities	Lack of broad-based representation on Healthy City Committee
Broad-based representation on Healthy City Committee	Larger cities
Committee action	
Technical support	
Positive media response	

Flynn BC, Rider MS, Ray DW: *Health Education Quarterly* 18(3):331-347, 1991.

in guiding the community's work in Healthy Cities (Rider et al., 1993). The manual incorporates the nine steps of the CITYNET Healthy Cities process, which, in turn, offer examples of implications for community health nursing.

In *Step 1, building the partnership* for Healthy Cities, the community health nurse can orient community leaders to the Healthy Cities process. This can be done by identifying key city leaders, politicians, and health providers and talking to them about the health benefits of becoming a Healthy City. In *Step 2, community commitment,* the nurse can answer policy makers' questions about what political commitment means to the community's health. The nurse also can meet with heads of community agencies to solicit their commitment to the Healthy Cities process. *Step 3* involves the *development of the Healthy City committee.* Based on the nurse's knowledge of key community people and populations at risk for problems, the community health nurse can contact community leaders and other citizens to serve on the committee. The nurse can ensure that the committee represents the various sectors of the community. The nurse may like to serve as a member of the committee, representing the public health sector. *Step 4* is focused on *leadership development* in Healthy Cities. The nurse recognizes that although leaders exist in every community, they may not understand their potential in health promotion. The community health nurse can recommend relevant consultants, speakers, conferences, workshops, and network sessions that are related to local concerns. *Step 5* is the *community assessment.* Community health nurses have skills in conducting community assessments, such as windshield surveys and needs assessments. They can be a resource to the committee or work as a member of a team that conducts the community assessment. *Step 6* involves *community-wide planning for health.* Here the community health nurse can use skiills in group dynamics to assist the Healthy City Committee in identifying their priorities and strategic planning for local health action. *Step 7* is *community action for health* and the community health nurse can redirect community health services toward local priorities and plans. For example, the nurse can facilitate this by expanding a community health service, such as an exercise program for the elderly. In *Step 8, providing data-based information to policy makers,* the community health nurse may be asked to testify or assist others in preparing testimony that will be given to the city council or county commissioners about issues identified by the Healthy City Committee. In *Step 9, monitoring and evaluating progress,* the community health nurse may be asked by the Healthy City Committee to provide the data relevant to community health services and to assist them in recommending policy changes. The community health nurse also may coordinate or be part of a research team conducting program evaluation research.

Although these are examples of the practice of community health nursing in Healthy Cities, the nurse must recognize that the goal is to promote the community's leadership for health. In other words, the community health nurse must not do for the community what it can do for itself. The role of the community health nurse and, for that matter, other health professionals in Healthy Cities, is to work in partnership with community leaders. John Ashton (1989), one of the founders of the European Healthy Cities project, summarized the role of health professionals in Healthy Cities as being "on tap, not on top."

 ## Clinical Application

Since the community health nurse works in partnership with the community in Healthy Cities, the examples of outcomes of Healthy Cities initiatives reflect that partnership rather than a specific nursing intervention. The principles of health promotion provide a framework for relating examples of outcomes in several Indiana cities that have used the CITYNET-Healthy Cities process.

An example of an outcome related to the first principle, *promoting healthy public policy,* is found in New Castle Healthy City. Healthy City Committee members provided testimony to the city council and drafted and supported an ordinance that was passed banning cigarette smoking in city buildings. An outcome related to the second principle, *creating supportive environments,* is found in Fort Wayne Healthy City. Healthy City Committee members collaborated in a community-wide program to address the fact that only 65% of Fort Wayne preschool children received immunizations. Access to immunization services was expanded to five sites throughout the city at three different times in a program called "Super Shot Saturday." An example of an outcome related to *strengthening community action* is the strategy to collect information from community residents about their health concerns at local health fairs. Several Healthy Cities Committees used this strategy to encourage community participation in establishing priorities for action. An example of an outcome related to *improving personal skills,* is Seymour Healthy City's family fitness walk. Finally, an example of *reorienting health services,* is the Clark County Community Health Clinic's expansion of services to the uninsured at one urban and two rural sites utilizing nurse practitioners. These services are focused on disease prevention and health promotion of patients with selected chronic illnesses.

Key Concepts

◆ Although Healthy Cities began in the mid-1980s in Canada and Europe, it is now an international movement of cities focused on mobilizing local resources and political, professional, and community members to improve the health of the community.

◆ Guiding the Healthy Cities movement are the principles of primary health care and health promotion.

◆ The models of community practice most frequently found in the Healthy Cities movement are locality development and social planning and an emphasis on partnerships with the community.

◆ Examples of Healthy Cities initiatives indicate that a broad range of health problems and issues are being addressed at the local level.

◆ The continuance of Healthy Cities is contingent upon a number of facilitators and barriers to the movement.

◆ As the Healthy Cities movement spreads worldwide, healthy public policies may become the norm for providing healthy environments in which to live.

◆ Implications of Healthy Cities for community health nursing can be organized by the steps of the CITYNET-Healthy Cities process.

◆ Outcomes of Healthy Cities suggest the successes of multisectoral community partnerships formed.

Critical Thinking Activities

1. Evaluate the effectiveness of a current approach to a health problem in your community (i.e., teen pregnancy). Describe how the approach would change with implementation of the CITYNET-Healthy Cities process. Compare and contrast the two approaches in addressing this problem.

2. Discuss the role of the community health nurse in health promotion.

3. Identify city council members, the President of the Chamber of Commerce, the director of Family Services, the Mayor, a religious leader, and other community leaders who are the "movers and shakers" in getting things done. Generate a list of questions that will help these leaders describe the major strengths and problems of the community. Interview several local leaders and summarize their responses.

4. You are asked by the health commissioner to organize a community coalition for orientation to the Healthy Cities process. Outline the Healthy Cities process.

5. Describe your philosophy of community leadership development for health promotion.

5. Debate the model that is most effective in health promotion: social planning, community development, or social action.

Bibliography

Arnstein S: A ladder of citizen participation, *J Am Institute of Planners* 35:216-224, 1969.

Ashton J: Making the healthy choices the easy choices, *Nutrition and Food Science*, Jul/Aug:2-5, 1987.

Ashton J: *Creating Healthy Cities.* Paper presented at Healthy Cities Indiana Network Session, Seymour, Ind, May, 1989.

Ashton J: *Healthy Cities*, Milton Keynes, UK, 1992, Open University Press.

Ashton J, Seymour H: *The new public health,* Philadelphia, 1988, Open University Press.

Bragh-Matzon K: Horsens. In Ashton J, editor: *Healthy Cities*, Milton Keynes, UK, 1992, Open University Press, pp 108-114.

Draper R, Curtice L, Hooper J, Goumans M: *WHO Healthy Cities Project: review of the first five years (1987-1992)*, Copenhagen, Denmark, 1993, WHO Regional Office for Europe.

Flynn BC: Healthy Cities: a model of community change, *Fam Community Health* 15(1):13-23, 1992.

Flynn BC: Partners for Healthy Cities, *Healthc Forum J* 37(3):55-56, 73, 1994.

Flynn BC, Dennis LI: Healthy families. In Altergott K, editor: *One world many families,* Minneapolis, 1993, National Council on Family Relations.

Flynn B, Ray D, Rider M: Empowering communities: action research through Healthy Cities, *Health Educ Q* 21(3):395-405, 1994.

Flynn BC, Rider MS, Ray DW: Healthy Cities: the Indiana model of community development in public health, *Health Educ Q* 18(3):331-347, 1991.

Hafey JM, Twiss JM, Folkers LF: California. In Ashton J, editor: *Healthy Cities*, Milton Keynes, UK, 1992, Open University Press, pp 186-194.

Hancock T: The Healthy City: utopias and realities. In Ashton J, editor: *Healthy Cities*, Milton Keynes, UK, 1992, Open University Press, pp 22-29.

Hancock T: Evolution, impact and significance of the Healthy Cities/healthy communities movement, *J Public Health Policy* 14(1):5-18, 1993.

Healthy lifestyles take hold in Halton, *The Ontario Prevention Clearinghouse Newsletter* 4(3):4, 1994.

Healthy People 2000: national health promotion and disease prevention objectives, Washington, DC, 1991, USDHHS, Public Health Service.

Minkler M: Improving health through community organization. In Glanz K, Lewis FM, Rimer BK, editors: *Health behavior and health education,* San Francisco, 1990, Jossey-Bass, pp 257-287.

Ottawa charter for health promotion, Copenhagen, Denmark, 1986, WHO Regional Office for Europe.

Pederson AP, Edwards RK, Kelner M, Marshall VW, Allison KR: *Co-ordinating healthy public policy: an analytic literature review and bibliography,* Canada, 1988, Minister of National Health and Welfare.

Primary Health Care, Geneva, Switzerland, 1978, WHO and UNICEF.

Rider MS, Flynn BC, Yuska TP, Ray DW, Rains J: *The CITYNET manual: how communities can (and do!) create healthy cities,* Indianapolis, 1993, Institute of Action Research for Community Health/Indiana University.

Rothman J, Tropman JE: Models of community organization and macro practice: their mixing and phasing. In Cox FM, Erlich JL, Rothman J, Tropman JE, editors: *Strategies of community organization,* ed 4, Itasca, Ill, 1987, Peacock.

Tsouros AD: *World Health Organization Healthy Cities Project: a project becomes a movement,* Copenhagen, Denmark, 1990, FADL Publishers.

Twenty steps for developing a Healthy Cities Project, Copenhagen, Denmark, 1992, WHO Regional Office for Europe.

World Health Organization: *Briefings on Multi-City Action Plans WHO Healthy Cities Project Phase II 1993-1997,* Copenhagen, Denmark, 1994, WHO Regional Office for Europe.

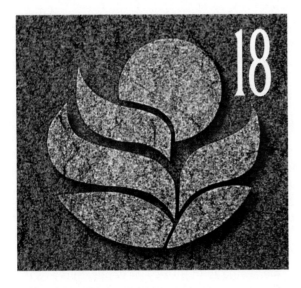

18

The Nursing Center: A Model of Community Health Nursing Practice

Sara E. Barger

Objectives

After reading this chapter, the student should be able to do the following:

◆ Describe the key components of the nursing center model.
◆ List at least three populations served by nursing centers.
◆ Identify at least five services provided by nursing centers.
◆ Identify at least three roles for nurses in nursing centers.
◆ Evaluate the risks and opportunities for nurses in nursing centers.
◆ Analyze the nursing center model for community health nursing practice.

Key Terms

advanced practice nurses (APNs)
business plan
direct reimbursement
nursing center
prescriptive authority
primary care

Outline

As America moves toward a reformed health care delivery system, critical concerns surround the following national goals: more access to care, improved quality of care, and reduced health care costs. Nurses who operate nursing centers find that they are well positioned to assist the nation in meeting these goals. In nursing centers, nurses are cost-effective providers who increase access to health care for people where they live, work, and play (*Nursing's Agenda for Health Care Reform,* 1991).

This chapter discusses the nursing center model and how it relates to community health nursing. For a clear understanding of the model, this examination of nursing centers focuses on the following: a historical perspective on their development; components of the contemporary nursing center model; nursing roles; populations served; classification of services provided; and the relationships of nursing center services to *Healthy People 2000* goals and *Healthy Communities 2000* standards. In addition, this chapter explores issues to be considered by those developing a nursing center, as well as areas for future research.

Because many authors have defined nursing centers, several definitions are offered in the box below. A review of all these definitions reveals a common theme. Phrases such as "nurse-conducted clinic," "nurse-anchored system," and "care that is managed by nurses" convey the theme that nurses are in charge of providing nursing care to patients or clients in a community setting. This theme is explored later as the contemporary conceptual model of a nursing center is discussed.

HISTORICAL PERSPECTIVE

The roots of nursing centers go back to the work of Lillian Wald in the Henry Street Nurses Settlement in New York City in 1893. The nurses in this center not only provided care to the sick and the poor, but also addressed issues related to preventing illness and promoting health. In 1916, Margaret Sanger opened the first birth control clinic in the United States. Her goal was to provide the poor with information about contraception and family planning (Aydelotte and Gregory, 1989).

 Definitions of Nursing Centers

"Nurse-conducted clinic (based on) a systems approach for effective delivery of health care and appropriate use of available health care resources" (Allison, 1973, p. 53)

"Nurse-anchored system of primary health care delivery as neighborhood health centers" (Kos and Rothberg, 1981, p. 20)

"Place where clients/patients receive care that is completely managed by nurses where education and research components are built in" (Lang, 1983, p. 1291)

One of the earliest nursing centers was the Frontier Nursing Service. In 1923, Mary Breckinridge surveyed a three-county area in Kentucky and "concluded that a decentralized service was needed, the supply of licensed doctors was inadequate, and the number of midwives could be reduced by three-fourths if they were young and well mounted [in horseback riding]" (Glass, 1989, p. 30). As a result of her study, a nursing center opened in Hyden in Leslie County in 1925 and a second center opened 1 month later. The centers provided sickness care, delivery, health education, social services, and advancement of economic independence. By 1930, there were six nursing centers (actually called "nursing centers"), each serving a 5-mile radius. The service was supported by a prospective payment system of not less than $1 from every householder that was payable annually in money or goods. Services included midwifery, bedside nursing, infant and preschool hygiene, and public health services, including immunizations and school hygiene (Glass, 1989).

Visiting nursing eventually gave way to public health nursing where nursing work and civic work were unified and involved not only the clients but also the family and the community. Then public health nursing led to the concept of nursing centers. Also important in the history of nursing centers is the impact of the development of the nurse practitioner's role in the late 1960s and early 1970s. With the advent of nurse practitioners, these nurses were prepared to "provide primary care as the client's first contact in illness-related care . . . with continued responsibility for the client's health maintenance, evaluation, and appropriate referral" (Aydelotte et al., 1987, p. 3).

Following the initial development of the nurse practitioner role, M. Lucille Kinlein established an independent nursing practice in 1971 to gain complete control of her professional practice. She stated, "I became convinced that the only way to identify precisely and meet satisfactorily the nursing needs of people was to change the setting in which I came into contact with persons in the need of nursing care" (Kinlein, 1972, p. 23). She described her services as providing direct physical and psychological care, emotional support, and health counseling in states of illness and health.

In 1978, O. Marie Henry, at the annual meeting of the American Public Health Association, urged the profession to develop nursing centers where the education of nursing students, the practice of patient care, and research to improve both practice and education would be planned and carried out. She stated, "Nursing would be the primary focus of the centers—nurses would have the responsibility for the administration of the setting and its funds and for coordinating all care provided to patients including that provided by other disciplines" (Henry, 1978).

During the 1970s, schools of nursing began establishing nursing centers for the purposes of providing educational experiences for students, practice opportunities for faculty, health services to the community,

tunities for faculty, health services to the community, and sites for nursing research. A survey of baccalaureate and higher-degree programs in nursing conducted in 1992 found 78 institutions reporting having a nursing center administered and operated by their school of nursing (Berlin et al., 1993).

Nursing centers are found in all regions of the United States.

MODEL OF A NURSING CENTER

The current conceptual model of a **nursing center** (Figure 18-1) has resulted from a blending of its historical roots in visiting nursing, public health nursing, the nurse practitioner movement, and the development of academic nursing centers. In 1987 a nursing center task force was convened by the American Nurses Association (ANA) to examine the concept. The definition of a nursing center is set forth in ANA's publication, *The Nursing Center: Concept and Design.* The definition reads as follows (Aydelotte et al., 1987. p. 1):

Nursing Centers—sometimes referred to as community nursing organizations, nurse managed centers, nursing clinics and community nursing centers—are organizations that give the client direct access to professional nursing services. Using nursing models of health, professional nurses in these centers diagnose and treat human responses to actual and potential health problems, and promote health and optimal functioning among target populations and communities. The services provided in these centers are holistic and client-centered, and are reimbursed at a reasonable fee level. Accountability and responsibility for client care and professional practice remain with the professional nurse. Overall accountability and responsibility remain with the nurse executive.

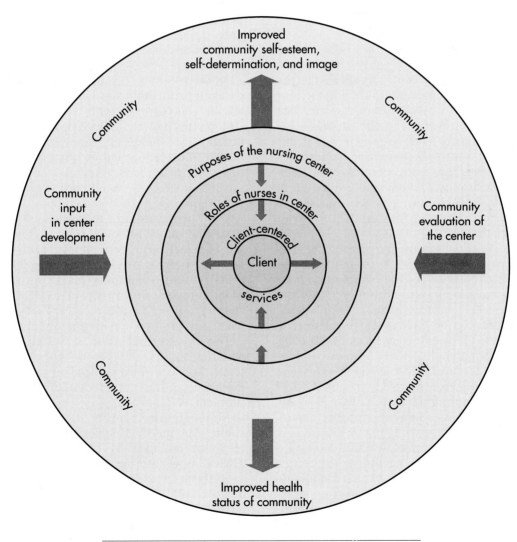

FIGURE 18-1

Contemporary nursing center model.

Key Points in Nursing Center Definition

An organization where:
- ◆ The client has direct access to nursing services.
- ◆ Nurses diagnose, treat, and promote health and optimal functioning.
- ◆ Services are client centered.
- ◆ Services are reimbursed.
- ◆ Accountability and responsibility for client care remain with the nurse.
- ◆ Overall accountability for the center remains with the nurse executive.

Roles of Nurses in Nursing Centers

Advanced practice nurse
Community health nurse
Nurse executive
Clinic nurse

Nursing centers are not limited to any particular organizational configuration. Nursing centers may be freestanding businesses or may be affiliated with universities or other service institutions such as home health agencies and hospitals. The primary characteristic of the organization is responsiveness to the health needs of the population.

The box above, left, highlights the key points in the nursing center definition.

This definition of a nursing center is reflected in the nursing center model in Figure 18-1. The larger community is represented by the outermost circle. The nursing center's responsiveness to the needs of the community occurs during its development and is ongoing. The need for a nursing center and its purposes are determined through an assessment of community needs and the community's review and evaluation of this assessment by a community advisory board. This initial input is reflected by the arrow on the left side of the outermost circle.

This input also is evident in the purposes of the center, the second circle in the model. These purposes will be determined by the needs of the community, both in the specific population groups needing services and the specific services needed by those populations. For example, if older adults have special unmet needs for health services, the center may focus on meeting the needs of that population. These purposes will also reflect the needs of the institution developing the center in that community. For example, a school of nursing located in the community may have a need for clinical experience for its students and practice opportunities for its faculty.

The purpose of the nursing center will determine what nursing practice roles are needed by the center (third circle in the model). Roles often seen in the center are shown in the box above, right. Because communities frequently identify the need for primary health care, advanced practice nursing roles are common in these centers. **Advanced practice nurses (APNs)** are nurses with additional education beyond their basic nursing program preparing them to provide an expanded level of health services to individuals, families, and communities. Nurse practitioners, nurse

midwives, and clinical nurse specialists are all advanced practice nurses.

Another important role is that of the community health nurse. These nurses synthesize nursing and public health practice in promoting and preserving the health of populations in the community. These nurses plan, implement, and evaluate health screenings, health promotion programs, and make home visits to targeted families with special needs.

Also, because centers require skilled management to plan, implement, and evaluate cost-effective services that meet community needs, a nurse executive is needed. This individual has additional educational preparation in leadership and management and is ultimately responsible for the viability of the center and its services.

As these centers continue to develop, it is expected that other nursing roles will develop as well. For example, clinic nurses, with basic nursing preparation, will be needed to interview clients, perform basic nursing assessments and laboratory tests, and provide health information. Other nursing roles, not yet defined, are likely to develop as communities continuously provide input about their health care needs and requirements.

The nursing roles of the center determine the services that can be provided (fourth circle in the model; see Figure 18-1). For example, primary health care can only be provided if APNs are in the center. Home visits require community health nurses. Although a more complete description of services follows in this chapter, nurses in these centers generally diagnose, treat, and promote health and optimal functioning.

The most central circle in the model is the client. Nursing centers' services are holistic and client centered. Services are organized to meet the client's total needs rather than focusing on a single specific problem.

Although the focus of the nursing center is the client, the model is incomplete without additional feedback provided by clients and the community. Therefore, clients' feedback is solicited regarding their satisfaction with nursing center services. Note the arrows from the client in the model. Also, feedback is solicited from the community through community surveys and input from the community advisory committee, as reflected by the arrow on the right side of the model's outer circle (see Figure 18-1). The ultimate success of the center is measured through improved health outcomes and improved self-esteem, self-determination, and image in the community.

Populations Served by Nursing Centers

General community
Elderly persons
Poor persons
Rural residents
Culturally diverse individuals and families
Homeless persons
University students and their families
Women
HIV-positive individuals
Migrants
Mentally ill persons
Developmentally disabled or handicapped clients
Victims of abuse
Prisoners

Table 18-1   Examples of Nursing Center Services by Levels of Prevention

Level of prevention	Examples of services
Primary	Exercise classes
	Nutrition classes
	Parenting classes
	Prenatal care
	Family planning
	Immunizations
Secondary	Weight control program
	Smoking cessation program
	Screening for chronic diseases
	Developmental screening
	Vision and hearing screening
	Primary care
Tertiary	Outpatient transfusion services
	Enterostomal therapy services
	Home health services
	HIV services

POPULATIONS SERVED BY NURSING CENTERS

Although nursing centers serve diverse populations (see box above), they have demonstrated a unique ability to provide access to health care for populations that have remained unserved or underserved by the traditional health care delivery system (Phillips and Steel, 1994). A study conducted by the National League for Nursing in 1990 found that centers were caring for an unusually high proportion of racial minorities, the very young and very old, and the poor—"groups that are considered among the potentially disadvantaged in terms of health care delivery" (Barger and Rosenfeld, 1993, p. 429).

These findings are further substantiated by descriptions in the literature of individual centers serving residents of low income housing (Lundeen, 1993), the homeless (Turner et al, 1989), and the elderly (Fielo and Crowe, 1992; Haq, 1993; Pulliam, 1991; Taira, 1991). Rural residents, another traditionally underserved population, have received health care from nursing centers (Barger, 1991; Lenz and Edwards, 1992). University students with limited resources and their families have found an excellent resource in nursing centers run by their schools of nursing (Bugle et al., 1990; VanAntwerp and Spaniolo, 1992).

Other nursing centers have provided specialty nursing services that targeted specific populations. These populations include women for prenatal care and delivery (Capan et al., 1993). Chronically mentally ill individuals (Connolly, 1991) and people with acquired immunodeficiency syndrome (AIDS) (Schroeder, 1993; Smerke, 1990) have found specialized nursing centers uniquely suited to meeting their needs.

In a study of nursing centers run by schools of nursing, 41 of 62 centers (66.1%) in the study reported that more than 15% of their clinic's client population consisted of special populations. These included frail elderly persons (over 85 years), culturally diverse people, substance abusers, the homeless, non–English-

speaking persons, abuse victims, mentally ill clients, persons positive for the human immunodeficiency virus (HIV), migrants, low-birth-weight and preterm infants, developmentally disabled persons, and prisoners (Berlin et al., 1993). These findings document that nursing centers offer access to health care to diverse populations.

SERVICES PROVIDED BY NURSING CENTERS

The services provided by nursing centers include a wide array of community health interventions. Because nursing center services have traditionally focused on prevention, they are described here using the levels of prevention model discussed in Chapter 11 on epidemiology. Table 18-1 provides examples of services within each level of prevention.

Primary Prevention

Primary prevention services are aimed at stopping disease before it occurs. Therefore, primary prevention includes both general health promotion and specific protection. General health promotion and wellness activities are conducted by virtually all nursing centers. These include health education, both to individuals and groups. Also, primary prevention includes specific measures that protect individuals against specific agents. The most common protective measure offered by nursing centers is immunization.

Secondary Prevention

Secondary prevention services are designed to detect disease early and treat it promptly. Activities that reduce risk factors also are classified as secondary prevention. Most nursing center activities fall into the area of secondary prevention, including risk reduction and screening services. Because screening tests only determine those persons likely to have the disease, those individuals screened positive require follow-up to determine if they actually have the disease. Early in their development, nursing centers referred these individuals to another health care provider for diagnosis, usually a physician. Now, however, many nursing centers also provide primary care.

Primary care is defined as the individual's initial contact for health care and the continuous care that most people need most of the time. It is accessible, comprehensive care that treats the whole person. Such care is community oriented, coordinated, consumer driven, and cost effective. In providing primary care, nursing centers treat minor illnesses such as upper respiratory infections and also monitor chronic diseases such as hypertension.

Tertiary Prevention

Tertiary prevention services focus on limitation of disability and rehabilitation when possible. Tertiary services can also be directed toward maintaining the highest quality of life possible when disease processes are irreversible. Although there are not as many nursing centers providing tertiary prevention services, those that do are frequently highly specialized. The examples in Table 18-1 document the critical services provided by nursing centers for those individuals coping with disabilities.

NURSING CENTERS AND *HEALTHY PEOPLE 2000* GOALS AND OBJECTIVES

The *Healthy People 2000* goals and objectives were developed to provide a national strategy for significantly improving health in the United States by the year 2000. This section discusses the populations served and services provided by nursing centers as they relate to those national goals and objectives.

Nursing Centers and *Healthy People 2000* Goals

The three overarching national goals that provide the structure for what needs to be done to improve the nation's health are listed in Table 18-2 along with the related services provided by nursing centers.

Goal I—Increase the Span of Healthy Life for Americans

The intent of this goal is to extend both the quantity and the quality of life of individuals so that they can live long, productive lives free from chronic diseases, preventable infections, and serious injury. Healthy people would have a full range of functional capacity at each life stage, maximizing their ability to have satisfying relationships, work, and play.

Nursing centers contribute to this goal by providing health education to individuals and groups on such

Table 18-2   Year 2000 Goals and Nursing Centers

U.S. year 2000 goals	Nursing center services
Increase the span of healthy life for Americans	Health education Aerobic exercise activities Screening tests Smoking cessation programs Chronic disease monitoring
Reduce health disparities among Americans	Primary care Prenatal services Immunizations
Achieve access to preventive services for all Americans	Prenatal services Parenting classes Family planning services Immunizations

From *Healthy People 2000: national health promotion and disease prevention objectives*, Washington, DC, 1991, USDHHS, Public Health Service.

topics as nutrition, weight control, and stress reduction. Smoking cessation programs and exercise classes also provide opportunities for individuals to reduce their risks and live healthier lives. Even those who already have been diagnosed with chronic diseases such as hypertension or diabetes can work closely with nurses in nursing centers to keep these problems under control. For example, clients with hypertension not only can have their blood pressure monitored by nurses in the center, but also can have medication monitored for both effect and difficulties, and can receive education about diet, stress, exercise, and even enroll in a smoking cessation program if needed.

Goal II—Reduce Health Disparities Among Americans

This goal focuses on the need to close the gap that exists in both health care and health status between the majority of the population and various underserved populations. These are population groups that have historically been disadvantaged economically, educationally, and politically. Generally, they include racial and ethnic minorities, people with low income, and people with disabilities. It is these same population groups that nursing centers have a rich history of serving. Two studies by the National League for Nursing (Barger and Rosenfeld, 1993) and the American Association of Colleges of Nursing (Berlin et al., 1993) confirm that nursing centers continue to serve an unusually high proportion of these disadvantaged groups. An important service provided to disadvantaged populations by these centers is primary care because they have frequently been denied access to even basic health care. Other important nursing center services for these groups are prenatal care and immunizations.

Goal III—Achieve Access to Preventive Services for All Americans

This goal places a high priority on access to prevention utilizing the approaches of health promotion, health protection, and preventive services. Many of the services provided by nursing centers fall within the categories of health promotion or preventive services. Health promotion services include nutrition education, aerobics classes, smoking cessation classes, and family planning. Preventive services in nursing centers include prenatal services, well-baby checkups, and the many screenings designed to provide early detection and the maximum degree of disability prevention that is possible when chronic diseases are detected early.

Efforts by nursing centers to increase access focus on reducing barriers to care. Thus, centers frequently use sliding fee scales and outreach workers to encourage families to seek care. Centers also may offer transportation or contract with other agencies for these services.

To determine the appropriate preventive interventions for different age groups and risk categories, nursing centers frequently follow the standards in the *Guide to Clinical Preventive Services* (Fisher, 1989). This report provides recommendations about preventive interventions, screening tests, counseling interventions, immunizations, and chemoprophylactic regimens for the prevention of 60 target conditions. The guide also identifies what should be included in periodic health examinations for all age groups. These recommendations are based on a comprehensive review of the related clinical research and therefore can be used by nursing centers with confidence.

Nursing Centers and the *Healthy People 2000* Objectives

In keeping with the three overarching national goals, the national health promotion and disease prevention objectives are organized within the same three categories just discussed: health promotion, health protection, and preventive services. An additional fourth category is surveillance and data systems. Under these categories, there are measurable national objectives for a total of 22 priority areas. Table 18-3 presents the 22 priority areas and indicates those that are addressed by nursing center services. This table documents that nursing centers provide services that address almost all the priority areas in the health promotion, health protection, and preventive services categories. With the exception of the priority area on surveillance and data systems, there are three types of objectives in the other priority areas:

Health status	Objectives to reduce death, disease, and disability
Risk reduction	Objectives to reduce the prevalence of risks to health or to increase behaviors known to reduce such risks
Services and protection	Objectives to increase comprehensiveness, accessibility, and quality of preventive services and preventive interventions

Table 18-3   *Healthy People 2000* Priority Areas Addressed by Nursing Centers

Priority areas	Nursing centers address this area
HEALTH PROMOTION	
1. Physical activity and fitness	X
2. Nutrition	X
3. Tobacco	X
4. Alcohol and other drugs	
5. Family planning	X
6. Mental health and mental disorders	X
7. Violent and abusive behavior	X
8. Educational and community-based programs	X
HEALTH PROTECTION	
9. Unintentional injuries	
10. Occupational safety and health	
11. Environmental health	
12. Food and drug safety	X
13. Oral health	X
PREVENTIVE SERVICES	
14. Maternal and infant health	X
15. Heart disease and stroke	X
16. Cancer	X
17. Diabetes and chronic disabling conditions	X
18. HIV infection	X
19. Sexually transmitted diseases	X
20. Immunization and infectious diseases	X
21. Clinical preventive services	X
SURVEILLANCE AND DATA SYSTEMS	
22. Surveillance and data systems	X

Services provided by nursing centers address each type of objective. For health status objectives aimed at reducing both morbidity and mortality, nursing centers provide primary care, prenatal care, and health screenings. Risk reduction objectives are addressed through the many educational programs provided by nursing centers on topics such as nutrition, weight control, and cardiovascular risk reduction. Aerobic exercise programs and smoking cessation programs also focus on risk reduction. Services and protection objectives are covered by all nursing center services because they frequently target populations with limited access to health care and who have not been receiving preventive health services.

In addressing the category of surveillance and data systems, nursing centers are selecting management information systems that enable them to collect data on clients served and services provided. They are also focusing on efficiency, effectiveness, and cost of services. Some centers have selected computerized systems designed for physicians' practices, and others have used a computerized version of the Omaha classification system, a system designed for community health nursing practice (Martin and Scheet, 1992).

DEVELOPING A NURSING CENTER

Because nursing centers are well positioned to do their part to save lives lost prematurely and needlessly and to improve the span of healthy life for the Americans they serve, nurses must have the necessary skills to develop nursing centers. At least five areas require in-depth exploration before beginning a nursing center: (1) integrating the center into the community; (2) determining services; (3) obtaining funding; (4) marketing; and (5) legal and regulatory issues. A sound **business plan** will be needed to ensure that all aspects of beginning a center have been considered. This document describes the development and direction of a proposed business and how the goals of the business will be achieved (Johnson et al., 1988). The business plan typically contains the following components (Vogel and Doleysh, 1994):

1. *Cover page.* The cover page includes the name, address, and phone number of the person beginning the center and the date.
2. *Executive summary.* This is a one- or two-page overview of the center.
3. *Table of contents.*
4. *Description of the business.* This describes what the center is and what services it will provide.
5. *Survey of the industry.* This describes the past, present, and future of the health care market.
6. *Market research and analysis.* This section describes existing competition and the size of the potential market share and identifies clients.
7. *Marketing plan.* This section plans for how the center will reach its clients.
8. *Management team.* This section provides an organizational chart for the center and a description of its management.
9. *Supporting professional assistance.* This lists other professionals, such as attorneys, accountants, and other professions to be used.
10. *Operations plan.* This describes how and where services will be carried out.
11. *Research and development.* This describes projected improvements and the development of new services.
12. *Overall schedule.* This is a time line for starting and developing the center.
13. *Critical risks and problems.* This section covers internal and external threats to the center and how they will be addressed.
14. *Financial plan.* This section includes the financial projections for the first 3 years. It includes a projected budget, cash flow forecast, and break-even point.
15. *Proposed financing of the center.* This section lists specific sources that will provide funding.

Planning Process Activities in *Healthy Communities 2000: Model Standards*

Assess and determine the role of one's health agency.
Assess the lead health agency's organizational capacity.
Develop an agency plan to build the necessary organizational capacity.
Assess the community's organizational and power structures.
Organize the community to build a stronger constituency for public health and establish a partnership for public health.
Assess the health needs and available community resources.
Determine local priorities.
Select outcome and process objectives that are compatible with local priorities and the *Healthy People 2000* objectives.
Develop community-wide intervention strategies.
Develop and implement a plan of action.
Monitor and evaluate the effort on a continuing basis.

From *Healthy Communities 2000: model standards*, ed 3, Washington, DC, 1991, American Public Health Association. Reprinted with permission.

16. *Legal structure of the center.* This may be sole proprietorship, partnership, or corporation, or the center may be part of a larger organization.
17. *Appendices and supporting documents.* This section includes additional documents to support the business plan.

Integrating the Center into the Community

During the initial planning for a nursing center, it is important to determine what the role of the center will be in the community. A series of steps or activities has been outlined in *Healthy Communities 2000: Model standards* (1991). (See box above.) The model standards assume that the public health agency serves as the lead healthy agency in assessing the community and determining its unmet health needs. Therefore, it is important to work with the local government public health agency to determine existing gaps in health services that could be met through a nursing center.

The nursing center's nurse executive can use these steps in developing a plan for nursing center services. In addition, the nurse executive should be involved in global planning for meeting the community's health needs to ensure that the nursing center fits within the greater plan for health services in the community.

It is important to enlist the community's help early in the planning process for the nursing center. A community needs assessment is completed that involves community agencies and individuals from the community. Focus groups, questionnaires, and interviews with service providers and health care consumers are used to collect data. In addition, existing community studies and epidemiological data are examined. These data are reviewed not just by the nurse executive, but by community agencies and individuals. This approach ensures accurate interpretation of the data and the development of services that are both useful and acceptable to the community.

To accomplish these goals for services, a community advisory board for the nursing center is established early in its development. Included on this board are influential community leaders, potential consumers of services, and community service providers. This group can help the administrator interpret the data from the community needs assessment to ensure that services are appropriate and needed. Later the board can assist in marketing the center and in providing feedback from the community about services provided by the nursing center.

Developing collaborative relationships with existing community agencies such as health departments, public aid departments, and other social services agencies is critical to the success of the nursing center. These agencies will refer their clients to the center and receive referrals from the center. Health departments can offer to provide support services such as immunizations and laboratory services to the nursing center. Health departments may also contract with the nursing center to provide specific services such as family planning, child health, and WIC (Women, Infants, and Children Supplemental Feeding Program) at expanded locations.

Also important to the success of the center is the development of cooperative relationships with community physicians. They need information about the nursing center and its services while it is being planned and when it is implemented. Frequently, centers have one or more physicians on their advisory board. Good working relationships with area physicians facilitate referrals of clients with medical problems to physicians and referral of clients with nursing needs to the nursing center.

Determining Services

The community needs assessment will identify gaps in health services in the community that could be filled by a nursing center. These may be specific services not sufficiently available in the total community or gaps in services to specific populations or a combination of both needs. An analysis of several studies on nursing centers finds an increasing trend toward offering primary care services (Barger and Bridges, 1990; Barger and Rosenfeld, 1993). This trend supports national and state efforts for health care reform. In addition to the types of nursing services discussed earlier in this chapter, other professional services such as those of a nutritionist, social worker, or psychologist may be offered at a nursing center as well. What is critical in the selection of services to be provided is a match between services not only needed but wanted by the community and the services offered by the center.

Hours of service must also be determined. In setting the hours when the center will be open, consideration is given to both the services of the center and the characteristics of the population being served. If a center is offering primary care, an expectation exists that there will be evening and/or weekend hours with access to services around the clock.

The center must also decide who will be served. Again, the decision is based on the community needs assessment. Options include the general population in the community or specific subgroups such as senior citizens, women and children, or economically disadvantaged clients. Although many nursing centers have focused on underserved or disadvantaged groups, these decisions can impact the economic viability of the center by limiting the revenue from the clients themselves.

Obtaining Funding

A critical component of the planning process for a nursing center is determining how it will be funded. The financial component of the business plan provides the information that forecasts how much is needed. Included here is the budget, with at least a 1-year projection, start-up balance sheet and income projection statement, a cash flow projection, and a break-even analysis (Vogel and Doleysh, 1994).

Sources of start-up funding include personal funds, borrowing funds, or grants from federal, state, or local agencies and foundations. The U.S. Public Health Service Division of Nursing has been a major source of start-up funding for nursing centers operated by schools of nursing. Other centers have obtained funding from the W.K. Kellogg and Robert Wood Johnson foundations.

However, any potential funder will be interested in the long-term economic viability of the nursing center. Therefore, grant proposals and the business plan will include how the center will be financed over the long term. There are at least five different ways to finance a nursing center: grants, fee for service, third-party reimbursement contracts, and charities (Elsberry and Nelson, 1993).

Grants are frequently identified as a way initially to fund a center. The funding agency or organization generally publishes guidelines of what it wants to support. Then a proposal is required identifying how the nursing center will accomplish the objectives of the granting organization. Most often these grants can be used to start new centers, projects, or programs but will not continue indefinitely. Also, the proposal usually must include a description of how the services will be continued after the grant.

In a *fee-for-service system*, the nursing center establishes a specific charge for each service the center offers. Frequently, however, these fees have been set lower than the actual cost of delivering the service, resulting in a financial loss for the center. Also, if fees are not collected from clients, there are not enough funds to keep the center open. Because nursing centers frequently have served economically disadvantaged groups, collecting an adequate amount of revenue from these populations has proved difficult.

In *third-party reimbursement,* the fee is not paid by the client but by a third party, typically an insurer, except in health maintenance organizations (HMOs), where there is a per capita annual fee that covers a package of services. Generally, the list of charges for different services in the fee-for-service system is the basis for what the third-party insurer is billed for services rendered to the client. Nevertheless, some third-party insurers refuse to pay nurses for services provided even when the same service would be reimbursed when provided by a physician at a higher cost.

Contracts are written agreements with another party to provide a special package of services to a group for an agreed-on fee. The services and fees are set before the services are provided, making contracts a predictable and reliable source of income. It should be noted that once a contract is finalized, the service must be provided for the contract period at the agreed-on cost. Contracts can provide predictable sources of income for a center.

Finally, funds can be raised for a nursing center from *charities.* Charities or community service organizations can contribute to the nursing center by raising funds for a specific project or for services to a specific population. In addition to providing financial assistance, their support can enhance the center's visibility and image in the community.

All these methods—grants, fee for service, third-party reimbursement, contracts, and charities—can be used to provide continued financial support for the center. Although each source could be used exclusively, it is more advantageous to use a combination of methods. Therefore, a diversified revenue stream using multiple sources of income is preferred.

Marketing

After the services have been determined and start-up funding obtained, a marketing plan is developed. Marketing is everything that is done to promote the nursing center from the moment the idea is conceived to the point at which consumers receive the service and begin to use the nursing center on a regular basis (Vogel and Doleysh, 1994). The marketing plan is a part of the business plan, but marketing never stops, even when the center is open and successful. The benefits of a planned marketing process are that it (1) generates clients, (2) provides trend analysis for growth decisions, (3) assesses the competition, and (4) assists in setting fees.

As part of the marketing plan, the center identifies specific promotion strategies to be used to promote clients' awareness and understanding of the service and to develop clients' perception of the need for the service and commitment to using the service (Vogel and Doleysh, 1994). Strategies frequently used by nursing centers include brochures, television and radio spots, and newspaper public interest pieces. Presentations are made to service organizations such as Rotary and Lions clubs. Personal contacts with physicians and other health care providers are important marketing strategies as well.

Although all these strategies are valuable, word of mouth is a major method of client recruitment. A study of nursing centers found that more than half the clients were recruited through the recommendations of other clients (Barger and Rosenfeld, 1993). This finding emphasizes the importance of satisfied customers.

Legal and Regulatory Issues

Nurses face three major legal and regulatory restrictions as they develop nursing centers: unnecessary restrictions on their scope of practice, prescriptive authority, and eligibility for reimbursement (Safriet, 1992).

Scope of Practice

Because many of the services provided in nursing centers are provided by APNs, state nurse practice acts that restrict the practice of these nurses ultimately limit the services provided in nursing centers. Many of these nurse practice acts were revised to include APNs before the many studies demonstrating that APNs are fully competent autonomous providers. Therefore, many include "mixed-regulator boards of differently licensed practitioners, variously defined mandates for physician participation in practice, and internally inconsistent scope of practice variations determined by practice settings" (Safriet, 1992, p. 454). In other words, it is required in some states but not in others that physicians supervise APNs. Also, many states that require physician supervision exempt those APNs who practice in rural or inner-city community health centers. Therefore, changes are needed to remove the restrictions to APNs' practice that are embedded in many state laws.

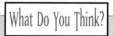

What Do You Think?

Debate continues regarding whether nursing centers require physician oversight.

Prescriptive Authority

State law also determines whether or not APNs have **prescriptive authority.** For nursing centers providing primary care, this authority is of critical importance. In January 1994, APNs in only three states had complete and independent (of any required physician supervision or collaboration) authority to prescribe, including controlled substances. In an additional 24 states, that authority to prescribe (including controlled substances) depends on some level of required physician supervision or collaboration. In another 16 states, APNs have the authority to prescribe (excluding controlled substances), and some level of physician supervision or collaboration is required. In eight states, APNs have dispensing authority (Pearson, 1994).

For centers in states with no legislative prescriptive authority, APNs attempt to follow the "normal standard" of practice for how nurse practitioners prescribe in that state. This usually means using physician presigned or cosigned prescriptions or calling in prescriptions under the name of the physician consultant. These practices increase the risk of liability for these nurses.

Eligibility for Reimbursement

Nursing centers must be able to receive direct reimbursement for nursing services. **Direct reimbursement** means that payment for services provided by nurses is made directly to the center rather than to another provider (typically a physician) who then pays the center. Whether or not APNs are able to be reimbursed directly by third-party insurers depends largely on state statute because states regulate the insurance industry (Safriet, 1992). In a January 1994 survey, APNs were found to receive third-party reimbursement in 34 states, but 10 of these were very limited (Pearson, 1994).

In contrast, federal reimbursement policy has been more favorable. Federal legislation grants authority for insurance carriers under the Federal Employees Health Benefits Plan to make direct payment to nurse practitioners, nurse midwives, and clinical nurse specialists. Nurse practitioners and clinical nurse specialists who practice in rural areas are eligible for direct Medicare reimbursement. Nurse practitioners are also eligible to receive reimbursement from Civilian Health and Medical Programs (CHAMPUS). The Health Care Financing Administration's regulations allow each state Medicaid agency to reimburse pediatric nurse practitioners and family nurse practitioners in accordance with state policies and regulations. As of January 1994, APNs received Medicaid reimbursement in 49 states and in 39 of these at 80% to 100% of a physician's rate of reimbursement (Pearson, 1994). The U.S. Department of Transportation allows nurse practitioners to conduct required physical examinations for truck drivers and be paid directly for these services.

The Rural Health Clinics Act of 1977 established a cost-based reimbursement mechanism for authorized rural health clinics. By law, the services of these clinics must be provided by nonphysician providers at least 50% of the time. Nursing centers located in rural areas designated as a health professions shortage area (HPSA) can seek designation as a rural health clinic.

A review of federal legislation for access to direct reimbursement for APNs and nursing centers reveals a more positive regulatory environment. Because both states and private insurers tend to follow the federal government's lead, federal reimbursement policy is critically important to understanding the future of nursing centers.

RESEARCH ON NURSING CENTERS

A review of the state of the art of research on nursing centers (Riesch, 1992a) found that researchers had examined "the location and demographic profiles of academic centers; student outcomes; client and patient outcomes such as knowledge, attitude, behavior, health status, and satisfaction with care; and cost effectiveness and quality of care" (Riesch, 1992a, p. 148). Nevertheless, major gaps in research were identified. For example, despite the number of academic nursing centers, only one study was found that examined student outcomes. In a review of the research on client health status, Riesch found that each study that examined health status had methodological flaws such as small samples, obscure instrumentation with poor reporting of psychometric properties, and lack of comparison groups. Only one study attempted to measure cost effectiveness, utilization outcomes, and quality of care.

After conducting a thorough review of the research on nursing centers, Riesch concluded that the studies (1) lacked a theoretical or conceptual framework; (2) used a variety of methods; (3) generally used small convenience samples mainly composed of low-income healthy females; (4) poorly defined the research variables; (5) lacked control conditions; (6) gathered data using only one method from only one center; (7) did not examine long-term or lag effects; (8) used mostly quantitative methods; and (9) did not replicate previous research.

To increase knowledge about nursing centers, multisite, multimethod, and clinical trial studies are needed that identify outcomes of nursing centers and analyze their cost effectiveness, efficiency, and quality of care. Riesch (1992b, p. 22) states:

Nursing's knowledge about the practice and outcomes from these centers and practices is scant. We know the clients and patients are satisfied with the care. We know how many and what types of persons avail themselves of the services. However, we know very little about the scientific adequacy of the practice in these centers, the cost of

 Research Brief

Barger SE, Rosenfeld P: Models in community health care: findings from a national study of community nursing centers, *Nurs Health Care* 14(8):426-431, 1993.

In a national study of 80 nursing centers conducted by the National League for Nursing, more than half were less than 5 years old and associated with a parent organization, frequently a school of nursing. Nurses employed in these nursing centers were better educated than their counterparts in other health care delivery settings, with two-thirds certified for advanced practice. Centers were found to be caring for an unusually high proportion of groups who are potentially disadvantaged in terms of health care delivery. Services frequently offered included primary care, health assessment, and screening services.

care, and the outcomes with respect to changes in knowledge, attitude, or behavior, functional ability, health status, or days lost from school or work. In terms of nursing practice, these are significant gaps in our knowledge.

Studies that provide information on these areas could be used to support needed legal and regulatory changes in the areas of scope of practice, prescriptive authority, and direct reimbursement.

Clinical Application

Two community health nurses who were faculty members in a university located in a rural area believed there was inadequate health care for certain populations in their community. They conducted a community needs assessment, including surveys of farm families, migrant families, and students. The assessment determined that there was inadequate access to primary health care for certain segments of the population, particularly uninsured rural farm families, migrant workers, and young families.

With the assistance of faculty and students in the university's college of business, the two faculty members developed a business plan for a nursing center. The plan enabled them to determine exactly what services would be offered, the staff needed to operate the center, the budget necessary for the center, and a marketing plan to let people know about the center. They projected their needs and plans over the next 5 years.

Their plan also included alternate methods of financing the center. They decided to apply for a grant from the U.S. Public Health Service Division of Nursing to start the nursing center. They knew that the grant would provide start-up funding, but they would need to implement their long-term financial plan from the beginning to ensure that the center would stay open after the grant.

After receiving the grant, the nurses located a building and used grant funds to renovate it. Equipment and supplies were ordered. Positions for staff were advertised and applicants interviewed. The nursing staff included family nurse practitioners, community health nurses, and clinic nurses. These nurses had different educational preparations, depending on the nursing role they would fill at the center. A physician consultant was also employed.

To ensure the center met the needs of the community, a community advisory board was formed and met regularly to provide input about services to be offered and how they should be offered. This board was an important link to the community to ensure that accessible, culturally sensitive care was provided.

The center opened with the full support of the community. One of the two nurses who started the center is the chief executive officer for the center. The second nurse coordinates clinical experiences for students. Nursing students enrolled in the university master's and baccalaureate programs have clinical experiences in the center. Students from the community college's associate degree nursing program also have experiences in the center. In addition, students from the fields of psychology, dietetics, and communicative disorders have educational experience in the nursing center.

As shown by this description, community health nurses who identify a problem in the health system of a community are able to implement change to the benefit of that community.

Key Concepts

♦ A nursing center is an organization where (1) the client has direct access to nursing services; (2) nurses diagnose, treat, and promote health and optimal functioning; (3) services are client centered; (4) services are reimbursed; (5) accountability and responsibility for client care remain with the nurse; and (6) overall accountability for the center remains with the nurse executive.

♦ Key nursing roles in a nursing center are advanced practice nurse, community health nurse, and nurse executive.

♦ Major populations served by nursing centers include the general community, elderly persons, poor persons, rural residents, culturally diverse individuals and families, homeless persons, university students and families, women, HIV-positive individuals, migrants, mentally ill clients, developmentally disabled or handicapped clients, victims of abuse, and prisoners.

♦ Major categories of services provided in nursing centers are health promotion and wellness activities, protective measures, risk reduction, screening, and primary care.

♦ Needed areas for research on nursing centers include quality of care, efficiency, cost effectiveness, and outcomes.

Critical Thinking Activities

1. Review your state's nurse practice act.
2. What is the regulatory environment the practice act provides for advanced practice nurses (APNs)?
3. Visit a nursing center in your region or state.
4. Estimate the probability of the center remaining open in the next decade. Use supporting evidence to justify your position.
5. What are the laws in your state on prescriptive authority and third-party reimbursement?
6. Determine your recommendations for change in these laws to be more supportive of APNs.
7. Hold a debate about the pros and cons of physician oversight for APNs. Develop a rationale to support your position.

Bibliography

Allison SE: A framework for nursing action in a nurse conducted diabetic management clinic, *J Nurs Adm* 3:53-60, 1973.

Andresen P, McDermott MA: Client satisfaction with student care in a nurse-managed center, *Nurse Educ* 17(3):21-23, 1992.

Aydelotte MK, Gregory MS: Nursing practice: innovative models. In *Nursing centers: meeting the demand for quality health care,* New York, 1989, National League for Nursing.

Aydelotte MK, Barger SE, Branstetter E, et al: *The nursing center: concept and design,* Kansas City, Mo, 1987, American Nurses Association.

Barger SE: The nursing center: a model for rural nursing practice, *Nurs Health Care* 12(6):290-294, 1991.

Barger SE, Bridges WC: An assessment of academic nursing centers, *Nurse Educ* 5(2):31-36, 1990.

Barger SE, Kline PM: Community health service programs in academe: unique learning opportunities for students, *Nurse Educ* 18(6):22-26, 1993.

Barger SE, Rosenfeld P: Models in community health care: findings from a national study of community nursing centers, *Nurs Health Care* 14(8):426-431, 1993.

Berlin LE, Bednash GD, Alsheimer O: *Institutional data systems: 1992-1993 special report on institutional resources and budgets in baccalaureate and graduate programs in nursing,* Washington, DC, 1993, American Association of Colleges of Nursing.

Bugle L, Frisch N, Woods T: The use of nursing diagnosis in a nurse-managed college health service, *J Am Coll Health* 38(4):191-192, 1990.

Capan P, Beard M, Mashburn M: Nurse-managed clinics provide access and improved health care, *Nurse Pract* 18(5):50-55, 1993.

Connolly PM: Services for the underserved: a nurse-managed center for the chronically mentally ill, *J Psychosoc Nurs Ment Health Serv* 29(1):15-20, 1991.

Elsberry N, Nelson F: How to plan financial support for nursing centers, *Nurs Health Care* 14(8):408-413, 1993.

Fielo SB, Crowe RL: A nursing center in Brooklyn, *Nurs Health Care* 13(9):488-493, 1992.

Fisher M, editor: *Guide to clinical preventive services: report of the US Preventive Services Task Force,* Baltimore, 1989, Williams & Wilkins.

Glass LK: The historical origins of nursing centers. In *Nursing centers: meeting the demand for quality health care,* New York, 1989, National League for Nursing.

Haq MB: Understanding older adult satisfaction with primary health care services at a nursing center, *Appl Nurs Res* 6(3):125-131, 1993.

Healthy Communities 2000: model standards, ed 3, Washington, DC, 1991, American Public Health Association.

Healthy People 2000: national health promotion and disease prevention objectives, Washington, DC, 1991, USDHHS, Public Health Service.

Henry OM: *Demonstration centers for nursing practice, education, and research.* Paper presented at the Association of Graduate Faculty of Public Health and Community Health Nursing, APHA Annual Meeting, Los Angeles, 1978.

Johnson JE, Sparks DG, Humphreys C: Writing a winning business plan, *J Nurs Adm* 18(10):15-19, 1988.

Kinlein ML: Independent nurse practitioner, *Nurs Outlook* 20(1): 22-24, 1972.

Kos BA, Rothberg JS: Evaluation of a freestanding nurse clinic. In Aiken LH, editor: *Health policy and nursing practice,* New York, 1981, McGraw-Hill.

Lang NM: Nurse-managed centers: will they thrive? *Am J Nurs* 83(9):1290-1293, 1983.

Lenz CL, Edwards J: Nurse-managed primary care: tapping the rural community power base, *J Nurs Adm* 22(9):57-61, 1992.

Lundeen SP: Comprehensive, collaborative, coordinated, community-based care: a community nursing center model, *Fam Community Health* 16(2):57-65, 1993.

Martin KS, Scheet NJ: *The Omaha system applications for community health nursing,* Philadelphia, 1992, Saunders.

Nursing's agenda for health care reform, New York, 1991, National League for Nursing.

Pappas CA, Scoy-Mosher CV: Establishing a profitable outpatient community nursing center, *J Nurs Adm* 18(5):31-33, 1988.

Pearson LJ: Annual update on how each state stands on legislative issues affecting advanced nursing practice, *Nurse Pract* 19(1):11-13, 17-18, 21-22, 24-27, 31-34, 39-40, 42-44, 50, 53, 1994.

Phillips DL, Steel JE: Factors influencing scope of practice in nursing centers, *J Prof Nurs* 10(2):84-90, 1994.

Pulliam L: Client satisfaction with a nurse-managed clinic, *Community Health Nurs* 8(2):97-112, 1991.

Riesch SK: Nursing centers. In Fitzpatrick JJ, Tauton RL, Jacox AK, editors: *Annual review of nursing research,* vol 10, New York, 1992a, Springer, p. 145-162.

Riesch SK: Nursing centers: an analysis of the anecdotal literature, *J Prof Nurs* 8(1):16-25, 1992b.

Safriet BJ: Health care dollars and regulatory sense: the role of advanced practice nursing, *Yale J Regulation* 9(2):417-488, 1992.

Schroeder C: Nursing's response to the crisis of access, costs, and quality in health care, *Adv Nurs Sci* 16(1):1-20, 1993.

Smerke JM: Healing and wholeness: a case study of a nurse-managed AIDS center. In *Perspectives in nursing: 1989-91,* NLN Pub No 41-2281, New York, 1990, National League for Nursing.

Taira F: Teaching independently living older adults about managing their medications, *Rehabil Nurs* 16(6):322-326, 1991.

Turner SL, Bauer G, McNair E, et al: The homeless experience: clinic building in a community health discovery-learning project, *Public Health Nurs* 6(2):97-101, 1989.

Van Antwerp C, Spaniola AM: Nursing services for children of families living in university housing, *J Pediatr Nurs* 7(3):211-215, 1992.

Vogel G, Doleysh N: *Entrepreneuring: a nurse's guide to starting a business,* ed 2, New York, 1994, National League for Nursing.

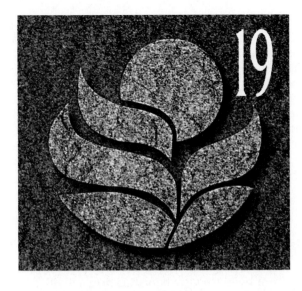

19

Case Management

Ann H. Cary

Objectives

After reading this chapter, the student should be able to do the following:

◆ Define continuity of care, case management, and advocacy.
◆ Describe the scope of practice, roles, and functions of a case manager.
◆ Compare and contrast the nursing process with processes of case management and advocacy.
◆ Identify methods to manage conflict, as well as the process of achieving collaboration.
◆ Define and explain the legal and ethical issues confronting case managers.

Key Terms

advocacy
affirming
amplification
autonomy
beneficence
capitation financing
case management
clarification
collaboration
constituency
coordination
critical path
informing
intercessor
justice
liability
mediator
negotiating
problem solving
promoter
supporting
verification

Outline

Case management has had a rich tradition in public health nursing while assuming more recent prominence in the acute care literature (Cohen and Cesta, 1993; Knollmueller, 1989). Nursing has maintained the leadership among health care professionals in coordinating resources to achieve health care outcomes based on quality, access, and cost. As health care delivery moves to capitation financing with an emphasis on pursuing the most efficient management of client outcomes, case management is expected to emerge as a strong determinant.

Capitation financing is a method of paying for the health care costs of clients based on a fixed amount per person annually rather than a fixed amount per each service to the client. For example, each client who joins a managed care delivery system may be allotted $4500 per year in anticipated health care costs. The goal of the system is to deliver quality care at or less than $4500 for each person in the system. By using primary, secondary, and tertiary prevention, systems using case management achieve the five "rights" of outcomes: the right *care* at the right *time* by the right *provider* in the right *setting* at the right *price* (American Nurses Association [ANA], 1992).

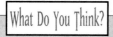

What Do You Think?

Case managers should ration health care services in the current delivery system.

CONCEPTS OF CASE MANAGEMENT
Definitions

Reviewing multiple definitions of **case management** helps to demonstrate the complexity of the process. Weil and Karls (1985) describe case management as a "set of logical steps and process of interaction within a service network which assures that a client receives needed services in a supportive, effective, efficient and cost-effective manner." (p. 4). Case management is defined by the American Hospital Association (AHA, 1986) as the process of planning, organizing, coordinating, and monitoring services and resources needed by clients while supporting the effective use of health and social services. Bower (1992) describes the continuity, quality, and cost containment aspects of case management as a health care delivery process whose goals are to provide quality health care, decrease fragmentation, enhance the client's quality of life, and contain costs. Secord (1987) defines case management as a systematic process of assessment, planning, service coordination, referrals, and monitoring that meets the multiple service needs of clients. The National Council on Aging (1987) states that case management involves assessment, planning care, arranging and monitoring service, and reassessing needs.

As a competency, case management is defined in the public health nursing literature (Kenyon et al., 1990) as the "ability to establish an appropriate plan of care based on assessment of the client/family and to coordinate the necessary resources and services for the client's benefit" (p. 36). Knowledge and skills required to achieve this competency include knowledge of community resources and financing mechanisms, written and oral communication and documentation, proficient negotiation and conflict resolution practices, critical thinking processes to identify and prioritize problems from provider and client and perspectives, and identification of best resources for the desired outcomes. Furthermore, case management is identified as one of the eleven competencies for practice in community health nursing.

The complexity of case management practice is further apparent by noting the **coordination** activities of multiple providers, payers, and settings throughout a client's continuum of care. Care provision by many disciplines, the client, family, significant others, and community organizations must be assessed, planned, implemented, adjusted, and evaluated in accordance with mutually designed goals. Although the community health nurse may be employed and located in one setting, the nurse will be influencing the selection and monitoring of care provided in other settings by formal and informal care providers. A particularly challenging problem is the fragmentation of services, which can result in overutilization, underutilization, gaps in care, and miscommunication; this may ultimately result in costly client outcomes. Parker et al. (1992) discuss the unique complexity of case management in rural settings, where fewer organized community-based systems, geographical distance to delivery, population density, economics, pace and style of life, values, and social organization differ from more urbanized environments. The complexity is further fueled by chaotic systems, changes in today's health care market in which providers, services, and coverage details are constantly manipulated.

Case Management and the Nursing Process

The community health nurse views the process of case management through the broader health status of the community. Clients and families in service represent the microcosm of health needs within the larger community. Through a nurse's case management activities, general community deficits in quality and quantity of health services often are discovered.

For example, the management of a severely disabled child by a nurse case manager may uncover the absence of respite services or parenting support and education resources in a community. While managing the disability and injury claims of a corporate site, the nurse may discover that alternative care referrals for home health visits and physical therapy are generally underutilized by the acute care providers in the community. Through a nurse's case management of brain-injured young adults, the absence of community standards and legislative policy for helmet use by bicyclists and motorcyclists may stimulate advocacy efforts for community policy implementation. Case management activities with individual clients and families will reveal the larger picture of health services and health status of the community. *Community assessment, policy development,* and *assurance* activities that frame the essential *core of public health* actions are often the logical next steps for a community health nurse's practice when observed at the individual and family intervention levels through case management. Clearly, the core components of case management and the nursing process are complementary (Table 19-1). Secord's (1987) illustration of case management remains an appropriate picture of the process that nurses use (Figure 19-1).

Characteristics and Roles

Case management can be labor intensive, time consuming, and costly. Because of the increasing number of clients with complex problems in nurses' caseloads, the intensity and duration of activities required to support the case management function may soon exceed the demands of direct caregiving. Management and clinicians in community health are exploring methods to make case management more efficient. In an effort to achieve efficiency, tasks and activities have been defined to describe the characteristics desired for case manager effectiveness (Weil and Karls, 1985):

1. The technical qualifications to understand and evaluate specific diagnoses, generally requiring clinical credentials (and experience) and financial analyses

Case Manager Roles

Facilitator: supports all parties to work toward mutual goals

Liaison: provides a formal communication link among all parties concerning the plan of care management

Coordinator: arranges, regulates, and coordinates needed health care services for clients at all necessary points of services

Broker: acts as an agent for provider services that are needed by clients to stay within coverage according to budget and cost limits of health care plan

Educator: educates client, family, and providers about case management process, delivery system, community health resources, and benefit coverage so that informed decisions can be made by all parties

Negotiator: negotiates the plan of care, services, and payment arrangements with providers; uses effective collaboration and team strategies

Monitor/reporter: provides information to parties on status of member and situations affecting patient safety, care quality, and patient outcome and on factors that alter costs and liability

Patient advocate: acts as advocate, provides information, and supports benefit changes that assist member, family, primary care provider, and capitated systems

Standardization monitor: formulates and monitors specific, time-sequenced critical path and CareMap (see text) plans that guide the type and timing of care to comply with predicted treatment outcomes for specific client and conditions; attempts to reduce variation in resource use and target deviations from standards so adjustments can occur in a timely manner

2. Conversance in language and terminology (able to understand and explain to others in simple terms)
3. Assertiveness and diplomacy with people at all levels
4. The ability to assess situations objectively to determine the appropriateness of case management

Table 19-1 The Nursing Process and Case Management

Nursing process	Case management process	Activities
Assessment	Case finding; identification of incentives for the target population; screening and intake; determination of eligibility; assessment	Develop networks with target population; disseminate written materials; seek referrals; apply screening tools according to program goals and objectives; use written and on-site screens; apply comprehensive assessment methods (physical, social, emotional, cognitive, economic, and self-care capacity); perform interdisciplinary, family, and client conferences.
Diagnosis	Identification of the problem	Determine conclusion based on assessment; use interdisciplinary team.
Planning/outcome	Problem prioritizing; planning to address care needs	Validate and prioritize problems with all participants; develop activities, timeframes, and options; gain client's consent to implement; have client choose options.
Implementation	Advocation of clients' interests; arrangement of delivery of service; monitoring of clients during service	Contact providers; negotiate services and price; coordinate service delivery; monitor for changes in client or service status.
Evaluation	Reassessment	Examine outcomes against goals; examine needs against service; examine costs; examine satisfaction of client, providers, and case manager.

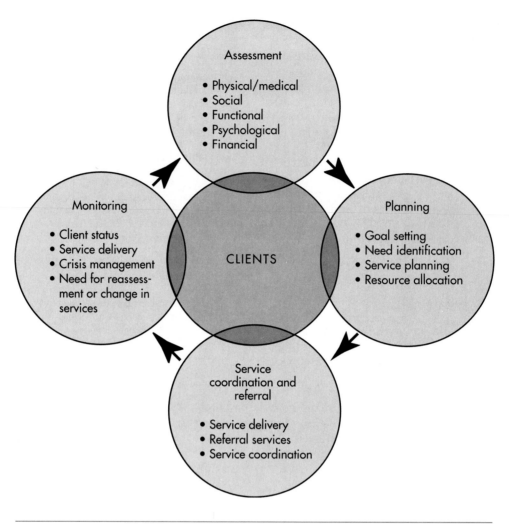

FIGURE 19-1

Core components of case management. (From Secord LJ: *Private case management for older persons and their families,* Excelsior, Minn, 1987, Interstudy).

5. Knowledge of available resources and the strengths and weaknesses of each
6. The ability to act as advocate for the client and payer in models relying on third-party payment
7. The ability to act as a counselor to clients in providing support, understanding, information, and intervention

Likewise, Coleman and Hagen (1991) have described the roles that case managers assume in the practice setting (see box on p. 359). The roles demanded of the community health nurse as case manager are vividly influenced by the forces that support or detract from the feasibility and creativity of possible solutions. Figure 19-2 presents factors that demand the attention of both the nurse and the client during the case management process.

Knowledge and Skill Requisites

Adoption of the case management role for community health nurses does not happen automatically with position. Knowledge and skills that are developed and

refined are essential to successful role implementation. Bower (1992) suggests knowledge domains useful for nurses and systems desiring to implement quality case management roles (see box on p. 361).

If a community health nurse seeks a case manager position, some of the skills and knowledge areas will need to be procured through orientation and mentoring experiences. Curriculum development in basic nursing education may need to be reevaluated for these knowledge requisites and practical experiences in case management.

Tools of Technology

Earlier, the five "rights" of case management were discussed: right care, time, provider, setting, and price. How does the community health nurse judge the effectiveness of case management? Case management plans have evolved through various names and methods (e.g., critical paths, critical pathways, CareMaps, multidisciplinary action plans, nursing care plans). Regardless of the title given, standards of patient care

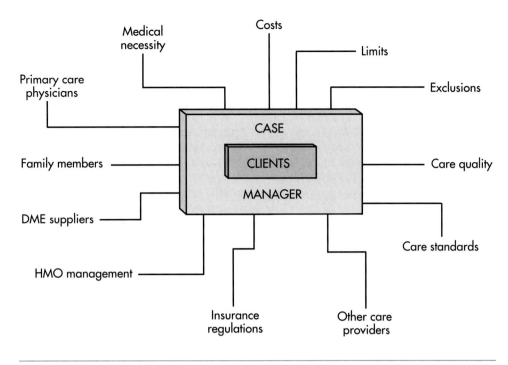

FIGURE 19-2

Forces affecting solutions in the case management process. (From Hicks LL, Stallmeyer JM, Coleman JR: *The role of the nurse in managed care,* Washington, DC, 1993, American Nurses Publishing.)

and standards of nursing practice serve as a core foundation of case management plans. Likewise, in multidisciplinary action plans, core professional standards of each discipline guide the development of the standardization process.

In 1985 the New England Medical Center in Boston instituted a system of critical path development to guide the case management process in the acute care

Knowledge Domains for Case Management

Knowledge of health care financial environment and the financial dimension of client populations that nurses manage

Clinical knowledge, skill, and maturity to direct quality-induced timing and sequencing of care activities

Care resources for clients within institutions and communities: facilitating the development of new resources and systems to meet clients' needs

Discharge planning for ideal timing and sequencing of care

Management skills: communication, delegation, persuasion, use of power, consultation, problem solving, conflict management, confrontation, negotiation, and management of change, marketing, group development, accountability, authority, advocacy, ethical decision making, and profit management

Teaching, counseling, and education skills

Program evaluation and research

Quality improvement techniques

Peer consultation and evaluation

Requirements of eligibility and benefit parameters by third-party payers

Legal issues

setting. A **critical path** is a case management tool composed of abbreviated versions of discipline-specific processes; it is used to achieve a measurable outcome for a specific client "case" (Zander et al., 1987). The critical path shows the key "incidents" that must be achieved in a timely manner to produce an appropriate length of stay. In the New England model, key incidents included consults, tests, activities, treatments, medication, diet, discharge planning, and teaching. The paths note the variances produced by clients. However, these are not revised unless a body of evidence is amassed to adjust the expected actions. CareMaps became the second generation of critical pathways of care that expanded beyond the activities. As described by Zander (1994), A CareMaps tool is a "cause-and-effect grid which identifies expected patient/family and staff behaviors against a timeline for a case-type or otherwise defined homogeneous population" (p. 4). The four components of the CareMaps tool are (1) index of problems with intermediate and outcome criteria, (2) timeline, (3) critical path, and (4) variance record. *Outcome* criteria are the measurable ends to be achieved based on the problems presented by the client's condition of health or illness. *Intermediate criteria* are incremental incidents of measure that serve to monitor progress toward outcomes. *Timelines* are landmarks of an episode of health or illness care from initial encounter to transfer of accountability. Timelines with standard nursing (and other disciplines) diagnoses and outcomes constitute the map. The timeline plan can be in hours, days, weeks, or months. *Variance* is the difference between what is expected and what is occurring with the client. Cohen and Cesta (1993) describe variances as *operational* (broken equipment, staffing mix, delays, lost documentation), health care *provider* (variance in provider practice, level of expertise/experience), *patient (client)* (refusal, nonavailability, change in status), and *unmet clinical quality* indicators. Variance data are useful in understanding why expected client outcomes and indicators have not been met. These data serve as an evaluation element that can be monitored for adjusting plans to clients' needs when flexibility is crucial or for establishing new CareMaps on contemporary changes in data.

The adaptation of the case management care plan process for community health nurses is a crucial skill for standardizing the process and outcome of care. It links multiple provider interventions to client responses and offers reasonable predictions for clients. Institutions report that sharing of case management plans with clients empowers them to assume responsibility for monitoring and adhering to the plan of care. Self-responsibility by clients truly incorporates autonomy and self-determination as the core of case management. As a community health nurse employed to function as a case manager, ample opportunity exists to develop, test, and revise CareMap prototypes for a target population experiencing health deficits.

Public Health and Community-based Models

Carondelet St. Mary's, in Tucson, Ariz., has developed a community nursing network (CNN) in which 15,000 enrollees are distributed among 17 community health centers. Professional nurse case managers assist older clients to attain healthier life-styles and maintain themselves in the community. Nurses have been successful in delivering services at a cost of less than $5 per month per Medicare enrollee. Through nurse case management services, this nursing health maintenance organization (HMO) has cut the number of inpatient days per 1000 enrollees by one-third at an average cost of $900 per day and a savings of $300,000 for every 1000 enrollees (ANA 1993; American Nurses Foundation [ANF], 1993).

Community-based statewide programs in New Jersey use case management methodologies to promote early identification, selection, evaluation, diagnosis, and treatment of children with potentially physically compromised needs. Local case management units provide coordinated and comprehensive care. Collaboration with existing local and regional agencies serving children supports this process. The nurse case manager (1) provides counseling and education to parents and children on problem identification and knowledge level, (2) develops individualized plans incorporating multidisciplinary services (education, social, medical development, rehabilitation), (3) procures appropriate community services, (4) acts as a family resource in crises and service concerns, (5) fa-

cilitates communication between child and family, and (6) monitors services for outcomes. Interdisciplinary teams include public health nurses and master's-prepared social workers for larger caseloads. A recommended caseload is 300 to 350 children per case manager (Bower, 1992).

The case management program for persons with acquired immunodeficiency syndrome (AIDS) pioneered at San Francisco General Hospital focuses on the support of community-based, out-patient services to reduce dependency on unnecessary and more costly services. It follows the public health model of minimizing hospitalizations and length of stay, utilizing community-based services, and brokering among a strong network of community services: housing, home, hospice delivery, and respite care. The San Francisco Department of Public Health used its positive reputation with the gay community to plan, develop, and evaluate care (Bower, 1992; Foster and Hall, 1986).

Liberty Mutual Insurance Company has used case management principles for more than 30 years in workers' compensation and has expanded services for employees whose conditions were noted as chronic or catastrophic. (See box below for examples of case-managed conditions.) Case managers coordinate all parties and services to reduce excessive expenses caused by lack of coordination, failure to use efficacious alternatives, duplication, and fragmentation (Bower, 1992).

Important guidance in developing a community-based case management program is found in the United States. Case management is a key component of federally financed and many state-financed delivery systems. The experiences of states over the past two decades provides testimony to the importance of case management for populations at risk. For older clients, state-derived case management provides objective advice and assistance with care needs and provides access to multidisciplinary providers and services. For payers (federal, state, clients), case management serves as a vehicle to ensure that funds are

 Examples of Case-managed Conditions

High-risk neonates
Severe head trauma
Spinal cord injury
Ventilator dependency
Coma
Multiple fractures
Acquired immunodeficiency syndrome (AIDS)
Severe burns
Cerebrovascular accident (CVA)
Amputations
Terminal illness
Substance abuse

allocated appropriately to those in greatest need. Case management serves a policy assurance and accountability function for communities. Within the states, the types of agencies designated to conduct case management are typified by district offices of state government, area agencies on aging, and county social services departments. States maintain the oversight responsibilities for case management agencies to (1) ensure compliance with program standards, contracts, reporting, and fiscal controls; (2) identify emerging problems and issues to be rectified by additional state policies; and (3) provide on-site technical assistance and consultation to improve performance. States' payment methods for case management include daily/monthly rates, hourly/quarterly rates, capped rates for services, and capped aggregate allocation to

 Research Brief

Erkel EA, Morgan EP, Staples MA, Assey VH, Michel Y: Case management and preventive services among infants from low-income families, *Public Health Nurs* 11(5):352-360, 1994.

An experimental approach to case management was tested to discover the use of child health clinic and immunization services by 98 Medicaid infants from low-income families. The experimental case management condition consisted of a single public health nurse (PHN) providing both case management and preventive child health services. The control condition consisted of multiple nurse providers of child health services to an infant and the segregation of case management delivery from child health services delivery.

Data were collected from health department clinical records to document the PHN interventions, child health clinic visits, immunizations, and demograhics. The health districts' protocols for case management of Medicaid infants and child preventive services were followed for the experimental and control groups. However, the infants in the experimental group received "continuous care" by one PHN, whereas the control-group infants received care from multiple PHN providers, or "fragmented care."

Differences between the preventive services obtained by infants receiving the two approaches were significant, although the study sample immunization rate of 62% is considerably below the national objective of 90% for 2-year-old children by the year 2000 (*Healthy People* 2000, 1991). Implications for nursing practice follow:

1. Case management delivery by a consistent provider who incorporates case management, delivery of preventive services, and home health visits can result in greater utilization of age-appropriate services by infants and their families.
2. The use of a consistent (singular) case manager can result in fewer nursing efforts (follow-up contacts) required to achieve adequacy of child preventive services.

cover both case management and provider costs (Congressional Research Service, 1993).

These models offer one solution to unnecessary health care expenditures; an estimated one-third of all health care ($2 billion in costs) administered in the United States is not needed (Lashley, 1993). Case management offers a method to reduce costs and access appropriate health care services. Imagine the impact on health status if these saved resources were shifted to primary prevention and health promotion activities.

◆ Advocacy, Conflict Management, and Collaboration Skills for Case Managers

Now that we have examined the concept, scope, role, and functions of case management and case managers, we can turn our attention to three specific skills essential to the role performance of the case manager: advocacy, conflict management, and collaboration.

ADVOCACY

For community health nurses, **advocacy** involves diverse activities, ranging from self-exploration to lobbying for health policy. Advocacy is essential for practice with clients and their families, communities, organizations, and colleagues on an interdisciplinary team. The functions of advocacy require scientific knowledge, expert communication, facilitation skills, and problem-solving and affirmation techniques. As the *Code of Nurses* (ANA, 1985) states, ". . . the goal of nursing actions is to support and enhance the client's responsibility and self-determination" (p. i). However, this goal is a contemporary one. As Nelson (1988) indicates, the perspective regarding the advocacy function has shifted through time. The nurse advocate has been described in earlier writings as one who acted on behalf of or interceded for the client. An example of the **intercessor** role is the community health nurse who calls for a well-child appointment for a mother visiting the family planning clinic when the mother is capable of making an appointment on her own.

The evolution of the advocate role to that of **mediator** by the nurse advocate is described as a response to the complex configuration of social change, reimbursers, and providers in the health care system (Winslow, 1984). Mediation is an activity in which a third party attempts to provide assistance to those who may be experiencing a conflict in obtaining what they desire. The goal of the nurse advocate as mediator is to assist parties to understand each other on many levels so that agreement on an action is possible. In the instance of a nurse as case manager for an HMO, mediation activities between an elderly client and the payer (HMO) could accomplish the following results: the client may understand the options for community-based skilled nursing care, and the payer may understand the client's desires for a less restrictive environment for care. Although the case manager as mediator does not *decide* the plan of action (in contrast to the role of arbitrator), he or she facilitates the decision-making processes between the parties so that the desired care can be reimbursed within the continuum of options.

In contemporary practice the nurse advocate places the client's rights as the focus of priority. The goal of **promoter** for the client's autonomy and self-determination may result in an optimal degree of independence in decision making. For example, when a group of young pregnant women is the collective "client," the nurse advocate's role may be to inform the group of the benefits and consequences of breast-feeding their infants. However, if the new mothers decide on formula feeding, the nurse advocate should support the group and continue to provide parenting, infant, and well-child services.

This proposition shows a different perspective of the nurse as advocate. It holds that the nurse's role as advocate may demand a variety of functions that are influenced by the client's physical, psychological, social, and environmental abilities. The nurse adapts the advocacy function to the client's dynamic capabilities as the client follows a trajectory of health states. Even clients who desire access to more substantial health promotion activities can benefit from a partnership with the nurse advocate. Examples of advocacy in such cases might include promoting a client group's access to on-site physical fitness programs in the occupational setting or supporting parents' and students' concerns about the high fat content of vending machine cuisine in the school system. With the cost of health care expected to exceed a trillion dollars annually before the year 2000 and consumers assuming a larger financial portion of the care they choose, the promoter role of advocacy for those clients capable of autonomy is expected to intensify.

Process of Advocacy

The goal of advocacy is to promote self-determination in a **constituency.** The constituency may be a client, family, peer, group, or community. The process of advocacy was defined by Kohnke (1982) to include informing and supporting; affirming is the third essential part of advocacy. All three activities are more complex than they may initially seem, and they require self-reflection by the nurse as well as skill development as the process unfolds. It is often easier for the nurse to inform, support, and affirm another person's decision when it is congruent with the nurse's values. When clients make decisions within their value systems that run counter to the nurse's values, however, the advocate may feel conflict in contributing to the process of informing, supporting, and affirming those decisions. Promoting self-determination in others demands a philosophy of free choice once the information necessary for decision making has been discussed.

Informing

Knowledge is essential, but not sufficient, to the outcome of decision making. The interpretation of knowledge is tempered by the client's values and meanings assigned to it. The interpretation of facts is the result of both objective and subjective processing of information. Subjective dimensions greatly influence client decisions.

Informing clients about the nature of their choices, the content of those choices, and the consequences to the client is not a one-way activity. The information exchange process is composed of interactions that reflect three subprocesses: amplification, clarification, and verification. **Amplification** occurs between the nurse and client to assess the needs and demands that will eventually frame the client's decision. Information is exchanged from both viewpoints. Although the exchange may be initiated at the objective, factual level, it will likely proceed to incorporate the subjective perspectives of both parties.

The information exchanged between the parties is important to consider. Guidelines include the nurse's need to do the following:

1. Assess the client's present understanding of the situation.
2. Provide correct information.
3. Communicate with the client's literacy level in mind, making the information as understandable as possible.
4. Utilize a variety of media and sources to increase the client's comprehension.
5. Discuss other factors that affect the decision, such as financial, legal, and ethical issues.
6. Discuss the possible consequences of a decision.

The tone of the amplification process can direct the remainder of the informational exchange. It is important to relate with clients in a manner that reflects the advocate's endorsement of their self-determination. Setting aside the time necessary to listen to clients is critical. Clients will sense they are part of a mutual process if the nurse can engage them during the information exchange with a message that says, "I respect your needs and desires as I share my knowledge with you." Nonverbal behaviors, including using direct eye contact, sitting at the client's level, arriving and concluding at a prescribed time, and employing verbal patterns that foster exchange (open-ended statements, questions, probes, reflections of feelings, paraphrasing), convey the interactive promotion of self-determination.

A client may not desire the exchange of information because of lack of self-esteem, fear of the information, or inability to comprehend the content of the communication. In such a case, the focus is to understand the client's desire for no information and to express to the client the consequences of such inaction. The nurse may invite the client to ask for the information exchange at a later time, when the client is ready, and can intermittently check with the client whether information exchange and amplification is desired. In these cases the nurse should document the implemented nursing actions to reflect the guidelines just discussed. This can reduce the basis for litigation and misunderstanding by other parties.

Clarification is a process in which the nurse and client strive to understand meanings in a common way. Clarification builds on the breadth and depth of the exchange developed in amplification to determine if the parties understand each other. During this process, misunderstandings and confusions are examined. The goal of clarification is to avoid confusion between the parties. To foster clarification, nurses can use certain verbal prompts:

"What do you understand about . . . ?"

"Please tell me more about how you . . . ."

"I don't think I am clear. Let me explain the situation in another way . . . . As an example . . . ."

"What other information would be helpful so that we both understand?"

Verification is the process used by the nurse advocate to establish accuracy and reality in the informing process. If the nurse discovers that a client is misinformed, the nurse may return to the clarification or amplification stage and begin the process again. Verification produces the chance for the advocate and client to examine "truth" from their perspectives, which may include knowledge, intuition, previous experiences, and anticipated consequences.

In reality, promoting a client's self-determination may take the advocate and client through the information exchange process several times as new dimensions or obstacles to an issue develop. Information exchange is a critical process for advocacy and is applicable to all advocacy constituents: individuals, families, groups, and communities.

Supporting

The second major process, **supporting,** involves upholding a client's right to make a choice and to act on the choice. People who become aware of clients' decisions fall into three general groups: supporters, dissenters, and obstructors. *Supporters* approve and support clients' actions. *Dissenters* do not approve and do not support clients. *Obstructors* cause difficulties while clients try to implement their decisions.

Kohnke (1982) points to the need for the nurse advocate to implement several actions that fulfill the supporting role. Assuring clients that they have the right and responsibility to make decisions and reassuring them that they do not have to change their decisions because of others' objections are important interventions.

Affirming

The third process in the advocacy role is **affirming.** It is based on an advocate's belief that a client's decision is consistent with the client's values and goals. The advocate validates that the client's behavior is purposeful and consistent with the choice that was made. The advocate expresses a dedication to the client's mission,

Table 19-2	Nursing Process and Advocacy Process
Nursing process	**Advocacy process**

Assessment/diagnosis	Information exchange
	  Gather data
	  Illuminate values

Planning/outcome	Generate alternatives and consequences
	Prioritize actions
Implementation	Decision making

	Support of client
	  Assure
	  Reassure

Evaluation	Affirmation
	  Evaluation
	  Reformulation

Communication that seeks to amplify, clarify, and verify knowledge, beliefs, and behaviors is used throughout both processes.

and a purposeful exchange of new information may occur so the client's choice remains viable. Recognizing that a client's needs may fluctuate with changing resources, the affirmation activity must encourage a process of reevaluation and rededication to promote self-determination.

The importance of affirmation activities cannot be emphasized strongly enough. Many advocacy activities stop with assuring and reassuring, but affirmation is often critical in promoting a client's self-determination. Table 19-2 compares the nursing process with the advocacy process.

The advocate's role in the decision-making process is not to tell the client which option is "correct" or "right." The advocate's role is to provide the opportunity for information exchange, arming clients with tools that can empower them in making the best decision from their perspective. Enabling the client to make an "informed decision" is a powerful tool for building self-confidence. It gives the client the responsibility for selecting the options and experiencing the success and consequences based on current data.

Clients are empowered in their decision making when they can recognize events that are beyond their control and can link chance occurrences with predictable events to make decisions they want. Sophisticated decision analysis techniques are beyond the scope of this book. Most involve mathematical calculations based on assigned values and are grounded in operation research literature.

Nurses can promote client decision making by using the information exchange process, promoting use of the nursing process, incorporating written techniques (contracts, lists), employing reflection and prioritization, and using role playing and sculpturing to "try on" and determine the "fit" of different options and consequences for the client. By engaging clients in the information-sharing process and   assisting them to recognize the progression of activities they experience as they build their "informed decision-making base," the nurse advocate is empowering clients with skills that can strengthen their autonomy and confidence in the future.

Advocacy is a comple.; process. The balance between "doing for" and "promoting autonomy" can be precarious and is influenced by the client's physical, emotional, and social capabilities. The goal of advocacy is to promote the ultimate degree of self-determination possible for the client given the client's current and potential status; for most clients, this goal can be realized.

When clients are comatose, unborn, or legally incompetent, nurse advocates have unique functions. The advocate's role is usually determined by the legal system; however, in some cases nurses must decide what roles they will play. These are areas requiring intensive self-exploration, research, and collaboration with professionals, family members, and significant others.

Skill Development

Skills needed by the nurse advocate are not unique to their profession. Nursing demands technical, relational, and problem-solving skills. Advocacy requires applying nursing skills to promote self-determination. However, several other skills are necessary and well defined.

Advocates must be open minded and aware of people, society, and social order (Kohnke, 1982). Knowledge of nursing and knowledge from other disciplines is essential for the advocacy role in establishing authority and developing skills. Highly developed communication skills and a strong sense of self-esteem and professional confidence are also needed (Webb, 1987). The capacity for assertiveness for personal rights and the rights of others is essential.

Systematic Problem Solving

The nursing process—assessment, diagnosis, planning, implementation, and evaluation of a problem—constitutes an example of a method of **problem solving** that can be used in the advocacy role. Advocates can be particularly helpful with clients in illuminating values and generating alternatives.

Illuminating Values

People's values affect their behavior, feelings, and goals. In the process of amplification, clarification, and validation, the advocate understands a client's values. Through the process of self-revelation, an emerging value (environment, people, cost, quality) may become more apparent to a client. This can have an im-

pact in two ways. The client may be able to focus on actions consistent with the value, or the value may lend confusion and assist the client in prioritizing action. Values can also change as new or relevant data are processed. The advocate's role is to assist clients in discovering their values, which can be particularly demanding in the information exchange and affirmation process.

Generating Alternatives

Clients and advocates may feel limited in their options if they generate solutions before completely analyzing the problems, needs, desires, and consequences. Several techniques can be used to generate alternatives, including brainstorming and a technique known as the problem-purpose-expansion method. In *brainstorming* the nurse, client, professionals, or significant others generate as many alternatives as possible, without critical evaluation. Brainstorming creates a list that can subsequently be examined for the critical elements the client seeks to preserve (e.g., environmental preferences, degree of control). The list can be analyzed according to the consequences, the probability of chance events occurring, and the effect of the alternatives on self and others.

The *problem-purpose-expansion method* is a way to broaden limited thinking (Volkema, 1983). It involves restating the problem and expanding the problem statement so that different solutions can be generated. For example, if the problem statement is to convince the insurance company to approve a longer hospital stay, the nurse and client have narrowed their options. However, if the problem statement is to make the client's convalescence as optimal and safe as possible, several solutions and options are available, such as the following:

Obtaining extended care institutional placement
Obtaining home health skilled services
Arranging physician home visits
Paying for custodial care
Paying for private skilled care
Obtaining informal caregiving

Impact of Advocacy

Advocacy empowers clients to participate in problem-solving processes and decisions about health care. Clients try to understand changing opportunities in the health care system for access, utilization, and continuity of care while nurse advocates promote client control of morale, life satisfaction, self-esteem, and adherence to therapeutic regimens (Kohler, 1988). Clients are part of larger systems: the family, the work environment, and the community. Each system interacts with the client to shape the available options through resources, needs, and desires. Each system also exhibits both confirming and conflicting goals and processes that need to be understood for client self-determination to be successful. For example, the practice of advocacy among minority groups may entail the ability to focus attention on the magnitude of problems caused by diseases affecting minority clients. Whether the client is an individual, family, group, or community, the advocacy function can promote the interest of self-determination that characterizes progressive societies.

Advocacy is not without opposition. Clients and advocates may find barriers to services, vendors, providers, and resources. A community may experience a shortage in nursing home beds, a child care facility may experience staffing shortages, a family may not have the financial resources to keep a child at home, and a client may find that the school system cannot fund a full-time nurse for its clinic. The reality of scarce resources constitutes a difficult barrier for advocates. However, it is often events such as these that stimulate a community's self-determination and innovative actions to correct gaps in service.

CONFLICT MANAGEMENT

Case managers help clients to manage conflicting needs and scarce resources. Techniques for managing conflict encompass the range of active communication skills. These skills are directed toward learning all parties' needs and desires, detecting their areas of agreement and disagreement, determining their abilities to collaborate, and assisting in discovering alternatives and valuable activities for reaching a goal. Mutual benefit with limited loss is a goal of conflict management.

Conflict and its management vary in intensity and energy in a number of ways. The effort needed to manage a conflict depends on different factors: the existence of evidence to support facts and objective/subjective perceptions of the parties involved.

Negotiating is a strategic process used to move conflicting parties toward an outcome. The outcome can vary from one in which one party enlarges its share at the other's expense *(distributive outcomes)* to one in which mutual advantages override individual gains *(integrative outcomes)*. Integrative outcomes are usually based on problem-solving and solution-generating techniques (Bisno, 1988).

The process of negotiation can be characterized in three stages: prenegotiation, negotiation, and aftermath. *Prenegotiations* are activities designed to have parties agree to collaborate. Parties must see the possibility of achieving an agreement and the costs of not achieving an agreement. Preparations must be made as to time, place, and ground rules concerning participants, procedures, and confidentiality.

The *negotiation* stage consists of phases in which parties must develop trust, credibility, distance from the issue (to limit the feeling of "one best way"), and the ability to retain personal dignity. Bisno (1988) characterizes the phases as the following:

Phase 1: Establishing the issues and agenda. This is accomplished by identifying, clarifying, presenting, and prioritizing the issues.

Phase 2: Advancing demands and uncovering interests. Negotiations center around presenting parties' interests and differentiating parties' demands and positions.

Phase 3: Bargaining and discovering new options. *Debates* include gathering facts based on reasoning that will generate understanding and promote relearning. *Bargaining* reduces differences on issues by giving or removing rewards or desired objects. Creating new solutions or options through brainstorming, reflective thinking, and problem-purpose-expansion techniques is important in achieving options that provide mutual benefits.

Phase 4: Working out an agreement. This may involve settling on some but not all points. Parties can agree to reexamine the issues later, and steps for implementation and follow-up must be clarified.

The *aftermath* is the period following an agreement in which parties are experiencing the consequences of their decisions. The reality of their decisions may lead to a reevaluation of their values.

Thomas and Kilmann (1974) postulate that in a conflict situation parties engage in behaviors that reflect the dimensions of assertiveness and cooperation. Assertiveness is the ability to present one's own needs. Cooperation is the ability to understand and meet the needs of others. Each person uses a predominant orientation and secondary orientation to engage in conflict (see box below). The importance of the Thomas-Kilmann categories is that one can use a repertoire of orientations and that each orientation can be valuable in a given situation.

Clearly, flexibility in conflict management behavior can facilitate an outcome that meets the client's goals. Helping parties to navigate the process of goal attainment requires effective personal relations, knowledge of the situation and alternatives, and a commitment to the process.

 Categories of Behaviors Used in Conflict Management

Competing	An individual pursues personal concerns at another's expense.
Accommodating	An individual neglects personal concerns to satisfy the concerns of another.
Avoiding	An individual pursues *neither* his or her concerns nor another's concerns.
Collaborating	An individual attempts to work with others toward solutions that satisfy the work of both parties.
Compromising	An individual attempts to find a mutually acceptable solution that partially satisfies both parties.

Modified from Thomas KW, Kilmann RH: *Thomas-Kilmann Conflict Mode Instrument,* New York, 1974, Xicom.

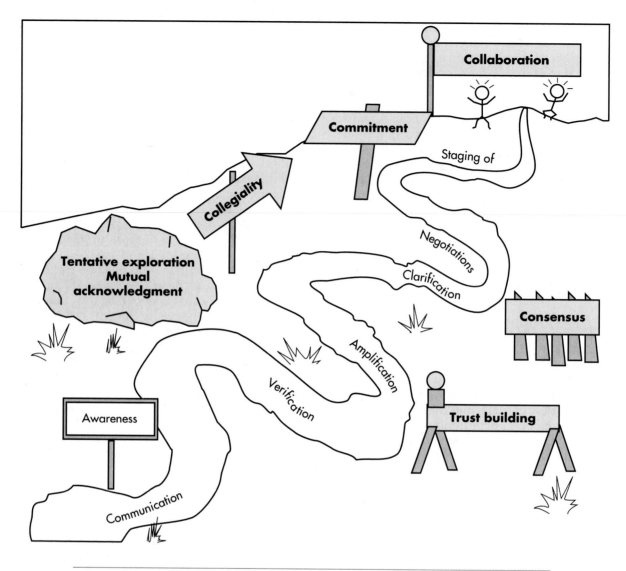

FIGURE 19-3

Collaboration is a sequential yet reciprocal process. (From Cary AH, Androwich I: Paper presented at the Association of Community Health Nursing Educators Spring Institute, Seattle, June 1989.)

COLLABORATION

In case management the activities of many disciplines are needed for success. Clients, the family, significant others, payers, and community organizations contribute to achieving the goal. **Collaboration** is achieved through a developmental process. It is sequential yet reciprocal (Cary and Androwich, 1989) and can be characterized by seven stages and activities (Figure 19-3).

The goal of communication in the collaborative development process is to promote amplification, clarification, and verification of all team members' perspectives. Although communication is an essential component in collaboration, it is not sufficient to result in or maintain collaboration. Although the collaboration model recognizes the contributions inherent in joint decision making, one member of the team should be accountable to the system and the client and should be responsible for monitoring the entire process.

Case managers are uniquely positioned to encounter conflict on a daily basis. Competing needs, resources, organizational demands, and professional role boundaries among resources present opportunities and pitfalls for conflict management and collaboration (see box on p. 369).

Teamwork and collaboration clearly demand knowledge and skills about clients, health status, resources, treatments, and community providers. The ability to assess clients' and families' complex needs encompasses knowledge of intrapersonal, interpersonal, medical, nursing, and social dimensions. The demonstration of team member and leadership skills in facilitating a goal-directed group process is essential. It is unlikely that any single professional possesses

Stages of Collaboration

AWARENESS

Make a conscious entry into a group process; focus on goals of convening together; generate definition of collaborative process and what it means to team members.

TENTATIVE EXPLORATION AND MUTUAL ACKNOWLEDGMENT

Exploration

Disclose professional skills for the desired process; disclose areas where contributions cannot be made; disclose values reflecting priorities: identify roles and disclose personal values, including time, energy, interest, and resources.

Mutual Acknowledgment

Clarify each member's potential contributions; verify the group's strengths and areas needing consultation; clarify member's work style, organizational supports, and barriers to collaborative efforts.

TRUST BUILDING

Determine the degree to which reliance on others can be achieved; examine congruence between words and behaviors; set interdependent goals; develop tolerance for ambiguity.

COLLEGIALITY

Define the relationships of members with each other; define the responsibilities and tasks of each; define entrance and exit conditions.

CONSENSUS

Determine the issues for which consensus is required; determine the process used for clarifying and decision making to reach consensus; determine the process for reevaluating consensus outcomes.

COMMITMENT

Realize the physical, emotional, and material actions directed toward the goal; clarify procedures for reevaluating commitments in light of goal demands and group standards for deviance.

COLLABORATION

Initiate a process of joint decision making reflecting the synergy that results from combining knowledge and skills.

Modified from Cary A, Androwich I: Paper presented at the Association of Communty Health Nursing Educators Spring Institute, Seattle, June 1989; and Mueller WJ, Kell B: *Coping with conflict*, Englewood Cliffs, NJ, 1972, Prentice Hall.

the expertise required in all dimensions. It is likely, however, that the synergy produced by all can result in successful outcomes.

ISSUES IN CASE MANAGEMENT

Legal Issues

Liability concerns of case managers exist when three conditions are met: (1) the provider had a duty to provide reasonable care, (2) a breach occurred through act or omission to act, and (3) the act or omission caused injury or damage to the client. Case managers must strive to diminish risks, practice wisely within acceptable standards, and limit legal defense costs through professional insurance coverage. Five general areas of risk are reviewed:

Liability for managing care (Hinden et al., 1994)

1. Inappropriate design or implementation of the case management system
2. Failure to obtain all pertinent records on which case management actions are based
3. Failure to have cases evaluated by appropriately experienced and credentialed clinicians
4. Failure to confer directly with the treating provider at the onset and throughout the client's care
5. Substituting a case manager's clinical judgment for that of the medical provider
6. Requiring the client or his or her provider to ac-

cept case management recommendation instead of any other treatment
7. Harassment of clinicians, clients, and family in seeking information and setting unreasonable deadlines for decisions or information
8. Claiming orally or in writing that the case management treatment plan is better than the provider's plan
9. Restricting access to otherwise necessary or appropriate care because of cost
10. Referring clients to treatment furnished by providers related to the case management entity without proper disclosure
11. Connecting case managers' compensation to reduced utilization and access

Negligent referrals (Hyatt, 1994)

1. Referral to a practitioner known to be incompetent
2. Substituting inadequate treatment for an adequate but more costly option
3. Curtailing treatment inappropriately when curtailment was substantial related to the injury
4. Referral to a facility or practitioner inappropriate for the client's needs

Experimental treatment and technology (Saue, 1994)

1. Failure to apply the contractual definition of "experimental" treatment found in the client's insurance policy
2. Failure to review sources of information referenced in the applicable insurance policy (e.g., Food and

Drug Administration [FDA] determination, published medical literature)

3. Failure to review the client's complete medical record
4. Failure to make a timely determination of benefits in light of timeliness of treatment
5. Failure to communicate coverage determination to the insured client or participant
6. Improper economic considerations determining the coverage

Confidentiality (Scheutzow, 1994)

1. Failure to deny access to sensitive information that is awarded special protection by state statute
2. Failure to protect access allowances to computerized medical records

Fraud and abuse (Sollins, 1994)

1. Making false statements of claims or causing incorrect claims to be filed
2. Falsifying adherence to *conditions of participation* of Medicare and Medicaid
3. Submitting claims for excessive, unnecessary, or poor quality services
4. Engaging in remuneration, bribes, kickbacks, or rebates in exchange for referral

Since 1986, 15 legal citings have been relevant to case management and managed care. Negligent referrals, provider liability, payer liability, breach of contract, and bad faith were the legal issues in these cases. As in any scope of nursing practice, proactive risk management strategies can lower the provider's exposure to legal liability.

Saue (1989) notes that court cases influence the legal considerations of case managers. When courts find that cost considerations affect medical care decisions, all parties to the decision will be liable for resulting damages. Guidelines to reduce risk exposure include the following:

1. Clear documentation of the extent of participation in decision making and reasons for decisions
2. Records demonstrating accurate and complete information on interactions and outcomes
3. Use of reasonable care in selecting referral sources, which may include verification of licensure of providers
4. Written agreements when arrangements are made to modify benefits other than those in the contract
5. Good communication with clients
6. Informing clients of their rights of appeal

Did You Know?

Family caregivers may be poorly prepared to assume high-technology care of the client at home. They often receive inadequate information about the client's illness trajectory, likely burdens and benefits of caregiving, and the complex and technical details of a plan of treatment.

Ethical Issues

Case managers as nursing professionals are guided in ethical practice by the *Professional Nursing Code of Ethics* (1985) and the contract expressed in the draft of the *Nursing Social Policy Statement* (ANA, 1995, p. 4):

Nursing is a caring-based practice in which processes of diagnosis and treatment are applied to the human experiences of health and illness. Nurses are guided by a philosophy of caring and advocacy. Nurses have a high regard for patient self-determination, independence and informed choice in decision making. Recognizing that responses to illness and disability may limit independence and self-determination, nurses focus on the rights of individuals, families and communities to define their own health-related goals and seek out health care that reflects their values.

This contractual philosophy of nursing practice is ideally suited to preserving the principles of autonomy, beneficence, and justice in case management processes. Banja (1994) describes how case managers may confront dilemmas in each of these areas.

Case management may hamper a client's **autonomy** of individual right to choose a provider if a particular provider is not approved by the case management system. If a new provider must be found who can be approved for coverage, continuity of care may be disrupted.

Beneficence can be influenced when excessive attention to cost containment supersedes or impairs the nurse's duty to provide measures to improve health or relieve suffering. "If cost containment goals are accomplished by diminishing services, at what point do health providers' behaviors subordinate the good of their (clients) to the interests of restraining expenditures?" (Banja, 1994 p. 39).

Justice as an ethical principle for case managers considers equitable distribution of health care with reasonable quality. Tiers of quality and expertise among provider groups can be created when quality providers refuse to accept reimbursement allowances from the managed system, leaving less experienced or lower-quality providers as the caregiver of choice for clients being managed.

The National Council on Aging (1987) reminds case managers of the client's rights in case management services:

1. Fair and comprehensive assessment of health, functional, psychosocial, and cognitive abilities
2. Right to access for needed health and social services
3. Right to be treated with respect and dignity
4. Opportunity to participate in developing a plan of services, preserving self-determination, and providing privacy and confidentiality
5. Right to know the cost of services before delivery
6. Right to be notified of any adjustment in service
7. Right to "deselect" from the case management program and service
8. Right to a grievance procedure if the client believes his or her rights have been violated in any manner

Standards of practice and care, codes of ethics, licensure laws, and organizational policies and procedures (e.g., ethics committees, risk management units) offer the case manager information and support in managing ethical conflicts and dilemmas in the case management system. Maintaining familiarity with ethical issues published in the case management literature can offer specific assistance for practicing case managers.

 # Clinical Application

The community health nurse from the public health department was conducting her regularly scheduled blood pressure clinic in a local apartment cluster. Mrs. B., a 45-year-old woman, had attended for the last 2 months. During one visit, Mrs. B. complained of feeling dizzy and forgetful. She could not remember which of her six medications she had taken during the last few days. Her blood pressure readings on reclining, sitting, and standing revealed gross elevation. The nurse and Mrs. B. discussed the danger of her present status and the need to seek medical attention. Mrs. B. called her physician from her apartment, and the nurse discussed the data findings with him. Reluctantly, Mrs. B. agreed to meet the physician in the emergency room, and the nurse, with Mrs. B.'s consent, arranged for her transportation.

While in the emergency room, Mrs. B. manifested the progressive signs and symptoms of a cerebrovascular accident (CVA, stroke). After hospitalization, she lost her capacity for expressive language and demonstrated hemiparesis and loss of bladder control. Her cognitive function became intermittently confused, and she was slow to recognize her physician and neighbors who came to visit. The clinic nurse contacted the discharge planner, a nurse from the health department's discharge-planning team contracted to the community hospital. She suggested that Mrs. B. be screened and assessed for care after her hospital stay as early as possible because she lived alone and family members resided out of town.

The discharge planner confirmed the referral and requested a written report from the clinic nurse. Mrs. B. met many of the screening criteria indicating she could benefit from the service. The discharge planner worked with the unit nurses, physician, social workers, speech therapist, physical therapist, client, family members (long distance by phone), the utilization review nurse, the insurance company, and the clinic nurse to determine Mrs. B.'s postdischarge prognosis, the desires that she and her family had for aftercare, and the appropriate reimbursable levels of care options. With the recommendations produced from the interdisciplinary and family conferences and with the client's and family's consent, the discharge planner initiated the referrals for home health care (skilled and supportive services) and Meals-on-Wheels. Family members agreed to come from out of town for 3 weeks to assist in Mrs. B.'s care and assess the adjustment to home supportive care. All supports were in place at the time of the client's discharge, and home health care (registered nurse, aide service) and Meals-on-Wheels were initiated within 6 hours of discharge. Therapies began within 48 hours.

Mrs. B. could be maintained at home with informal and formal caregiving systems in place. However, the situation and level of care were not static. It became apparent that family caregiving could not continue because members lived too far away. Mrs. B. had residual functional and cognitive deficits that would demand longer-term care. The home health agency nurse managing Mrs. B.'s care delivery communicated regularly with the insurance company to convey her status and prognosis. She held interdisciplinary team conferences with service providers and formulated community and institutional options for appropriate levels of care. Mrs. B. and family members were educated, advised, and supported to examine their goals and options and to formulate alternative options for remaining at home. The client and family selected a case management firm to guide them in the selection and access to care that would promote Mrs. B.'s optimal function.

The nurse case manager screened the client for eligibility for the service. A self-pay option augmented the benefit coverage. The case manager worked with the physician, home health nurse, therapists, social worker, client, and family to conduct a comprehensive assessment of current status and predicted prognosis. She presented her findings to the client and family, the home care nurse, and the insurance company. With the client's and family's permission, the case manager negotiated with the insurance company to reimburse for selected community-based services for 6 months as an alternative to institutionalization. She arranged for transportation, adult day care, cognitive stimulation sessions, environmental improvements to accommodate functional status, and an emergency response system device. With the assistance of church volunteers, support and monitoring of instrumental activities of daily living were provided. The original clinic nurse monitored the client's response during her weekly blood pressure clinics. The case manager coordinated, referred, monitored, and evaluated service delivery as related to the client's and family's goal to maintain the client in her residence. At the conclusion of the 6-month contract with the nurse case manager, the client was able to reduce the degree of formal support and assume more direction in her own management so that she could remain in the community. The case manager terminated her services with the client until a further need might be identified.

Key Concepts

- An important role of the community health nurse is that of client advocate.
- The goal of advocacy is to promote the client's self-determination.
- When performing in the advocacy role, conflicts may emerge regarding the full disclosure of information, territoriality, accountability to multiple parties, legal challenges to client's decisions, and competition for scarce resources.
- Amplification, clarification, and verification are three communication skills necessary in the advocacy process.
- Additional skills important in fulfilling the role of client advocate include the helping relationship, assertiveness, and problem solving.
- Problem solving is a systematic approach that includes understanding the values of each party and generating alternative solutions.
- Brainstorming and the problem-purpose-expansion method are two techniques to enhance the effectiveness of problem-solving skills.
- During conflict, negotiations can move conflicting parties toward an outcome.
- Prenegotiation, negotiation, and aftermath are three phases of managing a conflict.
- Each individual has a predominant orientation when engaging in conflict: competing, accommodating, avoiding, collaborating, or compromising.
- Collaboration may result by moving through seven stages: awareness, tentative exploration and mutual acknowledgment, trust building, collegiality, consensus, commitment, and collaboration.
- Continuity of care is a goal of community health nursing practice. It requires making linkages with services to improve the client's health status.
- As the structure of the health care system moves toward delivering more services in the community, the achievement of continuity of care will present a greater challenge.
- Case management is typically an interdisciplinary process in which the client is the focus of the plan.
- Documentation of case management activities and outcomes are essential to community health nursing practice.
- Case management and care management are synonymous terms for the systematic process of assessment, planning, service coordination, referral, and monitoring that meets the multiple service needs of clients.
- Community health nurses have within their scope of practice both advocacy and case management.
- Nurses functioning as advocates and case managers need to be aware of the ethical and legal issues confronting these components of their practice.
- Standardization of care for predictable outcomes can be achieved through critical paths, CareMaps, and multidisciplinary action plans.

Critical Thinking Activities

1. Observe a typical workday of a community health nurse, noting the types of activities that are done in coordination and case management, as well as the amount of time spent in these areas. Interview several staff members to determine whether they perceive that their time spent in case management is changing.

2. Initiating, monitoring, and evaluating resources are essential components of community health nursing practice. Describe a client situation and the case management process that might occur in the following practices:
   a. A school nurse in an elementary school and in a high school
   b. An occupational health nurse in a hospital and in a manufacturing plant
   c. A nurse working in a well-child clinic
   d. A case manager employed by a managed care organization

3. The values and beliefs held by a community health nurse influence the nurse's ability to be an advocate for clients. Discuss your values and beliefs about rationing health care and how they may impact on your ability to be a client advocate.

4. Read the following article: Kayser-Jones J, Davis A, Weiner CL, Higgins SS: An ethical analysis of an elder's treatment, *Nurs Outlook* 37(6):267, 1989. Discuss your reactions:
   a. "If I were in that situation, I believe I would . . ."
   b. Comment on the ethical issues and responses of the staff in the nursing home relative to the performance of the advocacy role.

Bibliography

Allen SA: Medicare case management, *Home Healthc Nurse* 12(3):21-27, 1994.

American Academy of Nursing: *Managed care and national health care reform: nurses can make it work,* Washington, DC, 1993, American Academy of Nursing.

American Hospital Association: *Glossary of terms and phrases for health care coalitions,* Chicago, 1986, AHA Office of Health Coalitions and Private Sector Initiatives.

American Hospital Association: *Case management: an aid to quality and continuity of care,* Chicago, 1987, AHA Council Report.

American Nurses Association: *Code for nurses with interpretive statements,* Pub No G-56, Kansas City, Mo, 1985, The Association.

American Nurses Association: *Standards of community health nursing practice,* Kansas City, Mo, 1986, The Association.

American Nurses Association: *Standards of home health nursing practice,* Kansas City, Mo, 1986, The Association.

American Nurses Association: *A statement on the scope of home health nursing practice,* Washington, DC, 1992, American Nurses Publishing.

American Nurses Association: *Innovation at the worksite,* draft, Washington, DC, 1992, The Association.

American Nurses Association: *Managed care: cornerstone for health care reform—a fact sheet,* Washington, DC, 1993.

American Nurses Association: *Nursing's social policy statement,* draft, Washington, DC, 1995, The Association.

American Nurses Foundation: *America's nurses: an untapped natural resource,* Washington, DC, 1993, The Foundation.

Arras JD, Dubler NN: Executive summary of project conclusions: the technical tether, an introduction to the ethical and social issues in high-tech home care, *Hastings Center Rep,* special supplement, New York, 1994.

Banez-Car M, McCoy N: Training for the transition to case management in home care, *Caring* 13(4):34-36, 1994.

Banja JD: Ethical challenges of managed care, *Case Manager* 5(3):37, 39-40, 1994.

Banja JD: Ethical dimensions of cultural diversity in case management, *Case Manager* 5(4):27-29, 1994.

Barkauskas VH: Case management within home care: old ideas and new themes, *Home Healthc Nurse* 12(1):8, 1994.

Bartling AC: Trends in managed care, *Healthcare Exec* 10(2):6-11, 1995.

Bisno H: *Managing conflict,* Beverly Hills, Calif, 1988, Sage.

Bower KA: *Case management by nurses,* Washington, DC, 1992, American Nurses Association.

Cary A, Androwich I: *A collaboration model: a synthesis of literature and a research survey.* Paper presented at the Association of Community Health Nursing Educators Spring Institute, Seattle, June 1989.

Cohen EL, Cesta TG: *Nursing case management: from concept to evaluation,* St Louis, 1993, Mosby.

Coleman JR, Hagen E: Collaborative practice: case managers and home care agency nurses, *Case Manager* 2(4):64-72, 1991.

Congressional Research Service: *Case management standards in state community-based long-term care programs for older persons with disabilities,* CRS-91-55, Washington, DC, 1993, CRS, Library of Congress.

Damron-Rodriguez J: Case management in two long-term care populations: a synthesis of research, *J Case Manage* 2(4):125-129, 1993.

Deal LW: The effectiveness of community health nursing interventions: a literature review, *Public Health Nurs* 11(5):315-323, 1994.

Erkel EA: The impact of case management in preventive services, *J Nurs Adm* 23(1):27-32, 1993.

Erkel EA, Morgan EP, Staples MA, Assey VH, Michel Y: Case management and preventive services among infants from low-income families, *Public Health Nurs* 11(5):352-360, 1994.

Feldman C, Olberding L, Shortridge L, Toole K, Zappin P: Decision making in case management of home health care clients, *J Nurs Adm* 23(1):33-38, 1993.

Feuer LC: Negotiating for all concerned, *Contin Care* 12(7):30, 33, 1993.

Foster J, Hall H: Public health and AIDS, *Caring* 5(6):4-11, 73-78, 1986.

Goodwin DR: Nursing case management activities, *J Nurs Adm* 24(2):29-34, 1994.

Gustafson DH: The total costs of illness: a metric for health care reform, *Hosp Health Services Admin* 40(1):154-171, 1995.

Healthy People 2000: national health promotion and disease prevention objectives, Washington, DC, 1992, DHHS, Public Health Service.

Helvie CO, Alexy BB: Using after-shelter case management to improve outcomes for families with children, *Public Health Rep* 107(5):585-588, 1992.

Hicks LL, Stallmeyer JM, Coleman JR: *The role of the nurse in managed care,* Washington, DC, 1993, American Nurses Publishing.

Hinden RA, Hyatt TK, Saue JM, Scheutzow SO, Sollins HL: Legal hazards on the case management highway, *Case Manager* 5(3):97-111, 1994.

Hyatt TK: Negligent referral, *Case Manager* 5(3):102, 106, 1994.

Kenyon V, Smith E, Hefty LV, Bell ML, McNeil J, Martaus T: Clinical competencies for community health nursing, *Public Health Nurs* 7(1):33-39, 1990.

Knollmueller RN: Case management: what's in a name? *Nurs Manage* 20(10):38-42, 1989.

Kohler P: Model of shared control, *J Gerontol Nurs* 14(7):21-25, 1988.

Kohnke MF: *Advocacy risk and reality,* St Louis, 1982, Mosby.

Lamb GS, Stempel JE: Nurse case management from the client's view: growing as insider-expert, *Nurs Outlook* 42(1):7-13, 1994.

Lashley M: The hidden benefits of case management, *Case Manager* 4(3):78-79, 1993.

Lowery SL: Qualifications for the successful case manager, *Case Manager* 3(4):66-72, 1992.

Lyon JC: Models of nursing care delivery and case management: clarification of terms, *Nurs Econ* 11(3):163-169, 1993.

Marschke P, Nolan MT: Research related to case management, *Nurs Admin Q* 17(3):16-21, 1993.

Mawn B, Bradley J: Standards of care for high-risk prenatal clients: the community nurse case management approach, *Public Health Nurs* 10(2):78-88, 1993.

Molloy SP: Defining case management, *Home Healthc Nurse* 12(3):51-54, 1994.

Mueller WJ, Kell B: *Coping with conflict,* Englewood Cliffs, NJ, 1972, Prentice Hall.

National Council on Aging: *Standards for case management,* Washington, DC, 1987, The Council.

National Institute of Community-Based Long-Term Care: *Care management standards: guidelines for practice,* Washington, DC, 1988, National Council on Aging.

Nelson ML: Advocacy in nursing, *Nurs Outlook* 36(3):136-141, 1988.

Parker M, Quinn J, Viehl M, McKinley AH, Polich CL, Hartwell S, VanHook R, Detzner DF: Issues in rural case management, *Fam Community Health* 14(4):40-60, 1992.

Redford LJ: Case management: the wave of the future, *J Case Manage* 1(1):5-8, 1992.

Romaine D: Case management challenges, present and future, *Cont Care* 14(1):24-31, 1995.

Saue JM: Legal issues related to case management. In Fisher K, Weisman E, editors: *Case management: guiding patients through the health care maze,* Chicago, 1989, JCAHO.

Salle SM: Experimental treatment and technology, *Case Manager* 5(3) 106-107, 1994.

Schaffer CL: Case management law, *Contin Care* 13(5):20-23, 1994.

Scheutzow SO: Confidentiality, *Case Manger* 5(3): 108-109, 1994.

Secord LJ: *Private case management for older persons and their families,* Excelsior, Minn, 1987, Interstudy.

Sollins HI: Fraud and abuse, *Case Manager* 5(3) 109-110, 1994.

Sowell RL, Meadows TM: An integrated care management model: developing standards, evaluation and outcome criteria, *Nurs Admin Q* 18(2):53-64, 1994.

Surles RC, Blanch AK, Shern DL, Donahue SA: Case management as a strategy for systems change, *Health Affairs* 11(3):271-272, 1992.

Thomas KW, Kilmann RH: *Thomas-Kilmann Conflict Mode Instrument,* New York, 1974; Xicom.

Vogler J, Ratliffe CE: Quality improvement and managed care as curriculum elements, *Nurs Educ* 18(3):29-33, 1993.

Volkema RJ: *Problem-purpose-expansion: a technique for reformulating problems,* 1983, University of Wisconsin (unpublished manuscript).

Webb C: Professionalism revisited, *Nurs Times* 83(35):39-41, 1987.

Weil M, Karls JM: Historical origins and recent developments. In Weils M, et al, editors: *Case management in human service practice,* San Francisco, 1985, Jossey-Bass.

Winslow GR: From loyalty to advocacy: a new metaphor for nursing, *Hastings Cent Rep* 14:32-40, 1984.

Zander K, editor: *The new definition,* South Natick, Mass, 1994, The Center for Case Management.

Zander K, Etheredge ML, Bower KA: *Nursing case management: blueprints for transformation,* Waban, Mass, Winslow Printing Systems.

Zander K, McGill R: Critical and anticipated recovery paths: only the beginning, *Nurs Manage* 25(8):34-37, 40, 1994.

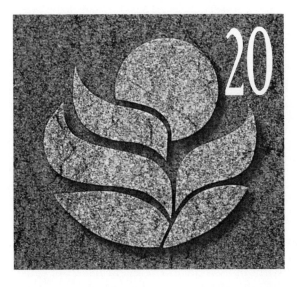

20

Disaster Management

Susan B. Hassmiller

Objectives ▼

After reading this chapter, the student should be able to do the following:

- ◆ Discuss types of disasters, including natural, man-made, and epidemics.
- ◆ Describe how disasters affect people and their communities.
- ◆ Discuss disaster management, including preparedness, response, and recovery.
- ◆ Discuss the community health nurses' role in the preparedness, response, and recovery phases of disaster management.
- ◆ Describe the priorities in a triage situation.
- ◆ Describe the steps for initiating and maintaining a clinic to care for the masses.
- ◆ Identify how the community, including voluntary, governmental, and community organizations, business, and labor, works together to prepare for, respond to, and recover from disasters.
- ◆ Describe the role of the American Red Cross in disaster management.

Key Terms ▼

community preparedness
delayed stress reaction
disaster
disaster action team (DAT)
disaster medical assistance
  teams (DMATs)
emergency support functions (ESFs)
Federal Emergency Management
  Agency (FEMA)
Federal Response Plan (FRP)
level I disaster
level II disaster
level III disaster
man-made disaster
National Disaster Medical
  System (NDMS)
natural disaster
personal preparedness
preparedness
professional preparedness
recovery
response
triage

The author acknowledges the following individuals for their thoughtful review and critique of this chapter: Laurie Willshire, RN; Jane Morgan; RN, and Judy Lee, RN, all disaster services associates who work for the national headquarters of the American Red Cross.

"We do not expect disasters, but they happen.... With living come natural calamities; with industrial and technological advances come accidents; with socioeconomic and political stagnation or change come dissatisfaction, terrorism, and war" (Waeckerle, 1991, p. 820). Disasters, man-made or natural, may be inevitable, but there are methods to prevent or manage the ways people and their communities respond to disasters. This chapter describes such management techniques throughout the preparedness, response, and recovery phases of disaster. The community health nurse's role throughout these phases is highlighted.

DISASTERS

As children, perhaps our first recollection of a natural disaster was hearing about Noah and the Great Flood in the Book of Genesis. The fairy tale fashion in which the story is invariably told in no way prepares one for the destruction and devastation that disasters truly leave behind. Disasters can affect one family at a time, as in a house fire, or in the case of a chemical leak in Bhopal, India, can kill 2500 people and injure 150,000 more (Taggart, 1985). According to the World Health Organization's (WHO's) Collaborating Centre for Research on the Epidemiology of Disasters, natural disasters between 1960 and 1989 affected 233 million people in China alone, claiming 727,849 lives and injuring 425,162. In 1990, one earthquake in Iran killed 40,000 people and created an instant homeless population of approximately 500,000.

Although the number of natural disasters per year has remained constant, the number of man-made disasters and ensuing deaths has risen sharply (Office of U.S. Foreign Disaster Assistance, 1990; Waters et al., 1992). The urbanization and overcrowding of cities have caused stressors that promote civil unrest and ensuing riots. In addition, the overcrowding of cities has forced populations to build their communities in areas that are more vulnerable to disasters, such as coastal and flood plains, earthquake zones, and barrier sea islands (Pickens, 1992). Finally, modern warfare has greatly increased the risk of injury and death from disaster.

The monetary amount to support disaster recovery efforts has also risen sharply, not only because of the number of people involved, but because of the amount of technology that must be restored. Americans are less self-sufficient than ever before and have become interdependent on technology, sometimes for their very existence. Americans also rely heavily on the social and economic systems within their community and can rapidly become devastated without its support. People who live on the brink of disaster every day, physically, emotionally and economically, are among the first to be "hard hit" when calamity strikes.

Defining Disasters

A **disaster** is any man-made or natural event that causes destruction and devastation that cannot be alleviated without assistance. The event need not cause injury or death to be considered a disaster. For example, a hurricane may cause millions of dollars in damage without causing a single death or injury. The box below lists examples of man-made and natural disasters.

International Decade for Natural Disaster Reduction

Although **natural disasters** will always occur, much can be done to prevent the further escalation of accidents, death, and destruction after impact. A concise, realistic, and well-rehearsed disaster plan, as well as sustained and open communication among involved organizations and workers, are both important in preventing further damage. In addition, many **man-made disasters** can be prevented. For example, consider how often substance abuse has been reported as the cause of major transportation accidents and fires.

To educate the world regarding disaster reduction and to end the fatalistic approach that so often accompanies disasters, the United Nations has declared the 1990s as the "Decade for Natural Disaster Reduc-

 Types of Disasters

NATURAL	MAN-MADE
Hurricanes	Conventional warfare
Tornados	Nonconventional warfare
Hailstorms	(e.g., nuclear, chemical)
Cyclones	Transportation accidents
Blizzards	Structural collapse
Drought	Explosions
Floods	Fires
Mudslides	Toxic materials
Avalanches	Pollution
Earthquakes	Civil unrest (e.g., riots,
Volcanic eruptions	demonstrations)
Communicable disease	Terrorist attacks
epidemics	

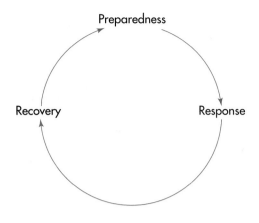

FIGURE 20-1

Disaster management cycle. (Modified from American Red Cross: *Disasters happen*, Washington, DC, 1993, American Red Cross.)

tion" (Pickens, 1992). Dr. Hiroshi Nakajima, Director-General of the WHO, has stated, "We cannot pursue our long-term strategies of 'Health For All' without paying attention to the global problem of disasters" (Pickens, 1992, p. 193). Dr. H.A. Hamad-Elneil, Director of the WHO's Emergency Relief Operations in Geneva, believes that health workers must play a lead role in disaster reduction, working alongside hydrologists, meteorologists, urban planners, engineers, and others at all stages of disaster management. Public health officials, in particular, can identify epidemiological risk factors associated with disease outbreaks (Pickens, 1992).

◆ *Three Stages of Disaster Involvement*

Disaster management requires attention to all three stages of a disaster: **preparedness, response,** and **recovery.** Figure 20-1 depicts the disaster management cycle. A key to disaster preparedness is that the plan must be kept realistic yet simple. The reasons for this are (1) no plan will ever exactly fit the disaster as it occurs, and (2) all plans must be implementable no matter what key members of the disaster team are there at the time (Public health responds to disaster, 1994). The remainder of this chapter elaborates on all three stages, including the role of the community health nurse.

PREPAREDNESS
Personal Preparedness

Great stress is placed on the nurse with client responsibilities who also becomes a disaster victim (Chubon, 1992). Conflicts arise between family and work-related responsibilities. For example, a mother whose child care needs go unmet will not be able to participate fully, if at all, in disaster relief efforts. In addition, the community health nurse who will be assisting in

Four Steps to Safety

FIND OUT WHAT COULD HAPPEN TO YOU

Determine what types of disasters are most likely to happen.
Learn about your communities' warning signals.
Ask about postdisaster pet care (shelters usually will not accept pets).
Review the disaster plans at your workplace, school, and other places where your family spends time.
Determine how to help elderly or disabled family members and neighbors.

CREATE A DISASTER PLAN

Discuss the types of disaster that are most likely to happen, and review what to do in each case.
Pick two places to meet, including outside your home and outside your neighborhood.
Choose an out-of-state friend to be your "family contact" to verify location of each family member. After a disaster, it is easier to call long distance.
Review evacuation plans, including care of pets. Identify ahead of time where to go if evacuation is necessary.

COMPLETE THIS CHECKLIST

Post emergency phone numbers by phones.
Teach everyone how and when to call 911.
Determine when and how to turn off water, gas, and electricity at the main switches.
Check adequacy of insurance coverage.
Locate and review use of fire extinguisher.
Install and maintain smoke detectors.
Conduct a home hazard hunt and fix potential hazards.
Stock emergency supplies and assemble a disaster supplies kit.
Become certified in first aid and cardiopulmonary resuscitation (CPR).
Locate all escape routes from your home. Find two ways out of each room.
Find the safe spots in your home for each type of disaster.

PRACTICE AND MAINTAIN YOUR PLAN

Review plan every 6 months.
Conduct fire and emergency evacuation drills.
Replace stored water every 3 months and stored food every 6 months.
Test and recharge fire extinguisher according to manufacturer's instructions.
Test your smoke detectors monthly and change the batteries at least once a year.

disaster relief efforts must be as healthy as possible, both physically and mentally. A disaster worker who is not well is of little service to his or her family, clients, and other disaster victims. **Personal preparedness** can help ease some of the conflicts that will arise and allows nurses to attend to client needs sooner than one may anticipate.

The American Red Cross and the **Federal Emergency Management Agency (FEMA),** two well-known authorities on disaster preparedness, response, and recovery, have devised a personal checklist to help individuals and families prepare for disasters before they strike (1992). The box above provides an adapted

Emergency Supplies Needed in Case of Disaster

A 3-day supply of water (1 gallon per person per day) and food that will not spoil

One change of clothing and footwear per person and one blanket or sleeping bag per person

A first-aid kit that includes your family's prescription medications

Emergency tools, including a battery-powered radio, flashlight, and plenty of extra batteries

Candles and matches

An extra set of car keys and a credit card, cash, or traveler's checks

Sanitation supplies, including toilet paper, soap, feminine hygiene items, and plastic garbage bags

Special items for infant, elderly, or disabled family members

An extra pair of glasses

version of their recommendations entitled *Four Steps to Safety.* Also, the box above lists emergency supplies that should be prepared and stored in a sturdy, easy-to-carry container. Important documents should always be kept in a waterproof container.

Professional Preparedness

Professional preparedness requires that nurses become aware of and understand the disaster plans at their workplace and community. Nurses who take disaster preparation seriously will take the time to read and understand workplace and community disaster plans and will participate in disaster drills and community mock disasters. The more adequately prepared nurses are, the more they will be able to function in a leadership capacity and assist others toward a smoother recovery phase. Personal items that are recommended for any nurse preparing to help in a disaster include the following (Switzer, 1985):

◆ A copy of their professional license
◆ Personal equipment, such as a stethoscope
◆ A flashlight and extra batteries
◆ Cash
◆ Warm clothing and a heavy jacket (or weather-appropriate clothing)
◆ Record-keeping materials
◆ Pocket-sized reference books

It must be remembered that disaster work is not "high tech." Field work, including shelter management, requires that nurses be creative and willing to improvise in delivering care. It is recommended that all workers be certified in first aid and cardiopulmonary resuscitation (CPR). In addition, the American Red Cross provides a comprehensive program of disaster training for health professionals to enable them to provide assistance within their own communities, as well as to other stricken communities and countries that would benefit from their expertise. The courses give nurses the tools to adapt their existing nursing skills to a disaster setting.

Community Preparedness

The level of **community preparedness** for a disaster is only as good as the people and organizations in the community make it. Some communities remain vigilant as to the possibility of a disaster hitting their community and stay prepared by having a solid disaster plan on paper and by participating in yearly mock disaster drills. Other communities are not as vigilant and depend on luck and the fact that they have never been hit before to see them through. Some organizations within the community may be more prepared than others. For example, most health care facilities have written disaster plans and require employees to perform mock drills every year, whereas many businesses do not have these requirements.

If possible, it is also important to review the disaster history of the community, including how past disasters have had an impact on the community's health care delivery system and how their particular organization fit into the plan. Understanding these aspects of past disasters have planning implications for future disasters. For example, it might be determined, according to disaster history, that the local disaster services committee has not appropriately used the county's community health nurses because of a lack of education regarding their roles. It might be beneficial for this committee to receive an educational program on what community health nurses do and what role they might best play in the event of a disaster. A solid disaster plan requires the multidisciplinary talents, coordination, and cooperation of many different organizations. Many community organizations and professionals are involved in disaster work including the clergy, morticians, police, fire and rescue, the mayor and other city officials, and the media. Working together cooperatively and with clear role definition before the disaster gives greater assurance that assistance will be delivered more smoothly once a disaster strikes.

Finally, it must be assured that the community has an adequate warning system, as well as a backup evacuation plan to remove individuals who hesitate to leave their homes from areas of danger. Individuals must be convinced that predisaster warnings are official, serious, and personally relevant before they are motivated to take action. Also, some people mistakenly believe that past experience with a particular type of disaster is preparation enough for the next one. Finally, individuals may refuse to leave their homes because they are fearful of personnel possessions becoming lost or destroyed from the disaster and from post-disaster looting. A face-to-face encounter with law-enforcement personnel or others in authority is often necessary to convince individuals to leave their homes and retreat to safer quarters.

Role of the Community Health Nurse in Disaster Preparedness

The role of the community health nurse in disaster preparedness is to facilitate preparation within the

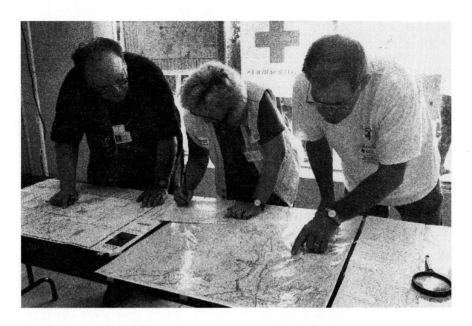

FIGURE 20-2

Understanding the community's disaster plan is a key role for community health nurses who seek greater involvement in disaster management. (Photo courtesy the American Red Cross. All rights reserved in all countries.)

community and place of employment (Figure 20-2). Within the employing organization, the nurse can help initiate or update the disaster plan, provide educational programs and material regarding disasters specific to the area, and organize disaster drills. The community health nurse is also in a unique position to provide an updated record of vulnerable populations within the community. For example, when calamity strikes, disaster workers must know what kinds of populations they are attempting to assist. If a tornado strikes a retirement village, the needs are quite different than if the tornado hits a church with predominantly young families or a center for physically disabled persons. In addition to knowing where special populations exist, the community health nurse should be involved in educating these populations about what impact the disaster might have on them. Individualized strategies should be reviewed, including the availability of specific resources, in the event of an emergency.

Finally, the nurse who leads a preparedness effort can help recruit others within the organization who will help if and when a response is required. Although there is no psychological profile of a disaster leader, it is wise to involve persons in this effort who have demonstrated flexibility, decisiveness, stamina, endurance, and emotional stability (Dinerman, 1990). The leader should also possess an intimate knowledge of the institution and familiarity with the individuals who work there. Persons with disaster management training, and especially those who have served on "real" disasters, make valuable members of any preparedness team as well. Demi and Miles (1984), in examining the role of nurses after the Hyatt Regency

skywalk collapse, found that nurses who were most effective in leadership roles generally had formal responsibilities in the disaster plan and who had previous disaster training and experiences.

Within the community the nurse might be involved in many roles. As a community advocate, the community health nurse should always seek to keep a safe environment. Recalling that disasters are not only natural but also man-made, the nurse in the community has an obligation to assess for and report environmental health hazards. For example, the nurse should be aware of and report unsafe equipment, faulty structures, and the beginning of disease epidemics such as measles or flu.

The community health nurse should also have an understanding of what community resources will be available after a disaster strikes and, most important, how the community will work together. A community-wide disaster plan will guide the nurse in understanding what "should" occur before, during, and after the response and his or her role within the plan. The community health nurse who seeks greater involvement or a more in-depth understanding of disaster management can become involved in any number of community organizations that are part of the official response team, such as the American Red Cross, Salvation Army, or Emergency Medical System/Ambulance Corps. The Red Cross offers classes on disaster health services and disaster mental health services in an effort to "help participants identify disaster health services preparedness measures that should take place on the local unit level and to become familiar with Red Cross disaster health services policies, regulations, and procedures that apply on locally administered disaster operations" (American Red Cross, 1989, p. 5). The Red Cross generally requires certification in a disaster health services or a disaster mental health services course before assigning an individual to a disaster site as a Red Cross representative.

For nurses who choose to work with agencies such as the Red Cross, many options for involvement exist. After several hours of disaster training, community health nurses may want to take the following steps: (1) place themselves on a local **disaster action team (DAT);** (2) act as a liaison with local hospitals; (3) determine health-related appropriateness for shelter sites; (4) plan with pharmacies, opticians, morticians, and other health personnel to facilitate services for disaster victims; (5) plan for and retain needed supplies; and (6) teach disaster nursing in the community. Another important job is keeping the nursing and medical protocols and intervention standards, whether they be with the Red Cross or employing institution, up to date and consistent with local public health standards (American Red Cross, 1989). Finally, community health nurses are needed for national and international disaster assignments as well.

Mass Casualty Drills or Mock Disasters

Mass casualty drills or mock disasters are valuable components of any preparedness plan. Whether the drills are carried forth in a desk-top manner or through realistic scenarios, the objectives are to do the following (Lehnhof, 1985):
1. Promote confidence.
2. Develop skills.
3. Coordinate activities.
4. Coordinate participants.

It is critical that those persons who will be involved in the actual disaster be involved in the drill (Berglin, 1990). It is especially important that the drill leader have special skills in disaster management and the ability to coordinate many organizations at one time. Finally, although a successful disaster drill has the capability of allowing participants to evaluate the rescue plan and make further recommendations, it should not create a misplaced sense of security (Waeckerle, 1991).

Agencies Involved in Disaster Preparedness

Many agencies within local communities contribute to disaster preparedness. Table 20-1 lists the preparedness responsibilities assumed by the American Red Cross, other voluntary organizations, business and labor organizations, and local government.

RESPONSE
Levels of Disaster and Agency Involvement

The response is determined by the level of disaster. Levels are not determined by the number of casualties per se, but by the amount of resources needed (Waeckerle, 1991). A **level I disaster** requires activation by the local emergency medical system in cooperation with local community organizations, such as the American Red Cross and Salvation Army (Sklar, 1987). A one-family fire would be an example of a level I disaster. A **level II disaster** requires more of a regional response necessitating several casualty protocols. The Hyatt Regency skywalk collapse, although many people were killed and injured, was a level II disaster because of its confinement to one building (Orr and Robinson, 1983).

Many agencies are involved in responding to a disaster. Table 20-2 lists the response responsibilities assumed by the American Red Cross, other voluntary organizations, business and labor organizations, and local government.

A **level III disaster** is one in which a federal emergency has been declared because of widespread destruction. In a presidentially declared disaster, state and federal authorities of all kinds must be prepared to respond under the coordination of FEMA. Hurricane Andrew, a hurricane that devastated south Florida and Homestead Air Force Base in 1992, was a level III disaster.

In any large-scale or major national disaster, not only do official agencies respond, but many other concerned citizens, including health professionals, come on their own to help as well. At times, so many people come "out of the woodwork" to help that role conflict, anger, frustration, and helplessness occur. Because of this, it is best that nurses attach themselves to an official agency with assigned disaster management responsibilities (Alson et al., 1993; Switzer, 1985).

Federal Response Plan

Once a federal emergency has been declared, the **Federal Response Plan (FRP)** also known as Public Law 93-288, may take effect depending on the specific needs of the disaster. The FRP is "based on the fundamental assumption that a significant disaster or emergency will overwhelm the capability of state and local governments to carry out the extensive emergency operations necessary to save lives and protect property" (FRP, 1993, p. 1). The box on p. 381 outlines the purpose of the FRP.

Within the FRP there are 12 **emergency support functions (ESFs),** each one headed by a primary agency. Each primary agency is responsible for coordinating efforts in a particular area with all its designated support agencies. In all, 26 federal agencies and the American Red Cross must respond if called. For example, in a presidentially declared disaster, all ongoing health and medical services fall under the auspices of the U.S. Public Health Service (PHS). The PHS divides its responsibilities among its own agencies as needed. The Centers for Disease Control and Prevention (CDC), for instance, may "assist in establishing surveillance systems to monitor the general population and special high-risk population segments; carry out field studies and investigations; monitor injury

Table 20-1   Disaster Preparedness Responsibilities by Agency

American Red Cross	Other voluntary organizations	Business and labor organizations	Local government
Participates with government in developing and testing community disaster plan. Designates persons to serve as representatives at government emergency operations centers and command posts.	Collaborates in developing and maintaining a local Voluntary Organizations Active in Disaster group to identify roles, resources, and plans for disasters.	Develops disaster plans for business locations and integrate their plans with the community disaster plan.	Coordinates the development of the community plan and conducts evaluation exercises.
Develops and tests local Red Cross disaster plans.	Identifies and train personnel for disaster response.	Develops procedures to facilitate continuity of operations in time of disaster.	Trains staff to carry out the plan.
Identifies and trains personnel for disaster response.	Identifies community issues and special populations for consideration in disaster preparedness.	Develops plans for assisting business employees after a disaster.	Passes legislation to mitigate the effects of potential disasters.
Collaborates with other voluntary agencies in developing and maintaining a local Voluntary Organizations Active in Disaster group to promote cooperation and coordinate resources and people for disaster work.	Makes plans to continue to serve regular clients after a disaster.	Identifies union and business facilities, resources, and people who may be able to support community disaster plans.	Designs measures to warn the population of disaster threats.
	Identifies facilities, resources, and people to serve in time of disaster.	Provides volunteers, financial contributions, and in-kind gifts to Red Cross and other voluntary organizations to support disaster preparedness.	Conducts building safety inspections.
Works with business and labor organizations to identify resources and people for disaster work.	Educates specific client groups on disaster preparedness.		Develops procedures to facilitate continuity of public safety operations in time of disaster.
Educates the public about hazards and ways to avoid, prepare for, and cope with their effects.		Educates employees and union members about disaster preparedness.	Identifies public facilities, resources, and public employees for disaster work.
Acquires material resources needed to ensure effective response.			Educates the public about disaster threats in the community and safety procedures.

From American Red Cross: *Disasters happen*, Washington, DC, 1993, American Red Cross. Used with the permission of the American Red Cross, Washington, DC, 1994.

and disease patterns and injury control measures and precautions" (FRP, 1993). Sheltering, feeding, giving emergency first aid, providing a disaster welfare information system, and coordinating bulk distribution of emergency relief supplies constitute the mass care of ESFs, of which the American Red Cross is the primary agency. The community health nurse could be involved with any of these response efforts within the local community or, with appropriate training, on a national basis.

The **National Disaster Medical System (NDMS)** is part of the ESF of health and medical services. In a presidentially declared disaster, including overseas war, the PHS can activate **disaster medical assistance**

 Purpose of the Federal Response Plan (FRP)

1. Establish fundamental assumptions and policies.
2. Establish a concept of operations that provides an interagency coordination mechanism to facilitate the immediate delivery of federal response assistance.
3. Incorporate the coordination mechanisms and structures of other appropriate federal plans and responsibilities into the overall response.
4. Assign specific functional responsibilities to appropriate federal departments and agencies.
5. Identify actions that participating federal departments and agencies will take in the overall federal response in coordination with the affected state.

Table 20-2   Disaster Response Responsibilities by Agency

American Red Cross	Other voluntary organizations	Business and labor organizations	Local government
Operates shelters.	Provides services that are identified in predisaster planning.	Takes action to protect employees and ensure the safety of the facility.	Provides for coordination of the overall relief effort.
Provides feeding services.	Provides regular services to ongoing client groups.	Advises public safety forces of hazardous conditions.	Advises the public on safety measures such as evacuation.
Provides individual and family assistance to meet immediate emergency needs. Services include providing the means to purchase groceries, clothing, and household items.	Identifies unanticipated needs and provide resources to meet those needs.	Identifies resources such as union halls, generators, and heavy equipment that are available to support the disaster response.	Provides public health services.
Provides disaster health services, including mental health support.	Acts as advocates for their client groups.	Provides volunteers, financial contributions, and gifts of goods and services to the relief effort.	Provides fire and police protection to the affected area.
Handles inquiries from concerned family members outside the area.	Coordinates services with all other groups involved with the disaster response.		Inspects facilities for safety and health codes.
Coordinates relief activities with other agencies, business, labor, and government.	Seeks and accept donations from those wanting to help.		Provides ongoing social services for the community.
Informs the public of services available.			Repairs public buildings, sewage and water systems, streets, and highways.
Seeks and accepts contributions from those wanting to help.			

From American Red Cross: *Disasters happen*, Washington, DC, 1993, American Red Cross. Used with permission of the American Red Cross, Washington, DC, 1994.

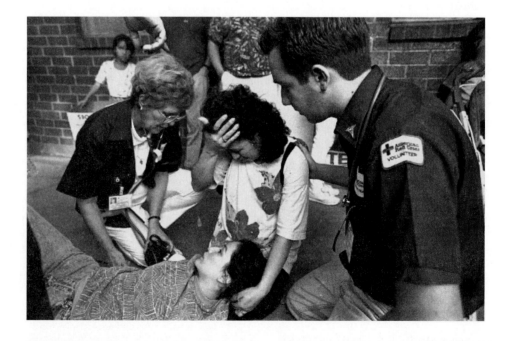

FIGURE 20-3

Individuals react to the same disaster in different ways. (Photo courtesy the American Red Cross. All rights reserved in all countries.)

Common Reactions to Disasters by Adults and Children

ADULTS

Extreme sense of urgency
Panic and fear
Disbelief
Disorientation and numbing
Reluctance to abandon property
Difficulty in making decisions
Need to help others
Anger and blaming
Blaming and scapegoating

Delayed Reactions

Insomnia
Headaches
Apathy and depression
Sense of powerlessness
Guilt
Moodiness and irritability
Jealousy and resentment
Domestic violence

CHILDREN

Regressive behaviors (bed-wetting, thumb sucking, crying, clinging to parents)
Fantasies that disaster never occurred
Nightmares
School-related problems, including inability to concentrate and refusal to go back to school

teams **(DMATs)** to an area to supplement local and state medical care needs. DMATs can also be activated by the assistant secretary for health at the request of a state health officer. Teams of specially trained civilian physicians, nurses, and other health care personnel can be sent to a disaster site within hours of activation. DMATs can provide triage and continuing medical care to victims until they can be evacuated to a national network of hospitals prearranged by the NDMS (FRP, 1993; Waeckerle, 1991). In reality, because of the nature of U.S. disasters since the initiation of the DMATs, these teams have been used primarily to staff community health outpatient clinics in the affected areas.

How Disasters Affect Communities

People in a community can be affected both physically and emotionally depending on the type, cause, and location of the disaster; its magnitude, extent of damage, and duration; and the amount of warning that was provided. For example, an earthquake may not result in any deaths; however, the structural damage to buildings and the continuous aftershocks, which may last for weeks, can cause intense psychological stress. In addition, the longer it takes for structural repairs and other cleanup, the longer the psychological effects can last.

Individuals react to the same disaster in different

ways depending on their age, cultural background, health status, social support structure, and general adaptability to crisis (Figure 20-3). The box at left lists common reactions of adults and children to disasters. The typical first reaction to being struck by a disaster, however, is an extreme sense of urgency (Chubon, 1992). Victims become obsessed with personal losses. Other initial reactions include fear, panic, disbelief, reluctance to abandon property, disorientation and numbing, difficulty in making decisions, need for information, seeking help for self and family, and offering help to other disaster victims (American Red Cross, 1991). Disturbances in bodily functions, such as gastrointestinal upsets, diarrhea, and nausea and vomiting, are also common (Richtmeier and Miller, 1985).

Anger, especially blaming and scapegoating, is common among victims soon after a disaster (Chubon, 1992; Cohen and Ahearn, 1980; Demi and Miles, 1983). Cohen and Ahearn (1980) note that anger and blaming stem from an increasing awareness of what has been lost, physical fatigue, emotional stress, and a continuing change in one's degree of personal comfort. Victims interviewed on television after a disaster often state that FEMA or the American Red Cross is simply not doing all that it can be doing. Some other responses that may occur later include difficulty sleeping, headaches, apathy and depression, moodiness and irritability, anxiety about the future, domestic violence, feelings of being overwhelmed, frustration and feelings of powerlessness over one's future, and guilt over not being able to prevent the disaster (American Red Cross, 1991). An exacerbation of an already existent chronic disease process is also common. For example, the emotional stress of being a disaster victim may make it difficult for persons with diabetes to gain control over their blood sugar levels.

Jealousy and resentment abound, even over fellow victims in the same community. Although poor persons typically are the most severely affected disaster victims, a group of nurses in South Carolina expressed anger after becoming victims of Hurricane Hugo because poor people were receiving added support and attention while the nurses continued to struggle for assistance (Chubon, 1992; Errington, 1989).

The effects on young children can be especially disruptive (Figure 20-4). Regressive behaviors such as thumb sucking, bed-wetting, crying, and clinging to parents can occur (American Red Cross, 1991). Fantasies that the disaster never occurred and nightmares are common as well. Finally, school-related problems may also occur, including an inability to concentrate and even refusal to go back to school.

An elderly person's reaction to disaster depends greatly on physical health, strength, mobility, self-sufficiency, and income source and amount (American Red Cross, 1993) (Figure 20-5). They react more deeply to loss of personal possessions because of the high sentimental value attached to the items and the limited time left to replace them. Anticipatory guidance may be needed related to elderly persons having

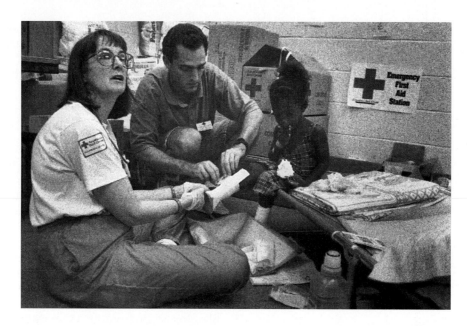

FIGURE 20-4

The effects of a disaster on young children can be especially disruptive. (Photo courtesy the American Red Cross. All rights reserved in all countries.)

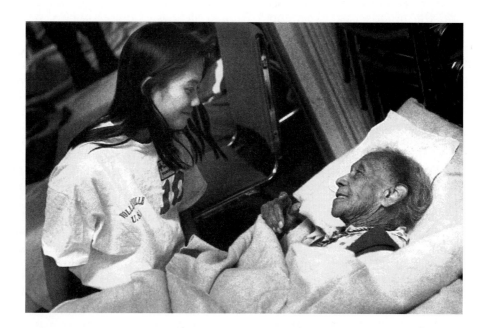

FIGURE 20-5

Elderly persons' reactions to a disaster depend greatly on their physical health, strength, mobility, self-sufficiency, and income source and amount. (Photo courtesy the American Red Cross. All rights reserved in all countries.)

Special Population Groups at Greatest Risk for Disruption from a Disaster

Persons with disabilities
Persons living on a low income, including homeless persons
Non-English-speaking persons and refugees
Persons living alone
Single-parent families
Persons new to the area
Institutionalized or chronically mental ill clients
Previous disaster victims or victims of traumatic events

either to move into a nursing home, either temporarily or permanently, or to make the adjustment to moving in with an adult child, depending on the extent of damage to their home or their compromised health. Elderly persons may cover up the seriousness of their losses out of fear of loss of independence (American Red Cross, 1993). The box above lists other populations at greatest risk for severe disruption from a disaster.

Role of the Community Health Nurse in Disaster Response

The role of the community health nurse during disaster depends greatly on the nurse's past experience, role in the institution's and community's preparedness, specialized training, and special interest. The most important attribute for anyone working in a disaster, however, is flexibility (Public health responds to disaster, 1994). One certain factor about disaster is that change is a constant (Gaffney et al., 1992).

Although valued for their expertise in community assessment, case finding and referring, prevention, health education, surveillance, and working with aggregates, at times the community health nurse is the first to arrive on the scene and must respond accordingly. In this situation, it is important to remember that all life-threatening problems take precedence. Once rescue workers begin to arrive at the scene, immediate plans for triage should begin.

Triage is the process of separating casualties and allocating treatment based on the victim's potential for survival. Highest priority is always given to victims who have life-threatening injuries but who have a high probability of survival once stabilized (Dixon, 1986). Second priority is given to victims who have injuries with systemic complications that are not yet life-threatening but who can wait up to 45 to 60 minutes for treatment. Last priority is given to those victims who have local injuries without immediate complications and who can wait several hours for medical attention.

Community health nurses working as members of an assessment team have the responsibility of feeding back accurate information to relief managers to facilitate rapid rescue and recovery. Many times nurses are required to make home visits to gather needed information, a task that comes quite naturally to the community health nurse. Types of information included in initial assessment reports include the following (Lillibridge et al., 1993):

1. Geographical extent of disaster's impact
2. Population at risk or affected
3. Presence of continuing hazards
4. Injuries and deaths
5. Availability of shelter
6. Current level of sanitation
7. Status of health care infrastructure

These assessments help to match available resources to a population's emergency needs. Lillibridge et al. (1993) also point out that disaster assessment priorities are related to the type of disaster that has occurred. For example, sudden-impact disasters, such as tornadoes and earthquakes, mainly involve ongoing hazards, injuries and deaths, shelter requirements, and potable water. Gradual-onset disasters, such as famines, primarily involve mortality rates, nutritional status, immunization status, and environmental health.

Lack of or inaccurate information regarding the scope of the disaster and its initial effects contributes to the misuse of resources. For example, after Hurricane Andrew, a well-meaning general public continued to ship thousands of pounds of clothing to South Florida, well beyond what the community would ever use. Much of the clothing eventually had to be burned because inadequate on-site personnel were available to sort and distribute the clothing, and the piles eventually became a public health nuisance. Local and regional emergency and public health resources can be readjusted as assessment reports continue to come in. Prioritizing needs that benefit the largest aggregate of imperiled individuals with the most correctable problems is consistent with the most basic tenets of triage (Waeckerle, 1991).

Ongoing assessments or surveillance reports are just as important as initial assessments. Surveillance reports indicate the continuing status of the affected population and the effectiveness of ongoing relief efforts. It continues to inform relief managers of needed resources. Nurses involved in ongoing surveillance use the following methods to gather information (Switzer, 1985):

1. Interview
2. Observation
3. Physical examination
4. Health and illness screening
5. Surveys (sample and special health)
6. Records (census, school, vital statistics, disease reporting)

Surveillance continues into the recovery phase of a disaster.

Shelter Management

Shelters are generally the responsibility of the local Red Cross chapter, although in level III disasters the military may be used to set up "tent cities" for the masses who are in need of temporary shelter. Community health nurses, because of their experience with delivering aggregate health promotion, disease prevention, and emotional support, make ideal shelter managers and team members. Although nurses may need to attend to physical health needs, especially among elderly and chronically ill persons, many of the predominant problems in shelters revolve around stress. Stress may be instigated by the shock of the disaster itself, loss of personal possessions, fear of the unknown, living in proximity to total strangers, and even boredom.

Common-sense approaches to working with victims dealing with stress work best. Basic measures that should be followed by the shelter nurse include (American Red Cross, 1991):

1. Listening to victims tell and retell their feelings related to the disaster and their current situation
2. Encouraging victims to share their feelings with one another if it seems appropriate to do so
3. Helping victims make decisions
4. Delegating tasks (e.g., reading, crafts, and playing games with children) to teenagers and others to help combat boredom
5. Providing the basic necessities (food, clothing, rest)
6. Attempting to recover or gain needed items (e.g., prescription glasses, medications)
7. Providing basic compassion and dignity (privacy when appropriate and if possible)
8. Referring to a mental health counselor if the situation warrants

The American Red Cross provides specialized training in disaster mental health services with the objective of "assisting the worker or client to understand disaster-related stress and grief reactions, develop adaptive coping and problem-solving skills, and return to a pre-disaster state of equilibrium or seek recommended further treatment" (1991, p. 5). Highly trained mental health counselors are always available in large-scale disasters as well, such as psychologists, psychiatrists, and psychiatric social workers and nurses. They are very important members of any disaster team, no matter what the level of disaster, and should be used as often as necessary.

Other shelter functions with which a community health nurse will be involved include assessing and referring, ensuring medical needs, providing first aid, serving meals, keeping patient records, ensuring emergency communications and transportation, and providing a safe environment (American Red Cross, 1989). The Red Cross provides training for shelter management and expects those trained to follow appropriate protocols.

International Relief Efforts

Countries other than the United States, especially those involved with political upheavals, suffer not only from natural disasters, but from man-made disasters as well. Civil strife leads to war, famines, and communicable disease outbreaks. Sometimes disaster or relief workers are sent to these international calamities at the request of the affected country's government. At other times, workers are not welcomed but instead may go with the support of the United Nations. When workers are not welcomed, their lives may be in danger, even though they go as peace-keeping agents of the Federation of Red Cross and Red Crescent Societies and the International Committee of Red Cross or as health representatives from the WHO. International disaster or relief workers generally have very intense training and preparation before embarking on a mission.

Psychological Stress of Disaster Workers

Psychological stress among victims, as well as workers, during disasters is well-documented (Cohen and Ahearn, 1980; Demi and Miles, 1983; Errington, 1989; Laube-Morgan, 1992). The degree of worker stress depends on the nature of the disaster, role in the disaster, individual stamina, and other environmental factors (Richtmeier and Miller, 1985). Environmental factors include noise, inadequate work space, physical danger, and stimulus overload, especially being exposed to death and trauma. Other sources of stress may evolve from workers not feeling they are doing enough to help, the burden of making life and death decisions, and the overall change in living patterns (Errington, 1989; Laube-Morgan, 1992).

When the nurse is from the same community in which disaster has struck, role conflict from organizational chaos, including the organization being cut off from usual support systems, also causes stress (Errington, 1989). Nothing has the potential for causing more stress and role conflict, however, than when the disaster nurse worker is also a victim of the disaster (Chubon, 1992; Laube-Morgan, 1992). Anger and resentment may occur as the job demands time away from one's own calamitous situation. Studies indicate, however, that nurses' emotional responses do not interfere with their effectiveness in helping others (Chubon, 1992; Laube, 1973).

Symptoms of early stress and burnout include minor tremors, nausea, loss of concentration, difficulty thinking, and problems with memory (Errington, 1989; Laube-Morgan, 1992). Suppressing feelings of guilt, powerlessness, anger, and other signs of stress

---

What Do You Think?

Is it appropriate for persons to drop off chronically ill family members, especially those with Alzheimer's disease, to Red Cross shelters for extended periods during the preparedness, response, and recovery phases of a disaster?

will eventually lead to symptoms such as irritability, fatigue, headaches, and distortions of bodily functions (Errington, 1989). It is normal to experience stress, but one must deal with it. The worst thing anyone can do is to deny that it exists.

Research Brief

Waters KA, Selander J, Stuart GW: Psychological adaptation of nurses post-disaster, *Iss Ment Health Nurs* 13:177-190, 1992.

This study of postdisaster stress (e.g., depression, anxiety, hostility, paranoia, somatic disorders) describes the responses of 25 nurses following Hurricane Hugo at 1, 4, and 12 months. Ten nurses remained at client's bedside during the disaster, five nurses volunteered to accompany clients to health care facilities out of the area, and 10 nurses left work to experience the disaster with their families. The two tools that were used to measure stress included the Impact of Events Scale (IES) and the Symptom Checklist. The research questions were as follows:

1. What is the relationship between the time lapsed after the disaster and the frequency of symptoms of psychological distress?
2. What is the relationship between family presence during the disaster and the frequency of symptoms of psychological distress?
3. Is there a relationship between the amount of damage inflicted by the disaster to one's home and the frequency of symptoms of psychological distress?

The findings regarding question 1 indicate that symptoms for all groups were significantly lower at 4 and 12 months compared with the 1-month scores. For question 2, the fewest symptoms were present for the home-with-family group, and the greatest symptoms were exhibited for the out-of-the-area group at 1 month, with a decrease in symptoms at 4 months for all groups. All groups had a reemergence of symptoms at 1 year, with the at-work group evidencing the greatest distress. Although there were no significant findings for question 3, the trend was that the more damage caused from the hurricane, the more the impact and the higher the symptom score. Among the many recommendations delineated by the authors to minimize the stress of nurses working during a disaster were (1) reduce patient census immediately, (2) attempt to staff with nurses who volunteer, (3) allow nurses to maintain telephone contact with their families or allow families to come to the nurses, (4) maintain adequate supplies of water, light, and nourishing food, (5) maintain a supportive environment, and (6) create an opportunity for debriefing, where nurses can discuss their personal feelings and experiences. The authors also recommend that the implications of requiring nurses to choose between work and family during times of disaster merit further study.

The American Red Cross (1993) recommends strategies for dealing with stress while working at the disaster. The strategies include the following:

1. Getting enough sleep
2. Taking time away from the disaster (e.g., breaks)
3. Avoiding alcohol
4. Eating frequently in small amounts
5. Using humor to break the tension and provide relief
6. Using positive self-talk
7. Not refusing defusing or debriefing time
8. Staying in touch with people at home
9. Keeping a journal
10. Providing mutual support

Delayed stress reactions, or those that occur once the disaster is over, include exhaustion and an inability to adjust to the slower pace of work or home. (American Red Cross, 1991). Other emotions out of the ordinary may be evident but are normal for someone who has been involved with a disaster. Disappointment may be felt as family members and friends do not seem as interested in what the worker has been through and as the homecoming, in general, does not live up to expectations. Frustration and conflict may occur because the worker's needs may be totally inconsistent from the family's and co-workers' needs. Frustration and conflict also occur as a result of having left the disaster site, when a real or perceived belief remains that much more could have been done (Gaffney et al., 1992). Issues or problems that once seemed pressing may now seem trivial. Anger may set in as others present problems that seem trivial compared with those that were faced by the victims left behind. Disaster workers may fantasize about returning to the disaster site, where they perceive their actions to have been more appreciated than at home or the office. Finally, mood swings are common and are part of a normal process to resolve conflicting feelings. Feelings or actions that persist or that the worker perceives are interfering with daily life should be dealt with by a trained mental health professional (American Red Cross, 1991).

RECOVERY

The stage of disaster known as recovery occurs as all involved agencies pull together to restore the economic and civic life of the community (American Red Cross, 1993). For example, the government takes the lead in rebuilding efforts, while the business community attempts to provide economic support. Many religious organizations help with rebuilding efforts as well. The Internal Revenue Service educates victims as to how to write off losses, and the Department of Housing and Urban Development provides grants for temporary housing. The CDC provides continuing surveillance and epidemiological services. Voluntary agencies continue to assess individual and community needs and meet those needs as they are able.

Role of the Community Health Nurse in Disaster Recovery

The role of the community health nurse in the recovery phase is as varied as in the preparedness and response phases of a disaster. Flexibility remains an important component of a successful recovery operation. Community cleanup efforts can incur a host of physical and psychological problems. For example, the physical stress of moving heavy objects can cause back injury, severe fatigue, and even death from heart attacks. In addition, the continuing threat of communicable disease will continue as long as the water supply remains threatened and the living conditions remain crowded (Gaffney et al., 1992). Community health nurses must remain vigilant in teaching proper hygiene and making sure immunization records are up to date.

Acute and chronic illnesses can be exacerbated by the prolonged effects of disaster. The psychological stress of cleanup and moving can bring about feelings of severe hopelessness, depression, and grief (Figure 20-6). Recovery can be impeded by short-term psychological effects eventually merging with the long-term results of living in adverse circumstances (Richman, 1993). In some cases, stress can lead to suicide and domestic abuse (Gaffney et al., 1992). In addition, although most people eventually recover from disasters, mental distress may persist in those vulnerable populations who continue to live in chronic adversity (Goenjian, 1993). Referrals to mental health professionals should continue as long as the need exists.

The community health nurse must also remain alert for environmental health hazards during the recovery phase of a disaster. Home visits may lead the nurse to uncover situations such as a faulty housing structure, lack of water supply, or lack of electricity. Objects that are dangerous and need to be removed may have been blown into the yard from a tornado or floated in from a flood. In addition, the nurse must be attentive to the dangers of live or dead animals and rodents that might be considered harmful to a person's health. An example of this would be finding snakes in and around homes once the waters from a flood start to recede. The role of case finding and referral remains critical during the recovery phase and in some cases will continue for a long time. In the end, all the nurses and organizations in the world can only provide partnerships with the victims of a disaster. Ultimately, it is up to each individual to recover on his or her own.

Wherever disaster calls there I shall go. I ask not for whom, but only where I am needed.

From the Creed of the Red Cross Nurse

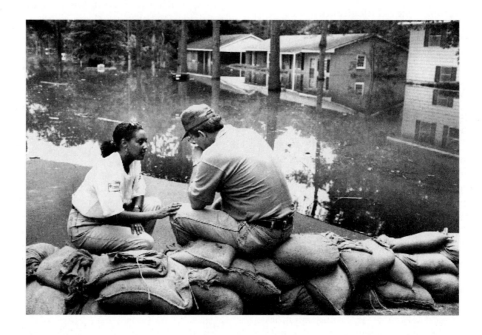

FIGURE 20-6

The psychological stress of cleanup and moving can bring about feelings of severe hopelessness, depression, and grief. (Photo courtesy the American Red Cross. All rights reserved in all countries.)

Clinical Application

Paula, a community health nurse in a midsize public health department in Lincoln, Nebraska, has been called to serve on her first national disaster assignment. She has taken both the disaster health and the disaster mental health training courses at the local American Red Cross chapter and has volunteered for the local disaster action team for the past 18 months. Although all of her experience so far has been with local level I disasters, she has looked forward to the challenge of working on a national assignment all year. Paula has made previous arrangements with her nursing supervisor to take approximately 3 weeks of vacation if and when she ever received the call to serve.

The director of nursing at Paula's local Red Cross chapter has informed Paula that a level III hurricane has hit south Miami and its surrounding areas. As part of the FRP, the Red Cross will be responsible for shelter management and mass feeding. The director asks Paula if she would feel comfortable helping to manage a shelter in an elementary school cafeteria in Homestead, Fla. Although Paula has only had one experience managing a shelter for 2 days in a local level I disaster, she believes she is up to the challenge. The director assures her that many experienced disaster workers will be there to assist her with her role. The Red Cross director reminds Paula that she has been well trained and that the most important attribute she can bring to the disaster is her flexibility. Paula is to fly to Miami International Airport this evening at 5 pm, spend the night at the Airport Hotel, and meet the designated Red Cross van at 8 am to be taken with six other nurses from around the United States to their designated areas of assignment.

Paula arrived at Kennedy Elementary School at 9 AM. The devastation that Paula encountered en route to the school had already had a negative effect on her psyche. Paula had never seen so much destruction and devastation in her life. She thought this is what it must be like in a war zone. However, once she entered the school and began to become oriented to what her role was to be for the next few weeks, she began to gain a sense of purpose and belonging. Paula understood why she had been chosen to serve in this particular school, since the vast majority of the shelter population only spoke Spanish, and Paula had stated on her disaster enrollment form that she was fluent in Spanish.

Paula was assigned to help with client intake. She was to assess every client as to their physical and mental state as they entered the shelter and determine their short-term and long-term needs. Many of Paula's clients were under great stress as they recalled to her the horrors of living through the storm. Paula always patiently listened to the disaster victims, referring many of her most distraught clients to the mental health counselor assigned to her school. She began to prioritize other needs as they arose. For example, she found that many clients left their medications behind and were in need of continuing therapy. Other needs included diapers and formulas for the babies, prescription glasses, and clothing. Paula's supervisor communicated with Paula regularly to determine client needs. The daily list that Paula's supervisor compiled was added to a master "need list." Once an accurate assessment of all the disaster victims began to be realized, donated items could be matched to the needs.

As the days went on, the stress level in Paula's shelter began to increase. Paula realized that the crowded living conditions and lack of privacy began to take a toll on the residents. The children in particular were bored and found it very confining to live in a shelter. In addition, the constant noise from the generators, sirens, and helicopters flying overhead was adding to the overstimulation that everyone was already experiencing, including the staff.

Around day 10 of Paula's assignment, she began to experience pounding headaches and was finding it difficult to concentrate. Paula believed she would be fine, but the mental health counselor told Paula she was experiencing a stress reaction. She assigned Paula to a debriefing/support group that met every evening at 7 PM. Once Paula began to share her feelings regarding her stress, her headaches began to disappear and she began to face each day feeling better about her role in helping her clients.

When Paula's 3 weeks were up, she began to have very mixed feelings about returning to Lincoln. She was glad to be going home but believed that much more could be done to help the disaster victims. After all, their lives would not return to normal for weeks or months. Although her co-workers praised her for meeting the challenge of working on a major national disaster, Paula thought they did not truly understand what she had been through. She could not adequately describe to them the devastation that her clients had been through and felt frustrated at some of their comments. She remembered that the on-site mental health counselor had encouraged her to keep a diary of her feelings, so she began to do so. After a short transition period, Paula began to meet the challenges of her job at the public health department with as much enthusiasm as she had before leaving for the disaster in Miami. She realized that disasters do happen, and she was glad that she had the opportunity to help. Paula now believes that she has gained much experience in working on a disaster and has since volunteered to be a member of her community's disaster planning committee. In addition, Paula feels confident that with her experience in disaster management, she will be an asset to any team that calls on her in the future.

Key Concepts

- The number of natural disasters has remained constant, but the number of man-made disasters and ensuing deaths continue to rise sharply.
- The dollar amount required to recover from a disaster has risen sharply because of the amount of technology that must be restored.
- The director general of the World Health Organization has made the decade of the 1990s the International Decade for Natural Disaster Reduction based on a worldwide need for disaster education and a curtailment of the fatalistic approach to disasters that so many people take.
- Professional preparedness entails an awareness and understanding of the disaster plan at work and in the community.
- To counteract a historical lack of use or misuse of community health nurses in disaster planning, response, and recovery, these nurses must become involved in their community's planning efforts.
- Disaster health and disaster mental health training from an official agency such as the American Red Cross helps prepare community health nurses for the many opportunities that await them in disaster preparedness, response, and recovery.
- The response to a disaster is determined by its assigned level. Levels are not determined by the number of casualties per se but by the amount of resources needed.
- Helping patients to maintain a safe environment and advocating for environmental safety measures in the community are key roles for the community health nurse during all phases of disaster management.
- Becoming knowledgeable about available community resources, especially for vulnerable populations, during the preparedness stage of disaster management ensures smoother response and recovery stages.
- The Federal Response Plan may be activated if a disaster is so significant in its effect that it will overwhelm the capability of state and local governments to carry out the extensive emergency operations needed for community restoration. In all, 26 federal agencies and the Red Cross have specific functions to carry out in such an event.
- People in a community react differently to a disaster depending on the type, cause, and location of the disaster; its magnitude, extent of damage, and duration; and the amount of warning that was provided. Individual variables that cause people to react differently include their age, cultural background, health status, social support structure, and general adaptability to a crisis.
- Great stress is exhibited by nurses who are caring for patients and who are disaster victims themselves.
- Disaster shelter nurses are exposed to a variety of physical and emotional complaints, including stress. Stress may be instigated by the shock of the disaster, loss of personal possessions, fear of the unknown, living in proximity to strangers, and boredom.
- The degree of worker stress during disasters depends on the nature of the disaster, role in the disaster, individual stamina, noise level, adequacy of work space, potential for physical danger, and stimulus overload, especially being exposed to death and trauma.
- Symptoms of worker stress during disasters include minor tremors, nausea, loss of concentration, difficulty thinking and remembering, irritability, fatigue, and other somatic disorders.
- A key attribute in aiding disaster victims is flexibility.
- The stage of disaster known as recovery occurs as all involved agencies pull together to restore the economic and civic life of the community.

Critical Thinking Activities

1. Select a vulnerable population within your community and determine what special needs the group would have in time of disaster. What community resources are currently available to help this group?
2. Describe the role of the community health nurse in the preparedness, response, and recovery stages of disaster.
3. Interview a community health nurse who has participated in a disaster to determine what role the nurse played and the reaction to that role.
4. Conduct an interview with an official from the fire department, civil defense, American Red Cross, or other agencies involved with disaster preparedness and response to determine your community's plan.
5. Discuss the advantages and disadvantages of serving on a disaster team, either in your own community or another community. Decide whether you would be a good candidate to serve on a disaster team.
6. Contact your local public health department to determine its role in a local disaster, including the role of the nurses who work there.
7. Find out the disaster plan for your place of employment.

Bibliography

Alson R, Alexander D, Leonard RB, Stringer LW: Analysis of medical treatment at a field hospital following hurricane Andrew, 1992, *Ann Emerg Med* 22(11):78-84, 1993.

American Red Cross: *Disaster health services. I. Instructor manual,* ARC Pub No 3076-1, Washington, DC, 1989, Red Cross.

American Red Cross: *Coping with disaster: emotional health issues for victims,* ARC Pub No 4475, Washington, DC, 1991, Red Cross.

American Red Cross: *Coping with disaster: returning home from a disaster assignment,* ARC Pub No 4473, Washington, DC, 1991, Red Cross.

American Red Cross: *Disaster mental health services,* ARC Pub No 3050M, Washington, DC, 1991, Red Cross.

American Red Cross: *Disaster mental health services. I.* ARC Pub No 3077-1A, Washington, DC, 1993, Red Cross.

Berglin SL: Emergency nurses in community disaster planning, *J Emerg Nurs* (16)4:290-292, 1990.

Chubon SJ: Home care during the aftermath of Hurricane Hugo, *Public Health Nurs* (9)2:97-102, 1992.

Cohen RE, Ahearn FL: *Handbook for mental health care of disaster victims,* Baltimore, 1980. Johns Hopkins University Press.

Demi AS, Miles MS: Understanding psychologic reactions to disaster, *J Emerg Nurs* 9:11-16, 1983.

Demi AS, Miles MS: An examination of nursing leadership following a disaster, *Topics Clin Nurs* 6:63-78, 1984.

Dinerman N: Disaster preparedness: observations and perspectives, *J Emerg Nurs* (16)4:252-254, 1990.

Dixon M: Disaster planning, medical response: organization and preparation, *AAOHN J* 34:580-584, 1986.

Errington G: Stress among disaster nurses and relief workers, *Int Nurs Rev* 36(3): 80, 90-91, 1989.

Federal Emergency Management Agency and American Red Cross: *Your family disaster plan,* FEMA L-191, ARC 4466, Washington, DC, 1992, The Agency and Red Cross.

Federal Emergency Management Agency: *Federal response plan,* FEMA-229(1), Washington, DC, 1992.

Gaffney JK, Schodorf L, Jones G: DMATs respond to Andrew and Iniki, *J Emerg Med Services* November 1992, pp 76-79.

Goenjian A: A mental health relief program in Armenia after the 1988 earthquake, *Br J Psychiatry* 163:230-239, 1993.

Hogan J, Pega P, Forkapa B: A civilian-sponsored DMAT: a community's collaboration among three hospitals, *J Emerg Nurs* 16(4):245-247, 1990.

Kates RW, Hass JE, Amaral DJ, Olson RA, Ramos R, Olson R: Human impact of the Managua earthquake, *Science,* 182:981-990, 1973.

Lander JF, Alexander RH, Downing TW: *Inventory of natural hazards data resources in federal government,* Washington, DC, 1979, US Department of Commerce, US Department of the Interior.

Laube J: Psychological reactions of nurses in disaster, *Nurs Res* 22:343-347, 1973.

Laube-Morgan J: The professional's psychological response in disaster: implications for practice, *J Psychosoc Nurs* 30(2):17-22, 1992.

Lehnhof DB: Planning mass casualty drills. In Garcia LM, editor: *Disaster nursing: planning, assessment, and intervention,* Rockville, Md, 1985, Aspen.

Lillibridge SR, Noji EK, Frederick MB: Disaster assessment: the emergency health evaluation of a population affected by a disaster, *Ann Emerg Med* 22(11):72-77, 1993.

Office of US Foreign Disaster Assistance: *Disaster history: significant data on major disasters worldwide, 1990-present.* Washington, DC, 1990, The Office.

Orr SM, Robinson WA: The Hyatt Regency skywalk collapse: an EMS-based disaster response, *Ann Emerg Med* 12:601-605, 1983.

Pickens S: The decade for natural disaster reduction: the role of health care workers, *Nurs Health Care* (13)4:192-195, 1992.

Public health responds to disaster: the Los Angeles earthquake, *Nation's Health,* March 1994, pp 1, 6-7.

Richman N: After the flood, *Am J Public Health* 83(11):1522-1524, 1993.

Richtmeier JL, Miller JR: Psychological aspects of disaster situations. In Garcia LM, editor: *Disaster nursing: planning, assessment, and intervention,* Rockville, Md, 1985, Aspen.

Sklar DP: Casualty patterns and disasters, *J World Assoc Emerg Disaster Med* 3:49-51, 1987.

Switzer KH: Functioning in a community health setting. In Garcia LM, editor: *Disaster nursing: planning, assessment, and intervention,* Rockville, MD, 1985, Aspen.

Taggart SB: Background and historical perspective. In Garcia LM, editor: *Disaster nursing: planning, assessment, and intervention,* Rockville, Md, 1985, Aspen.

Waeckerle JF: Disaster planning and response, *N Engl J Med* 324(12):815-821, 1991.

Waters KA, Selander J, Stuart GW: Psychological adaption of nurses post-disaster, *Issues Ment Health Nurs* 13:177-190, 1992.

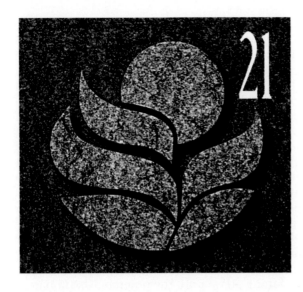

21

Program Management

Marcia Stanhope

Objectives ▼

After reading this chapter, the student should be able to do the following:

◆ Compare the program management process to the nursing process.
◆ Analyze the program planning process and its application to community health nursing.
◆ Compare and contrast a program planning method to use in community health nursing practice.
◆ Identify the benefits of program planning.
◆ Analyze the components of program evaluation and application to community health nursing.
◆ Identify evaluation methods and techniques.
◆ Name program evaluation sources.
◆ Describe types of program evaluation measures.
◆ Describe types of cost studies applied to program management.

Outline ▼

Key Terms ▼

assessment of need
case register
cost accounting
cost benefit
cost effectiveness
cost efficiency
cost studies
evaluation
evaluation of program effectiveness
formative evaluation
health index
health planning
health program planning
needs assessment
outcome
planning
process
program
program evaluation
strategic planning
structure
summative evaluation
tracer method

Program management consists of assessing, planning, implementing, and evaluating the processes involved in the life of a program. This chapter focuses primarily on planning and evaluation. Although presented in separate discussions, these factors are interrelated, dependent processes that work together to bring about a successful program (U.S. Department of Health and Human Services [DHHS], 1989). This chapter does not deal with implementation because most chapters in the text focus on implementation. The program management process parallels the nursing process. One is applied to a program, whereas the other is applied to clients.

The process of program management, as with the nursing process, consists of a rational decision-making system designed to help nurses know when to make a decision to develop a program (problem identification), to know where they want to be at the end of the program (assessment), how to decide what to do to have a successful program (planning), how to develop a plan to go from where they are to where they want to be (implementation), how to know they are getting there (formative evaluation), and what to measure to know what they are doing is appropriate (summative evaluation) (DHHS, 1989).

With more emphasis on accountability for nursing actions on client outcomes, the introduction of prospective payment systems, and health care reform, the focus of nursing is changing. Planning for nursing services is essential today if the nursing discipline is to survive in the field of health care delivery.

This chapter examines how nurses can act instead of react by planning programs that can be evaluated for their effectiveness in meeting their social purpose. This discussion focuses on the historical development of health planning and evaluation, a generic program planning and evaluation method, the benefits of planning and evaluation, the elements of planning and evaluation, and cost studies applied to program evaluation.

DEFINITIONS AND GOALS

A **program** is an organized response designed to meet the assessed needs of individuals, families, groups, or communities by reducing or eliminating one or more health problems. Examples of specific programs in public health nursing are home health programs, immunization programs, health risk screening programs for industrial workers, and family planning clinic programs. These specific programs are usually conducted under the direction of a total program plan of the local health department. More broadly based group and community programs are the community school health program, the occupational health and safety program, the environmental health program, and community programs directed at specific illnesses through special interest groups (e.g., American Heart Association, American Cancer Society, March of Dimes).

Planning is defined as the selecting and carrying out of a series of actions designed to achieve stated goals (Kropf, 1995). The goal of planning is to ensure the acceptability, equality, efficiency, and effectiveness of services. **Evaluation** is defined as the methods used to determine whether a service is needed and likely to be used, whether it is conducted as planned, and whether the service actually helps people in need (Posavac and Carey, 1989). Evaluation for the purpose of assessing whether objectives are met or planned activities are completed is referred to as **formative evaluation.** This type of evaluation begins with an assessment of the need for the program. Evaluation to assess program outcomes or as a follow-up of the results of the program activities is called **summative evaluation.**

Program evaluation is an ongoing process from the initial planning phase until the program is terminated. The major goals of program evaluation are to determine the relevance, progress, efficiency, effectiveness, and impact of program activities to the clients served (Veney and Kaluzny, 1991).

HISTORICAL OVERVIEW OF HEALTH CARE PLANNING AND EVALUATION

As the health care delivery system has grown in the past 60 years, emphasis in **health planning** and evaluation has increased. Factors that have fostered increased interest in planning and evaluation are advances in health care technology and consumer education, increased health care expectations, third-party payers, budget pressures, increased professional conflicts, focus on preventive care, new focus on health care as a business, unionization of health care workers, urbanization, increased health risks, personnel shortages, and increased health care costs.

In the 1920s the American Public Health Association's Committees on Administrative Practice and Evaluation emphasized the need for public health officers to engage in better program planning to change the haphazard method by which public health programs were begun (Pickett and Hanlon, 1990). During this period the Committee on Costs of Medical Care studied the economic and social aspects of health services. The committee recognized the need for comprehensive health care planning, citing the rising costs and the unequal distribution of health services across the nation (Committee on the Costs of Medical Care, 1970; Kovner, 1995). As a result of the committee report, a few states began to coordinate medical services for their residents. However, regionalized planning for health services nationwide was not attempted until the American Hospital Association established its Committee on Postwar Planning in 1944.

The post–World War II era also brought an interest in evaluating program effectiveness. As government and third-party payers began to finance health care services and money became more plentiful, public demand for health services grew. As a result, numbers and kinds of health care agencies increased; laws were passed to increase the scope of and control over health care, and the health care delivery system was beginning to be held accountable for its actions (Pickett and Hanlon, 1990). The federal government's first attempt to legislate health planning was the passage of the Hospital Survey and Construction Act in 1946 (also called the Hill-Burton Act).

The 1960s were marked by the Great Society programs of President Johnson. The social, economic, and health programs that grew out of the Great Society concept were designed primarily to meet peoples' needs and to show that the federal government could deliver services to the public efficiently. For example, the *Community Mental Health Centers Act* of 1963 (P.L. 88-464) gave state governments the authority to plan mental health programs to meet population needs. This legislation clearly defined the roles of consumers and professionals as advisors in the planning process for all future health planning legislation. In 1965 the Regional Medical Program legislation (P.L. 89-239) was passed to upgrade the quality of tertiary health care services to consumers. This legislation required health providers and consumers to work together in groups to address a number of issues in health care, such as heart disease, cancer, kidney disease, and cerebrovascular accidents. Thus the phrase "partnership for health" was coined.

During this time the Office of Health Planning was established in the Department of Health, Education, and Welfare (now the Department of Health and Human Services, or DHHS). Because the scope and functioning of the Office of Health Planning was limited and had no direct authority for national health planning, the Eighty-Ninth Congress passed the Comprehensive Health Planning (CHP) and Public Health Services amendments in 1966, P.L. 89-749, in an attempt to develop a national health planning system. This was the law that provided grants for planning, development, and implementation of a variety of public health services (Rikach et al., 1992).

The CHP amendments also provided a format for the development of later planning legislation. From the CHP experience, the states and federal government developed a method for organizing planning within states. Data on existing needs and resources were collected, procedures for reviewing facilities and program changes were established, and methods for cooperation between governmental and health care agencies were developed.

Although the CHP legislation proved inadequate for comprehensive health planning, the strengths of the planning legislation led Congress to pass the National Health Planning and Resources Development Act (P.L. 93-641) in 1974. This act was a landmark in health care legislation because of its specific directions regarding the structure, process, and functions of a national health planning system.

Although P.L. 93-641 provided a more comprehensive structure and more power over federal program funds than the CHP amendments of 1966, there still existed limited authority to carry out some of the more critical tasks of improving the health of residents, increasing accessibility and quality of services, restraining costs, and preventing unnecessary duplication of services. Power over the private health care sector continued to be essentially nonexistent.

As *new federalism* became the catch phrase of the 1980s and emphasis was placed on cost shifting, cost reduction, and more competition within the health care system, President Ronald Reagan proposed doing away with the federal government's role in health planning. In 1981, with cutbacks in federal spending, states began the takeover or dismantling of their own health planning systems as established under P.L. 93-641. Today the national health planning system has come to a halt. The federal, state, and consumer partnership for health is nonexistent.

In 1993, with President Clinton's emphasis on health care reform, the decision was made that the government would continue not to be involved in health planning but would use its power to set limits on health insurance costs and limit overall health care expenditures. In this way it would influence health planning decisions made by the private health care agencies and providers (Kropf, 1995).

The process of health planning today is in the control of hospitals, physicians, health maintenance organizations (HMOs), pharmaceutical companies, equipment companies, and insurance companies (Kropf, 1995; Sofaer, 1988). The outcome of the national and state health care reform effort is often influenced by the political party in power. The community health nurse must be involved in aspects of health planning for the community in which he or she lives to influence the direction of health care reform.

In addition, internal health care agency planning is necessary to meet the goals and objectives of providing efficient, effective health care services to the consumer at reasonable cost. Pickett and Hanlon (1990) emphasized the responsibility of community health personnel to participate in internal planning and evaluation to solve the problems of a client population. Internal health care agency planning is often affected by the health care planning within the community as well as national health care planning.

BENEFITS OF PROGRAM PLANNING

Systematic planning for meeting client needs benefits clients, nurses, and the employing agencies. Planning focuses attention on what the organization and health provider are attempting to do for clients. Planning assists in identifying the resources and activities that are essential in meeting the objectives of client services. Planning reduces role ambiguity (uncertainty) by assigning responsibility to specific providers to meet program objectives.

Planning also reduces uncertainty within the program environment and enhances the abilities of the provider and the agency to cope with the external environment. Everyone involved with the program can anticipate what will be needed to implement the program, what will occur during implementation, and what the program outcomes will be. Planning helps the provider and the agency anticipate events. Finally, planning allows for quality decision making and better control over the actual program results. Today this type of planning is referred to as **strategic planning** and involves the successful matching of client needs with specific provider strengths and competencies and agency resources.

Planning usually reflects the planner's desire to reduce the gap between the program goals and the realities of program implementation and to minimize unanticipated occurrences during program implementation. Inherent in the planning process is the desire to implement a reality-based program that can be readily evaluated.

THE PLANNING PROCESS

Health program planning is affected by governmental control over licensure and funding, by the social structure, and by the cultural and belief system in which the program must function. Program planning is essential to meet federal, state, and local government mandates for funding, philanthropic organization funding guidelines, and internal agency requirements.

Planning programs and planning for the evaluation of programs are two of the most important activities for community health nurses to ensure successful program implementation. Whether the program being planned is a national health insurance program such as Medicare, a state health care program such as early childhood developmental screening programs, or a local program such as vision screening for elementary schoolchildren, the essential elements of planning are the same.

Needs assessment is a key ingredient in the planning process. The target population for any program must be identified and involved in program development. If the client population does not recognize the need for a health services program, that program is destined to fail regardless of the commitment of health providers and the program's resources.

A number of tools are available for assisting planners in needs assessment. Some of the major tools used for needs assessment are census data, key informants, community forums, surveys of existing community agencies, surveys of community residents, and statistical indicators.

Several procedural methods can be applied to plan program offerings. A few of these methods are the Planning, Programming, and Budgeting System; Program Evaluation Review Technique; Critical Path Method; Multi-Attribute Utility Method; and Program Planning Method.

Table 21-1   Basic Planning Process

Basic planning	Elements
1. Formulation	Client identifies problems
2. Conceptualization	Provider group identifies possible solutions
3. Detailing	Client, provider analyze available solutions
4. Evaluation	Clients, providers, administrators select best plan
5. Implementation	Best plan presented to administrators for funding

Nutt (1984) describes a basic planning process that is reflected in the steps of most planning methods. The **process** includes five planning stages for program development: formulation, conceptualization, detailing, evaluation, and implementation (Table 21-1).

Formulation

The initial and most critical step in planning for a health program is defining the problem and assessing client need. This stage in the planning process can be *preactive*, projecting a future need; *reactive*, defining the problem based on past needs identified by the consumer or the sponsoring agency; *inactive*, defining the problem based on the existing health state of the population to be served; or *interactive*, describing the problem using past and present data to project future population needs (Achoff, 1982).

Program planners must verify the existence of a current health problem that is being ignored or being unsuccessfully treated in a client group. These data will provide the rationale to establish a new program or revise existing programs to meet the needs of the client group. The **assessment of need** is defined as a systematic appraisal of type, depth, and scope of problems as perceived by clients, health providers, or both.

The needs assessment process includes six steps (Figure 21-1): (1) identify the client population, (2) identify the needs to be met, (3) specify the size and distribution of the client population, (4) set boundaries for the client group, (5) clarify the perspectives on the program, and (6) identify the program resources (Posavac and Carey, 1989; Rossi and Freeman, 1989).

The *client population* may be identified as a community or group, as families or individuals. The client population should be defined specifically by its biological and psychosocial characteristics, by geographical location, and by the problems to be addressed. For example, in a community with a large number of preschool children who require immunizations to enter school, the client population may be described as all children between ages 4 and 6 years residing in Cen-

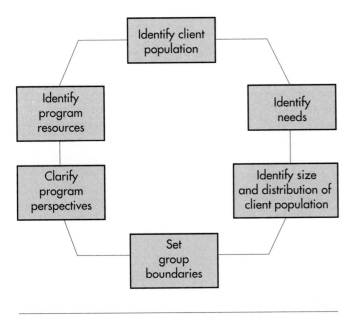

FIGURE 21-1

Steps in the needs assessment process.

tral County who have not had up-to-date immunizations.

The *needs to be met* for the client population must be identified by both the client and the health provider. *If the client population does not recognize the need, the program will usually fail.* A health education program may be necessary to alert the population to the existing need. In the example of the need for immunization of preschool children, public service announcements on television and radio and in newspapers may be used to alert parents to laws requiring immunizations, to the continued existence of communicable diseases, and to communicable diseases, such as smallpox, that have been successfully eradicated by immunization programs. A good example of the use of media is the 1990 outbreak of rubella in Los Angeles. Local and national television was used to bring attention to the problem, to encourage parents to have children immunized, and to encourage other communities to launch campaigns to prevent other outbreaks.

Specifying the size and distribution of a client population for a program involves more than counting the number of persons in the community who may be eligible for the program. More specifically, it involves determining the number of persons with the problem who are unserved by existing programs and the number of eligible persons who have and have not taken advantage of existing services. For an example, consider again the community need of a preschool immunization program. In planning the program, the estimates of numbers of preschool children in the county may be obtained from census data or birth certificates. One then must determine the number of children unserved and the number of children who have not used services for which they are eligible.

Boundaries for the client population are primarily established by defining the size and distribution of the client population. The boundaries will stipulate who is included and who is excluded in the health program. If the fictional immunization program were designed to serve only preschool children of low-income families, all other preschool children would be excluded.

Perspectives on the program might differ among health providers, agency administrators, policy makers, and potential clients. Collecting data on the opinions and attitudes of all persons directly or indirectly involved with the program's success is essential to determining the program's feasibility, the need to redefine the problems, or the decision to develop a new program or expand an existing program. For example, policy makers in the 1970s determined that neighborhood health clinics were the answer to providing service for low-income residents. They discovered that their perspectives were not the same as those of most health providers or clients, who were not supportive of developing neighborhood clinics. The neighborhood health clinic concept failed because the clients would not use them. If the policy makers had explored the perspectives of the clients when planning the program, they might have chosen another option.

Before implementing a health program, one must also *assess available resources.* Program resources include personnel, facilities, equipment, and financing. The numbers and kinds of personnel available to implement a program must be determined. The availability of supplies and up-to-date equipment is as essential a resource for implementing a program as the source and amount of funds. If any one of the essential resources is unavailable, the program is likely to be inadequate to meet the needs of the client population.

Needs Assessment Tools

A number of tools exist to assist the program planner in the needs assessment process. The major tools, used for needs assessment, summarized in Table 21-2, are census data, key informants, community forums, surveys of existing community agencies with similar programs, surveys of residents of the community to be served (client population), and statistical indicators (Rossi and Freeman, 1989).

Conceptualization

The need and demand for a program are determined through the formulation process. The conceptualization stage of planning creates options for solving the problem and considers several solutions. Each option for program solution is examined for its uncertainties and consequences, leading to a set of outcomes.

When considering alternative solutions to the problem, some will have more risk or uncertainties than others. One must decide between the solution that involves more risk and the solution that is free of risk. A "do nothing" decision is always the decision with the least risk to the provider. When choosing a solution, one looks at the probability of achieving the desired outcome. After careful thought about each possible

Table 21-2 Summary of Needs Assessment Tools

Name	Definition	Advantages	Disadvantages
Community forum	Community, group, organization, open meeting	Low cost Learn perspectives of large number of persons	Limited data Limited expression of views Discourages less powerful Becomes arena to discuss political issues
Key informant	Identify, select, and question knowledgeable leaders	Provides picture of services needed	Bias of leaders Community characteristics may be incorrectly perceived by informants
Indicators approach	Existing data used to determine problem	Excellent data on problems and location of client groups Observations made at regular intervals show trends New problems can be identified	Data may be obsolete Growth and change in population may make data outdated
Survey of existing agencies	Estimates of client population via services used at similar community agencies	Easy method to estimate size of client group Know extent of services offered in existing programs	Records and data may be unreliable All cases of need may not be reported Exaggeration of services may occur
Surveys/census	Measurement of total or sample client population by interview or questionnaire	Direct and accurate data on client population and their problems	Expensive Technically demanding Need many interviews or observations

solution to the problem, one should rethink the solutions. The information collected from census data, key informants, community forums, surveys of existing community agencies, and statistical indicators should be used to develop these alternative solutions.

Decision trees are useful graphic aids that will give a picture of the solutions and the consequences and risks of each. Such a pictorial graph of the process of identifying a solution helps clients and administrators to understand why one solution may be chosen over another. Figure 21-2 shows the process of conceptualization using a decision tree.

Although in the immunization example the best consequence would be for families to provide for immunizations, one must consider the value of this action to the parents, the odds that immunizations will occur if a formal clinic is not established, the cost to the parents versus the taxpayer, and the cost to the community. Costs to the community include the possibility of increased incidence of communicable disease or mortality, and increased need for more expensive services to treat the diseases if children are not immunized. If the parents provide the immunizations, costs to the taxpayer and to the community are low.

Detailing

In this phase the provider, with client input, determines the possibilities of solving a problem using one of the solutions identified. The provider details the costs, resources, and program activities needed to choose one of the solutions from the conceptualization phase. For each of the three proposed alternatives in Figure 21-2, the program planner must list activities that would need to be implemented to use each of the alternatives. To illustrate, consider again the immunizations scenario. Using the proposed solution of encouraging the *parents* to provide the immunizations, the best consequence, examples of activities include developing a script for a health education program and implementing a TV program to encourage parents to take children to their physician. If the second, third, or fourth best consequence was chosen, offering a clinic 8 hours per day at the health department and providing a mobile clinic to each day-care center for 4 hours each day to provide the immunizations would be possible activities.

For each of the alternatives, the program planner lists the resources needed to implement each activity. The resources to be considered include all costs of personnel, supplies, equipment, facilities, and acceptability to the clients and the administrators of the program. In the example, personnel could include nurses, volunteers, and clerks; supplies might include handouts, bandaids, medications, records, and consent forms; equipment might include syringes, needles, stethoscopes, and blood pressure cuffs; and facilities might include a TV studio for a media blitz on the education program and examination tables, chairs, and emergency carts. Finally, the costs of each solution

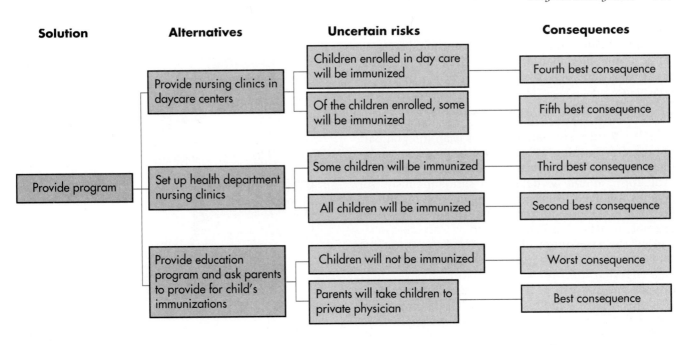

Solution **Alternatives** **Uncertain risks** **Consequences**

Provide program

- Provide nursing clinics in daycare centers
  - Children enrolled in day care will be immunized → Fourth best consequence
  - Of the children enrolled, some will be immunized → Fifth best consequence
- Set up health department nursing clinics
  - Some children will be immunized → Third best consequence
  - All children will be immunized → Second best consequence
- Provide education program and ask parents to provide for child's immunizations
  - Children will not be immunized → Worst consequence
  - Parents will take children to private physician → Best consequence

FIGURE 21-2

Ranking of solutions to problem: providing a preschool immunization program to low-income children, using a decision tree.

must be considered by determining the costs of personnel, supplies, equipment, and facilities for each solution. As indicated, clients should review each solution for acceptability.

Evaluation

In the evaluative phase, each alternative would be weighed to judge the costs, benefits, and acceptability to the client, community, and provider. The information outlined in the detailing phase would be used to rank the solutions for choice by client and provider based on cost, benefit, and acceptance. Consideration must be given to the solution that will provide the desired outcomes. Looking at available information might suggest whether each of the options had been tried before in another place or by someone else. The results from other sources would be helpful in deciding whether a chosen solution would be useful.

Implementation

In the implementation phase, the clients, providers, and administrators select the best plan to solve the original problem. In this phase, change theory is useful to help create an environment in which the best solution may be supported by funding. Providing reasons why a particular solution was chosen will help the provider to obtain the approval of the administration for the plan. Involving clients and administrators throughout the planning process helps to promote acceptance of the plan.

PROGRAM EVALUATION
Benefits of Program Evaluation

The major benefit of program evaluation is that it determines and demonstrates whether the program is fulfilling its purpose. It should answer the questions: Are the needs for which the program was designed being met? Are the problems it was designed to solve being solved? This is critical information for funding agencies, top-level decision makers, accreditation reviews, and the community at large. Evaluation data may be used to justify expanding the program, reducing the program, or even closing it.

Quality assurance programs are prime examples of program evaluation in health care delivery. Evaluation data are used to justify the continued existence of programs in community health.

Program evaluation focuses on goal attainment and the efficiency and effectiveness of program activities. Many methods of program evaluation are described in the literature. The primary method of evaluation used in health care today in Donabedian's Evaluative Framework. The **tracer method** and **case register** are other methods applied to program evaluation.

Program records and community indexes serve as the major source of information for program evaluation. Surveys, interviews, observations, and tests are ways to assess consumer and participant response to health programs. Cost studies help identify program benefits and effectiveness.

As economic resources become scarce, nursing and the health care system must be able to justify their existence, prove that their services are responsive to consumer needs, and show their professional concern for accountability. Planning and evaluation will assist in meeting these objectives.

Planning for the Evaluative Process

Planning for the evaluative process is an integral part of program planning. When plans for program implementation are being developed, the plan for program evaluation should be developed simultaneously. All persons involved in program implementation should be a part of the plan for program evaluation. This is an example of what has been defined as formative evaluation: the assessment of need. The basic questions to be answered, after careful consideration of the data collected from census, key informants, community forums, surveys, or health statistics indicators, are Will the objectives and resources of this program meet the identified needs of the client population? and Is the program relevant? Once need has been established and the planning process for designing the program has been instituted, the community health nurse must plan for program evaluation. As a part of the

Research Brief

Finnegan J et al: Process evaluation of a home based program to reduce diet-related cancer risk: the "Win at Home Series," *Health Educ Q* 19(2):233, 1992.

An experimental study was designed to perform a process evaluation of a home-based learning program to reduce diet-related cancer risk. The study involved two communities in Minnesota, each with a population of 20,000. The intervention, the home-based program, in one community lasted 1 year. The intervention included a mass media campaign, food demonstrations and product labeling in grocery stores, and a community organization strategy involving local leaders in an advisory capacity.

The purpose of the process evaluation was to look at recruitment, salience, use of the course, knowledge of participants, and implementation of recommended diet changes. The study showed:

1. Women, college graduates and those over age 44 were more likely to enroll in the program.
2. Most participants learned about the program through mass media first and second through interpersonal sources.
3. The level of participation predicted knowledge gained about nutrition.
4. If the course seemed to meet the needs (salient) of the participants, they were more likely to change their behavior.
5. More than half the participants shared the program with someone else who usually needed it more than the participants.

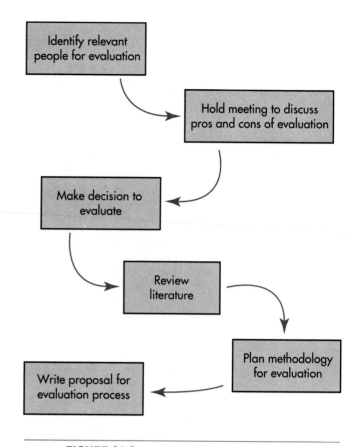

FIGURE 21-3

Six steps in planning for program evaluation.

planning process, Posavac and Carey (1989) describe six steps to use for continuing program evaluation (Figure 21-3).

The first step is to identify the relevant people for evaluation. Program personnel, program sponsors, and the clients of the program should be included in planning for evaluation.

The second step is to arrange preliminary meetings to discuss the questions of whether the group wants an evaluation, and if so, why, what kind, and when. If the program planners and others agree on an evaluation, the resources for conducting the program evaluation must be identified. Evaluation is necessary even though some may not be interested in it. Public health nurses can be instrumental in helping others to see that without evaluation, money to support programs will not be available or need for a new nurse to help with the work cannot be justified.

The third step comes after the relevant people have met and considered the questions in the previous steps. They are ready to decide whether the evaluation should be carried out. Even though evaluation may be desired, the decision to conduct the evaluation may be an administrative one, based on availability of resources or determined by the existing circumstances. For example, if a program evaluation were attempted in a situation in which program personnel wanted it and clients chose to be uncooperative, evaluation efforts would fail.

The fourth step is to examine the literature for suggestions about the appropriate methods and techniques and their usefulness in program evaluation. This step is particularly helpful if the organization has chosen an evaluator who is external to the program. If the evaluation is internal, the evaluators may be unfamiliar with the literature.

The external evaluator may make suggestions regarding the questions to be answered in the evaluation process. If the literature has been reviewed by the public health nurse and others affected by the evaluation, they can determine whether the evaluation suggestions are appropriate for their situation.

The fifth step is to plan the methodology, including decisions about what items will be measured, how they will be measured, and on what population.

The sixth and final step is to write a plan that outlines the purpose and goals of the overall program, the type of evaluation to be done, the operational measure to be used to evaluate the program goals, the choice of internal or external evaluators, the available resources for conducting the evaluation, and the readiness of the organization, personnel, and clients for program evaluation.

Aspects of Evaluation

The aspects of program evaluation include the following: (1) evaluation of relevance, the need for the program; (2) progress, the tracking of program activities to meet program objectives; (3) efficiency, the relationship between program outcomes and the resources expended; (4) effectiveness, the ability to meet program objectives and the results of program efforts; and (5) impact, the long-term changes in the client population (Kaluzny and Veney, 1991).

Relevance

Evaluation of relevance is an important component of the initial planning phase. As money, providers, facilities, and supplies for delivering health care services are more closely monitored, the automatic assumption that all health care delivery programs are needed is an error. The needs assessment done by the public health nurse will determine whether the program is needed.

Progress

The monitoring of program activities, such as hours of services, numbers of providers used, numbers of referrals made, and amount of money spent to meet program objectives, provides an evaluation of the progress of the program. This type of evaluation is an example of formative evaluation and occurs on an ongoing basis while the program is in existence. This provides an opportunity to make effective day-to-day management decisions about the operations of the program. Progress evaluation occurs primarily during implementation. The community health nurse who completes a daily or weekly log of clinical activities (i.e., number of clients seen in clinic or visited at home, number of phone contacts, number of referrals made) is contributing to progress evaluation of the nursing service.

Efficiency

If the reason for evaluation is to examine the efficiency of a program, it may occur on an ongoing basis as formative evaluation or at the completion of the program as a summative evaluation. The evaluator may be able to determine whether the program provides better benefits at a lower cost than a similar program or whether the benefits to the clients or numbers of clients served justify the cost of the program.

Effectiveness and Impact

An **evaluation of program effectiveness** may help the community health nurse evaluator determine both client and provider satisfaction with the program activities, as well as whether the program met its stated objectives. However, if *evaluation of impact* is the goal, long-term effects such as changes in morbidity and mortality must be investigated. Both effectiveness and impact evaluations are usually summative evaluation functions primarily performed as end-of-program activities.

The Evaluative Process

The evaluative process initially described by Suchman (1967) and modified by Rossi and Freeman (1989) is explained here. It is very similar to steps in the planning process. The first step in the evaluative process is *goal setting*. The value and beliefs of the agency, the providers, and the clients provide the basis for goal setting and should be considered at every step of the evaluation process. In the preschool immunization scenario, the fact that children should not be exposed to early childhood diseases would lead to a program goal to decrease the incidence of early childhood diseases in the county where the program is planned.

The second step is *determining goal measurement*. In the case of the previous goal, disease incidence would be an appropriate goal measurement. The third step is *identifying goal-attaining activities*. This would include such activities as media presentations urging parents to have their children immunized. The fourth step is *making the activities operational*, that is, actually administering the immunizations. The fifth step is *measuring the goal effect*, which consists of reviewing the records and summarizing the incidence of early childhood disease before and after the program. The final step is *evaluation of the program*, determining whether the program goal was achieved. Keep in mind that only one program goal is used in this example. Most programs have multiple goals (Figure 21-4).

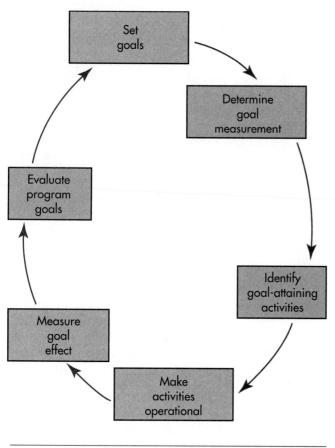

FIGURE 21-4

The evaluative process.

Formulation of Objectives

The most important step in the evaluative process is the formulation of program objectives. The objectives set the stage for conducting the program and provide the mechanism for evaluating the activities and the total program. The following discussion helps in the development of clear, concise objectives. Development of program objectives coincides with the initial phases of program planning.

Specification of Objectives (Goals)

If the objectives are too general, program evaluation becomes impossible. The objectives must be specific and stated so that anyone reading them could conduct the program without further instruction. To be truly effective, objectives must be very specific and should begin with a general program goal and move on to specific objectives that will help meet the program goal.

Useful program objectives include a statement of the specific behaviors, accomplishments, and success criteria for the program. Each program objective requires *a strong, action-oriented verb to specify the behavior, a statement of a single purpose, a statement of a single result, and a time frame for achieving the expected result.* In this continuing example, a program objective that meets these criteria may be to decrease *(action verb)* the inci-

dence of early childhood disease in Center County *(result)* by providing immunization clinics in all schools *(purpose)* between August and December of 1999 *(time frame).*

As objectives are developed, an operational indicator for each objective should be considered so the evaluator knows when and if the objective has been met. For instance, an operational indicator for the previous objective would be a 10% to 25% decrease in the incidence rates of the most frequently occurring childhood vaccine-preventable illnesses in Center County. Such indicators provide a target for persons involved with program implementation.

Levels of Program Objectives

It is customary for objectives to be stated in levels from general to specific. The first level consists of general and broad objectives that are sometimes called goals. Their purpose is to focus on the major reason for the program.

A general program objective (goal) may be to reduce the incidence of low-birth-weight babies in Center County in 1999 by improving access to prenatal care. The specific objectives, or subgoals, describe a measurable behavior, the circumstances under which the behavior is observed, and the minimal acceptable standard for the performance of the behavior. A specific objective for this program may be to open a prenatal clinic in each health department within the county by January 1997 to serve the population within each census tract of the county.

Specific program activities are then planned to meet each specific objective; resources, such as number of nurses, equipment, supplies, and location, are planned for each of the objectives. It is assumed that as each specific objective is met, the general program objective will also be achieved. Remember that several specific objectives are required to meet a general program objective or goal.

Sources of Program Evaluation

Major sources of information for program evaluation are program participants, program records, and community indexes. The program participants, or consumers of the service, have a unique and valuable role in program evaluation. Whether the clients, for whom the program was designed, accept the services will determine to a large extent whether the program achieves its purpose. Thus, their reactions, feelings, and judgments about the program are very important to the evaluation.

To assess the response of participants in a program, the evaluator may use a written survey in the form of a questionnaire or an attitude scale. Interviews and observations are other ways of obtaining feedback about a program. Attitude scales are probably used most often, and they are usually phrased in terms of whether the program met its objectives. The client sat-

Healthy People 2000: Example of National Health Objective Combining Health Status, Risk Reduction and Service Goal, and Possible Activities to Meet Objectives

9.1 Reduce **(action verb)** deaths caused by unintentional injuries **(result)** to no more than 29.3 per 100,000 people **(target)** by increasing the use of helmets to at least 80% of motorcyclists and at least 50% of bicyclists **(objective indicator)** by extending to 50 state laws requiring helmet use for all ages **(purpose)** by the year 2000 **(time frame)**.

Healthy Communities 2000: Example of Activities to Evaluate Objective 9.1 to Reduce Deaths Caused by Unintentional Injuries

FOCUS OF OBJECTIVE
Deaths from injuries

OBJECTIVE
Reduce deaths caused by unintentional injuries

EVALUATION INDICATOR
Change in unintentional injury
Number of hospital admissions (increasing or decreasing)
State law changed
Percentage wearing helmets

isfaction survey is an example of an attitude scale often used in the health care delivery system to evaluate the attainment of program objectives.

The second major source of information for program evaluation is program records, especially clinical records. Clinical records provide the evaluator with information about the care given to the client and the results of that care. To determine whether a program goal has been met, one might summarize the data from a group of records. For example, if one overall goal is to reduce the incidence of low-birth-weight babies through prenatal care, records would be reviewed to obtain the number of mothers who received prenatal care and the number of low-birth-weight babies born to them.

A third major source of evaluation is a community **health index.** Health and illness indicators, such as mortality and morbidity data, are probably cited more frequently than any other single index for program evaluation. Health and illness indicators are useful in evaluating the impact of health care programs. Incidence and prevalence are also valuable indexes used to measure program effectiveness and impact (see Chapter 11 for further discussion of rates and ratios).

> ### Did You Know?
>
> *Healthy People 2000*, the national program to improve the health of all Americans in 10 years, used key informants, census data, statistical indicators, forums, and surveys of existing programs to establish the goals and objectives of the program.

An example of a national program based on a needs assessment of the U.S. population is the national health objectives program called *Healthy People 2000* (1991). *Healthy People 2000* has three overall goals and 300 specific health status objectives, which include an action verb, a result, a time frame (10 years), and an operational indicator (see Appendix A-1). Each health status objective is accompanied by a risk

reduction objective, which further defines the result of the health status objective, and a services objective, which gives the purpose of the objective (see the example in box above, left).

Healthy Communities 2000: Model Standards (1991) suggests activities to evaluate the national health objectives (see the example in box above, right).

ADVANCED PLANNING METHODS AND EVALUATION MODELS

After the need and demand for a program have been determined through the needs assessment process, the next step in the development of the program is to choose a procedural method that will assist the community health nurse in planning the program to be offered. *The following is offered for students who are more advanced in their career and need to consider several methods of program planning plus more extensive evaluation models for program management.*

Five planning methods are discussed in this section (1) the Planning, Programming, and Budgeting System (PPBS), (2) the Program Planning Methods (PPM), (3) the Program Evaluation Review Technique (PERT), (4) the Critical Path Method (CPM), and (5) the Multi-Attribute Utility Method (MAUT).

PPM and PPBS are more general approaches to program planning, whereas PERT, CPM, and MAUT offer guidelines for identifying and tracking specific program activities essential to program success. All of these approaches establish the basis for program evaluation.

Planning, Programming, and Budgeting System

Planning, Programming, and Budgeting System (PPBS) is a procedural tool initially developed for use by the Department of Defense and other governmental agencies. PPBS is an outcome-oriented accounting system, the effect of which is to determine the most efficient method of resource allocation to attain measurable objectives.

The steps involved in PPBS are (1) setting program goals, (2) defining measurable program objectives,

(3) identifying and evaluating alternatives to accomplish program objectives, (4) choosing the method for accomplishing the objectives, and (5) developing a program budget with justification for minimizing costs while maximizing program benefits (Figure 21-5).

PPBS is an economic method of describing a program plan. In PPBS, *planning* represents formulation of objectives and conceptualization or identification of alternatives and methods for accomplishing objectives; *programming* represents detailing of resources (personnel, facilities, equipment, and financing) for each identified alternative; and *budgeting* represents the assignment of dollar values to resources required for the program implementation, or the evaluation of program costs and benefits.

PPBS is widely used for planning broad-scale governmental programs. It is a system that can also be used to plan programs for an agency or for client groups. For example, PPBS could be used to develop the annual program plan for the health department or a prenatal program for the local community. A community health nurse could also use this method to develop a health education program for the school population on sexually transmitted diseases. PPBS's use of objectives that are operationally defined by nursing standards or performance criteria is a system that lends itself to effective program evaluation.

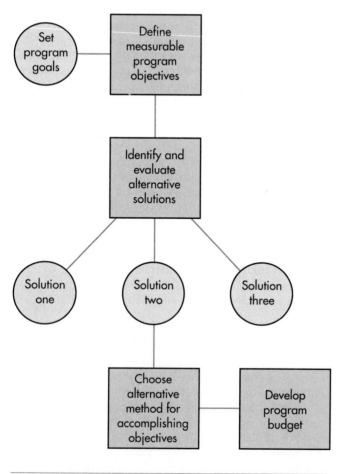

FIGURE 21-5

Planning, programming, and budgeting system.

Program Planning Method

PPM, or Program Planning Method, is a technique employing the nominal group technique of Delbecq and Van de Van (1971). It can be used by the community health nurse to involve clients more directly in the planning process. This is a five-stage process to identify program needs and focuses on three levels of planning groups comprised of clients, providers, and administrators. The client or consumer group relays a list of problems to the provider group, who in turn aids the client group in presenting the solution to the problem to the administrative group (Nutt, 1984).

The stages of PPM are compared with Nutt's planning process in Table 21-3. The PPM *stage one* involves problem diagnosis. Each client in the group works with all other members of the group to develop a written problem list, one problem at a time. After all problems have been shared and recorded, they are discussed by the total client group. Following the discussion, clients select the problems with the highest priority by voting on the ranking of each problem.

In the *second stage* of PPM the expert provider group identifies solutions or each of the problems identified by the clients. In the *third stage* the client and provider groups present their problems and suggested solutions to the administrative group to determine the possibilities of developing a program to meet one or more of the problems, using one or more of the solutions. In this phase, clients and providers are seeking acceptance from the administrators who control the program resources. *Phase four* of PPM involves identifying the alternative solutions to the problem and analyzing the pros and cons of each. *Phase five* involves the client, providers, and administrators in selecting the best plan for program implementation. In this phase the link between the planned solutions and the problem are evaluated, pointing out strengths and limitations of the proposed program plan.

The community health nurse may use this technique for developing school health services within the total community or in one school. This method may also be used by the nurse working with a senior citizens group to identify their priority needs for nursing or physician clinic services at the health department. It is important to note that this method is used to get consensus among all persons involved in the program—clients, providers, and administrators. Consensus is most helpful in having a successful program.

Program Evaluation Review Technique

The Program Evaluation Review Technique (PERT) is a network programming method developed in the 1950s through a joint effort of the United States Navy, Lockheed Aircraft Corporation, and Booz-Allen and Hamilton, Inc. The method was developed for planning and controlling the program activities involved in developing the Polaris missile.

The PERT method is primarily useful for large-scale projects that require planning, scheduling, and controlling a large number of activities. PERT is men-

Table 21-3   Planning Methods Compared With Basic Planning Process

Basic planning	PPBS	PPM	PERT/CPM	MAUT
1. Formulation	Identify the goals and define in measurable terms	Problems identified by client	Identify program activities	Identify target population and program objectives
2. Conceptualization	Identify alternatives	Provider group identifies solution	Explore time and events required to meet program activities	Identify alternative problem solutions
3. Detailing	Evaluate alternatives for use of resources	Analyze available solutions	Determine sequencing of events and resources to meet activities	Identify criteria for choice; rank, rate, and weight; calculate value
4. Evaluation	Choose method for accomplishing objectives and develop budget to evaluate costs vs. benefits	Clients, providers, administrators select best plan	Select appropriate events	Choose best alternatives
5. Implementation		Best plan presented to administrators for funding		

tioned here to introduce the reader to the concept of network planning. PERT as a planning method has been used successfully in hospitals to plan for the development of nursing services such as primary care services, and for designing projects such as the installing and use of computers for organizing and providing nursing services.

The major objectives of PERT are to (1) focus attention on the key developmental parts of a program; (2) identify potential program problems that could interfere with movement toward program goals; (3) evaluate program progress toward goal attainment; (4) provide a prompt reporting method; and (5) facilitate decision-making (Nutt, 1984; Rakich, et al., 1994).

PERT involves the concepts of *time* and *events*. The basic tool used in the technique is the *network* or *flow plan*, which is a series of circles, ovals, or squares representing the program events, or goals, and their interrelationships with the activities of the program. The program activities are the time-consuming events of the program and are represented by arrows that connect the program accomplishments or goals (Figure 21-6). Note in the flow plan that it may take several activities to attain a program event (goal) and that some events (goals) must be accomplished before other events may be attained. The interrelationship of several program events (subgoals) may be essential to attain the ultimate program event (goal).

Another element in PERT is the estimate of the time it will take to implement activities leading to program goals. In PERT, three estimates of activity time are given: the optimistic time it will take to complete activities, given minimal difficulties; the most likely time it will take to complete activities, given past experi-

ences with normal development of such activities; and the pessimistic time it will take to complete activities, given maximum difficulties. From the time estimates, a simple formula can be applied to indicate the probability of completing a project in a given time period. The numbers appearing along the arrows in Figure 21-6 are the estimated numbers of days required for completion of activities leading to a particular event.

Critical Path Method

Critical Path Method (CPM) is a network programming planning method that is described by some authors as a technique in itself and by others as an element of PERT (Rakich, et al., 1994).

CPM is a technique that focuses the program planner's attention on the program activities, the sequencing of activities for the best use of time and resources, and the estimated time it will take to complete the project from beginning to end. Using this method the planner can determine the amount of time it will take to accomplish each activity and can identify those activities that may take longer. The planner can then determine the amounts of resources needed (personnel, money, facilities, and supplies) to accomplish tasks at given points in time along the program's *critical path*.

CPM allows for frequent review of progress by program planners. Problems can be identified early in the program implementation, and corrective action can be taken or alternative activities can be substituted for activities that are not meeting program requirements. The amount of time and resources being used during program implementation can be assessed, and time and resources can be increased or decreased as neces-

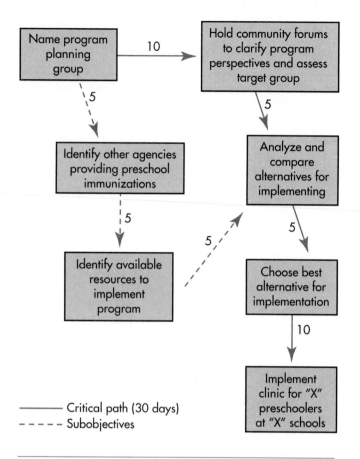

———— Critical path (30 days)
– – – – Subobjectives

FIGURE 21-6

Simplified PERT network, for planning a preschool immunization program. Numbers represent days required for completion of activities.

sary and can be compared to initial estimates of program need.

Hospital nursing services and home health agencies are beginning to use CPM to develop protocols for caring for clients with specific health problems, (e.g., breast cancer, hypertension, or total hip replacement). The CPM protocols identify the estimated number of days the client will be in the hospital and nursing care activities for each day the client is hospitalized, from admission to discharge. The CPM extends to the home, estimating nursing care activities and rehabilitation in the home (see Chapter 19). Nurses must document reasons why activities may not have been accomplished. These notes are used to change nursing care plans and set new goals for clients.

PERT and CPM embody the five generic stages of planning described by Nutt. However, these two methods focus on specific activities, times, and events essential to program success. The emphasis in these two models is on detailing and evaluation (Table 21-3).

The Multi-Attribute Technique

The Multi-Attribute Utility Technique (MAUT) is a planning method based on decision theory (Edwards, Guttentag, and Snapper, 1975). This method can be adapted for making decisions about the care of a sin-

gle client or about national health care programs. The purpose of MAUT is to separate all elements of a decision and to evaluate each element separately for its impact on the overall decision.

Ten basic steps to MAUT method are described by Edwards, Guttentag, and Snapper (1975):

1. *Identify the person or aggregate whose utilities are to be maximized.* In other words, who is the client for whom the program is being planned?

2. *Identify the issue(s) or decision(s) to which the utilities are relevant.* This step involves the identification of the program objectives.

3. *Identify the entities to be evaluated.* The program planner identifies the available options or action alternatives to accomplish the program goals.

4. *Identify the relevant dimensions of value.* The program planner places a value on competing options or alternatives or identifies criteria to be considered to make a choice between them.

5. *Rank the value dimensions in order of importance.* The program planner will decide which of the criteria are most important and which are least important for meeting program goals.

6. *Rate dimensions in importance.* In this step the program planner assigns an arbitrary rating of 10 to the least important criteria. In considering the next least important criteria, the planner decides how many times more important it is than the least important criteria. If it is considered twice as important, the dimension will be assigned a 20. If it is only considered half again as important, it will be assigned a 15. If it is considered four times as important, it will be assigned a 40. The process is continued until all dimensions have been rated.

7. *Add the importance rate, divide each by the sum, and multiply by 100.* Edwards refers to this process as "normalizing" the weights. This is considered a purely mechanical step that provides the program planner with a clearer picture of the relative values of the criteria. However, if too many criteria are identified in Step 4, the computational process underestimates the value of some actions and overestimates the value of others. To avoid this problem, it is recommended that the number of criteria be kept between 6 and 15. Therefore, in this initial process the planner can be concerned with only general criteria for choosing action alternatives.

8. *Measure the location of the entity being evaluated on each dimension.* The planner may ask a colleague or expert to estimate on a scale of 0 to 100 the probability that a given option from Step 3 will maximize the value of the criteria from Step 4. An option thought to have a low probability of meeting the criteria may be assigned a value of 20, whereas an option thought to have a high probability may be assigned a value of 80.

9. *Calculate utilities for entities.* The program planner will obtain the usefulness of each identified action alternative by multiplying the weight for each criterion (Step 7) by the rating of an option for each

criterion (Step 8) and adding the products. The sum of the products for each action is termed the aggregate utility.

10. *Decide on best alternative to meet program objective.* The action alternative with the highest aggregate utility is considered the best decision for meeting the program objectives. If cost was not considered as one of the criteria on which to evaluate the action alternatives, then the usefulness of each option may need to be considered in relation to cost.

If money is no object, then the option with the highest utility is the best decision. However, if the highest utility option exceeds the budget, the next highest utility option may be the alternative to choose. An example of the application of MAUT to a program decision in community health nursing is given at the end of this discussion. The steps of MAUT relate closely to the basic planning process described by Nutt (1984) as shown in Table 21-3.

Steps 1 and 2 of MAUT relate to problem formulation. Step 3 involves conceptualization of the program alternatives, and Steps 4 through 9 focus on detailing and the implications of each option. Step 10 involves the evaluation phase of planning or the choice of the best solution as identified in Steps 4 through 9. Placing quantitative values on solutions to meet program needs is most helpful in the implementation phase of planning (e.g., convincing administrators of the need for such a program). However, caution must be taken in using all planning methods since the best solution reflects the bias of the planner.

Evaluation Models and Techniques
Structure-Process-Outcome Evaluation

The method for evaluation of programs by Donabedian (1982) was initially directed primarily toward medical care but is applicable to the broader area of health care. He described three approaches to assessment of health care: structure, process, and outcome.

Structure refers to settings in which care occurs and includes materials, equipment, qualification of the staff, and organizational structure (Donabedian, 1982). This approach to evaluation is based on the assumption that, given a proper setting with good equipment, good care will follow; but this assumption is not strongly supported.

Process refers too whether the care that was given was "good" (Donabedian, 1982), competent, or preferential. Use of process in program evaluation may consist of observation of practice but more likely consists of review of records. The review may focus on pathology reports to ascertain whether the number of surgeries was strongly indicated or questionable. The review could focus on whether documentation of preventive teaching was on the clinical record. Audits using specific criteria are examples of the use of process.

Outcome refers to client recovery and restoration of function and survival (Donabedian, 1982) but is also used in the sense of changes in health status or changes in health-related knowledge, attitude, and behavior. Thus program outcomes may be expressed in terms of mortality, morbidity, and disability for given populations, such as infants, but could be expressed in a broader sense through health promotion behaviors such as weight control, exercise, and abstinence from tobacco and alcohol.

Donabedian (1982) supports the use of the process approach when possible, followed by outcome, and then by structure. Process and outcome are used more than structure in the evaluation of care. Donabedian's model of evaluating program quality is a popular model and is widely used for evaluation in the health care field. It can be useful in evaluating program effectiveness. Health Care Financing Administration and other third party payers are currently placing more emphasis on outcome evaluation. It is essential that nurses begin to develop outcome criteria for client interventions.

Tracer Method

The board on Medicine of the National Academy of Sciences developed a program to evaluate health service delivery called the tracer method (Kessner and Kalk, 1973). The tracer method of evaluation of programs is based on the premise that health status and care can be evaluated by viewing specific health problems called *tracers*. Just as radioactive tracers are used to study the thyroid gland, specific health problems are selected to evaluate the delivery of health and nursing services. Examples of conditions selected as tracers are middle ear infection and associated hearing loss, vision disorders, iron deficiency anemia, hypertension, urinary tract infections, and cervical cancer. This program can be used to (1) compare health status among different population groups, (2) compare health status in relation to social, economic, medical care, nursing care, and behavioral variables, and (3) compare various arrangements for health care delivery. The application of this method to the study of health care for children has been reported by Kessner and Kalk (1973) and is discussed by Veney and Kaluzny (1991).

The tracer method is a useful technique for looking at efficiency, effectiveness, and impact of a program.

Case Register

Systematic registration of contagious disease has been a practice for many years. Denmark began a national register of tuberculosis in 1921 (Horwitz, 1979). Its contribution to the reduction in the incidence of contagious diseases has been widely recognized (Clemesen, 1979). Case registers are also used for acute and chronic disease (e.g., cancer and myocardial infarction).

Registers collate information from defined groups, and the information may be used for evaluation and planning of services, disease prevention, provision of care, and monitoring changes in patterns and care of diseases. The method is described here because of its use in evaluation of services. Information obtained by the community registers in Europe on myocardial infarction is a good example of the way a case register is used (Keil, 1979). The following are questions that were asked about cases of myocardial infarction for the community registers:

1. What is the incidence of disease? What differences in incidence are there between one community and another?
2. What percentage of clients recover? What percentage die?
3. Where does death occur?
4. How long do clients wait before calling a doctor?
5. How long is it before they see a doctor?
6. How many cases are associated with other major risk factors?
7. How many cases are associated with environmental factors such as water hardness or air pollution?
8. What happens after clients leave the hospital and when they return to work? Are there rehabilitation programs?
9. How many had been seen by a physician shortly before the problem occurred?
10. What prevention measures are taken for persons considered susceptible?

The answers to these questions before and after implementation of a given program would give information about the impact of the program. A tuberculosis register indicates the degree to which infection is being controlled. Cancer registers make state, regional, national, and international comparisons possible, and they provide clues to causes of disease.

COST STUDIES APPLIED TO PROGRAM MANAGEMENT

Although cost must be considered in planning and evaluating, it is particularly significant in programs involving nursing services. The major types of cost studies primarily applied to health care industry are cost accounting, cost benefit, cost efficiency, and cost effectiveness. A discussion of the types of cost studies is presented to give the reader an idea of the kinds of questions that can be answered with such studies. Nurses must be willing to answer these questions to help show the actual costs of nursing programs and the relevance of the programs to the clients they have served.

Cost Accounting

Cost accounting studies are performed to find the actual cost of a program. A question answered by this method could be, "What is the cost of providing a family planning program in Anytown, USA?" To answer the question, the total costs of equipment, facilities (rental), personnel (salaries and benefits), and supplies used over a period are calculated. The total program costs are divided by the number of clients participating in the program during that time. The total program cost per client is the end product. Thus, a cost accounting study can provide data about total program costs and about total cost per client, which makes program management easier. A simple example of cost accounting is what one does each month when balancing a checkbook. One looks at the costs of providing food, shelter, and clothing for a family versus the family income.

Cost Benefit

Cost benefit studies are a way of assessing the desirability of a program by placing a specific dollar amount on all costs and benefits. If benefits outweigh the costs, the program is said to have a *net positive impact*. The major problem with cost benefit analysis is placing a quantifiable value on all benefits of the program. Can a dollar value be placed on human life, on safety, on the relief of pain and suffering, or on prevention of illness? These are all program benefits. If an attempt is made to perform cost benefit analysis of a hospice program, can a dollar amount be placed on the family and client support and comfort provided or on the relief of pain of the terminally ill client? Can such benefits be weighed against costs to justify continuing the program? Or should the program be continued despite costs?

It is recognized that public health programs have net positive impacts because preventing morbidity with illness prevention programs such as hypertension screenings averts or reduces the future cost of chronic long-term illnesses such as cerebrovascular accident (stroke) or cardiovascular disease. To initiate a cost benefit study for a program, it must be decided which costs and which benefits are to be included, how the costs and benefits are to be valued, and what constraints are to be considered—legal, ethical, social, and economic. For example, in a home health care program funded by the state health department to offer care to clients with acquired immunodeficiency syndrome (AIDS), the mortality rate would continue to be high because a cure is not available. Would the program be considered to have a low cost benefit ratio (negative impact) because clients cannot be cured? The program would be considered to have a high cost benefit ratio (positive net impact) if the cost of home health care services were less expensive than providing similar care in the hospital. The benefits of the program would include the reduction in costs to the client and reduction in need for hospital services (Rossi and Freeman, 1989).

In *Healthy People 2000*, information is presented on the cost and benefit of prevention of illness versus an available medical intervention if the illness had been prevented from occurring (Table 21-4). The cost per client to use the intervention is considered a negative net impact because the nation has had to spend money on illness that could be prevented and there have been lost work productivity and lost lives (increased mortality) as a result of the preventable illness.

Table 21-4   *Healthy People* 2000: The Economics of Prevention—Costs of Treatment for Selected Preventable Conditions

Condition	Overall magnitude	Avoidable intervention*	Cost per patient†
Heart disease	7 million with coronary artery disease 500,000 deaths/yr 284,000 bypass procedures/yr	Coronary bypass surgery	$30,000
Cancer	1 million new cases/yr 510,000 deaths/yr	Lung cancer treatment Cervical cancer treatment	$29,000 $28,000
Cerebrovascular accident (stroke)	600,000 strokes/yr 150,000 deaths/yr	Hemiplegia treatment and rehabilitation	$22,000
Injuries	2.3 million hospitalizations/yr 142,500 deaths/yr 177,000 persons with spinal cord injuries in United States	Quadriplegia treatment and rehabilitation Hip fracture treatment and rehabilitation Severe head injury treatment and rehabilitation	$570,000 (lifetime) $40,000 $310,000
Human immunodeficiency virus (HIV) infection	1-1.5 million infected 118,000 AIDS cases (as of January 1990)	AIDS treatment	$75,000 (lifetime)
Alcoholism	18.5 million abuse alcohol 105,000 alcohol-related deaths/yr	Liver transplant	$250,000
Drug abuse	Regular users 1-3 million, cocaine 900,000, IV drugs 500,000, heroin Drug-exposed babies 375,000	Treatment of cocaine-exposed baby	$66,000 (5 years)
Low-birth-weight baby (LBWB)	260,000 LBWBs born/yr 23,000 deaths/yr	Neonatal intensive care for LBWB	$10,000
Inadequate immunization	Lacking basic immunization series 20%-30%, aged 2 and younger 3%, aged 6 and older	Congenital rubella syndrome treatment	$354,000 (lifetime)

From *Healthy People* 2000: *national health promotion and disease prevention objectives*, Washington, DC, 1991, USDHHS, Public Health Services.
*Examples (other interventions may apply).
†Representative first-year costs, except as noted. Not indicated are nonmedical costs, such as lost productivity to society.

Cost Effectiveness

Cost effectiveness analysis, a measure of the quality of a program as it relates to cost, is the most frequently used analysis in nursing. Cost effectiveness is a subset of cost benefit analysis and is designed to provide an estimate of costs incurred in achieving a given outcome. A cost effectiveness study can answer several questions: Did the program meet its objectives? Were the clients and nurses satisfied with the effects of the interventions? Are things better as a result of the interventions? (Kaluzny and Veney, 1991). In cost benefit analysis, both costs and outcomes are quantitative, whereas in cost effectiveness analysis the outcomes are qualitative and quantitative. Outcome measures addressed by cost effectiveness might increase client knowledge after health teaching, changes in the client's condition after treatment, differences in graduates of two nursing programs with similar goals, and the ability of two hearing screening programs to detect hearing loss.

A cost effectiveness study requires collection of baseline data on clients before the program is implemented and evaluation after the program is completed. The box on p. 410 shows the procedure for completing a cost effectiveness study.

There are several potential outcomes of a cost effectiveness study. For example, a community health nurse is interested in comparing two methods for implementing a program to teach diabetic clients self-care techniques. The nurse chooses self-teaching modules and a group formal instruction program for comparison. There are several potential outcomes of comparing the two teaching methods. Of the potential outcomes in a cost effectiveness study, the program of choice would be the most effective teaching method for the least cost. However, if the most costly program demonstrates superior effectiveness, it may be chosen. If the least costly program is of poor quality, a more costly program would be appropriate.

Steps in Cost Effectiveness Analysis

Step I	Identify the program goals or client outcome to be achieved.
Step II	Identify at least two alternative means of achieving the desired outcomes.
Step III	Collect baseline data on clients.
Step IV	Determine the costs associated with each program activity.
Step V	Determine the activities each group of clients will receive.
Step VI	Determine the client changes after the activities are completed.
Step VII	Combine the costs (step IV), amount of activity (step V), and outcome information (step VI) to express costs relative to outcomes of program goals.
Step VIII	Compare cost outcome information for each goal to present cost effectiveness analysis.

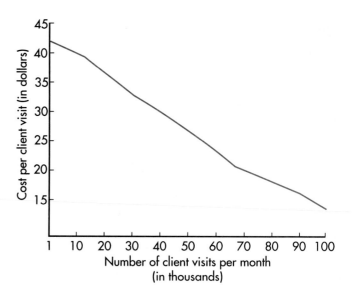

FIGURE 21-7

Cost per client visit at a home health agency.

Cost Efficiency

Cost efficiency analysis is the actual cost of performing a number of program services. To determine cost efficiency of a program, its productivity must be analyzed. Productivity is the relationship between what the nurse does and how much it costs him or her to do it.

To determine the nurse's activities with a group of clients, one is primarily concerned with a nurse's workload, including direct client care and indirect care activities such as charting, phone calls, client care conferences, and travel. The functions are then related to the client load, client need, and the number of nurses available to meet the needs of all clients served by a program.

Figure 21-7 shows an example of the cost efficiency of a home health agency. The graph indicates that as the number of client visits per year increases, the cost per client visit decreases. The graph assumes that the number of nurses from the beginning to the end of the time period is the same, that the nurses' workloads were essential to provide home health ser- vices, that caseloads were assigned based on staff mix and client need, and that organized structure was conducive to nurses being highly productive.

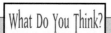

What Do You Think?

The combination of prenatal care programs, delivered by community health nurses, and the Women, Infants, and Children (WIC) supplemental nutritional programs produces better pregnancy and postnatal outcomes for mothers and babies than traditional medical care.

All **cost studies** have three major tasks: financial, research, and statistical. The financial tasks involve identifying total program costs and breaking them down into smaller parts. To identify the costs of a nurse's participation in a teaching program, the costs for facilities, equipment, supplies, and salaries would have to be examined. All costs associated with the program, such as the nurse's time and use of facilities, equipment, and supplies, should be compared with the total program costs. The statistical tasks involve the identification of appropriate quantifiable measures for analyzing data, and the research tasks involve setting up an appropriate study design to answer the questions of benefit, efficiency, or effectiveness.

Nurses with varying educational backgrounds may be involved in cost studies with the assistance of people knowledgeable in research statistics and accounting techniques. Nurses with undergraduate degrees may be involved in the actual implementation of a cost study, whereas nurses with graduate degrees may be involved in planning, designing, implementing, analyzing, and evaluating study results related to program management.

Cost studies are essential to show the worth of nursing in the marketplace of the future, and nurses should be familiar with the results of cost studies so that sound decisions may be made about future program management. Nurses must be ready to identify appropriate program outcomes, client outcomes, the roles that graduates have in health care delivery, and the requirements to perform nursing procedures so that appropriate decisions about program management will be made based on adequate information.

Clinical Application

The following is a real-life example of the application of the program management process by an undergraduate community health nursing student. This activity resulted in the development and implementation of a nurse-managed clinic for the homeless. This example shows how students as well as providers can make a difference in health care delivery. It also shows that no mystery surrounds the program management process.

Eva was listening to the radio one Sunday afternoon and heard an announcement about the opening of a soup kitchen within the community for the growing homeless population. She was beginning her community health nursing course and wanted to find a creative clinical experience that would benefit herself as well as others.

The announcement gave her an idea. Although it mentioned food, clothing, shelter, and social services, nothing was said about health care. She contacted the pastor of the church who was planning to open the soup kitchen to discuss the issue (*formulation* and *assessment*). She found him most receptive to the idea of developing a solution to the health care needs of the homeless. In her assessment, Eva found that no other health services were available to the homeless in the community. She looked at national data to estimate needs and size of the population. She talked with the community health nursing faculty to discuss potential solutions to the problem. She talked to members of the homeless population to get their perceptions of their needs.

On completing her assessment, Eva *conceptualized* the solutions. Several solutions were possible: work with the health department, attempt to provide better care through the local medical center, or open a clinic on site at the soup kitchen where most of the people gathered so that transportation would not be a problem.

After considering the solutions, Eva *detailed* the plan looking at the resources needed for opening a clinic at the soup kitchen. She considered supplies, equipment, facilities, and acceptability to the clients. She also considered the time involved, the activities required to implement a program, and funding sources.

In *evaluating* the possibilities, Eva considered the cost, the client and community benefits, and acceptability to clients, self, faculty, and the church. Although it would have been easier for her to choose to work with the health department or the medical center, she knew that the solution most acceptable to the clients would be to have a clinic located at the soup kitchen. The clinic would be more accessible, transportation would not be needed, and health services through the clinic could possibly prevent more costly hospital and emergency care (*value*).

Eva presented her plan to the faculty and the church. She convinced them that it would not be a costly endeavor. She had nurses in the community who volunteered to help, she had a carpenter who would donate his time to build an examining room in the back of the soup kitchen, and she had equipment promised to her by community physicians. The client assessment indicated that a first-aid and health assessment clinic was what was needed most. With approval from all (*implementation*), Eva began the clinic in 1981, seeing 25 to 35 clients a week, 1 hour per day for 5 days per week.

Eva evaluated the *relevance* of the program via the needs assessment process. She tracked the *progress* of the program by keeping records of her activities. She kept track of the resources in relation to the number of persons served (*efficiency*) and used these data to convince the church and the college of nursing to fund the ongoing clinic operation after she graduated. A *summative evaluation* of the clinic was completed by the faculty at the end of 4 years. The program's *impact* was outstanding. The clinic had grown. The client demand was high; most of the health problems could be handled at the clinic, which eliminated the cost burden to the community for more expensive health care; and it was highly acceptable to the clients (*effectiveness*). This clinic began as a service to 25 people for 1 hour per day. Today this clinic is open all day, 5 days per week, has more than 900 clients per year, and provides for more than 5000 client visits per year. The success of this clinic shows the effect that one community health nursing student can have on a community.

Key Concepts

- Planning and evaluation are essential elements of program management and vital to the survival of the nursing discipline in health care delivery.
- A program is an organized response designed to meet the assessed needs of individuals, families, groups, or communities by reducing or eliminating one or more health problems.
- Planning is defined as selecting and carrying out a series of actions designed to achieve a stated goal.

Continued.

Key Concepts—cont'd

- Evaluation is defined as the methods used to determine if a service is needed and will be used, whether a program to meet that need is carried out as planned, and whether the service actually helps the people it intended to help.
- To develop quality programs, planning should include four essential elements: problem diagnosis and assessment of need, identification of problem solutions, analysis and comparison of alternative methods, and selection of the best plan and planning methods.
- The initial and most critical step in planning a health program is assessment of need.
- Some of the major tools used in needs assessment are census data, community forums, surveys of existing community agencies, surveys of community residents, and statistical indicators.
- The major benefit of program evaluation is to determine whether a program is fulfilling its stated goals. Quality assurance programs are prime examples of program evaluation.
- Plans for program implementation and program evaluation should be developed at the same time.
- Program records and community indexes serve as major sources of information for program evaluation.
- Planning programs and planning for their evaluation are two of the most important ways in which community health nurses can ensure successful program implementation.
- Cost studies help identify program management benefits, effectiveness, and efficiency.
- The program management process, as with the nursing process, is a rational decision-making process.
- The health care delivery system has grown in the past 60 years, making health planning and evaluation very important.

- Comprehensive health planning grew out of a need to control costs.
- Program planning helps nurses and agencies focus attention on services that clients need.
- Planning helps everyone involved understand their role in providing services to clients.
- The assessment of need process provides an evaluation of the relevance that a new service may have to clients.
- A decision tree is a useful tool to choose the best alternative for solving a problem.
- Setting goals and writing objectives to meet the goals are necessary to evaluate program outcomes.
- *Healthy People 2000* is an example of a national zprogram based on needs assessment that has stated goals and objectives on which the program can be evaluated.
- Cost accounting studies are similar to balancing a checkbook and help to determine the actual cost of a program.
- Cost benefit studies are used to assess the desirability of a program by examining costs and benefits, such as the value of human life.
- Cost effectiveness studies measure the quality of a program as it relates to cost.
- Cost efficiency studies examine the actual cost of performing program services and focus on productivity versus cost.
- Program planning models include PPBS, PERT, CPM, and MAUT.
- Program evaluation includes assessing structure, process, and outcomes of care.
- Tracer methods and case registers are two methods of program evaluation.
- Critical path method of evaluating care is a popular model.

Critical Thinking Activities

1. Choose the definitions that best describe your concept of programs, planning, and evaluation.
2. Apply the program planning process to an identified clinical problem for a client group with whom you are working in the community.
   a. Assess the client need.
   b. Choose tools appropriate to the assessment of needs.
   c. Analyze the overall planning process of arriving at decisions about program implementation.
   d. Summarize the benefits for program planning that are applicable to your situation.
3. Given the situation just described, choose three or four of your classmates to work with on the following projects.
   a. Plan for evaluation of the program in activity 2.

Critical Thinking Activities—cont'd

   b. Apply the evaluative process to the situation.

   c. Name the measures you will use to gather data for evaluating your program.

   d. Name the sources you will tap to gain information for program evaluation.

   e. Analyze the benefits of program evaluation that are applicable to your situation.

4. Talk with a community health nurse or administrator about the application of program planning and evaluation processes at the local agency. Compare their answers to your readings.

Bibliography

Achoff R: Our changing concept of planning, *J Nurs Adm* 35:40, 1982.

Barentson P: *Critical path planning: present and future technique*, Princeton, NJ, 1970, Brendon Systems Press.

Begley C, et al: Evaluation of a primary health care program for the poor, *Community Health* 14(2):107, 1989.

Blaney D, Hobson C: *Cost-effective nursing practice: guidelines for nurse managers*, Philadelphia, 1988, Lippincott.

Brownson R, et al: The role of data-driven planning and coalition development in preventing cardiovascular disease, *Public Health Rep* 107(1):32-36, 1992.

Budgen C: Modeling a method for program development, *J Nurs Adm* 17(12):19, 1987.

Clemmesen J: Registration in the study of human cancer. In Holland WW, Karhausen L, editors: *Health care and epidemiology*, Boston, 1979, Hall.

Commission on Hospital Care: *Hospital care in the United States*, New York, 1947, Commonwealth Fund.

Committee on the Costs of Medical Care: *Medical care for the American people*, Chicago, 1932, University of Chicago Press. Reprinted, Washington, DC, 1970, Department of Health, Education, and Welfare.

Dean D, et al: A report of a collaborative process between a university and a church, *Fam Community Health* 10(4):13, 1988.

Delbecq A, Van de Ven A: A group process model for problem identification and program planning, *J Appl Behav Sci* 7(4):466-492, 1971.

Donabedian A: *Explorations in quality assessment and monitoring*, vol 2, Ann Arbor, Mich, 1982, Health Administration Press.

Downey A, et al: Health promotion model for "heart smart": the medical school, university, and community, *Health Values* 13(6):31, 1989.

Edwards W, Guttentag M, Snapper K: A decision-theoretic approach to evaluation research. In Struening E, Guttentag M, editors: *Handbook of evaluative research*, Beverly Hills, Calif, 1975, Sage.

Fagin C: Strategic planning—outline of plan, *J Prof Nurs* 3(2):79, 1987.

Finnegan J, et al: Process evaluation of a home-based program to reduce diet-related cancer risk: the "Win at Home Series," *Health Educ Q* 19(2):233, 1992.

Fortmann S, et al: Effect of community health education on plasma cholesterol levels and diet: the Stanford five-city project, *Am J Epidemiol* 137(10):1039-1041, 1993.

Friedman L, et al: Cost-effectiveness of a self-care program, *Nurs Econ* 6(4):173, 1988.

Garofalo K: Worksite wellness—rewarding healthy behaviors, *AAOHN J* 42(5):236-240, 1994.

Glasgow R, et al: Implementing a year-long worksite-based incentive program for smoking cessation, *Am J Health Promotion* 5(3):192-193, 1991.

Hargreaves M, et al: Changing community health behaviors: a model for program development and management, *Health Values* 10(6):34, 1986.

Healthy People 2000: national health promotion and disease prevention objectives, Washington, DC, 1991, USDHHS, Public Health Services.

Healthy Communities 2000: model standards, ed 3, Washington, DC, 1991, American Public Health Association.

Horwitz O: Epidemiological parameters for public health evaluation of a chronic disease. In Holland WW, Karhausen L, editors: *Health care and epidemiology*, Boston, 1979, Hall.

Jason L, et al: A large-scale, short-term, media-based weight loss program, *Am J Health Promotion* 5(6):432-433, 1991.

Johnson J, et al: Writing a winning business plan, *J Nurs Adm* 18(10):15, 1988.

Jones K: Feasibility analysis of preferred provider organizations, *J Nurs Adm* 20(1):28, 1990.

Kaluzny A, Veney J: Evaluating health care programs and services. In Williams S, Torrens P, editors: *Introduction to health services*, New York, 1993, Wiley.

Keil U: Community registers of myocardial infarction as an example of epidemiological register studies. In Holland WW, Karhausen L, editors: *Health care and epidemiology*, Boston, 1979, Hall.

Kessner DM, Kalk CE: *Contacts in health status: a strategy for evaluating health services*, vol 2, Washington, DC, 1973, Institute of Medicine, National Academy of Sciences.

Konrad T, DeFriese G: On the subject of sampling . . ., *Am J Health Promotion* 5(2):147-153, 1990.

Kovner A, editor: *Health care delivery in the United States*, New York, 1995, Springer.

Kropf R: Planning for health services. In Kovner A, editor: *Health care delivery in the United States*, New York, 1990, Springer.

Krueger JC: Establishing priorities for evaluation and evaluation research, *Nurs Res* 29:115, 1980.

Litwack L, Linc L, Bower D: *Evaluation in nursing: principles and practice*, New York, 1985, National League for Nursing.

London J: On the right path, *Health Prog* 1993, pp 36-38.

Lowe J, et al: Quality assurance methods for managing employee health-promotion programs: a case study in smoking cessation, *Health Values* 13(2):1, 1989.

Martin J: The array of community services for people with AIDS, *Caring* 8(11):18, 1989.

McAlvanah M: Long range planning—who has the time? *Pediatr Nurs* 14(3):247, 1988.

Morris F: A comparison of three allied health manpower projection methodologies, *J Allied Health* 16(1):59, 1987.

Nash M: Strategic planning: the practical vision, *J Nurs Adm* 18(4):12, 1988.

Nutt P: *Planning methods for health and related organizations*, New York, 1984, Wiley.

Pentz M: Community organizations and school liaisons: how to get programs started, *J Sch Health* 56(9):382, 1986.

Phaneuf MC: Future direction for evaluation and evaluation research in health care, *Nurs Res* 29:123, 1980.

Pickett G, Hanlon J: *Public health administration and practice*, St Louis, 1990, Mosby.

Posavac EJ, Carey RG: *Program evaluation: methods and case studies*, Englewood Cliffs, NJ, 1989, Prentice Hall.

Public Law 79-725: *Hospital survey and construction act*, Aug 13, 1946.

Public Law 89-749: *Comprehensive health planning and public services amendments of 1966*, Nov 3, 1966.

Public Law 93-641: *National health planning and resources development act*, Jan 4, 1975.

Rikach J, Longest B, Darr K: *Managing health services organizations*, Health Professions Press, 1994, Baltimore.

Rikach J, et al: *Managing health services organizations,* Baltimore, 1992, Health Professions Press.

Roman D: The PERT system: an appraisal of program evaluation review technique. In Schulberg H, Sheldon A, Baker F, editors: *Program evaluation in the health fields,* New York, 1969, Behavioral Publications.

Rossi P, Freeman H: *Evaluation: a systematic approach,* Beverly Hills, Calif, 1989, Sage.

Schultz P, Magilvy J: Assessing community health needs of elderly populations: comparison of three strategies, *J Adv Nurs* 13(2):193, 1988.

Smith J, Sorrell V: Developing wellness programs: a nurse-managed stay well center for senior citizens, *Clin Nurs Specialist* 3(4):198, 1989.

Sofaer S: Community health planning in the US: a post mortem, *Fam Community Health* 10(4):1, 1988.

Steckler A, et al: Measuring the diffusion of innovative health promotion programs, *Am J Health Promotion* 6(3):214-215, 1992.

Suchman EA: *Evaluative research,* New York, 1967, Russell Sage Foundation.

US Department of Health and Human Services: *Program management: a guide for improving program decisions,* Atlanta, 1989, Centers for Disease Control.

Valdiserri R: Applying the criteria for the development of health promotion and education programs to AIDS risk reduction programs for gay men, *J Community Health* 12(4):199, 1987.

Veney J, Kaluzny A: *Evaluation and decision making for health service programs,* Englewood Cliffs, NJ, 1991, Prentice Hall.

Warner K, Luce B: *Cost-benefit and cost-effectiveness analysis in health care,* Ann Arbor, Mich, 1982, Health Administration Press.

Weiner J, Trocchio J: Protecting children's health, *Health Prog* 1992, pp 28-31.

Wiest J, Levy F: *A management guide to PERT.CPM,* Englewood Cliffs, NJ, 1969, Prentice Hall.

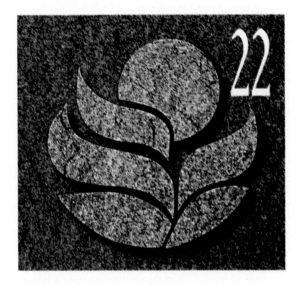

22

Quality Management

Judith Lupo Wold*

Objectives ▼

After reading this chapter, the student should be able to do the following:

- ◆ Define Total Quality Management (TQM)/Continuous Quality Improvement (CQI).
- ◆ State the goals of TQM/CQI in a health care system.
- ◆ Define quality assurance/improvement.
- ◆ State the role of QA/QI in continuous quality improvement.
- ◆ Discuss the historical development of the quality process in nursing.
- ◆ Evaluate approaches and techniques for implementing continuous quality improvement.
- ◆ Describe a model quality assurance/improvement program.
- ◆ Identify the purposes for the types of records kept in community health agencies.
- ◆ Explain a method for documentation of client care in community health nursing.

Outline ▼

Key Terms ▼

academic degrees
accountability
accreditation
audit process
certification
charter
concurrent audit
Continuous Quality Improvement (CQI)
credentialing
evaluative studies
licensure
malpractice litigation
mandatory nurse licensure
Phaneuf Nursing Audit
Plan/Do/Check/Act Cycle
Professional Review Organizations (PROs)
Professional Standards Review Organization (PSRO)
quality
quality assurance/improvement (QA/QI)
quality care
quasi-voluntary
recognition
records
retrospective audit
risk management
staff review committees
Total Quality Management (TQM)
utilization review

*Contents of this chapter may reflect contributions by Kathleen Blomquist from edition 2 and Marcia Stanhope from editions 1 and 3 of this text.

Demand for quality in all areas seems to be a rallying point for today's society. In addition to the demand for quality, the public wants health care delivered at a lower cost, with greater accessibility, accountability, efficiency, and effectiveness. Total Quality Management (TQM)/Continuous Quality Improvement (CQI), a management style that encompasses quality assurance, or quality control, is one method used to assure that the client is getting quality care at top value for money spent. Although relatively new in the healthcare arena, the concept of TQM/CQI has been tried and proven over time in the industrial sector. The terms total quality management, continuous quality improvement, total quality, and organization-wide quality improvement often are used synonomously. These terms refer to a management philosophy that focuses on the processes by which work is done with the goal of continously improving those processes. By obtaining factual information about work processes (e.g., all the steps in certifying a child for the Women, Infants, and Children's (WIC) program) it is possible to discover which steps are unnecessary (i.e., non–value adding) and to eliminate the steps (Tindall and Stewart, 1993).

Both consumers and providers have a vested interest in the quality of the health care system. According to Jonas (1986), the health care provider has three basic reasons to be concerned about health care quality:

1. The principle of nonmaleficence—above all, do no harm—has been a basic principle of the health care system since the writing of the Hippocratic Oath.
2. The principle of beneficence—do good work—is a basic principle of professionalism.
3. The strong social work ethic in our culture places a high value on "doing a good job."

Jonas says that in health care there is a direct link between doing a good job and individual and professional survival. Healthcare providers pride themselves on individual achievement and responsibility for good patient outcomes.

Because of prospective payment mechanisms and consumer demands for quality nursing, objective and systematic evaluation of nursing care has become a priority within the nursing profession. Since nursing is committed to direct accountability, is evolving as a scientific discipline, and is concerned about how costs of health services limit access, it demands delivery and evaluation of quality service aimed at superior patient outcomes (Lang and Clinton, 1984; Maciorowski et al., 1985; Martin et al., 1993).

Records are maintained on all clients of the health care system to provide complete information about the client and to show the quality of care being given to the client within the system. Records are one necessary part of a continuous quality improvement process, as are the tools and methods for evaluating quality.

DEFINITIONS AND GOALS

Quality can be defined as a continuous striving for excellence and a conformance to specifications or guidelines (Davis, 1994). **Total Quality Management/Continuous Quality Improvement (TQM/CQI),** used here synonymously, is a process driven–customer oriented philosophy of management that embodies leadership, teamwork, employee empowerment, individual responsibility, and continuous improvement of system *processes* that lead to improved outcomes (Berwick, 1989). Under TQM/CQI quality is defined as customer satisfaction. **Quality assurance/improvement (QA/QI)** is the promise or guarantee that certain *standards* of excellence are being met in the delivery of care (Lalonde, 1988). The quality assurance, or quality control, process (1) sets standards for care, (2) evaluates care provided, based on the standards, and (3) takes action to bring about change when care does not meet standards (Bull, 1985; Maibusch, 1984). Quality assurance is concerned with the accountability of the provider and is only one tool in achieving optimum client outcomes (Davis, 1994). **Accountability** means being responsible for care and answerable to the client (Meisenheimer, 1989). Under QA/QI, quality may have varying definitions.

Quality traditionally has been a prime issue in the delivery of healthcare, and quality assurance programs historically have had the major role in assuring this accountability. According to Jonas (1986), the goals of quality assurance and improvement are (1) to ensure the delivery of quality client care and (2) to demonstrate the efforts of the health provider to provide the best possible results. However, standards are a static measurement and do not provide incentive for improvement beyond that standard (Tindall and Stewart, 1993). Under a CQI philosophy, quality assurance and improvement is but one of the many tools employed to ensure that the health care agency fulfills what the client believes to be the requirements for the service. The focus of quality assurance is finding what providers have done wrong in the past (i.e., deviations from a standard of care found through a chart audit). Continuous quality improvement focuses on the sources of variation in the *ongoing process* of health care delivery (i.e., steps in the appointment process) and seeks to improve the process (Tindall and Stewart, 1993).

The process of health care includes two major components: technical interventions and interpersonal relationships between practitioner and client. Both are important in providing quality care, and both can be evaluated (Donabedian, 1990). Hart (1993) feels that TQM/CQI exists on a continuum with manufacturing and professional services at opposite ends. While the industrial and healthcare perspectives on quality are similar, the industrial model does not recognize the intricacies of the practitioner-client relationship, and because of its focus on process as cause of poor outcomes, it downplays both practitioner knowledge and skills and the need for practitioner retraining or censure in case of a standard's violation. A variety of approaches and techniques are used in quality programs. Approaches are methods used to ensure quality, and techniques are tools for measuring deviations from quality (Weitzman, 1990).

The term quality assurance and improvement will be used in place of quality assurance in this chapter to more accurately reflect the most recent advancements in this field (Schmele, 1993). Traditional approaches to quality have included a focus on assessing or measuring performance, assuring performance conforms to standards, and providing remediation if those standards are not met. Such a definition of quality is too narrow in health care systems that try to meet the needs of many clients, both internal and external to the agency (Donabedian, 1990). Many agencies are employing some of the TQM/CQI concepts, such as client satisfaction questionnaires, but have not adopted the entire management philosophy. However, because QA/QI methods traditionally have been used and are still in use in many agencies, the QA/QI concept will be covered fully.

HISTORICAL DEVELOPMENT

Approaches to the improvement of quality care have been evident in nursing since the days of Florence Nightingale. In 1860 Nightingale called for the development of a uniform method to collect and present hospital statistics to improve hospital treatment. Nightingale was a pioneer in setting standards for nursing care. The impetus for establishing nursing schools in the United States came in the late 1800s from a desire to set standards that would upgrade nursing care. In the early 1900s efforts were begun to set similar standards for all nursing schools. From 1912 to 1930 the interest in quality nursing education led to the development of nursing organizations involved in accrediting nursing programs. Licensure has been a major issue in nursing since 1892. By 1923 all states had permissive or mandatory laws directing nursing practice.

After World War II, the attention of the emerging nursing profession focused on establishing a scientific method of practice. The nursing process was the chosen method and included evaluation of how the activities of nurses helped clients (Maibusch, 1984). Quality assurance and improvement involves the evaluative step in the nursing process.

The 1950s brought the development of tools to measure quality assurance. One of the first tools was the **Phaneuf Nursing Audit** (1965), which has been used extensively in community health nursing practice.

In 1966 the American Nurses Association (ANA) created the Divisions on Practice in its bylaws. As a result of this, in 1972 the Congress for Nursing Practice was charged with developing standards to be used to institute quality assurance programs. The Standards for Community Health Nursing Practice were distributed to ANA Community Health Nursing Division members in 1973. In 1986 the standards were revised; these revised standards can be found in Chapter 10.

In 1972 the Joint Commission on Accreditation of Hospitals (JCAH) clearly stated the responsibilities of nursing in its description of standards for nursing services. The JCAH called on the nursing industry to clearly plan, document, and evaluate nursing care provided. In the mid-1980s JCAH became the Joint Commission on Accreditation of Health Care Organizations (JCAHO) and began developing quality control standards for home health nursing and for hospital nursing. JCAHO presently is beginning to incorporate continuous quality improvement principles in its standards.

Also in 1972, the Social Security Act (Public Law 92-603) was amended to establish the **Professional Standards Review Organization (PSRO)** and to mandate the process review of the delivery of health care to clients of Medicare, Medicaid, and maternal and child health programs. The PSRO program was modified to become the **Professional Review Organizations (PROs)** by 1983 Social Security Amendments. The purpose of the PROs is to monitor implementation of the prospective reimbursement system for Medicare clients. How PROs will function under health care remains to be seen. Although PSROs were only for physicians, PROs have made quality improvement a primary issue for all health care professionals.

In response to a growing malpractice crisis in this country the government responded with the National Health Quality Improvement Act of 1986. Not funded until 1989, the two major provisions of the act encouraged consumers to become informed about their practitioner's practice record and created a national clearinghouse of information on the malpractice records of providers. The emphasis of this act continued to be on structure and not process or outcome (NAHQ, 1993).

Efforts to strengthen community health nursing practice include the development of frameworks for community health nursing practice by both the ANA (1982) and the American Public Health Association (1980). A discussion of these two models and of the Consensus Conference on the Essentials of Public Health Nursing Practice and Education, 1984 can be found in Chapter 10. The quality of community health nursing education is a major concern of the Association of Community Health Nursing Educators, which was established in 1978. In 1991 and 1993, three reports published by this organization identified the curriculum content required to prepare community nursing students for practice (ACHNE, 1991, 1993). Quality assurance and improvement programs remain the enforcer of standards of care for many agencies who have not elected to engage in a program of continuous quality improvement.

APPROACHES TO QUALITY IMPROVEMENT

Two basic approaches exist in quality improvement: general and specific. The general approach involves a large governing or official body's evaluation of a person's or agency's ability to meet criteria or standards. Specific approaches to quality improvement are methods used to manage a specific health care delivery system in an attempt to deliver care with outcomes that are acceptable to the consumer. Quality assurance and improvement programs that evaluate provider and client interaction through compliance with standards historically have been used alone to monitor quality care. In a TQM/CQI management approach, quality assurance and improvement methods are an integral, but not the only, tool for assuring quality or customer satisfaction.

General Approaches

General approaches to protect the public by assuring a level of competency among health care professionals are credentialing, licensure, accreditation, certification, charter, recognition, and academic degrees. All of these approaches are covered more thoroughly in most fundamentals texts but are discussed here briefly as a review.

Credentialing generally is defined as the formal recognition of a person as a professional with technical competence (Cary, 1989) or of an agency that has met minimum standards of performance. These mechanisms are used to evaluate the agency structure through which care is provided and the outcomes of care given by the provider. Credentialing can be mandatory or voluntary. Mandatory credentialing requires statutory laws. State nurse practice acts are examples of mandatory credentialing. Voluntary credentialing is performed by an agency or institution. Certification examinations offered to nurses by the ANA are examples of voluntary credentialing. Licensing, certification, and accreditation are all examples of credentialing.

Licensure is one of the oldest general quality assurance approaches in the United States and Canada. Individual licensure is a contract between the profession and the state. Under this contract the profession is granted control over entry into and exit from the profession and over quality of professional practice.

The licensing process requires that written regulations define the scope and limits of the professional's practice. Job descriptions based on these regulations set minimum and maximum limits on the functions and responsibilities of the practitioner. Licensure of nurses has been mandated by law since 1903. Today all 50 states have **mandatory nurse licensure,** which requires all who practice nursing for compensation to be licensed.

Accreditation, a voluntary approach to quality control, is used for institutions. Since 1954 the National League for Nursing (NLN), a voluntary organization, has established standards for inspecting nursing education programs. In 1966 community health–home health program standards were established by the NLN for the purpose of accrediting these programs. In addition, state boards of nursing accredit basic nursing programs so that their graduates are eligible for the licensing examination.

The accreditation function may be classified as quasi-voluntary. Although appearing to be a voluntary participatory program, accreditation often is linked to governmental regulation that encourages programs to participate in the accrediting process. Examples include the federal Medicare regulations restricting payments to accredited public health and home health care agencies and JCAHO for other health care providers.

Accreditation provides a means for effective peer review and an opportunity for an in-depth review of program strengths and limitations (Cary, 1989). In the past the accreditation process primarily evaluated an agency's physical structure, organizational structure, and personnel qualification. However, beginning in 1990 more emphasis was placed on evaluation of the outcomes of care and on the educational qualifications of the person providing the care.

Certification, another general approach to quality, combines features of licensure and accreditation. **Certification** usually is a voluntary process within professions. Educational achievements, experience, and performance on an examination determine a person's qualifications for functioning in an identified specialty area, such as community health nursing. An example of certification is the ANA certification program which includes a number of certification areas. To become a certified community health nurse, one must have a baccalaureate degree in nursing and 2 years of practice as a community health nurse immediately before application.

Although usually a voluntary process, certification also can be a **quasi-voluntary** process. For example, to function as a nurse practitioner in some states, one must show proof of educational credentials and take an examination to be "certified" to practice within the boundaries of the state.

There are major concerns about certification as a quality assurance mechanism. Data are lacking about the clinical competence of the practitioner at the time of certification because clinical competency usually is measured by written test. There are also insufficient data about the quality of the practitioner's work following the certification process. Except for occupational health nurses and nurse anesthetists, certification has not been recognized by employers as an achievement beyond basic preparation, so financial rewards are few. Although the nursing profession has accepted the certification process as a mechanism for recognizing competence and excellence, certifiers must help nurses communicate the significance of certified nurses in health care delivery to the public.

Charter, recognition, and **academic degrees** are other general approaches to quality assurance. *Charter* is the mechanism by which a state governmental agency, under state laws, grants corporate status to institutions with or without rights to award degrees (i.e., university-based nursing programs). *Recognition* is defined as a process whereby one agency accepts the credentialing status of and the credentials conferred by another. An example is when state boards of nursing accept nurse practitioner credentials that are awarded by the ANA or by one of the specialty credentialing agencies. *Academic degrees* are titles awarded to individuals recognized by degree-granting institutions as having completed a predetermined plan in a branch of learning. There are four academic degrees awarded in nursing, with some variations at each degree level: Associate of Arts/Science; Bachelor of Science in Nursing; the master's degrees—Master of Science in Nursing and Master of Nursing; and the doctoral degree—Doctor of Philosophy, Doctor of Nursing Science, Doctorate of Science in Nursing, and Doctor of Nursing.

Specific Approaches

Historically, quality assurance programs conducted by healthcare agencies have been a measurement or assessment of the performance of individuals and their conformance to standards set forth by accrediting agencies. Total quality management/continuous quality improvement is a management philosophy and method that incorporates many tools, including QA, to maximize customer satisfaction by delivery of quality care. **Quality care** has four components, which include: "(1) professional performance, (2) efficient use of resources, (3) minimal risk to the client of illness or injury associated with care, and (4) patient satisfaction" (Davis, 1994, p. 6). TQM/CQI seeks to eliminate errors in process before negative outcomes can occur rather than waiting until after the fact to correct individual performance.

Health care agencies only recently have paid heed to the tenets of TQM/CQI although Donabedian's early conceptualizations of quality bear a striking resemblance to writings of industry's TQM leaders. This management philosophy has been incorporated into Japanese industry since the post-World War II era when W. Edwards Deming was invited to Japan to help rebuild its broken economy. In addition to Deming, names associated with the total quality concept are Walter Stewart, who first published in this area, Joseph M. Juran, Armand F. Feigenbaum, Phillip B. Crosby, Genichi Taguchi, and Kaoru Ishikawa. Unlike traditional QA programs, the focus of CQI is the "process" of delivering health care. This process focus avoids assigning personal blame for less than perfect outcomes. Applying TQM in health care allows management to look at the contribution of all systems to outcomes of the organization. Additional distinguishing characteristics of TQM/CQI are the following (McLaughlin and Kaluzny, 1994, p. 4):

1. Empowering clinicians and managers to analyze and improve processes
2. Adopting a norm that customer preferences are the primary determinants of quality, and the term customer includes both the patient and provider in the process
3. Developing a multidisciplinary approach that goes beyond conventional departmental and professional lines
4. Providing the motivation for a rational, data-based, cooperative approach to process analysis and change

Deming's guidelines are summarized by his 14-point program (see box below). As expressed in Deming's first point, an organization must have purpose and values. Health care has a clear idea of its values and has been committed to quality in the past as witnessed by our codes of ethics and volumes of standards of care. However, in order for the TQM/CQI process to be successful, a cultural change must occur within an oragnization and top management must be totally in favor of TQM/CQI for the process to be successful. With respect to health care, a paradigm shift

---

Deming's 14-Point Program

1. Create and publish to all employees a statement of the aims and purposes of the company or other organization. The management must demonstrate constantly their commitment to this statement.
2. Learn the new philosophy, top management and everybody.
3. Understand the purpose of inspection, for improvement of processes and reduction of cost.
4. End the practice of awarding business on the basis of price tag alone.
5. Improve constantly and forever the system of production and service.
6. Institute training.
7. Teach and institute leadership.
8. Drive out fear. Create trust. Create a climate for innovation.
9. Optimize toward the aims and purposes of the company the efforts of teams, groups, staff areas.
10. Eliminate exhortations for the work force.
11a. Eliminate numerical quotes for production. Instead, learn and institute methods for improvement.
11b. Eliminate management by objective. Instead, learn the capabilities of processes and how to improve them.
12. Remove barriers that rob people of pride of workmanship.
13. Encourage education and self-improvement for everyone.
14. Take action to accomplish the transformation.

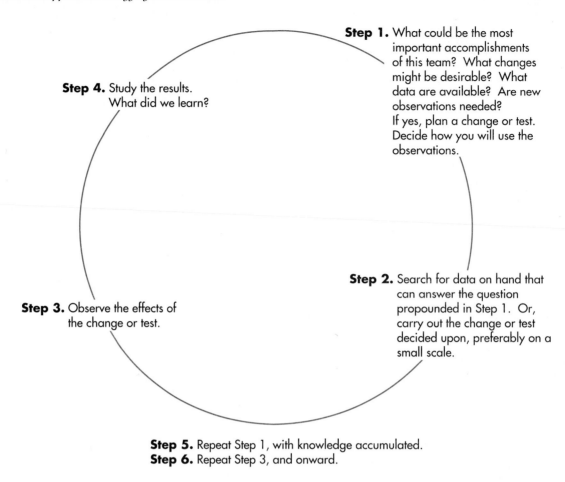

Step 1. What could be the most important accomplishments of this team? What changes might be desirable? What data are available? Are new observations needed?
If yes, plan a change or test. Decide how you will use the observations.

Step 2. Search for data on hand that can answer the question propounded in Step 1. Or, carry out the change or test decided upon, preferably on a small scale.

Step 3. Observe the effects of the change or test.

Step 4. Study the results. What did we learn?

Step 5. Repeat Step 1, with knowledge accumulated.
Step 6. Repeat Step 3, and onward.

FIGURE 22-1

Shewhart's P/D/C/A Cycle. (Reprinted from *Out of Crisis* by W. Edwards Deming by permission of MIT and The W. Edwards Deming Institute. Published by MIT, Center for Advanced Engineering Study, Cambridge, Mass 02139. Copyright 1986 by W. Edwards Deming.)

from individual provider responsibility to team responsibility for the delivery of quality healthcare has to occur (Kaluzny et al., 1992). A customer orientation focused on positive health outcomes and perceived satisfaction must be a guiding principle. To this end, customer satisfaction surveys must be done for both internal and external users of services.

Personnel policies that are motivating and continuous training/learning opportunities are crucial to any quality improvement program. Deming's eighth point speaks to driving out fear. Fear in this context means the fear of being fired for being innovative, or taking risks. In the CQI process, individuals are not blamed for failures in the system and therefore are motivated through the group to continually look for problems and improve system performance.

TQM/CQI exists best in a flat organizational structure. This organization operates with a multidisciplinary team approach and a separate but parallel management quality council that monitors strategy and implementation. Teams are empowered to solve problems and locate opportunities for system improvement. Shewhart's **Plan/Do/Check/Act Cycle,** seen in Figure 22-1, serves as a guideline for the team ap-

proach to problem solving. A suggested way to start the problem-solving process with a team in Step 1 is "brainstorming" (Al-Assaf, 1993). Brainstorming is getting everyone's input about a possible process situation with no critique of suggestions made by any team member. Following through to Step 2, since TQI organizations are data driven, ongoing statistics are collected. Variations from the mean or norm are detected through consistent use of tools, such as the flow chart, the Pareto Chart, cause-and-effect diagrams, checksheets, histograms, control charts, regression, and other statistical analyses (i.e., quality assurance data and techniques, risk management data, risk-adjusted outcome measures, and cost-effectiveness analysis) (McLaughlin and Kaluzny, 1994). Steps 3, 4, and 5 are self-explanatory.

Joseph Juran builds on Deming's initial quality work and is a proponent of building quality into all processes. The Juran Trilogy, provides an effective comparison of the tasks of quality planning, quality control, and quality improvement. Quality planning involves determining who the clients are, the needs of those clients, the service that fulfills that need, and the process to produce that service. Quality control evalu-

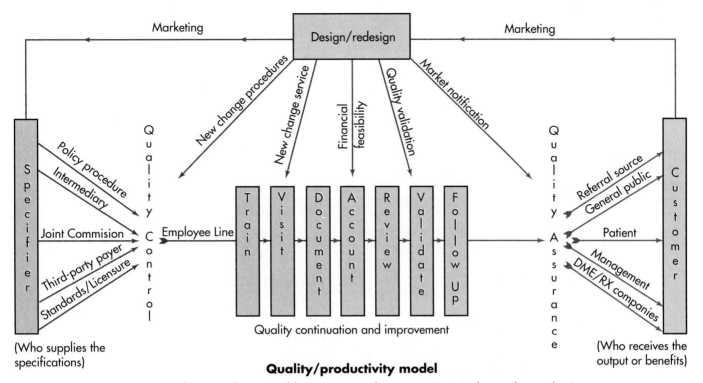

Quality/productivity model

1. Quality control: Measurable process stated in written terms (policy and procedure)
2. Quality assurance: Standard by which the measurable process is validated (audits)
3. Quality continuation: Constant self-measurement by known standards
4. Quality improvement: Culmination of control, assurance, and continuation

DME, Durable medical equipment; Rx, treatment.
NOTE: Model modified from work of W. Edwards Deming—Japan Management, 1950.

FIGURE 22-2

Quality Productivity Model. (Reprinted from *Total Quality Management for Home Care* by ER Davis by permission of Aspen Publishers. Copyright 1994 by Aspen Publishers, Inc.)

ates the performance of that service, compares it to the service goals, and then makes corrections if necessary. Quality improvement (QI) makes sure the infrastructures exists to empower individuals to identify improvement projects. Management of QI establishes project teams and provides those teams with the resources needed to carry out improvement projects (Juran, 1989).

TQM/CQI IN COMMUNITY HEALTH SETTINGS

Public Health Agencies are able to implement TQM/CQI because of the existing guidelines provided by the 1991 American Public Health Association (APHA) Model Standards. These guidelines "link standards to meeting the health goals for the nation in the year 2000" (Kaluzny et al., 1992, p. 258). Healthy People 2000 and APHA Model Standards provide not only a prioritized list of health objectives for the nation but the most current statistics and scientific knowledge about health promotion and disease prevention. Addi-

tionally, the Assessment Protocol for Excellence in Public Health (APEX-PH) (APHA, 1990) provides not only a method of assessing community needs but also a method of assessing how well departments are operating to meet existing standards. As health care reform evolves, public health facilities may be faced with competing in an open market and may move more rapidly toward more corporate forms of management.

Because of the competition that exists in this arena, home health agencies have made progress in adopting quality improvement programs. Congruent with the TQM/CQI philosophy, meeting customer expectations is a must for home health agencies. Davis (1994) presents a quality productivity model for home health based on Deming's work (Figure 22-2). Under the first step, labeled as specifier, Davis makes clear that straightforward definitions of requirements and processes are necessary before embarking on a CQI process. This reinforces the need for the continuing learning process called for under Deming's 14 points. The model then proceeds with quality control, quality assurance, and quality continuation processes that should result in quality improvement. Quality control is a proactive process and flows from specifiers being written in measurable terms and taught to all employees. Quality assurance activities are implemented through a proactive quality continuation sequence. QA retrospectively validates measures of policies, procedures, and standards set forth under quality control. In addition to the QA function an ongoing effort is underway to eliminate errors before they happen. QA can serve to alert the organization to unwanted trends. The quality continuation sequence continues as an "alignment of quality policy, procedure, practice, hiring criteria, training, rewards, and recognition" (Davis, 1994, p. 11). Quality improvement is the result of all preceding activities and must be an ongoing process with continuing higher standards for achievement reintroduced into the system.

Using QA/QI in TQM/CQI

Though the methods differ, the objective of both TQM/CQI and QA/QI programs is quality outcomes for clients. QA/QI methods and tools help agencies conform to standards required by external accrediting agencies. QA/QI provides a way to identify examples of substandard care and improve that care when standards are not met (Harris, 1990). Whereas QA is focused on problem detection, TQM/CQI focuses on problem prevention and continuous improvement. A basic tenet of the total quality philosophy is that quality cannot be inspected in, it must be built in. According to Tindall and Stewart (1993) under QA/QI, there is generally little attention paid to prevention of errors/problems and minimal ownership of quality issues. Further the QA process may come to a halt until another problem is found. Kaluzny, McLaughlin and Simpson (1992, p. 259) point out differences in traditional management models that use performance standards versus those that use TQM/CQI (see Table 22-1).

Since common ground exists between TQM/CQI and QA/QI, positive aspects of a known quality assurance program can be integrated into a total quality approach. Strengths of quality assurance include a history of expertise in development of evaluation of structures, identification of high-priority problems and development of knowledge in quality assessment and information systems. These strengths can be used to advantage in a continuous quality improvement effort.

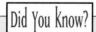

Did You Know?

Total quality management is a concept that gives direction for managing a system of care, whereas quality assurance focuses on the care a client receives within the system.

Table 22-1   Traditional Management Compared to TQM Model

Traditional model	TQM model
Legal or professional authority	Collective or managerial responsibility
Specialized accountability	Process accountability
Administrative authority	Participation
Meeting standards	Meeting process and performance expectations
Longer planning horizon	Shorter planning horizon
Quality Assurance	Continuous improvement

Traditional Quality Assurance

Traditional quality assurance programs can fit well with the continuous quality improvement process. Organizations may implement only parts of the total quality management process, so it is important to understand existing traditional QA programs. The overall goal of specific quality assurance approaches is to monitor the process and outcomes of client care. The goals are (1) to identify problems between provider and client, (2) to intervene in problem cases, (3) to provide feedback regarding interaction between client and provider, and (4) to provide documentation of interactions between provider and client.

The specific approaches often are implemented voluntarily by agencies and provider groups interested in the quality of interactions in their setting. However, the state and federal governments require mandatory programs within public health agencies. For instance, periodic utilization review, peer reviews (audits), and other quality control measures are required in public health agencies that receive funds from state taxes, Medicaid, Medicare, and other public funding sources. Examples of specific approaches to quality control are agency staff review committees (peer review), utilization review committees, research studies, PRO monitoring, client satisfaction surveys, risk management, and malpractice litigation.

Staff Review Committee

Staff review committees are the most common specific approach to quality assurance in the United States. Staff, or peer review, committees are designed to monitor client-specific aspects of certain levels of care. The audit is the major tool used to ascertain quality of care.

The **audit process** (Figure 22-3) consists of six steps: (1) selection of a topic for study, (2) selection of explicit criteria for quality care, (3) review of records to determine whether criteria are met, (4) peer review of all cases that do not meet criteria, (5) specific recommendations to correct problems, and (6) follow-up to determine whether problems have been eliminated (LoGerfo and Brook, 1984).

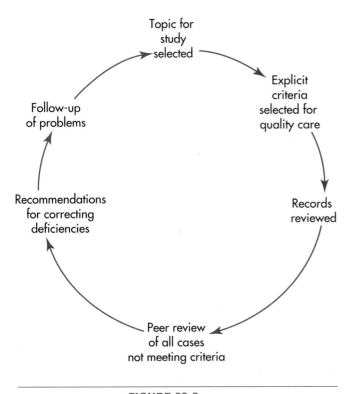

FIGURE 22-3

The Audit Process.

Two types of audits are used in nursing peer review: concurrent and retrospective. The **concurrent audit** is a process audit that evaluates the quality of ongoing care by looking at the nursing process. Concurrent audit is used by Medicare and Medicaid to evaluate care being received by public health/home health clients. The advantages of this method are (1) identification of problems at the time care is given, (2) provision of a mechanism for identifying and meeting client needs during care, (3) implementation of measures to fulfill professional responsibilities, and (4) provision of a mechanism for communicating on behalf of the client. The disadvantages of the concurrent audit are that (1) it is time consuming; (2) it is more costly to implement than the retrospective audit; and (3) because care is ongoing, it does not present the total picture of care that the client ultimately will receive.

The **retrospective audit,** or outcome audit, evaluates quality of care through appraisal of the nursing process after the client's discharge from the health care system. The advantages of the retrospective audit are that it provides (1) comparison of actual practice to standards of care, (2) analysis of actual practice findings, (3) a total picture of care given, and (4) more accurate data for planning corrective action. Disadvantages of the retrospective audit method are (1) the focus of evaluation is directed away from ongoing care and (2) client problems are identified after discharge, so corrective action can only be used to improve the care of future clients.

Utilization Review

The purpose of **utilization review** is to assure that care actually is needed and that the cost is appropriate (Davis, 1994). LoGerfo and Brook (1984) described three types of utilization review: (1) prospective—an assessment of the necessity of care before giving service; (2) concurrent—a review of the necessity of services while care is being given; and (3) retrospective—an analysis of the necessity of the services received by the client after the care has been given. Each of these reviews provides an assessment of the appropriateness of the cost of care. Prospectively, care can be denied and money saved. Concurrently, services can be cut if they are not deemed essential. Retrospectively, payment can be denied to the provider if the care was not necessary.

Utilization review began in the middle part of this century out of concern for increasing health care costs. The first committees were developed by insurance companies and professional groups. Utilization review committees became mandatory under the 1965 Medicare Law as a way to control hospital costs (Davis, 1994).

The utilization review process includes development of explicit criteria regarding the need for services and the length of service. Utilization review has been used primarily in hospitals to establish the need for client admission and to determine the length of hospital stay. In community health, especially home health care, utilization review establishes criteria for admission to agency service, the number of visits a client may receive, the eligibility for client services, such as a nursing aide or physical therapist, and discharge.

Utilization review has several advantages: (1) it assists clients to avoid unnecessary care; (2) it may encourage the consideration of alternative care options, such as home health care rather than hospitalization; (3) it can provide guidelines for staff and program development; and (4) it provides for agency accountability to the consumer. The major disadvantage of utilization review is that not all clients fit the classic picture presented by the "explicit criteria" used to determine approval or denial of care. For example, an elderly female client was admitted to a home health care agency for management after hospital discharge. The client was paraplegic as a result of a cerebrovascular accident. After several weeks of physical and speech therapy, the client showed little sign of progress. The utilization review committee considered the client's condition to be stable and did not recognize the continued need for management to prevent future complications; therefore, Medicare payment was denied.

Appeal mechanisms have been built into the utilization review process used by Medicare and Medicaid. The appeal allows providers and clients to present additional data that may help to reverse the original decision to deny payment.

Risk Management

Risk management committees often are a part of the quality assurance/improvement program of a community agency. The goal of risk management is to reduce the liability on the part of the agency and the number of grievances brought against the agency. The risk management committee reviews all risks to which an agency is exposed. It reviews client and personnel safety policies and procedures and determines whether personnel are following the rules. Examples of problems reviewed by a risk management committee would include administering incorrect vaccination dosage, pediatric client injury caused by a fall from an examining table, or injury to the community health nurse as a result of an accident while making a home visit. Incident reports are reviewed by the risk management committee for appropriate, accurate, and thorough documentation of any problem that occurs relating to clients or personnel. In addition patterns are identified that may require changes in policy or staff development to correct the problem. As a part of risk management, grievance procedures are established for both clients and personnel.

Professional Review Organizations

The Professional Standards Review Organization (PSRO) was established in 1972 in an amendment to the Social Security Act (Public Law 92-603) as a publicly mandated utilization and peer review program. This law provided that medical, hospital, and nursing home care under Medicare, Medicaid, and Title V Maternal and Child Health Programs would be reviewed for appropriateness and necessity and such care would be reimbursed accordingly.

In 1983 Congress passed the Peer Review Improvement Act (PL 97-248), creating PROs. PROs replaced PSROs and are directed by the federal government to reduce hospital admissions for procedures that can be performed safely and effectively in an ambulatory surgical setting on an outpatient basis, and reduce inappropriate or unnecessary admissions or invasive procedures by specific practitioners or hospitals. Quality measures include reduction of unnecessary admissions caused by previous substandard care, avoidable complications and deaths, and unnecessary surgery or invasive procedures (Gremaldi and Micheletti, 1985).

Institutions contract with PROs for quality reviews. PROs are local (usually state) organizations that establish criteria for care based on local patterns of practice. They can be for-profit or not-for-profit organizations. They have access to physicians or may include physicians in their membership. PROs must define their operational objectives and are required to consult with nurses and other nonphysician health care providers when reviewing the activities of those professionals. PROs monitor access to care and cost of care. Professionals working under the regulation of PROs should develop accurate and complete documentation procedures to ensure compliance with the criteria of the PRO.

The federally mandated quality review process has produced much debate about its limitations and benefits. Limitations of the process incude jeopardizing professional autonomy because decision making regarding care includes professionals, consumers, and government representatives. Another limitation of this process is the development of a costly control mechanism whereby client care activities may be determined by cost rather than by professional criteria. The benefit of the PSRO/PRO system has been the challenge to health care professionals to develop standards and to institute peer review mechanisms to increase accountability for care provided (Bull, 1985; Gremaldi and Micheletti, 1985; Lieski, 1985).

In 1985 PRO authority was expanded to include review of services offered by health maintenance organizations and competitive medical plans. In addition the Medicare Quality Assurance Act was passed to strengthen quality assurance programs and to improve access to posthospital care. This act required hospitals receiving Medicare payments to provide to Medicare beneficiaries written forms of discharge planning supervised by registered nurses and social workers.

> ## What Do You Think?
>
> Quality assurance efforts focus on the quality of care received by Medicare and Medicaid clients. Little is done to assure quality of the privately insured and the uninsured.

Evaluative Studies

Evaluative studies for quality health care have increased throughout the twentieth century. The purpose of such studies is to show the effect of nursing and health care interventions on client populations. Three major models have been used to evaluate quality: Donabedian's structure-process-outcome, the tracer, and the sentinel.

Donabedian's (1982, 1985, 1990) model introduced three major methods for evaluating quality care. The first method is structure, evaluating the setting and instruments used to provide care. Examples of structure are facilities, equipment, characteristics of the administrative organization, client mix, and the qualifications of health providers. The second is process, evaluating activities as they relate to standards and expectations of health providers in the management of client care. The third is outcome, the net change that occurs as a result of health care or the net result of health care. The three methods may be used separately to evaluate a part of care. However, to get an overall picture of quality of care they should be used together.

The tracer method described by Kessner and Kalk

(1973) is a measure of both process and outcome of care. This method is more effective in evaluating health care of groups rather than of individual clients, and it is more effective in evaluating care delivered by an institution than by an individual provider.

Kessner and Kalk (1973) described the following essential characteristics for implementing the tracer method: a tracer, or a problem, that has a definite impact on the client's level of functioning; well-defined and easily diagnosed characteristics; population prevalence high enough to permit adequate data collection; a known variation resulting from use of effective health care; well-defined management techniques in either prevention, diagnosis, treatment, or rehabilitation; and understood (documented) effects of nonmedical factors on the tracer. Stevens (1985) provided a classification system for selecting client groups for tracer outcome studies in nursing: (1) a particular disease, (2) similar treatment, (3) similar needs, (4) similar community, (5) similar life-style, and (6) similar illness stage. The tracer method provides nurses with data to show the differences in outcomes as a result of nursing care standards.

The sentinel method of quality evaluation is based on epidemiological principles (Rutstein et al., 1976). This method is an outcome measure for examining specific instances of client care. The characteristics of this method are as follows: (1) cases of unnecessary disease, disability, complications, and death are counted; (2) the circumstances surrounding the unnecessary event, or the sentinel, are examined in detail; (3) a review of morbidity and mortality is used as an index to determine the critical increase in the untimely event, which may reflect changes in quality of care; and (4) health status indicators, such as changes in social, economic, political, and environmental factors that may have an effect on health outcomes, are reviewed. Changes in the sentinel indicate potential problems for others. For example, increases in encephalitis in certain communities may result from increases in mosquito populations.

Client Satisfaction

Client satisfaction is another approach to measuring quality of care. Client satisfaction can be assessed using in-person or telephone interviews and mailed questionnaires. In community health nursing, satisfaction surveys are used to access care received during a specific agency admission, to assess the client's personal nursing care, or to assess the total care that the client received from all services.

Satisfaction surveys may measure the interventions of client care, attitudes about the care received and the providers of care, and perceptions of the situation (environment) in which the care was received. Clients often are more critical of interpersonal and situational components of care than of the interventions of care.

Satisfaction surveys are an essential aspect of quality assessment. The survey data provides clues to reasons for client compliance or noncompliance with plans of care. The surveys also provide data about health-seeking behaviors, the probability of malpractice litigation, and the likelihood of continuing client-provider-agency relationships. The NLN (CHHA/CHS, 1985) provides an example of a client satisfaction survey (Discharged Patient Questionnaire) that can be used in a community health agency.

Malpractice Litigation

Malpractice litigation is a specific approach to quality assurance imposed on the health care delivery system by the legal system. Malpractice litigation typically results from client dissatisfaction with the provider and with the content of the care received. Nursing is not immune from malpractice litigation. Community health nursing must continue to have a sound quality assurance program that ensures quality care. This will reduce the risk of quality control measures being imposed by an external source, such as the legal system.

MODEL QUALITY ASSURANCE/QUALITY IMPROVEMENT PROGRAM

The primary purpose of a quality assurance/quality improvement program is to ensure that the results of an organized activity are consistent with the expectations. All personnel affected by a quality assurance program should be involved in its development and implementation. Although administration and management are responsible for the quality of services, the key to that quality is the knowledge, skills, and attitudes of the personnel who deliver the service (Porter, 1988).

In 1977 the ANA introduced a model for a quality assurance program. Figure 22-4 depicts the model, which identifies seven basic components of a quality assurance program. A quality assurance program answers the following questions about health care services and nursing care: (1) What is being done now? (2) Why is it being done? (3) Is it being done well? (4) Can it be done better? (5) Should it be done at all? (6) Are there improved ways to deliver the service? (7) How much is it costing? (8) Should certain activities be abandoned and/or replaced? (Gottlieb, 1988).

The ANA model and Donabedian's framework for evaluating health care programs using the components of structure, process, and outcome can be used in developing a quality assurance program. Today outcome is the most important ingredient of a program. Outcome now is the key to evaluation of providers and agencies by accrediting bodies, by insurance companies, and by Medicare and Medicaid through PROs and other accrediting agencies.

Structure

The philosophy and objectives of an agency serve to define the structural standards of the agency. Evaluation of structure is a specific approach to quality ap-

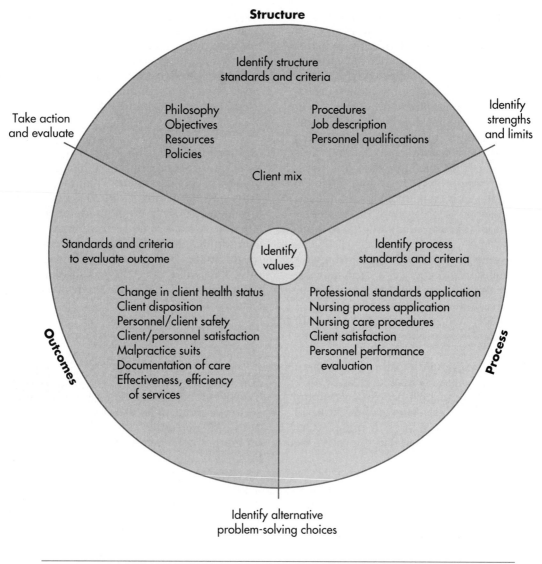

Structure

Identify structure
standards and criteria

Take action
and evaluate

Identify
strengths
and limits

Philosophy
Objectives
Resources
Policies

Procedures
Job description
Personnel qualifications

Client mix

Identify
values

Standards and criteria
to evaluate outcome

Identify process
standards and criteria

Change in client health status
Client disposition
Personnel/client safety
Client/personnel satisfaction
Malpractice suits
Documentation of care
Effectiveness, efficiency
of services

Professional standards application
Nursing process application
Nursing care procedures
Client satisfaction
Personnel performance
evaluation

Outcomes

Process

Identify alternative
problem-solving choices

FIGURE 22-4

Model quality assurance program.

praisal. In evaluating the structure of an organization, the evaluator determines whether the agency is adhering to the stated philosophy and objectives. Is the agency providing services to populations across the life span? Are primary, secondary, and/or tertiary preventive services offered? Standards of structure are defined by the licensing or accrediting agency, for example, the NLN standards for accrediting home health agencies (CHHA/CHS, 1986).

Values identification, the first step in a quality assurance program, serves to define the beliefs of the agency about humanity, nursing, the community, and health. The beliefs of the community, the population to be served, and the providers of care are equally important to the agency beliefs, and all need to be considered to provide quality service.

Identification of standards and criteria for quality assurance begins with writing the philosophy and objectives of the organization. These program objectives are being written in the 1990s to define the intended

results of nursing care, descriptions of client behaviors, and/or change in health status to be demonstrated on discharge (Rinke and Wilson, 1988).

Once objectives are formulated, the required resources are identified to accomplish the objectives. Need for the resources of personnel, supplies and equipment, facilities, and finances are described. Once resources are determined, policies, procedures, and job descriptions are formulated to serve as behavioral guides to the employees of the agency. These documents should reflect the essential nursing and other health provider qualifications needed to implement the services of the agency.

Standards of structure are evaluated internally by a committee composed of administrative, management, and staff members for the purpose of doing a self-study. Standards of structure also are evaluated by a utilization review committee often composed of an external advisory group with community representatives for all services offered through an agency, such as a nurse, a physical therapist, a speech pathologist, a physician, a board member, and an administrator from a sister agency. The data from these committees identify the strengths and weaknesses of the agency structure.

Process

The evaluation of process standards is a specific appraisal of the quality of care being given by agency providers, such as nurses. Agencies use a variety of methods to determine criteria for evaluating provider activities: conceptual models, such as a developmental model or Neuman's Systems Model; the standards of care of the provider's professional organization, such as the ANA community health nursing standards; or the nursing process. The activities of the nurse are evaluated to see whether they correspond with nursing care procedures defined by the agency.

The primary approaches used for process evaluation include the peer review committee and the client satisfaction survey. The techniques used for process evaluation are direct observation, questionnaire, interview, written audit, and videotape of client and provider encounters.

Although many audit instruments have been developed, Schmele has developed and tested an instrument based on the nursing process and applied in the community setting: The Schmele Instrument to Measure the Process of Nursing Practice in Community Nursing Service. This is a three-part instrument that includes data from direct observation, from the record audit, and from the client by means of survey questionnaire. Each technique involves evaluation of the four steps of the nursing process (Schmele, 1985; Meisenheimer, 1989). A copy of a second instrument developed by Schmele to measure the process of nursing practice in Home Health (SIMP-H) appears in Appendix C.3.

Once data are collected to evaluate nursing process standards, the peer review committee reviews the data to identify strengths and weaknesses in the quality of care delivered. The peer review committee usually is an internal committee composed of representatives of the nursing staff who are trained to administer audit instruments and conduct client interviews.

Outcome

The evaluation of outcome standards, or the end result of nursing care, is one of the more difficult tasks facing nursing today. The ability to identify changes in the client's health status as a result of nursing care will give nursing data that show the contribution of nursing to the health care delivery system. Research studies using the tracer method or the sentinel method to identify client outcomes and client satisfaction surveys are approaches that may be used to measure outcome standards. Techniques that can be used to measure outcome standards are client admission data on the level of dependence, the acuity of problems, and discharge data that may show changes in levels of dependence and activity.

From these data, strengths and weaknesses in nursing care delivery can be determined. The most common measurement methods used are direct physical observations and interviews. Rissner (1975) developed a client satisfaction survey to evaluate client attitudes and the content of nursing care in a primary setting. The survey has been adapted for use in home health by Reeder (Meisenheimer, 1989).

Instruments also have been developed to measure general health status indicators in home health (Choi et al., 1987; Gould, 1985; Padilla and Grant, 1987). The Omaha Visiting Nurses Association Problem Classification System includes nursing diagnosis, protocols of care, and a problem-rating scale to measure nursing care outcomes. Community health nursing has been involved primarily in evaluating program outcomes to justify program expenditures rather than in evaluating client outcomes.

 Research Brief

Martin KS, Scheer NJ, Stegman MR: Home health clients: characteristics, outcomes of care and nursing interventions. *Am Public Health* 83(2):1730-34, 1993.

Using the Omaha System to measure nursing outcomes, this study examined 2403 recipients of home health services in four agencies in Wisconsin, New Jersey, and Nebraska. Nurses, trained in the Omaha system schemata, abstracted data from random samples of records throughout the data collection period on client problems, problem specific knowledge, behavior, status outcome changes, and interventions. Findings of the study showed that nurses conducted 70% of all visits, identified 9107 problems and provided 96,000 interventions. Client status improved by .52 points on three, five-point subscales designed to measure problem specific outcome. This study offers evidence that the Omaha System is useful in quantifying nursing practice outcomes in a community setting.

Outcome evaluation assumes that health care has a positive effect on client status. The major problem with outcome evaluation is determining which nursing care activities are primarily responsible for causing changes in client status. In community health nursing there are multiple uncontrolled factors in the field, such as environment and family relationships, that have an effect on client status, and often it is difficult to determine whether these factors are the cause of changes in client status or whether nursing interventions have the most effect. NLN has published useful guides for developing outcome criteria (Rinke, 1987).

Types of problems studied in a quality assurance

Table 22-2 Quality Assurance Measures

Structure	Process	Outcome
Internal agency committees	**Peer review committees**	**Internal Agency**
Self-study	Prospective audit	Evaluative studies
Review agency documents	Concurrent audit	Survey health status
	Retrospective audit	
External agency	**Client**	**Client**
Regulatory audit	Satisfaction survey	Satisfaction survey
Utilization review		Malpractice suits

program include: reasons for client death, client injury, personnel and client safety and agency liability, causes of increased costs, denied reimbursement by third-party payers, client complaints, inefficient service, staff noncompliance with standards of structure, lack of resources, unnecessary staff work and overtime, documentation of care, and client health status. Table 22-2 summarizes quality assurance measures.

Evaluation, Interpretation, and Action

Interpreting the findings of a quality care evaluation is an essential component of the process. It allows for the identification of discrepancies between the quality care standards of the agency and the actual practice of the nurse or other health providers. These patterns reflect the total agency's functioning over time and generate information for decisions to be made about the strengths and limitations of the agency. Regular intervals for evaluation should be established within the agency, and periodic reports should be written so that the combined results of structure, process, and outcome efforts can be analyzed, and health care delivery patterns and problems can be identified. These reports should be used to establish an ongoing picture of changes that occur within an agency to justify community nursing services. Identification and choices of possible courses of action to correct the weaknesses within the agency should involve both the administration and the staff. The courses of action chosen should be based on their significance, economic benefit, and timeliness. For example, if there is a nursing problem dealing with the recording of client health education, the agency administration and staff may analyze the problem to see why it is occurring. Reasons for recording inadequacies given by the nurses include a lack of time to do paperwork properly, case overloads that reduce the amount of time spent with clients, and lack of available resources for health education. If such reasons are given, it would not be appropriate for management to deal with the problem by providing a staff development program on the importance of doing and recording aggregate health education. It would be more important to assess how to provide the time and resources necessary for the nurses to offer health education to the clients. Economically, it may be more beneficial to provide dictating equipment and clerical assistance so that nurses can dicate notes and other paperwork, thereby providing more client contact time, or it may be more beneficial economically to employ an additional nurse and reduce caseloads.

Taking action is the final step in the quality assurance/quality improvement model. Once the alternative courses of action are chosen to correct problems, actions must be implemented for change to occur in the overall operation of the agency. Follow-up and evaluation of actions taken must occur for improvement in quality of care to occur. Although health provider evaluation will continue to be included in a quality improvement effort, the focus of a continuous quality improvement effort emphasizes the process and not the person. The assumption here is that health care professionals and other employees customarily want to do the best job possible for the client, and problems or variations in a process should not be automatically attributed to their behavior (Laffel and Blumenthal, 1993). Although frequent feedback should be given to all employees, the hallmark of quality improvement is continuous learning. Staff development must be ongoing for all employees.

Documentation is essential to the evaluation of quality care in any organization. The following section focuses on the kinds of documentation that normally occur in a community health agency.

RECORDS
Purposes

Records are an integral part of the communication structure of the health care organization. Accurate and complete records are required by law and must be kept by all agencies, governmental and nongovernmental. In most states, the state departments of health stipulate the kind and content requirements of records for community health agencies.

Records provide complete information about the client, indicate the extent and quality of services being rendered, resolve legal issues in malpractice suits, and provide information for education and research.

Community Health Agency Records

Within the community health agency many types of records are kept and are used to predict population trends in a community, to identify health needs and problems, to prepare and justify budgets, and to make administrative decisions. The kinds of records kept by the community health agency may include reports of accidents, births, census, chronic disease, communicable disease, mortality, life expectancy, morbidity, child and spouse abuse, occupational illness and injury, and environmental health.

Other types of records kept within the agency are records used to maintain administrative contact and control of the organization. Three types of records make up this category: clinical, service, and financial. The clinical record is the client health record. The provider service records include information about the numbers of clinic patients seen daily, the immunizations given, home visits made daily, transportation and mileage, the provider's time spent with the client, and the amount and kinds of supplies used. The service record is completed on a daily basis by each provider and is summarized monthly and annually to indicate trends in health care activities and costs relative to personnel time, transportation, maintenance, and supplies. The provider service records are used to correlate with the agency's financial records of salaries, overhead, and transportation costs, and they serve as the basis for the cost accounting system (Pickett and Hanlon, 1990). These records are basic to peer review and audit.

Three additional kinds of service records seen in the community health agency are the central index system, the annual implementation plan, and the annual summary of agency activities. The central index system is a data-filing system that indicates the services requested, services offered, active and inactive clients of the agency, and a profile of the agency's clients.

The annual implementation plan is developed at the beginning of each fiscal year to define the short-term and long-term goals of the agency. The annual imple-

mentation plan serves as the basis for the agency's annual summary. The annual summary reflects the success of the agency in meeting the annual objectives, changes in population trends and health status during the year, the actual versus the projected budget requirements, the number of services offered, the number of clients served, and the plans and changes recommended for the future. This plan serves as the basis for the evaluation of agency structure.

As an outgrowth of quality assurance efforts in the health care system, comprehensive methods are being designed to document and measure client progress and client outcome from agency admission through discharge. An example of such a method is the client classification system developed at the Visiting Nurses Association of Omaha, Nebraska (Martin, 1982). This comprehensive method for evaluating client care has several components: a classification system for assessing and categorizing client problems, a data base, a nursing problem list, and anticipated outcome criteria for the classified problem. Such schemes are viewed as having the potential to improve the delivery of nursing care, documentation, and the descriptions of client care. Briefly, implementation of comprehensive documentation methods will enhance nursing assessment, planning, implementation and evaluation of client care, and it will allow for the organization of pertinent client information for more effective and efficient nurse productivity and communication.

 ## Clinical Application

Catherine, a community health nursing student, has been asked to be a member of the health care team designated to monitor the quality of service provided to the clients and community of the health care agency. As a member of this committee she is interested in identifying the current system used to monitor quality.

To prepare for her role in planning and implementing a quality assurance/quality improvement program she reads the federal and state regulations to identify those elements which, by law, must be included in the QA/QI program. She finds that Medicare now has specific tools to measure outcomes of client care. She learns that when the Medicare evaluator visits the agency, Catherine will be making home visits with the evaluator to observe directly the physical appearance of the client.

At the first meeting, the student is interested in the relationship between philosophy and objectives of the agency. Does the philosophy reflect beliefs about the clients to be served by the agency, the type of nursing care and services to be delivered, the population or the community to be served and, finally, beliefs about health care versus illness care? Are the objectives of the agency reflective of the stated beliefs in the philosophy? For example, does the phi-

losophy indicate beliefs about client education or research? If so, are there agency objectives that address providing health education or enhancing research related to better client care?

Once the committee establishes from the philosophy and objectives that the agency's goal is to deliver primary health care services to the total population of the community, Catherine is interested in the standards of care used to deliver quality health care. In nursing, are the ANA standards for community health nursing used to evaluate nursing care given? Are the nurses employed by the agency qualified to fulfill their job descriptions through education, experience, or both?

Then the committee looks at the employment criteria of the agency. Do the criteria reflect the beliefs of the agency about nursing and the agency goals? Do the agency's policies and procedures assist the nurse in meeting the stated standards of care?

Given the structure of the agency, how is the process of care evaluated? Does the agency use prospective, concurrent, or retrospective audits to evaluate the process of care given? Are the audits designed to measure the standards of care used by the agency? How is the data used after it is collected? Is there any evidence that the evaluation makes a dif-

Continued

Clinical Application—cont'd

ference? Has the process of care changed as a result of the evaluation.

After the structure and process elements are identified, the committee members and the student are interested in the outcome elements. How is health outcome defined by the agency: client satisfaction, change in health status, number of malpractice suits, or number of Medicare payments received? How is the data used to make a difference in future quality outcomes?

After answering these questions with the committee, Catherine decides she would like to perform a self-evaluation or, preferably, have a peer review by fellow students to determine the quality of care she has given through the semester. She uses the client satisfaction survey in Appendix J.1 to determine how the clients feel about the services she has delivered. She applies the SIMP audit instrument (see Appendix C.3) to review and evaluate several records of clients she has cared for. She interprets the data, makes adjustments in her care, and shares findings with her faculty advisor. Catherine feels good about the process and outcomes of her clients' care. She has functioned under the agency policies and knows that she has contributed to the overall quality of care as defined by the agency structure.

Key Concepts

- The health care delivery system is the largest employing industry in the United States; society is demanding increased efficiency and effectiveness from the system. Quality control is the tool used to ensure effectiveness and efficiency.

- Objective and systematic evaluation of nursing care has became a priority within the profession for several reasons, including the effects of cost on health care accessibility, consumer demands for better quality care, and increasing involvement of nurses in public and health agency policy formulation.

- Total Quality Management/Continuous Quality Improvement is a management philosophy new to the health care arena. It is prevention oriented and process focused. Its primary focus is to deliver quality health care. Quality is defined as customer satisfaction.

- Quality assurance and improvement is the monitoring of the activities of client care to determine the degree of excellence attained in implementation of the activities.

- Quality assurance has been a concern of the profession since the 1860s, when Florence Nightingale called for a uniform format to gather and disseminate hospital statistics.

- Licensure has been a major issue in nursing since 1892.

- Two major categories of approaches exist in quality assurance and improvement today—general and specific approaches.

- Accreditation is an approach to quality control used for institutions, whereas licensure is used primarily for individuals.

- Certification combines features of both licensing and accreditation.

- Three major models have been used to evaluate quality: Donabedian's structure-process-outcome model, the sentinel model, and the tracer model.

- Seven basic components of a quality assurance program are (1) identifying values; (2) identifying structure, process, and outcome standards and criteria; (3) selecting measurement techniques; (4) interpreting the strengths and weaknesses of the care given; (5) identifying alternative courses of action; (6) choosing specific courses of action; and (7) taking action.

- Records are an integral part of the communication structure of a health care organization. Accurate and complete records are by law required of all agencies, whether governmental or nongovernmental.

- Quality assurance and improvement mechanisms in health care delivery are the mechanisms for controlling the system and requesting accountability from individual providers within the system. Records help establish a total picture of the contribution of the agency to the client community.

Critical Thinking Activities

1. Write your own definition of TQM/CQI; compare your definition with the one given in the text. Are they the same or different? Give justification for your answer.
2. How does traditional QA/QI fit into the TQM/CQI effort. Explain the relative importance of a continuing QA/QI effort.
3. Interview a nurse who is a coordinator of (or is responsible for) quality assurance and improvement in a local health agency. Ask the following questions and add others you may wish to have answered.
   a. Does the agency subscribe to the TQM/CQI approach to management?
   b. If not, is the agency incorporating elements of the TQM/CQI process as outlined by Deming in his 14 points?
   c. Is a traditional method of QA used to assure quality?
   d. Describe the components of the QA/QI program.
   e. How are records used in your QA/QI effort.
   f. Discuss the approaches and techniques that are used to implement the QA/QI program.
   g. How has the QA/QI program changed in the health agency over the past 20 years?
   h. What influence has the QA/QI program had on decreasing problems attributable to process? to provider accountability?
   i. List and describe the types of records usually kept in a community health agency. Explain the purpose of each type of record.

Bibliography

Al-Assaf AF: Data management for total quality. In Al-Assaf AF, Schmele JA, editors: *The textbook of total quality in healthcare,* Delray Beach, Fla, 1993, St Lucie Press, pp 123-156.

American Nurses Association: *Quality model: a plan for implementation of the standards of nursing practice,* Kansas City, Mo, 1977, The Association.

American Nurses Association: *A conceptual model of community health nursing,* Kansas City, Mo, 1982, The Association.

American Nurses Association: *The key to your professional future: professional certification,* Kansas City, Mo, 1990, The Association.

American Nurses Association Committee for the study of credentialing a new approach, vols 1 and 2, Kansas City, Mo, 1979, The Association.

American Nurses Association Congress on Nursing Practice: *Standards of nursing practice,* Kansas City, Mo, 1973, The Association.

American Public Health Association: *The definition and role of public health nursing in the delivery of health care,* Washington, DC, 1980. The Association.

Assessment protocol for excellence in public health (APEX-PH), Washington, DC, 1990, American Public Health Association.

Association of Community Health Nursing Educators: *Essential components of master's level practice in community health nursing,* Lexington, Ky, 1991, The Association.

Association of Community Health Nursing Educators: *Essentials of baccalaureate education,* Louisville, Ky, 1991, The Association.

Association of Community Health Nursing Educators: *Perspectives on doctoral education in community health nursing,* Lexington, Ky, 1993, The Association.

Berwick DM: Continuous improvement as an ideal in healthcare, *N Engl J Med* 320:53-56, 1989.

Bull MJ: Quality assurance: its origins, transformations, and prospects. In Meisenheimer CG, editor: *Quality assurance: a complete guide to effective programs,* Rockville, Md, 1985, Aspen Publishers.

Cary A: Credentialing: opportunities and responsibilities in nursing. In Lambert C, Lambert V: *Perspectives in nursing,* Norwalk, Conn, 1989, Appleton & Lange.

Chernin S, Ayer T: The outcome audit: assuring quality care, *Caring* 9(2):8, 1990.

Choi T, Josten L, Christensen ML, et al: Health specific family coping index for noninstitutional care. In Rinke L, editor: *Outcome measures in home care,* vol 1, New York, 1987, National League for Nursing.

Chu N, Schmele J: Using the ANA Standards as a basis for performance evaluation in the home health setting. *J Nurs Quality Assurance* 4(3):25, 1990.

Council of Home Health Agencies and Community Health Services: *Accreditation of home health agencies and community nursing services: criteria and guide for preparing reports,* New York, 1986, National League for Nursing.

Council of Home Health Agencies and Community Health Services: *Administrator's handbook for the structure, operation, and expansion of home health agencies,* New York, 1985 and 1988, National League for Nursing.

Daley J: Mortality and other outcome data. In Longo, Bohr, editors: *Quantitative methods in quality management: a guide to practitioners,* Chicago, 1991, American Hospital Association.

Davis ER: *Total quality management for homecare,* Gaithersburg, Md, 1994, Aspen Publishers.

Decker F, Stevens L, Vancini M, Wedeking L, et al: Using patient outcomes to evaluate community health nursing, *Nurs Outlook* 27(4):278, 1979.

Decker CM: Quality assurance: accent on monitoring, *Nurs Manag* 16:20, 1985.

Deming WE: *Out of the Crisis,* Cambridge, Mass, 1986, MIT, Center for Advanced Engineering Study.

Dolbie S, Creason N: Outcome criteria for the patient using intravenous antibiotic therapy at home, *Home Healthcare Nurse* 6(4):23, 1988.

Donabedian A: *The criteria and standards of quality,* vol 2, *Exploration in quality assessment and monitoring,* Ann Arbor, Mich, 1982, Health Administration Press.

Donabedian A: *Explorations in quality assessment and monitoring,* vol 3, Ann Arbor, Mich, 1985, Health Administration Press.

Donabedian A: The seven pillars of quality, *Arch Pathol Lab Med* 114:1115-1118, 1990.

Fosbinder D: Setting standards and evaluating nursing performance with a single tool, *J Nurs Adm* 19(10):23, 1989.

Gottlieb H: Quality assurance: a blueprint for improved patient care and service, *Home Healthcare Nurs* 6(3):11, 1988.

Gould J: Standardized home health nursing plans: a quality assurance look, *QRB* 11(11):334, 1985.

Gremaldi PL, Micheletti JA: PRO objectives and quality criteria, *Hospitals* 59:64, 1985.

Harris JS: The bridge for quality assurance to quality improvement. *J Occ Med* 1990; 17:1175.

Hart C: *Handout Northern Telecom,* University Quality Forum, Research Park Triangle, NC, 1993.

Health Care Financing Administration: *HCF research report: PSRO program evaluation,* Washington, DC, 1979.

Healthy Communities 2000: Model standards, guidelines for community attainment of the year 2000 national health objectives, ed 3, Washington, DC, 1991, American Public Health Association.

Horn BJ, Swain MA: *Development of criterion measures of nursing care, vols I and II, Final report to the National Center for Health Services Research for HS D1649,* Springfield, Va, 1977, National Technical Information Service.

Jonas S: Measurement and control of the quality of health care. In Jonas S, editor: *Health care delivery in the United States,* New York, 1986, Springer Publishing.

Juran JM: *Juran on leadership for quality,* New York, 1989, Free Press.

Kaluzny AD, Mclaughlin CP, Simpson K: Applying total quality management concepts in public health organizations, *Public Health Rep* 107(3):257-264, 1992.

Kessner DM, Kalk CE: Assessing health quality—the case for tracers, *N Engl J Med* 288:189, 1973.

Kreidler M, Bobo NK, Solem GS, Dannemiller, Vishnia D, et al: Developing standards and criteria: family health nurse specialists in a nursing center, *J Nurs Quality Assurance* 4(1):73, 1989.

Laffel G, Blumenthal D: The case for using industrial quality management science in health care organizations. In Al-Assaf AF, Schmele JA, editors: *The textbook of total quality in healthcare,* Delray Beach, Fla, 1993, St Lucie Press, pp 40-50.

Lalonde B: Assuring the quality home care via the assessment of client outcomes, *Caring* 7(1):20, 1988.

Lang NM, Clinton JF: *Assessment of quality of nursing care,* vol 2, *Annual review of nursing research,* New York, 1984, Springer-Verlag.

Lieski AM: Standards: the basis of a quality assurance program. In Meisenheimer CG, editor: *A complete guide to effective programs,* Rockville, Md, 1985, Aspen Publishers.

LoGerfo J, Brook R: Evaluation of health services and quality of care. In Williams S, Torrens P, editors: *Introduction to health services,* New York, 1984, John Wiley & Sons.

Lohr K, Harris-Wehling J: Medicare: a strategy for quality assurance, a recapitulation of the study and definition of quality of care, *QRB* 17(1):6, 1991.

Maciorowski LF, Larson E, Keane A: Quality assurance: evaluate thyself, *J Nurs Adm* 15:38, 1985.

Maibusch RM: Evolution of quality assurance for nursing in hospitals. In Schrolder PS, Maibusch RM, editors: *Nursing quality assurance,* Rockville, Md, 1984, Aspen Publishers.

Martin KS, Scheer NJ, Stegman MR: Home health clients: characteristics, outcomes of care, and nursing interventions, *Am J Public Health* 83(12):1730, 1993.

Martin K: A client classification system adaptable for computerization, *Nurs Outlook* 30:515, 1982.

McLaughlin CP, Kaluzny AD: Defining total quality management/continuous quality improvement. In McLaughlin CP, Kaluzny AD, editors: *Continuous quality improvement in healthcare: theory, implementation and applications,* Gaithersburg, Md, 1994, Aspen Publishers, pp 3-10.

Meisenheimer C: *Quality assurance for home health care,* Rockville, Md, 1989, Aspen Publishers.

Miller J: Evaluating structure, process and outcome indicators in ambulatory care: the AMBUQUAL approach, *J Nurs Quality Assurance* 4(1):40, 1989.

NAHQ: *Risk management: NAHQ guide to quality management,* Skokie, Ill, 1993, NAHQ Press.

National League for Nursing: *Historical perspective of NLN's participation in the ANA credentialing study,* NLN accreditation update, Report No. 1, New York, Oct, 1979, The League.

National League for Nursing Accreditation Division for Home Health Care and Community Health: *Accreditation criteria, standards, and substantiating evidences,* New York, 1987, The League.

Office of Professional Standards Review: *PSRO program manual,* Washington, DC, 1974, Department of Health, Education, and Welfare.

Padilla G, Grant M: Quality of life as a cancer nursing outcome variable. In Rinke L, editor: *Outcome measures in Home Care,* vol 1:169, 1987.

Peters D, Poe S: Using monitoring in a home care quality assurance program, *J Nurs Quality Assurance* 2(2):32, 1988.

Phaneuf M: A nursing audit method, *Nurs Outlook* 5:42-45, 1965.

Phaneuf M: *The nursing audit: profile for excellence,* New York, 1976, Appleton-Century-Crofts.

Phaneuf MC, Wandelt MA: Quality assurance in nursing, *Nurs Forum* 13(4):329, 1974.

Phaneuf M, Wandelt M: Three methods of process oriented nursing evaluation, *QRB* 7(8):20, 1981.

Pickett G, Hanlon J: *Public health administration and practice,* St Louis, 1990, Mosby.

Porter A: Assuring quality through staff nurse performance, *Nurs Clin North Am* 23(3):649, 1988.

Public Law 97-248, Tax Equity and Fiscal Responsibility Act of 1982.

Rinke L, Wilson A: Client oriented project objectives, *Caring* 7(1):25, 1988.

Rissner N: Development of an instrument to measure patient satisfaction with nurses and nursing care in primary care settings, *Nurs Res* 24(1):45, 1975.

Rutstein DD, Berenberg W, Chalmers TC, Child CG, Fishman AP, Perrin EB, et al: Measuring the quality of medical care: a clinical method, *N Engl J Med* 294:582, 1976.

Schmele JA: Research and total quality. In Al-Assaf AF and Schmele JA, editors: *The textbook of total quality management,* Delraz Beach, Fla, 1993, St Lucie Press, pp 239-257.

Schmele J: A method for evaluating nursing practice in a community setting, *QRB* 11(4):115, 1985.

Schmele J, Allen M: A comparison of four nursing process measures of quality in home health, *Journal of Nursing Quality Assurance* 4(4):26, 1990.

Schmele J, Foss S: A process method for clinical practice evaluation in the home health setting, *Journal of Nursing Quality Assurance* 3(3):54, 1990.

Stanhope M, Murdock M: *A psychometric measure of the Phaneuf Nursing Audit.* Paper presented at the American Public Health Association Annual Meeting, Los Angeles, November, 1981

Stevens B: *The nurse as executive,* 1985, Contemporary Publishing.

Tindall BS, Stewart DW: Integration of total quality and quality assurance. In Al-Assaf AF, Schmele JA, editors: *The textbook of total quality in healthcare,* Delray Beach, Fla, 1993, St Lucie Press, pp 209-220.

USPHS: *Essentials of public health nursing practice and education consensus conference,* Washington, DC, 1984, US Government Printing Office.

Wagner D: Who defines quality: consumers or professional? *Caring* 7(10):27, 1988.

Wandelt M, Ager J: *Quality patient care scale,* New York, 1975, Appleton-Century-Crofts.

Wandelt M, Stewart D: *Slater nursing competencies rating scale,* New York, 1975, Appleton-Century-Crofts.

Weid L: *Medical records, medical education and patient care,* Chicago, 1970, Year Book, Medical Publishers.

Weidmann J, North H: Implementing the Omaha Classification system in a public health agency, *Nurs Clin North Am* 22(4):971, 1987.

Weitzman B: The quality of care: assessment and assurance. In Kovner A, editor: *Health care delivery in the United States,* New York, 1990, Springer Publishing.

Werner J: PSROs and hospital accreditation. In McCloskey J, Grace H, editors: *Current issues in nursing,* Oxford, England, 1984, Blackwell Scientific Publications.

Wright D: An introduction to the evaluation of nursing care: a review of the literature, *J Adv Nurs* 9:457, 1984.

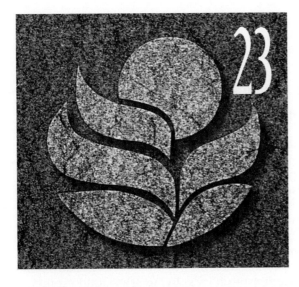

23

Group Approaches in Community Health

Peggye Guess Lassiter

Objectives ▼

After reading this chapter, the student should be able to do the following:

◆ Describe member interaction and group purpose as the major elements of a group.
◆ Describe the effect of cohesion on group effectiveness.
◆ Identify the influence of group norms on group members.
◆ Articulate the usefulness of groups in promoting individual health.
◆ Describe nursing behaviors that assist groups in promoting health for individuals.
◆ Identify the groups constituting a community and illustrate links between them.
◆ Describe the role of the community health nurse working with established groups toward community health goals.

Key Terms ▼

cohesion
communication structure
conflict
established groups
formal groups
group
group culture
group purpose
group structure
informal groups
leadership
maintenance functions
maintenance norms
member interaction
norms
reality norms
role structure
selected membership groups
task function
task norm

Outline ▼

Working with groups is an important skill in community nursing. Groups are an effective and powerful way to initiate and implement changes for individuals, families, organizations, and the community. People naturally form groups in the home setting; in turn, the community's health is dramatically influenced by smaller groups in the community. The community health nurse who works with groups must have an understanding of group concepts, practice in group work, and an appreciation of the use of group process.

Groups form for various reasons. They may form for a clearly stated purpose or goal, or they may form naturally as individuals are attracted to each other by shared values, interests, activities, or personal characteristics.

Community groups represent the collective interests, needs, and values of individuals; they provide a link between the individual and the larger social system. Individual attitudes are developed in families and friendships; throughout life, membership in other groups influences thoughts, choices, behaviors, and values as people socialize and interact. Through groups, people may express personal views and relate them to the views of others. Groups serve as communication networks and may be viewed as an organization of community parts.

Groups can bring about changes to improve the health and well-being of individuals and communities, and some individual changes for health are difficult or impossible to achieve without group support and encouragement.

All nurses have group experience. In daily practice, nurses routinely plan and use health-focused action with clients, other nurses, and other health care workers. Nurses often participate in groups in which they are encouraged to observe their own responses to members and leaders. Such study and experience enrich a nurse's knowledge of how to apply group concepts in a variety of group settings.

As discussed in Chapter 13, community health nurses often use groups to communicate health information in a cost-effective way to a number of clients who meet together, rather than repeating the information several times to individuals. During a time of decreasing resources, groups are an increasingly popular format for community health nursing intervention.

Identifying groups and their goals, member characteristics, and their place in the community structure is an important first step toward understanding the community and assessing its health. Through community groups, nurses help people to identify priority health needs and capabilities and to make valuable changes in their own communities.

GROUP CONCEPTS

The basic group concepts described in this section may be used in nursing practice to identify community groups and their contributions to community life and to assist groups in working toward community and individual health goals.

Group Definition

A **group** is a collection of interacting individuals who have a common purpose or purposes. Each member influences and is in turn influenced by every other member to some extent. Key elements in this definition of group are **member interaction** and **group purpose** (Figure 23-1).

The following examples illustrate member interaction and group purposes. Families are a unique and familiar example of community groups. Family purposes are numerous, including providing psychological support and socialization for their members. Usually, families share kinship bonds, living space, and economic resources. Interactions are diverse and frequent.

A second example is groups formed in response to particular community needs, problems, or opportunities. For example, in one community, residents banded together to form a neighborhood association to protect their health and welfare. This neighborhood of upper middle-class homes was located in an unincorporated area. Over 3 years the residents were threatened with multiple environmental hazards, including a forest fire (fire hydrants had been overlooked in developing part of the area), establishment of a small airport near the homes, and construction of an interstate highway adjacent to the homes. To protect their interests, residents formed a neighborhood association and elected officers to represent their interests in a constructive manner.

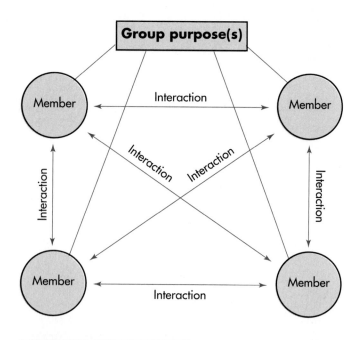

FIGURE 23-1

A group is a collection of interacting individuals who have a common purpose or purposes.

Other groups in the community occur spontaneously because of mutual attraction between individuals and obvious and keenly felt personal needs. Young and single adults sharing similar desires for socialization and recreation are likely to form loosely structured groups. Through parties and other social meetings, the young adults establish new ways of behaving and relating. They select partners, test ideas and attitudes, and establish their identity within a group of people with similar developmental needs. Their unstated purpose is to test and become familiar with adult roles.

A fourth example is health-promoting groups, which are formed as people meet in the community and health care settings and discover common challenges to their physical and emotional well-being. The purposes of health-promoting groups are to improve members' health and deal with specific threats to health. Chapters of Alcoholics Anonymous, Parents without Partners, and La Leche League illustrate health-promoting groups. Members both give and receive personal support and participate in group problem solving and education. These groups may be one of two types: established groups or selected membership groups. Both types of groups are discussed later in this chapter.

How do purpose and interaction vary in these four examples? Some groups, such as the neighborhood association and La Leche League, have an obvious purpose that can be easily stated by members. For families, social groupings, and many spontaneously formed groups, the purposes are unstated. However, the purpose can be determined by studying their activities as a group over time. Purpose and member interaction are important components of all groups.

Group Purpose

When the need for a particular health change is identified and group work is selected as the most effective way to make it happen, a clear statement and presentation of the proposed group's purpose are essential. A clear purpose helps in establishing criteria for member selection.

A clear statement of purpose proved valuable in forming a new group in one city's housing development. The local department of social services had received numerous reports of child abuse and neglect. Routine home visits for well-child care documented high stress between parents and their offspring, and some parents requested guidance from the community health nurse in child discipline. The community health nurse proposed that a parent group address this community need. Nurses who were involved selected the following purpose for the group: dealing with kids for child and parent satisfaction. The purpose indicated both the process (to help parents deal with kids) and the desired outcome (satisfaction for parents and children). As potential members were approached, this statement of purpose for the group helped the individuals decide whether or not they wanted to join.

When a group makes a public appeal for members and accepts everyone who wants to join, the membership is self-selected, based on the stated group purpose. In this type of recruitment, publicity must reach those in need of particular health changes. Prospective members often want to discuss the purpose with leaders or clarify questions concerning the purpose at the first group meeting. Their commitment to the health group is partly based on individual goals and how well the group goal satisfies their personal objectives.

Cohesion

Cohesion is the amount of attraction between individual members and between each member and the group. Individuals in a highly cohesive group identify themselves as a unit, work toward common goals, are willing to endure frustration for the sake of the group, and defend the group against outside criticism. Attraction increases when members feel accepted and liked by others, see similar qualities in each other, and believe they share similar attitudes and values (Figure 23-2). Members' traits that increase group cohesion and productivity include (1) compatible personal and group goals, (2) attraction to group goals, (3) attraction to other selected members, (4) an appropriate mix of leading and following skills, and (5) good problem-solving skills.

Anything a member does that deliberately contributes to the group's purpose is termed a **task function.** Members with task-directed abilities become more attractive to the group. These traits include strong problem-solving skills, access to material resources, and skills in directing. Of equal importance

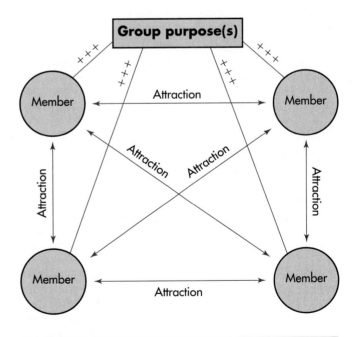

FIGURE 23-2

Cohesion is the measure of attraction between members and member attraction to group purpose(s).

are abilities to affirm and support individuals in the group; these functions are called **maintenance functions** because they help other members to stay with the group and feel accepted. The ability to help people resolve conflicts and ensure social and environmental comfort is also a maintenance function. Both task and maintenance functions are necessary to group progress. Naturally, those members who supply such group requirements are attractive, and an abundance of such traits within the membership tends to increase group cohesion.

Other group members' traits may decrease cohesion and productivity. These include (1) conflicts between personal and group goals, (2) lack of interest in group goals and activities, (3) poor problem-solving and communication abilities, (4) lack of leadership skills, (5) disagreement about types of leadership, (6) aversion to other members, and (7) behaviors and attributes that are poorly understood by others.

Usually, the more alike group members are, the stronger a group's attraction, whereas differences tend to decrease attractiveness. Members' perceptions of differences can create marked competition and jealousy. At the same time, personal differences can increase group cohesion if they support complementary functioning or provide contrasting viewpoints necessary for decision making. This only underlines that cohesion factors are complex; many factors influence member attraction to each other and to the group's goal. In either case, group productivity and member satisfaction are positively affected by high group cohesion. Two examples illustrate factors that influence group cohesion.

A community health nurse initiated and provided beginning leadership for a group of clients who had been treated for burns. Ten residents, all from one town, had been discharged after 3 months in the local burn unit. The stated purpose for the group was to assist members in the difficult transition from hospital to home. Each individual had been treated for extensive burns in an intensive care treatment center; each had relied heavily on health workers for physical, social, and emotional rehabilitation; and each had faced the challenge of resuming work and family roles. Individuals shared some similar experiences and hopes for the future but varied in the amount of trauma and stress experienced. They also differed widely in psychological readiness for return to ordinary daily routines. One woman was able to return quickly to her job as cashier in a large supermarket. The strength of her determination to overcome public reaction to her scars, coupled with an ability to "use the right words" and an empathy for others, distinguished her from others in the group. These differences proved very attractive to other members, inspiring them to work toward a return to their own roles in life. Other members saw her differences as attainable. The cohesion for this group was provided by the members' attraction to the common purpose of returning to successful life patterns and managing relations with others. Each

member also believed that interaction with others with similar burn experiences could help them reach that goal. This example shows that certain member experiences, such as crises or traumas, may help individuals identify with each other and may increase member attraction.

Being different from the general population and similar to the other group members is, for some, a compelling force for membership in the group. (Others are repelled by the group because they do not want to be identified by an aversive characteristic, such as disfigurement.) Empathy for another's pain, learned only through mutual experience, may provide each individual with a required perspective for problem solving or affirming another's view. The nurse in this example helped members use common experiences and learn from their differences. The group was effective.

Differences created tension in one self-help group for victims of spouse abuse; in this group, nurses met a severe challenge stemming from the differences they presented as nonvictims. The community health nurses had been invited by professional staff to assist the group in its process toward the goal of "learning to manage: safety, health, and independence." Victim members of the group believed that the nurses could not truly understand the intensely personal and devastating injury each had experienced and told the nurses so. They isolated the nurses from membership but tolerated their presence. Attraction of the group diminished, and attendance at meetings fell. Discussion of superficial issues occupied group time as the victim members avoided topics of member safety and violence in general. Differences between the nurses and victims hampered group cohesion; the group was not effectively addressing its goal, and members felt isolated.

In response to this deterioration, the nurses encouraged all members to describe experiences seen as threatening to self-respect in their family and work roles. The nurses revealed some of their own struggles for responsible self-direction and control. Revealing their vulnerability made the nurses more attractive to the group. The members were able to accept the nurses, whom they now saw as more similar to themselves. They promptly refocused their efforts on the purpose of the group.

Group members supported one another to assert individual rights for safety, to locate employment, to make necessary living arrangements for independence from the abuser, and to identify needs for personal interactional changes. The clear purpose of maintaining member safety, combined with the new, broader common goal of asserting one's self-respect, contributed to successful group work.

Members' attraction to the group also depends on the nature of the group. Factors include the group programs, size, type of organization, and position in the community. When goals are perceived clearly by individuals and group activities are believed to be effective, attraction to the group is increased.

The concept of cohesion helps to explain group productivity. Some cohesion is necessary for people to remain with a group and accomplish the set goals. Attractiveness positively influences members' motivation and commitment to work on the group task. Cohesion for groups may be increased as members better understand the experiences of others and are able to identify common ideas and reactions to various issues. Nurses facilitate this process by pointing out similarities, contrasting supportive differences, or helping members redefine differences in ways that make those dissimilarities compatible.

 Research Brief

Spink KS, Carson AV: Group cohesion effects in exercise class, *Small Group Res* 25(1):26-42, 1994.

Two Canadian studies, one with university aerobics classes and a second with participants in private exercise clubs, report a significant relationship between member perception of group cohesion and individual adherence to group exercise programs. Both studies use the Group Environment Questionnaire to measure perceptions of group cohesiveness. This questionnaire contained scales to assess individual attraction to group task and to social interaction. Adherence was measured by attendance in the exercise programs of more than 4 weeks.

In both studies, adherents were discriminated from drop-outs by measures of group cohesion perception. For university groups, measures of *task* cohesion were more discriminating, whereas for private fitness club groups, measures of *social* cohesion were more discriminating.

Findings of the studies support the following views:
1. Perceptions of cohesiveness operate in exercise groups.
2. Perceptions of cohesiveness in exercise classes play an important role in the adherence behavior of individual participants.
3. Task and social factors of cohesion vary by setting and moderate the cohesion/adherence relationship.
4. A team-building approach may enhance cohesiveness and adherence among group participants in different programs for health behavior change.

Norms

Norms are standards that guide, control, and regulate individuals and communities. The group **norms** set the standards for group members' behaviors, attitudes, and even perceptions. All groups have norms and mechanisms whereby conformity is accomplished (Sampson and Marthas, 1990). Group norms serve three functions: (1) to ensure movement toward the group's purpose or tasks, (2) to maintain the group through various supports to members, and (3) to influence members' perceptions and interpretations of reality.

Even though certain norms keep the group focused on its task, a certain amount of diversion is permitted as long as members respect central goals and feel committed to return to them. This commitment to return to the central goals is the **task norm;** its strength determines the group's keeping to its work.

Maintenance norms create group pressures to affirm members and maintain their comfort. Individuals in groups seem most productive and at ease when their psychological and social well-being is nurtured. Maintenance behaviors include identifying the social and psychological tensions of members and taking steps to support those members at high stress times. Health supportive maintenance norms may direct the group's attention to conditions such as temperature, space, and seating to ensure the physical comfort of the group during meeting times. This attention to arrangements may include meeting in places that are easily accessible and comfortable to the participants, providing refreshments, and scheduling meetings at convenient times.

A third and equally important function of group norms relates to members' perceptions of reality. Daily behavior is largely based on the way each aspect of life is understood. Through socialization, individuals learn how to gather information, assign meaning, and react to situations in a way that satisfies needs. Decision-making and action-taking processes are influenced by the meanings ascribed by a group's **reality norms.** Individuals look to others to reinforce or to challenge and correct their ideas of what is real. Groups serve to examine the life situations confronting individuals. As individuals gather information, attempt to understand that information, make decisions, and consider the facts and their implications, they can take responsible action, not only in relation to themselves and their group, but also for the community.

All of these groups norms (task, maintenance, and reality norms) are combined to form a **group culture.** Although working with a group does not mean dictating its norms, the nurse can support helpful rules, attitudes, and behaviors. Only when these rules, attitudes, and behaviors become part of the life of the group, independent of the nurse, are they norms.

Figure 23-3 shows that reality norms influence members to see relevant situations in the same way as other members see them. They may feel strong normative pressures to support members who are considering change. Benne (1976), describing how small groups contribute to planned changes, pointed out that people develop their values by internalizing their particular small groups' norms, especially their families' norms. "Changes in value orientations of individuals may be accomplished by seeking and finding significant membership in a small group with norms that are different in some respects from the normative ori-

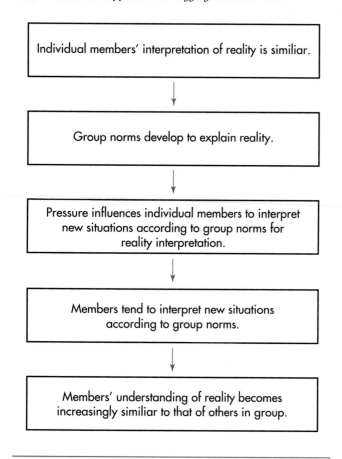

FIGURE 23-3

Influence of group reality norms on individual members.

entation these individuals bring to a group" (Benne, 1976, p. 76).

To illustrate, suppose a group of individuals with diabetes defines an uncontrollable diet as harmful; its members will begin to try to influence one another to maintain diet control. The role of the nurse in this group would be to provide accurate information about diet and the disease process, including cause and effect between food intake and disease. The nurse would also continually display a belief that health through diet control is attainable and desirable.

When members of any group have similar backgrounds, their scope of knowledge may be limited. For example, female members in a spouse abuse group may believe that men are exploitive and harmful based on common childhood and marriage experiences. Such a stereotypical view of men could be reinforced by similar perceptions in other members; this might lead to continuing anger, fear of interactions with men, and a hostile or helpless approach to family affairs. Nurses or group members who have known men in loving, helpful, and collaborative ways can describe their different and positive perceptions of men, thereby adding information and challenging beliefs. Thus the group functions to influence members' perceptions and interpretations of reality. The health and condition of the individual improves as members' perceptions of reality become based on a full range of data and as cause-and-effect factors are understood.

Nurses bring an important perspective to groups in which similar backgrounds limit the understanding and interpretation of personal concerns.

Leadership

Leadership is a complex concept. It consists of behaviors that guide or direct members and determine and influence group action. Positive leadership defines or negotiates the group's purpose(s), selects and helps implement tasks that accomplish the purpose, maintains an environment that affirms and supports members, and balances efforts between task and maintenance. An effective leader attends to member communications and interactions as they unfold in the here-and-now. Attention to both spoken and body language provides leaders and members continuous feedback, alerting members to changing group needs and encouraging members to take responsibility and pride in their own involvement.

Groups can only be effective when leadership is clearly executed. Such leading may be concentrated in one or a few persons or may be shared by many. Generally, shared leadership increases productivity, cohesion, and satisfying interactions among members. A democratic approach to leading is most effective when there are many alternatives, much information is needed, and issues of values and ethics are involved (Sampson and Marthas, 1990).

After initiating or establishing a group, a nurse may facilitate leadership within and among members, frequently relinquishing central control and encouraging members to determine the ultimate leadership pattern for their group. Of course, nurses differ widely in preference for leadership style. In some settings and circumstances, a single authority seems necessary, for example, when members have limited skills or limited time or when groups claim discomfort with shared responsibility for leading.

Experiences with committees, work teams, and client groups promote self-confidence and increasing appreciation of the leading capabilities of others. Practice teaches that getting selected tasks done is only one group outcome. A second, equally valuable, result is watching members become more competent and able to share more and more responsibility. Shared leadership limits power seekers and supports group wholeness, flexibility, and freedom.

Leadership behaviors and definitions are listed in the box on p. 439. Sources of leader influence are knowledge, ability, access to needed resources, personal attractiveness, status or position in the community or organization, and ability to control sanctions for others.

Leadership is typically described as patriarchal, paternal, or democratic; each of these styles has a particular effect on members' interaction, satisfaction, and productivity. Groups may reflect one or a combination of styles.

When one person has the final authority for group direction and movement, the leadership style is patriarchal or paternal. *Patriarchal leadership* may control

Examples of Leadership Behaviors

Advising—introducing direction based on knowledgeable opinion.

Analyzing—reviewing what has occurred as encouragement to examine behavior and its meaning.

Clarifying—checking out meanings of interaction and communication through questions and restatement.

Confronting—presenting behavior and its effects to the individual and group to challenge existing perceptions.

Evaluating—analyzing the effect or outcome of action or the worth of an idea according to some standard.

Initiating—introducing topics, beginning work, or changing the focus of a group.

Questioning—bringing about analysis of a view or views by questions that support examination.

Reflecting behavior—giving feedback on how behavior appears to others.

Reflecting feelings—naming the feelings that may be behind what is said or done.

Suggesting—proposing or bringing an idea to a group.

Summarizing—restating discussion or group action in brief form, highlighting important points.

Supporting—giving the kind of emotionally comforting feedback that helps a person or group continue ongoing actions.

---

members through rewards and threats, often keeping them in the dark about the goals and rationale behind prescribed actions. Paternal leadership wins the respect and dependence of its followers by parental-like devotion to members' needs. The leader controls group movement and progress through interpersonal power. Patriarchal and paternal styles of leadership are authoritarian. These styles are effective for groups such as a disaster team, in which the immediate task accomplishment or high productivity is the goal. However, group morale and cohesiveness are typically low under these styles of leadership, and members may fail to learn how to function independently. In addition, issues of authority and control may disrupt productivity if the group members challenge the power of the leader.

Paternal leadership was effective in the following situation. Mary Jones, a community health nurse, called her neighbors together to alert them to the threat of drug traffic in the neighborhood. The residents agreed with Mary that several recent drug-related arrests in the area signaled a need for community concern. No one knew what to do, but all believed quick action was necessary. Mary had experience in organizing people, knew of local resources, and thought that information, education, and residents' collaboration with police could substantially control the local drug traffic problem. She organized the neighborhood group, assigned and monitored their tasks, and praised them as progress was made toward the goal of keeping the area free of drug sales.

Democratic leadership is cooperative in nature and promotes and supports members' involvement in all aspects of decision making and planning. Members in-

fluence each other as they explore goals, plan steps toward the goals, implement those steps, and evaluate progress.

A more common experience for nurses is illustrated in the following example. A committee of nurses for a small community health organization met weekly to improve nursing services. Tom initiated a revision of the written standards. Several members of the group felt threatened by Tom's idea. They feared that their daily work would change and that a resulting evaluation using new standards would find them inferior or necessitate that they alter familiar procedures. Jane supported updating the standards. She also recognized the necessity of continuing support and affirmation of each nurse's worth on the committee. While Tom pushed the committee toward revising the standards, she often interrupted to ask members to respond and to make suggestions, noting to the group the excellent contributions. Sara provided a touch of humor whenever group tension became high. Amber provided a critical, questioning support to the decision-making process and encouraged the members to evaluate each step. In these and other ways, group members shared leadership tasks. Some served predominantly to push the group toward its objective, whereas others facilitated that movement by maintaining member involvement through support. For this group, the chairperson served as convener but did not dominate in leader activities. The members accomplished the work of writing and implementing an audit for new nursing standards in a democratic leadership style.

Group Structure

Structure describes the particular arrangement of group parts as they combine to make up the group as a whole. A **communication structure** identifies message pathways and member participation in sending and receiving messages. People who are active in receiving and sending messages and who serve as channels for messages are important in the structure. These "central" individuals influence the group because of their access to and interpretive control over communication flow. Communication and role structures are interrelated.

Role structure describes the expected behaviors of members in relation to each other as the group interacts. The role assumed by each member serves a purpose in the life of that group. Examples of roles are leader, follower, task specialist, maintenance specialist, evaluator, peacemaker, and gatekeeper (see the box on p. 440). Members' roles in the group may be described by their predominant actions. Identification of communication patterns helps to determine roles because people occupying particular roles characteristically use certain kinds of communication.

Group structure emerges from various member influences, including the members' understanding and support of the group purpose. Nurses assess the group structure as it relates to goal accomplishment. Many groups also consider their own structure, assess its

Examples of Group Role Behaviors

Evaluator—analyzes the effect or outcome of action or the worth of ideas according to some standard.
Follower—seeks and accepts the authority or direction of others.
Gatekeeper—controls outsiders' access to the group.
Leader—guides and directs group activity.
Maintenance specialist—provides physical and psychological support for group members, thereby holding the group together.
Peacemaker—attempts to reconcile conflict between members or takes action in response to influences that disrupt the group process and threaten its existence.
Task specialist—focuses or directs movement toward the main work of the group.

usefulness in relation to member comfort and productivity, and then plan for a different division of tasks that is agreeable to the whole.

In the earlier example of nurses working on standards of nursing service, Tom served a role as task specialist, Jane as maintenance specialist, and Amber as evaluator. These members consistently occupied particular roles and were expected by others to maintain their behavior to serve the purposes of the group.

A person occupying a gatekeeper's role controls outsiders' access to the group. Gatekeepers either facilitate or block communication between outsiders and group members. Identification of those in gatekeeper roles is crucial when established groups are used for community health. The gatekeeper usually confronts the nurse after beginning contacts are attempted. An invitation to communicate further with group members is extended only after the nurse and gatekeeper determine mutual benefits and possible risks from continued contact between the nurse and the group.

PROMOTING INDIVIDUALS' HEALTH THROUGH GROUP WORK

Health behavior is influenced greatly by the groups to which people belong. Individuals live within a social structure of significant others such as family members, friends, co-workers, and acquaintances. The patterns and directions of everyday activities are learned in a family, and these are later reinforced or challenged by new groups. These groups constitute the context in which values, beliefs, and attitudes are formed; individuals usually consider the responses of others in all types of decisions regarding personal welfare.

The following example illustrates the effects of a person's social network on health behavior. Mary Berton was worried about a lump she had recently discovered in her breast. She first asked her husband, Lew, to confirm its presence, which he did. He agreed that she should arrange for a diagnostic evaluation, and an appointment was arranged. Mary talked with

Lew about the possible consequences of malignancy, and she noted Lew's concern for her safety. She was fearful of radical surgery and its impact on her relationship to Lew, but she did not discuss that with him. Mary telephoned two close friends from her workplace and asked them to meet her for coffee. Although they thought it was premature to fret about the lump being malignant, they discussed all they knew about treatment for breast cancer, including the trials, defeats, and successes of three mutual friends who had had surgery for breast cancer. Each of the friends had reacted differently to her own situation, and Mary's friends retold familiar details. The retelling seemed important to understanding the current situation and helping Mary sort out her feelings. She was assisted in facing the reality of risk, recognizing the need to follow through with diagnostic procedures, selecting able medical sources, and managing her emotional stress.

Mary's friends' and her husband's responses to her situation influenced her assessment, decision making, and subsequent behavior. The work done by Mary and her social network in response to her health need was important. It illustrates a common mechanism among individuals and the groups to which they belong. The groups described in this example are Mary's family group, which includes Mary and Lew, and Mary's friendship group, of which those who met for coffee are a subset.

Groups who will support an individual's health changes are unavailable to some people because of their social or emotional isolation. Isolated individuals may have low self-esteem, be mentally ill, or occupy positions of low status in their family or community. They may be disadvantaged, gifted, or deviant, or they may simply live in a rural area or be engaged in solitary work. These individuals benefit greatly through newly organized groups established for specific purposes.

Although social support is basic to health, the absence of negative social interactions is of equal importance to well-being. Groups sometimes oppose health. Friends who use addictive drugs are a clear example of such a group. It may be impossible for an individual to quit drug use while associating with such friends. To effect a lasting behavior change, an addicted individual needs support and new friends who do not abuse drugs. In such circumstances the individual must leave his or her group of associates, even if he or

Did You Know?

The absence of negative social interactions is as important as social support for emotional functioning. Four negative interactions are: ineffective helping, excessive helping, negative regulation, and unpleasant interactions (Schuster et al., 1990).

she must move from the neighborhood where they gather.

As community nurses increase their knowledge of group concepts, develop skills in working with varied groups, and learn to employ the power in groups for individual changes, they will become available, visible, and sought for group work.

Choosing Groups for Health Change

Nurses frequently use groups to help individuals within a community after studying the overall needs of the community and its people. Such a study is based on client contacts, expressed concerns from various community spokespersons, health statistics for the area, health resources availability, and the community's general well-being. These data point to the community's strengths and critical needs. Just as other nursing interventions are based on the assessment of needs and knowledge of effective treatment, group formation is determined by the assessment of priority community needs for individual health change.

At times community health nurses work with existing groups, and at other times they form new groups. Initiation of change and recruitment of a community health nurse may come not just from the nurse, but from individuals, the affected group(s), or a related organization. A decision about whether to work in established groups or to begin new ones is based on the clients' needs, the purpose of existing groups, and the membership ties in existing groups.

Established Groups

There are advantages to using **established groups** for individual health change. Membership ties already exist, and the structure already in place can be used. It is not necessary to find new members because compatible individuals already form a working group. Established groups usually have operating methods that have already proved successful; an approach for a new goal is built on this history. Members are aware of each others' strengths, limitations, and preferred styles of interaction. Members' comfort levels, stemming from their experience together, facilitate their focus on the new goal.

Established groups have a strong potential for influencing members. Ties between members have been enhanced through successful group endeavors. Their bonds are usually multidimensional because of the length of time they have spent together. Such rich ties support group change efforts for individuals' health.

Before deciding to work with particular established groups, the nurse must judge whether introducing a new focus is compatible with existing group purposes. In some cases, individual health goals will enhance existing group purposes, and the nurse is an important resource for bringing information for health, behavior, and group process.

How can the community nurse enter existing groups and direct their attention to individual health needs? One nurse employed by an industrial firm noted the deleterious effect of managerial stress on several individuals. They had elevated blood pressure, stomach pain, and emotional tension. The nurse learned that the employees with stress were all members of a jogging team that met weekly for conversation in addition to regular workouts. The other joggers readily accepted the offer to work together on individual stress management, recognizing that their fellow members were facing high-stress circumstances and the accompanying danger to health. High-level health had been a value shared by all team members, and although jogging was seen as an enjoyable and health-promoting activity, they had never talked about a shared purpose for improved health. In this circumstance the nurse observed a need for stress reduction, thought that the individuals at risk would be able to achieve stress reduction if supported through a group process from valued friends, and proposed that a new purpose be added to the jogging team's activities.

Selected Membership Groups

In some situations using existing groups is undesirable or impossible. The nurse then begins a selection process and brings a new group into existence. Nurses are familiar with group work in which members are selected because of their health. For instance, individuals with diabetes are brought together to consider diet management and physical care and to share in problem-solving remedies; community residents are brought together for social support and rehabilitation following treatment for mental illness; or isolated elderly persons are brought together for socialization and hot meals.

Members' attributes are an important consideration in composing a new group. Members are attracted to others from similar backgrounds, with similar experiences, and with common interests and abilities. Selecting members so that common ties or interests balance out dissimilar traits is therefore an important consideration.

Membership ties are influential; even in newly formed groups, people bring emotional and social ties from previous and parallel group memberships. People are influenced by the interaction in the newly formed group and by their alliance with other important groups to which they belong. Memory serves to keep the norms and role expectations from one group present in a person as he or she moves from one group to another. Individual behavior is then influenced not only by the membership, purpose, attraction, norms, leadership, and structure of the group, but also by those processes remembered from other valued group memberships. Consideration of the multiple influences on members helps to determine an appropriate grouping for each situation and its particular dimensions.

When the nurse is able to arrange it, the membership for **selected membership groups** should contain one or more individuals with expressive and problem-solving skills and others who are comfortable in supportive roles. Many people demonstrate abilities in task and maintenance functions, and others have undeveloped potential for such functions. Support and training for group effectiveness within the unit build cohesion. As members perform increasingly valuable functions for the group, they become more attracted to it and more attractive to others.

The size of the group influences effectiveness; generally, eight to 12 people are considered a good number for group work focused on individual health changes. Groups of up to 25 members may be effective when their focus is on community needs, such as the group discussed previously who formed a neighborhood association. Large groups often divide and assign tasks to the smaller subgroups, with the original large groups meeting less frequently for reporting and evaluation.

Recruitment and selection of the most appropriate members for any group can be facilitated by setting member criteria. The criteria usually suggest a mixture of member traits, allowing for balance for the processes of decision making and growth.

Beginning Interactions

Once a group forms, work begins on the stated purpose. Early meetings require further clarification of both individual and group goals. Members with varying degrees of openness present themselves and their backgrounds. They begin to interact with each other by seeking and giving information about themselves and their circumstances and simultaneously demonstrating their capabilities in problem solving and group participation. The nurse assists by supporting ideas and feelings, inviting participation, giving information, seeking and providing clarification, and suggesting structure. Subsequent steps are then planned not only according to the nurse's skill and preference, but also according to the group composition and the skills brought by members.

Nurses in the beginning groups should place priority on helping members interact with a degree of satisfaction. This requires close attention to maintenance tasks of attending, eliciting information, clarifying, and recognizing contributions of members. Attending includes simple responses to people, such as listening carefully to their speech and noting their mood, dress, and informal conversation as they enter the meeting. Attending behavior communicates recognition and acceptance of the person and his or her presentations to the group.

A beginning format that focuses on whatever brought each member to the group provides recognition and helps the individual acknowledge similar and different perspectives. Members may be asked to describe what each hopes to accomplish in the group and what experiences each has previously had in groups. Member-to-member exchanges are encouraged; individuals are recognized and supported as they take on leadership functions.

Even in these beginning sessions, roles and a structure for the new group begin to take shape. Members try out familiar roles and test their individual abilities. Those approaches to member support, leadership, and decision making that are comfortable and productive become normative ways for the group to work. The nurse helps by creatively evaluating the appropriateness of style and productivity of roles. The work of the group is begun even as the goals for health change are examined carefully and are realistically accepted. During this early period, members' attractions to each other and to the group begin to develop.

Conflict

Although **conflict** occurs normally in all human relations, people generally see conflict as the opposite of harmony, a state of interference to guard against. This view is an unfortunate one because the tensions of difference and potential conflict actually help groups work toward their purposes. Understanding common causes of conflict, conflict management approaches, and conflict resolution models is especially important in this decade of challenges to health and health care systems and increasingly violent expressions of community conflict.

Conflict arises whenever individuals perceive that their concerns have been or are about to be frustrated (Sitkin and Bies, 1993). Conflict signals that antagonistic points of view must be considered and that one must reexamine beliefs and assumptions underlying relationships. Some sources of concern for people are security, control of self and others, respect between parties, and access to limited resources; in groups, members express frustrations about trust, closeness and separation, and dependence and independence. These themes of interpersonal conflict operate to some extent in all interactions; they are not unique to groups. Within a group, because of members' regular and committed associations toward a common purpose, such issues are key; responding to them appropriately encourages personal growth and the facing of frustrations in the group.

Thomas (1992) differentiates two potentially positive dimensions of response to conflict: *assertiveness* (attempting to satisfy one's own concerns) and *cooperativeness* (attempting to satisfy the others' concerns). Behaviors that reflect either assertiveness or cooperativeness and also hold the potential to satisfy the frustrated parties include confrontation, competition, compromise, reconciliation, and collaboration. Avoidance, forcing with power, capitulation, and excluding a member are conflict responses that fail to satisfy the concerns of frustrated parties.

Resolving conflict within groups depends on open

communication among all parties, diffusion of negative feelings and perceptions, focusing on the issue(s), fair procedures, and a structured approach to process. The following model describes steps that support and encourage participants to acknowledge and resolve conflicts:

1. Give a full description of concerns and divergent views.
2. Clarify assumptions on the conflict issue.
3. Specify underlying factors, including beliefs, individual desires, and expectations.
4. Identify the real issue(s).
5. Jointly search for a collaborative resolution through a problem-solving approach.
6. Finalize resolution agreement (either a full agreement or a compromise in which each party is satisfied on important points.

Conflict can be overwhelming, especially when members believe that the expression of controversy is unacceptable or unresolvable. Conflict suppressed over time tends to build up and finally explode out of proportion to the current frustration. A group that repeatedly avoids the expression of conflict becomes fragile, unable to adapt to growth within the group, and helpless to face challenges. Conflict may be destructive if contentious parties fail to respect the other's rights and beliefs.

Conflict-acknowledging and problem-solving approaches that respect others and represent self-concerns are first learned in families and other small groups. These lessons teach some to embrace conflict as a natural occurrence that supports growth and change. Other individuals learn to avoid conflict or to disregard others in the promotion of self. Individuals may evaluate conflict management styles and refine skills in collaborative groups that support expression and resolution of conflict.

Conflict management theory has long held that collaboration produces superior outcomes in conflict resolution; full participation of concerned parties, respecting the concerns of each and working toward full consensus, is commended. Thomas (1992) and L. Brown (1992) critiqued a value shift portrayed in conflict management literature; some recent writings suggest that collaboration is impractical, requiring a long-term commitment to change at the individual, group, and institutional levels. Hindrances to collaboration cited are competitive incentives, individuals having insufficient problem-solving skills, shortness of time, and lack of trust between parties (Thomas, 1992). Management strategies considered more practical than full collaboration include restructuring of settings, helping concerned parties reframe frustration as less stressful, and increasing competitive incentives. Although some circumstances undoubtedly warrant these less visionary responses to conflict, collaboration more completely resolves frustration and differences.

The following example illustrates conflict resolution through collaboration. A small church in a rural town initiated a project for youth recreation because fast driving around the countryside was the primary form of recreation for the teens. A roadway was frequently used as a speedway by the restless youth. The church enlisted the high-school principal and the community health nurse to work with a project group. All supported the development of a local youth center and worked energetically toward the goal.

After 2 months of steady cooperation, many arguments began to erupt at meetings. Conflict about the supervision of the proposed center, the site for the physical plant, and numerous smaller concerns seemed to dominate planning time. The group consisted of active, aggressive members; four individuals seemed to dominate the discussions and to resist argument resolution. After several frustrating meetings, the nurse asked the group to explore each person's concerns and individual views on the direction and interaction of their work together. Welcoming an opportunity to relieve tension, members described their hopes, misgivings, and frustrated expectations related to the project. Each person elaborated on his or her assumptions about who would do what and how work should proceed. From this full discussion, the real issue became clear to all: disagreement related to members' functions in the project. The four dominant individuals expressed personal wishes to direct the planning and displayed aggravation when these attempts were thwarted. Other members described supportive and task functions but did not seek dominance in leadership functions. The open analysis of role structure made it clear to the members that arguments grew out of competition for directing roles rather than from true disagreements about the recreation project. Members searched for a collaborative resolution to the issue. They reached agreement to divide the work into several task areas to be led by separate area directors. Members expressed relief that basic agreement about the purpose remained intact, and they were able to modify their role expectations to accommodate all members. They joked together about being a collection of bosses and renewed their productive work.

Strategies for Change

Efforts toward established health goals are facilitated by community health nurses through their considerable knowledge of health and health risks for individuals, groups, and communities. Skill in problem solving for change is an important complement for accomplishing health goals.

What Do You Think?

Collaboration is the most effective approach to conflict resolution.

Change, whether welcome or not, is disruptive to the client. Even though moving from a familiar way of being and interacting with others is uncomfortable (and resisted), all human systems do change over time because of development within the system and adaptation to outside stimuli. A change for one person in a group has an impact on every other member. The disruption of growth, new opportunities, and threats to security trigger a fertile period for reevaluating, selecting new directions, improving, and maturing. Change creates opportunity for learning that is more than mastery of new information and identification of appropriate adjustment resources.

As discussed throughout this chapter, healthful change requires knowledge, practice of new skills, examination of attitudes and values about the change, and adjustment of roles in one's personal group or network. Helping people accomplish needed changes is ideally done within the small group context.

Basic teaching helps members understand the known association among environment, body response, wellness, and pathological states that are pertinent to desired changes. Together, group members focus on the reality of the problems and ways to understand them. A group reaches its full potential for effecting individual change when members work actively and directly through discussion and other approaches to problem solving.

Expectant-parent groups illustrate a type of community group in which teaching is a highly appropriate method. Participants need to understand facts concerning pregnancy, labor and delivery, self-care and infant care, parenting, and adjusting to change. They also need an opportunity to practice the skills required in anticipated tasks and to explore their attitudes and emotional responses to the anticipated family changes. Specific learning activities in the group might include demonstration and practice for baby baths and situation enactment of family activity after the baby comes home. Such experiential learning activities, which require interaction among members and involve topics highly relevant to the goal of change, are useful.

One approach for improved health involves analyzing both supportive and interfering forces that affect movement toward the particular change proposed for improved health, including sources such as important individuals within the family, work, and community groups. These forces are identified during group meetings when group members learn from each other and the nurse how to help overcome interferences and promote facilitative factors.

With the support of a group, people often make needed changes for health that they are unable to accomplish on their own or with the help of just one individual. Skillful use of group methods can help the client analyze the problem, help sustain motivation for change, support the client during vulnerable periods, and provide quick interpersonal feedback for success and failure. The discomfort associated with change is greatly mitigated through the relationships with others in beneficial groups.

Evaluation of Group Progress

Evaluation of individual and group progress toward health goals is important. (A Guide for Evaluation of Group Effectiveness is shown in Appendix E.3). Action steps toward the goal are identified early in the planning stage. These small steps may be responses to learning objectives (listed action steps designed to support facilitative forces and deal with resistive forces), or they may reflect the group's problem-solving plan. These action steps and the indicators of achievement are discussed and written in a group record. Celebration is built into the group's evaluation system to help individuals recognize and reinforce each step toward the health goal. Celebration may include concrete rewards such as special foods and drinks, or it may be the personal expression of joy and member-to-member approval. Celebration for group accomplishments marks progress, rewards members, and motivates each person to continue.

COMMUNITY GROUPS AND THEIR CONTRIBUTION TO COMMUNITY LIFE

An understanding of group concepts provides a starting point for identifying community groups and how they function as components of the community. Because individuals develop, refine, and change their ideas within the context of the groups to which they belong, groups are vital to community well-being. Groups help identify community problems and are key in the management of interactions within the community and between the community and larger society.

Community groups may be informal (e.g., social networks, friendships, neighborhood groups) or formal (e.g., school, church, business groups). **Formal groups** have a defined membership and specific purpose. They may or may not have an official place in the community's organization. In **informal groups,** the ties between members are multiple, and the purposes are unwritten yet understood by members. Informal groups can be identified through interviews with key spokespersons. Information about when and why they gather is learned through interviews or observing gatherings to which the nurse is invited. Informal groups often are recognized in the news when they are distinguished for community action or service. Formal groups usually can be identified in a variety of community media with meetings announced and business reported publicly. Membership lists, goals, and mission statements are usually written and available to interested persons.

Typically, residents willingly describe the informal and formal groups in their communities after they learn the nurse's purpose for entering and studying their community.

Group communication and member interactions across groups influence the overall harmony and free exchange in the community. Many communities encourage cooperation among groups through interagency councils, and many naturally occurring links among groups exist through family, friendships, and other relationships. Local extended-family groups, club relationships, work, and other acquaintance networks may influence the activities of seemingly separate groups in the larger community.

The community health nurse discerns goals for the community and for various groups through media reports, from community informants, and from local archives. These goals tell of resources and visions for change as perceived by the people living and working in the local community. Data may be organized according to the opinions and behaviors of the groups identified. Such information about community groups and assessment data are used with community representatives to plan desired interventions. Groups are both units of community analysis and vehicles for change.

The small group has the potential to influence and change the larger social community of which it is a part. The social system depends on groups for governing, making policy, determining community needs, taking steps to alleviate those needs, and evaluating program outcomes. The small group is a mechanism for interrelatedness between community subsystems, certain subsystems and their counterparts in the larger social structure, and factions within subsystems. Change in the composition and function of strategic small groups may produce change for the wider social system that depends on small groups for direction and guidance (Benne, 1976).

WORKING WITH GROUPS TOWARD COMMUNITY HEALTH GOALS

Collaboration with Community Partners

Community health nurses use their understanding of group principles to work with community groups to make needed health changes. The groupings appropriate for this work include both established, community-sanctioned groups and groups for which nurses select members representing diverse community sectors.

Existing community groups formed for community-wide purposes such as elected executive groups, health-planning groups, better-business clubs, women's action groups, school boards, and neighborhood councils are excellent resources for community health assessment because part of their ongoing purpose is to determine and respond to community needs. In addition, they are already established as part of the community structure. When a group representing one community sector is selected for community health intervention, the total community structure is studied. Data about family ties, experiences with resource centers, and lifelong contacts to other sector groups are evaluated. Groups reflect existing community values, strengths, and normative forces.

How might community health nurses help established groups to work toward community goals? The same interventions recommended for groups formed for individual health change are beneficial to community health-focused groups. Such interventions include the following: building cohesion through clarifying goals and individual attraction to groups, building member commitment and participation, keeping the group focused on the goal, maintaining members through recognition and encouragement, maintaining member self-esteem during conflict and confrontation, analyzing forces affecting movement toward the goal, and evaluating progress. On entering established groups, nurses seek to assess the leadership, communications, and normative structures. This facilitates group planning, problem solving, intervention, and evaluation. The steps for community health changes parallel those of decision making and problem solving in other methodologies.

One community health nurse, Mrs. Winter, was asked to meet with a neighborhood council to help them study and "do something about" the number of homeless living on the streets. Mrs. Winter was known to residents from a local clinic, and they knew she also consulted at a shelter for the homeless in an adjacent community. When the council invited her, they stated that "our intent is to be part of the solution rather than part of the problem." Mrs. Winter accepted the invitation to visit. She learned that the neighborhood council had addressed concerns of the neighborhood for 20 years—protecting zoning guidelines, setting up a recreational program for teens, organizing an afterschool program for latch-key children, and generally representing the homeowners of the area. The neighborhood was composed of low-income families who took great pride in their homes. After meeting with the council and listening to their description of the situation, Mrs. Winter agreed to help and she joined the council.

As the first step in addressing the problem, the council conducted a comprehensive problem analysis on the homeless situation. All known causes and outcomes of homeless persons on the street were identified, and the relationships between each factor and the problem were documented from literature and from the local history. Mrs. Winter lent her expertise in health planning and her knowledge of the homeless and health risks. She suggested negotiation between the council and the local coalition for the homeless, recognizing that planning would be most relevant if homeless individuals participated. The council was cohesive and committed to the purpose, had developed working operations, and did not need help with group process. They made adjustments in their usual group operation to use the knowledge and health-planning skills of Mrs. Winter.

Interventions for the homeless included establishment of temporary shelter at homes on a rotating basis, provision of daily meals through the city council or churches, and joining the area coalition for the homeless. This example shows how an established, competent group addressed a new goal successfully by building on existing strengths in partnership with the community health nurse.

Community groupings, because of their interactive roles, seem to be logical and natural ways for people who work together for community health change. As the decision-making and problem-solving capabilities of community groups are strengthened, the groups become more able representatives for the whole community. Community health nurses improve the community's health by working with groups toward that goal.

National Issues

Nurses collaborate with diverse segments of the U.S. population in health care reform. At times, work is done in interdisciplinary groups; at other times, it is done with consumers, communtiy spokespersons, and health care workers. Individuals who share common beliefs on how reform should be shaped work through coalitions to build a persuasive argument to legislators. Ultimately, legislators work in committees to influence their colleagues and draft bills that will successfully pass. At national and state levels, professional organizations such as the American Nurses Association and the American Public Health Association organize legislative influence groups to articulate and promote nursing, public health, and health care reform interests. At local levels, nurses work with other disciplines and consumers of health care to work out differences, often through debate and compromise, negotiating for consensus on issues. Collaboration required for success at each of these levels highlights the importance of group work. Such a demanding and necessary task as planning for and selling a changed health care system teaches the dramatic relevance of cooperation. Only through respect and consideration of disparate points of view can true negotiation for change be accomplished. Health care reform must address critical health care issues while attending to the perspective of providers, consumers, and financiers of care.

 ## Clinical Application

Community health assessment in a small rural county revealed a rate of chronic diseases that was much higher than the rates for the neighboring urban county and for the state as a whole. Individuals and their families received health care supervision in the local clinics and through nursing visits to them in their home. However, the chronically ill persons still were not managing their pain and mobility problems to their own satisfaction. Community health nurses set up an initial group meeting, inviting all the persons with chronic illness in the county seat. The invitation was published in the county newspaper and all local church bulletins. Free transporation was provided by the auxiliary club at one county church. Thirty individuals came to the first meeting and indicated great dissatisfaction with their health and an interest in working with the nurses on a better approach to their chronic diseases.

At the first meeting, three groups were organized, which would meet regularly for 6 weeks each. Members selected a group based on their scheduling needs and friendship ties. The nurse then met with each group to facilitate the process of setting goals and selecting a variety of group-work intervention steps toward the goal.

One group decided to review each member's individual health care plan and assist in finding needed resources, thereby encouraging aggregate members to continue their participation. Another group thought that the stress related to their chronic condition was their major concern. They requested a course in stress management, which a community resident taught. Group learning experiences were facilitated by the community health nurse. The third group's primary concern was that many residents with chronic disease failed to use existing health care services. Because they thought that lack of transportation was a key causative factor for underuse of services, they decided to seek transportation from members of the Ruritan Club. Because the group had strong family links to the Ruritans and because their arguments were convincing, they were able to establish a carpool at no cost to residents needing rides to health care services. Interventions were planned and implemented by resident and nurse partnerships.

Follow-up evaluation showed that individuals were more successfully managing pain and mobility; clients attributed these changes to the collective group efforts. Group meetings did not change the rate of chronic illness; they did successfully intervene to address specific health concerns, whereas the nurse working alone or with individuals could not accomplish these interventions as effectively or as efficiently. This nursing intervention was effective for individuals and for the rural community.

Key Concepts

◆ Working with groups is an important skill for community health nurses. Groups are an effective and powerful vehicle for initiating and implementing healthful changes.

◆ A group is a collection of interacting individuals with a common purpose. Each member influences and is influenced by other group members to varying degrees.

◆ Group cohesion is enhanced by commonly shared characteristics among members and diminished by differences among members.

◆ Cohesion is the measure of attraction between members and the group. Cohesion or the lack of it affects the group's function.

◆ Norms are standards that guide and regulate individuals and communities. These norms are unwritten and often unspoken and serve to ensure group movement to a goal, to maintain the group, and to influence group members' perceptions and interpretations of reality.

◆ Some diversity of member backgrounds is usually a positive influence on a group.

◆ Leadership is an important and complex group concept, Leadership is described as patriarchal, paternal, or democratic.

◆ Group structure emerges from various member influences, including members' understanding and support of the group purpose.

◆ Conflicts in groups may develop from competition for roles or member disagreement about the roles ascribed to them.

◆ Health behavior is greatly influenced by the groups to which people belong and for which they value membership.

◆ An understanding of group concepts provides a basis for identifying community groups and their goals, characteristics, and norms. Community health nurses use their understanding of group principles to work with community groups toward needed health changes.

Critical Thinking Activities

1. Consider three groups of which you are a member. What is the stated purpose of each one? Are you aware of unstated but clearly understood purposes? What is the nature of member interaction in each group? How do purpose and interaction differ in the three groups?

2. Observe two working groups in session from the community, a health care agency, or a school. Notice the overall attractiveness of each group through the eyes of its members.

a. List actions that nurses may take to assist groups in various aspects of their work, such as member selection, purpose clarification, arrangements for comfort in participation, and group problem solving.

b. Observe a nurse working with a health promotion group. Does he or she function in the way you anticipated? What nursing behavior facilitated the group process?

3. List the areas of skill and knowledge most likely to be expected of the nurse by the community residents' groups.

4. Identify areas of conflict in a work group to which you belong. Describe how one of these expressed or potential conflicts could be managed. Use the steps for conflict resolution outlined in this chapter What role would you take? Practice conflict-acknowledging and problem-solving behaviors in the next conflict you encounter.

5. Using the references in the chapter bibliography, identify your most frequently used style of conflict management.

Bibliography

Abraham IL, et al: Therapeutic work with depressed elderly, *Nurs Clin North Am* 26(3):635-50, 1991.

Benne KD: The current state of planned changing in persons, groups, communities, and societies. In Bennis WG, et al, editors: *The planning of change*, ed 3, New York, 1976, Holt, Rinehart, & Winston.

Boulding KE: Conflict resolution and control. In Gamson WA, editor: *Simsoc: simulated society*, ed 4, New York, 1991, Free Press.

Brown L: Normative conflict management theories: past, present and future, *J Organizational Behav* 13(3):303-309, 1992.

Brown Y: The crisis of pregnancy loss: a team approach to support, *Birth* 19(2):82-91, 1992.

Bulechek GM: Support groups. In Kinney CK, et al, editors: *Nursing interventions: essential nursing treatments*, Philadelphia, 1992, Saunders.

Coser L: The functions of conflict. In Gamson WA, editor: *Simsoc: simulated society*, ed 4, New York, 1991, Free Press.

Cottrell LS: The competent community. In Kaplan BH, et al, editors:

Further explorations in social psychiatry, New York, 1976, Basic Books.

Dahl RA: Conflict: a paradigm. In Gamson WA, editor: *Simsoc: simulated society,* ed 4, New York, 1991, Free Press.

DelPo EG, Koontz MA: Group therapy with mothers of incest victims: structure, leader attributes, and countertransference, Part 1, *Arch Psychiatr Nurs* 5(2):64-69, 1991a.

DelPo EG, Koontz MA: Group therapy with mothers of incest victims: therapeutic strategies, recurrent themes, interventions and outcomes. Part 2, *Arch Psychiatr Nurs* 5(2):70-75, 1991b.

Glanz K, et al: *Health behavior and health education,* San Francisco, 1990, Jossey-Bass.

Jones MA, et al: A paradigm for effective resolution of interpersonal conflict, *Nurs Manage* 2(12):64B, F, J-L, 1990.

Kirchmeyer C, Cohen A: Multicultural groups: their performance and reactions with constructive conflict, *Group Organizational Manage* 17(2):153-170, 1992.

Krasnoff MJ: Perspective: participation in a multidisciplinary women's health study group, *J Womens Health* 1(3):185-187, 1992.

Lassiter PG: A community development perspective for rural nursing, *Fam Community Health* 14(4):29-39, 1992.

Mayers A, Spiegel L: A parental support group in a pediatric AIDS clinic: its usefulness and limitations, *Health Soc Work* 17(3):183-191, 1992.

McClure BA: Conflict within a childrens' group: suggestions for facilitating its expression and resolution strategies, *Sch Counselor* 39(4):268-272, 1992.

Miller CR: Group therapy for women: benefits of ethnocultural diversity, *J Women's Health* 1(3):189-191, 1992.

Mondros J, et al: The use of groups to manage conflict, *Soc Work Groups* 15(4):43-57, 1992.

Newton G: Self-help groups: can they help? In Spradley BW, editor: *Readings in community health nursing,* Philadelphia, 1991, Lippincott.

O'Connor K, et al: The experience and effects of conflict in continuing work groups, *Small Group Res* 24(3):362-382, 1993.

Ramsey PW: Characteristics, processes and effectiveness of community support groups: a review of the literature, *Fam Community Health* 15(3):38-48, 1992.

Sampson EE, Marthas M: *Group process for the health professions,* ed 3, Albany, NY, 1990, Delmar.

Schopler JH, Galinsky MJ: Support groups as open systems: a model for practice and research, *Health Soc Work* 18(3):195-207, 1993.

Schuster TL, et al: Supportive interactions, negative interactions and depressed mood, *Am J Community Psychol* 18(3):423-438, 1990.

Sitkin SB, Bies RJ: Social accounts in conflict situations: using explanations to manage conflict, *Hum Relations* 46(3):349-370, 1993.

Spink KS, Carson AV: Group cohesion effects in exercise class, *Small Group Res* 25(1):26-42, 1994.

Staples NR, Schwartz M: Anorexia nervosa support group: providing transitional support, *J Psychosoc Nurs Ment Health Serv* 28(2):6-10, 1990.

Thomas KW: Conflict and conflict management: reflections and update, *J Organizational Behav* 13(3):265-274, 1992.

Tommasini NR: The impact of a staff support group on the work environment of a specialty unit, *Arch Psychiatr Nurs* 6(1):40-47, 1992.

Unger R: Conflict management in group psychotherapy, *Small Group Res* 21(3):349-357, 1990.

van Servellen G, et al: Methodological concerns in evaluating psychiatric nursing care modalities and a proposed standard group protocol format for nurse-led groups, *Arch Psychiatr Nurs* 6(2):117-24, 1992.

Wheeler CE, Chinn PL: *Peace and power: a handbook of feminist process,* New York, 1991, National League for Nursing.

Witteman H: Group member satisfaction: a conflict related account, *Small Group Res* 22(1):24-58, 1991.

Part Five   Issues and Approaches in Family and Individual Health Care

The family is a major influence on the individual's concept of health and illness. It is within the family that a person's sense of self-esteem and personal competence is developed. The action taken by or for the person with a health problem depends on this sense of self-worth and the family's definition of illness. The environmental, social, cultural, and economic factors, as well as the resources of the community to meet health needs, influence the family's health risks and reaction to health. The goals of the nation for the year 2000 name the individual as the primary target for changing the overall health of the nation. Through family support the individual may develop the responsibility to participate in activities that will lead to a healthier life-style.

Major health problems of individuals can be identified and related to their developmental phase. This factor becomes evident when age-specific morbidity data are reviewed. Community health nurses can influence the actions and reactions to health of all individuals in the community from birth through senescence. The community health nurse can influence the health of children by introducing healthy parenting behaviors, risk factor appraisal, and age appropriate interventions.

Women and men are faced with many life changes and challenges, some of which are gender specific. Previous life-styles and increases in stress from social, environmental, and economic constraints often result in risk for major health problems during adulthood.

The community health nurses' primary function with persons of all ages should be to promote quality and quantity of life. As the elderly segment of the population continues to grow, the health care delivery system and nursing must address and plan strategies to cope with increasing longevity, chronic health problems, and technological advances, as well as twenty-first century economic, social, and health issues.

Chapters 24 through 26 discuss family development, health risks, and assessment. Chapters 27 through 30 explore the major developmental tasks, health needs, risk factors, and issues for individuals from birth through senescence. Chapter 31 focuses attention on the needs of a special population, the physically compromised. Community health nursing interventions must be refined to assist this group in meeting their health care needs. ▼

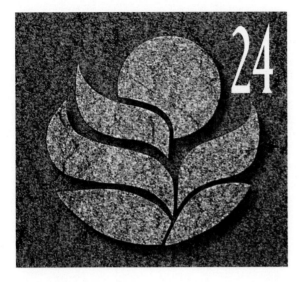

24 Family Theories and Development

Marcia Stanhope*

Objectives ▼

After reading this chapter, the student should be able to do the following:

◆ Analyze various approaches to defining the family.
◆ Discuss the various types of family and household structures.
◆ Identify family demographic trends that have implications for community health nursing practice.
◆ Identify and discuss family adult roles.
◆ Identify and discuss the functions common to most families.
◆ Identify and discuss family health functions and tasks.
◆ Analyze the family development conceptual approach to studying families.
◆ Discuss the developmental tasks involved in the processes of separation and divorce.
◆ Discuss the application of the developmental framework to community nursing practice with adoptive, single-parent, re-married, and vulnerable families.

Key Terms ▼

adoptive families
adoptive parents
cohabitation
critical transition points
developmental task
divorce
family
family demography
family development
family functions
family life cycle
family structure
household
marriage
nuclear family
primary relationship
remarriage
remarried family
roles
role sharing
separation
siblings
single-parent family
stepfamily
stepparent
transition points

Outline ▼

Continued.

*The author acknowledges the contribution of Rosemary Johnson to this chapter's content.

Outline—cont'd ▼

The family, as society's most significant unit of social behavior, has been experiencing considerable changes. These changes have affected the family's development: how it is structured and how it functions and interacts both internally and within the community. Demographic and socioeconomic changes, which had their beginnings in the late 1700s, have continued throughout the twentieth century, resulting in considerable consequences for families in the United States. Demographic trends that have affected the family are related to age at time of first marriage; fertility patterns and birth rates; increases in the numbers of single, divorced, and remarried persons in society; larger numbers of children experiencing family divorce or living with a never-married parent; and a growing elderly population.

Although general societal and familial expectations surround family roles and functions, trends in marriage and family influence the types of roles found in families and the structures and functions carried out by the family. Each family tends to modify family roles and role behaviors in relation to the family structure and in relation to the internal and external environment of the family unit. All families, regardless of their structure, have certain functions that are performed to maintain the integrity of the family unit and to meet the family's needs, individual members' needs, and society's expectations.

DEFINING THE FAMILY

Traditionally, the family has been defined in relation to the **nuclear family** (mother, father, and young children), in which the original parents remained together throughout the family life cycle and were monogamous. Thus the traditional family pattern is characterized as a "legal, lifelong, sexually exclusive marriage between one man and one woman, with children, where the male is primary provider and ultimate authority" (Macklin, 1988, p. 317).

There are six major premises related to the traditional monogamous family: (1) romantic love forms the basis for a successful marriage; (2) sexual activity should be confined to marital relationships; (3) a person should have only one partner of the opposite sex; (4) masculine and feminine sex roles should be clearly defined; (5) children should be raised in a nuclear family setting; and (6) the nuclear family is the most effective unit for family living and social functioning (Gutknecht et al., 1983).

The traditional nuclear family, as a continuing unit with original parents, is no longer the predominant family structure in American society. The family as an intact unit has become more transient. This transient nature has resulted in changes in family structure, membership goals, and in some instances, the family's reason for being. A consequence of family changes and the emergence of other family forms has been the increased difficulty in defining the family. The way the family is defined determines to some extent how the family's functions and roles in society are described.

The following definitions show several ways in which families are defined today. A family is defined as follows:

1. A system of interdependent members who possess two attributes: membership in the family and interaction with other members (Janosik and Green, 1992).
2. A unique social group bound together by generational ties, emotions, caregiving, established goals, altruistic orientation, and a nurturing form of governance (Bentler et al., 1989).
3. Two or more persons joined together by bonds of sharing and emotional closeness and who identify themselves as family (Friedman, 1992, p. 9).
4. A group of two or more persons related by birth, marriage, or adoption and residing together in a household (National Center for Health Statistics, 1990a).

Some family theorists have openly challenged attempts to define families formally because of the many exceptions and varieties. One approach is to conceptualize the family as a primary relationship. This approach is considered particularly useful for community health nursing practice. The **primary relationship** consists of at least two persons interacting in continuing fashion within an immediate situation as well as within a larger environment (Scanzoni et al., 1989). The primary relationship approach includes legal marriages, two natural-parent families, and other family structures.

Definitions of the family range from viewing the family as having a single, exclusive structure to perceiving the family as a household unit representing various types of family structures. A broad definition of the family is needed in community health nursing because community health nurses work with families that represent both traditional and less traditional family structures. Developing a definition of the family for research purposes is even more problematic, especially in relation to family membership, family behavior, family goals, and family life. The following definition represents Johnson's (1992) perspective on the family; the **family** is represented by two or more individuals, belonging to the same or different kinship groups, who are involved in a continuous living arrangement, usually residing in the same household, experiencing common emotional bonds, and sharing certain obligations toward each other and toward others.

CONCEPTUAL FRAMEWORKS

A conceptual framework is essential for guiding the community health nurse in the process of assisting families in their health-promoting efforts. Several frameworks are introduced here, with further discussion of each applied to community health nursing throughout the chapter.

Role Theory

Community health nurses need to understand the family and its roles to offer clients important insights into the family's behavior among its members and within the community and society. Roles within a family both affect and are affected by its health status. Individuals within a family have shared role expectations about how each member will behave (e.g., the father goes to work each day, children go to school). These role (behavioral) expectations imply that there are common experiences among those who are in a role (Bomar, 1992).

The box above provides the nurse with those concepts that are important to understand in order to assess the family and how its members behave. Understanding these concepts is valuable to the nurse in (1) understanding the roles each family member plays, (2) recognizing the behavioral expectations of family members, (3) identifying various sources of stress and interpreting meaning to the family, (4) identifying in-

Definitions of Important Role Theory Concepts

Family role—learned repetitive behaviors by which each member fulfills the expectations of his or her role position (e.g., father, mother, sister, brother, significant other).
Role stress—emotional discomfort because of intense demands related to expected behaviors.
Role strain—an individual's feelings of frustration and anxiety that result in inappropriate behaviors.
Role conflict—a source of emotional discomfort when multiple roles, with intense demands, become competitive with one another (e.g., mother, nurse).
Role incongruity—stress and strain develop when the individual self-preceptors are in disagreement with role expectations.
Role ambiguity—stress and strain occur when the expected role is not defined well.
Role overload—strain occurs when the individual cannot meet role expectations.
Role sharing—the implementing of family activities by individual members without regard to gender.
Role negotiation—agreement among family members as to the appropriate behaviors within a role position.
Role modeling—the demonstration of behaviors associated with a role; provides a standard by which others can learn a role.
Complementary roles—one or more roles fit together so that family activities can be accomplished (e.g., mother/father sharing child socialization).
Role transition—a change from one role to another.

Data from Bomar P: *Nurses and family health promotion: concepts, assessment and interventions*, Philadelphia, 1992, Saunders; Hardy M, Conway M: *Role theory perspective for health professionals*, East Norwalk, Conn, 1978, Appleton-Century-Crofts; and Smith AD, Reid WJ: *Role-sharing marriage*, New York, 1986, Columbia University Press.

appropriate behaviors of family members that may affect their health, (5) determining the adaptation to multiple roles, (6) identifying incompatibility between the role (of mother) and the person (mother) filling the role, (7) assessing roles when the behaviors are not clearly defined, and (8) identifying family members who cannot meet role expectations. Collecting data about these concepts assists the nurse in working with the family to reduce stress and strain. Role sharing, modeling, negotiation, and encouraging complementary roles are concepts the nurse can use to reduce family stress and strain and subsequently enhance the family's health status (Bomar, 1992).

Systems Framework

Systems theory was introduced by von Bertalanffy more than 50 years ago as a method of thinking about the order of the environment. This framework has been applied to families. In systems theory, families are described as units comprised of members whose interactional patterns become the focus of attention. The family is viewed as a whole, with boundaries that are affected by and permeated by the external environment. The family as an organizational structure is

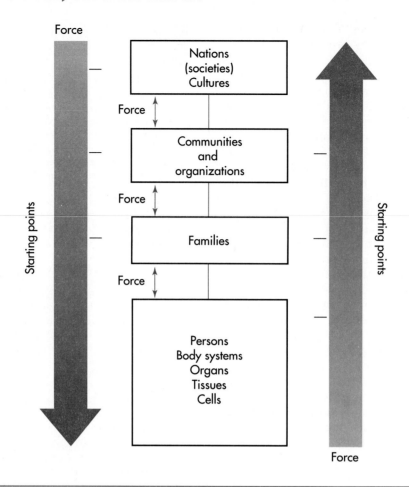

FIGURE 24-1

Family health and community health: a systems perspective. (Modified from Blum HL: *Expanding health care horizons from a general systems concept of health to a national health policy*, Oakland, Calif, 1976, Third Party Associates.)

a subsystem of the community and of society. Interaction of family members is directed toward maintaining homeostasis through a feedback mechanism of input from members and from the external environment, throughput, and output from members to the external environment. Feedback may be positive or negative, and it affects the control or adaptation of the family to its environment.

Application of this framework helps the community health nurse to understand (1) family interaction patterns, (2) family norms and expectations, (3) effectiveness of interaction patterns, (4) decision-making processes, (5) family adaptation in individual needs, (6) family expectations of its members, and (7) family adaptation to the community. The following situation, illustrated in Figure 24-1, provides an example of how systems theory is applied to families in interaction with society and communities.

Hypothetically, assume that numerous cultural systems decide that the values of peace and general human welfare take priority over war and full domestic employment, and that there is a resulting national policy that the manufacturing of armed services aircraft will cease. Some communities would experience

a loss of income and possible population loss of engineers and skilled workers. Likewise, the families of aerospace engineers previously employed by such aircraft industries would experience economic and emotional stress. They also might experience possible role changes if, for example, the spouse had to seek employment or a child had to drop out of college. Additional changes might be the loss of health insurance and other benefits. Consequences for the individual engineer could be the loss of self-esteem, the need to learn new skills, the need to adjust to changing lifestyles, and family poverty.

The final outcome for one or more family members could be the development of digressive social behaviors or stress-related illnesses. At this point, the spread of disequilibrium upward through the hierarchy of systems might be observed, as the behaviors of the individual family members begin to affect the health status and coping behavior of the family. The family's ability or inability to cope adequately and to adjust with or without consequential family disorganization has obvious consequences for the community. Family disorganization places demands on the community's health and human services resources and reduces the availability of productive, contributing family members in the community. Multiple families experiencing states of disorganization eventually would affect the general health status of the community.

Structural-Functional Framework

Within the structural-functional framework, the family is viewed as a social system with members who have specific roles and functions. General assumptions in the structural-functional approach include the following (Friedman, 1992; Leslie and Korman, 1989):

1. The family is a social system with functional requirements.
2. The family is a small group possessing certain generic features common to all small groups.
3. The family as a social system accomplishes functions that serve both the individual and society.
4. Individual members behave according to internal norms and values learned within the family.

Studying the family from a structural-functional perspective also includes analyzing the family as a system with boundaries that regulate input from and output to the environment. The boundaries facilitate or interfere with adaptation. The family as a social system consists of individuals organized into a single unit so that change in any family member inevitably results in changes in the entire family system (Friedman, 1992).

The structural-functional approach provides a framework for assessing family structure and functions, such as the socialization process of family members for roles and behaviors necessary for living and interacting in society; the socialization process for family members in relation to cultural and social norms; values, rights and privileges assigned to family roles; enactment of family roles; focus of authority and decision making in the family; development of coping behaviors; development of family subsystems; and communication patterns. Other examples of the structural-functional approach include the family health estate, the interrelationship between family and individual health, and the relationship between family health and community health.

Interactional Framework

The interactional approaches focuses on the family as a unit of interacting personalities and examines the symbolic communication processes by which family members relate to one another. Within the family, each member occupies a position or positions to which a number of roles are assigned. Family members define their role expectations in each situation through their perceptions of the role's demands. Family members judge their own behavior by assessing and interpreting the actions of others toward them. The responses of others in the family serve to challenge or reinforce the family members' perceptions of the norms or of role expectations (Bomar, 1992; Schuaneveldt, 1967).

Central to the interactional approach is the process of role taking. Every role exists in relation to some other role, and interaction represents a dynamic process of testing perceptions about each other's roles. Through family interaction, the result of the testing process is stabilization or modification of roles. The ability to predict other family members' expectations for one's role enables each member to have some knowledge of how to react in the role. It also indicates how other members will react to the performance in the role.

Assessment of the family within an interactional framework would emphasize (1) interaction between and among family members and (2) family communication patterns about health and illness behaviors appropriate for different roles. Using this theory specifically, the nurse would want to assess (1) the effectiveness of communications among members, (2) the ability to establish communication between nurse and the family, (3) the clarity and conciseness of messages between members, (4) similarities between the nonverbal and verbal communications, and (5) the directions of the interaction (Bomar, 1992).

Developmental Framework

One framework generated for studying families, which has been used in conjunction with other conceptual approaches, is the developmental framework. Developmental theory focuses on common general features of family life and provides a longitudinal view of the **family life cycle** (FLC). The family developmental framework identifies points in a family's development where changes occur in the status and roles of family members. Increasingly, variation in family structure such as single-parent families, remarried families, and vulnerable families is being studied from the developmental perspective.

The family development framework contributes to the community health nurse's understanding of families at different points in their FLC. A major strength of this approach is that it provides a basis for forecasting what a family will be experiencing at any period in the FLC, for example, role transitions and family constellation changes.

The developmental approach can be used successfully in practice with a variety of family structures, but the nurse must recognize that in every family there are individual and family developmental tasks to be accomplished that are unique to that particular family. Implicit in this approach is the need to be aware of the internal and external environmental forces (psychosocial, cultural, economic) that influence the family's development.

Knowledge about family life stages and the accompanying tasks gives the community health nurse a focus for family assessment, planning, intervention, and evaluation. Assessing the family's developmental stage and the family's performance of the tasks appropriate for that stage provides the nurse with guidelines for analyzing the family's development and health promotion needs. Anticipatory guidance can be used to prepare the family to cope with predictable role and position changes. The developmental approach also identifies periods in the FLC when problems may emerge because of limited or strained personal, emotional, and financial resources. Consequently, the family may need to be made aware of available support resources in the extended family or in the community.

Although anticipating what to expect is helpful when working with families, the nurse must recognize that not all families move through the FLC in the same way because of the variations among families. The nurse still can predict important aspects about the overall pattern of a family's developmental activities by knowing (1) where the family is in its development history and FLC; (2) the number, age, and way in which family members in the household are related; and (3) the family's ethnic, religious, and socioeconomic characteristics. (See pp. 463 to 465 for further discussion.)

FAMILY STRUCTURES

The social significance of the family has been founded in its mediating function between society and individual family members. The family has the dual responsibility of meeting the needs of family members and at the same time meeting the needs of the society with which it is associated. Social expectations for family members in the form of obligations and responsibilities are modified by the family to fit the needs and abilities of its members. The family, in turn, prepares and assists family members to meet societal responsibilities and obligations. Some recent trends affecting marriage and the family are becoming well established, whereas others remain tenuous.

Traditional and Other Family Structures

Each family, regardless of its structural system, has the potential for serving societal needs in one way or another. In addition, all families tend to be similar in attempting to provide for family needs, including the need to exchange affection; to provide reasonable stability; to provide financial resources for food, clothing, and shelter; to offer educational opportunities; and to make health services available and accessible.

Families with whom the community health nurse works represent a variety of structures and living arrangements. The community health nurse is responsible for assisting the family to promote its health, to meet family health needs, and to cope with health problems within the context of the existing family structure and life-style. Thus, community health nurses must be knowledgeable about family structures, functions, processes, and roles. In addition, they must be aware of and must understand their own values and attitudes pertaining to the family and varying family life-styles.

Family structure refers to the characteristics (gender, age, number) of the individual members who make up the family unit. More specifically, the structure of a family represents the positions occupied by the individuals who are engaged in regular, recurring interactions and relationships within that family unit. Many people envision a family structure in which they will be married, have children, live in a single-family household, prefer heterosexuality, and desire permanence and sexual exclusivity. However, increasing numbers of people are choosing other family life-styles at some point in their lives. As social norms have become more tolerant of a range and variety of choices in relation to managing one's life, there is no longer a general consensus that the traditional nuclear family model is the only "right" model. As a consequence, there is a growing number of family and household types. There is also an increasing awareness that more variation exists within particular family structures as well as among them. For example, the single-mother household may be represented by the unmarried, teenaged mother with an infant (unplanned pregnancy); the divorced mother with one or more children; or the single, career-oriented woman in her late thirties who elects to have a baby and remain single.

Thus far, attention has focused on the changing family structure, but what about the family career of the individual? An individual may participate in a number of family life-course experiences or trajectories over a lifetime (Figure 24-2). For example, a child may spend the early, formative years in the family of origin (mother, father, sibling); experience some years in a single-parent family because the parents divorce; and participate in a stepfamily relationship when the single parent (of custody) remarries. This same child as an adult may experience several family types. As an adult, the individual may cohabit while completing a desired education, marry and have a commuter-type marriage while developing a career, divorce and become the custodial parent, eventually cohabit with another partner, and finally marry another partner who also has children.

Although variations of the traditional nuclear family have existed throughout history, the increase in differing family structures is becoming more recognized and pronounced. There are many reasons that an increasing number of families diverge from the traditional family structure. A typology of family and household structures is presented in the box on p. 457. **Household** is defined as a single dwelling (apartment or house) occupied by an individual or a group of two or more individuals (related or unrelated). Thus, two or more individuals residing in the same dwelling may be defined as a family unit by some or as a household unit by others.

Over time the community health nurse will work with many families representing various structures and living arrangements. For example, one type of family living arrangement may be found among dual-career families in which spouses maintain separate

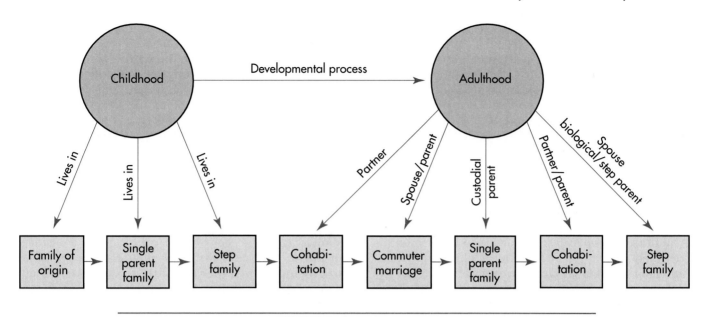

FIGURE 24-2

Family career of an individual.

Family and Household Structures

MARRIED FAMILY

Traditional nuclear family
Dual-career family
  Spouses reside in same household
  Commuter marriage
Husband/father away from family
Stepfamily
  Stepmother family
  Stepfather family
Adoptive family
Foster family
Voluntary childlessness

SINGLE-PARENT FAMILY

Never married
  Voluntary singlehood (with children—biological or adopted)
  Involuntary singlehood (with children)
Formerly married
  Widow (with children)
  Divorced (with children)
    Custodial parent
    Joint custody of children
    Binuclear family

MULTIADULT HOUSEHOLD (WITH/WITHOUT CHILDREN)

Cohabiting couple
Communes
Affiliated family
Extended family
New extended family
Home sharing individuals
Same-sex partners
Fictive kin

residences for the purpose of pursuing their individual careers. Families experiencing *commuter marriages* may need assistance in reducing stresses associated with spousal separation, temporary or long-term parental absences, and financial management associated with maintaining two households.

Some couples deliberately elect not to have children *(voluntary childlessness)*. They may tend to associate few advantages with parenthood and view greater couple intimacy as a more satisfying relationship. Voluntary childlessness has implications for social policy. Childlessness is perceived as noncompliance with the dominant social norm prescribing children. Thus, a social policy is needed that will increase the public's awareness of choice as well as enhance freedom of choice (Janosik and Green, 1992).

Singlehood may be voluntary or involuntary and permanent or temporary. Included in the group of singles are single parents, both women and men. The status of single parent may result from divorce, or from conception or adoption outside of marriage. Adults pursuing the singlehood track may need health education related to nutrition, emotional and sexual well-being, budgeting, preparation for retirement and old age, and other "living alone skills." Single parents may need assistance with parenting skills, and if employed, access to evening and weekend home visits, clinics, and group classes.

The placement of a child in another family setting, the *foster home,* may be for an unknown period. The foster care population is represented by children from economically deprived backgrounds (usually single-parent, female-headed households), children experiencing emotional and physical disabilities or abuse, and teenagers having conflictual relationships with their parents or difficulties with other authority figures (Eastman, 1982). The foster parent(s) may need guidance regarding parenting skills appropriate to the individual child's needs, assisting the child to adjust to a new home and family environment, and providing appropriate health care.

Same-sex partner households may or may not include children. Many same-sex partners have been in a heterosexual marriage at one time or another and have children from that marriage. In addition, some same-sex (homosexual) partners elect to have a baby through natural means, artificial insemination, or adoption (Macklin, 1988). These families may need assistance with parenting skills, health guidance, and helping the child to cope with social attitudes about same-sex partner households.

Voluntary *group living* is predicted to become an increasingly viable option for older adults. It is one solution for providing companionship and care for elderly persons as health and income decline. In "share-a-home" arrangements, older persons pool their resources, share household and care responsibilities, and possibly employ a manager. In the *affiliated family,* older nonkin are integrated into a younger family unit. The *fictive kin* family structure is common to low-income and minority cultures. Nonkin members of various ages are incorporated into the family structure for various economic and social reasons. Much of the work with these types of families can be conducted on a group basis.

Trends in the Family Life Cycle

During the preindustrial European period, the family was functional, patriarchal, and community dependent. Marriage was founded on rational and economic grounds, and there was little affection between family members. The affectionate, private, male-dominant nuclear family developed with the industrialized society. This nuclear family was a social and emotional unit. The permanent, exclusive affectionate bond between the spouses formed the foundation for the family. Today, families tend to be partial to the individualized, open, equal-value pattern in which independence, close emotional ties with persons outside the family, and individual interests are emphasized. The family continues to evolve, maintaining many of its traditional functions and structures while adapting to changing economic circumstances and social ideologies (Macklin, 1988).

Did You Know?

In 1993 the U.S. Congress passed legislation to require employers to give workers official leave for family events, such as fathers for the birth of their children.

The historical study of families in the early settlements in the United States finds that most of the fam-

ily structures currently in existence were present then. The difference is the numbers found in each of the structures: the nuclear intact household, single-parent family, blended family, extended family, three-generational family, dual-job family, and other structures. Prospects for families for the twenty-first century are numerous. New family structures that currently are experimental will emerge as everyday "natural" families; for example, families in which the members are not related by blood or marriage, but who provide the services, caring, love, intimacy, and interaction needed by all persons to experience a quality life. These family structures will bring together people from different generations as well as persons of similar ages. The baby-boom cohort, with a history of low fertility rates, will find new relatives available to care for them in the years 2010 to 2020 when they reach late adulthood. New "like" families will be needed in increasing numbers to provide homelike environments and care (Sussman, 1987). Other trends and prospects are as follows (Macklin, 1988; Settles, 1987; Sussman 1987):

1. The continued presence and existence of multiple family structures will result in changes in federal regulations related to a family's qualifications for service programs.
2. Court decisions will continue to accept broader definitions of the family than current traditional and legal definitions.
3. Middle-age adults may find themselves "squeezed" between the prolonged dependency of adult children remaining in the home of origin for longer periods of time and elderly parents and grandparents entering into their homes on a somewhat permanent basis.
4. People will move from one type of household to another more frequently than in the past.
5. People will have more complicated family histories and complicated kinship relationships resulting from divorce and remarriage.
6. Women will continue to bear most of the costs associated with technological and family changes.
7. There will be an increase in the number of women socialized to be career- or work-oriented in adulthood, particularly for personal reasons.
8. Redefinition of family roles toward equality will continue even though attempts have been made to maintain traditional roles.
9. An important function of the family will continue to be providing for individual life transitions.
10. The primary relationship between parents and children will continue to be the most enduring of family relationships.

FAMILY DEMOGRAPHY

Family demography is the study of the structure of families and households and the events that alter the structure (Teachman et al., 1987). Changes in family and household structures can be explained by the events that alter status or position within the structure. For example, the position of being a married parent is changed by the divorce process, and the family structure is altered to one of a single-divorced parent with children.

An important use of family demography is forecasting such as planning for the number of houses, types of housing, and sizes of residences needed in the future. Such forecasts become increasingly important as family and household structures change. To account for the variations in the number, timing, and sequencing of family-related events, various social, economic, and demographic influences must be examined. The following is a brief summary of the demographic changes that must be considered in working with family units.

Marriage

At present more than 90% of Americans marry, but it is predicted that by the year 2000 this percentage may drop to 85% (Macklin, 1988). Since 1987, **marriages** have declined annually except for 1988, when marriages increased during that year. Although the total first marriage rates rose in 1987, the total remarriages declined for both men and women (National Center for Health Statistics, 1994).

The marriage rates for divorced men and women were higher than the rates for their single and widowed counterparts. Factors associated with age differentials at the time of marriage are education, labor force participation, income, and premarital fertility. Educational and occupational aspirations tend to influence the postponement of marriage, whereas dating or early heterosexual involvement and sexual experimentation may lead to early marriages for both males and females. Many early marriages are accompanied by a premarital pregnancy, although willingness to have an abortion or to experience a premarital birth may delay marriage (National Centers for Health Statistics, 1994).

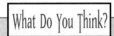

What Do You Think?

Two unmarried persons living together, with emotional bonds, are considered a family unit.

Cohabitation

From 1970 to 1987 the number of unmarried heterosexual couples sharing the same household rose considerably, with the greatest increase occurring in the middle-age group. There were considerably more widowed women than widowed men who were **cohabitating.**

Singles

In 1993, 22% of the population 18 years of age and older were single. Since 1970 the number of men and women who are single has steadily increased. It has been predicted that 8% to 9% of the adults in their twenties will experience a lifetime of singlehood. Also, there is an increased likelihood that an individual may be single several times in a lifetime: before marriage, after divorce, after remarriage and divorce, and after death of a spouse (Macklin, 1988; National Center for Health Statistics, 1994).

An interesting phenomenon is the number of young single adults who remain in their parent's home or return to their home of origin after a period of absence. More males than females were in this type of living arrangement (U.S. Bureau of the Census, 1994).

Divorce

Between 1970 and 1987 the ratio of the population 18 years of age and older undergoing divorce increased more than 100%. In 1988 the median length of a marriage for a divorcing couple was 7 years (National Center for Health Statistics, 1994). Approximately one-third of the divorces occurred before the fourth year of marriage. Some of the factors associated with marital disruption are less than a high school education, a premarital birth or premarital pregnancy, marrying during the teen years or in the early twenties, and husband's frequent unemployment (Teachman et al., 1987).

Remarriage

More than 75% of people who divorce remarry. In 1988 the marriage rate for divorced women was 47% higher than the rate for single women marrying, and 14 times higher than the rate for widows remarrying. The marriage rate for divorced men was 137% higher than the rate for single men and more than four times the rate for widowers. One-half of divorced and one half of widowed men remarried within 2.2 years of the date their last marriage ended. The median interval of **remarriage** for divorced women was 2.5 years, and 4.6 years for widows (National Center for Health Statistics, 1994). Studies support that there is greater diversity in remarriage experiences than in first marriages; for example, men and women in remarriages tend to differ in age by a greater margin than do men and women in first marriages (Furstenberg and Spannier, 1984).

Children of Divorce

Each year in the United States, more than 2 million couples divorce, and more than 1 million children are affected. Nearly 10 million children under age 18 years lived with a biological parent and a stepparent or with two parents who were remarried. Seventy percent of these children lived with their biological mother and stepfather, and 30% lived with both natural parents (born after mother remarried). Nearly one-half of all the children from maritally disrupted families have not seen one of their biological parents, usually the father, in the previous 5 years. Only one child in six whose parents were separated or divorced saw the outside biological parent about once a week (Furstenberg and Spannier, 1994).

One-Parent Families

In 1990 there were over 7 million single-parent, female-headed households with children, and approximately 2 million single-parent, male-headed households (U.S. Bureau of the Census, 1994). It has been predicted that by the age of 17, 70% of the white children born in 1980 will have spent at least some time with only one parent. The same prediction has been made for 94% of African-American children (Espenshade, 1987).

Children in Poverty

The federal poverty income guidelines for 1995 range from $7,476 for one person to $25,392 for a family of eight, exclusive of Alaska and Hawaii, which have higher ranges. The poverty level income for a family unit of two is $10,032, for three $12,600, and for four $15,156. For families of a larger size, $2,568 should be added for each additional family member (Social Security Bulletin, 1995). These guidelines are important because they determine whether a child or family is eligible for community services such as Women, Infants, and Children (WIC) programs and Medicaid.

In 1970 almost 15% of children under 18 years of age lived in families with incomes below the poverty level. That percentage increased to 21% in 1992. In 1990, 7.2 million children living in poverty were in female-headed families with no husband present (U.S. Bureau of the Census, 1994). Forty-six percent of single-mother households fall below the poverty level (Health US, 1993; 1994).

Working Women

Women presently make up a large proportion of the work force. Sixty-one percent of the households consisting of married couples with children have two wage earners in the family. Seventy percent of the working mothers hold full-time jobs (Family Service of America, 1987). Thus, there has been a steady increase across all marital statuses, from 1970 to 1988, in the number of women with children who are in the work force.

Elderly Persons

In 1920, less than 5% of the U.S. population was 65 years of age or older. At present, older people represent 12% of the population (Health US, 1993; 1994), and it is predicted that by the year 2050, the proportion will be 24% to 35%. The majority of these persons will be women. The living conditions for older women are

 Research Brief

Burley K: Gender differences and similarities in coping responses to anticipated work-family conflict, *Psychol Rep* 74:115-123, 1994.

The current, most frequently occurring family structure is the dual-earner couple. This has resulted because of changing sex-role attitudes and the economic recession. This life-style is highly stressful for couples because of multiple role demands. This study sought to identify gender differences in anticipated work-family conflict and anticipated coping mechanisms to manage conflict and to explore the role that coping processes play in mediating the relationship between gender and work-family conflicts.

Participants in the study were 256 university students. The study results showed that gender was significantly related to anticipated work-family conflict, with women expecting to experience substantially less than men. It was also found that gender plays a role in the extent and use of coping strategies to manage family conflict. However, coping strategies such as behaviors relating to reduction of the tension, support, and modifying the roles did not account for the relationship between gender and work-family conflict.

The nurse can use these findings to increase awareness and sensitivity to potential work-family conflicts and to help families work together to balance career and family life.

quite different than for older men. There are more elderly women than men, almost twice as many men as women live with a spouse, and there are over three times as many widows as widowers. In addition, a much higher proportion of elderly women live alone compared with men, and more than twice as many women as men live below the poverty level.

It is important for community health nurses to keep themselves informed and up to date regarding demographic trends. Such knowledge is essential so that nurses can identify high-risk populations such as the many children living in poverty, children of working mothers who care for themselves, and elderly women living alone. Implications exist for planning health care services for groups such as the elderly persons, children living in poverty, and unmarried mothers; developing community resources for adequate child care and numerous counseling services; and becoming politically active in relation to the appropriate allocation of scarce funds and resources for health services needed by a growing, diverse population.

FAMILY ROLES AND FUNCTIONS

Implicit in the study of the family are the concepts of roles and functions. The current trends in marriage and the family influence the types of roles found in families, the enactment of those roles, and the functions carried out by the family. The nurse working with families must be knowledgeable about family roles and functions and their modifying factors.

Family Roles

In every family, each member holds a recognized position or status, such as husband, wife, son, or daughter. Each family member usually occupies several positions simultaneously (husband, worker, grandfather, etc.). Individuals are guided by **roles** that are "expectations of behavior, obligations, and rights that are associated with a given position in a family or social group" (Duvall and Miller, 1985, p. 77). Individuals acquire the knowledge and develop the skills, attitudes, and competence to function in a given position through the process of socialization. Unfortunately, an individual may be thrust into a position without adequate preparation for the associated roles, for example, the young teenager who becomes a mother.

No two individuals occupying the same position will enact their role exactly the same way, although societal expectations ensure some similarities. The extent of one's commitment to or conflict about a role is affected by the socialization process. Social and cultural factors that influence role fulfillment include rates of social change, ambiguities, contradictions, modifications, and alternatives in prevailing role definitions. For example, the women's movement has caused some men to experience difficulties in defining their roles, while some women assume a defensive posture regarding their role as full-time homemaker.

Social class, race/ethnicity, and age/generation have significant implications for role conception and performance. Among the poor population in society, a married woman with a husband present usually has few rights but has demanding domestic and economic obligations to the family. The upper-class wife usually has great freedom and serves as the manager for employed assistants who provide domestic services. Among urban, professional families, the wife may be pursuing her own career full time, sharing authority with her husband and delegating some of the homemaking and childrearing responsibilities to others. Generally, married full-time working women still perform most of the household and child care activities with varying amounts of assistance from their husbands. In addition to societal and cultural expectations about the behavior of family members, each family also has expectations. These expectations may or may not be congruent with those of society. Each family tends to modify family roles and role behaviors in relation to the family structure and to forces internal and external to the family unit.

Family Adult Roles

The enactment of family adult roles, and the behaviors associated with them, will vary. The following describes typical family adult roles (Nye, 1976):

1. *Child socialization.* Encompasses the processes and activities in the family that contribute to the development of the child's social and mental capacities.
2. *Child care.* Involves provision of physical and emotional care to the child for the purpose of developing a healthy individual.
3. *Provider role.* Includes the production of goods and services needed by the family or the obtaining of them through the exchange of goods and services.
4. *Housekeeper role.* Involves preparing and maintaining the goods and services for the family's use. This role also includes services in the home that contribute to the pleasure and comfort of the family members.
5. *Kinship role.* Includes the maintenance of contact with kin and implies assistance during periods of crisis.
6. *Sexual roles.* Require mutual participation of both partners, with the implicit assumption that both partners enjoy the sexual relations.
7. *Therapeutic role.* Entails assisting the family member to cope with problems and providing emotional support, as well as handling intrafamily problems.
8. *Recreational role.* Involves providing for family recreation and aspects of relaxation, entertainment, and personal development.

Although husbands and wives participate in the family adult roles in different ways and to a different extent, some couples are subscribing to the new values of equality at work and at home. **Role sharing** has been defined as "both partners having equal claims to the bread winning role and equal responsibilities for the care of the home and children, including the obligations to contribute equally or equitably to the family expenses" (Smith and Reid, 1986, p. 6).

Sibling Roles

Siblings are both instigators of socialization in the family and recipients of the socialization process. They contribute to one another's (sibling) identity formation by serving as defenders and protectors of each other, interpreting the outside world, teaching others about equity, building coalitions, bargaining, negotiating, and mutually regulating each other's behavior. Siblings also provide direct services to each other by serving as a buffer between a sibling and the parents and by providing resources such as lending money and other material goods. As a subgroup within the family, siblings assist in establishing and maintaining family norms and contribute to the development of the family's culture. Aldous (1978) has examined sibling role behavior from a life cycle perspective (Table 24-1). The life cycle approach identifies sibling roles starting with preschool-age siblings and concluding with elderly siblings.

The preceding adult and sibling roles are viewed as part of formal family roles. In addition to formal family roles, there are also informal family roles, such as scapegoat, placater or pleaser, martyr or sacrificer, encourager, blamer or know-it-all, follower, or initiator of change.

Table 24-1   Life Cycle Sibling Role Behavior

Sibling age	Role behaviors
Preschool	Handle competition for parents' attention Handle grievances toward each other resulting from parental differential treatment
School age	Develop an affectional sibling structure Engage in role making with siblings Function as discipline to siblings Develop power patterns within sibling subsystem Provide gender role socialization
Adolescent	Learn from each other how to relate to peers of opposite gender Serve as reminder to younger siblings that adolescent tasks can be mastered Supply younger siblings with current information on content of adolescent tasks Become advisor and confidant to siblings Provide support and understanding that can ease parent-adolescent conflicts Serve as mediator within family and also between family and broader community
Adult	Maintain sibling contacts through obligatory parental contacts Maintain sibling bond Perform kin-keeping functions after death of parents
Elderly	Reestablish sibling relationships (if necessary) Provide comfort and support

Modified from Aldous J: *Family careers: developmental change in families,* New York, 1978, Wiley.

Family Functions

All families have certain functions that are performed to maintain the integrity of the family unit and to meet the family unit's needs, the individual family member's needs, and society's expectations. Duvall and Miller (1985) identified six **family functions** that are generally applicable to all types of family structures:

1. *Generating affection.* Affection is generated between spouses, between parents and children, and among members of the generations.
2. *Providing personal security and acceptance.* The family provides a home base with a stability that allows the family members to develop naturally in their own way at their own pace.
3. *Giving satisfaction and a sense of purpose.* In the family setting the family members enjoy life with each other through satisfying activities.
4. *Ensuring continuity of companionship.* In most cases, family associations that provide sympathetic companionship and encouragement can be expected to endure.
5. *Providing social placement and socialization.* The family serves as the transmitter of culture from one gen-

eration to the next and prepares family members for their place in the social hierarchy.
6. *Imposing controls and a sense of what is right.* Within the family, members first learn the rules, rights, obligations, and responsibilities characteristic of human societies.

Family Health Functions

In addition to the functions just listed, a basic family function is to protect the health of the family members and to provide supportive, nurturing care during periods of illness. The family is the primary social system within which the individual develops, is nurtured, and becomes socialized, and it is where personal growth and anatomy are fostered. The family contributes to the health of individual family members by supporting the biophysical and psychosocial development of the members. It is within the family unit that members develop their concept of health and establish their health habits. The family as a social unit develops a system of values, beliefs, and attitudes about health and illness that are imparted to and demonstrated through the health-illness behaviors of the family members (family health estate). The family also functions as the primary source for transmitting health-related cultural traits to the next generation. Through the family, members learn the beliefs and practices of the larger society concerning health and illness (Johnson, 1992).

How the family carries out its health care responsibilities, and its ability to do so are influenced by factors such as the family's structure, division of labor, socioeconomic status, and ethnicity.

The list of health-related functions and tasks in the box below is applicable to most families, but the extent to which these functions and tasks will be ob-

---

 Family Health Functions and Tasks

Provision of adequate food, shelter, and clothing
Maintenance of health-supporting physical home environment
Maintenance of health-supporting psychosocial home environment
Provision of resources for maintenance of personal hygiene
Provision for meeting spiritual needs
Health education
Health promotion (nutrition, exercise, etc.)
Health-illness decision making
Recognition of developmental disruptions
Recognition of health disruptions
Seeking health care
Seeking illness care
Seeking dental care
First aid
Supervision of medications (prescribed and over the counter)
Illness care (short term and long term)
Rehabilitation care
Involvement with community's health

served for every family varies in accordance with the previously mentioned family characteristics. The community health nurse supports the family in its ability to perform health-related tasks, contributes by assisting the family in strengthening its resources for carrying out these responsibilities, and intervenes more directly as necessitated by the family situation.

FAMILY DEVELOPMENT THEORY

Family development refers to the process of progressive structural changes over time. This includes the taking on and discarding of roles by family members as they seek to meet changing requirements for survival and adapt to recurring life stresses as a family (Janosik and Green, 1992). Family development theory focuses on common, general features of family life through a longitudinal view of the FLC. It assumes that there are successive phases and patterns that occur within the experience of family living over the years. Family development theory divides family life over time into a series of stages or phases that are qualitatively and quantitatively different from the preceding and succeeding stages. This assumes that a high degree of interdependence exists among the family members. As a consequence of this interdependence, families change each time members are added to or subtracted from the family (Duvall and Miller, 1985; Friedman, 1992). These changes, referred to as **critical transition points,** also result in changes in the status and roles of family members. The family operates through roles that shift and alter during the course of the family's life. The healthy family performs all roles appropriately according to family members' ages, competencies, and needs during the FLC.

Family development is unique as a framework for studying families. The FLC provides the basis for the study of families over time, emphasizes family members' and families' developmental tasks at every stage of development, identifies family stresses at critical developmental periods, and recognizes the need for services and programs for families throughout their FLCs (Duvall, 1988).

The family development framework, as originally formulated, focuses essentially on the FLC of the nuclear family from the wedding, to the birth of children, to the death of the surviving spouse. In recent decades, it has become apparent that not everyone fits into this normative FLC pattern. As stated by Duvall and Miller (1985), "Families express their individuality in the distinctive ways in which they proceed through the universal life cycle. Each family history has its own unique design" (p. 21).

At all times during the course of the family's development, an interrelationship exists among individual, family system, and intergenerational development. There are four kinds of action in the family's developmental history; movement of family members through their own unique life cycle, interaction among members' life cycles, developmental movement of the family system through the FLC, and the interweaving of intergenerational FLCs (e.g., young parent in a family of procreation who is, at the same time, an adult child in a family of origin).

Family Developmental Frameworks

As originally conceived, the FLC, also referred to as the *family career,* consists of stages related to the child's entry into and exit from the family. Events related to the child's stages in the family were considered to be **transitional** points for the family because role relationships among family members were significantly altered by those events (Figure 24-2).

Duvall and Miller (1985) categorized the family life cycle into eight stages: (1) married couple without children, (2) childbearing family in which the oldest child is 30 months of age, (3) family with preschool children (oldest 2.5 to 6 years of age), (4) family with school age children (oldest 6 to 13 years), (5) family with teenagers (oldest 13 years to 20 years), (6) family launching young adults (time from first and last child leaving home), (7) middle-age parents (residing alone to retirement), and (8) aging family members (retirement to death of both spouses). These are summarized in Table 24-2.

Assumptions of the family developmental framework can be summarized as follows (Aldous, 1978):
1. Families develop and change over time in similar and consistent ways.
2. Humans initiate actions as they mature and interact with others as well as reacting to environmental pressures.
3. The family and family members must perform certain time-specific tasks set by themselves, and they must perform tasks determined by culture and society.
4. Families tend to have a beginning and an end.

Since the early work of the family development theorists in the 1940s, considerable research and conceptualization regarding family development has continued. Over the past decade, increasing concern has been expressed about the need to minimize the emphasis placed on the FLC stages and to increase the focus on the transitional process from one stage to another. Family development includes two interrelated types of change: (1) change in the role content of family positions, essentially because of changes in age norms for those positions (e.g., moving from parent of infant, to parent of adolescent, to parent of adult children), and (2) change in interactional patterns in the family (e.g., changes in spousal interactions when a couple become parents) (Olson and Lavee, 1989).

Barnhill and Longo (1978) formulated the key principles of the transition points for various FLC stages (Table 24-3). Although it is readily apparent that this approach to transitions in the FLC focuses essentially on the entrance and exit of children in the family, this type of model could be used to develop transition points for different family structures.

Table 24-2   Family Developmental Tasks

Family stages	Developmental tasks
Beginning family	Establishing a marriage Relating to kin network Family planning
Early childbearing family	Stabilizing the family unit Reconciling family members' conflicting developmental tasks Facilitating developmental needs of mother, father, and infant
Family with pre-school child(ren)	Nurturing and socializing children Maintaining a stable marriage
Family with school-age child(ren)	Socializing children Promoting school achievement Maintaining satisfactory marital relationship
Family with teenager(s)	Balancing teenage freedom and responsibility Maintaining open parent-child communication Maintaining a stable marital relationship Building a foundation for future family stages
Launching family	Releasing children as young adults Readjusting the marriage Assisting aging parents
Middle-age family	Strengthening the marital relationship Sustaining relationships with parents and children Providing a healthy environment Cultivating leisure-time activities
Aging family	Adjusting to retirement Maintaining satisfactory living arrangement Adjusting to reduced income Adjusting to health problems Adjusting to death of spouse

Modified from Friedman MM: *Family nursing: theory and assessment*, East Norwalk, Conn, 1992, Appleton & Lange.

Family Developmental Tasks

A family **developmental task** is defined as a "growth responsibility that arises at a certain stage in the life of a family, the successful achievement of which leads to present satisfaction, approval, and success with later tasks." Failure in completing the tasks can lead to family unhappiness, societal disapproval, and difficulty with later developmental tasks (Duvall and Miller, 1985, p. 61). Tasks are considered accomplished if the family's biological needs are met, societal obligations are fulfilled, and the family's own values and aspirations are satisfied. The developmental tasks basic to most families, such as physical maintenance and socialization of family members, tend to be congruent with the family functions discussed previously. Although specific family developmental tasks were identified for each FLC stage, many tasks are common to several stages. Examples include providing adequate housing, facilities, and equipment; meeting family expenses; sharing responsibilities for household management and child care; maintaining mutually satisfying intimate family communications; relating to relatives; engaging in community participation; maintaining family morale; and developing mature roles within the family (Duvall and Miller, 1985). Examples of family developmental tasks by stage appear in Table 24-2. Some of the developmental tasks are more relevant for intact families (mother, father, children residing together) than for some other types of family structures.

The achievement of family developmental tasks at each family stage is interrelated with the accomplishment of developmental tasks by individual family members. Achievement of family developmental tasks assist the individual members to accomplish their tasks. This in turn enables the family to complete its task(s). In addition, individual family members must accomplish many of their individual developmental tasks to be able to fulfill their family roles adequately (Aldous, 1978; Duvall and Miller, 1985; Havighurst, 1974; Stevenson, 1977).

The following example illustrates the interrelationship of the tasks and also demonstrates the complex nature of the family at this stage of development. When an adolescent becomes pregnant, in addition to working on the developmental tasks common to adolescence, she is confronted with the developmental tasks associated with pregnancy. Pregnancy-associated developmental tasks are (1) development of an emotional attachment to the fetus during the first trimester; (2) differentiation of the self and the fetus during the third trimester; (3) acceptance and resolution of the relationship with the pregnant woman's mother; and (4) resolution of dependency issues in relation to the woman's mother and husband/partner (if present). Successful accomplishment of these tasks should contribute to the development of a coherent sense of oneself as a person and as a parent. Thus the adolescent is confronted with a double set of developmental tasks that are not necessarily compatible. The adolescent also is confronted with premature entry into the parental role and possible premature exit from the educational role.

The tasks of the other family members become more complex because certain roles shift as a result of the pregnancy. The parents may become grandparents prematurely, and the siblings become aunts and uncles. If the adolescent decides to keep the baby and remain in the family of origin, the family unit size and composition will change.

The family development approach assists community health nurses in understanding and anticipating clinical problems in the family as well as identifying family strengths. The framework can serve as a guide in assessing the family's developmental stage, the ex-

Table 24-3 Family Life Cycle Stage Transitions

Transition points	Issues
Commitment (late courtship, wedding, honeymoon, parenthood)	Moving away from family of origin Developing lifetime commitment to new family
Developing new parent roles	Shift from spouse to parent (within conjugal and extended families) Role transitions for numerous family members
Accepting new personality	Accepting normal dependency of newborn Allowing development of new individual personality (as child passes from infancy to childhood)
Introducing child to institutions outside the family	Dealing with individual's adjustment to establishing independent relationships with school, church, etc.
Accepting adolescence	Developing a sexual identity for adolescent and individual integration into peer group culture
Experimenting with independence	Lessening of ties with family of origin Allowing adult strivings to emerge
Preparations to launch	Accepting independent adult role of first child
Letting go/facing each other again	Letting go of children and facing each other as spouses alone again Children leaving parents to themselves Developing new roles: grandparents, parents
Accepting retirement and old age	New life-style, excluding career plans, goals, and responsibilities Plan for caring for older and younger generations

Modified from Barnhill LR, Longo D: *Fam Proc* 17(4):469-478, 1978; by Johnson R: In Stanhope M, Lancaster J, editors: *Community health nursing: process and practice for promoting health,* ed 3, St Louis, 1992, Mosby.

tent to which the family is fulfilling the tasks associated with the respective stage, the family's developmental history, and the availability of resources essential for performing the developmental tasks. One example of the application of the family development framework to community health nursing intervention is its appropriateness for use in anticipatory guidance. Family members can be assisted by preparing them to cope with FLC role transitions and by making them aware of supporting community resources. For example, the early childbearing family may experience stress from the arrival of a new baby. The community health nurse can plan to share with the parents changes that they should expect in their lives and schedules (i.e., sleep, rest, feeding schedule, emotions, new demands on time). A community resource that the nurse could refer them to is a parenting group.

In summary, developmental theory as a framework assists the community health nurse to (Duvall and Miller, 1985):

1. Keep the family in focus throughout its life cycle.
2. See family members in interaction with one another.
3. Observe the ways in which family members and the family unit influence each other.
4. Recognize what a given family is experiencing at a particular time.
5. Identify critical periods of growth and development for both the individual family members and the family.

6. Recognize the commonalities and variations among the life cycles of families.
7. Respect the way in which culture and families influence each other.
8. Forecast what a family will be experiencing at any period of its life cycle.

DEVELOPMENTAL THEORY AND NONTRADITIONAL FAMILY STRUCTURES

Increasingly, the life course of many families is not following the typical life cycle of the nuclear family. Greater numbers of families are demonstrating variations in childbearing and childrearing patterns, frequency in marital disruption before widowhood, and in reconstituting family structures. The developmental framework helps to understand these family life changes. These family changes result in developmental crises that must be resolved for families to continue to function normally.

Adoptive Family

Adoptive parents, as with their nonadoptive counterparts, must adapt to the increased personal and interpersonal strains that accompany parenthood. In addition, adoptive parents encounter other developmental transitional issues and stresses; examples of these are described in Table 24-4. Although numerous stresses are associated with the transition to adoptive

Table 24-4 Transition to Adoptive Parenthood

Developmental issues	Stresses
No role models	Difficulty developing realistic expectations about the transition to adoptive parenthood
	Preparation for parenting tends to be based on experiences with own parents
Timing of transition role	Uncertainty about the transition to parenthood—may be anywhere from a few months to 6 to 7 years
	Absence of usual pregnancy cues makes it difficult for others to alter perceptions and expectations of couple becoming parents
In-depth evaluation process	Proving their worthiness to be parents
	Process perceived as intrusive and anxiety arousing
Timing of adoption placement	Extent of attachment bonds between child and biological or foster parents
Biological risk associated with adoption	Background of child (genetic, parents' behavior, prenatal/birth complications)
Telling child about adoption	Makes explicit that adoptive parents are not biological parents
	Introduces image of natural parents into adoptive family system
	Threatens exclusiveness of relationship between adoptive parent and child

Modified from Brodzinky DM, Huffman L: *Marr Fam Rev* 12(3-4):267-286, 1988; and Di Guilio JF: *Soc Casework* 68(9):561-566, 1987; by Johnson R: In Stanhope M, Lancaster J, editors: *Community health nursing: process and practice for promoting health*, ed 3. St Louis, 1992, Mosby.

parenthood, protective factors are also related to the transition.

Adoptive families need ongoing services to help them cope with adoptive issues in general. They also may need assistance with parenting skills that are specific to their needs as adoptive parents. Finally, family life education programs should be made available to explain the similarities and differences between adoptive and biological parenthood at various stages in the family's and child's life cycle (Di Guilio, 1987).

Separation

Separation is one set of transitions in the total process of moving from family organization in marriage to family reorganization in divorce and remarriage. Not all separations end in divorce. Major developmental role transitions in the family system occur in separation, divorce, and remarriage. At these times, families experience adjustment, restructuring, and consolidation. In the adjustment phase, families attempt to handle their stresses by avoidance, elimination, or assimilation (incorporating the stress into the existing family structure in a way that reduces stress). The restructuring phase consists of families establishing new patterns of interaction that recognize that the marital relationship no longer is present. During the consolidation phase, new role patterns are incorporated into new family structures, resulting in a testing of members to see how they fit into the family structure and to see how a family fits into the community. During this dynamic adjustment and adaptation process, the family and family members pursue strategies designed to regain or maintain the themes they

value in family life (Ahrons and Rodgers, 1987). It should be remembered that adults of all ages experience separation.

Divorce

Divorce is an event that moves individuals from a condition of being legally married to a state of being legally divorced. The divorce experience begins before the actual divorce, its effects extend into the future, and each family member is affected by it. Divorce is viewed as a developmental crisis and necessitates focusing on the normal family patterns resulting from the crisis. It is possible that defining divorce as a societal institution in the United States is at hand, even though sociocultural norms are poorly defined for divorce at present. The directions taken by families regarding divorce are related to their history, the current family situation, and family members' desired goals for the future (Ahrons and Rodgers, 1987).

Some of the postdivorce developmental tasks are a continuation of the tasks initiated during the separation transition phases (see box on p. 467, top, left). Additional tasks are handling the legal problems of the divorce and interpreting the meaning of the divorce to other family members, extended family, and friends (Duvall and Miller, 1985).

Single-Parent Family

The three most common family patterns in the United States at present are **nuclear, single-parent,** and **remarried families.** This discussion of single-parent families focuses essentially on the separated or divorced female as head of the household because that

Developmental Transition Phases of Separation

PRESEPARATION

Gradual emotional separation
Continue to enact public/social roles
Avoid exposing state of relationship to the public
Initiator usually experiences guilt
Assentor usually experiences anger

EARLY SEPARATION

State of emotional and social anomie
Emotional ambivalence (feelings vacillate)
Ambiguity of separation itself
Status of family undefined

MIDSEPARATION

Emotional distress still felt
Faced with a deficit in structure (two separate households)
Realignment of family member relationships
Conflict between meeting own needs and children's needs
Convert anxieties into "other-directed" anger
Restructure tasks to meet children's health and nutritional needs (may require outside support)
Try to form a coparenting relationship
Seek support from friends, relatives, etc.

LATE SEPARATION

Old patterns replaced by new ones: family reorganization
Trial-and-error period for meeting needs
Power struggles of the marriage become more exaggerated
Reassessment of economic condition of family and friendships
Create a sense of family for all family members

Modified from Ahrons CR, Rodgers RH: *Divorced families: a multidisciplinary developmental view*, New York, 1987, Norton; by Johnson R: In Stanhope M, Lancaster J, editors: *Community health nursing: process and practices for promoting health*, ed 3, St Louis, 1992, Mosby.

Developmental Tasks for Single-Mother Families

ESTABLISHMENT OF SINGLE-PARENT FAMILY

Developing new patterns of power, communication, and affection
Altering childrearing patterns
Developing new social networks
Fulfilling physical maintenance tasks
Coping with disrupted intimacy and sexual aspects of the marital relationship

WOMAN CONTINUING, INSTITUTING, OR REINSTITUTING OCCUPATIONAL CAREER

Developing new family physical maintenance arrangements
Restructuring relationships with younger children
Emphasizing affectional relationship with children
Maintaining morale of children
Providing children with needed extra nurturance
Reestablishing self-esteem (mother) through outside involvement

Modified from Aldous J: *Family careers: developmental changes in families*, New York, 1978, Wiley; by Johnson R: In Stanhope M, Lancaster J, editors: *Community health nursing: process and practice for promoting health*, ed 3, St Louis, 1992, Mosby.

family structure continues to predominate for divorced single-parent families.

Aldous (1978) identified six developmental stages for single female-parent families (i.e., divorced women): (1) establishment of the single-parent family; (2) the woman continuing, instituting, or reinstituting her occupational career; (3) the family with adolescents; (4) the family with young adults; (5) the woman in middle years; and (6) the woman's retirement from her career and/or assuming responsibilities for parents. The box (above, right) depicts some of the developmental tasks associated with the first two stages of the single-parent family. Many of the tasks related to the last four stages tend to be comparable to the tasks that have been identified for most families, with the exception of tasks related to the spouse.

Many of the family tasks delineated for the single mother family would apply to the single-father family as well. While the single mother may have to learn about and assume responsibility for tasks around the home that the husband formerly carried out (e.g., home repairs, yard work), similarly, the single father may face some of the same problems, especially problems related to child care (e.g., child's nutritional and health care needs).

The community health nurse working with the single-parent family will need to be prepared to assist the parent and children with developmental tasks through the provision of professional support, anticipatory guidance and problem solving, and the development of support systems and social networks. One of the major problems for single-parent families is task overload. This problem is very apparent in the single-mother family with young children because the major task of raising children becomes the responsibility of one parent rather than two parents. A problem for the children is not only the absence from the home of one of the parents, but also the perceived loss of both parents if the mother seeks employment outside the home at the same time that the divorce is occurring.

Remarried Family

There are several synonyms for the term remarried family: merging, blended, restructured, reconstituted, synergistic, and stepfamily. The terms **remarried family** and **stepfamily** are used interchangeably in this section because of the selected developmental issues that are discussed.

At present, there is no widely accepted, concrete model of behavioral stages related to how a remarried family, with children involved, should function normally. Stepfamilies as well as community health nurses tend to develop their ideas about the expected family roles on models of the biological nuclear fam-

Table 24-5   Remarried Family Formation: Developmental Issues

Steps	Prerequisite attitude	Developmental issues
1. Entering the new relationship	Recovery from loss of first marriage (adequate "emotional divorce")	Recommitment to marriage and to forming a family with readiness to deal with the complexity and ambiguity
2. Conceptualizing and planning new marriage and family	Accepting one's own fears and those of new spouse and children about remarriage and forming a stepfamily Accepting need for time and patience for adjustment to complexity and ambiguity of: 1. Multiple new roles 2. Boundaries; space, time, membership, authority 3. Affective issues: guilt, loyalty conflicts, desire for mutuality, unresolved past hurts	a. Work on openness in the new relationships to avoid pseudomutuality b. Plan for maintenance of cooperative coparental relationships with ex-spouses c. Plan to help children deal with fears, loyalty conflicts, and membership in two systems d. Realignment of relationships with extended family to include new spouse and children e. Plan maintenance of connections for children with extended family of ex-spouses
3. Remarriage and reconstitution of family	Final resolution of attachment to previous spouse and ideal of "intact" family Acceptance of a different model of family with permeable boundaries	a. Restructuring family boundaries to allow for inclusion of new spouse/stepparent b. Realignment of relationships throughout subsystems to permit interweaving of several systems c. Making room for relationships of all children with biological (noncustodial) parents, grandparents, and other extended family d. Sharing memories and histories to enhance stepfamily integration

From Carter E, McGoldrick M, editors: *The changing family life cycle: a framework for family therapists*, New York, 1988, Gardner Press.

ily. In remarriages, family members need to develop a concept of family that is acceptable to the spouses and to the stepfamily (Keshet, 1988). Stepfamilies, as with some adoptive families, find children and adults, once strangers, becoming instant relatives without the shared experience of developing their parent-child relationship over time. In remarried families that include children, many habitualized family behaviors may no longer apply. As a result, these families must solve problems unknown to other types of families. Some of the major structural elements associated with the stepfamily follow (Visher and Visher, 1979):

1. Permeability of the family's boundaries—shifting boundaries and membership
2. Presence of family members with interpersonal bonds associated with another previous family constellation
3. Presence of at least two individuals who experienced the rupturing of spousal and/or parent-child bonds
4. Possible presence of another natural parent with power outside the stepfamily boundary
5. New relationships that are more difficult to negotiate because they do not develop slowly as in the early stages of the nuclear family life cycle—they possibly begin in the school-age or adolescent period
6. Rapid engagement of family members in instant multiple roles

Table 24-5 provides a format for conceptualizing the development of a remarried family. The developmental steps in the formation of the remarried family build on the successful resolution of the developmental issues involved in the divorce process.

A model for stepfamily development constructed by Mills (1984) could be used as a guide by the community health nurse in assessing, guiding, and evaluating the family's task accomplishments relevant to the stepfamily cycle. An adequate model for the stepfamily should stress the ways in which the stepfamily functions that are unique to that type of family structure. For example, the model should focus on the developmental tasks appropriate for the stepparent-stepchild relationship while taking into account that this relationship will differ with different children. The **stepparent** eventually may be able to develop a parental role with a young stepchild but may never fully achieve the parental role with a teenager. This may be because of the lack of a common family his-

Table 24-6 Stepfamily Developmental Tasks

Stages	Tasks
1. Setting goals	Develop desired long-term goals for the family structure based on the needs of all the family members (focus on satisfactions to be gained in the stepfamily).
	Explore possible roles for the stepparent in relation to the stepchildren (the stepparent may or may not work toward a parental goal).
2. Parental limit setting	Biological parent (in stepfamily) in charge of setting and enforcing limits for biological child.
	Stepparent sets limits in accordance with biological parents' rules.
	In the family where both spouses have children, the couple will need to accept the existence of different rules for different children.
3. Stepparent bonding	Create periods of time free from limit setting for stepparent nurturing of the stepchild to allow stepparent-child bonding appropriate to child's age.
4. Blending family rules	Stepfamily develops own new rules and traditions.
	Negotiate regarding the stepparent parental role (if there is to be one—this begins only after the initial bonding phase completed).
	Disagreement regarding rules resolved by the biological parent.
	Biological parent accommodates the stepparent regarding rules to the extent that the stepparent contributes positively to the child's development.
5. Stepfamily's relations in the binuclear family	Stepparent supports the child's relationship with the same-sex parent in the other household.
	Differentiate between the two binuclear households.

Modified from Mills D: A model for stepfamily development, *Fam Rel* 33:365, 1984; by Johnson R: In Stanhope M, Lancaster J, editors: *Community health nursing: process and practice for promoting health*, ed 3, St Louis, 1992, Mosby.

tory (for the stepparent and teenager) over most of the teenager's life and also because of the teenager's needs in relation to the developmental task of seeking more autonomy from the family. General characteristics of the model are as follows: (1) both spouses, working as a pair, should assume conscious executive control of the family; (2) with the cooperation of the biological parent, the stepparent can select from a variety of possible roles (e.g., friend, parent) the role most appropriate for the stepparent-stepchild relationship; and (3) the stepfamily will need to select the family structure that best satisfies the individual needs of all its members. This structure may change considerably over time.

Table 24-6 presents the developmental stages and tasks in the Mills model. The developmental tasks are implemented sequentially so that each task can build on the process initiated in the preceding stages. All the tasks should continue throughout the stepfamily development process.

Certain themes emerge when considering the stepfamily structure: (1) no clearly delineated sociocultural norms exist for enactment of family roles in the stepfamily; (2) there are identifiable developmental tasks for the remarried family; (3) the boundaries of the stepfamily are permeable and sometimes changing as family members (i.e., children) move in and out of the family; (4) most of the concerns related to the stepfamily center around the stepparent-stepchild relationship; (5) the individuals in the remarried family engage in instant multiple roles and relationships; and (6) this family type experiences its own unique FLC.

VULNERABLE FAMILIES—AN ANALYSIS

In every community health nurse's caseload, there are one or more families who have experienced generational poverty as well as multiple problems of a physiological, psychological, and social nature. This is the family (to be referred to as a vulnerable family) that has never experienced financial stability; has been a long-time client of public agencies; has experienced frequent, if not continuous, states of disorganization; and whose FLC represents an endless succession of crises. The family members of the vulnerable family usually possess deep-seated assumptions about themselves as related to the broader society: (1) they are not needed or wanted; (2) they really have no right to exist; (3) there is nothing they can do; and (4) they are being destroyed by society itself. The adults may develop a conviction that regardless of what they do to get a job or try to keep it, their efforts are useless. For this reason, they may view illegal options as the only opportunity for economic gains, and consequently they may develop a pervasive sense of impotence, rage, and despair. The important struggle is for survival.

Certain factors are related to the vulerable family that the community health nurse should remember when preparing to work with the family: (1) the family should be viewed across a three-generational time frame that includes members of the immediate family and the extended family; (2) the vulnerable family is subject to more abrupt loss of membership through such events as desertion, death, and imprisonment; and (3) the vulnerable family seems to have less calendar time in which to experience the various developmental stages. The shortened duration of the FLC frequently results in (1) inadequate time to achieve the developmental tasks of each family life stage, (2) more blurring of the boundaries of the life stages of this family, and (3) difficulty with the subsequent stages because the previous developmental tasks have not been resolved. The community health nurse can assume that the vulnerable family has developed a variant family structure for the purpose of surviving and carrying out essential functions.

If the community health nurse adopts a developmental framework to guide the nursing process with the vulnerable family, it is important to know that a three-stage FLC framework probably will be the most appropriate. The three stages are (1) the unattached young adult (includes late adolescence), (2) the family with children, and (3) the family in later life. The following discussion focuses on these three stages.

It generally is assumed for most young adults that the major developmental tasks for the unattached young adult are to develop an identity, make a commitment to work/career and marriage, and gradually to disengage from the family. By contrast, the adolescent (i.e., young adult) in the vulnerable family may not grow away from the family gradually but may be forced to leave the family and become independent. Another possibility may be that the adolescent/young adult will remain with the family as a source of income. This phenomenon of being forced to leave home prematurely may occur with children as young as 10 or 11 years of age. Another developmental problem for the young adult is that without viable work options, it is difficult to make a commitment to work. This is particularly important for the young adult male who may infrequently have observed adult males functioning in a stable work role. Because of limited job opportunities and limited opportunities to see an adult male functioning in a stable parental role, the young adult male may function as a transient participant in heterosexual relationships.

The young adult female tends to perceive her role as a mother and develops her identity with that role. When two young adults do get married or decide to live together for a time, the relationship generally is unstable. There have been few models representative of a stable married couple, except those on television, and these are difficult for the young adults to identify with. As the couple moves into another stage of FLC (family with children), the arrival of children coupled with unemployment results in additional problems for the family. The family may receive outside public assistance, with the result that the father becomes more peripheral to the family. Another pattern that may develop is that the parents remain primarily identified with their adolescent peer groups, and avoid the adult parenting roles. By way of contrast, if the adult has not had an opportunity to develop an identity through the satisfactory fulfillment of the child and/or adolescent roles and developmental tasks, the individual may view the parental role as a source of identity.

Within the vulnerable family, one of the children may emerge as a surrogate parent to help with the siblings. In addition, the school-age children may not receive adequate attention from the mother or father, resulting in the inadequate development of cognitive, affective, and communication skills that would enable them to benefit adequately from their learning experiences in the school system. As more children are born over a longer period, the childrearing stage tends to be protracted. As a result, the older children frequently are discharged from their peer groups. That is, they turn to their peer groups for needs fulfillment because their parents are too busy caring for younger siblings to give them the needed attention.

During the FLC stage of the vulnerable family in later life, the forward progress of the generational process may come to a standstill or may break down, especially if the household is three generational. The adult daughter's mother may make the grandchild one of her children, the adult daughter remains a daughter instead of a mother, and family roles become very confused. The family system becomes a system for survival and homeostasis and not for change and growth. The death of the grandmother can have a devastating effect on the family, both emotionally and developmentally. At this time the oldest daughter, who was unable to become a mother in terms of fulfilling the role, may be able to move into that role now because of the death of her mother. Thus the new mother role occupant begins to repeat the life cycle of the vulnerable family.

The community health nurse can combine theories about the family system's development, family roles, functions, and interactions with knowledge about vulnerable families. The emerging framework should generate a working plan that will guide the assessment of the family, assist the involvement of the family in the planning process, and provide direction for the intervention strategies and evaluation.

The community health nurse should realize that the family members may distrust professionals because of past experiences with public agencies. The nurse also should make clear to the family the kind and extent of assistance that can be expected from the nurse and the agency. It is very important that the nurse retain a flexible perspective on the family and avoid viewing the family within a middle-class family developmental model of structure, roles, and functions. The community health nurse can view the nursing process with the vulnerable family as a socializing experience for the family members in which they participate in problem solving and informed decision making, identify their strengths and resources, plan their care, and evaluate the outcomes of their health care efforts.

Clinical Application

Nancy approached her community health nursing experience knowing that her caseload would include families in the community. As she reviewed her assignment, she discovered that the five families with whom she would be working included a nuclear family of mother, father, and two school-aged children; a single mother with a toddler; and a stepfamily with mother, stepfather, stepgrandmothers, and two teenage siblings, one from each prior marriage.

Nancy first *assessed* the families' development. She found that all families were meeting the appropriate tasks for each developmental stage except the single mother. Nancy assessed the demographics of this family and found that Mrs. Rodgers' income was lowered as a result of her divorce; she was having difficulty fulfilling the physical maintenance tasks of rent, food, and day care for her child. This was affecting her ability to show affection toward the child. Mrs. Rodgers and her child were now among the families whose life events had placed them in poverty.

As Nancy *planned* her care for Mrs. Rodgers, she considered providing anticipatory guidance regarding Mrs. Rodgers' developmental tasks and her needs to be able to meet her tasks. Nancy also considered providing guidance to Mrs. Rodgers about her toddler's tasks and the toddler's need for affection from the mother to survive this life crisis successfully. Nancy sought out community resources available to help Mrs. Rodgers and discovered that she was eligible for rent subsidy, day-care subsidy, and food stamps through social services. Mrs. Rodgers also was eligible to receive a Medicaid card for preventive and illness care services for herself and her child. Nancy also discovered a single-parent self-help group to refer Mrs. Rodgers to for needed emotional support.

Nancy knew that her role in *implementing* the plan would include advocating for Mrs. Rodgers with the community resources and serving as educator, facilitator, and supporter in guiding her through this crisis. Nancy planned to include Mrs. Rodgers in establishing goals for resolving this developmental crisis and the transition to family stability.

During each visit, Nancy *evaluated* Mrs. Rodgers' progress toward meeting her individual and family developmental tasks, her compliance with the interventions, and progress toward mutually agreed-on goals.

Key Concepts

- Family development is one theoretical framework used to study families. This approach emphasizes how families change over time and focuses on interactions and relationships among family members.
- Demographic trends affecting the family's structure and development are age at time of first marriage; fertility patterns and birth rates; increase in the number of individuals engaging in singlehood, divorce, and remarriage; increase in the number of dependent children experiencing divorce in the family or living with a never-married parent; and an increase in the number of elderly persons.
- Implicit in the developmental approach to the study of family are the concepts of family roles and functions. Knowledge in the areas is essential to adequately assess the family and to effectively plan, intervene, and evaluate care with the family.
- A family developmental task is a responsibility for growth that arises at a certain stage in the family life cycle (FLC). Successful accomplishment of the task leads to satisfaction, approval, and success with future tasks.

- The family's culture affects the enactment of family roles, the timing of developmental tasks, and the meaning attached to the different stages of the FLC.
- The family developmental framework identifies points in a family's development at which changes occur in family members' status and roles.
- Increasingly, variations in family structure, such as single-parent families, remarried families, and vulnerable families, are being studied from the developmental perspective.
- Traditionally, families have been defined as a nuclear family: mother, father, and young children.
- There are a variety of family definitions, such as a group of two or more, a unique social group, and two or more persons joined together by emotional bonds.
- Role theory provides insight into how family members behave toward one another, society, and the community.
- Systems theory describes families as a unit of the whole composed of members whose interactional patterns are the focus of attention.

Continued.

Key Concepts—cont'd

Members have boundaries that are affected by the external environment.

◆ Structural functional frameworks view the family as a social system with members who have specific roles and functions.

◆ Interactional framework focuses on the family as a unit of interacting personalities and examines the communication processes by which family members relate to one another.

◆ Conceptual frameworks are essential for guiding the community health nurse in the process of assisting families in their health-promoting efforts.

◆ Family structure refers to the characteristics, gender, age, and number of the individual members who make up the family unit.

◆ Household is defined as a single dwelling occupied by an individual or a group of two or more individuals, related or unrelated.

◆ Family demography is the study of the structures of families and households and the events that alter the family, such as marriage, singlehood, divorce, remarriage, children of divorce, poverty, working women, and elderly persons.

◆ Family members hold a recognized position or status, such as father, mother, and child.

◆ Family health status affects family role relationships.

◆ Mills' model for stepfamily development can be used to help assess, guide, and evaluate the stepfamily's task accomplishment.

Critical Thinking Activities

1. Select six or more health professionals and other human service workers and ask them to define a family. The health professionals should include community health nurses and physicians, and the human service workers should represent social workers, teachers, and others. Analyze the responses for commonalities and differences.

2. Form small groups and discuss the implications of family demography and demographic trends for community health nursing.

3. Develop a typology of the different family structures and household arrangements representative of the community. This information may be available from various sources, such as the health department, schools, other social and welfare agencies, and census data.

4. Interview several individuals who represent different family structures and family living arrangements. Ask them to define a family and to identify their family roles and functions. Analyze the responses for commonalities and differences. Analyze the implications of your survey and your knowledge about family structures for community health nursing. (If there are several persons carrying out this activity, pool all responses and proceed with the analysis.)

5. Select several families representing first marriages and remarriages who have more than one child in the family. The children in the families should be old enough to talk about their relationships with their siblings. Ask the children about their relationship with their brother(s) and/or sister(s). The discussion should include the children's ideas about how their siblings help them, how they help their siblings, and their perceptions about sibling difficulties. Analyze the responses for commonalities and differences regarding age and gender of the respondents and sibling relationships (biological sibling, stepsibling, half-sibling).

6. As a group project, each student/community health nurse should select several families and interview the family, as a unit, about (a) their perceptions of their health-related functions and tasks, (b) their health promotion behaviors, and (c) their values and attitudes about health promotion. The families selected should represent different ethnic/racial and socioeconomic backgrounds.

7. Form five discussion groups and discuss the use of the developmental approach as a guide for the nursing process used by the community health nurses in working with the (a) nuclear family, (b) adoptive family, (c) single-parent family, (d) remarried family, and (e) vulnerable family. Each group should select one family type to discuss. As a group, analyze the similarities and variations in the application of the developmental framework to the nursing process with each family.

8. As a group, discuss your attitudes about working with the different family/household types discussed in the chapter.

Bibliography

Ahrons CR, Rodgers RH: *Divorced families: a multidisciplinary developmental view*, New York, 1987, Norton.

Aldous J: *Family careers: developmental change in families*, New York, 1978, Wiley.

Atwater L: Long-term cohabitation without a legal ceremony is equally valid and desirable. In Feldman H, Feldman M, editors: *Current controversies in marriage and family*, Beverly Hills, Calif, 1985, Sage.

Barnhill LR, Longo D: Fixation and regression in the family life, *Fam Proc* 17:469-478, 1978.

Bentler I, et al: The family realm: theoretical contributions for understanding its uniqueness, *J Marr Fam* 51:805-816, 1989.

Blum HL: *Expanding health care horizons: from a general systems concept of health to a national health policy*, Oakland, Calif, 1976, Third Party Associates.

Bomar P: *Nurses and family health promotion: concepts, assessment and interventions*, Philadelphia, 1992, Saunders.

Bozett FW: Gay men as fathers. In Hanson SM, Bozett FW, editors: *Dimensions of fatherhood*, Beverly Hills, Calif, 1985, Sage.

Brodzinsky DM, Huffman L: Transition to adoptive parenthood, *Marr Fam Rev* 12(3-4):267-286, 1988.

Butler EW, Meints J: Notes on nontemporary singles. In Gutknecht RB, Butler EW, Criswell L, Meints J, editors: *Family, self, and society: emerging issues, alternatives, and interventions*, Lanham, Md, 1983, University Press of America.

Carter E, McGoldrick M: The family life cycle and family therapy: an overview. In Carter E, McGoldrick M, editors: *The changing family life cycle: a framework for family therapists*, New York, 1988, Gardner Press.

Crane PT: Processes surrounding the decision to remain permanently voluntarily childless. In Gutknecht DB, Butler EW, Criswell L, Meints J, editors: *Family, self, and society: emerging issues, alternatives, and interventions*, Lanham, Md, 1983, University Press of America.

Demick J, Wapner S: Open and closed adoption: a developmental conceptualization, *Fam Proc* 27:229-249, 1988.

Di Guilio JF: Assuming the adoptive parent role, *Soc Casework* 68(9):561-566, 1987.

Duvall EM: Family development's first forty years, *Fam Rel* 37:127-134, 1988.

Duvall E, Miller B: *Marriage and family development*, ed 6, New York, 1985, Harper & Row.

Eastman KS: Foster parenthood: a nonnormative parenting arrangement, *Marr Fam Rev* 5:95-120, 1982.

Espenshade TJ: Marital careers of American women: a cohort life table analysis. In Bongaarts J, Burch TK, Wachter KW, editors: *Family demography: methods and their application*, New York, 1987, Oxford University Press.

Family Service of America: *The state of families*, Milwaukee, 1987, Family Service of America.

Friedman MM: *Family nursing: theory and assessment*, East Norwalk, Conn, 1992, Appleton-Lange.

Furstenberg FF, Spannier GB: *Recycling the family: remarriage after divorce*, Beverly Hills, Calif, 1984, Sage.

Gerstel N, Gross HE: Commuter marriages: a review, *Marr Fam Rev* 5:71-93, 1982.

Gutknecht DB, Butler EW, Criswell L, Meints J: Alternative life styles: implications for family, self, and society. In Gutknecht DB, Butler EW, Criswell L, Meints J, editors: *Family, self, and society: emerging issues, alternatives, and interventions*, Lanham, Md, 1983, University Press of America.

Hanson SMH: Single custodial fathers. In Hanson SMH, Bozett FW, editors: *Dimensions of fatherhood*, Beverly Hills, Calif, 1985, Sage.

Hardy M, Conway M: *Role theory perspective for health professionals*, East Norwalk, Conn, 1986, Appleton-Century-Crofts.

Havighurst R: *Developmental task and education*, ed 3, New York, 1974, David McKay.

Hill R, Mattessich P: Family development theory and life span development. In Baltes P, Brim O, editors: *Life span development and behavior*, vol 2, New York, 1979, Academic Press.

Janosik E, Green E: *Family life: process and practice*, Boston, 1992, Jones & Bartlett.

Johnson R: Family development. In Stanhope M, Lancaster J, editors: *Community health nursing: process and practice for promoting health*, ed 3, St Louis, 1992, Mosby.

Jorgensen SR: The American family of the future: what choices will we have? In Gutnecht DB, Butler EW, Criswell L, Meints J, editors: *Family, self, and society: emerging issues, alternatives, and interventions*, Lanham, Md, 1983, University Press of America.

Keshet JK: The remarried couple: stresses and successes. In Beer WR, editor: *Relative strangers: studies of stepfamily processes*, Totowa, NJ, 1988, Rowman & Littlefield.

Keyfitz N: Form and substance in family demography. In Bongaarts J, Burch TK, Wachter KW, editors: *Family demography: methods and their application*, New York, 1987, Oxford University Press.

Leslie G, Korman S: *The family in social context*, New York, 1989, Oxford University Press.

Macklin ED: Nontraditional family forms. In Sussman MB, Steinmetz SK, editors: *Handbook of marriage and the family*, New York, 1988, Plenum.

Marciano TD: Homosexual marriages and parenthood should not be allowed. In Feldman H, Feldman M, editors: *Current controversies in marriage and family*, Beverly Hills, Calif, 1985, Sage.

Mills D: A model for stepfamily development, *Fam Rel* 33:365-372, 1984.

National Center for Health Statistics: *Advance report of final marriage statistics, 1987*, Washington, DC, 1987, US Department of Health and Human Services.

National Center for Health Statistics: *Advance report of final natality statistics, 1987*, Washington, DC, 1989a, US Department of Health and Human Services.

National Center for Health Statistics: *Children of divorce*, DHHS Pub No PHS 89-1924, Hyattsville, Md, 1989b, US Department of Health and Human Services.

National Center for Health Statistics: *Advance report of final divorce statistics, 1987*, Washington, DC, 1990a, US Department of Health and Human Services.

National Center for Health Statistics: *Births, marriages, divorces, and deaths for 1989*, Washington, DC, 1990b, US Department of Health and Human Services.

National Center for Health Statistics: *Health US: 1993*, Hyattsville, Md, 1994, Public Health Service.

Nye FJ: *Role structure and analysis of the family*, Beverly Hills, Calif, 1976, Sage.

Olson DH, Lavee Y: Family systems and family stress: a family life cycle perspective. In Kreppner K, Lerner RM, editors: *Family systems and life span development*, Hillsdale, NJ, 1989, Lawrence Erlbaum Associates.

Parrot A, Ellis MJ: Homosexuals should be allowed to marry and have children. In Feldman H, Feldman M: *Current controversies in marriage and family*, Beverly Hills, Calif, 1985, Sage.

Pitkin JR, Masnick GS: The relationship between heads and nonheads in the household population: an extension of the headship rate method. In Bongaarts J, Burch TK, Wachter KW, editors: *Family demography: methods and their application*, New York, 1987, Oxford University Press.

Renvoize J: *Going solo: single mothers by choice*, Boston, 1985, Routledge & Kegan.

Rexroat C, Shehan C: The family life cycle and spouses time in housework, *J Marr Fam* 49:737-750, 1987.

Scanzoni J, Polonko K, Teachman J, Thompson L: *The sexual bond: rethinking families and close relationships*, Newbury Park, Calif, 1989, Sage.

Schuaneveldt JD: The interactional framework in the study of the family. In Nye FI, Berardo FM, editors: *Emerging conceptual frameworks in family analysis*, New York, 1967, Macmillan.

Settles BH: A perspective on tomorrow's families. In Sussman MB, Steinmetz SK, editors: *Handbook of marriage and the family*, New York, 1987, Plenum.

Shapiro ER: Individual change and family development: individualization as a family process. In Falicov CJ, editor: *Family transitions: continuity and change over the life cycle*, New York, 1988, Guilford.

Shostak AB: Singlehood. In Sussman MB, Steinmetz SK, editors: *Handbook of marriage and the family*, New York, 1987, Plenum.

Smith AD, Reid WJ: *Role-sharing marriage*, New York, 1986, Columbia University Press.

Social Security Bulletin: *Federal poverty guidelines 1989*, vol 52, no 3, Washington, DC, 1989, Social Security Administration.

Stevenson J: *Issues and crises during middlescence*, New York, 1977, Appleton-Century-Crofts.

Sussman MB: From the catbird seat: observations on marriage and the family. In Sussman MB, Steinmetz SK, editors: *Handbook of marriage and the family*, New York, 1987, Plenum.

Teachman JD, Polonko KA, Scanzoni J: Demography of the family. In Sussman MB, Steinmetz SK, editors: *Handbook of marriage and the family*, New York, 1987, Plenum.

US Bureau of the Census: *Household and family characteristics: March 1985*, Current Population Report Series P-20, No 411, Washington DC, 1986, US Department of Commerce.

US Bureau of the Census: *Statistical abstract of the United States 1994*, ed 114, Washington, DC, US Department of Commerce.

Valentine D: The experience of pregnancy: a developmental process, *Fam Rel* 31:243-248, 1982.

Visher E, Visher J: *Stepfamilies: a guide to working with stepparents and stepchildren*, New York, 1979, Brunner/Mazel.

Watkins SC, Menken JA, Bongaarts J: Demographic foundations for family change, *Am Soc Rev* 52:346-358, 1987.

Willekens F: The marital status life table. In Bongaarts J, Burch TK, Watcher KW, editors: *Family demography: methods and their application*, New York, 1987, Oxford University Press.

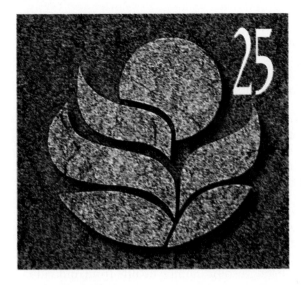

25

Family Health Risks

Carol Loveland-Cherry

Objectives ▼

After reading this chapter, the student should be able to do the following:

◆ Analyze the various approaches to defining and conceptualizing family health.
◆ Analyze the major risks to family health.
◆ Analyze the interrelationship among individual health, family health, and community health.
◆ Explain the relevance of knowledge about family structures, roles, and functions for family-focused community health nursing process.
◆ Explain the application of the nursing process (assessing, planning, implementing, evaluation) for reducing family health risks and promoting family health.

Outline ▼

Key Terms ▼

adaptive model
biologic risk
clinical model
contracting
economic risk
empowerment
eudaimonistic model
family crisis
family health
health risk appraisal
health risk reduction
health risks
home visits
in-home phase
initiation phase
life-event risk
life-style risk
postvisit phase
previsit phase
role-performance model
social risk
termination phase

The importance of the family in promoting the health of individuals and communities is well established (Bomar, 1989; Feetham et al., 1990; Gilliss et al., 1989; Nightingale et al., 1978; Turk and Kerns, 1985). Acknowledgment of the family as a client unit has been a basic assumption underlying the practice of community health nursing. But how does family health fit into the picture of larger health schema, such as *Healthy People 2000?* Does family have a contribution to make? And, from the opposite perspective, are our broader health goals sensitive to the needs of the family?

In establishing health objectives for the nation, an emphasis has been placed on both health promotion and risk reduction. The notion is that reducing the risks to segments of the population is a direct way of improving the health of the general population. Specific risks have been identified and related to specific objectives. Although none of the objectives directly address families, it is clear that the family is both an important environment affecting the health of individuals and a unit whose health is basic to that of the community and larger population. It is within the family that health behavior, including health values, health habits, and health risk perceptions are developed, organized, and performed (Baranowski and Nader, 1985; Doherty and McCubbin, 1985; Litman, 1974). Individuals' health behaviors are affected by and acted out within the context of not only the family environment but also that of the larger community and society. In turn, the larger community and society are made up of and depend upon the functioning of individuals for continued well-being. For example, traditional indices of morbidity and mortality are computed on the basis of aggregated data about individuals (see Chapter 11 on epidemiology).

In order to intervene effectively and appropriately with families to reduce their health risk and thereby promote their health, it is necessary to understand family structure and functioning, family theory, nursing theory, and models of health risk (see Chapter 10, Organizing Frameworks; Chapter 14, Community Health Promotion; and Chapter 24, Family Development). However, it is necessary to go beyond the individual and the family and understand the complex environment in which the family exists. Increasing evidence of the impact of social, biological, economic, and life events on health necessitates a broader approach to addressing health risks for families. Pender (1987) identifies six categories of risk factors: genetics, age, biologic characteristics, personal health habits, life-style, and environment.

In this chapter, health risks in these six categories for families are identified and analyzed, and approaches to reducing these risks are discussed. We will also explore options for structuring community health nursing interventions with families to decrease health risks and to promote their health and well-being.

EARLY APPROACHES TO FAMILY HEALTH RISKS
Health of Families

Early consideration of the family in health and illness focused on three major areas: (1) the impact of illness on families, (2) the role of the family in the etiology of disease, and (3) the role of the family in utilization of services. In his classic review of the family as an important unit, Litman (1974) pointed out the important role that the family plays in health and illness as a primary unit of health care and emphasized that the interrelationship among health, health behavior, and family "is a highly dynamic one in which each may have a dramatic effect on the other" (Litman, 1974, p. 495). Mauksch (1974) proposed the idea of distinguishing family health from individual health. Pratt's (1976) examination of the role of the family in health and illness expanded the literature to include the role of family health in promoting behavior. Pratt proposed the "energized family" as being an ideal family type most effective in meeting health needs. The energized family is characterized by promotion of freedom and change, varied and active contact with other groups and organizations, flexible role relationships, egalitarian power structure, and a high degree of autonomy in family members. Doherty and McCubbin (1985) proposed a family health and illness cycle with six phases: (1) family health promotion and risk reduction, (2) family vulnerability and illness onset, (3) family illness appraisal, (4) family acute response, (5) family and health care system interaction, and (6) family adaptation to illness.

Health of the Nation

Paralleling the focus in family studies on health, increased attention was being given to ways to improve the health of the nation. As the result of major public health and scientific advances, the leading causes of morbidity and mortality shifted from infectious diseases to chronic diseases, accidents and, violence, all of which have strong life-style and environmental components. A population-based study in Alemeda County, California, (Belloc and Breslow, 1972) demonstrated relationships between seven life-style habits and morbidity and mortality. These habits included (1) sleeping 7 to 8 eight hours daily, (2) eating breakfast almost every day, (3) never or rarely eating between meals, (4) being at or near recommended height-adjusted weight, (5) never smoking cigarettes, (6) moderate or no use of alcohol, and (7) regular physical activity. A growing body of literature supported the notion that life-style and the environment interact with hereditary tendencies for disease. In response to these findings and the limited effect of medical interventions on the growing incidence and prevalence of injuries and chronic disease, the government launched a major effort to address the health status of the population. Part of this effort was a report by the Division of Health Promotion and Disease Prevention of the Institute of Medicine that examined the critical components of the physical, socioeconomic, and family environments related to decreasing risk and promoting health (Nightengale et al., 1978). Subsequently, the Surgeon General's Report on Health Promotion and Disease Prevention (Califano, 1979) delineated the risks to good health. Health Objectives for the nation were established and then evaluated and restated for the year 2000 (Healthy People 2000, 1991).

Within this context, the notion of "risk," a factor predisposing or increasing the likelihood of ill health, took on increased importance. Specific attention was paid to those "environmental and behavioral influences capable of provoking ill health with or without previous predisposition" (Califano, 1979, p. 13). The reduction of health risks is a major approach to improving the health of the nation. Although the family is considered an important environment related to achieving important health objectives, limited attention and research has been given to family health risk.

CONCEPTS IN FAMILY HEALTH RISK

Individuals participate in behaviors for two different basic motivations. One of these underlying forces is health promotion—"behaviors directed toward increasing the level of well-being and actualizing the health potential of individuals, families, communities and society" (Pender, 1987, p. 4). In contrast, health protecting behaviors are those "directed toward decreasing the probability of specific illness or dysfunction in individuals, families, and communities, including active protection against unnecessary stressors" (Pender, 1987, p. 4). It can be argued that the same behavior may be undertaken from either of the two perspectives. Health risk is conceptually congruent with the notion of health protecting behaviors.

Understanding family health risk requires an examination of several related concepts: family health, family health risk, risk appraisal, risk reduction, life events, life-style, and family crisis. Although health is a vague term that can be defined from a number of perspectives, it usually is defined by the individual within the context of his or her own culture and value system. Similarly, illness is the experience of a disease process.

Family Health

Family theorists refer to healthy families, but generally do not define **family health.** Based on the various family theoretical perspectives (see Chapter 10, Organizing Frameworks; Chapter 14, Illness Prevention; Chapter 24, Family Development; and Chapter 26, Family Assessment), definitions of healthy families can be derived within the guidelines of any one of the frameworks. For example, within the perspective of the developmental framework, family health can be defined as possessing the abilities and resources to accomplish family developmental tasks. Thus, the accomplishment of stage-specific tasks is one indicator of family health.

From the perspective of Neuman's model (1989), family health would be defined in terms of system stability as characterized by five interacting sets of factors: physiological, psychological, sociocultural, developmental, and spiritual. These sets of factors are evaluated in light of three critical dimensions related to the family's ability to interact with stressors from its environment in effective ways (see Chapter 10, Organizing Frameworks). Family system stability is thus indicated by measuring the integrity of flexible lines of defense for families, including role enactment, rule implementation, decision-making mechanisms, processes for resource allocation, and bonding patterns; the normal line of defense for families, including communication patterns, problem-solving mechanisms, mechanisms for meeting family needs for intimacy and affection, and ways of dealing with loss and change; and the lines of resistance (core characteristics, such as interrelatedness, values and beliefs, and interdependence).

Another dimension of family health can be identified by using Smith's (1983) four models of health: **clinical model, role-performance model, adaptive model,** and **eudaimonistic model** (see Table 25-1).

The following clinical example applies these models to one family's situation.

The Harris family consists of Mr. and Mrs. Harris, 12-year-old Kevin, and 6-year-old Leisha. Kevin was recently diagnosed with insulin dependent diabetes mellitus (IDDM) and the family was referred by the endocrinology clinic for community health nursing service to work with the family in adjusting to the diagnosis.

The focus in a clinical model approach might be to identify realistic perceptions of health risks for Kevin and to teach the parents how to recognize and deal with symptoms of complications. Assessment would include completing a family health/illness history, determining Mr. and Mrs. Harris' perceptions and knowledge of diabetes mellitus, identifying the family's health care resources, and recognizing their concerns about caring for a child with a chronic disease.

Assessment in the role-performance model would include exploring with the family their feelings about their abilities and resources to accomplish developmental tasks. This family is in the developmental stage of families with school-aged children, based on the age of the oldest child. Developmental tasks for families in this stage include:
1. Providing suitable housing and health care for the family.
2. Meeting family costs and making adjustments when the wife/mother works.
3. Allocating and monitoring responsibilities for maintaining the home.
4. Continuing socialization through wider community participation.

Table 25-1   Smith's Four Models of Health

Model	View of health	Assessment	Nursing goals
Clinical	*Individual* The absence of disease *Family* The absence of disease or dysfunction	Includes family health/illness history; family's definition of health and illness; family's value of health; family's knowledge of health promotion and illness prevention/treatment; family practices related to nutrition, sleep/rest, exercise, and recreation; use of alcohol, tobacco, drugs; family processes for determining illness and whether and how professional care will be sought	To promote family's physical, mental, and social health; to provide comfort in the family; to prevent deterioration of family system
Role-Performance	*Individual* Effective performance of roles *Family* Effective meeting of family functions and developmental tasks	Includes family's current developmental stage/history; family's role structure, socialization patterns, resources for meeting functions and developmental tasks; family's perceptions of family functioning	To promote effective performance of family functions; to promote achievement of developmental tasks; to assist in identifying and mobilizing support systems and resources
Adaptive	*Individual* Condition of the whole person engaged in effective interaction with physical/social environment *Family* Condition of the whole family engaged in effective interaction with physical/social environment; family/environment fit	Includes the identification of family coping patterns, social networks, and support systems; family's perceptions of their environment; family's flexibility in altering behaviors, roles, rules, and perceptions when needed	To promote the family's adaptation and health-directed patterning with the environment
Eudaimonistic	*Individual* Complete development of individual's potential for general well-being and self-realization *Family* Development of family's well-being and maximum potential	Includes family's values and goals; family interaction patterns; family patterns of recreation and relaxation; family cohesion; family promotion of autonomy	To clarify family's values; to assist in identifying and prioritizing family's goals; to assist family in implementing plans to meet goals

Modified from Smith JA: *The idea of health: implications for the nursing professional,* New York, 1983, Teachers College Press, Columbia University.

5. Encouraging husband-wife, parent-child, and child-child communication.
6. Rearing children with appropriate parenting skills in two-parent, one-parent, or reconstituted family households.
7. Demonstrating interest in children's schooling and in their acquisition of basic skills and knowledge.
8. Recognizing achievement and growth of individual family members and building solid values and morals in the family (Duvall and Miller, 1985, p. 217).

Assessment in the adaptive model would focus on identifying with the family the kinds of changes that have occurred since Kevin's diagnosis and the differ-

ent or new demands that have resulted. The nurse would work with the family members to help them adapt to having a child with a chronic illness and to repattern their lives to deal with the related increased and different demands on the family. By pointing out the knowledge and skills that the family already has and the ways to adapt them to the changes in the family system, the nurse builds on family competencies. Another potential intervention would be to identify appropriate services in the community, such as support groups, and summer camps for children with diabetes mellitus.

In the eudaimonistic model, the nurse could work with the family in reassessing family goals and ways to meet them. The diagnosis of a family member with a chronic condition indicates assessment of family values and goals, such as socialization and education of children, family recreation, and patterns of interaction. At some point it might be appropriate to inform the family about how they could offer support to other families in similar circumstances.

Based on the assessment, the nurse can assist the family in identifying areas of strength and areas where external resources may be necessary.

Health Risk

A number of factors contribute to the experience of healthy/unhealthy outcomes. Clearly, not everyone exposed to the same event will have the same outcome. The factors that determine/influence whether or not disease or other unhealthy results occur are called **health risks.** This notion of controlling health risks is central to disease prevention and health promotion (Califano, 1979). Health risks can be classified into general categories. Califano (1979) identifies four major categories: inherited biological risk, environmental risk, behavioral risk, and age-related risk. Each of these categories of risk will be discussed in terms of family health risk in the following section. Although risk factors can singly influence outcomes, the cumulated risks are synergistic; their combined effect is more than the sum of the individual effects. For example, a family history of cardiovascular disease is a single risk factor that is potentiated by smoking, a behavioral risk. This combination of risks is greater for males than females (up to a certain age). Thus, the combined effect of a family history, smoking, and being male is greater than merely adding the probabilities of each of the three individual risk factors.

Health Risk Appraisal

Health risk appraisal refers to the process of assessing the presence of specific factors within each of the categories that have been identified as being associated with an increased likelihood of an illness, such as cancer, or an unhealthy event, such as an automobile accident. A number of techniques have been developed to accomplish health risk appraisal, including computer software programs and paper and pencil instruments. The general approach is to determine whether or not a risk factor is present and to what degree. Based on scientific evidence, each factor is weighted and a total summated score is derived.

Health Risk Reduction

Health risk reduction is based on the assumption that decreasing the number of risks or the magnitude of risk will result in a lower probability of the undesired event, for example, substance abuse in adolescents.

Reduction of health risks can be accomplished through a variety of approaches, usually specific to the theoretical and research knowledge relevant to the particular risk.

Life Events

Life events can increase the risk for illness and disability. These events can be categorized as either normative or nonnormative. Normative events are those that generally are expected to occur at a particular stage of development or of the lifespan. Normative events can be identified from the Family Developmental Framework. Examples of normative events are a child leaving home to go to college, retirement from work, and starting a first job. Nonnormative events, in contrast, are those that are *not* anticipated to occur with any predictability (e.g., loss of a job). Further, life events and the accumulation of such events can, under certain conditions, result in a family crisis.

Family Crisis

A crisis exists when the family is not able to cope with the event and becomes disorganized/dysfunctional. When the demands of the situation exceed the resources of the family, a **family crisis** is said to exist. When families experience a crisis or crisis-producing event, they attempt to marshal their resources to deal with the demands created by the situation. Burr and Klein and associates (1994) differentiate between family resources and family coping strategies. The former are the resources that a family has available to them. The latter are the "active processes and behaviors families actually try to do to help them manage, adapt, or deal with the stressful situation" (Burr et al., 1994, p. 129). Thus, if a family were to experience an unexpected illness in the main wage earner, family resources might include financial assistance from relatives or emotional support. Family coping strategies, in contrast, would include whether the family asked a relative to loan them emergency funds or talked with relatives about the worries they were experiencing. Based on the existing literature, Burr and Klein and colleagues developed a three-level classification of coping strategies with seven major categories, 20 subcategories, and 41 sub-subcategories. While the last level is too extensive to present here, the seven major categories and 20 subcategories are listed in Table 25-2.

MAJOR FAMILY HEALTH RISKS

Risks to families' health arise in several major areas: biologic risk, social risk, economic risk, life-style risk, and life events leading to crisis. In most instances, no one of these five areas is sufficient to be a single threat to family health; rather a combination of risks from

Table 25-2 Burr and Klein's Conceptual Framework of Coping Strategies

Highly abstract strategies	Moderately abstract strategies
1. Cognitive	1. Be accepting of the situation and others.
	2. Gain useful knowledge.
	3. Change how the situation is viewed or defined (reframe the situation).
2. Emotional	4. Express feelings and affection.
	5. Avoid or resolve negative feelings and disabling expressions of emotion.
	6. Be sensitive to others' emotional needs.
3. Relationships	7. Increase cohesion (togetherness).
	8. Increase adaptability.
	9. Develop increased trust.
	10. Increase cooperation.
	11. Increase tolerance of each other.
4. Communication	12. Be open and honest.
	13. Listen to each other.
	14. Be sensitive to nonverbal communication.
5. Community	15. Seek help and support from others.
	16. Fulfill expectations in organizations.
6. Spiritual	17. Be more involved in religious activities.
	18. Increase faith or seek help from God.
7. Individual Development	19. Develop autonomy, independence, and self-sufficiency.
	20. Keep active in hobbies.

From Burr WR, Klein SR, Burr RG, et al: *Reexamining family stress: new theory and research*, Thousand Oaks, Calif, 1994, Sage Publications.

two or more categories is more usual. For example, there may be a familial history of cardiovascular disease, but often the health risk is compounded by an unhealthy life-style. An understanding of each of these categories provides the basis for a comprehensive perspective on family health risk assessment and intervention.

Beginning with the Surgeon General's report (Califano, 1979), an emphasis in health promotion and disease prevention has focused on these life-style patterns. *Healthy People 2000* targets areas in health promotion, health protection, preventive services, and surveillance and data systems and sets age-related objectives (Healthy People 2000, 1991). Included in the area of health promotion are physical activity and fitness, nutrition, tobacco use, use of alcohol and other drugs, family planning, mental health and mental disorders, violent and abuse behavior. Health protection activities include issues related to unintentional injuries, occupational safety and health, environmental health, food and drug safety, and oral health. Preventive services relate to reducing risk related to illness and include maternal and infant health, heart disease and stroke, cancer, diabetes and chronic disabling conditions, HIV infection, sexually transmitted diseases, immunization and infectious diseases, and clinical preventive services. The interrelationships among the various groups of risk are clear when the objectives for the nation are considered.

Biologic Risk

The family plays an important role both in the development and in the management of a disease or condition. A number of illnesses have a familial component that can be accounted for either from a genetic basis or established life-style patterns. These formulated factors contribute to the **biologic risk** for certain conditions. Patterns of cardiovascular disease, for example, often can be traced through many generations of families. Such families are said to be at risk for cardiovascular disease. How or whether cardiovascular disease is manifested in a family is often influenced by the life-style of the family. Consistent research evidence supports the positive mediating effects of diet, exercise, and stress management on preventing or delaying cardiovascular disease. A propensity for hypertension can be managed by following a low-sodium diet, maintaining a normal weight, regular exercise, and effective stress management techniques, such as meditation. Diabetes mellitus is another disease with a strong genetic pattern and the family plays a major role in the management of the condition. Family patterns of obesity is a condition that increases the risk for individuals for a number of conditions, among them, coronary heart disease, hypertension, diabetes, some types of cancer, and gallbladder disease (Healthy People 2000, 1991).

Another form of biologic risk experienced by families is susceptibility for certain illnesses. Generally, if a family maintains a level of general health, individual members are less at risk for contracting certain infectious diseases. This protection can be extended by maintaining health practices, such as current immunizations, adequate nutrition, and adequate rest (see Chapter 39, Communicable Disease Risk and Prevention).

Social Risk

The importance of **social risks** to families' health is gaining increased recognition (see Chapter 7, Cultural Diversity; and Chapter 8, Environmental Health). Living in high-crime neighborhoods, living in communities without adequate recreational or health resources, living in communities that have major chemical noise, or other contaminants, or other high-stress environments increases a family's health risk. One social stress that has been identified is discrimination, whether racial, cultural, or other. The psychological burden resulting from discrimination is a stressor in and of itself and also compounds the effects of other stressors. The implication of these examples of risky social situations is that they contribute to the stressors experienced by the families. If adequate resources and coping processes are not available, breakdowns in health can occur.

Economic Risk

It is well established that the poor are at greater risk for health problems (see Chapter 33, Poverty and Homelessness). **Economic risk** is determined by the relationship between family financial resources and demands on those resources. Having adequate financial resources means that a family is able to purchase necessary commodities related to health. These includes adequate housing, clothing, food, education, and health/illness care. The amount of money that a family has available needs to be considered relative to expenditures, as well as social factors. A family may have an income well above the poverty level but because of a devastating illness in a family member, may not be able to meet financial demands. Likewise, families from ethnic populations frequently experience discrimination in finding housing, and even if they do they may not be welcome and may be harassed, resulting in increased stress. Unfortunately, not all families have access to health care insurance. Approximately 15% of the population in this country lived in poverty in 1993 (Pyen, 1995) and nearly 42% of American children grow up in low-income families ($27,380 for a family of four) and about 23% in poverty ($14,800 or less for a family of four). For families at the poverty level, programs like Medicaid are available to pay for health and illness care; families in the upper-income brackets can either afford to pay for health care out-of-pocket, purchase health insurance, or are in employment situations that have health care

benefits. An increasing number of families have major wage earners in jobs that do not have health benefits, do not have a sufficient income to purchase health care, and earn too much to qualify for any public assistance programs. Consequently, many families have financial resources that allow them to maintain a subsistence level, but that limit the quality of their purchasing power. Illness care may be available but not preventive care; food high in fat and calories may be affordable, while fresh fruit and vegetables are not. A Department of Agriculture study found that for "every $1.00 spent on a pregnant woman in its Women, Infants and Children (WIC) program, $1.77 to $3.13 is saved in Medicaid costs during her child's first 60 days of life" (Greer, March 5, 1995, p. 6).

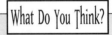

What Do You Think?

Government priority to funding health risk reduction and health promotion programs, including assistance programs, would have greater benefit to the population's health than funding for illness activities.

Life-Style Risk

Personal health habits continue to contribute to the major causes of morbidity and mortality in this country (see Chapter 14, Illness Prevention). The pattern of personal health habits and risk behaviors defines individual and family **life-style risk.** The family is the basic unit within which health behavior, including health values, health habits, and health risk perceptions is developed, organized, and performed. Families maintain major responsibility for determining what food is purchased and prepared, setting sleep patterns, planning family activities, setting and monitoring norms about health and health risk behaviors, determining when a family member is ill, when health care should be obtained, and carrying out treatment regimens. Diet has been identified as a element in 5 of the 10 leading causes of death in the United States (Healthy People 2000, 1991). General guidelines from the U.S. Departments of Health and Human Services and Agriculture include eating a variety of foods; maintaining healthy weight; choosing a diet low in fat, saturated fat, and cholesterol; including plenty of vegetables, fruits, and grain products; moderate use of sugars, moderate use of salt and sodium; and if alcohol is consumed, only in moderation.

Multiple health benefits of regular physical activity have been identified; regular physical exercise is effective in health promotion, disease prevention, and health maintenance. Among the benefits of regular physical activity are increased muscle strength, endurance, and flexibility; management of weight; prevention of colon cancer, stroke, and back injury; prevention and management of coronary heart disease, hypertension, diabetes, osteoporosis, and depression (Healthy People 2000, 1991). Families structure time and activities and can be helped to select between those that are sedentary and those that provide moderate, regular physical activity.

Substance use is a major contributor to morbidity and mortality in the United States. Tobacco use has been identified as the single most preventable cause of death in this country; it has been associated with several types of cancer, coronary heart disease, low birth weight, prematurity, sudden infant death syndrome, and chronic obstructive pulmonary disease. Further, passive smoking has been linked to disease in nonsmokers and children. Drug use, including alcohol, is a major social and health problem. Alcohol use is a factor in approximately 50% of homicides, suicides, and motor vehicle deaths (Healthy People 2000, 1991). Drug use is associated with transmission of the HIV virus, fetal alcohol syndrome, liver disease, unwanted pregnancy, delinquency, school failure, violence, and crime. The literature consistently identifies the impact of family factors, such as family closeness, families doing activities together, and behavior modeled in the family in decreasing the risk of children for substance use (Dielman et al., 1990; Glynn, 1984; Volk et al., 1989).

Did You Know?

Adolescents from families that have close, supportive interactions, clearly set and enforced rules, and parents who are involved with their children have decreased risk for alcohol use/misuse. These family patterns can be enhanced through family-focused intervention sessions in the home.

Although violence and abusive behavior are not limited to families, the amount of intrafamilial violence is thought to be underestimated. The obvious difficulties in collecting sensitive data from families make it difficult to obtain accurate statistics on family violence, but estimates of 28% of cohabiting couples report use of physical violence, 3.6% of parents report child abuse, and an incidence of elder abuse of 2.5 to 7 per 1000. Evidence supports the intergenerational nature of violence and abuse; abusers were often abused as children.

Life-Event Risk

Transitions, movement from one stage or condition to another, are times of potential risk for families. Tran-

sitions present new situations and demands for families. These experiences often require that families change behaviors, schedules, and patterns of communication; make new decisions; reallocate family roles; learn new skills; and identify and learn to use new resources. The demands that transitions place on families have implications for the health of the family unit and individual family members and can be considered as **life-event risk.** How well prepared families are to deal with transitions is affected by the nature of the event. If the event is a normative, or anticipated, event, then it is possible for families to identify needed resources, make plans, learn new skills, or otherwise prepare for the event and its consequences. This kind of anticipatory preparation can increase the family's coping processes and lessen stress and negative outcomes. If, on the other hand, the event is nonnormative or unexpected, families have little or no time to prepare and the outcome can be increased stress, crisis, or even dysfunction.

A number of normative events have been identified for families. The developmental family framework (see Chapter 24, Family Development) organizes these events within a staged model and identifies important transition points. The developmental model provides a useful framework for use in identifying normative events and preparing families to cope successfully with related demands. The developmental tasks associated with each stage define the types of skills families need to acquire. The kinds of normative events families experience usually are related to the addition or loss of a family member: the birth or adoption of a child, the death of a grandparent, a child moving out of the home to go to school or take a job, the mar-riage of a child. There are health-related responsibilities associated with each of these tasks. For example, the birth or adoption of a child requires that families learn about human growth and development, parenting, immunizations, management of childhood illnesses, normal childhood nutrition, and safety issues.

Nonnormative events present different kinds of issues for families. The nature of unexpected events can be either positive or negative. A job promotion or inheriting a substantial sum of money may be unexpected, but are usually positive events. More often nonnormative events are unpleasant, such as a major illness, divorce, the death of a child, or loss of the main family income.

Regardless of whether a life event is normative or nonnormative, it is often a source of stress for families. Several theoretical frameworks have been developed to examine the processes of family stress and coping. Perhaps, the most widely used and developed is the ABC-X model and its evolution over time. The model was originally formulated by Hill (1949) and was based on work with families separated by war. Within the model, crisis (X) was proposed to be a product of the nature of the event (A), the family's definition of the event (B), and the resources available to the family (C). McCubbin extended the model to the Double ABC-X Model to encompass the period after the initial crisis and introduced the idea of pile-up of stressors. Adaptation or maladaptation is proposed to be predicted by the pile-up of stressors (Aa), the family's perception of the crisis (Bb), and new resources and coping strategies (Cc).

Burr and associates (1994) recently challenged this linear view of families and stress and coping. They advocate a more systems-oriented conceptualization of family stress. They point out that families develop a series of processes to manage or transform inputs to the system (e.g., energy, time) to outputs (e.g., cohesion, growth, love) known as "rules of transformation." Over time, families develop these patterns in sufficient quantity and variety to handle most changes and challenges; this is referred to as "requisite variety of rules of transformation." It is when families do not have an adequate variety of rules to allow them to respond to an event that the event then becomes stressful. Rather than proceeding to deal with the situation, they fall into a pattern of trying to figure out what it is they need to do and the usual tasks of the family are not adequately addressed. Rules that were implicit in the family are now reconsidered and explicated.

Further, the reformulation of family stress theory proposes three levels of stress: Level I is change "in the fairly specific patterns of behavior and transformation processes" (e.g., change in who does which household chores); Level II is change "in processes that are at a higher level of abstraction" (e.g., change in what are defined as family chores); and Level III are changes in highly abstract processes (e.g., family values) (Burr et al., 1994, pp. 44-45). There are analogous coping strategies to address each level of stress that families go through sequentially, if necessary.

Based on results of a study of 50 families who had experienced a variety of stressors, Burr and co-workers (1994) examined the changes experienced under stress in nine areas of family life: marital satisfaction, family rituals and celebrations, quality of communication, family cohesion, functional quality of the executive subsystem, quality of the emotional atmosphere, management of daily routines and chores, contention, and normal family development versus changed or arrested development. The results of the study supported that families did use the proposed strategies, both the helpful ones and the harmful ones, with significant differences between men and women on 10 of the 80 strategies. Women tended to use a wider range of strategies and men tended to use more of the harmful strategies. The results supported the sequential, developmental nature of families' use of strategies in acute stressor situations, but not in chronic stressor situations. Thus, the pattern was evident in stresses, such as bankruptcy, but not in families with a child with a chronic condition.

Results of this work provide direction for community health nursing intervention with families over the lifespan. The three levels share similarities with Neuman's (1989) flexible lines of defense (Level I change), normal line of defense (Level II change), and lines of resistance (Level III change). Based on Neuman's model, primary prevention strategies (e.g., parenting classes) would be appropriate for dealing with Level I change; secondary prevention strategies (e.g., crisis intervention) for dealing with Level II change; and tertiary prevention strategies (e.g., family therapy) for dealing with Level III change.

COMMUNITY HEALTH NURSING APPROACHES TO FAMILY HEALTH RISK REDUCTION
Family Health Risk Appraisal

Assessment of family health risk requires multiple approaches to address the many components of risk. As in any assessment, the first and most important task is to get to know the family, their strengths and needs (see Chapter 26, Family Nursing Assessment, for an in-depth discussion). Pender (1987) presents guides for health protection and health promotion for both individuals and families. In the family version, Pender includes family structure; community affiliations; communication patterns, decision-making patterns, family values, goals, and strengths; major sources of stress; family developmental or situational transitions; concerns or challenges; self-care patterns; sense of purpose; actualization efforts; relationships; environmental control; information-seeking patterns; use of health-promotion facilities/services; consistency among family values, goals, and health actions; and family health goals. This section will focus on appraisal of family health risks within the five identified areas of biologic, social, economic, life-style and life events risk.

Biologic Health Risk

One of the most effective techniques for assessing the patterns of health and illness in families is the use of the family genogram (Bahr, 1990). See Chapter 26, Family Nursing Assessment, for further discussion and example of a genogram.

A genogram is a schematic representation of a family that depicts the family unit of immediate interest and includes several generations using a series of circles, squares, and connecting lines. Basic information on composition of the family, relationships in the family, and patterns of health and illness can be obtained by completing the genogram with the family. As shown in Figure 25-1, a square indicates a male, a circle indicates a female, and an "x" through either a square or a circle indicates a death. Marriage is indicated by a solid horizontal line and offspring/children by a solid vertical line. A broken horizontal line indicates a divorce or separation. Dates of birth, marriage, death, and other important events can be indicated

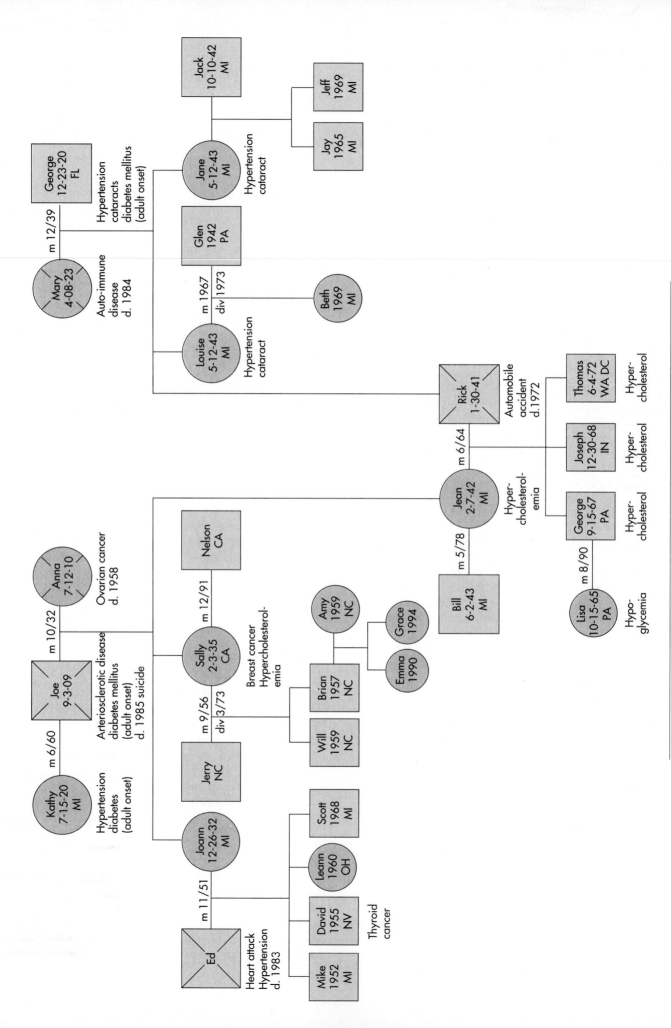

FIGURE 25-1   Family genogram—the Graham family.

where appropriate. Major illness or conditions can be listed for each individual.

The genogram in Figure 25-1 was completed for the Graham family. Some of the interesting patterns that can be seen from the genogram are the repeated recurrence of hypertension, adult onset diabetes, cancer, and hypercholesterolemia. Completion of a genogram requires interviews with the family members. Bahr suggests that a family chronology, a time-line of family events over 3 generations, be completed to extend the genogram.

A more intensive and quantitative assessment of a family's biologic risk can be achieved through the use of a standardized family risk assessment. Because such assessments involve other areas in addition to biologic risk, one will be described later in this section following description of assessment of other types of risk.

Social Health Risk

Assessment of social health risk is less well defined and developed. Information on relationships that the family has with others such as relatives and neighbors, their connections with other social units, church, school, work, clubs, and organizations, and the flow of energy, positive or negative, can be assessed through the use of an ecomap. See Chapter 26, Family Nursing Assessment, for further discussion and example of an ecomap.

An ecomap is merely a visual representation of the family's interactions with other groups and organizations, accomplished using a series of circles and lines. The family of interest is represented by a circle in the middle of a page; other groups and organizations are then indicated by other circles; lines, representing the flow of energy, are drawn between the family circle and the circles representing other groups and organizations. An arrow head at the end of each line indicates the direction of the flow of energy (into or out of the family), and the boldness/darkness of the line indicates the intensity of the energy. Thus, an ecomap drawn for the Graham family (Fig. 25-2) indicates that much of the family energy goes into work (also a source of stress) for the parents. In contrast, major sources of energy for the Grahams are their immediate and extended families and friends.

Other aspects of social risk include characteristics of the neighborhood and community where the family lives. If the nurse has worked in the general geographic area, he or she already may have done a community assessment (see Chapter 15, Community as Client) and have a working knowledge of the neighborhood and community. It is important, however, for information to be obtained from the family in order to understand their perceptions.

Information about the origins of the family is useful to understand other social resources and stressors. Information about how long the family has lived in their current location and the origin and immigration patterns of their family and ancestors provides insight into the pressures they experience.

Economic Health Risk

Financial information often is considered private by families. It is not necessary to know actual family income except in certain instances when it is necessary to determine eligibility for programs or benefits. What is useful to know is whether or not the family's resources are adequate to meet the demands. In terms of health risk, it is important to understand the resources that families have to obtain health/illness care; adequate shelter, clothing, and food; and access to recreational resources. Families with limited resources may qualify for programs, such as Medicaid, Aid to Dependent Families, WIC, or Maternal Support Systems/Infant Support Systems (see Chapters 27, Children's Health; Chapter 28, Women's Health; Chapter 29, Men's Health; Chapter 30, Elder Health; Chapter 31, The Physically Compromised; Chapter 32, Vulnerability: An Introduction; and Chapter 33, Poverty and Homelessness). Families with wage earners with health/medical benefits and those with sufficient income usually are able to afford adequate health care. Unfortunately, there is a growing number of families whose main wage earner is employed but receives no health/medical benefits.

Life-Style Health Risk

Families are the major source of factors that can promote or inhibit positive life-styles. They regulate time and energy and the boundaries of the system (Kantor and Lehr, 1977). A number of tools exist for assessing individuals' life-style risk, but few are available for assessing family life-style patterns. Although assessment of individual life-style contributes to determining the life-style risk of a family, it is important to look at risks for the family as a unit. One approach is to identify family patterns for each of the life-style components included in *Healthy People 2000*. Within the areas of health promotion, health protection, and preventive services, life-style can be assessed on several dimensions. Based on the literature in health behavior research, the critical dimensions include value placed on the behavior, knowledge of the behavior and its consequences, efficacy of the behavior, self-efficacy for the behavior, barriers to performing the behavior, and benefits of the behavior. In terms of specific behaviors, it is important to assess the frequency, the intensity, and the regularity of the behavior. It also is important to evaluate the resources available to the family for implementing the behavior. Thus, items for assessment of physical activity would include the value a family places on physical activity, the hours that a family spends in exercise, the kinds of exercise the family does, and resources available for exercise.

Life-Event Health Risk

As discussed earlier, both normative and nonnormative life events pose potential risks to the health of families. Even events that generally are viewed as being positive require changes and can place stress on a

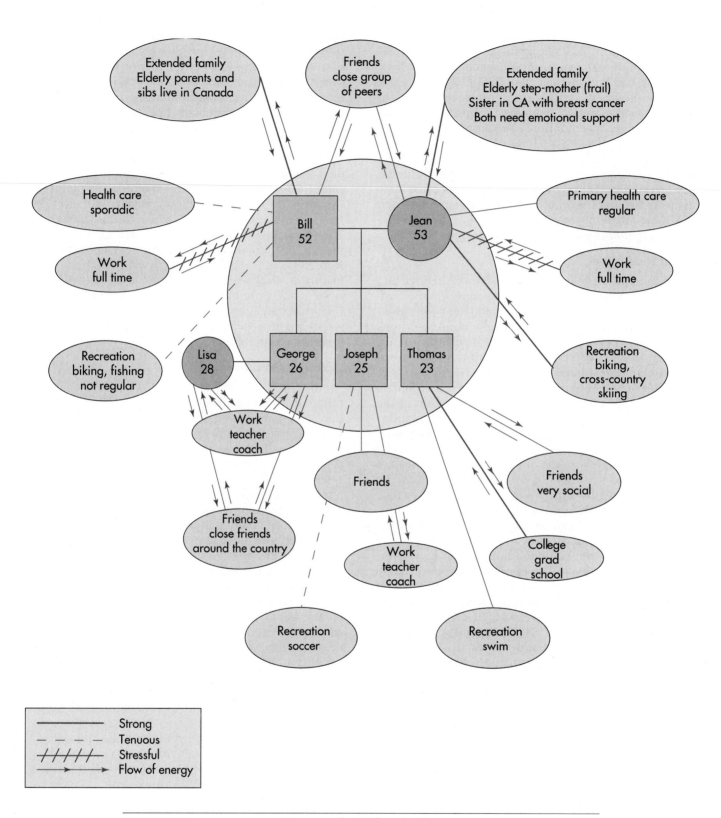

FIGURE 25-2   Ecomap—the Graham family.

family. The normative event of the birth of a child, for instance, requires considerable changes in family structures and roles. Further, family functions are expanded from previous levels, requiring families to add new skills and establish additional resources. These changes in turn can result in strain, and, if adequate resources are not able to be mobilized, stress. Therefore, in order to adequately assess the risks associated with life risks, both normative and nonnormative events occurring in the family need to be considered.

Family Home Visits

Community health nurses work with families in a variety of settings including clinics, schools, support groups, and offices. But, in particular, an important aspect of community health nursing's role in reducing health risks and promoting the health of populations has been the tradition of providing services to individual families in their homes.

Purposes

Home visits give a more accurate assessment of the family structure, the natural or home environment, and behavior in that environment. Home visits also provide opportunities to identify both barriers and supports for reaching family health promotion goals. The nurse can work with the client first hand to adapt interventions to meet realistic resources. Meeting the family on their home ground also may contribute to the family's sense of control and active participation in meeting their health needs. The majority of these studies have focused on the maternal-child population (Barkauskas, 1983; Bradley and Martin, 1994; Brooten et al., 1986; Larson, 1980; Lowe, 1970; McNeil and Holland, 1972; Olds et al., 1986; Siegel et al., 1980).

A home visit may be more than just an alternative setting for service; it may be an intervention modality. If the home visit is to be a valuable and effective intervention, careful and systematic planning must occur. Mayers (1973) cautions that the process of home visits may become more a patterned response set, or ritual, rather than a vital exchange with productive outcomes.

Advantages and Disadvantages

Recently, the effectiveness of providing large portions of health promotion services in this mode has been critically reexamined by agencies, including health departments and visiting nurses associations (VNAs) (Oda, 1989; Wasik et al., 1990). Advantages include convenience for the client, client control of the setting, provision of an option for those clients unwilling or unable to travel, the ability to individualize services, and a natural, relaxed environment for the discussion of concerns and needs (Barkauskas, 1983; Wasik et al., 1990). Costs were the major disadvantage identified by Barkauskas (1983). The cost of previsit

preparation, travel to and from the home, time spent with one client and postvisit preparation is high. In a study comparing teaching to new mothers in groups and home visits, the group approach was found to be more effective in terms of knowledge and cost by approximately one third that of home visits (McNeil and Holland, 1972). Many agencies have actively explored alternative modes of providing service to families, particularly group interventions (see Chapter 23, Group Management). The important issue is determining which families would most benefit from them and how home visits can most effectively be structured and scheduled. With increasing demands for home health care, the home visit is again becoming a prominent mode for delivery of nursing services.

 Research Brief

Bradley PJ, Martin J: The impact of home visits on enrollment patterns in pregnancy-related services among low-income women, *Public Health Nurs* 11(6):392-398, 1994.

The purpose of this retrospective study was to evaluate the impact of home visits on enrollment in pregnancy-related services for a group of urban, low-income, high-risk women. During the home visits, the care coordinator (a nurse or a social worker) did a complete assessment and developed a plan of care to guide subsequent home visits. The women were followed through pregnancy and for at least 3 months postpartum. Data on enrollment patterns in prenatal care, WIC, Medicaid, and Food Stamps were collected from care-coordination records.

The results supported the effectiveness of the home visits in influencing women to enroll in pregnancy-related services. Recommendations included:

1. Outreach efforts to reach highest-risk women in the first trimester should be intensified. Other evidence support the benefit of early participation in programs, such as prenatal care, WIC, Food Stamps, and Medicaid on infant birthweight.
2. Further research is needed to determine the impact of care-coordination services and home visits on pregnancy outcomes and their cost-effectiveness. Medicaid reimburses for care-coordination in 24 states; the cost-effectiveness of these services needs to be evaluated.

Process

The components of a home visit are summarized in Table 25-3 and are elaborated on in the following sections.

Initiation Phase. Usually, a home visit is initiated as the result of a referral from a health or social agency.

Table 25-3   Phases and Activities of a Home Visit

Phase	Activity
I Initiation Phase	Clarify source of referral for visit Clarify purpose for home visit Share information on reason and purpose of home visit with family
II Previsit Phase	Initiate contact with family Establish shared perception of purpose with family Determine family's willingness for home visit Schedule home visit Review referral and/or family record
III In-Home Phase	Introduction of self and professional identity Social interaction to establish rapport Establish nurse-client relationship Implement nursing process
IV Termination Phase	Review visit with family Plan for future visits
V Postvisit Phase	Record visit Plan for next visit

However, a family may request services or the nurse may initiate the home visit as a result of case-finding activities. The **initiation phase** is the first contact between the nurse and the family. This provides the foundation for an effective therapeutic relationship. Subsequent home visits should be based on need and mutual agreement between the nurse and the family. Frequently, nurses are not sure of the reason for the visit. This carries with it the potential for the visit to be compromised and to come aimlessly or abruptly to a premature halt. Regardless of the impetus for making a home visit, it is essential that the nurse be clear about the purpose for the visit and that this perception or understanding be shared with the family.

Previsit Phase. The **previsit phase** has several components. For the most part, these are best accomplished in the following order:

◆ First, if at all possible, the family should be contacted by telephone prior to the home visit to introduce oneself, to identify the reason for the contact, and to schedule the home visit. Leavitt (1982) suggests that a first telephone contact should be brief, with an outside limit of 15 minutes. The nurse should give name and professional identity, for example: "This is Karen Smith. I'm a community health nurse from the Middle County Health Department."

◆ The family should be informed of how they came to the attention of the community health nurse, for example as the result of a referral or a contact from observations or records in the school setting. If a re-

ferral has been received, it is important and useful to ascertain whether or not the family is aware of the referral. This will establish a perspective of valuing the client's input and involvement in care.

◆ Next, a brief summary of the nurse's given information allows the family to know the extent of the nurse's knowledge about the family. For example, the nurse might say, "I understand that your baby was discharged from the hospital yesterday and that you requested some assistance with caring for the child at home."

◆ A visit should be scheduled for as soon as is possible and appropriate for the nurse and the family. Letting the family know agency hours available for visits, the approximate length of the visit, and the purpose of the visit are helpful to the family in determining when to set the visit. Although the length of the visit may vary, depending on circumstances, approximately 45 minutes is usual (Kallins, 1967).

◆ If possible, the visit should be arranged when as many as possible of the family members will be available for the entire visit. It is also important for the nurse to tell the client about any fee for the visit and subsequent visits and potential methods for payment.

◆ The telephone call can terminate with a review by the nurse of the time, place, and purpose for the visit and a means for the family to contact the nurse in case they need to verify or change the time for the visit or to ask questions. If the family does not have a telephone, another method for setting up the visit can be used. The most obvious is dropping off a note at the family home or sending a letter or postcard informing the family of when and why the home visit will occur with a means for the family to contact the nurse if necessary.

Of course, the possibility always exists that the family may refuse to agree to a home visit. Less experienced nurses or students may interpret this as a personal rejection when it is not. Families regulate when and which outsiders are allowed entry into their territory (Kantor and Lehr, 1977). The nurse needs to explore the reasons for the refusal; there may be a misunderstanding about the reason for a visit or there may be a lack of information about services. The contact may be terminated as requested, if the nurse determines that either the situation has been resolved or services have been obtained from another source, and if the family understands that services are available and how to contact the agency if desired. However, the nurse should leave open the possibility of future contact. There are instances when the nurse will be mandated to persist in requesting a home visit because of legal obligations, such as follow-up of certain communicable diseases.

Before visiting the family, it can be useful for the nurse to review the referral or, if not a first visit, the family record. If there is a time lapse between the contact and the visit, a brief telephone call to confirm the time often prevents the nurse from finding no one at home for the visit.

In-Home Phase. The actual visit to the home constitutes the **in-home phase** and affords the nurse the opportunity to assess the family's neighborhood. An issue that may arise either in approaching the family home or once the family has opened the door to the nurse is that of personal safety. Nurses need to examine personal fears and objective threats to determine if safety is indeed an issue. Certain precautions can be taken in known high-risk situations. Agencies may provide escorts for nurses or have them visit in pairs, readily identifiable uniforms may be required, or a sign-out process indicating timing and location of home visits may be used routinely. The nurse needs to use caution; if a reasonable question about the safety of making the visit exists, the visit should not be made.

"Pride, the ethic of self-sufficiency, territoriality, and privacy" are issues for nurses making home visits with families (Leavitt, 1984, p. 288). The nurse needs to be aware that families may feel that they are being "checked up on," are seen as being inadequate or dysfunctional, or that their privacy is being impinged upon. Nursing services, especially those from health departments, have been identified by the public as being "public services" for needy families or those with insufficient funds to pay for care. These potential areas of concern underline the needs for sensitivity on the part of the nurse, the need for clarity in information regarding the reason for visits, and the need to establish collaborative, trusting relationships with the family.

The changing nature of the American family can make it difficult to schedule visits during what have been traditional agency hours. The number of working single-parent or dual-wage earner two-parent families is increasing, which means that families are busy, with many more demands on their time. Even if one parent is at home during the usual work day, the ideal is to work with the entire family unit. This often is not possible because of conflict between agency hours and school or work schedules. It may be possible to schedule a visit at the beginning or end of a day to meet with working or school-age members. In some parts of the country agencies are reconsidering traditional hours and Monday through Friday visits.

Families may or may not be able to control interruptions during the visit. Telephones ring, pets join in the visit, people come and go, televisions are left on. The nurse can ask that for a limited time televisions be turned off or other disruptive activities be limited (Leavitt, 1982). Families may be so used to the background noises and routine activities that they do not recognize them as being potentially disruptive.

The actual home visit includes several components. Once at the family home, the nurse needs to again provide personal identification and professional affiliation. This is part of the introductory phase. Then there should be a brief social period to allow the client to assess the nurse and to establish rapport (Leahy et al., 1982).

The major portion of the home visit is concerned with establishing the relationship and implementing the nursing process. Assessment, intervention, and evaluation are ongoing. It is important that the nurse be realistic about what can be accomplished in a home visit. In some situations, one visit may be all that is possible or appropriate. In this instance, needs and resources for meeting needs are explored with the family and a determination is made as to whether further services are desired or indicated. If they are indicated and the current agency is not appropriate, the nurse can assist the family in identifying other services available in the community and can help in initiating any referrals. Although it is not unusual to have only one home visit with a family, often multiple visits are made (Guilino and LaMonica, 1986). The frequency and intensity of home visits vary with not only the needs of the family, but also with eligibility for services and agency policies and priorities. It is realistic to expect initial assessment and at least the beginning of building a relationship to occur on a first visit.

Termination Phase. When the purpose of the visit has been accomplished, the nurse reviews with the family what has occurred and been accomplished as the major focus of the **termination phase.** This provides a basis for planning any further home visits. Ideally, termination of the visit and, ultimately, of service begins at the first contact, with the establishment of a goal or purpose. If communication has been clear to this point, the family and nurse can now plan for future visits, specifically, the next visit. Planning for future visits is part of another issue: setting goals and planning service. Contracting is a constructive approach to working with clients and is receiving increasing attention by health professionals. The purpose and components of contracting with clients will be discussed in the next section.

Postvisit Phase. Even though the nurse has now concluded the home visit and left the client's home, responsibility for the visit is not complete until the interaction has been recorded. A major task of the **postvisit phase** is documentation of the visit and services provided. Agencies may or may not organize their records by families. That is, the basic record may be a "family" folder or record with all members included in one record, or each family member receiving services may have a separate record, with family members' records cross-referenced. In reality the concept of a family-focused record often breaks down. History and background usually are given to some extent for the family, but often the focus shifts to individual health histories and, consequently, nursing diagnoses, goals, and interventions are directed towards individual family members rather than the family unit. Record systems and formats will vary from agency to agency. The nurse needs to become familiar with the particular system used in the agency. All systems should include the following elements: a data base; nursing diagnoses and problem list; a plan, including specific goals; actual actions and interventions; and evaluation. These are the basic elements needed for legal and clinical purposes. The format may consist of narrative, flow sheets, problem oriented medical records (POMR), subjective, objective, assessment plan (SOAP) or a combination of formats. It is important that recording be current, dated, and signed.

Be sure to use theoretical frameworks that are appropriate to the *family*-centered nursing process. For example, a nursing diagnosis of "ineffective mothering skill related to lack of knowledge of normal growth and development" is an individual-focused nursing diagnosis. "Inability for family to accomplish stage-appropriate task of providing safe environment for preschooler related to lack of knowledge and resources" is a family-focused nursing diagnosis based on knowledge of the developmental approach to families. At times it may be necessary to present information for a specific family member. However, the emphasis should be on the individual as a member of, and within the context of, the family.

Contracting with Families

Increasingly, health professionals look at working with clients in a more interactive, collaborative style. This approach is consistent with a more knowledgeable public and the recent self-care movement. **Contracting** which is an agreement between two or more parties, involves a shift in responsibility and control to a shared effort by client and professional versus that of the professional alone. The ANA Standards of Community Health Nursing Practice (1986) explicitly state the rights of clients to participate actively in planning their own health care; these same standards designate that "in partnership with the family and individual" the community health nurse collects, interprets, and analyzes data; formulates and validates diagnoses; formulates plans and implements interventions; and evaluates process and revision of the plan. This active involvement of the client is reflected in several of the existing nursing models, particularly those of Rogers (1970), King (1981), and Orem (1995). Contracting is one strategy aimed at promoting a collaborative working relationship, in this instance, one specifically focused on health risk reduction and health promotion.

Contracting is one way of formally involving the family in the nursing process and explaining their roles. Some nurses are reluctant to use the term contracting but discuss it in terms of mutual goal setting. Some of this reluctance may be related to the potential legal ramifications of a contract, whether formal or informal. There may be concern about possible liability in terms of services agreed upon versus those re-

ceived or attainment of agreed-upon outcomes. In some cases, the connection of the term contracting, with a compliance may be contrary to a philosophy of an interactive partnership between nurse and client.

Thus, an important issue that needs to be considered at this point is the purpose and/or philosophy that underlies the nurse's use of contracting with families. A large body of literature addresses the noncompliant client or family. Edel identifies the concept of compliance as applying to relationships between "those who have power and those over whom they exercise it" (Edel, 1985, p. 183). These relationships are described as vertical, with one party dominating the other. This approach contradicts the collaborative relationship. If contracting is viewed only as another approach to increasing compliance, the basic premises of the concept are violated. Contracting addresses the issue of control by client versus control by the professional (Boehm, 1983; Hayes and Davis, 1980).

Purposes

The purpose of the agreement is to enhance and support the clients' active role in health care by defining clients' and professionals' roles in accomplishing health-related goals (Herje, 1980). Sloan and Schommer (1975) differentiate between a legal contract and a nursing contract. The former is defined as a written, binding agreement and the latter as a working agreement that is continuously renegotiable and may or may not be written. A nursing contract may be either a contingency or noncontingency one (Boehm, 1983). A contingency contract states a specific reward for the client after completion of the client's portion of the contract; a noncontingency contract does not specify rewards. The implied rewards are the positive consequences of reaching the goals specified in the contract.

In the instance of family health risk reduction, it is essential that the contract be made with all responsible and appropriate members of the family. Involving only one individual is invalid if the goal is family health risk reduction, which requires a total family system effort and change. Scheduling a visit with all family members present may require extra effort; if meeting with the entire family is not possible, each family member can review a contract, give input, and sign it. This allows for active participation by all family members without the necessity of finding a time when everyone involved can be present.

The Process of Contracting

Contracting is a learned skill on the part of both the nurse and the family. All parties involved need to know the purpose and process of contracting. Leavitt (1982) identifies three general phases: beginning, working, and termination. The three phases can be further specified into seven sets of activities. The phases and activities are summarized in Table 25-4.

The first activity involves both the family and the nurse in data collection and analysis of the data. An

Table 25-4   Phases and Activities in Contracting

Phase	Activity
I Beginning Phase	Mutual data collection and exploration of needs and problems
	Mutual establishing of goals
	Mutual exploration of resources
	Mutual development of a plan
II Working Phase	Mutual division of responsibilities
	Mutual setting of time limits
	Mutual implementation of plan
	Mutual evaluation and renegotiation
III Termination Phase	Mutual termination of contract

important aspect of this step is obtaining the family's perspective of the situation and its needs and problems. The nurse can present his or her observations and validate them with the family and also obtain the family's view. Leavitt (1982) suggests that the initial contract be based on the most obvious and/or concrete of the family's needs; more subtle problems can be added as the family and nurse build their working relationship.

It is important that goals be mutually set and realistic. A pitfall for nurses and clients who are new to contracting is to set overly ambitious goals. The nurse should recognize that there may be discrepancies between professional priorities and those of the client and determine whether negotiation is required. Because contracting is a process characterized by renegotiation, the goals are not static.

Throughout the process, the nurse and family need to continually learn and recognize what each can contribute to meeting health needs. This exploration of resources allows both parties to become cognizant of their own and others' strengths and requires a review of the nurse's skills and knowledge, family support systems, and community resources.

Developing a plan to meet the goals involves specifying activities, prioritizing goals, and selecting a starting point. Next the nurse and the family need to decide who will be responsible for which activities. Structuring time limits involves deciding on a deadline for accomplishing or evaluating progress towards accomplishing a goal and the frequency of contacts. At the agreed-upon time, the nurse and family together evaluate the progress to date in both process and outcome. Based on the evaluation, the contract can be modified, renegotiated, or terminated.

Advantages and Disadvantages of Contracting

Contracting takes time and effort and may require the family and nurse to reorient their roles. Increased control on the part of the family also means increased responsibility. Some nurses may have difficulty relinquishing the role of the controlling expert professional. Contracts will not always be successful and contracting

is neither appropriate nor possible in some cases. Some clients do not want to have this kind of involvement; they prefer to defer to the "authority" of the professional. Included in this group are individuals with minimal cognitive skills, those who are involved in an emergency situation, those who are unwilling to be more active in their care, and those who do not see control or authority for health concerns within their domain (Herje, 1980). Some of these clients may learn to contract; some never will.

The use of the nursing process does not necessarily provide an active role for the family as a client; it assumes that needs exist based only on professional judgment and that changes can and should be made within the family unit. Contracting is one alternative approach that depends on the value of input from the nurse and the family, competency of the family, responsibility on the part of the family, and the dynamic nature of the process, which not only allows for but also requires continual renegotiation. Although it may not be appropriate in all situations or with all families, contracting can give direction and structure to health risk reduction and health promotion in families.

Enabling and Empowering Families

Help-giving interventions do not always have positive outcomes for clients. If families do not perceive a situation as a problem or need, offers of help may cause resentment. Help giving also may have negative consequences if there is not a match between what is expected and what is offered. Nurses' failure to recognize families' competencies and to define an active role for families can lead to dependency and lack of growth for families. This can be frustrating for both the nurse and the family. For families to become active participants, they need to feel a sense of personal competence, as well as "a desire for and, willingness to take action, the public domain" (Zimmerman and Rappaport, 1988, p. 746). Recently, approaches for assisting individuals and families to assume an active role in their health care have focused on empowerment (Dunst and Trivette, 1987; Hegar and Hunzeker, 1988; Pinderhughes, 1983; Rappaport, 1987). Definitions of **empowerment** reflect three characteristics we would expect to find in the *empowered* family seeking help: (1) access and control over needed resources, (2) decision-making and problem-solving abilities, and (3) acquisition of instrumental behavior needed to interact effectively with others to obtain resources (Dunst and Trivette, 1987, p. 445). The last characteristic refers to the fact that families may need to learn how to identify sources of help, how to contact agencies, how to ask critical questions, and how to negotiate with agencies to have family needs met. These characteristics generally reflect a process by which people (individuals, families, organizations, or communities) "gain mastery over their affairs" (Rappaport, 1987, p. 122).

Empowerment requires a viewpoint that often conflicts with the perspective of many helping professions, including nursing; empowerment's underlying assumption is one of a partnership between the professional and the client versus one in which the professional is dominant. First, families are assumed to be either competent or capable of becoming competent. This implies that the professional is not an unchallengeable authority who is in control. Second, an environment that creates opportunities for competencies to be used is necessary. Finally, families need to identify that their actions result in behavior change. Dunst and Trivette (1987) propose that different models of helping result in very different outcomes. The compensatory model recognizes the client's responsibility for the need/problem and emphasizes the client's responsibility for solving the problem. This model is proposed to lead clients to acquire behaviors that increase independence and autonomy and a sense of self-efficacy resulting in enhanced well-being. This model has the potential to guide interventions that are empowering to families.

Specifically, a community health nursing intervention that incorporates the principles of empowerment identified by Dunst and Trivette (1987) would be directed toward the building of nurse-family partnerships that emphasize health risk reduction and health promotion. The nurse's approach to the family should be positive and focused on competencies rather than on problems or deficits. The interventions need to be consistent with family cultural norms and the family's perception of the problem. Rather than making decisions for the family, the nurse would support the family in primary decision-making and bolster their self-esteem by recognizing and using family strengths and support networks. Interventions promoting family behaviors increase family competency and decrease the need for outside help, resulting in families seeing themselves as being actively responsible for bringing about desired changes. The goal of an empowering approach is to create a partnership between the nurse and the family characterized by cooperation and shared responsibility.

COMMUNITY RESOURCES

Families have varied and complex needs and problems. The community health nurse often mobilizes a number of resources in order to effectively and appropriately meet family health promotion needs. Although the specific resources vary from community to community, general types can be identified. A number of governmental resources, such as Medicare, Medicaid, Aid to Families of Dependent Children, Supplementary Security Income, Food Stamps, and WIC are available in most communities. These programs primarily provide support for basic needs (e.g., illness/health care, nutritional needs, funds for housing and clothing) and funds are based on the meeting of eligibility criteria.

In addition to governmental agencies providing health-related services to families, most communities have a number of voluntary (nongovernmental) programs. Local chapters of such organizations as Cancer Society, Heart Association, Lung Association, and Muscular Dystrophy Association, to mention a few, provide educational and support services and some direct services to individuals and families regarding specific conditions. These agencies provide primary prevention and health promotion services, as well as screening programs and assistance, once the disease or condition is diagnosed. Local social service agencies, such as Catholic Social Services, provide direct services, such as counseling to families. Other voluntary organizations provide direct service (e.g., shelters for the homeless or battered individuals, substance abuse counseling and treatment, Meals on Wheels, transportation, clothing, food, furniture).

Health resources in the community may be proprietary, voluntary, or public. In addition to private health care providers, community health nurses should be aware of voluntary and public clinics, screening programs, and health promotion programs.

Identifying resources in a community requires time and effort. One obvious and valuable source is the telephone book. Often community service organizations, such as the Chamber of Commerce and the local health department, publish community resource listings. Regardless of how the resource is identified, the community health nurse must be familiar with the type of service offered and any requirements or costs involved. If this information is not available, the community health nurse can contact the resource.

Locating and using these systems often requires skills and patience that many families lack. Community health nurses work with families to identify community resources and as a client advocate in assisting families to learn to use resources. This may involve sharing information with families, rehearsing with families what questions to ask, preparing required materials, making the initial contact, and arranging transportation. Finally, the appropriateness and effectiveness of resources should be evaluated with families after referrals.

Clinical Application

The initial referral for community health nursing service to a family provides limited information and the situation that develops may be much more complex than anticipated. The following example, based on an actual case, illustrates the issues and approaches outlined in this chapter.

A referral was received at the Middle County Health Department indicating that Amy Cress, age 16, had been referred by the school counselor at the local high school for prenatal supervision. Amy was 4 months pregnant, in apparently good health, in the tenth grade and living at home with her mother, stepfather and younger sister. The family lived in a rural area outside of a small farming community. The father of the baby also lived in the community and continued to see Amy on a regular basis. The referral information provided the community health nurse with a beginning, but limited, assessment of the family situation. A home visit would allow for a more extensive assessment of the family within the four models of health: clinical, role-performance, adaptive, and eudaimonistic.

The community health nurse phoned the home to make an appointment for a home visit. Amy's mother answered the phone and indicated that Amy was at school during the day. The nurse introduced herself and explained that the counselor at the high school had talked with Amy about the possibility of having a community health nurse from the health department help her to learn more about her pregnancy, labor and delivery, and caring for a new infant. Amy's mother sounded both relieved and enthusiastic about having the nurse visit. Although Amy was in school during the day, she could arrange to be at home so the nurse could meet her at the end of the agency working day. An appointment was made for later in the week to meet with Amy and her mother. At this point, the initiation and previsit phases of the home visit process were completed by the nurse.

At the first home visit, it became apparent that Amy and her mother were interested in continuing community health nursing service. During her visit with Amy and her mother, the nurse added to her assessment by exploring with them what they saw as problems and concerns. This is consistent with an approach focused on empowerment. Amy and her mother identified a number of questions and concerns. How could Amy finish her education and care for a child? What would labor and delivery be like? How could Amy and her boyfriend avoid unplanned pregnancies in the future? How could the family members be supportive and yet have their own needs met? To extend the assessment to the entire family system, a second visit was scheduled to include Amy's boyfriend and father.

During the second visit, additional areas related to clinical health of the family, in terms of acute or chronic conditions, were assessed using a family genogram. Because it was apparent that there was a potential conflict between individual and family development needs that had implications for the adaptive processes of the family, time was spent identifying both family needs and individual needs and how best to meet these needs. A contract was negotiated to continue visiting with Amy, but the visits would occur at school during a study period. The focus would be on prenatal teaching on the nurse's part, with Amy agreeing to attend a group for pregnant students offered at the school. Visits also were arranged with Amy's mother to discuss her concerns. These approaches reflected acknowledgment of the family's abilities to be actively and competently involved in resolving problems they had identified.

Over time, the contract was modified and expanded to include well-child supervision during the year following the birth of a healthy baby boy. Additionally, during this time Amy's maternal grandfather, who had been recently widowed, became ill and unable to live alone. The grandfather moved into the family home and the family became a four-generation unit. Amy's mother discussed a number of conflicts about caring for her father, assisting with the care of her grandson until Amy finished school and could make other arrangements, having time for her other daughter, and continuing to develop her relationship with her husband in a fairly new marriage (she had been widowed three years earlier). Although the focus of nursing assessment and intervention continued to be on increasing the skills and resources of the family, the contract was evaluated to determine both effectiveness and needs for revision to meet the changing needs of the family.

The contract was modified to include working with Amy's mother to renew her child care skills, providing health supervision for the grandfather, and identifying a schedule for the family that allowed time for the mother and stepfather to have some time alone. The complexity of the family's needs meant that the contract was modified frequently and that not all plans worked. Amy's mother eventually indicated that alternative care was needed for the grandfather and, based on a variety of options identified by the nurse and the mother, an adult foster home was located and a placement made. Conflict arose between Amy's and her boyfriend's individual developmental needs as adolescents and family developmental tasks to be accomplished. Plans and responsibilities had to be renegotiated. With much effort, some pain, and a great deal of commitment to each other, the family moved to a pattern described by Smith (1983) as role-sharing in incorporating the adolescent mother and child into the household. Successful completion of developmental tasks of confirming of pregnancy to the family, committing to a new system, redefining re-

Continued.

Clinical Application—cont'd

lationships, and role sharing characterized the evolution of this family. The family has yet to deal with whether or not Amy and her son will continue to live in the family home when she finishes the beautician training she enrolled in after high school. Amy's mother has indicated a desire to have Amy, her son, and the baby's father live separately, with or without marriage.

This family situation is not an unusual one and mirrors many of the problems and needs of contemporary families. The skills required of the community health nurse are many and varied. Knowledge of family structure, function, developmental tasks, family support systems, health promotion over the lifespan, and community resources have been essential at various points in working with this family.

Key Concepts

- The importance of the family as a major client system for community health nursing in reducing health risks and promoting health of individuals and populations is well documented; the family system is a basic unit within which health behavior, including health values, health habits, and health risk perceptions, is developed, organized, and performed.

- Knowledge of family structure and functioning, family theory, nursing theory, and models of health behavior are fundamental to implementing the nursing process with families in the community. However, community health nurses need to go beyond the individual and family and understand the complex environment in which the family functions to be effective in reducing family health risks. Categories of risk factors that are important to family health are biologic risk, life-style risk, social risk, life-event risk, and economic risk.

- A number of factors contribute to the experience of healthy/unhealthy outcomes. Not everyone exposed to the same event will have the same outcome. The factors that influence whether or not disease or other unhealthy results occur are called health risks. The cumulated risks are synergistic; their combined effect is more than the sum of the individual effects.

- An important aspect of community health nursing's role in reducing health risk and promoting the health of populations has been the tradition of providing services to individual families in their homes.

- Home visits afford the opportunity to gain a more accurate assessment of the family structure and behavior in the natural environment. Home visits also provide opportunities to make observations of the home environment and to identify both barriers and supports to reducing health risks and for reaching family health goals.

- Increasingly, health professionals have come to look toward working with clients in a more interactive, collaborative style.

- Contracting, which is an agreement between two or more parties, involves a shift in responsibility and control to a shared effort by client and professional versus that of professional alone.

- Families have varied and complex needs and problems. The community health nurse often mobilizes a number of resources to effectively and appropriately meet family health needs.

Critical Thinking Activities

1. Select one of the Year 2000 objectives and identify how Biologic Risk, Social Risk, Economic Risk, Lifestyle Risk, and Life-event Risk contribute to family health risk for that objective.

2. Select three to four families (hypothetically or from actual situations) representative of different ethnic and socioeconomic backgrounds. Complete a family genogram and ecomap for each family and identify and compare major health risks.

3. Select one or more agencies in which community health nurses work and examine the agency's and community health nursing's philosophies and ob-

Critical Thinking Activities—cont'd

jectives with emphasis on individual care, family care, illness care, risk reduction and health promotion.

4. Identify three community health problems in your community and discuss the implications of these problems for the health of families. Identify three health problems common to families in your community and discuss the implications of the problems for the health and/or health care resources of the community.

Bibliography

American Nurses Association, Council of Community Health Nurses: *Standards of community health nursing practice,* Kansas City, Mo, 1986, American Nurses Association.

Bahr KS: Student responses to genogram and family chronology, *Family Relations* 39(3):243-249, 1990.

Baranowski T, Nader PR: Family health behavior. In Turt DC, Kerns RD, editors: *Health illness, and families: a life-span perspective,* New York, 1985, John Wiley and Sons.

Barkauskas VH: Effectiveness of public health nurse home visits to primiparous mothers and their infants, *AJPH* 73(5):573-580, 1983.

Belloc NB, Breslow L: Relationship of physical health in a general population survey, *Am J Epidemiol* 93:329-336, 1972.

Berg CL, Helgeson D: That first home visit, *J Community Health Nurs* 1(3):207-215, 1984.

Boehm S: Patient contracting. In Fitzpartick JJ, Taunton RI, Benoliel JQ, editors: *Annual review of Nursing Research,* vol 7, New York, 1983, Springer.

Bomar PJ, editor: *Nurses and family health promotion: concepts, assessment, and interventions,* Baltimore, 1989, Williams & Wilkins.

Bradley PJ, Martin J: The impact of home visits on enrollment patterns in pregnancy-related services among low-income women, *Public Health Nurs* 11(6):392-398, 1994.

Brooten D, Kumar S, Brown LP, Butts P, Finkler SA, Sachs S, Gibbons A, Papadopoulos M: A randomized clinical trial of early hospital discharge and home follow-up of very-low-birth weight infants, *N Engl J Med* 314:924-938, 1986.

Burr WR, Klein SR, Burr RG, et al: *Reexamining family stress: new theory and research,* Thousand Oaks, Calif, 1994, Sage Publications.

Califano JA Jr: *Healthy people: the Surgeon General's report on health promotion and disease prevention,* Washington, DC, 1979, US Government Printing Office, (Stock No 017-001-00416-2).

Dielman TE, Butchart AT, Shope JT, Miller M: Environmental correlates of adolescent substance abuse: implications for prevention programs, *Int J Addict* 25:855-880, 1990.

Doherty WJ, McCubbin HI: Family and health care: an emerging arena of theory, research and clinical intervention, *Family Relations* 34(1):5-11, 1985.

Dunst CM, Trivette CM: Enabling and empowering families: conceptual and intervention issues, *School Psychology Review* 16(4):183-85, 1987.

Duvall EM, Miller BC: *Marriage and family development,* ed 6, New York, 1985, Harper & Row.

Edel MK: Noncompliance: an appropriate nursing diagnosis? *Nurs Outlook* 33(4):183-85, 1985.

Feetham SL, Meister SB, Bell JM, Gilliss CL, editors: *The nursing of families: theory/research/education/practice,* Newbury Park, 1993, Sage Publications.

Gilliss C, Highley BL, Roberts BM, Martinson IM, editors: *Toward a science of family nursing,* Menlo Park, Calif, 1989, Addison-Wesley.

Glynn TJ: Adolescent drug use and the family environment: a review, *J Drug Issues* 14:271-295, 1984.

Greer C: Something is robbing our children of their future, *Parade Magazine* pp 4-6, March 5, 1995.

Guilino C, LaMonica G: Public health nursing: a study of role implementation, *Public Health Nurs* 3(2):80-91, 1986.

Hayes WS, Davis LL: What is a health care contract? *Health Values: Achieving High Level Wellness* 4(2):82-89, 1980.

Healthy People 2000: national health promotion and disease prevention objectives, Washington, DC, 1991, USDHHS, Public Health Service.

Hegar RL, Hunzeker JM: Moving toward empowerment-based practice in public child welfare, *Social Work* 33:499-502, 1988.

Helgeson DM, Berg CL: Contracting: a method of health promotion, *J Community Health Nurs* 2(4):199-207, 1985.

Herje PA: Hows and whys of patient contracting, *Nurse Educator* 5(1):30-34, 1980.

Hill R: *Families under stress,* New York, 1949, Harper.

Kallins EL: *The textbook of public health nursing,* St Louis, 1967, Mosby.

Kantor D, Lehr W: *Inside the family,* San Francisco, 1977, Jossey-Bass.

King IM: *A theory for nursing: systems, concepts, process,* New York, 1981, John Wiley & Sons.

Larson CP: Efficacy of prenatal and postpartum visits on child health and development, *Pediatrics* 66:183-190, 1980.

Leahy KM, Cobb MM, Jones MC: *Public health nursing,* ed 4, New York, 1982, McGraw-Hill.

Leavitt MB: *Families at risk: primary prevention in nursing practice,* Boston, 1982, Little, Brown, & Company.

Litman TJ: The family as a basic unit in health and medical care: a social behavioral overview, *Soc Sci Med* 8:495-519, 1974.

Lowe ML: Effectiveness of teaching as measured by compliance with medical recommendations, *Nurs Res* 19:59-63, 1970.

Mauksch HO: A social science basis for conceptualizing family health, *Soc Sci Med* 8:521-528, 1974.

Mayers M: Home visit—ritual or therapy? *Nurs Outlook* 21(5):328-331, 1973.

McNeil HJ, Holland SS: A comparative study of public health nurse teaching in groups and in home visits, *AJPH* 62(12):1629-1637, 1972.

Neuman B: *The Neuman systems model,* ed 2, Norwalk, Conn, 1989, Appleton & Lange.

Nightingale EO, Cureton M, Kalmar V, Trudeau MB: *Perspectives on health promotion and disease prevention in the United States,* Washington, DC, 1978, Institute of Medicine, National Academy of Sciences.

Oda DS: Home visits: effective or obsolete nursing practice? *Nurs Res* 38(2):121-123, 1989.

Olds DL, Henderson CR Jr, Tatelbaum R, Chamberlain R: Improving the life-course development of socially disadvantaged mothers: a randomized trail of nurse home visitation, *AJPH* 78(11):1436-1445, 1988.

Orem DE: *Nursing: concepts of practice,* ed 5, St Louis, 1995, Mosby.

Pender NJ: *Health promotion in nursing practice,* ed 2, Norwalk, Conn, 1987, Appleton & Lange.

Pratt L: *Family structure and effective health behavior,* Boston, 1976, Houghton Mifflin.

Pinderhughes EB: Empowerment for clients and for ourselves, *Social Casework: The Journal of Contemporary Social Work* 64:331-338, 1983.

Pyen CW: Wide disparity exists in poverty guidelines for property tax breaks, *The Ann Arbor News* pp C1, C2, March 19, 1995.

Rappaport J: Terms of empowerment/exemplars of prevention: toward a theory for community psychology, *Am J Community Psychol* 15(2):121-148, 1987.

Rogers M: *An introduction to the theoretical basis of nursing,* Philadelphia, 1970, FA Davis.

Siegel E, Bauman KE, Schaefer ES, et al: Hospital and home support during infancy: impact on maternal attachment, child abuse and neglect, and health care utilization, *Pediatrics* 66:183-190, 1980.

Sloan MR, Schommer BT: The process of contracting in community nursing. In Spradley BW, editor: *Contemporary community nursing,* Boston, 1975, Little, Brown, & Company.

Smith JA: *The idea of health, implications for the nursing professional,* New York, 1983, Teachers College Press, Columbia University.

Smith LA: A conceptual model of families incorporating an adolescent mother and child into the household, *Adv Nurs Sci* 6(1):45-59, 1983.

Turk DC, Kerns RD, editors: *Health, illness, and families: a life-span perspective,* New York, 1985, John Wiley & Sons.

United States General Accounting Office: *Home visiting: a promising early intervention strategy for at-risk families,* Washington, DC, 1990, United States General Accounting Office, (GAO/HRD-90-83).

Volk RJ, Edwards DW, Lewis RA, Sprenkle DH: Family systems of adolescent substance abusers, *Family Relations* 38(3):266-272, 1989.

Wasik BH, Bryant DM, Lyons CM: *Home visiting: procedures for helping families,* Newbury Park, Calif, 1990, Sage Publications.

Zimmerman MA, Rappaport J: Citizen participation, perceived control, and psychological empowerment, *Am J Community Psychol* 16(5):725-750, 1988.

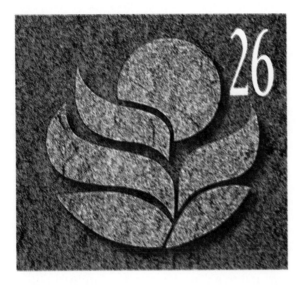

26 Family Nursing Assessment

Shirley M. H. Hanson ◆ Joanna Rowe Kaakinen

Objectives

After reading this chapter, the student should be able to do the following:

◆ Explain the importance of family nursing in the community-based setting.
◆ Define family, family nursing, family health, and healthy versus nonhealthy families.
◆ Explain the various steps of the family nursing process.
◆ Summarize the importance of the assessment to the intervention outcomes.
◆ Compare and contrast the four ways to view family nursing.
◆ Compare and contrast two different models and approaches that can be used for family assessment and intervention.
◆ Explain one assessment model and approach in detail.
◆ Summarize how the genogram and ecomap can be used for family assessment.
◆ Describe the various barriers to family nursing.
◆ Share the implications for family policy.

Outline

Family nursing is practiced in all settings. The trend in the health care delivery system has been to move much of health care delivery to community-based settings. Family nursing is a specialty area that has a strong theoretical base and is more than just "common sense" or viewing the family as the context for individual health care. **Family nursing** is nurses and families working together to ensure that each family member successfully adapts to health and illness. There are many barriers in the current health care delivery system that inhibit the practice of family nursing.

The overall purpose of this chapter is to present strategies to practice family nursing in community-based settings. Specific emphasis is placed on family health assessment, since this lays the foundation for the other aspects of the family nursing process. Two assessment instruments derived from family nursing theory are presented, along with a discussion of the use of genograms and ecomaps. The chapter concludes with a discussion of the future of family nursing and the importance of the nurse's role in establishing family policy.

BARRIERS TO PRACTICING FAMILY NURSING

Two significant barriers to practicing family nursing are the narrow definitions of both *family* and *healthy family* used by health care providers and social policy makers. Other barriers are summarized by Hanson and Boyd (1996) and Gillis (1993):

1. Until the last decade, the majority of practicing nurses had very little exposure to family concepts during their undergraduate education and continued to practice using the individual paradigm. Family nursing was viewed as "common sense" and not a theory-based nursing approach.
2. There has been a lack of good comprehensive family assessment models, instruments, and strategies in nursing.
3. Nursing has strong historical ties with the medical model that views the family as context and not central to individual health care.
4. The traditional charting system in health care has been oriented to the individual.
5. The medical and nursing diagnostic systems used in health care are disease centered, and diseases are focused on individuals.
6. Insurance carriers traditionally have based reimbursement and coverage on individual bases, not on the family unit.
7. The hours during which health care systems provide services to families are at times of day when family members cannot accompany one another.

These and other obstacles to family focused nursing practice are slowly shifting, and nurses must continue to lobby for changes that are more conducive to caring for the family as a whole.

WHAT IS FAMILY?

The definition of **family** is critical to the practice of family nursing. Family traditionally has been defined using the legal concepts of relationships, such as biologic/genetic blood ties, adoption, guardianship, or marriage. Since the 1980s a broader definition of family has been used that moves beyond the traditional blood, marriage, and legal constrictions. The definition for family used in this chapter is ". . . two or more individuals who depend on one another for emotional, physical and/or economical support. The members of the family are self-defined" (Hanson and Boyd, 1996).

Nurses should ask clients to identify people whom they consider to be family and then include those members in health care planning. The family may range from traditional notions of the family, the nuclear and extended family, to such "postmodern" family structures as single-parent, step, extended, and same-gender families.

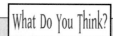

What Do You Think?

There are people in our society who believe the definition of family should be and is expanding and should include two-parent, single-parent, remarried, gay, adoptive, foster, and many other alternative family forms. That is, families are what people define them to be and the government with its health, legal, and economic sanctions should be supportive of all family groups.

WHAT IS FAMILY HEALTH?

Despite the focus on family health within nursing, the construct of family health lacks consensus and precision. Anderson and Tomlinson (1992, p. 58) said, "the analysis of family health include simultaneously both health and illness and the individual and the collective."

The term family health is often used interchangeably with the concepts of family functioning, healthy families, or familial health. Hanson (1985a, 1985b) defined **family health** as ". . . a dynamic changing relative state of well-being which includes the biological, psychological, sociological, cultural, and spiritual factors of the family system."

This multidisciplinary approach refers to individual members, as well as the family unit as a whole. An individual's health (wellness and illness continuum) affects the entire family's functioning; in turn, the family's functioning affects individuals' health. Thus, assessment of family health involves simultaneous assessment of individual family members and the family system as a whole.

Healthy versus Nonhealthy Families

Terms related to healthy versus nonhealthy families have varied throughout time in the literature. Health professionals have tended to classify clients and their families into two groups: good families and bad families who are in need of psychosocial evaluation and intervention (Satariano and Briggs, 1993). Family health then has come to imply mental health rather than physical health. Currently, the popular term for nonhealthy families is dysfunctional families, also called noncompliant, resistant, or unmotivated, phrases that denote enmeshed families who are not functioning well with each other or the world. The label dysfunctional family, however, does not allow for family change and intervention, and it needs to be dropped from the nursing vernacular. Labeling families as dysfunctional implies that nothing in the family system is working and that they are a "bad" family. The catch-all term dysfunctional is so nonspecific that no guidance is provided to assist the family and health care provider in creating a plan of intervention. Families are neither all good nor all bad. Basing family nursing diagnoses on specific family behaviors and strengths provides a structured constructive avenue for intervention.

Did You Know?

Some people believe American families are in decline, whereas others believe that families are healthy. According to a report from the National Commission on Children, people are both discouraged and encouraged about the status of America's families. The contradictions in this report are partially due to a disparity between people's perceptions of their own families (healthy) and the perception of families outside their own (unhealthy or dysfunctional).

Family strengths is the term often used to speak about healthy families (Otto, 1963; Pratt, 1976; Stinnett et al., 1979). Beavers (1985) wrote about beliefs that are associated with healthy couples, believing that family health was associated with the attributes of the healthy couple. In sum, there has been a lot of research about healthy families but it is clear that they all fall into the category of relational needs (Gershwin and Nilsen, 1989). This presumes that in healthy families the basic survival needs are met. The traits ascribed to healthy families are based on attachment and are affectional in nature (Carter and McGoldrick, 1980).

Curran (1983, 1985) reported traits of healthy families, as well as family stressors, that are useful for nurses to include in their assessment. Characteristics of families who are healthy and functioning well in society are listed in the box above, right.

Characteristics of Healthy Families

1. The family tends to communicate well and listen to all members.
2. The family affirms and supports all of its members.
3. Teaching respect for others is valued by the family.
4. The family members have a sense of trust.
5. The family plays together and humor is present.
6. All members interact with each other and a balance in the interactions is noted among the members.
7. The family shares leisure time together.
8. The family has a shared sense of responsibility.
9. The family has traditions and rituals.
10. The family shares a religious core.
11. Privacy of members is honored by the family.
12. The family opens it boundaries to admit and seek help with problems.

Modified from Curran D: *Traits and the healthy family*, Minneapolis, 1983, Winston Press, Harper & Row.

WAYS TO VIEW FAMILY NURSING

Central to the practice of family nursing is viewing the family as more than just the context for the individual. There are four approaches or ways to view families that have legitimate implications for nursing assessment and intervention. The approach that nurses use is determined by many factors, including the health care setting, family circumstances, and nurse resources.

The first approach to family nursing care views *family as the context* and has a traditional focus that places the individual in the foreground and the family as background. The family as context serves as either a resource or a stressor to individual health and illness. A nurse using this focus might ask an individual client: "How has your diagnosis of insulin dependent diabetes affected your family?" "Will your need for medication at night be a problem for your family?"

The second approach to family nursing conceptualizes *family as the client*. The family is in the foreground and individuals are in the background. The family is seen as the *sum* of individual family members. The focus is concentrated on each and every individual as they affect the whole family. From this perspective, a nurse might ask a family member who has just become ill: "Tell me about what has been going on with your own health and how you perceive each family member responding to your mother's recent diagnosis of liver cancer."

The third approach to care focuses on the *family as a system*. The focus is on the family as client, and it is viewed as an interactional system in which the whole is more than the sum of its parts. This approach focuses on the individual and family simultaneously. The interactions between family members become the target for nursing interventions; for example, the direct interactions between the parental dyad or the indirect interaction between the parental dyad and the child. The systems approach to family always implies that when something happens to one family member, the other members of the family system are affected. Questions nurses ask when approaching a family as system are: "What has changed between you and your spouse since your child's head injury?" or "How do you feel your son's long-term rehabilitation will affect the ways in which your family is functioning and getting along with each other?"

The fourth approach to family care views the *family as a component of society* and the family is seen as one of many institutions in society, along with health, educational, religious, or economic institutions. The family is a basic or primary unit of society, as are all the other units, and they are all a part of the larger system of society. The family as a whole interacts with other institutions to receive, exchange or give communication and services. Community health nursing has drawn many of its tenets from this perspective as it focuses on the interface between families and community agencies.

FAMILY NURSING PROCESS

The family nursing process is a dynamic systematic organized method of critically thinking about the family. It is problem solving with the family to assist successful adaptation of the family to identified health care needs. The family nursing process is the application of the generic nursing process grounded in knowledge of family nursing and family theory.

The **family nursing process,** suggested by these authors, consists of the following steps adapted specifically with family as the focus group (Carnevali and Thomas, 1993, p. 10):

1. Collection of a family nursing data base (general or focused). Data collection is focused on both identification of problem areas and strengths of the family. Often this and the following step of diagnostic reasoning become integrated so that assessment and analysis of the data collected occur concurrently. Nurses make inferences and conclusions about the data they collect, which in turn directs more data collection or demarcates the problem areas.

2. Diagnostic reasoning and generation of specific family nursing diagnosis. In this analytic step, nurses make clinical judgments about which problems can be resolved by nursing intervention, which problems need to be referred to other professionals, and which areas of concern the family is successfully adapting to on its own without intervention. The problems that require nursing intervention are specifically stated as family nursing diagnoses. The family nursing diagnosis provides direction for the collaboration of the nurse and the family in designing a plan of action. Diagnostic statements for the family as a whole can be derived from any of the common taxonomies that contain statements related to families: North American Nursing Diagnosis Association (NANDA) (Carpenito,1993); Diagnostic and Statistical Manual of Mental Disorders (DSM IV) (American Psychiatric Association, 1994); International Classification of Diseases (ICD) (International Classification of Diseases, 1991); or the Omaha System (Martin and Scheet, 1992).

3. Collection of prognostic nursing and medical data and generation of data-supported nursing prognosis for each family nursing diagnosis. The nursing prognosis is a nursing judgment, based on the holistic view of the family and its members, that predicts the probability of the family's ability to respond to the current situation. The predictive or prognostic statement outlines the most successful course of action on which to focus the interventions.

4. Treatment planning based on both family nursing diagnosis and prognosis, plus additional data on daily living and family resources/deficits should affect planned nursing actions. The nurse and family work in a partnership to design and contract a plan of action based on identified family strengths. The goal of the plan of action is to have the family successfully manage its health care concerns.

5. Implementation of family-negotiated plans of action. The specific family and nursing interventions are carried out by the designated party to achieve the goals they agreed on.

6. Evaluation of family/family members' responses to plans of action, effects of family diagnosis, prognosis, and previous treatment. The evaluation phase is based on family outcomes, not on effectiveness of the interventions. Modification of family nursing diagnoses and plans occurs as necessary, based on formative evaluation.

7. Termination of the nurse-family partnership is included in the plan of action and is implemented based on the evaluation.

A more detailed discussion of the family nursing process occurs in the following sections demonstrating how to implement the process.

Collection of Data

The first step in the traditional nursing process is assessment, a comprehensive data-collection process. Shaw (1993) claims that the assessment process is the most critical step in the nursing process because it directs the whole problem-solving process. The selection of the appropriate assessment tool is made by the nurse based on areas of concern identified by the referral source and the theoretical framework of the nurse. Two family assessment tools are discussed in detail later in this chapter.

Identification of a potential problem area. Data collection begins with the identification of a potential problem area identified by a variety of sources that include the family, the physician, a school nurse, or a case worker. The identification of a problem, actual or potential, triggers the nurse to establish contact with a family. Several examples follow:

1. A family is referred to the home health agency because of the birth of the newest family member. In that district, all births are automatically followed up with a home visit.
2. A family calls the Visiting Nurse Association to request assistance in providing care to a family member who has a terminal health care problem.
3. The school nurse is asked to conduct a family assessment by a teacher who noticed that a student has frequent absences and significant behavior changes are evident in the classroom.
4. A physician requests a family assessment with a child who has been diagnosed with failure to thrive.

The initial source of referral has identified an actual or potential family health care problem. The specific problem or the central issue may not have been identified at this point. One of the most important pieces of information provided by the referral source is the focus or the cluster of cues/symptoms that leads someone to believe a problem might exist. The cluster of cues helps to focus the assessment process and selection of the appropriate family assessment tools.

As soon as the referral occurs, the nurse begins the assessment process and data collection. Sources of pre-encounter data collected before the family interview by the nurse include the following:

1. Referral source. The referral source provides important data that helps the nurse focus the initial interview with the family. The information collected from the referral source includes the cues/symptoms that lead them to identify that a problem area exists for this family. Demographic information may be obtained from the referral source. Both subjective and objective information are helpful in the assessment process.

2. Family. A family may identify a health care concern and seek assistance. During the initial intake or screening procedure, valuable information can be collected that provides the focus for the assessment interview between the nurse and the family.

Information is collected by the nurse during the interaction with the family member on the phone while making arrangements for the initial appointment. Information that may be noted might include family members' views of the problem, surprise that the referral was made, reluctance to set up the meeting, avoidance in setting up the interview, or recognition that a referral was made or that a probable health care concern is prevalent.

3. Previous records. Previous records may be available for review prior to the first meeting between the nurse and the family. Often a record release for information signed by an adult family member is necessary to obtain family or individual records.

Setting up the meeting with the family. Prior to contacting the family to arrange for the initial appointment,

the nurse decides the best place to conduct the interview. Often this decision is dictated by the type of agency with which the nurse works; for example, home health is conducted in the home, or the mental health agency may choose to have the family meet in the neighborhood clinic office.

The advantages of conducting the interview in the family home are many. The everyday environment of the family can be viewed by the nurse during the visit. An important reason to conduct home interviews is to emphasize that the problem is the responsibility of the whole family and not one family member. The family members are likely to feel more relaxed and demonstrate typical family interactions in their own environment. The convenience of conducting the interview in the home may increase the probability of having more family members present. Two important disadvantages of conducting the interview in the home are (1) the home may be the only sanctuary or safe place for the family or its members to be away from the scrutiny of others; and (2) to conduct an interview in the personal space of the family requires skilled communication ability on the part of the nurse.

Conducting the family interview in the office or clinic allows for easier access to consult other health care providers. Another advantage of using the clinic may be that the family situation is so intense that a more formal, less personal setting may be necessary for the family to begin discussion of emotionally charged issues. A disadvantage of conducting the family interview in the office is that it may reinforce a possible cultural gap between the family and the nurse by not seeing the everyday family environment.

After the decision is made regarding the location of the family interview, the appointment should be arranged with the family. The nurse needs to be confident and organized when making the initial contact. After the introduction, the nurse succinctly states the reason for requesting the family visit. All family members are encouraged to attend the interview. Several possible times for the appointment can be offered to allow the family to select the most convenient time for all members to be present; often this occurs in the late afternoon or evening.

Purpose of the family interview. The purpose of the initial family interview is to identify the health concerns of the family. The central issues often are not the same as the problem for which the family was referred, as the following case study illustrates:

The Raggs family is referred to the home health clinic by a physician for medication management after Sam, the 73-year-old husband, was discharged from the hospital with the diagnosis of insulin dependent diabetes. He has a 13-year history of noninsulin dependent diabetes. The potential area of concern that prompted the referral was the actual administration of insulin. After the initial interview, the nurse finds that administration of the medication is not the central issue for Sam and his wife, Rose, but rather the nutritional management of the disease. The assumption of the referral source was that the family knew how to manage the dietary aspects of diabetes because Sam had noninsulin diabetes for 13 years. In this particular case, the focus needed to be on nutritional management rather than medication administration.

Family Nursing Diagnosis

The family nursing diagnosis is based on the nurse determining the central issue of concern with the family. It is paramount for the nurse to state the specific family nursing diagnosis because it structures the remaining steps in the family nursing process. The **family nursing diagnosis** is a public statement of the problem and the specific reason that brings the nurse and family together to solve a family health care need. If the family nursing diagnosis is misidentified, the family and the nurse will collect evidence, design interventions, and implement plans of care that do not meet the family's needs. A key factor in identifying the correct family nursing diagnosis is asking broad-based questions that allow for data collection in multiple option tracks concurrently. The following two scenarios demonstrate the importance of identifying the central issue of concern and accurately making the family nursing diagnosis.

Scenario 1: The hypothesized central issue for the Raggs family was identified by the referral source: Is insulin being administered correctly by the Raggs family? Based on this central issue, evidence was collected and the family nursing diagnosis identified was "Lack of family knowledge related to the administration of insulin secondary to new diagnosis of insulin dependent diabetes as evidenced by: (1) verbal statements of concern about giving the injection, (2) difficulty drawing up the accurate amount of insulin, and (3) questions about the storage of insulin. This nursing diagnosis focuses further data collection and the plan for interventions on: (1) the psychomotor skills necessary to give the insulin injection, (2) the correct amount of insulin to give according to blood glucose level, and (3) the correct storage and handling of the medication and the equipment."

Based on this family nursing diagnosis, from an individual as client, the nurse made the conclusion that the most important facet to concentrate on was the ability of the family to administer medication. The data collection process and the nurse's thinking were focused on a single problem, not the whole impact of this health issue on the family. The identification of other family health care needs may occur, but the identification will be delayed, which may cause potential harm.

Scenario 2: The real central issue for the Raggs family identified by the nurse conducting the assessment is "What is the best way to assure that the Raggs family understands the relationship of insulin dependent diabetes and the administration of medication?" After collecting evidence, the family nursing diagnosis was "Lack of family knowledge related to health care management of a family member who has been newly diagnosed with insulin dependent diabetes."

Asking a broader based question, from a family as client perspective, allows the nurse to view the whole picture of the family dealing with this specific health concern and directs the data-collection process. More evidence was collected in this case scenario because more options for possible interventions were considered concurrently in the data-collection process. Areas of data collection for this nursing diagnosis were (1) administration of medication, (2) nutritional management, (3) blood glucose monitoring, (4) activity exercise, and (5) knowledge of pathophysiology of diabetes. The nurse was able to collect data looking at the family in a more holistic fashion. The central issue for the family centered around nutritional management, which ultimately affects the administration of medication.

The major difference between the two scenarios presented above was the way in which the nurse framed the question. In the first scenario the nurse asked a question that allowed for only one aspect of the family and the health care concern to be considered at a time. This type of step-by-step problem-solving process is tedious, time consuming, and has a high probability for error in the identification of the most pressing family nursing diagnosis. In the second scenario, the nurse asked a question that allowed for critical thinking about several options concurrently.

An important part of defining the family nursing process is continuous **reflective questioning,** which helps to keep the central issue in focus and allows for modification of the family nursing diagnosis (Alfaro-Lefevre, 1994). Reflective questions that are helpful include: (1) Am I continuing to focus on the central issue? (2) Am I sure that I am understanding the information correctly? (3) Is everyone involved focused on the central issue? (4) Have I collected enough information to be drawing inferences or conclusions? and (5) Have I made any assumptions that might not be true or valid?

The family nursing diagnoses should not be limited to the few that are endorsed by NANDA (Carpenito, 1993). The taxonomies presented earlier are other useful tools for coming up with family nursing diagnoses. However, nurses are encouraged to state the family nursing diagnosis in the NANDA format and forward frequently occurring family nursing diagnoses to NANDA for inclusion in the listing. After the family nursing diagnosis has been identified and verified with the family, the next step is the family nursing prognosis.

Family Nursing Prognosis

The family prognosis is a realistic statement about the ability of the family to adapt successfully to the nursing diagnosis, given the strengths of the family, the pattern of family response in similar situations, and the trajectory of the family health care problem. In essence, the prognosis statement represents the nurse's judgment of the evidence presented in the family assessment process. **Family nursing prognosis** "is a prediction of the possible or probable course of events and outcomes associated with a particular family health status or family situation under various circumstances, treatment options or lack of treatment" (Carnevali and Thomas, 1993, p. 80).

The family prognosis contains information about "areas where changes can occur, types of outcomes and trajectory of change" (Carnevali and Thomas, 1993, p. 80). The treatment plan is based on predicting the areas in which the family can change to achieve successful adaptation.

The areas of change may be focused on the family's response to the situation, the family system process, and the family function most affected, or family components, such as roles, communication, decision-making, or stress and coping. The trajectory is the prediction of the course of events or the pattern of change given information known about the family. The types of outcomes that the nurse considers include (1) prevention of a potential problem, (2) minimization of the problem, (3) stabilization of the problem, or (4) deterioration of the problem.

A case example showing the importance of the prognosis statement from a family as a system viewpoint follows.

The home hospice nurse has been working with the Brush family for 3 weeks. The Brush family consists of the following members, all of whom live in the home:

Dylan—Father   Myra—Mother
William—10 yrs. old   Jessica—7 yrs. old
Beatrice—Grandmother, Myra's mother

Beatrice was diagnosed with terminal liver cancer 4 weeks ago. The Brush family all agreed that Beatrice should live with them and be cared for until her death in their home. Beatrice has other children who live in the same city. The hospice nurse in collaboration with the Brush family has identified several family nursing diagnoses, but the following family nursing diagnosis is of major importance because it affects the lives of all family members: Family role conflict related to the maternal grandmother moving into her daughter's home after being diagnosed with terminal liver cancer. The daughter evidenced her role conflict by stating, "sometimes I do not know who I am: daughter, nurse, mother, or wife."

Prognosis: Prognosis for resolving the role conflict experienced by Myra can be minimized successfully by working with the family to spread the caregiver role among the extended family members, to negotiate certain tasks and who performs them, and providing for respite care. One of the strengths of the family is agreement that caring for the dying grandmother in the home is the "right" ethical choice for them. The disruption to the family and their expected roles will be short term, since the grandmother will probably not live for more than 4 months. Home hospice has been contacted and is involved in the care management. The family has a strong internal and external support system. The extended family is willing to be involved in the care of Beatrice.

The prognosis is critical because it serves as the foundation for the interventions or strategies of action the family and nurse design in response to the identified family nursing diagnosis. In the case example above, the area of change is family roles and the expected behaviors of each family member. The trajectory of the course of events is short term, but Myra's role conflict may escalate as her caregiver role becomes more intense as her mother gets worse. The type of outcome is to mobilize resources to minimize Myra's role conflict.

Planning, Implementation, and Evaluation

After the prognosis statement is formulated, it is essential for the nurse to determine if the family's responses to the problem require nursing intervention or should be referred to a different professional. The planning phase is a form of contracting with families. The contract, or plan of action, includes establishing goals, plans of action, determining who does what in the plan, and building in evaluation steps. The contract or written plan of care (1) ensures involvement of each person, (2) involves people in their own care, and (3) increases autonomy and self-esteem of the family members.

Once the nurse determines that the identified central issues are appropriate for nursing, the planning and intervention aspects of the family nursing process assist the family members to be part of the solution. The degree of involvement of each family member varies and needs to be negotiated among the family members with the help of the nurse. The types of plans, the implementation, and evaluation process are specific to the family and the family nursing diagnosis. The plan, implementation, and evaluation will be designed based on the evidence collected in the assessment and the prognosis statement.

During the planning stage, it is important for the nurse to recognize that the family has the right to make its own health decisions. The role of the nurse is to offer guidance to the family, provide information, and assist in the planning process. An important part of the planning phase is to determine who does what. The nurse may assist the family by (1) providing direct care that the family cannot; (2) removing barriers to needed services, which facilitates the family functioning; and (3) improving the capacity of the family to act on its own behalf and assume responsibility (Friedman, 1992, p. 42).

In the reflective critical thinking process, the nurse should ask the following questions while assisting the family in designing the plan of action:

1. Will the proposed approaches result in increased dependence or increased independence on the part of the family?
2. Is this action within the information and skill level of the family members or their own resources?
3. Will this action diminish or strengthen the coping ability of the family? (Dyer, 1973)
4. Does the family and/or its members have sufficient commitment and motivation to adhere to the plan?
5. Are there adequate resources available to carry out the plan? (Friedman, 1992, p. 48)

Building the plan of action for the family on family strengths increases the probability that the family will achieve the desired outcome. Once the plan has been developed and all individuals involved have approved or committed to the plan, the plan is put into effect. Data collection continues throughout the implementation phase and is part of the formative evaluation process. When a plan is not working well, the nurse and the family should work together to determine the barriers to implementation. Friedman (1992) identified that family apathy and indecision are often barriers to implementation. Family apathy may occur because of value differences between the nurse and the family; the family may be overcome with a sense of hopelessness; the problems may be viewed by the family as too overwhelming, and the family may have a fear of failure. Additional factors to be considered include the following issues: the family may be indecisive because they cannot determine which course of action is better; the family may have an unexpressed fear or concern; or the family may have a pattern of de facto decision making (Wright and Levac, 1993).

The evaluation process contains both formative (ongoing) and summative (ending) evaluation components. The evaluation is based on the family outcomes and response to the plan, not the success of the interventions. An important part of the plan is the termination of the relationship between the nurse and the family.

Termination of the Nurse-Family Relationship

The termination phase is the exiting of the nurse from the family system. When termination is built into the plan, the family benefits from a smooth transition process. The family is given credit for the outcomes of the plan they helped design. Strategies often used in the termination component are to reduce frequency of sessions with the nurse, extend invitations to the family for follow-up, and make referrals when appropriate. The termination should include a summative evaluation meeting in which the nurse and family put a formal closure to their relationship (Herriott, 1982; Yalom, 1985).

When termination occurs suddenly, it is important for the nurse to determine the forces bringing about the closure. The family may be initiating the termination prematurely, which requires a renegotiation process, or the insurance or agency requirements may be placing a financial constraint on the amount of time the nurse can work with a family. Regardless of how termination comes about, it is an important aspect in the family nursing process.

The family nursing process summarized in this section represents a critical thinking approach to working with families. The assessment aspect of the nursing process is a crucial component to successful intervention and is described in detail in the next section.

FAMILY NURSING ASSESSMENT: MODELS AND STRATEGIES

Assessing and intervening for family health is a systematic process requiring a conceptual framework and an approach that provides data as a foundation for action.

Two family assessment models and approaches are presented: the Family Assessment Intervention Model and the Family Systems Stressor Strength Inventory (FS³I) (Berkey and Hanson, 1991; Hanson and Mischke, 1996; Mischke-Berkey et al., 1989) and the

Research Brief

Boyd ST, Hanson SMH: Theoretical and research foundations. In Hanson SMH, Boyd ST, editors: *Family health care nursing: theory, practice and research*, Philadelphia, FA Davis (in press).

There are many issues pertaining to family nursing assessment and intervention that need to be studied. Although family social science has been around for the last 25 years, the field focused their previous work on the theoretical foundations of family and just recently looked at family health and the application of theory to practice. Concurrently, nursing research is also about 25 years old and has focused largely on individuals rather than on the family as a unit. The merger of family social science and family therapy into nursing to form a new specialty called family nursing has only received attention in the last 5 years. Much work yet needs to be done by family nursing researchers. Considerations for research include the following:

1. Development of additional family nursing assessment models. At the present time there are three major models: Mischke-Berkey and Hanson (1991), Friedman (1992), and Wright and Leahey (1994), all of which have a very different focus and yield different data.

2. Field test the existing family nursing assessment models. The existing three models mentioned above have received very little field testing for clinical or research utility.

3. Develop measurement instruments that are psychometrically tested specifically for nursing of families. In fact, very little measurement instrumentation has been developed by and for nurses or for use with families as a unit.

4. Field test existing family measurement instruments for their adaptability to family nursing and family health. There are hundreds of instruments purportedly developed for use in family social science, but they have not been adapted for clinical use in health care.

5. Further work needs to be done on diagnostic taxonomies that focus on families as a unit of analysis/care. Presently the health care model is driven by individual diagnostic taxonomies, which influence the kind of care nurses give families.

6. There is a need for a paradigm shift from individual health care to family health care. Most students of nursing are not educated in family assessment. Nursing educators need to find ways to teach more effective ways of teaching family concepts to nursing students of all levels.

Friedman Family Assessment Model and Short Form (Friedman, 1992). The Calgary Family Assessment and Intervention Models (CFAM and CFIM) (Wright and Leahey, 1984, 1994) is another general theoretical approach presented elsewhere in the nursing literature. Nurses are encouraged to select the model and strategy that provide the best fit to their particular philosophy and practice, or nurses can use a combination of both.

The Family Assessment Intervention Model and the Family Systems Stressor Strength Inventory

The **Family Assessment Intervention Model** is based on an extension of Betty Neuman's Health Care Systems Model and uses a family as client approach (Berkey and Hanson, 1991; Neuman, 1989; Reed, 1993).

In this model, families are subject to the tensions produced when stressors (see arrows in Figure 26-1), in the form of problems, penetrate through their de-

fense system. The family's reaction depends on how deeply the stressor penetrates the family unit and how capable the family is of adapting to maintain its stability. The lines of resistance protect the family's basic structure, which includes the family's functions and energy resources. The core contains the patterns of family interactions and unit strengths. The basic family structure must be protected at all costs or the family will cease to exist. Reconstitution or adaptation is the work the family undertakes to preserve or restore impaired family stability after stressors penetrate the family lines of defense, altering usual family functions. The model addresses three areas: (1) health promotion, wellness activities, problem identification, and family factors at lines of defense and resistance; (2) family reaction and stability at lines of defense and resistance; and (3) restoration of family stability and family functioning at levels of prevention. The basic assumptions for this family-focused model are listed in the box on p. 506.

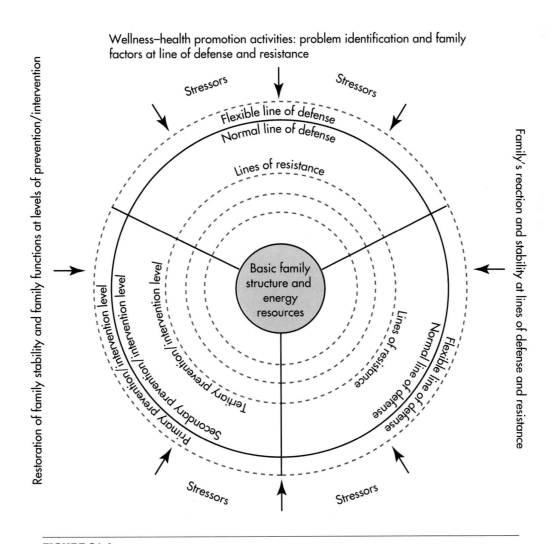

FIGURE 26-1

Family assessment intervention model. (From Mischke-Berkey KM, Warner P, Hanson SMH: In PJ Bomar, editor, *Nurses and family health promotion: concepts, assessment, and interventions,* Philadelphia, 1989, WB Saunders.)

Basic Assumptions for Family Assessment and Intervention Model

1. Though each family as a family system is unique, each system is a composite of common, known factors or innate characteristics within a normal, given range of response contained within a basic structure.

2. Many known, unknown, and universal environmental stressors exist. Each differs in its potential for disturbing a family's usual stability level, or normal line of defense. The particular interrelationships of family variables—physiological, psychological, sociocultural, developmental, and spiritual—at any time can affect the degree to which a family is protected by the flexible line of defense against possible reaction to one or more stressors.

3. Over time, each family/family system has evolved a normal range of response to the environment, referred to as a normal line of defense, or usual wellness/stability state.

4. When the cushioning, accordion-like effect of the flexible line of defense is no longer capable of protecting the family/family system against an environmental stressor, the stressor breaks through the normal line of defense. The interrelationships of variables—physiological, psychological, sociocultural, developmental, and spiritual—determine the nature and degree of the system reaction or possible reaction to the stressor.

5. The family, whether in a state of wellness or illness, is a dynamic composite of the interrelationships of variables—physiological, psychological, sociocultural, developmental, and spiritual. Wellness is on a continuum of available energy to support the system in its optimal state.

6. Implicit within each family system is a set of internal resistance factors, known as lines of resistance, that function to stabilize and return the family to the usual wellness state (normal line of defense), or possibly to a higher level of stability, following an environmental stressor reaction.

7. *Primary prevention* relates to general knowledge that is applied in family assessment and intervention in identification and mitigation of risk factors associated with environmental stressors to prevent possible reaction.

8. *Secondary prevention* relates to symptomatology following reaction to stressors, appropriate ranking of intervention priorities, and early treatment to reduce their noxious effects.

9. *Tertiary prevention* relates to the adjustive and restructive processes taking place as reconstitution begins and maintenance factors move the client back in a circular manner toward primary prevention. Primary prevention coexists with tertiary (e.g., a family recovering from mental illness of one of its members, still needs primary prevention R/T other aspects of health, such as nutrition, sleep/rest, immunizations, seat belt use, etc.).

10. The family is in dynamic, constant energy exchange with the environment.

Modified from Berkey KM, Hanson SMH: *Pocket guide to family assessment and intervention,* St Louis, 1991, Mosby, pp 23-24.
Neuman B: The Neuman systems model. In Neuman B, editor: *The Neuman systems model,* ed 2, Norwalk, Conn, 1989, Appleton & Lange.

An assessment instrument based on this model was developed and named the **Family Systems Stressor Strength Inventory (FS³I)** (Berkey and Hanson, 1991). The FS³I is a family health assessment/measurement instrument that provides for quantitative and qualitative input by all family members and the nurse. It focuses on identifying stressful situations occurring in families and the strengths families use to maintain health functioning despite their problems. The FS³I is divided into three sections: (1) Family Systems Stressors: General, (2) Family Stressors: Specific, and (3) Family System Strengths. A sample FS³I form is shown in Figures 26-2, 26-3, and 26-4. The forms are completed using data concerning the Jeddi Family, which is discussed in the Clinical Application section at the conclusion of this chapter.

The data collected by this instrument determine the level of prevention/intervention needed: primary, secondary, and tertiary (Pender et al., 1992). The primary prevention mode focuses on movement of the individual and family toward a positively balanced state of increased health or health promotion activities. Primary interventions include providing families with information about their strengths, supporting their coping and functioning capabilities, and encouraging attempts toward wellness through family education. Secondary prevention modes address actions necessary to attain system stability after the family system has been invaded by stressors or problems. Secondary interventions include helping the family to handle their problems, helping them find and use appropriate treatment, and intervening in crisis. The tertiary prevention mode encompasses those actions instituted to maintain systems stability. Tertiary intervention strategies are initiated after treatment has been completed and may include coordination of care following discharge from the hospital or rehabilitation services.

In summary, the FS³I focuses on two concepts of family health: family stressors and family strengths. It provides nurses with entrée into the family system to gather data useful for nursing intervention.

The Friedman Family Assessment Model

The **Friedman Family Assessment Model** (Friedman, 1992) draws heavily on the structural-functional framework, as well as on developmental and systems theory. The scope of this model is very broad. It takes a macroscopic approach to family assessment, which views families as a subsystem of larger society. The family is conceptualized as an open social system. The family's structure (organization) and functions (activities and purposes) and the family's relationship to other social systems are the focus of this approach.

This assessment approach is important for family nurses because it enables them to assess the family system as a whole, as part of the whole of society, and as an interaction system. The general assumptions for this model are listed in the box on p. 509.

The guidelines for the Friedman Assessment Model consist of six broad categories of interview questions: (1) identifying data; (2) developmental family stage and history; (3) environmental data; (4) family structure, including communication, power structures, role structures, and family values; (5) family functions, in-

Directions: Graph the scores from each family member inventory by placing an **X** at the appropriate location. (Use first name initial for each different entry and a different color code for each family member.)

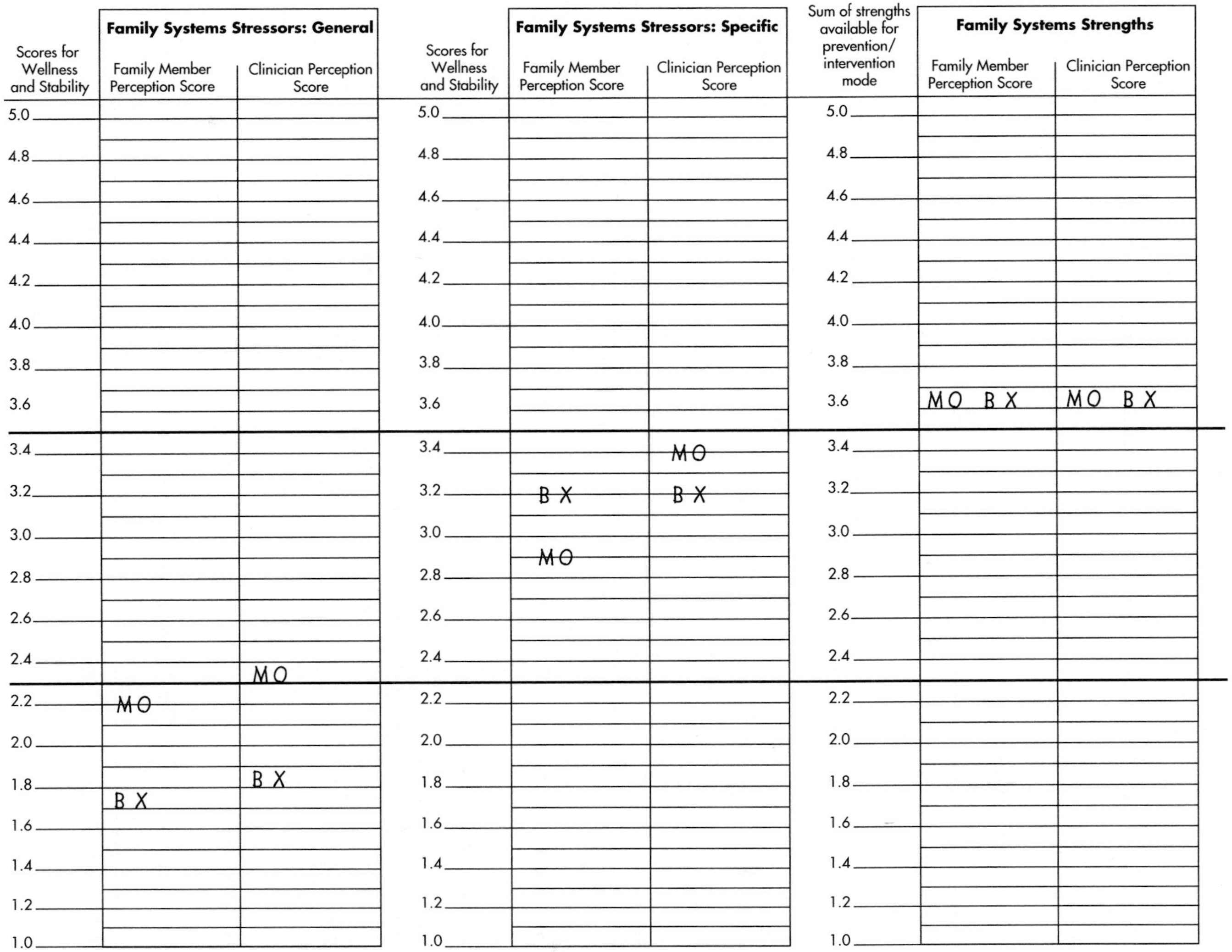

Scores for Wellness and Stability	Family Systems Stressors: General		Scores for Wellness and Stability	Family Systems Stressors: Specific		Sum of strengths available for prevention/ intervention mode	Family Systems Strengths	
	Family Member Perception Score	Clinician Perception Score		Family Member Perception Score	Clinician Perception Score		Family Member Perception Score	Clinician Perception Score
5.0			5.0			5.0		
4.8			4.8			4.8		
4.6			4.6			4.6		
4.4			4.4			4.4		
4.2			4.2			4.2		
4.0			4.0			4.0		
3.8			3.8			3.8		
3.6			3.6			3.6	M O B X	M O B X
3.4			3.4		M O	3.4		
3.2			3.2	B X	B X	3.2		
3.0			3.0	M O		3.0		
2.8			2.8			2.8		
2.6			2.6			2.6		
2.4		M O	2.4			2.4		
2.2	M O		2.2			2.2		
2.0			2.0			2.0		
1.8	B X	B X	1.8			1.8		
1.6			1.6			1.6		
1.4			1.4			1.4		
1.2			1.2			1.2		
1.0			1.0			1.0		

- **PRIMARY** Prevention/Intervention Mode: Flexible Line   1.0 - 2.3
- **SECONDARY** Prevention/Intervention Mode: Normal Line   2.4 - 3.6
- **TERTIARY** Prevention/Intervention Mode: Resistance Lines   3.7 - 5.0

- Breakdown of numerical scores for stressor penetration are suggested values

FIGURE 26-2

FS³I quantitative summary of the Jeddi family.

Part I: Family Systems Stressors: General

Summarize general stressors and remarks of family and clinician. Prioritize stressors according to importance to family members.

Ben: General stressors are: lower self-image, dieting, and adopting new child.

Mare: General stressors are: Guilt for not doing more; adopting new child.

Tom: lower self-image; dieting; housekeeping; lack of shared responsibility; knee problem.

Part II: Family Systems Stressors: Specific

A. Summarize specific stressor and remarks of family and clinician.

Both Ben and Mare feel the adoption of new child is the most important stressor; specifically,

Mare is concerned about time management relative to cooking healthy meals for the family. Nurse

sees these stressors higher than Ben and Mare.

B. Summarize differences (if discrepancies exist) between how family members and clinician view effects of stressful situation on family.

Both Ben and Mare see this stressor similarly, but Mare also sees several other related family

stressors, particularly the lack of shared responsibilities.

C. Summarize overall family functioning.

Family is functioning well overall with this stressor, but as the adoption gets closer the

stress level will continue to rise; both are perfectionists and first time parents. They

communicate well and are now open to help from the outside.

D. Summarize overall significant physical health status for family members.

Ben: OK, but stressed.

Mare: Stressed and concerned about knee problem which increases her emotional lability.

Tom: Healthy; small for age in both height and weight; mild developmental delay.

E. Summarize overall significant mental health status for family members.

The family members are stressed, but not in a crisis mode. They talk openly about concerns, and

they help each other emotionally.

Part III: Family Systems Strengths

Summarize family systems strengths, as well as family and clinician remarks that facilitate family health and stability.

The major strengths are open, honest communication between Ben and Mare and their experience with

solving problems, both together and independently. They recently have opened their closed family

boundary to help from extended family, friends, and professionals.

FIGURE 26-3
FS³I qualitative summary of the Jeddi family.

Diagnosis: general and specific family system stressors	Prognosis goals: family and clinician	Family systems: strengths supporting family care plan	Prevention/Intervention mode		Outcomes: evaluation and replanning
			Primary, secondary, or tertiary	Prevention/intervention activities	
1. Family life cycle transition: Stress related to adoption of 4-year-old boy from Russia.	1. Excellent prognosis with anticipatory guidance, information, and history of problem solving.	Family communication. Family commitment to adoption.	Primary	1a. Offer educational material on families with preschool child and adopting issues found when adopting older child. 1b. Introduce family to adoption support groups and networks. 1c. Have family identify resources in the event of developing needs related to new family member.	1a. Discuss normal family stressors. 1b. Attend support group. 1c. Written list of possible resources.
2. Family nutrition management: Stress related to adoption, ongoing eating patterns, and family health problems.	2. Good prognosis because they had faced this problem before. Investigate prior problems family had with last cook. Poor self-images will take time to affect.	Family communication. Family known problem solvers.	Secondary	2a. Provide sources to contact where family can hire a cook. 2b. Investigate why they did not follow through with their last cook. 2c. Education on nutrition for 4-yr-old.	2a. and b. Contact and hire a cook. 2c. Design healthy family meal plan for 1 month.

FIGURE 26-4

FS³I Family care plan for the Jeddi family.

Assumptions Underlying Friedman's Family Assessment Model

1. The family is a social system with functional requirements.
2. A family is a small group possessing certain generic features common to all small groups.
3. The family as a social system accomplishes functions that serve the individual in addition to the society.
4. Individuals act in accordance with a set of internalized norms and values that are learned primarily in the family through socialization.

Modified from Friedman MM: *Family nursing: theory and practice,* ed 3, Norwalk, Conn, 1992, Appleton & Lange, p 74.

cluding affective, socialization, and health care; and (6) family coping. Each category has several subcategories. Both a long and a short form of this assessment tool are available. The short form is applied to a sample family in the clinical application of this chapter.

In summary, this approach was developed to provide guidelines for family nurses who are interviewing a family to gain an overall view of what is going on in the family. The possible questions are quite extensive and it may not be possible to collect all the data at one visit. All the categories may not be pertinent for every family.

Summary of Family Assessment Models

Each family nursing assessment model and approach is unique and creates a different data base upon which to plan interventions. The *Family Assessment Intervention Model and the Family Systems Stressor Strength Inventory (FS³I)* measure very specific dimensions and give a microscopic view of family health. The *Friedman Family Assessment Model* is more broad and general. It is particularly useful for viewing families in the context of their communities. Examples of completed family assessment tools are in the clinical application section of this chapter.

GENOGRAMS AND ECOMAPS

The genogram and ecomap are essential components of any family assessment; they should be used concurrently with either one or both of the assessment approaches just described.

Outline for Brief Genogram Interview

For each person on the genogram the following information may be included. The nurse should determine which of the following information is relevant to include on the genogram, depending on the issues the family is concerned about.

first name
age
date of birth
occupation
health problems
cause of death
dates of marriages, divorces, separations, dates of commitments, dates of cohabitation, and remarriages
education level
ethnic or religious background

Modified from McGoldrick M, Gerson R: *Genograms in family assessments*, New York, 1985, WW Norton, pp 157-158.

 Genogram Interpretive Categories

The following areas are important to observe in the family genogram:

1. Family Structure: nuclear, blended, single-parent household, gay-lesbian relationship, co-habitation, divorces, separations
2. Sibling Subsystem Group: birth order, gender, distance between age of children
3. Pattern of Repetition: look for patterns of repetition across the generations relative to family structure, family behaviors, family health problems, patterns of relationships, family violence, abuse issues, and poverty
4. Life events: look for similar types of events across generations, family transitions, family traumas

Modified from McGoldrick M, Gerson R: *Genograms in family assessment*, New York, 1985, WW Norton, pp 159-160.

Genogram

The **genogram** displays pertinent family information in a family tree format that shows family members and their relationships over at least three generations (McGoldrick and Gerson, 1985). The genogram shows family history and patterns of health-related information (Bowen, 1985), providing a rich source of information from which to plan interventions. The identified patient (IP) and the family are highlighted on the genogram. Genograms enhance nurses' capacities to make clinical hypotheses and connect them to family context and history.

A sample of a three-generation genogram is depicted in Figure 26-5 and is discussed in the Clinical Application section of this chapter. The symbols most often used in a genogram are shown in Figure 26-6. An outline for a brief genogram interview is located in the box above, left, with genogram interpretive categories above, right. The health history for all family members (morbidity, mortality, onset of illness) is important information for family nurses and can be the focus of analysis of the family genogram. Most families are cooperative and interested in completing their genogram. A genogram does not have to be completed in one sitting and becomes a part of the ongoing health care record.

Ecomap

The **ecomap** is a visual representation of the family unit in relation to the community around them (Hartman, 1978). An example of a completed ecomap is depicted in Figure 26-7, and the case of the Jeddi family is discussed in the Clinical Application section at the conclusion of this chapter. The ecomap serves as a tool to organize and present a great deal of factual information and thus allows the nurse to have a more holistic and integrated perception of the family situation. The ecomap shows the nature of the relationships between family members and between family members and the world around them; it is "an overview of the family in their situation, picturing both the important nurturant and stress-producing connections between the family and the world" (Ross and Cobb, 1990, p. 176). The nurse starts with a blank ecomap, which consists of a large circle with smaller circles around it. The identified patient and their family are placed in the center of the large circle in a genogram format. The outer smaller circles around the family unit represent "significant people, agencies, or institutions in the family's context" (Wright and Leahey, 1984, p. 36) that interact with the different family members. The nature, quality of the relationships, and direction of energy flow between the family members and the subsystems are depicted by different connection lines.

The ecomap serves as a tool to organize and present information, allowing the nurses to have a more holistic and integrated perception of the family situation. Not only does it portray the present situation, but it can be used to set goals for the future by encouraging connection and exchange with individuals and agencies in the community. A more detailed discussion of ecomapping can be found in Hartman (1978), McGoldrick and Gerson (1985) and Ross and Cobb (1990).

FUTURE IMPLICATIONS FOR NURSING AND FAMILY POLICY

Family Nursing

Family nursing practice is an evolving area of nursing (Kirschling et al., 1994) and will continue to be a significant aspect of health care in the future, especially with the current focus of health care reform in the United States. The barriers confronting the practice of family nursing need to be integral aspects addressed in the new health care delivery system.

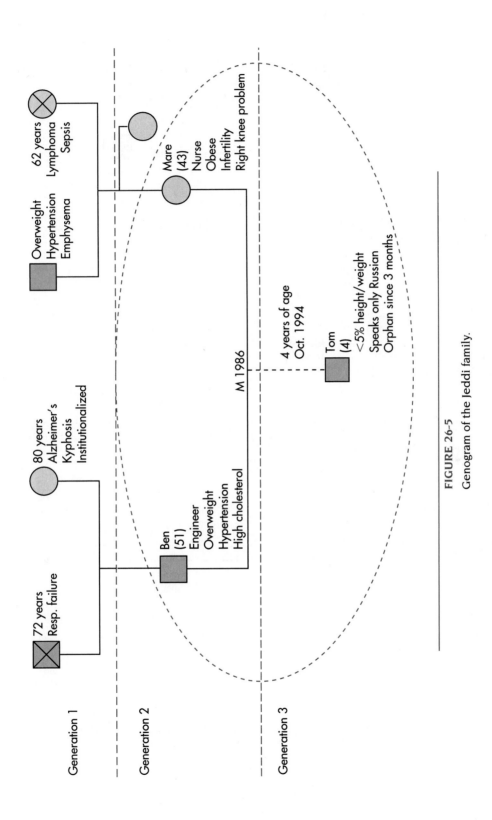

FIGURE 26-5
Genogram of the Jeddi family.

Symbols to describe basic family membership and structure.

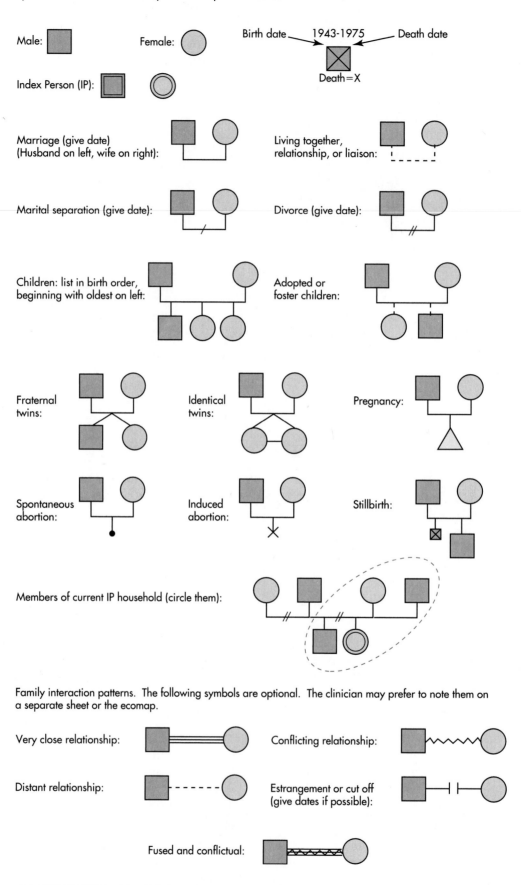

FIGURE 26-6

Genogram symbols. (Modified from McGoldrick M, Gerson R: *Genograms in family assessment,* New York, 1985, WW Norton.

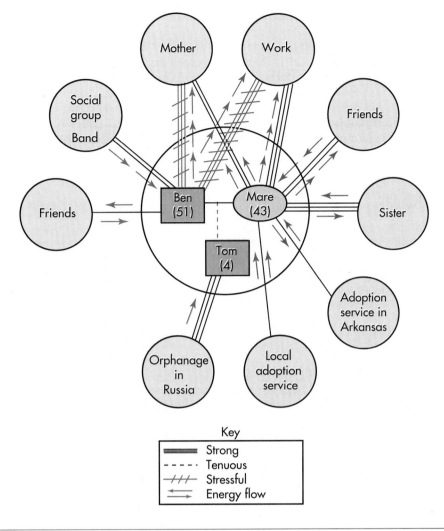

FIGURE 26-7

Ecomap of the Jeddi family.

Family Policy

Most nursing research has focused on the individual, not family health care. Research pertaining to family and mental health is further advanced than that regarding family and physical health (Campbell, 1985). Recently nursing has awakened to the connection between family dynamics and health and illness. More family-centered research needs to be done by family nurses.

Family nursing education is being included more in nursing curricula than in the past in both the United States and Canada. Recent studies in family nursing education (Hanson and Heims, 1993; Hanson et al., 1992) reported these findings: (1) more family content is being included in undergraduate and graduate nursing curricula but could be made more explicit; (2) an eclectic approach to family assessment is taught rather than the use of specific models; and (3) many clinical practicums are still focused on individuals rather than families as a whole. For family nursing to be practiced in community-based settings more nurses need to be educated in family nursing.

As professionals, nurses are accountable for participating in the development of legislation and family policy. Governmental actions that have a direct or indirect impact on families are considered family policy. All governmental actions, whether at the local, county, state, or national level, affect the family either directly or indirectly. The range of social policy decisions that affect families is vast and includes such areas as health care access and coverage, low-income housing, social security, welfare, food stamps, pension plans, affirmative action, and education. "Although all governmental policies affect families, in both negative and positive ways, the United States has no overall, official explicit family policy" (Zimmerman, 1992, p. 4).

Most governmental policy indirectly affects families. Much debate has taken place within governmental bodies regarding the definition of family. An argument often cited for the lack of more explicit family policies related to the financial burden that would occur if the definition of family was too broad.

The National Health Promotion and Disease Prevention Objectives outlined in both *Healthy People 2000* (Healthy People 2000, 1991) and *Healthy Communities 2000* (Healthy Communities 2000, 1991) have direct and indirect consequences and outcomes that affect families. Equally important today is the role that families will be assigned in the new health care reform. Because families are a primary source for health care beliefs and delivery, it is paramount that the issues of families and their place in the health care reform be overt. "All policies impact families, strengthening or diminishing their ability to sustain themselves and to prepare the next generation" (Elliott, 1993, p. ii). According to Jocelyn Elders, former U.S. Surgeon General, "poverty, unplanned pregnancies, drug and alcohol abuse, and family violence have become the central issues of public health in the 1990s" (Elders and Tuteur, 1993, p. 2).

 ## Clinical Application

The Jeddi family is a real family in a real situation. They came to the attention of the nurse when the family was referred to the county home health agency for a baseline family assessment with their impending adoption of Tom, a 4-year-old boy from Russia. This upper-middle-class, Caucasian family consists of Ben (age 51), Mare (age 43), and Tom, the 4-year-old son they will adopt. See Figure 26-5 for the Jeddi family genogram and Figure 26-7 for the Jeddi family ecomap.

Ben and Mare have been married for 8 years. Ben has a PhD in chemical engineering and does consulting work. His business is located in the caretaker apartment located in the basement of their home. Mare has a PhD, is a pediatric nurse, and teaches at a private university. They are adopting a 4-year-old boy from Russia. Mare has a diagnosis of infertility after 2 years of trying to have a biological child and extensive testing. The infertility issue was a significant loss for both Ben and Mare. The couple considered in vitro fertilization. Mare decided against this approach because she felt the risks of failure of pregnancy and miscarriage were too great. Ben felt that this was Mare's decision to make because it more directly involved her physical and mental health. He supported Mare's decision to not pursue in vitro fertilization.

Mare initiated the discussions about adoption. The decision to adopt a child was reached in May of this year after a year and a half of discussion and investigation. Initially, Ben was not equally committed to the concept of adoption and had a longer grieving process over their inability to have a child together than Mare. The issue of biological heritage and the loss of blood lineage were more significant to Ben. The significant issue for Mare was the loss of being a parent and raising a child.

The couple investigated several adoption agencies and attended potential adoptive parent classes a year and a half ago. At that time, Ben was not ready to make a commitment to adoption. The topic of adoption repeatedly was discussed by the couple over the course of the next year. In January 1994, the couple again seriously considered adoption. Mare investigated several adoption agencies again because she was not satisfied with the one they selected the last time. A local adoption agency was found to be supportive and informative for them. The couple attended an information meeting. After much intense emotional discussion, the couple pursued more information about adoption with the support personnel from the agency. At the end of May, Ben and Mare decided they wanted to adopt a child and completed the application process.

Both Ben and Mare feel this was an emotional time for them. After they made their decision to adopt, the next steps were to decide from which country they wanted to adopt a child, the child's age, and which child. They decided that given their life-styles and personalities that they wanted to adopt an older child between 3 and 5 years of age and not an infant. Ben wanted to adopt a son. Mare was not selective of the gender. The issue of race was important to Ben because he felt that he might have difficulty bonding with a child of darker skin as his own family. Because of Ben's immediate family origins from Finland, they decided to adopt a child from Eastern Europe. Russia was selected because of its historical ties with Finland.

Mare reviewed video tapes of 40 children and selected the top male children for them to select from. Mare is a pediatric nurse and was determined to be the one to make the decisions about health. After viewing the films numerous times and reviewing a medical examination, Tom was the young child of choice. Ben and Mare made a formal petition to adopt Tom.

The process has taken 6 months. They are currently waiting for the final paper work to arrive from the Russian government, which is expected in the next few days. They are in the midst of preparing their home for the arrival of Tom. They will both travel to Russia in 2 weeks to pick him up, complete the formal adoption process in Russia, and travel home together as a new family.

They are nervous and excited about the adoption. They are concerned about how Tom will adjust to them and the move to America. They are concerned about how adopting a 4-year-old will change their life-style. The preparation of their home for the arrival of Tom has been time consuming. The arrangements for travel to Russia are being finalized. Ben

Clinical Application—cont'd

had studied Russian for 2 years 20 years ago; both are currently taking individual language tutoring in Russian. Ben and Mare currently work full-time. Mare plans to continue working full-time after they adopt Tom, but she does have a reduced workload for the next 4 months. They plan to have Tom attend preschool full-time.

The initial assessment of the Jeddi family involved the use of two assessment approaches with their respective instruments, guidelines, a genogram, and an ecomap. A summary of the findings from this assessment follows.

Family Systems Stressor Strength Inventory
The FS³I is presented, which focused on the Jeddi family stressors and strengths to create a plan of action. Ben and Mare were interviewed together in their home by the nurse. Each person completed the FS³I, which provided individual and composite scores. Figure 26-5 presents the completed genogram. Figure 26-7 shows the Jeddi family ecomap. Figure 26-2 provides the scoring for the quantitative summary of stressors and strengths. A qualitative summary (Figure 26-3) presents a brief picture of the family stresses and strengths and served as the guide for the family care plan (Figure 26-4).

The general stressors of the family were the impending adoption of Tom, issues of family nutrition and dieting, and lowered self-image for both Ben and Mare. Mare was found to have a higher general stress level than Ben. She states that in addition to the above stressors she is concerned about stress relative to housekeeping issues, an ongoing physical problem with her knee, and guilt for not accomplishing more than she presently is able. Ben noted that issues related to his mother, who has Alzheimer's disease and lives in an assisted living center, cause him additional stress. The nurse rated their general and specific stressors higher than both Ben and Mare.

The specific stressor identified by Ben that is causing him the most stress is the impending adoption of Tom. He is concerned about time management with work and a new family member. The additional stress of his mother's care is requiring a lot of his time. She is well taken care of in an assisted living center, but he is concerned about her advancing dementia. At present he is actively involved in renting out his mother's home.

The specific stressor identified by Mare was how she is going to manage food preparations and meal times after they adopt Tom. She stated that cooking and meal preparation are currently a big problem for her. Mare stated that Ben does not help with food preparation or clean up now. They both eat on different schedules. She is concerned about family dinners and feels this will be an important time for them with Tom. Food preparation is not a new issue for them. She stated that she feels pressured and "like a

failure" because she does not manage this aspect of their family life well now, without the addition of Tom. In the past the family has hired a cook which was an "excellent solution" for them. They have been without a cook for 2 years now since their previous cook moved out of state.

The strengths of this family are many. They scored their individual strengths inventory almost identically, which demonstrates a similar perception of their family unit. Both Ben and Mare viewed their family and each other as experienced problem solvers. They have good, open communication between them and feel that the adoption of Tom has brought them even closer together. They recognized that much of their current stress is related to the unknown about Tom. They feel that once they meet Tom that they will be able to work together to solve their problems.

The nurse concluded that this family has the strengths they need to adapt to their new family life cycle of a family with a preschooler. In looking at the ecomap, the family is found to be well supported by resources. They are responsive to information provided to them and to ideas suggested by others for them to consider in their problem solving.

Friedman Family Assessment Form
 Identifying Data
 Ben and Mare Jeddi
 Portland, Maine
 Type of family: Nuclear
 Ethnic background: Ben comes from a Finnish
        background
        Mare has no particular ethnic
        identity
 Religious: no affiliation
 Social Class: upper middle class
 Leisure activities: travel, gardening, music
 Occupations: Ben, consulting chemical engineer
       Mare, pediatric nurse and university
       faculty

Developmental Stage and History of Family
The family's present developmental stage cannot be defined in the conventional family life cycle. Ben and Mare have been married for 8 years, so they do not fit the categories for beginning families or families with children. However, they are in transition with the adoption of a 4-year-old boy. The family will fit into the classical family life cycle stage of family with preschooler.

Ben comes from a nuclear family of origin, however, his parents were divorced after 30 years of marriage. Mare comes from a nuclear family of origin.

Environmental Data
The family live in an upper-middle-class urban neighborhood that is ethnically diverse. They are within close distance of schools, hospitals, fire department, and shopping areas. The neighborhood is clean and

Continued.

Clinical Application—cont'd

considered relatively safe since there have been few burglaries in the neighborhood. Both attend the neighborhood community meetings. The family is centrally located only eight blocks from freeways around town, two miles from downtown, and five blocks from a bus route. Ben works in the home, where the basement caretaker apartment has been converted into his office and labs. Mare works at the University which is four miles away. She often rides her bike to work.

Their home is a 75-year-old brick house that has four levels. It is situated on the edge of a hollow. The home is well kept, but is old. Both Ben and Mare enjoy their home and spend a lot of time there. They are slowly remodeling. The house is safe, but with the adoption of a 4-year-old boy, several safety factors need to be addressed. There is no medicine cabinet in the bathroom and medicines are easily within reach of a 4-year-old. The cleaning solutions are kept under the sinks in the kitchen and the bathroom. The patio above the garage does have a railing, but a 4-year-old may be tempted to walk on it. A fire plan needs to be made for the family because all the bedrooms are on the top floor, which is three levels above the ground.

Family Structure

Communication is a strength of this family. There is an open relationship and communication pattern between Ben and Mare. Both are very verbal and expressive about their feelings, opinions, and needs. Because of this openness, they state that there is often conflict and arguing between them. However, they feel that they are good at conflict resolution. At times however, the argument does get out of control and takes a personal attack format. When they realize this, usually Mare suggests that they take up the conversation at a later time when they can both approach the topic more calmly. They are not worried about arguing in front of their son. They feel that their open, honest communication will be helpful in raising their son.

The decision making of the family is by consensus for important issues that affect the lives of both members. Otherwise, the decision-making style is accommodation. The power and decision making is more situational in that whoever has more experience with certain issues influences the decisions. For example, Mare is a nurse and has the referent power in health-related issues. Ben is a chemical engineer. He has referent power for concerns about fixing things in the house or with cars. Both state that a strength of their family is that they are both known problem solvers.

The role structure is typical relative to gender. Mare does the cooking, laundry, house cleaning, shopping, and kinship roles. Ben does the lawn mowing, carries out the garbage and services the cars.

Mare feels that she has more roles and expected behaviors of her than Ben does. They both work full-time outside the home. Both state they are concerned about role overload and time management issues with the adoption of their 4-year-old. Mare knows that she will be the primary care giver, but is not sure how much or in what way Ben will assist with these new role requirements. Ben is concerned about how much time the new child will demand and his ability to juggle all his work responsibilities and family responsibilities.

The family values are clear and shared by both Ben and Mare; they include: education; open, honest communication; family; health; diversity; caring and compassion for others.

Family Functions

Affective Function. Ben and Mare have a close, caring relationship and demonstrate a reciprocal emotional relationship. They are a close cohesive family. They are excited about expanding their family with the adoption of Thomas. They each state that the other is a major support person in their lives. The family has closed boundaries, but does look to extended family members for needed support. They express concern about their son's adjustment to them as parents because he has lived in an orphanage in Russia since the age of 3 months. They have investigated as much as possible about how other children adapt to their new situations. They plan to go to Russia to pick up their son, which will give them access to information about rules and rituals he is familiar with in the orphanage, and they plan to institute them in their home.

Socialization Function. Ben and Mare talk about the importance of their parenting their son. They openly have discussed discipline and have decided that they will use time out. They plan to be involved in the child-rearing practices of their son. Their son will be in full-time preschool. They plan to be active in the education process of their son.

Health Care Function. The family has a primary care physician for Ben and Mare, but they have not selected a pediatrician for their son. Ben sees the physician regularly for management of hypertension and high cholesterol. Mare rarely sees the doctor. They have a medical report for their son. He appears to be in good health, except he is below the fifth percentile for height and weight. He is current on immunizations, except hepatitis. They both have dental cleaning and exams every 6 months. They value health, yet both are overweight. Mare is obese. A major concern for Mare is a regular meal preparation for their son. At present, Ben and Mare do not eat dinner together on a regular basis. In the past they have hired a cook to assure that healthful meals were available, especially with Mare working full-time.

Clinical Application—cont'd

Family Coping

The short-term stressors for this family are the imminent adoption of their 4-year-old son from Russia in 3 weeks. They are concerned about his adaptation to his new environment, his ability to learn English, and how their lives will change with this adoption. Long-term stressors are not an issue at this time.

The family has a large repertoire of successful coping strategies. They have a pattern of problem solving issues to the best of their ability. They are seeking out information and garnering support from people and resources acceptable to them. They are a well-adjusted family unit. The family is open to education and information.

Summary of Assessments

In summary, both assessment approaches provided important information for the nurse and family to create the plan of action presented in the family care plan in the FS³I (Figure 26-4). There was some overlap of information, but the whole picture of the family was enhanced by merging data from both assessment tools.

Key Concepts

- Family nursing is a specialty area that has a strong theoretical base and is more than just common sense.
- Two significant barriers to practicing family nursing are the narrow definitions of both family and family health.
- Nurses should ask clients whom they consider to be family and then include those members in the nurse's health care plan.
- Throughout history health professionals have tended to classify clients and their families into good families and bad families.
- There are four approaches to viewing families: family as context, family as client, family as a system, and family as a component of society.
- The family nursing process is a dynamic, systematic, organized method of critically thinking about the family.
- The purpose of the initial family interview is to identify the health concerns of the family.
- The family nursing diagnosis is based on the nurse determining the actual issue of concern within the family.
- An important part of defining the family nursing process is continuous reflective questioning.
- The family prognosis is a realistic statement about the ability of the family to successfully adapt to the nursing diagnosis.
- It is essential in the beginning of the planning step to determine if the family's respose to the problem requires nursing intervention or should be referred to a different professional.
- It is important for the nurse to recognize that the family has the right to make its own health decisions.
- The nurse, in working with families, must evaluate the family outcomes and response to the plan, not the success of the interventions.
- Two family assessment models and approaches are the Family Assessment Intervention Model and the Family Systems Stressor Inventory.
- The Friedman Family assessment model takes a macroscopic approach to family assessment, which views families as a subsystem of a larger society.
- Family systems stressor inventory measures very specific dimensions and gives a microscopic view of health.
- The whole family picture is enhanced by merging data from both assessment tools.
- Genograms and ecomaps are essential components of any family assessment.

Critical Thinking Activities

1. Talk with your own family. Ask them how they define family.
2. Talk with a community health nurse, a home health nurse, and a pediatric nurse. Ask them how they define family nursing.
3. Discuss how family assessment fits into community health nursing with a community health nurse.
4. In an interview with a community health nurse, identify barriers to practicing family nursing in a community based setting. How do they compare to those listed in the chapter?
5. What kind of difficulties have you experienced when arranging for a family assessment interview with a client?
6. Describe and compare the Family Stressor and Strength Inventory Assessment Tool and the Friedman Family Assessment Instrument to those used in the agency in which you are doing your clinical practice.
7. Draw a family genogram and ecomap for your client family. Discuss how they are used in family nursing with your community health nurse preceptor.

Bibliography

Alfaro-LeFevre R: *Applying nursing process: a step-by-step process,* ed 3, Philadelphia, 1994, JB Lippincott.

Anderson KH, Tomlinson PS: The family health system as an emerging paradigmatic view for nursing, *Image: J Nurs Scholarship* 24:57-63, 1992.

Beavers W: *Successful marriage: a family systems approach to couple therapy,* New York, 1985, Norton.

Berkey KM, Hanson SMH: *Pocket Guide to family assessment and intervention,* St Louis, 1991, Mosby.

Bowen M: *Family therapy in clinical practice,* New York, 1985, John Wiley & Sons.

Boyd ST, Hanson SMH: Theoretical and research foundations. In Hanson SMH, Boyd ST, editors: *Family health care nursing: theory, practice and research,* Philadelphia, 1996, FA Davis.

Campbell T: *Family's impact on health: a critical review and annotated bibliography,* Washington, DC, 1985, US Government Printing Office, (DHHS Publication No ADM861461).

Carnevali D, Thomas M: *Diagnostic reasoning and treatment decision making in nursing,* Philadelphia, 1993, JB Lippincott.

Carpenito L: *Nursing diagnosis: application to clinical practice,* ed 5, Philadelphia, 1993, JB Lippincott.

Carter E, McGoldrick M: The family life cycle and family therapy: an overview. In Carter E, McGoldrick M, editors: *The family life cycle: a framework for family therapy,* New York, 1980, Gardner Press, pp 3-28.

Curran D: *Traits and the healthy family,* Minneapolis, 1983, Winston Press, Harper & Row.

Curran D: *Stress and the healthy family,* Minneapolis, 1985, Winston Press, Harper & Row.

Diagnostic and Statistical Manual of Mental Disorders (DSM-IV), ed 4, Washington, DC, 1994, American Psychiatric Association.

Dyer W: Working with groups. In Reinhardt A, Quinn M, editors: *Family-centered community nursing,* St Louis, 1973, Mosby.

Elders J, Tutuer J: Public health. In Elliott B, editor: *Vision 2010: families and health care,* Minneapolis, 1993, National Council on Family Relations.

Elliott B: *Vision 2010: families and health care,* Minneapolis, 1993, National Council on Family Relations.

Friedman MM: *Family nursing: theory and practice,* ed 3, Norwalk Conn, 1992, Appleton & Lange.

Gershwin MW, Nilsen JM: Healthy families: forms and processes. In Gilliss CL, Highley BC, Roberts BM, Martinson IM, editors: *Toward a science of family nursing,* Reading, Mass, 1989, Addison-Wesley.

Gillis CL: Father nursing research, theory and practice. In Wegner GD, Alexander RJ, editors: *Readings in Family Nursing,* Philadelphia, 1993, JB Lippincott.

Hanson SMH: *Defining family health.* Unpublished paper presented at the Annual Conference of the Oregon Council of Family Relations, 1985a, Portland, Ore.

Hanson SMH: *Family health inventory: a measurement.* Paper presented at the National Council of Family Relations, 1985b, Dallas.

Hanson SMH, Boyd S: *Family health care nursing: theory, practice and research,* Philadelphia, 1996, FA Davis.

Hanson SMH, Heims ML: Family nursing curricula in US schools of nursing, *Fam Relations* 31(7):303-308, 1993.

Hanson SMH, Heims ML, Julian DJ: Education for family health care professionals: nursing as a paradigm, *Family Relations* 41:49-53, 1992.

Hanson SMH, Mischke K: Family health assessment and intervention. In Bomar PJ, editor: *Nurses and family health promotion: concepts, assessment and interventions,* ed 2, Philadelphia, 1996, WB Saunders.

Hartman A: Diagrammatic assessment of family relationships, *Social Casework* 59:465-476, 1978.

Healthy Communities 2000: model standards: guidelines for community attainment of year 2000 national health objectives, Washington, DC, 1991, American Public Health Association.

Healthy People 2000: national health promotion and disease prevention objectives, Washington, DC, 1991, USDHHS, Public Health Service.

Herriott P: *Termination of the nurse-client relationship.* Unpublished manuscript, North Carolina Memorial Hospital, 1982, Chapel Hill.

International Classification of Diseases, ed 4, Washington, DC, 1991, US Department of Health and Human Services, (DHHS [PHS] No 91-1260).

Kirschling JM, Gilliss CL, Krentz L, Camburn CD, Clough RS, Duncan MT, Hendricks J, Howard JKH, Roberts C, Smith-Young J, Tice KS, Young T: "Success" in family nursing: experts describe phenomena, *Nurs Health Care* 15:186-189, 1994.

Martin K, Scheet M: *The Omaha system: application for community health nursing,* Philadelphia, 1992, WB Saunders.

McGoldrick M, Gerson R: *Genograms in family assessment,* New York, 1985, WW Norton.

Mischke-Berkey K, Warner P, Hanson SMH: Family health assessment and intervention. In Bomar PJ, editor: *Nurses and family health promotion: concepts, assessment, and interventions,* Philadelphia, 1989, WB Saunders, pp 115-154.

Neuman B: The Neuman systems model. In Neuman B, editor: *The Neuman systems model,* ed 2, Norwalk, Conn, 1989, Appleton & Lange, pp 3-50.

Otto H: Criteria for assessing family strengths, *Fam Process* 2:329-338, 1963.

Pender N, Barkauskas V, Hayman L, Rice V, Anderson E: Health promotion and disease prevention: toward excellence in nursing practice and education, *Nurs Outlook* 40:106-109, 1992.

Pratt L: *Family structure and effective health behavior: the energized family,* Boston, 1976, Houghton Mifflin.

Reed KS: *Betty Neuman: The Neuman systems model,* Newbury Park, Calif, 1993, Sage.

Ross B, Cobb KL: *Family nursing: a nursing process approach,* Redwood City, Calif, 1990, Addison-Wesley Nursing.

Satariano HJ, Briggs NJ: The good family syndrome. In Wegner GD,

Alexander RJ, editors: *Readings in family nursing,* Philadelphia, 1993, JB Lippincott.

Stinnett N, Chesser B, DeFrain J, editors: *Building family strengths: blue prints for action,* Lincoln, Neb, 1979, University of Nebraska Press.

Wright LM, Leahey M: *Nurses and families: a guide to family assessment and intervention,* Philadelphia, 1984, FA Davis.

Wright LM, Leahey M: *Nurses and families: a guide to family assessment and intervention,* ed 2, Philadelphia, 1994, FA Davis.

Wright LM, Levac AM: The nonexistence of noncompliant families: the influence of Humberta Maturana, *Journal of Advanced Nursing* 17:913-917, 1993. (Also in Feetham SL, Meister SB, Bell JM, Gillis CL, editors: *The nursing of families: theory/research education/practice,* Newbury Park, Calif, 1993, Sage Publications, pp 111-117.)

Yalom I: *The theory and practice of group psychotherapy,* ed 3, New York, 1985, Basic Books.

Zimmerman S: *Family policies and family well-being: the role of political culture,* Newbury Park, Calif, 1992, Sage International.

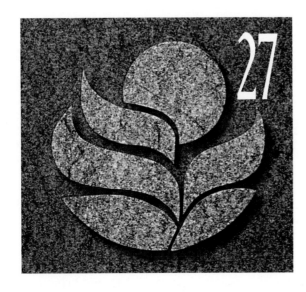

27 Children's Health

Marcia Cowan*

Objectives ▼

After reading this chapter, the student should be able to do the following:

◆ Identify significant physical and psychosocial developmental factors characteristic of the child and adolescent population.
◆ Identify the role of the community health nurse and discuss appropriate nursing interventions that promote and maintain the health of children and adolescents.
◆ Identify major health problems of children and adolescents.
◆ Identify the role of the community health nurse with specific at-risk populations in the community.
◆ Identify ways to promote child and adolescent health within the community.

Key Terms ▼

accommodation
assimilation
attention deficit disorder (ADD)
cognitive development
development
growth
homeless child syndrome
immunizations
infancy
neonatal period
preschool period
psychosocial development
secondhand smoke
sudden infant death syndrome (SIDS)
toddler period

*The author acknowledges the contribution of Nancy Dickenson-Hazard for the chapter in previous editions of this book, from which this chapter is revised.

Children are one third of our population and all of our future; their health is our foundation. Community health nurses have two major responsibilities in the area of child and adolescent health. The nurse is responsible for direct services to children and their families, including assessment, management of care, education, and counseling. Nurses are also involved in the assessment of the community and the establishment of programs to ensure a healthy environment for its children.

The role of the community health nurse offers the opportunity to teach health promotion, prevention, and health maintenance to children and caregivers and to provide family-centered care in the ambulatory setting. This chapter provides information on the assessment of child health within the family and community and activities to promote well-being. The content includes principles of growth and development from birth through adolescence and major health problems seen in this population. Families are vital to the growth and development of children, and family functioning is presented as a framework for nursing assessment and interventions. The chapter also focuses on the unique needs of children and families within the community based on *Healthy People 2000* objectives.

CHILD DEVELOPMENT
Physical Growth and Development

Growth is the quantitative or measurable aspects of the individual's size; **development** is the qualitative or observable aspects of changes in the individual. Progression through phases of growth and development are influenced by heredity and environmental factors. A unique feature of the pediatric population is the ongoing process of growth and development, resulting in physical, cognitive, and emotional changes. Health visits or well-child checkups are scheduled at key ages to monitor these processes. Nursing assessments include growth and health status, developmen-

Table 27-1   Guidelines for Well-Child Care

| | Age | | | | | | | | | | | | |
| | Months | | | | | | | Years | | | | | |
	2	4	6	9	12	15	18	2	3	4-6	8-10	12-14	16-18
Physical examination	•	•	•	•	•	•	•	•	•	•	•	•	•
Height/weight	•	•	•	•	•	•	•	•	•	•	•	•	•
Head circumference	•	•	•	•	•	•	•						
Blood pressure								•	•	•	•	•	•
Vision	s	s	s	s	s	s	s	s	s	•	•	•	•
Hearing	s	s	s	s	s	s	s	s	s	•	•	•	•
Developmental	•	•	•	•	•	•	•	•	•	•	•	•	•
Hematocrit/hemoglobin				•						•		•	
Urinalysis										•		•	
Tuberculosis skin test					•					•			
Lead level					•					•			
Anticipatory guidance:													
Feeding/nutrition	•	•	•	•	•	•	•	•	•	•	•	•	•
Growth/development	•	•	•	•	•	•	•	•	•	•	•	•	•
Behavior	•	•	•	•	•	•	•	•	•	•	•	•	•
Safety/poisons/injury	•	•	•	•	•	•	•	•	•	•	•	•	•
Sexual behaviors											a	a	a
Substance abuse											a	a	a
Physical activity										a	a	a	a

Modified from *American Academy of Pediatrics: Guidelines for health supervision. II,* Elk Grove Village, Ill, 1992, The Academy.

S, Subjectively determined by behavioral observations; *blank,* formal assessment as determined by history; *a,* as appropriate for age.

tal level, and the quality of the parent-child relationship. Table 27-1 identifies recommendations for schedules and components of well-child assessments as recommended by the American Academy of Pediatrics (AAP) and the *Guide to Clinical Preventive Services.* The nurse needs to be aware of issues of concern at each age. Assessment strategies and tools, common concerns and problems, and specific interventions for each age group are further discussed in Appendixes E and F.

In 1990 the U.S. Department of Health and Human Services (DHHS) and Public Health Service (PHS) released the report *Healthy People 2000: national health promotion and disease prevention objectives,* setting targets to improve health status, reduce risks, and improve health care services in the United States. One of the key objectives identified in the objectives is to increase the percentage of primary care providers who routinely screen children for vision, hearing, speech, and development to 80%. Community health nurses are in a position to achieve this objective.

Focus of Assessments

Neonates. The **neonatal period** is the time from birth to 1 month of age. Physiological stabilization and rapid growth highlight this time as the neonate completes the transition to extrauterine life. Weight gain averages $\frac{1}{2}$ to 1 ounce per day. Early discharge from the hospital at 24 hours of age often gives the community health nurse responsibility for assessing physical status, monitoring family adaptation, referring to community resources as indicated, and teaching infant

care (Table 27-2). The nurse should be aware of factors that place the infant at risk and danger signs indicating need for referral and management (see the box on p. 524).

Infants. **Infancy** extends from 1 month to 1 year. During this time, rapid growth continues as infants usually double the birth weight by 6 months and triple the birth weight by 1 year. Length usually increases by 10 to 12 inches (25 to 30 cm). Nurses identify and intervene in situations when the infant is at risk because of health or socioeconomic problems. Nursing interventions include monitoring of growth and development, with particular attention to areas of feeding, sleeping, elimination, and neuromotor development (Table 27-3).

Toddlers and Preschoolers. The **toddler period** is the second and third years of life. The **preschool period** encompasses ages 3 to 5 years. Slowing and stabilization of growth are hallmarks of this period, as reflected by changes in appetite and eating patterns. Increased physical abilities and expansion of cognitive skills enable increasing independence. Nursing interventions include monitoring of growth and neuromotor development, assessment of feeding and sleeping patterns, and initiation of dental and skeletal assessment (Table 27-4).

School-age Children. Physical growth is typically slow and steady until the preadolescent growth spurt. The growth spurt usually occurs between the ages of 9

Table 27-2 Assessing the Neonate

Assessment	Activity	Nursing implications
Apgar scoring	Observe and score newborn appearance, pulse, grimace, activity, and respiration.	Identify deviations. Influence management of well-infant care.
Gestational age	Indications of physical maturity; note number of weeks in utero.	Influence nutrition, education, development, care, and referral needs.
Physiological changes	Observe norms of: Average birth weight: 3400 with 100 to 200 g weekly gain by 1 month Average birth length: 49 cm with 1.2 to 2.5 cm monthly gain Average head circumference: 33 to 35 cm with 1.5 cm monthly gain	Periodically monitor weight, height, head and chest circumference, and vital signs. Influence infant care management and nutritional planning.
Reflex activity	Observe and assess for absence, asymmetry, or abnormal persistence.	Identify deviations.
Sensory function	Observe and assess for response to tactile, auditory, and taste stimulation and visual activity.	Identify deviations. Offer anticipatory guidance and education for parents.
Normal variations	Observe and assess for normal variations and minor abnormalities (see Appendix E.4).	Identify deviations. Offer anticipatory guidance and education for parents.

Danger Signs in the Newborn

Family history for major disease	Full, bulging fontanel
Gestational or delivery complications	Microcephaly
Abnormal positioning of neonate	Convulsions, jitteriness, irritability
Congenital malformations	Lethargy
Rapid or difficult respirations	Fever or hypothermia
Rapid, slow, or irregular pulse rate	Paralysis
Abnormal cry	Jaundice
Unusual cough	Pallor
Cyanosis	Petechiae
Sweating	Behavior or appearance change
Vomiting bile	Excessive salivation
Delayed or inadequate voiding	Diarrhea
Bleeding, especially cord and circumcision	No meconium passage in 48 hours
Single umbilical artery	Cord odor or exudate

Modified from Chow MP et al: *Handbook of pediatric primary care*, ed 2, New York, 1984, Wiley; and Behrman RE, Vaughan VC, editors: *Nelson textbook of pediatrics*, ed 13, Philadelphia, 1987, Saunders.

to 14 years for girls and 12 to 16 years for boys. During this time, neuromuscular and cognitive skills are refined and expanded. Sexual growth begins with the appearance of secondary sex characteristics (see Appendix F.7). Nursing interventions include monitoring and assessment of growth and sexual development, skeletal system, dental health, sleep and eating patterns, developing motor and cognitive skills, immunization status, and hearing and vision screening (Table 27-5). Nurses also encourage children and adolescents to take responsibility for their own health needs.

Health Assessment Tools

Growth Charts. Measurements of height, weight, and head circumference (until age 2 years) are recorded at each health visit to document the rate of growth. Measurements are plotted on standard growth curves and compared with normals for the age (see pediatric text for examples). It is important to note the child's pattern of growth rather than individual measurements. Most healthy children will follow the same percentile over time (see Appendix F.1).

Table 27-3   Assessing the Infant

Assessment	Activity	Nursing implications
Physiological stability	Monitor vital signs routinely.	Offer anticipatory guidance. Refer deviations.
Sleep patterns	Obtain history of patterns, comparing with normal of 16 hours with short alert (7 to 10 minutes) span for newborn; 10 hours at night, with 2- 3-hour day naps at 3 months; and 12 hours at night, with 1- 2-hour day naps at 12 months.	Provide anticipatory guidance for encouraging appropriate sleep/wake patterns.
Elimination patterns	Obtain history of patterns, comparing with normal of first meconium stools by 48 hours of life; soft, easily passed stools on a regular basis; and 6 to 8 wet diapers per day.	Identify elimination problems. Educate parents.
Feeding patterns	Obtain history of feeding patterns and techniques.	Identify and intervene with feeding problems. Educate and support parents.
Neuromotor development	Observe and obtain history relevant to normal cephalocaudal progression, from reflexive to purposeful and voluntary.	Identify developmental problems. Provide anticipatory guidance and education on techniques of promoting development.

Table 27-4 Assessing the Toddler and Preschool Child

Assessment	Activity	Nursing implications
Physical growth	Monitor growth, comparing with normal of annual weight gain of 5 pounds and height increases of 3 to 4 inches annually.	Identify deviant growth patterns. Provide anticipatory guidance regarding normal growth.
Skeletal development	Observe closure of anterior fontanel around 18 months and normal progression from bowlegs (12 to 18 months) to knock-knees (18 to 24 months) to normal.	Initiate orthopedic screening. Identify deviant skeletal problems. Provide education and reassurance regarding normal variations.
Dental growth	Inspect number and condition of teeth, comparing with normal of first tooth eruption about 6 months, 20 primary teeth by age 2, addition of molars between ages 3 to 8, and loss of first primary tooth at ages 5 to 6.	Identify dental problems. Provide education regarding early preventive dental care.
Sleep patterns	Obtain sleep history, comparing with normal of 8 to 12 hours of night sleep by 3 years, afternoon nap until 3 years, and establishment of bedtime routine.	Provide guidance regarding routine and common problems. Identify deviant sleep behaviors.
Feeding patterns	Obtain dietary history; assess development of feeding skills; food preferences and food jags are common at these ages.	Provide nutritional guidance. Identify eating problems and nutritional problems.
Motor skills	Observe gross and fine skills; screen motor development by use of tools and history.	Provide anticipatory guidance on development and safety. Identify problems in motor development.

Table 27-5 Assessing the School-Age Child and Adolescent

Assessment	Activity	Nursing implications
Physical growth	Monitor growth with weight and height increases occurring with growth spurts: Girls: 9 1/2 to 14 years (peak at age 12) Boys 10 1/2 to 16 years (peak at age 14) Assess secondary sex characteristics (Tanner staging).	Provide anticipatory guidance regarding normal growth patterns. Identify deviant growth patterns.
Skeletal development	Observe pattern of growth, progressing from leg lengthening to widening of thighs, to broadening of shoulders and trunk lengthening. Skeletal mass doubles during adolescence.	Initiate orthopedic screening. Identify deviant patterns. Provide anticipatory guidance and reassurance regarding normal variations.
Dental growth	Inspect number and condition of teeth, noting loss of deciduous teeth and eruption of permanent teeth.	Provide education on preventative dental care. Identify dental problems.
Sleep patterns	Obtain history of sleep requirements. Ideal sleep is 9 hours a night with regularity of schedule.	Identify deviant sleep patterns. Provide counseling on meeting sleep requirements.
Eating patterns	Obtain diet history. Caloric needs increase with periods of increased growth.	Provide education regarding healthful diet. Identify eating disorders and obesity.
Motor/cognitive skills	Observe motor competency, noting increasing coordination of fine and gross motor skills. Assess school performance and intellectual competency, noting transition from concrete to abstract conceptualization. Note move from egocentrism.	Provide anticipatory guidance regarding safety, independence, peer pressure, and conformity.

Table 27-6   Assessment Tools

Test	Focus	Ages	Summary
Denver II	Developmental screen	Birth to 6 years	Screening of gross motor, fine motor, adaptive/language, and personal/social skills
Revised Denver Prescreening Developmental Questionnaire	Developmental screen	3 months to 6 years	Parent questionnaire; short form of the Denver to identify children who need further testing.
Developmental Profile II	Developmental screen	Birth to 9 years	Structured interview with parent; screens physical/motor, self-help, social, academic, and communication skills
Preschool Readiness Experimental Screening Scale	Preschool readiness	4 to 5 years	Addresses school-related skills and maturation
Early Language Milestone Scale	Speech and language screening	Birth to 36 months	Screening tool for general speech/language development; includes visual, auditory receptive, and auditory expressive areas; combines history, direct testing, and observation
Denver Articulation Screening Examination	Speech and language screening	2 to 6 years	Word imitation to screen articulation and intelligibility of speech
Brazelton Neonatal Behavioral Assessment Scale	Infant behavior, state, and temperament patterns	Birth to 1 month	Assessment of reflexes and behavioral responses; tests for state and individual characteristics to identify abnormalities and provides parent education
Infant Temperament Questionnaire	Temperament	1 to 12 months	Child's temperamental characteristics identified based on parental responses; assess the following aspects of temperament: activity, rhythmicity, adaptability, approach, sensory threshold, intensity, mood, distractibility, and persistence
Toddler Development Scale		1 to 3 years	
Behavioral Style Questionnaire		3 to 7 years	
Middle Childhood Questionnaire		8 to 12 years	

Developmental Assessment. Children generally follow predictable patterns of development. Developmental standards have been established based on age levels at which children master key motor, language, adaptive, and social behaviors. Developmental screening tests assess how an individual child compares to the average standard and are used to identify children requiring further evaluation and intervention. Table 27-6 provides an overview of frequently used tools in the pediatric setting.

Temperament and Behavioral Assessments. Behavioral characteristics or temperament have an important role in how a child interacts with others and the environment. Nurses use information about temperament and behavior to help parents understand the child and the individual needs, which may have a positive influence on the parent-child relationship. Table 27-6 lists tools to assess these characteristics.

Psychosocial Development

The child's growth process includes not only physical development but also **psychosocial development.** The work of Erik Erikson focuses on the interaction of emotional, cultural, and social forces on personality development. Personality development culminates in the achievement of ego identity, which involves accepting oneself and having the skills for healthy functioning in society. Erikson believed that development is a continual process that occurs in distinct stages. At each stage, a developmental crisis requires resolution. Although a child never completely finishes all the developmental tasks in a given stage, some degree of mastery and comfort must be achieved before proceeding successfully to the next stage. As internal conflicts are resolved, there is new orientation to self and society. This sets the stage for the next conflict, however; each crisis emerges from the mastery of the previous stage. All new development is rooted in prior experiences. Difficulty with resolution of the crisis will cause problems progressing through the subsequent stages.

The first five stages deal with the tasks of childhood and adolescence; the last three stages, of Erikson's model deal with adulthood.

Trust versus mistrust involves the period of infancy. The infant learns to trust both self and the environment based on the consistency with which needs are met. If needs are met inconsistently, the infant feels a sense of confusion and mistrust. Resolution depends on the quality of interaction and attachment between the parent and infant.

Autonomy versus shame and doubt encompasses early childhood and involves the child's developing physical and mental skills. Resolution is supported as parents allow increasing independence and acquisition of skills. When parents have appropriate expectations and encourage autonomy, the child develops a sense of control over self and environment. If not allowed the opportunity for mastery, the child feels inadequate.

Initiative versus guilt occurs during preschool and early school years. The child achieves mastery through initiation of activity and asking questions. This stage also includes incorporation of adult standards and learning to take responsibility for one's own actions. Restriction may lead to a sense of guilt about thoughts and actions.

Industry versus inferiority occurs as the child moves from initiating to completion of projects. This occurs during middle and late childhood. Competition and peer involvement increase during this time. The child uses expanding cognitive skills to become a productive member of a group. The status in the group and self-esteem are challenged if the child feels that he or she is not "good enough."

Identity versus identity diffusion is the classic task of adolescence. The conflict is to achieve a sense of self and a set of values and belief system. This is accomplished by "trying on" various roles and receiving responses from others. Identity diffusion results when the adolescent is unable to acquire a sense of self or direction or to find a way to "fit" into the *surrounding* world (Table 27-7) (Mott et al., 1990)

Cognitive Development

The work of Jean Piaget is widely used to understand the process of **cognitive development.** According to Piaget, learning results from active manipulation of objects and information, followed by a mental processing of the event. As the child interacts with the environment, new objects and problems are discovered. The child creates mental schemes or thought patterns to understand the encounter. The scheme is the action pattern and the mental basis for the action. It permits the child to receive information from the world, make sense of it, and predict future events. Development occurs as the schemes increase in scope and complexity.

Assimilation is the process of integrating new experiences into existing schemes. When new information cannot fit into the existing schemes, the child must modify schemes or develop new schemes. This process is **accommodation.** The general thought process or mental activity is an operation (Mott et al., 1990).

Piaget identified four stages of cognitive development that represent increasing problem-solving ability. A transition period with combinations of behaviors exists between the stages. The nurse must understand characteristics of cognitive ability at each stage to work effectively with the child and family.

The *sensorimotor period* from birth to age 2 years involves the operations object permanence, causality, and symbolism. The infant moves through progressive stages from an inability to remember objects not seen to an ability to locate an object if only a part of it is visible. The toddler later learns to locate a totally hidden object, but not if moved from the location to another. Finally, the toddler can locate the object after a series of moves without actually seeing the moves to achieve object permanence. By similar progressions, the concept of cause and effect emerges. The infant moves from simply recreating accidentally discovered effects (such as kicking movements) to moving a toy, to increasingly complex behaviors to cause events (such as winding up a toy to make it move). Symbolic representation involves a progression from using the same actions on all objects to using an object to represent another correctly (e.g., offering a doll a drink from a toy cup) (Zuckerman and Frank, 1992).

During the *preoperational stage* from ages 2 to 7 years, children are magical thinkers. They are unable to separate stories and fantasy from reality. This stage is divided into two periods. The first period, the *preconceptual stage* from ages 2 to 4 years, is characterized by increasing symbolism in play and language. The child is unable to take the perspective of another or imagine how another might feel or think. The second period is the *intuitive phase* from ages 4 to 7 years. The child is very literal in understanding of words and is apt to confuse coincidental occurrences with causation. During this phase the child can only deal with one aspect of an object at a time, enabling very simple classification or grouping (Shonkoff, 1992).

Age	Psychosocial conflict	Resolution
Birth to 1 year	Trust/mistrust	Sense of hope
2 to 3 years	Autonomy/shame or doubt	Self confidence and self-control
4 to 5 years	Initiative/guilt	Independence
6 to 11 years	Industry/inferiority	Competence
12 to 18 years	Identity/identify diffusion	Sense of self/loyalty

Table 27-7   Erikson's Stages of Ego Development

Table 27-8   Piaget's Stages of Cognitive Development

Stage	Age	Characteristics	Example
Sensorimotor	Birth to 8 months 8 to 18 months 18 to 24 months	Reflex behaviors become purposeful. Object permanence: objects and people exist when not present. Symbolism: objects can represent other objects; words can represent objects. Beginning of mental representation: thinks before doing action.	Moves fist while grasping rattle; repeats action to shake rattle for the sound it makes. Looks for hidden toy or cries for mother when she leaves. Gets an object from another room; knows mentally what object is even if not seen and can think about getting it before acting.
Preoperational	2 to 7 years	Self awareness: aware of self as separate from events in environment; develops a sense of vulnerability. Egocentric: is unable to take other's view. Symbolism: language is literal; blending of real world and fantasy; increasing complexity of symbolic play. Irreversibility: cannot reverse an action or situation. Finalism: every event has direct cause and every question has direct answer. Centration: only focuses on one aspect of situation. Magical thinking: not a clear sense of what is real; confuses coincidence with causation.	Questions to learn about environment. Develops fears as unable to separate reality from things seen on television or heard. Learns from imitation. Nightmares seem "real." Cannot retrace steps of situation to look for lost thing. Changing shape changes toy (e.g., rolling out a ball of clay makes it bigger). Fascination with monsters and super-heroes to cope with sense of vulnerability.
Concrete operations	7 to 11 years	Learns by manipulation of objects. Classification: orders objects by characteristics Conservation: understands that properties of objects remain the same despite change of appearance. Egocentricity: considers other viewpoint. Internal regulation: able to send messages to self.	Has better understanding of time, place, and number. Enjoys collections because of the ability to group and classify. Ability to understand beyond the literal meanings of words. Increasing use of humor, riddles, and jokes. Participates in group games; peer relationships important. Increasing ability to apply relationships, build on previous experiences, and make inferences as long as the ideas involve concrete or physical objects.
Formal operations	11 years to adolescence	Hypothesizes: uses propositional thinking, which does not require experience with the problem. Considers alternative explanation for same phenomenon. Considers alternate frames of reference. Test hypothesis with deductive reasoning. Synthesizes and integrates concepts to other schemes. Works with abstract ideas. Reflective, futuristic thinking.	Ability to perform scientific process. Follows train of thought to a logical conclusion. Idealism may interfere with reality. Begins to form personal rules and values.

The *concrete operations stage* from age 7 to 11 years enable new skills but only with directly perceived information. The child is unable to perform mental operations requiring abstract thinking. The understanding of the concept of relations is evidenced by the ability to classify objects by characteristics, order a series of objects, and understand that the properties of objects remain the same even if the appearance is altered (Levine, 1991).

Formal operations, beginning approximately at age 11 years, enable the child to work with abstract ideas and use inductive and deductive reasoning to solve problems. With this stage comes the ability to construct new thoughts and ideas from previously obtained information and to form hypotheses. Development of formal operations continues through adolescence and into adulthood, although some people never completely progress through this stage (Felice, 1992). Table 27-8 summarizes these concepts.

An understanding of cognitive abilities of the child enables the nurse to plan appropriate teaching strategies. A teaching session on nutrition, including superheroes and incorporating imitation as a strategy to choose healthful food, would be appropriate for a 4-year-old child who is in the preoperational stage. An 8-year-old child has the ability to understand food groups and composition of a healthy diet; these skills would guide the content and approach used to offer nutrition information. Concrete thinkers need visual methods of teaching, such as pictures and diagrams, and would benefit from "hands on" experiences. Those with formal operation capabilities would be able to form and test hypotheses.

Piaget's theory offers information to help parents understand and cope with the child's behavior. Parents are often distressed because the infant cries with separation and is afraid of strangers between 7 to 9 months of age. Offering information about the development of object permanence and the ability to handle several pieces of information at the same time is reassuring. Separation anxiety or protest results from the infant's ability to remember that the parent exists even though not seen, which is a newly emerging skill at this age. Stranger anxiety or awareness occurs because the infant is able to compare two sets of information simultaneously, familiar and unfamiliar people. It is helpful for parents to understand the behavior as a normal part of cognitive development.

NUTRITION

Promoting good nutrition and dietary habits is one of the most important components of maintaining child health. The first 6 years of life are the most important for developing sound eating habits for the lifetime. The quality of nutrition has been widely accepted as an important determinent of growth and development. It is now becoming recognized for an important role in disease prevention. Atherosclerosis begins during childhood. Other diseases, such as obesity, dia-

betes, osteoporosis, and cancer, may have early beginnings as well (Cohn and Deckelbaum, 1993). *Healthy People 2000* objectives include reducing obesity, improving the quality of the American diet, and increasing cardiovascular fitness. Educating children and their families is an appropriate way to accomplish these objectives.

Factors Influencing Nutrition

The child and family both provide a wide range of variables that influence nutritional habits. Ethnic, racial, cultural, and socioeconomic factors influence what the parents eat and how they feed their child. The child brings individual issues to the nutritional arena, such as slow eating, picky patterns, food preferences, allergies, acute or chronic health problems, and changes with acceleration and deceleration of growth. The parent's perception of the child's nutritional status is often influenced by the same variables and often leaves the parent with unrealistic expectations of what the child should eat. Table 27-9 offers guidelines to daily requirements for all ages.

Nutritional Assessment

Physical growth serves as an excellent barometer of adequacy of the diet. Measurements of height and weight, and if less than 2 years old, head circumference, plotted on appropriate growth curves at regular intervals allow assessment of growth patterns. Good nutritional intake supports physical growth at a steady rate.

A 24-hour dietary recall by the parent is another good screening tool to assess the amount and variety of food intake. If the recall is fairly typical for the child, the nurse can compare the intake with basic recommendations for the child's age. It is important to determine the family's and child's concerns regarding diet. It is also helpful to determine the family's meal patterns. An important part of nutritional adequacy is an assessment of the child's and family's activities. Behavior problems that occur during meals may also be an issue.

Nutrition During Infancy

The first year of life is critical for growth of all major organ systems of the body. Most of the brain growth that occurs during the lifespan occurs during infancy. The digestive and renal systems are immature at birth and during the first part of infancy, and certain nutrients are not handled well. Energy needs are high. Nutrition during this time influences how an infant will grow and thrive.

Types of Infant Feeding

Breast milk is the preferred method of infant feeding. Breast milk provides appropriate nutrients for the

Table 27-9 Daily Dietary Guidelines: Childhood to Adolescence

	1 to 3 years	4 to 6 years	7 to 12 years	Adolescent

MILK/DAIRY
1/2 cup milk =
  1 oz cheese or
  1/2 cup yogurt or
  1/2 cup pudding
	Servings/day: 2
	
	Serving size:
	1/2 cup
		Servings/day: 2
		
		Serving size:
		3/4 cup
			Servings/day: 2 or 3
			
			Serving size: 1 cup
				Servings/day: 2 or 3
				
				Serving size: 1 cup

PROTEIN
1 oz lean meat =
  1 egg or
  1 oz cheese or
  2 tablespoons peanut butter or
  1/4 cup cottage cheese or
  1/2 cup dried peas or beans
	Servings/day: 2
	
	Serving size: 1 oz.
		Servings/day: 2
		
		Serving size:
		2 oz
			Servings/day: 2
			
			Serving size: 2 oz
				Servings/day: 2 or 3
				
				Serving size: 2 oz

VEGETABLES/FRUITS
1 sm fruit =
  1/2 cup juice or
  1/2 cup fruit
	Servings/day:
	4 or 5
	Serving size: 3 or
	4 tablespoons
	(1/4 cup)
		Servings/day:
		4 or 5
		Serving size:
		4 to 6 table-
		spoons
		(1/2 cup)
			Servings/day: at least 5
			Serving size:
			1/3 to 1/2 cup
				Servings/day: at least 5
				Serving size: 1/2 cup

BREADS/CEREALS
1 slice =
  1/2 cup cereal or
  1 oz cold cereal or
  1/2 cup pasta or
  2 or 3 crackers
	Servings/day:
	3 or 4
	
	Serving size:
	1/2 slice
		Servings/day: 4
		
		Serving size:
		1/2 slice
			Servings/day: 6 to 11
			
			Serving size: 1 slice
				Servings/day: 6 to 11
				
				Serving size: 1 slice

Modified from Barness L: *Pediatr Rev* 15:8, 1994; Tennessee Department of Health–Division of Supplemental Food Programs.

infant, as well as antibodies. Breast-fed infants have a lower incidence of illness and allergies. If breast-feeding is not chosen, commercially prepared formulas are an acceptable alternative. Although evaporated milk with added sugar has been used in the past as a low-cost alternative to breast milk, it is now discouraged. Errors in mixing and the lack of vitamins and minerals have been problematic.

The method of feeding is a choice that parents should make with guidance and education. The advantages and disadvantages of breast, formula, and combination feeding should be discussed with the parents.

Nurses should be prepared to instruct, encourage, reassure, and support parents in the feeding method of their choice. For breast-feeding, teaching topics include comfortable positioning, appropriate techniques, feeding frequency, the let-down reflex, care of breasts, and length of feedings. In addition, assessing the mother's feelings about nursing her infant, providing support and encouragement, and the presence or absence of family support are important to success. For bottle-feeding, parents require instruction regarding preparation and care of equipment and formula, positioning, frequency, amount, and feelings about the method of feeding.

Supplements

Current recommendations from the AAP indicate that the iron in breast milk is highly available to the infant. Breast-fed infants do not require iron supplementation. Infants who are not breast-fed should be given a commercial formula that is fortified with iron. Addition of iron to formula has reduced the incidence of anemia and does not cause gastrointestinal symptoms. After 4 to 6 months of age, iron needs are further met by the introduction of iron-fortified cereals.

Fluoride at 0.25 mg per day is recommended for infants who drink ready-to-feed formula or formula mixed with water from a supply containing less than 0.3 parts per million (ppm) of fluoride. Fluoride is currently started at 6 months of age and maintained until 16 years of age. Fluoride is no longer recommended for breast-fed infants whose mothers have a fluoridated water supply (Wilson, 1994).

Introduction of Solid Foods

Current trends include the introduction of solids between 4 and 6 months of age. There is no nutritional, developmental, or psychological advantage to starting earlier. No studies have demonstrated that cereal helps a baby sleep longer. Parents need to understand the risks of feeding solids too early. The incidence of constipation is greater when solid food intake is too high. Early introduction of solids may lead to overfeeding and obesity. There is a greater possibility of food allergy because immunoglobulin A (IgA) production is insufficient for solid foods until closer to 6 months. If the infant decreases milk intake because of filling on solids, an imbalance of nutrients may occur.

Once parents have decided to start solids, nurses can assist them in developing a program for introducing appropriate food in sensible amounts and in the best sequence. Dry cereal fortified with iron is an appropriate starter food because of the ease of digestion (see Appendix E.9).

At 1 year of age, the infant may be given whole milk. Skim, low-fat, and 2% milk are not recommended for babies less than 2 years old because of insufficient fat and caloric content.

Nutrition During Childhood

The ability and desire to self-feed begins at approximately 1 year of age. The parent role begins to shift at this time to providing a balanced, healthy range of foods as the child assumes more independence. Growth velocity and caloric needs decrease during this time. Nurses can best assist parents by offering information on daily needs and healthy food choices. Suggestions for children might include the following:

- Frequent, small meals may be better accepted.
- Offer a balanced diet incorporating variety and food preferences.
- Limit milk intake to the recommendations for age.
- Consider the child's development and safety; avoid nuts, popcorn, grapes, and similar foods to minimize risk of aspiration in young children.
- Encourage children to participate in food selection and preparation, based on developmental capabilities.
- Generally, vitamin and iron supplements are not necessary.
- Avoid using food as a punishment or reward.

Fat content in the diet should be restricted to less than 30% beginning at age 2 years, with no more than 10% of the total calories coming from saturated fats. Studies indicate that children as young as ages 2 to 6 years have diets higher in total fats and saturated fats than recommended. In general, the family diet does not contain enough fiber-rich foods or fruits and vegetables. Diets of school-age children have been shown to be deficient in calcium. Children also need regular participation in physical activity. Observations of children indicate that they are too sedentary (Cohn and Deckelbaum, 1993). The entire family may benefit from suggestions to modify the diet:

- Choose low-fat protein sources: plant proteins, such as beans, peas, and whole-grain products, or lean cuts of meat, chicken, or fish, trimming visible fat.
- Broil, bake, stir-fry, or poach foods rather than fry them.
- Use polyunsaturated and monosaturated fats found in nuts, seeds, nut butters, wheat germ, and vegetable oils.
- Decrease salt, sugar, and fats.
- Increase complex carbohydrates: breads, grains, and cereals.
- Increase fruits and vegetables to at least five servings per day, especially green and orange vegetables and citrus fruits.
- Use low-fat dairy products.
- Increase calcium intake through low-fat dairy products, calcium-fortified products, and supplements, if necessary.
- Maintain regular activity (e.g., exercise, sports, household chores) and limit TV.

Remind parents that they are teaching children lifelong strategies to prevent illness and promote good health (Wilson, 1994).

Adolescent Nutritional Needs

The preadolescent and adolescent years are a time of increased growth that is accompanied by increases in appetite and nutritional requirements. Caloric and protein requirements increase for boys ages 11 to 18 years. Girls have an increased protein need but a decreased caloric need during the same age span. In addition, the iron needed by the adolescent is nearly double that needed by adults, and iodine, calcium, niacin, and thiamine requirements also increase (Pipes and Trahms, 1993).

Adolescent nutritional needs are influenced not only by the physical alterations that are occurring, but also by the psychosocial adjustments. Teenagers are often free to eat when and where they choose. It is a time when eating habits acquired from the family are dropped, snacking outside the home is a major source of nutrition, and fad foods and diets are prominent (Torre, 1977).

The factors of accelerated growth and poor eating habits make the adolescent at risk for poor nutritional health. Adolescents have been found to demonstrate the most unsatisfactory nutritional status of all age groups. Deficiencies in iron, vitamins, calcium, riboflavin, and thiamin are most common (Wilson, 1994).

Nurses have a responsibility to intervene and initiate activities that promote improved nutritional status. Such activities include the following:

- Provision of information on good nutrition in individual or group sessions
- Diet assessment
- Educational activities that focus on:
  - Effects of fad foods and diets
  - Supplying of "at risk" nutrients
  - Provision of a daily food guide (see Table 27-9)
  - Suggested snacks and "on the run" foods that supply essential nutrients
  - Relationship of good nutrition to healthy appearance

IMMUNIZATIONS

Routine **immunization** of children have been extremely successful in the prevention of selected diseases. The ultimate challenge is making sure children receive immunizations. The *Healthy People 2000* goals include the immunization for the nine childhood diseases of 90% of 2-year-old children in the United States by the year 2000. Immunization rates have improved since 1989, largely because of efforts of health organizations to educate health care providers, parents, and government. In 1993, 71% of civilian children under age 2 years were up to date on diphtheria–tetanus toxoid–pertussis (DTP), polio, and measles-mumps-rubella (MMR) vaccines. Only 60% had received *Haemophilus influenzae* and 16% received hepatitis B vaccines. However immunization rates for the first quarter of 1994 showed a slight decline (*MMWR*, 1995).

Cost and convenience are two critical issues in determining whether children are immunized. Successful programs combine low-cost or free immunizations provided at convenient times and locations. It is important to urge parents to obtain immunizations for their children, focusing on the issue at every opportunity.

The goal of immunization is to protect by using immunizing agents to stimulate antibody formation (see Chapter 39 for types of immunity). Immunizing agents for active immunity are in the form of toxoids and vaccines. Toxoid is a bacterial toxin (e.g., tetanus, diphtheria) that has been heat or chemically treated to decrease the virulence but not the antibody-producing ability. Vaccines are suspensions of attenuated (live) or inactivated (killed) microorganisms. Examples include pertussis (inactivated bacteria); measles, mumps, and rubella and oral polio (live attenuated virus); and hepatitis B (inactivated virus).

The neonate receives placental transfer of maternal antibodies. This natural passive immunity lasts about 2 months. Protection is temporary and only applies to diseases to which the mother has sufficient antibodies. The immune system of both term and preterm infants is capable of adequate antibody response to immunizations 2 months after birth. Generally, this is the recommended age to start immunizations (exception: the hepatitis B series may begin at birth).

The interval between immunizations is important to the immune response. After the first injection, antibodies are produced slowly and in small concentrations (primary response). Subsequent injections with the same antigen are recognized by the body, and antibodies are produced much faster and in higher concentration (secondary response). Because of this secondary response, once an initial immunization series has been started, *it does not need to be restarted if interrupted, regardless of the length of time elapsed*. Once the initial series is completed, boosters are required at the appropriate time intervals to maintain an adequate concentration level of antibodies.

Recommendations

Immunization recommendations rapidly change as new information and products are available. Two major organizations are responsible for guidelines: the AAP and PHS Advisory Committee on Immunization Practices (ACIP). Tables 27-10 and 27-11 list current recommendations. Originally the guidelines differed in several areas, causing confusion for health care providers and families. In January 1995 the recommendations were coordinated. The main goal of the guidelines is to provide flexibility to ensure that the largest number of children will be immunized. The recommendations reflect that flexibility by using age ranges rather than specific ages. All health care providers are urged to determine immunization status at every encounter with children and to update immunizations whenever possible. (See Appendix D.3 for immunizing agents, contraindications, and side effects.)

Contraindications

There are relatively few contraindications to giving immunizations. In general, minor acute illnesses are not contraindications. Immunizations should be deferred with moderate or acute febrile illnesses, since the reactions may mask the symptoms of the illness or the side effects of the immunization may be accentuated by the illness.

People with the following conditions are not routinely immunized and require medical consultation: pregnancy, generalized malignancy, immunosuppressive therapy or immunodeficient disease, sensitivity to components of the agent, or recent immune serum globulin, plasma, or blood administration.

Legislation

The National Childhood Vaccine Injury Act became effective in 1988. It requires providers to advise parents and patients about the risks and benefits of the immunizing agent and possible side effects. Informed consent is recommended. Vaccine information statements are available for this purpose. Provisions for reporting specific compensable adverse reactions to specific vaccines are also covered in this act (Kleiman, 1991).

Vaccines for Children (VFC), an entitlement program enacted in 1995, is designed to provide free vaccines to eligible children. This program includes children on Medicaid, those without health insurance, Native Americans, and those whose health insurance does not cover immunizations (Katz, 1994). Although this program is limited in scope, it reflects a commitment to child health and a beginning to an expanding focus on prevention.

Table 27-10   Immunization Schedule: Range of Ages for Routine Immunizations

Vaccine	Births	2 months	4 months	6 months	12 months	15 months	18 months	4 to 6 years	11 to 12 years	14 to 16 years
HBV	HBV #1	HBV #2		HBV #3						
DTP		DTP #1*	DTP #2*	DTP #3*	DTP #4† or DTaP‡			DTP #5 or DTaP‡	Td	
Hib		Hib #1*	Hib #2*	Hib #3*	Hib #4*					
OPV		OPV #1	OPV #2	OPV #3				OPV #4		
MMR					MMR #1			MMR #2		

Modified from American Academy of Pediatrics: *Report of the Committee on Infectious Diseases*, ed 23, 1994, and *Recommended childhood immunization schedule, United States*, Elk Grove Village, Ill, 1995, The Academy.

HBV, Hepatitis B virus; *DTP*, diphtheria–tetanus toxoid–pertussis; *DTaP*, diphtheria–tetanus toxoid–acellular pertussis; *Hib*, *Haemophilus influenzae* type b conjugate vaccine; *OPV*, oral polio vaccine; *MMR*, measles-mumps-rubella; *Td*, adult tetanus–diphtheria toxoid (used after age 7).

*DPT and Hib combination vaccine may be given when DTP and Hib are administered simultaneously.

†DTP #4 may be given as early as 12 months if 6 months have elapsed since DTP #3.

‡DTaP preparations are only recommended for use as the fourth or fifth dose for children 15 months or older.

Table 27-11   Recommended Immunization Schedules for Children Not Immunized in First Year of Life

Time interval/age	Immunization	Comment
YOUNGER THAN 7 YEARS		
First visit	DTP, Hib, HBV, MMR, OPV	MMR if child is older than 12 months; tuberculosis testing may be done at the same visit. Hib is not indicated if the child is older than 60 months.
Interval after first visit:		
1 month	DTP, HBV	
2 months	DTP, Hib, OPV	Second dose of Hib is not indicated if child older than 15 months when first dose given.
At least 8 months	DTP or DaTP, HBV, OPV	DaTP is not used for child younger than 15 months and is not used for the primary series.
4 to 6 years old	DTP or DaTP, OPV	DPT or DaTP is not necessary if the fourth dose was given after the fourth birthday; OPV is not necessary if the third dose was given after the fourth birthday.
11 to 12 years old	MMR	
14-16 years old	Td	Repeat every 10 years throughout life.
7 YEARS AND OLDER		
First visit	HBV, OPV, MMR, Td	
Interval after first visit:		
2 months	HBV, OPV, Td	
8 to 14 months	HBV, OPV, Td	
11 to 12 years old	MMR	Minimal interval between doses of MMR is 1 month.
10 years after last Td	Td	Repeat every 10 years throughout life.

Modified from American Academy of Pediatrics: *Report of the Committee on Infectious Diseases,* ed 23, Elk Grove Village, Ill, 1994, The Academy.
For abbreviations, see footnote to Table 27-10.

Table 27-12   Leading Injury Causes of Death by Age

Less than 1 year old	1 to 4 years old	5 to 14 years old	15 to 20 years old
Aspiration	Fires/burns	Pedestrian	Motor vehicle
Homicide	Drowning	Motor vehicle	Suicide
Motor vehicle	Motor vehicle	Drowning	Homicide

Modified from Baker SP, et al: *The injury fact book,* ed 2, New York, 1992, Oxford Press.

MAJOR HEALTH PROBLEMS
Injuries and Accidents

Injuries and accidents represent the single most important cause of disease, disability, and death among children. Injuries compose one half of all childhood and three fourths of all adolescent deaths in the United States. One out of five children per year will experience a serious problem related to accidents or injuries. The critical issue is that most are preventable (Wilson, 1994).

The *Healthy People 2000* objectives address reducing injuries in all areas, including motor vehicle accidents, falls, burns, drowning, and head injuries. The key to changing behaviors is providing age-appropriate counseling about safety.

Motor vehicle accidents are the leading cause of death among the pediatric population. One fourth of those deaths are caused by inappropriate use of restraints (Nachem, 1984). Motor vehicle accidents not

only include automobile collisions but also pedestrian injury. Drowning and burns account for most of the other deaths; poisonings and falls also contribute heavily. Development is an important issue in identifying risks to children. Table 27-12 lists the leading injury causes of death by age.

Infants

Infants have the second highest injury rate of all groups of children, second only to adolescents. The infant's small size contributes to the type of injury. The small airway may be easily occluded. The small body fits through places where the head may be entrapped. Infants are handled on high surfaces for the convenience of the caregiver, placing them at great risk for falls. In motor vehicle accidents, their small size is a great disadvantage and increases the risk for crushing or being propelled into surfaces. Their immature motor skills do not allow escape from injury, placing them at risk for drowning, suffocation, and burns.

Toddlers and Preschoolers

This population experiences many falls and poisonings as well as motor vehicle accidents. They have a high level of activity and increasing motor skills, making supervision difficult. They are extremely inquisitive and have relatively immature logic abilities.

School-age Children

The school-age group has the lowest injury death rate. At this age, it is difficult to judge speed and distance, placing them at greatest risk for pedestrian and bicycle accidents. Peer pressure often inhibits the use of protective devices such as helmets and limb pads. Sports and athletic injuries are increased in this age group.

Adolescents

Injury accounts for 75% of all deaths occurring during adolescence. Risk taking becomes more conscious at this time, especially among males. The death and serious injury rates for males are three times higher than for females. Adolescents are at the highest risk of any age group for motor vehicle deaths, drowning, and intentional injuries. Use of weapons and drug and alcohol abuse play an important role in injuries in this age group (Wilson, 1994). Youth gangs are more violent and seem to be increasing in prevalence. Suicide is the second leading cause of death among youth between ages 15 and 24 (Brent et al., 1992). Poor social adjustment, psychiatric problems, and family disorganization increase the risk for suicide.

Injury and Accident Prevention

The nurse has a major role in the prevention of accidents and injuries. The nurse is responsible for identification of risk factors by assessing the characteristics of the child, family, and environment. Interventions include anticipatory guidance, environmental modification, and safety education. Education should focus on age-appropriate interventions based on knowledge of leading causes of death and risk factors. Topics to consider are listed in the box below (see also Appendix E.11).

Acute Illness

Infection is the largest single cause of illness in infants and children. Infectious diseases, whether bacterial or viral in origin, are usually associated with a variety of symptoms: fever, upper respiratory symptoms, generalized discomfort and malaise, loss of appetite, rash, vomiting, and diarrhea. Most are self-limited and can be handled by the family on an outpatient basis with appropriate interventions to prevent complications. The nurse may need to identify whether the child can be managed at home, based on the severity of symptoms and the family's ability to provide care. The nurse may be involved in developing a home management plan, including administration of medications or therapy and evaluation of the effectiveness of that plan. Also, the nurse teaches the family about the illness and prevention of its spread. Nursing interventions for home management of a child with a gastrointestinal virus are shown in the box on p. 536.

Infectious diseases may be more serious in younger children and infants. Neonates, because of immunological immaturity, are more susceptible to bacterial illness and dissemination to multiple organ systems or sepsis. Children of all ages are at risk for invasion of the spinal fluid or meningitis. The morbidity and mortality of these forms of infection vary with the age of the child, causative organism, severity of the illness, and the onset of treatment. The nursing role includes early identification and referral (see pediatric text for signs and symptoms of sepsis and meningitis), supporting the family during the treatment phase, and follow-up care as indicated. Preventive measures include family education in hygiene and identification of environmental sources of infection.

 Research Brief

Jones ME: Injury prevention: a survey of clinical practice, J *Pediatr Health Care* 6:3, 1992.

A study was done to determine what education and training pediatric nurse practitioners (PNPs) receive about injury prevention and what activities they perform related to injury prevention. Sixty-four PNPs in the greater New York area were surveyed. Information was obtained on demographics, education, training in injury prevention, and relevant clinical activities. Results indicated that 97% of the respondents received training on childhood injuries, but few routinely incorporated that information into clinical practice. Information was given only by 30% about car restraints, 15% about smoke detectors, and 7% about firearms.

The following implications for nursing practice were made. Efforts should be made to increase the nursing awareness of the scope of the problem of injuries and the importance of educating families. In conjunction with the *Healthy People* 2000 priorities, surveys should be completed now and again in the year 2000 to verify improvement.

 Injury Prevention Topics

Car restraints/seat belts
Preventing falls
Safe driving practices
Gun control
Preventing fires/burns
Preventing drowing/water safety
Sports safety
Decreasing gang activities
Poison prevention
Bicycle safety
Pedestrian safety
Substance abuse prevention

Nursing Inverventions for Home Management of Gastrointestinal Virus in Children

Education regarding expected course of the illness: virus usually self-limited with vomiting lasting 1 to 2 days and diarrhea lasting 7 to 10 days

Progressive diet management: nothing by mouth (NPO) for 3 to 4 hours: sips of oral electrolyte solution every 5 to 10 minutes for 2 hours; clear liquids (primarily oral electrolyte solution) for the rest of the day; bland, easily digested foods (BRAT diet: bread, rice, applesauce, toast) for the next 24 to 48 hours

Fever management with antipyretic agent if needed

Monitoring for signs of dehydration and instructions on seeking further care: urinates less than usual; parched, dry mouth and mucous membranes; poor skin turgor; sunken eyes with no tears; irritability; lethargy

Prevention of spread: instructions on handwashing technique

Sudden Infant Death Syndrome

Sudden death may occur in infants with a specific disorder such as meningitis or a chronic illness. When no specific cause of death can be determined, the death is labeled **sudden infant death syndrome (SIDS).** Each year, more than 5000 infants die of SIDS in the United States, making it the most common cause of death during the first year of life. Few factors can be used to predict the occurrence. Most deaths occur between 1 and 5 months of age, although it may occur up to age 1 year. Only a small number of infants experienced a previous episode of cyanosis or apnea. Cardiorespiratory monitoring has not been shown to decrease the incidence. There is an increased occurrence in preterm and low-birth-weight infants and possibly in infants with upper respiratory tract infections. SIDS occurs more frequently in male infants and in low socioeconomic groups. Maternal cigarette smoking doubles the risk. The risk to siblings is unclear at present. Evidence indicates that the prone sleeping position may increase the risk, as well as tightly swaddling infants. No test exists to identify infants who may die, making this a frustrating clinical problem (Carroll and Loughlin, 1994).

When an infant dies, the family requires tremendous support. The nurse should focus on providing empathetic support and assisting the family in coping, progressing through the grief process, and dealing with siblings and other family members. Referral to support groups may be helpful.

Nursing interventions include teaching the following prevention strategies:

◆ Supine or side-lying position for healthy infants
◆ Decreased parental smoking
◆ Improved access to prenatal and postnatal health care
◆ Teaching and close follow-up care for high-risk groups
◆ Improved compliance in use of monitoring for selected infants

<table>
<tr><td>

Did You Know?

No studies have shown the effectiveness of home cardiorespiratory monitoring for the prevention of SIDS deaths. Research is needed to improve technology to enhance results and to encourage compliance.

</td></tr>
</table>

Chronic Health Problems

Improved medical technology has increased the number of children surviving with chronic health problems. Examples include Down syndrome, spina bifida, cerebral palsy, asthma, diabetes, congenital heart disease, cancer, hemophilia, bronchopulmonary dysplasia, and acquired immunodeficiency syndrome (AIDS). Despite the differences in the specific diagnoses, the families have complex needs and similar problems. A number of variables are used to assess each child and family. Is the condition stable or life-threatening; what is the actual health status? What is the degree of impairment to the child's ability to develop? What type and what frequency of treatments and therapy are required? How often are health care visits and hospitalizations required? To what degree are the family routines disrupted? The commonalities include the following:

◆ All children and adolescents with chronic health problems need routine health maintenance care. Often in the struggle to handle the illness, monitoring for physical growth and development, immunizations, nutritional needs, dental health, behavioral and developmental concerns, and self-care teaching are neglected. Many of the same issues of health promotion and health maintenance of all pediatric patients need to be addressed with this population.

◆ Ongoing medical care specific to the health problem needs to be provided. Examples include monitoring for complications of the health problem, specific medications, dietary adjustments, and therapies such as speech, physical, or occupational therapy. Ongoing evaluation of the effectiveness of treatment protocols is critical.

◆ Care is often provided by multiple specialists. A need exists for coordination in scheduling visits, tests, or procedures, as well as the treatment regimen.

◆ Skilled care procedures are often required and may include suctioning, positioning, medications, feeding techniques, breathing treatments, physical therapy, and use of appliances.

◆ Equipment needs are often complex and may include monitors, oxygen, ventilators, positioning or ambulation devices, infusion pumps, and suction machines.

◆ Educational needs are often complex. Communication between the family and team of health care

Nursing Interventions for Insulin-Dependent Diabetes Mellitus in Children

Follow-up care to evaluate child for disease control and to ensure that family is coping well with management of care.
Family teaching, including:
  Disease process, complications, insulin action
  Insulin therapy: technique, storage, dose adjustment
  Glucose monitoring: technique, frequency of readings, interpretation of results
  Diet regulation: diet developed to consider family diet, food preferences, and schedules: diet plan, timing meals and snacks, allowing for occasional treats and modifications for "special times"
  Exercise planning: type, intensity, duration, monitoring, relationship of diet and insulin to exercise, coordination with family patterns and school activity
  Smoking prevention: additive effects to vascular disease
  Skin care and hygiene to prevent infections
  Emergency management of hypoglycemia and hyperglycemia
Coordination of specialty services; eye care, endocrinology, nutritionist, primary care provider
Referral to support groups, camps for psychosocial needs
Referral for qualification for state or federal programs (e.g., Children's Specialty Services)

 Nursing Interventions for Attention Deficit Disorder in Children

Assessment: history, physical examination, parent/family assessment, learning and psychoeducational evaluations
Behavioral modifications at home and school: teaching families techniques to support clear expectations, consistent routines, positive reinforcement for appropriate behavior, timeout for negative behaviors
Classroom modifications: consulting with family and teachers to meet individual needs for remediation or alternate instruction methods if necessary; structure activities to respond to child's needs
Referral to family therapy/support groups/mental health services to assist development of positive coping behaviors
Medications: consulting with physician to monitor for therapeutic and adverse effects
Follow-up: assess at 3- to 6-month intervals when stable; dynamic process affected by relationships with others; behaviors will change with age; problem may persist through adulthood

Modified from Murphy MA, Hagerman RJ: J *Pediatr Health Care* 6:1, 1992.

providers and teachers is essential to meet the child's health and educational needs.

♦ Safe transportation to health care services and school must be available. Several barriers exist, including family resources, location, ability to be fitted appropriately in car restraint systems, and the amount and size of supportive equipment.

♦ Financial rsources may not be adequate to meet the needs.

♦ Behavioral issues include the effect of the condition on the child's behavior and on other family members. Chronic health problems may cause stress on relationships.

Nursing interventions in the primary care setting with a child diagnosed with insulin-dependent diabetes serve as a model for pediatric chronic health problems. Several problems may be identified within the Omaha Problem Classification Scheme, including actual or potential nutrition, physical activity, prescribed medication regimen, technical procedures, pain, and income. The box above lists examples of nursing management.

Alterations in Behavior

Behavioral problems in the child and adolescent are highly variable and may include eating disorders, attentional problems, substance abuse, elimination problems, conduct disorders and delinquency, sleep disorders, and school maladaptation. A healthy self-concept is supported by positive interactions with others. Maladaptive behaviors may provide negative feedback, which may generate low self-esteem. A child's coping mechanisms are influenced by the individual developmental level, temperament, previous stress experiences, role models, and support of parents

and peers. Maladaptive coping mechanisms present as dysfunctional behaviors. Inappropriate behaviors may lead to further physical or developmental problems.

The common areas of behavior problems are the interplay of self-concept and self-esteem and the need for a family-centered approach to management. Multidisciplinary teams often are involved in care.

Attention deficit disorder (ADD) interventions are presented as a model for nursing management of a behavior problem (see box above). ADD is a combination of inattention, impulsiveness, and hyperactivity not appropriate for age. It frequently includes low self-esteem, mood lability, low frustration tolerance, temper outbursts, and poor academic skills. The evaluation is based on symptoms, and the diagnosis is made by excluding other disorders. Symptoms vary with severity of the problem, and interventions range from simple to complex. A familial tendency exists; several members of a family may be affected. Treatment involves a family focus and includes health professionals and educators (Murphy and Hagerman, 1992).

ROLE OF THE COMMUNITY HEALTH NURSE IN CHILDREN'S HEALTH

A major goal of the *Healthy People 2000* objectives is improving access to health care for children, specifically increasing preventive services and immunizations. The community health nurse is in an key position to bring about this goal. Community health nurses may practice in a variety of settings, including community health centers, school-based clinics, or through home health programs. They may provide care through well-child clinics, immunization programs, federally mandated programs such as the Early and Periodic Screening, Diagnosis and Treatment pro-

Components of Family Assessment

Composition of family
    Members
    Roles
Values and beliefs
Parenting skills
    Parent history: childhood experiences
    Caregiving abilities: physical/psychosocial
    Discipline
Mechanisms of functioning
    Decision making
    Distribution of responsibilities
Emotional relationships
Availability of resources
    Economic resources
    Social support
    Emotional support
Communication patterns
Coping Patterns: responses to crisis/stress
Enviroment
    Structural safety
    Appropriateness of stimulation

gram or Women, Infants, and Children program, or specific state-funded programs. Nurses share the ability to provide health supervision and well-child care. The nursing process and a knowledge base of the factors unique to this population provide a framework of care.

The nursing assessment includes a health history of individual and family health and illness patterns. A complete history is usually obtained at the first encounter, with interim history obtained at subsequent visits. The nurse assesses the adequacy of growth, nutritional status, and concerns about diet. A physical examination is performed, the extent of which varies with the purpose of the visit. For well-child care, a complete assessment, including vital signs, hearing, vision, dental screening, and laboratory tests, is done. Developmental and behavioral assessments enable early detection of problems and are an important component of health supervision. The nurse identifies psychosocial and emotional concerns of the child and family. Family assessment enables the nurse to identify problems that may interfere with parenting abilities. Environmental and safety issues are identified (see box above).

The nursing plan of care and interventions include three major components. The first is the mangement of actual or potential health problems. The second involves both education and anticipatory guidance. This enables families to understand what to expect in the areas of growth and development as well as social, emotional, and cognitive changes. The nurse offers information to promote healthy life-styles and to prevent health problems and accidents. A third role is case management or coordination of care. For example, the nurse serves to coordinate referrals to com-

munity agencies, other health care services or providers, or assistance programs. The box lists examples of community resources.

Evaluation of care has always been a critial part of the nursing process. It is now a necessity in the current health care environment with health care payers requiring justification of the cost of health care services. Nurses identify and document positive outcomes from the interventions. This may include objectives such as increased knowledge or observable changes in behaviors.

NEEDS OF CHILDREN WITHIN THE COMMUNITY

Nursing, through development and coordination of community-based services and through formation of public policies, promotes the well-being of children within the community. Assessments are made to identify the needs and target populations at risk. Programs based on the needs of specific at-risk populations are developed for the delivery of health care. Three strategies for common pediatric concerns are identified to model nursing interventions in the community. *Healthy People 2000* priorities serve as an organizing framework for the development of services targeting the pediatric population. Programs may include health promotion, protection, or prevention services.

Strategies for Child Care in the Community

Nurses are in a position to work with groups of families or children through programs targeting the health care needs of those at risk. Strategies include programs based in the home, targeted at the needs of homeless persons, or centered in day-care or school settings.

Home-based Service Programs

Home-based service programs vary in goals and target populations. In general, home visiting programs increase utilization of available community resources by bringing the services into the home or neighborhood or by promoting awareness of resources (see the box on p. 539, top, left). By working on problems within the home setting, families can strengthen problem-solving abilities. Home visitor programs may offer the following services based on needs of the community:

◆ Monitoring the health status of vulnerable populations
◆ Child-rearing education
◆ Counseling services
◆ Social support
◆ Clinical services
◆ Safety instruction

Programs may consist of professional and trained lay people forming a team to provide services. Home-based programs have been shown to decrease preterm and low-birth-weight deliveries, improve parenting capabilities, enhance the development of disabled children, promote early hospital discharge, and de-

Community Resources for Children's Health Care

Children's service clinics
Women, Infants, and Children (WIC) programs
Infectious disase clinics
Family violence/child abuse centers
Head Start
Crisis hotlines
Early Intervention/Developmental Services
Breast-feeding support groups
Family planning clinics
Medicaid
Well-child clinics
Immunization clinics
Children's Specialty Services
School health programs
Parents Anonymous
Community education classes
Childbirth education classes
Parent support groups
Youth employment/training programs

Components of the Home Assessment

INTERACTION AND RELATIONSHIPS

Interaction with home visitor
  Ease of family members
  Accurate representation of the normal relationships
Interaction/relationships observed between family members
  Express positive responses to the child
  Family members talk to child and respond to child
  Age-appropriate discipline and restriction

ENVIRONMENT

Age/type of building
Adequacy of sanitation facilities: waste disposal, washing facilities
Adequate refrigeration
Type of heating and cooling systems, routinely maintained
Adequate space
Safety
  Fire/burns: smoke detector, fire extinguisher, hot water temperature less than 120° to 130° F, fire plan established, limit exposure to sources of burns (fireplaces, heating units)
  Falls/injury: hazards identified and limited (e.g., stairs, windows), firearms absent or secured, toys and furniture safe
Poison prevention: hazards identified and limited, ipecac syrup, emergency procedure

DEVELOPMENTAL OPPORTUNITIES

Toys, games, books appropriate for age
Controlled use of television and radio
Family expectations of child appropriate
Child given age-appropriate responsibilities
Family encourages and supports activities to develop skills

crease health care costs (Olds, 1991). Specific programs might include home visiting programs to support the transition from hospital to home for preterm infants or programs to prevent home accidents and injury.

Interventions are based on assessment of the needs of the child and family. Areas to be assessed include interactions and relationships, environment, and developmental appropriateness (see box, above, right).

Programs for Homeless Families

Actual numbers of homeless children and adolescents are difficult to determine. Estimates vary from 200,000 to 800,000 children and adolescents. Families compose the fastest-growing segment of the homeless population; 25% to 40% of homeless persons are families, often a single mother with two or three children. The longer the duration and the amount of disruption of support systems determine the effects of homelessness on health. Children in homeless situations are often not immunized and suffer from poor nutrition. There is limited or no access to health care. Often there is increased exposure to environmental hazards, as well as violence and substance abuse. The combination of health problems, environmental dangers, and stress is referred to as the **homeless child syndrome** (Redlener, 1991).

Children experience chronic illness, such as tuberculosis, asthma, anemia, and chronic otitis media. Hospitalizations are more frequent in this population. Behavioral problems may exist, such as sleep disorders, withdrawal, aggression, or depression. School performance problems may arise from lack of regular attendance. Many homeless children demonstrate developmental delays because of the lack of an appropriate environment to foster development.

The community health nure may be involved in outreach programs combining health care workers and community members to take the health care services to the homeless (see box on pg. 540, top, left). Identifying a consistent team to provide continuity of care on a regular basis is important. The family is often removed from its network of neighbors, friends, and relatives, as well as the usual health care providers. Emphasis should be placed on preventive and follow-up care as well as immediate problems. Services include physical examination, behavioral and developmental assessments, nutritional support, screening tests, and immunizations.

Day Care and School

Day-care centers and schools provide an environmental framework for the child and adolescent population. More than 7 million children under age 6 years are enrolled in day care. Studies have shown that these children are 18 times more likely to acquire infectious diseases (Brunell, 1994). Most of these experiences for the older child and adolescent involve school. The community health nurse can establish programs and serve as a resource to day-care centers and schools.

Nurses can provide information regarding illness and injury prevention for child care providers and teachers to improve health and safety. Centers and schools may need assistance in developing standards

Responsibilities of the Outreach Team

COMMUNITY HEALTH NURSE

Develop and maintain trusting relationship with families.
Follow up acutely ill family members.
  Review medicines and treatment plans.
  Facilitate referrals and follow-up on referrals.
  Provide feedback to health care teams.
Perform field assessments and triage to clinic.
Provide health education and disease prevention.
Continue assessment and follow-up for child abuse and neglect in high-risk families.

COMMUNITY WORKER

Develop and maintain trusting relationship with families.
Help family set priorities and develop goals to meet them.
Assist families in progress toward meeting goals.
Provide family advocacy with public agencies (welfare, WIC, housing authority).
Provide family advocacy with health agencies.

From Wood D: *Pediatr Heath Care* 3:4, 1989.

Healthy People 2000 Priorities for Children

Health promotion: breast-feeding support programs, parenting skills classes, prevention of tobacco use, parent support groups, screening for families at risk for child abuse/neglect, nutrition education programs
Health protection: injury prevention counseling, toy safety seminars, playground safety, sports physical examinations and safety instruction, dental screenings, fluoride supplementation, car seat loan programs
Preventive services: WIC programs, family planning services, immunization programs, lead screening, hearing and vision screening

for hygiene, sanitation, and disinfection to prevent the spread of disease. This may include handwashing, food preparation, and cleaning of toys and equipment. Requirements for immunizations of both children and staff may need to be established. Guidelines for care of sick children should be developed. Staff members may benefit from educational programs on topics such as infectious diseases, cardiopulmonary resuscitation (CPR), behavior management and discipline, or other concerns they may have.

Within the school, health education should be incorporated into the school curriculum for older children and adolescents. The students should be encouraged to participate in identifying the content and presentation of the material. Topics may include sports participation, self-care, and health-related topics, such as prevention of disease.

Education for families of the children may focus on coping strategies, such as division of responsibilities, identification of frustrations, and dealing with behaviors that signify stress and tension. Nurses are in a key position to consult with these populations and serve as a resource for program development.

Service Programs for Children in the Community

Types of services offered based on the priorities from *Healthy People 2000* objectives include health promotion, health protection, and preventive services. Many health care needs of children and adolescents fall within these priorities. The box (above, right) lists examples. To address these priorities, the nurse may be involved in community assessment, political action, and establishment of programs. Three program ideas with strong implications regarding the health of children are presented next as models.

Smoking Prevention

Smoking has been identified as the most important preventable cause of morbidity and mortality in the United States, but 50 million Americans smoke. Smoking is associated with cardiovascular disease, cancer, and lung disease. Parents often do not understand or believe the effects of smoking on children. Children exposed to **secondhand smoke** experience increased episodes of ear and upper respiratory tract infections. Children of smokers are more likely to smoke. Teenagers who become smokers are rarely able to quit (Rasco, 1992). The *Healthy People 2000* objectives include decreasing both the number of children and adolescents who smoke and the number of children exposed to tobacco smoke.

The number of teenagers smoking has not decreased since 1980, with the age of onset of smoking becoming younger. Statistics show that as many as 6 million teenagers and 100,000 preteens smoke on a daily basis. Tobacco industry advertising has increased through use of ads, billboards, and sponsorship of sporting events. Cigarette ads appear in "teen" magazines, and companies offer logo products that appeal to children. More than 80% of a group of 6-year-old children were able to associate a picture of Joe Camel with cigarettes. Although 46 states have laws prohibiting the sale of cigarettes to minors, restrictions are not enforced. Minors are able to purchase tobacco products 46% to 88% of the time (MacKenzie et al., 1994).

Interventions to discourage smoking focus on the parent, the child or adolescent, and public policy. Parents should be offered educational programs dealing with the negative effects of smoking on children, as well as "stop smoking" interventions and ways to create a "smoke-free" environment. Behavior modification techniques should be incorporated.

Antismoking programs directed to children and teenagers are more successful if the focus is on short-term rather than long-term effects. Developmentally, it is difficult to project themselves into the future to imagine the consequences of smoking. The immediate health risks and the cosmetic effects should be emphasized. Teaching should include how advertising puts pressure on people to smoke. Music, sports, and other activities, as well as stress reduction techniques, should be encouraged. Teaching social skills to resist peer pressure is critical.

Nurses should become politically active in the area of smoking. Banning tobacco advertising, enforcing restrictions of sales to minors, increasing funds for antismoking education, and restricting public smoking may reduce the incidence of smoking.

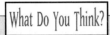

Taxes should be increased on tobacco products to provide funding for health care programs.

Reduction of Gun Violence

In 1994 13 children were killed and 30 were wounded each day in the United States in gun-related accidents, suicides, and homicides. Often with each event, other children are affected by witnessing gun violence or knowing the victims. More than 135,000 children are carrying guns to school, many obtained in their own homes. At least 50% of U.S. families report owning guns, many of which are stored loaded. In a national survey, one-third of teens and preteens reported that they could obtain a gun (Havens and Zink, 1994).

Consequences of gun violence are serious. Permanent, debilitating physical injuries are sustained. Little is known about the emotional impact of being a victim of or witnessing acts of violence, but it has been proposed that the effects are long-lasting. The financial burden of treatment and rehabilitation is high and often not completely compensated.

Some of the factors associated with gun violence include access to firearms, substance abuse, poverty, and cultural acceptance of violent behavior. Interventions must begin early and address each of these factors.

Nurses can actively participate in efforts to reduce gun violence among young people. Numerous legislative actions have been proposed limiting the sale of handguns to minors and restricting possession of guns in schools. The recently passed Brady Bill authorized a waiting period for handgun purchases, raised licensing

Guidelines for Playground Safety

Playgrounds should be surrounded by a barrier to protect children from traffic.

Activity centers should be distributed to avoid crowding in one area.

Finishes should meet Consumer Product Safety Commission regulations for lead.

Durable materials should be used.

Sand, gravel, wood chips, and wood mulch are acceptable surfaces for limiting the shock of falls.

Equipment should be inspected regularly for protrusions that could puncture skin or entagle clothes.

The following are not recommended: multiple-occupancy swings, animal swings, rope swings, and trampolines.

fees for gun dealers, and required police notification of multiple gun purchases. Nurses can urge legislators to support gun control legislation. Nurses can collaborate with schools to develop programs to discourage violence among children. Community programs focusing on gun storage, promoting safety at school, and managing aggressive behavior need to be offered. Families may need support in supervising their children after school. Community efforts to enhance family stability and promote self-esteem are vital to decreasing violence (Havens and Zink, 1994).

Promotion of Safe Playgrounds

Schools, day-care centers, and community groups often need guidance toward developing safe places for children to play. An average of 15 deaths per year occur on playground equipment, with 191,000 reported injuries. The most frequent injuries are falls, with three-fourths involving head injuries. The U.S. Consumer Product Safety Commission has published guidelines for playground safety. Guidelines include structure, materials, surfaces, and maintenance of equipment. Suggestions as to the developmental capabilities of specific ages are incorporated, as well as recommendations for disabled children. Nurses can use these guidelines to assist the community to establish standards for play areas. The box above summarizes these guidelines (Swartz, 1992).

Clinical Application

John D. is a 9-year-old child brought to the clinic by his mother for follow-up of an emergency room visit 5 nights ago for an episode of asthma. John has a history of recurrent episodes of wheezing and respiratory distress occurring on a regular basis since age 4. Until 4 or 5 months ago, John has been under good control using a combination of bronchodilator and cromolyn sodium inhalers on a prescribed protocol, based on peak flow meter readings. Mrs. D. reports

that over the past few months, John has been uncooperative about his asthma. He refuses to use his flow meter and would not use his maintenance medication at school. During this episode, he even refuses to use his bronchodilator at school, even though he is still "sick." Mrs. D. is very frustrated and states that she just "can't understand him at all." She reports no changes at home or at school. John is an excellent student, gets along well with peers, participates in many activities

Continued.

Clinical Application—cont'd

and sports, and normally is very cooperative with both parents. He frequently "picks on" his sister, but his mother perceives this as normal. Mrs. D. does admit that since the weather has been so rainy, she has smoked inside the house a few times.

The clinic nurse reviews this information with the nurse practitioner who is John's health care provider. They review findings from his assessment. Physical examination is unremarkable except for evidence of an upper respiratory tract infection and peak flow readings in the clinic of 60% to 80% of his expected baseline. His medication orders from the emergency room are appropriate for his condition and include albuterol and cromolyn sodium inhalations three to four times a day using a spacer device. John is fairly knowledgeable about his asthma and treatment regimen but has "forgotten" some of the information he learned when he first started his treatment. He admits that he does not go to the office to use his inhalers at school but does not reveal why.

The clinic nurse identifies problems in the phsyiological domain of respiration and health-reslated behaviors of prescribed medication and technical procedures. After talking with John, she thinks the real issue is in the area of health care supervision. Understanding of psychosocial development leads her to realize that John is dealing with issues of industry versus inferiority. Peer involvement is important to him. Children at this time are competitive and want to be the best. His status with his friends and self-esteem are threatened by being different or not "as good" as others. The nurse also recognizes that John is learning from examples offered by role models. When his mother smokes inside the home, she is modeling noncompliance with the treatment plan, as well as offering a trigger to his asthma. The nurse discusses her concerns with John and his mother, and a plan is formulated.

Mrs. D. agrees to resume her efforts to decrease smoking and to smoke only outside the home. The nurse reviews information with John regarding the dynamics of asthma, appropriate medication use, purpose of peak flow readings, asthma triggers, early warning signs, and intervention strategies. She uses materials that incorporate humor and games, as well as illustrations and charts that are appropriate for his level of concrete thinking. She refers them to a regional asthma support program through the American Lung Association.

The nurse also suggests that Mrs. D. and John explore ways for him to use his inhalers at school by either making his use less conspicuous or involving his friends positively in his treatment. John prefers to make arrangements at school to use the inhalers with privacy. Mrs. D. thinks the principal and teachers will be helpful. Mrs. D. and John arrange a contract regarding use of his peak flow meter. For compliance on a daily basis, John will select a "fun" activity every 2 weeks.

At the follow-up visit 2 weeks later, Mrs.D. reports that " things are great." John is back to his baseline maintenance therapy with peak flows about 80% consistenly. John reports that he is using his inhaler at school in a special, private place without any problem. He is excited about receiving a letter from a "pen pal" from the asthma support program. He is planning on attending an asthma summer camp where "everybody has asthma and my sister won't be there."

Using principles of psychosocial and cognitive development, the nurse is able to understand the client and plan appropriate interventions. This information assists the family in maintaining optimal health even when the child has a chronic illness. Resources available within the community can offer support.

Key Concepts

♦ Physical growth and development is an ongoing process resulting in physical, cognitive, and emotional changes that affect health status.

♦ Psychosocial development is subject to the interaction of emotional, cultural, and social forces. Resolution of crises at each stage of development is important for mastery of skills needed to accept oneself and to function in society.

♦ Cognitive development follows an orderly process of increasing complexity of thought and action patterns. Understanding the child's

cognitive level is the basis for effective interventions.

♦ Good nutrition is essential for healthy growth and development and influences disease prevention in later life. The adolescent population is at greatest risk for poor nutritional health.

♦ Immunizations are successful in prevention of selected diseases. Barriers to immunizing children are cost and convenience.

♦ Accidents and injuries are the major cause of health problems in the child and adolescent population. Most are preventable. Nurses have

Key Concepts—cont'd

a major role in anticipatory guidance and prevention.

- ◆ Community health nurses are involved in strategies to meet the needs of the pediatric population in the community. Home-based service programs have been successful in providing cre for at-risk populations. Children of homeless families are at risk for health problems, environmental dangers, and stress. Community programs to provide health care

for homeless persons may decrease those risks. A third strategy is using day care and school as a framework for offering education and services to groups of children, adolescents, and their families.

- ◆ Service programs aimed at decreasing smoking, reducing gun violence, and promoting community playground safety are important aspects of the *Healthy People 2000* initiative and help to ensure a safer future for children.

Critical Thinking Activities

1. Develop a plan of immunization for a 5½-year-old child who has had one DTP, Hib, and OPV.
2. Administer the Denver II to a 9-month-old infant. Develop a plan of anticipatory guidance.
3. Develop a plan of nursing care for a family who has experienced a SIDS death.
4. Develop a plan of nursing care for a family who has a 12-year-old child with spina bifida and a family with a 12-year-old child with leukemia. Note the commonalities.
5. Develop a nutritional program for (a) mothers who are breast-feeding their infants, (b) a group of 5-year-olds in a kindergarten class, and (c) a group of high-school sophomores. What factors do these programs have in common? How do they differ?
6. Administer a safety survey (TIPP program from the American Academy of Pediatrics or develop your own) to assess the home environment of a 6-month-old infant and a 5-year-old child. Develop a plan of education and anticipatory guidance for the family.

Bibliography

Alpern GD, Boll TJ, Shearer MS: *Developmental profile, II,* Los Angeles, 1982, Wesler Psychological Services.

American Academy of Pediatrics, Committee on Nutrition: *Pediatric nutrition handbook,* ed 2, Elk Grove Village, Ill, 1985, The Academy.

American Academy of Pediatrics: *Report of the Committee on Infectious Diseases,* ed 23, Elk Grove Village, Ill, 1994, The Academy.

Baker SP, O'Neill B, Ginsberg MJ, Li G: *The injury fact book,* ed 2, New York, 1992, Oxford Press.

Barness L: Nutrition update, *Pediatr Rev* 15:8, 1994.

Brazelton TB: *Neonatal behavioral assessment scale,* Philadelphia, 1973, Lippincott.

Brazelton TB: *Touchpoints,* New York, 1992, Addison-Wesley.

Brent DA, Puig-Antech J, Rabinovitch H: Major psychiatric disorders in childhood and adolescence. In Levine MD, Carey WB, editors: *Developmental-behavioral pediatrics,* ed 2, Philadelphia, 1992, Saunders.

Brunell PA, editor: New CEC natinal program to improve quality of day care setting, *Infect Dis Watch* 4:1, 1994.

Carey WB: Temperament: a tool for coping with problem behavior, *Contemp Pediatr* 1:139, 1989.

Carroll JL, Loughlin GM: Sudden infant death syndrome. In Oski FA, DeAngelis CD, Feigin RD, et al: *Principles and practice of pediatrics,* ed 2, Philadelphia, 1994, Lippincott.

Centers for Disease Control and Prevention: *General recommendations on immunizations: recommenations of the Advisory Committee on Immunization Practices, MMWR* 43(RR-1), 1994.

Chow MP et al: *Handbook of pediatric primary care,* ed 2, New York, 1984, Wiley.

Cohn L, Deckelbaum RJ: Early childhood nutrition: eating today for tomorrow's health, *Pediatr Basics* 66:3, 1993.

Drumwright AF: *Denver Articulation Screening Exam,* Denver, 1971, Denver Developmental Materials.

Felice ME: Adolescence. In Levine MD, Carey WB, editors: *Developmental-behavioral pediatrics,* ed 2, Philadelphia, 1992, Saunders.

Frankenburg WK, Dodds J, Archer P, et al: *Denver II,* Denver, 1990, Denver Developmental Materials.

Frankenburg WK, Fandal AW, Thorton SM: Revision of the Denver Preschool Screening Developmental Questionnaire, *J Pediatr* 110:653, 1987.

Friedman MM: *Family nursing: theory and assessment,* East Norwalk, Conn, 1994, Appleton & Lange.

Havens DMH, Zink RL: President Clinton's childhood immunization program, *J Pediatr Health Care* 7:6, 1993.

Havens DMH, Zink RL: A pediatric nurse practitioner call to arms: new solutions needed for nation's growing public health problem, *J Pediatr Health Care* 8:3, 1994.

Healthy People 2000: national health promotion and disease prevention objectives, Washington, DC, 1992, DHHS, Public Health Service.

Immunizations, *MMWR* 44:8, 1995.

Katz S: Experts speak out at symposium on navigating the waters of the Nation Vaccines for Children Program, *Pediatr News* 22:8, 1994.

Kleiman MB: Immunizations. In Green M, Haggerty RJ, editors: *Ambulatory pediatrics,* ed 4, Philadelphia, 1991, Saunders.

Levine MD: Middle childhood. In Levine MD, Carey WB, editors: *Developmental-behavioral pediatrics,* ed 2, Philadelphia, 1992, Saunders.

MacKenzie TD, Bartecchi CE, Schrier MD: The human costs of tobacco use, *N Engl J Med* 330:14, 1994.

Millonig VL: *The pediatric nurse practitioner certification review guide,* Potomac, Md, 1990, Health Leadership Associates.

Mott SR, James SR, Sperhac AM: *Nursing care of children and families,* ed 2, Redwood City, Calif, 1990, Addison-Wesley.

Murphy MA, Hagerman RJ: Attention deficit hyperactivity disorder in childen: diagnosis, treatment and follow up, *J Pediatr Health Care* 6:1, 1992.

Nachem B: Children still aren't being buckled up, *Matern Child Nurs* 9:320, 1984.

Olds DL: Nonphysician home visits. In Green M, Haggerty RJ, editors: *Ambulatory pediatrics*, ed 4, Philadelphia, 1991, Saunders.

Pipes PL, Trahms CM: *Nutrition in infancy and childhood*, ed 5, St Louis, 1993, Mosby.

Popenoe D: The family transformed, *Fam Affairs* 2:1, 1989.

Rasco C: Discouraging smoking: interventions for pediatric nurse practitioners, *J Pediatr Health Care* 6:4, 1992.

Redlener I: Health care for homeless children: special circumstances. In Green M, Haggerty RJ, editors: *Ambulatory Pediatrics*, ed 4, Philadelphia, 1991, Saunders.

Rogers WB, Rogers RA: A new simplified Preschool Readiness Experimental Scale (PRESS), *Clin Pediatr* 11:558, 1972.

Shonkoff JP: Preschool. In Levine MD, Carey WB, editors: *Developmental-behavioral pediatrics*, ed 2, Philadelphia, 1992, Saunders.

Shulsinger E: Needs of sheltered homeless children, *J Pediatr Health Care* 4:136, 1990.

Swartz MK: Playground safety, *J Pediatr Health Care* 6:3, 1992.

Thomas HS: Conceptual underpinnings of the family support movement, *J Pediatr Health Care* 8:2, 1994.

Torre CT: Nutritional needs of adolescents, *Matern Child Nurs* 2:105, 1977.

Wilson MH: Prevention of diseases. In Oski FA, DeAngelis, CD, Feigin RD, et al: *Principles and practice of pediatrics*, ed 2, Philadelphia, 1994; Lippincott.

Wood D: Homeless children, *J Pediatr Health Care* 3:4, 1989.

Zuckerman BS, Frank DA: Infancy and toddler years. In Levine MD, Carey WB, editors: *Developmental-behavioral pediatrics*, ed 2, Philadelphia, 1992, Saunders.

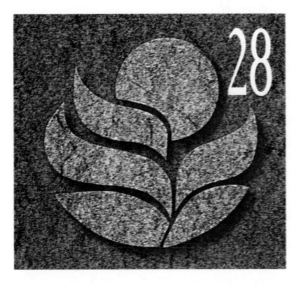

28

Women's Health

Linda Corson Jones ◆ Shirleen Trabeaux

Objectives _____ ▼

After reading this chapter, the student should be able to do the following:

◆ Differentiate the traditional and expanded scope of women's health.
◆ Describe the health status of women in the United States.
◆ Discuss the development of women.
◆ Discuss the major health problems of women.
◆ Identify the health needs of special populations of women.
◆ Explore issues related to women's access and use of health services.
◆ Identify legislation that influences women's health services.

Outline _____ ▼

Key Terms _____ ▼

breast self-examination (BSE)
caregiver burden
clinical breast examination
heterosexism
homophobia
mammography
menopause
osteoporosis
Papanicolaou (Pap) test
perimenopause
postmenopause
preconceptional counseling
urinary incontinence (UI)

Women's health primarily focuses on women's psychosocial and physiological well-being, functional abilities, and experiences of symptoms and health problems. This broad emphasis on women's health is in distinct contrast to viewing women in terms of their reproductive health or their role in parenting children. Women's health recognizes that the health of women is related to the biological, social, and cultural dimensions of women's lives. Moreover, women's normal life events or rites of passages, such as menstruation, childbirth, and menopause, are considered part of normal female development, rather than syndromes or diseases requiring only medical treatment.

Although the importance of women's health began gaining national recognition during the last two decades, questions continue to be raised about the health and well-being of American women. In recent years, various national groups have asked critical questions about the health of American women and the services available to women. Although progress has been made in treating women, who make up 52% of the population, continuing issues related to women's health exist. These issues include questions related to areas of health care neglect, shortcomings of health services available to women, and the need to understand the key health problems of women.

Important health issues related to women are still not well understood. The rate of breast cancer deaths has increased, yet no one knows why (Sharp, 1990). Heart disease is a major killer of women, but until recently virtually all research has been conducted on men. Women are the fastest-growing high-risk group for developing human immunodeficiency virus (HIV), yet only in the last few years have national HIV treatment studies included women. Most types of depression are twice as common in women as they are in men. Sexual and physical violence remain significant health problems.

This chapter examines ways community health nurses can assist women, from youth through older adulthood, to meet health needs. The health status of women in the United States and worldwide is discussed. The relatively new but growing body of literature that documents the distinctive nature of women's development is explored. Major health issues of women, such as heart disease, cancer, HIV, reproductive health, depression, midlife, and aging, are presented. The community health nursing role is emphasized, with tools for assessment and strategies for implementation included. The pivotal role of women in ensuring the family's and community's health is highlighted in the discussion of women's use of health services. Factors influencing women's access to health services, including inequities in services, economic and employment issues, family considerations, health behaviors of women, and health care providers' attitudes, are considered. Health policy, including major legislation affecting women's health services and future directions for women's health, is discussed.

STATUS OF WOMEN

The Fifth International Congress on Women's Health Issues in 1992 affirmed that health is primarily determined by adequate economic and social conditions that ensure adequate food, water, shelter, and other necessary resources (Dan, 1994). Unfortunately, millions of people, particularly women, do not have these basic resources. Within all societies, most poor people are women. Women compose half of the world's population and head one third of all households in the world, but most individuals who live in poverty are women and children.

In the United States, the situation for women is also bleak. Men are more likely to be employed than women, and women are more likely to be employed in lower-paying service sector jobs. Women are also less likely to have job-sponsored medical benefits, such as medical leave and insurance; they are more likely to depend on assistance programs such as Medicaid and Medicare. When women do perform the same work as men, they earn less than 80% of the salaries of men (Wuest, 1993).

In the United States, two-thirds of all poor adults are women. More than half of individuals with incomes in the lowest fifth of the nation are women. Of those individuals living below the poverty level, most are single mothers with children. See the box below for factors contributing to the "feminization of poverty."

Although women have made some strides in their efforts to achieve economic equality during the last decade, progress has been slow. Because women's economic stability is closely linked to health outcomes, it is essential that work continue in improving women's access to and control over their resources. As advocates for women, community health nurses can play a vital role in the advancement of women and the improvement of women's health. Nurses can become key mobilizers in empowering women and communities to take charge of their health and ensure that resources be developed that benefit both genders.

 Factors Contributing to the "Feminization of Poverty"

Gender wage gap
Number of single female–headed households
Teenage birth rate
Welfare system providing subsistence below the poverty level
Lack of adequate affordable child care
Lack of enforcement of child support payments
Budget cuts in social programs
Women assuming the principal caretaker role in the family

Modified from Sidel R: J *Public Health Policy* 12:37-49, 1991.

DEVELOPMENT OF WOMEN

Major theories of human development are based on the work of men such as Erikson, Freud, Piaget, and Kohlberg. According to Gilligan (1982), a female psychologist and researcher, an inherent gender bias exists in the work of these classic human developmental theorists because their research was based on males. Consequently, theories of men's development became the accepted normal adult development for all. When the research findings did not easily apply to women, it was assumed that the problem was with the female gender and not with the research. For example, in Erikson's now classic stages of psychological development, the stage of "identity formation" is identified as crucial in the development of a normal healthy adult. To achieve "identity formation," an individual must separate and become autonomous from others. As a result of Erikson's work, many developmental psychologists continue to define normal development in terms of autonomy, independence, and separation (Gilligan, 1982). As a result of the research of women, such as Gilligan (1979, 1982) and Chodorow (1978), another developmental psychologist, our understanding of human development has expanded. These researchers found that a female's identity is not found through independence and separation but instead in the relationships that she forms with others.

Until the 1960s the classic developmental theories, on which modern developmental psychology is based, were unchallenged. Three factors led women to challenge the male-dominated human development theories. First, in the 1960s the feminist movement pushed women's issues to the forefront. Second, the number of women psychologists increased significantly in the 1970s. Finally, female psychologists began to conduct research with women.

As the evolution of women's developmental theory advances, we will learn more about qualities important to women's development, such as nurturance and intimacy. Through an understanding of the importance of relationships and responsibilities to women, the nurse can support women.

HEALTH OF WOMEN

Women have a longer life expectancy than men. In 1993 the life expectancy for a woman was approximately 79 years, compared with 72 years for a man. Projections for the year 2000 show the life expectancy for women and men to increase to 80 years and 73 years, respectively (National Center for Health Statistics [NCHS], 1993b). Women over 50 years are the fastest-growing segment of the U.S. population. Projections are that the number of women over 45 years will increase by 32%, while the number of women of reproductive age will grow by only 4% (Garner, 1991).

Some experts believe that in the future, sex differences in mortality will not be as great between men and women. A decline in cardiovascular mortality rates among males will result in an increased life expectancy for men. It is also forecast that the life expectancy of women will decline as they assume many of the poor health habits traditionally associated with men, such as cigarette smoking and alcohol use. In addition, as women become more integrated into the labor force, they will be increasingly exposed to occupational hazards and job stressors.

Although women may live longer than men, they experience more morbidity and use health services at higher rates than men. In the National Health Interview Survey, men and women were compared for the acute and chronic conditions (NCHS, 1993a). For nearly every acute condition except injuries, women exceeded men. In addition, women experienced a number of chronic conditions at a higher rate than men, including arthritis, cataracts, orthopedic problems, diabetes, hemorrhoids, hypertension, chronic bronchitis, asthma, and chronic sinusitis. Men experienced higher rates of visual and hearing problems, ulcer and abdominal hernia, heart disease, and emphysema than did women. In this national survey, response to illness was also addressed. Men experienced higher rates of bed-disability days, but women reported higher rates of work or school loss days. In response to illness, men made more outpatient hospital visits than women, whereas women used more telephone calls and office visits than men. Even when hospitalization for childbirth was excluded, women were hospitalized more frequently than men. People were also asked to rate their health as excellent, very good, good, fair, or poor. Fewer women rated their health as excellent (36%) compared with men (42%).

The three major causes of mortality in women are heart disease, cancer, and cerebrovascular disease. The three major chronic conditions women experience are heart conditions, arthritis, and hypertension; these conditions increase with age.

Heart Disease

Heart disease is the leading cause of death among women over 50 and the second leading cause of death among women ages 35 to 39 years (American Heart Association [AHA], 1994). Although women are less likely to have heart attacks than men, they are more likely to die from heart attacks.

Over the last 30 years, initiatives to help women prevent heart disease in their spouses have been replaced more recently with initiatives to help women prevent heart disease in themselves. Although a number of researchers are now studying women and heart disease, our traditional knowledge base (including diagnosis and therapeutics) is based on studies using males (Pittman and Kirkpatrick, 1994). Women may experience heart disease different from men. Men with heart disease may initially have acute myocardial infarction, but women with heart disease are more likely to report chest pain (Holm et al., 1993). In addition, women may delay seeking treatment, expecting that heart disease involves much more pain than they experience. In addition, women's complaints may not be taken seriously by health care providers, who may attribute symptoms to stress. Thus, women may be misdiagnosed until their condition warrants emergency surgery (Hawthorne, 1994).

It is important for the community health nurse to teach clients about symptoms of heart disease. Angina may be manifested as chest pain radiating down one or both arms. In addition, angina may be experienced as pressure, chest fullness lasting several minutes, a choking sensation, lightheadedness, fainting, and shortness of breath pain (Holm et al., 1993).

Some standard diagnostic tests, such as treadmill exercises and thallium scan, were developed for males. Therefore, they are not as reliable or as sensitive for women. Drugs typically prescribed for women with heart disease, such as beta blockers, nitrates and calcium channel blockers, were not originally tested with women (Holm et al., 1993). Women may respond to these drugs differently from men.

Women may also experience cardiac surgery differently from men. Because coronary artery disease develops 10 to 20 years later in women than men, women who require cardiac surgery are much older than their male counterparts. This may be one of the reasons that women have higher operative mortality rates than men. One study found that whereas men viewed surgery as a major event in their lives, women viewed the surgery as a part of growing old. These differences in perceptions influence postsurgical recovery. Postoperatively, more men participated in cardiac rehabilitation than women. Women were less likely to follow discharge instructions; they allowed family responsibility and level of fatigue to guide their postoperative activity (Hawthorne, 1994).

Community health nurses can play a key role in the prevention and early detection of heart disease. Cessation of smoking is the most important factor in decreasing the morbidity and mortality of heart disease in women (Das and Banka, 1992). For women who smoke and take oral contraceptives, the risk of heart disease increases significantly (Hanson, 1994). One study found that women who take oral contraceptives and do not smoke have a coronary heart disease risk of 0.9 per 1000 women, whereas in women who take oral contraceptives and smoke fewer than 15 cigarettes, the risk rises to 3.5. Smoking more than 15 cigarettes a day increases the risk of coronary heart disease to 20.8 (Croft and Hannaford, 1989). Women over 35 years old who smoke cigarettes and take oral contraceptives are at the greatest risk of developing heart disease (Hanson, 1994). Women who continue to smoke should be informed of other contraceptive methods available to them. In addition, the community health nurse can provide information about other key prevention strategies to prevent heart disease, including following a diet low in cholesterol, triglyc-

erides, and saturated fat; participating in regular exercise; and preventing and treating hypertension.

Postmenopausal women are at risk for heart disease because of decreased levels of estrogen (Leaf, 1990). Hormone replacement therapy (HRT) reduces the risk of death from heart disease by 50% (Barrett-Conner and Bush, 1991). The U.S. Preventive Services Task Force (1989) recommends that all women be counseled about HRT. For some women, however, estrogen replacement therapy is contraindicated. The community health nurse should be aware of the benefits and contraindications of this therapy. Contraindications include unexplained vaginal bleeding, active liver disease, chronic impaired liver functions, recent vascular thrombosis, and breast or endometrial cancer.

Cancer

Cancer is the second leading cause of death for women. The most common types of cancer in women are lung, breast, colorectal, ovarian, and pancreatic. Many women have a great fear and incorrect information about the incidence, diagnosis, and treatment of cancer. Community health nurses have an opportunity to educate women about the risk factors, signs and symptoms, and treatment of cancers.

Lung cancer is the leading cause of cancer deaths among women, surpassing breast and colorectal cancer (Knobf and Morra, 1993). Most lung cancer is preventable; smoking causes most lung cancer.

More women between ages 25 and 35 smoke than any other age group. African-American women in this age group are more likely to smoke than white women (NCHS, 1993a). It is projected that after 1995, African-American women will have the highest prevalence of smoking (Shervington, 1994). The quit rate for African-American smokers is significantly less than for whites.

The U.S. Preventive Services Task Force does not recommend screening asymptomatic individuals for lung cancer. The task force recommends that all individuals should be counseled about the use of tobacco products. For long-term prevention of lung cancer, community health nurses can help reduce the number of young women who smoke. To be effective, smoking cessation programs for young women need to consider some of the powerful forces that encourage young women to initiate and continue smoking. For a number of years, cigarette advertisements have promoted smoking in women through an emphasis on slimness (e.g., Virginia Slims). This has resulted in many young women associating smoking with maintaining an acceptable body weight.

Nurses need to target young African-American women for education about the dangers of smoking. Oakley (1994) described smoking as "increasingly a marker for poverty" that is a powerful "strategy for calming the nerves and coping with stress" (p. 432). Findings from research studies focusing on African-American women's attitudes and practices regarding smoking offer insights that are important in planning smoking cessation programs (Lacey et al., 1993; Shervington, 1994). Many women identified only minimal risks of smoking. Barriers to smoking cessation were closely linked to their difficult life situations. Barriers include living in highly stressful environments; feeling isolated and without social support; and choosing smoking as an affordable, attainable legal pleasure given limited financial resources. Women stated that in order for smoking cessation programs to be effective, this cannot be a single focus or the primary focus of the intervention. Instead, smoking needs to be addressed within a more comprehensive program that has other purposes meaningful to their lives, such as dealing with disappointments, handling stress, and obtaining resources.

Breast cancer is the second leading cause of death from cancer among women and the most frequently diagnosed cancer. Breast cancer incidence has risen dramatically since 1982 (Miller et al., 1993). Although earlier detection and better reporting may account for some of the increase in incidence, other causes of this increase are not known. The mortality rate from breast cancer has changed little since 1930 (Garfinkel, 1993). The 5-year survival among women with localized breast cancer has improved from 78% in 1940 to 91% in 1990. Once cancer spreads, cancer survival rate drops to 71% (Price, 1994). Therefore, early detection of breast cancer is the most important strategy to increase breast cancer survival.

Risk factors for breast cancer that have been identified are listed in the box below. It has been estimated that many cases of breast cancer cannot be explained by these established risk factors. Moreover, most risk factors cannot be reduced by change in behavior. The major risk factor is advancing age; breast cancer increases significantly for women over 50 years old. Although researchers of epidemiological and animal studies reported a link between dietary fat and the development of breast cancer, this has not been confirmed in prospective human studies.

 Risk Factors Associated with Breast Cancer

MAJOR RISK FACTORS
Over 50 years old
Family history (mother, sister, or daughter)
Previous breast cancer

MODEST RISK FACTORS
First pregnancy after 30 years of age
Nulliparity
Menarche before 12 years old
Menopause after 55 years old
Proliferative atypical breast hyperplasia
History of ovarian or endometrial cancer
Obesity after menopause
High socioeconomic status

Although breast cancer occurs most frequently in women of higher socioeconomic status, economically disadvantaged women have the highest mortality rate (Price, 1994). The high mortality rate among these women may be related to lack of information about the disease and inadequate health care, which often results in late-stage diagnosis and delayed treatment. Economically disadvantaged women are much less likely to have regular mammograms (Price, 1994).

Early detection remains the primary factor in survival for women with breast cancer. All women should receive age-appropriate periodic screening and education. This includes a combination of **mammography, clinical breast examination,** and **breast self-examination (BSE)** teaching. An objective of *Healthy People 2000* is to increase to at least 80% the proportion of women 40 years and over who have ever had a clinical breast examination and a mammogram.

The community health nurse should teach asymptomatic women the risk factors for breast cancer, the importance of practicing monthly BSE, and the value of clinical breast examination and mammography. During the National Health Survey, women were asked about BSE (NCHS, 1993a). Knowledge of BSE was highest among college graduates (94%) and lowest among women who had not completed high school (77%). Actual practice of BSE did not show any clear association with educational level. Among women 65 years and older, white women (82%) were more likely to know the procedure than African-American women (68%).

Although the efficacy of screening mammography for women between ages 50 and 69 is well documented, the usefulness of mammography for women aged 40 to 49 has provoked considerable debate. In December 1993 the National Cancer Institute (NCI) issued a statement that studies have not shown a significant reduction in mortality through routine mammography screening for women under age 50. Therefore, they recommended that women ages 50 and over have routine screening, consisting of mammography and clinical breast examination, every 1 to 2 years (Kaluzny et al., 1994). They projected that through this screening, breast cancer mortality can be reduced by approximately 30%. The American Cancer Society (ACS), on the other hand, continues to recommend that annual mammography begin by age 40 years and consist of annual clinical examination, with screening mammography performed at 1- to 2-year intervals. For women 50 years of age and over, mammography should be performed annually (Dodd, 1993). The ACS guidelines have been widely accepted by at least 12 health care professional organizations.

Despite much mass media publicity about the high rates of breast cancer and the importance of early detection, many women do not adhere to recommended screening guidelines for BSE, clinical breast examination, and mammography. During the 1990 National Health Survey, only about two-thirds of women aged 50 to 59 reported ever having had a mammogram (NCHS, 1993a). In 1994 the Agency for Health Care Policy and Research (AHCPR) released a comprehensive review of research surrounding clinical breast examination and mammography and excellent recommendations for health care providers. The report recognizes that women may lack information or harbor fears of embarrassment and pain about being examined. A nurse's recommendation to seek breast cancer screening can be very powerful. A number of studies report that more than 90% of women had a mammography after their health care provider recommended it (Breen and Kessler, 1994).

Nurses will find the AHCPR practice guidelines helpful in counseling women about mammography. Nurses need to inform women that mammography is the most sensitive and specific screening test for breast cancer currently available. Women need to understand the importance of routine screening for asymptomatic women. In addition, women need to understand the difference between screening and diagnostic mammography. Women with breast signs or symptoms such as a mass, skin changes, and nipple discharge should request diagnostic rather than screening mammography. Women need to be informed that the procedure can be uncomfortable or painful. If possible, women should schedule mammography when they are not experiencing cyclical breast tenderness or conditions that increase breast density. Women's privacy should be respected; women should not be required to travel or to wait in a public area while wearing an examination gown.

Older women have been identified as a group who are less likely to participate in breast cancer screening. They are less likely to perform BSE, to obtain clinical breast examinations, and to seek mammograms. Lack of knowledge about cancer, particularly the fact that risk of cancer increases with age, is cited by elderly women as the reason for not participating in screening. Older women are not as likely as middle-aged women to view themselves at risk for breast cancer (Champion, 1992). A nursing study reported that the nursing literature and popular media have inadequately addressed the degree of risk and the special needs of the older woman. Most nursing studies do not include older women in their samples. Typically, photography and artwork accompanying articles on breast cancer depict younger women. Messages on breast cancer do not acknowledge the older woman's degree of risks. Thus, a myth has been created that older women are not vulnerable to this disease. Community health nurses need to target older women for breast cancer teaching and screening. Educational initiatives should be culturally sensitive. In addition, pictorial and written materials should be designed for all ages.

The incidence of reproductive cancers increases with age. Women over 40 years old are at increased risk for cervical, uterine, and ovarian cancer (Garner, 1991). Ovarian cancer causes more deaths than any other gynecological cancer, accounting for 6% of all cancers in women. **Postmenopausal** women have the highest incidence and mortality rates from ovarian cancer. The 5-year survival rate is about 30% to 35%, decreasing to 4% in women diagnosed with advanced disease. Symptoms of ovarian cancer usually do not occur until the disease has progressed to an advanced stage. Consequently, most women with ovarian cancer receive the diagnosis during an advanced stage. A major risk factor is family history. Although a woman's lifetime risk of developing ovarian cancer is 1 in 70 or 1.4%, this can be as high as 50% when there is a positive family history (Averette et al., 1993). Other risk factors for ovarian cancer include nulliparity, late first pregnancy, infertility, late menopause, high-fat diet, higher socioeconomic status, a family history of ovarian cancer, and occupational exposure to talc and asbestos. The periodic pelvic examination is the only reliable screening test available. One test that has attracted great attention from the popular media is the CA-125 blood test. This tumor marker test has limited specificity for detecting ovarian cancer. The CA-125 is not recommended for screening the general population because it is elevated in some healthy women and women with pelvic inflammatory disease, endometriosis, and fibroids (Averette et al., 1993).

About one-third of gynecological cancers include uterine cancers (cervical and endometrial). Endometrial cancer occurs most often in postmenopausal women. Risk factors include nulliparity, late menopause, early menarche, obesity, high socioeconomic status, and a family history of breast cancer. Symptoms of endometrial cancer include abnormal vaginal bleeding and an enlarged uterus. The **Papanicolaou (Pap) test** is a poor screening test for endometrial cancer; endometrial biopsy is an accurate diagnostic method for endometrial cancer. There are insufficient data, however, to justify screening of the general population of postmenopausal women with endometrial biopsies (Averette et al., 1993).

With early detection, appropriate treatment, and adequate follow-up, cervical cancer is one of the most preventable diseases. Major risk factors for cervical cancer include low socioeconomic status, a history of multiple sexual partners, early onset of sexual activity, and use of oral contraceptives. Moreover, sexually transmitted viral diseases, such as herpes and human papilloma, have recently been recognized as playing a possible role in the development of cervical cancer (Kelley et al., 1992).

Early symptoms of cervical cancer can include vaginal bleeding or discharge, symptoms often associated with douching and sexual intercourse. The principal screening test for cervical cancer is the Pap test. It is responsible for a dramatic reduction of cervical cancer during the last two decades. Women should be asked if they have recently received an examination and should be encouraged to seek gynecological care. All women should be educated about the importance of having regular gynecological examinations.

Only 50% of women 18 years and over report having an annual Pap test (NCHS, 1993a). An objective of *Healthy People 2000* is to increase to at least 95% the proportion of women 18 years and over who have ever had a Pap test and to at least 85% those who have received a Pap test in the preceding 1 to 3 years. The U.S. Preventive Services Task Force recommendations call for Pap tests to begin when the female first engages in sexual intercourse or by age 18 years. The test should be performed every 1 to 3 years on females who have been or are sexually active. The ACS (1994) recommends that after a woman has had three or more annual examinations with normal results, the Pap test may be performed less frequently at the discretion of her health care provider. The American College of Obstetricians and Gynecologists (ACOG, 1993) recommends a yearly Pap test. They cite several reasons for having a yearly test: (1) there has been an increased incidence in intraepithelial neoplasia in the last 10 years; (2) Pap tests have a high false-negative rate; and (3) many women further extend the recommended time between examinations.

Did You Know?

Women who receive a Pap test are significantly more likely to receive other screening tests, such as mammography, colorectal screening, and cholesterol tests. Nurses may use the Pap test as a "sentinel" marker of whether a woman has received screening for other medical problems (Hueston and Stiles, 1994).

Human Immunodeficiency Virus

HIV is a major health problem and cause of death among women. Worldwide, more than 3 million women are HIV infected. As the number of women with HIV doubles every 1 to 2 years, HIV is approaching the top five leading causes of death among women.

Many women are at risk because they are not aware of the modes of transmission of HIV and do not acknowledge their risk behaviors (Sipes, 1995). The highest HIV seroprevalence rates in women are found in women of childbearing age. Injection drug use is the main risk factor for women, accounting for more than 50% of cases (Ickovics and Rodin, 1992). Intravenous (IV) drug use has increased among females, making the IV route the most high risk. Heterosexual contact with injection drug users, hemophiliacs, and bisexual partners account for 30% of cases.

More than 70% of women with HIV are African-American or Hispanic. Although membership in an ethnic group is not a risk factor, this overrepresentation is believed to be linked to the disproportionate numbers of minority members engaged in high-risk behaviors. Most HIV-infected women are clustered within urban areas where poverty and drug abuse are prevalent.

Research findings point to several distinctions about women with HIV. Generally, women with HIV have many more coexisting problems than men, including malnutrition, other sexually transmitted diseases (STDs), substance abuse, lack of social support, and poor access to health care (Smeltzer and Whipple, 1991). The disease progression of HIV differs between women and men (Sipes, 1995). For example, *Pneumocystis carinii* pneumonia and Kaposi's sarcoma are often seen as AIDS-defining markers in men with acquired immunodeficiency syndrome (AIDS); they occur less often among women. Vaginal fungal infections, especially caused by *Candida albicans*, are frequently the AIDS-defining events in women (Sipes, 1995). Women with HIV are also prone to cervical neoplasias and pelvic inflammatory disease (Ickovics and Rodin, 1992). Sex differences in the clinical manifestations of AIDS may contribute to women receiving a later diagnosis or a misdiagnosis. The problem of early recognition of HIV infection in women may result in insufficient or incorrect health care treatment (Ickovics and Rodin, 1992). The community health nurse should know gender differences in HIV and educate their clients.

Because women of childbearing age comprise the largest at-risk group for becoming infected with HIV, attention to pregnancy and perinatal transmission of HIV are paramount. The most common route by which a child acquires HIV is from an infected mother. Estimates of the rate of perinatal transmission have ranged from 20% to 40% (Lambert, 1990).

The community health nurse should discuss a number of issues with HIV-seropositive women, including the possibility of vertical transmission to the fetus and the unknown effect of the pregnancy on their own HIV disease state (Sherr, 1991). It is recommended that all HIV-seropositive pregnant women receive counseling, with abortion and sterilization services offered (Arras, 1990). HIV-seropositive status, however, may not be a decisive factor for a woman deciding to continue or terminate her pregnancy. In fact, a number of surveys have found that most women choose to continue their pregnancy despite their HIV status (National Research Council, 1990; Stratton et al., 1992). Complex social, cultural, and psychological factors often determine whether a woman becomes pregnant and influences the degree of commitment she has to the pregnancy (Smeltzer and Whipple, 1991). Community health nurses need to recognize the powerful cultural dynamics that surround the life choices that HIV-seropositive women make for themselves, their children, and families (Smeltzer and Whipple, 1991;

Williams, 1990). They must be prepared to assist and support women's decisions.

HIV is often a family illness, resulting in extraordinary needs that embrace all domains—physical, psychosocial, spiritual, and economic. The lives of these families are frequently complicated by the death of one or more parents and a child because of HIV illness. In addition, the same circumstances that may have led the mother to become HIV infected may undermine her ability to provide care for her HIV-infected infant and her other children. Many of these families experience other difficulties: poverty, isolation, poor education, unemployment, inadequate housing, and drug use. The creation of health care that demonstrates appreciation and respect for HIV-infected families is a challenge.

Women and Weight Control

Americans, particularly women, spend a great deal of time, money, and effort in pursuit of the slender body. For women, obesity is highly stigmatized in our culture. Research has consistently documented that more women than men are dissatisfied with their bodies. Often, women of normal weight and even underweight women view their bodies as too large. Moreover, females begin developing a fear of obesity in childhood.

In our culture, thinness symbolizes competence, success, control, and sexual attractiveness. Our culture's preoccupation with thinness and shape of women can be seen in the popular media "waif" models. Conversely, people may associate obesity with laziness and a lack of willpower.

Approximately 27% of women are obese, a condition characterized by excessive body fat (Vickers, 1993). Obesity is greater among African-American women (44%) than among white women (25%). The prevalence of obesity and the associated risks of obesity in the development of diabetes, hypertension, cardiovascular disease, and other medical problems makes this condition a major health problem among women. The community health nurse can provide education regarding weight and obesity's risks to health.

Because obesity in women is so highly stigmatized in Western culture, women are at highest risk for suffering adverse social and psychological consequences of obesity. These consequences can include social and economic discrimination. More women enter weight treatment programs for their perceived loss of attractiveness rather than for health concerns.

In the last 20 years, reports of disordered eating have noticeably increased. Many girls and women are dissatisfied with their current shape and weight, but only a small number of these actually develop serious eating disorders. The most common eating disorders seen in women are anorexia nervosa and bulimia. *Anorexia* is defined as fear of gaining weight and disturbances in perception of body. Excessive weight loss

is the most noticeable clue. Individuals with anorexia rarely complain of weight loss because they view themselves as normal or overweight. Many of these women struggle with psychological problems, including depression, obsessive symptoms, and social phobias. *Bulimia* is characterized by persistent concern with body shape and weight, recurrent episodes of binge eating, a loss of control during these binges, and use of extreme methods to prevent weight gain, such as purging, strict dieting, fasting, or vigorous exercise. Unlike anorexia, bulimia is observed across all weight categories, with most women being within a normal weight range. Although bulimia is considered less dangerous medically than anorexia, electrolyte imbalance and dehydration can create serious physical complications, such as cardiac arrhythmias.

Community health nurses are in a prime position to incorporate assessment for eating disorders and referral for treatment into their routine clinical practices. The goal of the community health nurse is not only to identify those women with eating disorders, but also those women at risk for developing problems in this area. Through a thorough physical and psychosocial assessment, as well as a history of dietary practice, the nurse will be able to identify women with eating disorders and provide appropriate referrals.

Arthritis

Arthritis is the most prevalent chronic condition experienced by women; it is twice as common in women than men. The rate of arthritis increases significantly with age. Many arthritic diseases exist; the most common form of arthritis is degenerative joint disease, or osteoarthritis. About 25% of women with arthritis experience some limitations in activity because of their condition. Women with arthritis often suffer from chronic, often debilitating, pain. The monetary cost of managing this pain can be devastating to an older woman's meager income (Shaul, 1994). Other areas of concern include obtaining adequate sleep, dealing with medications, maintaining energy, and experiencing depression/anxiety (Buckley et al., 1990; Sotosky et al., 1992). Community health nurses can encourage women to prevent progression of osteoarthritis by teaching about the relationship between extra body weight and increased "wear and tear" on joints. In addition, women should be cautioned to protect their joints from repeated trauma. Physical therapy may be helpful in reducing pain and disability.

Osteoporosis

Osteoporosis is a major health problem for postmenopausal and elderly women. Osteoporosis causes between 1.3 and 1.5 million spinal, hip, and forearm fractures annually (Polan, 1994). The most common fracture associated with osteoporosis is compression fracture of the vertebrae. These fractures may result in curvature of the spine and reduced thoracic volume, leading to a compromised respiratory system. Hip fractures are the second most common fractures associated with osteoporosis. The incidence of this type of fracture increases with age.

The health consequences of osteoporosis are tremendous. Individuals may face pain, surgery, hospitalization, loss of independence, and decreased quality of life. Of the women who survive a hip fracture, 50% will never be able to walk without aid, and 25% will be forced into long-term care (Polan, 1994). It is the leading cause of loss of independent living for women (Birge, 1993).

Two groups of variables contribute to the risk of developing osteoporosis. The first group includes factors that women cannot control: 50 years and over, being Caucasian or Asian, having a petite or slim bone structure, being menopausal or having experienced an early menopause, and having a family history of osteoporosis (Ali and Twibell, 1994). The second group consists of variables that women can change: inadequate intake of calcium, limited exercise, smoking, and excessive alcohol use. Prevention of osteoporosis includes maintaining a desirable weight; maintaining an adequate intake of dietary calcium, phosphorus, and vitamin D; and participating in regular weight-bearing exercise. Researchers have found that women begin experiencing significant bone loss as early as 35 years old. Therefore, premenopausal women should be encouraged to take 1000 mg of calcium daily; postmenopausal women need calcium supplementation of 1500 mg a day and a vitamin D supplement. Weight-bearing exercises and estrogen replacement therapy are also recommended (Birge, 1993).

Prevention efforts for osteoporosis should be targeted at young girls as they develop health promotion behaviors. It is believed that women increase bone mass through their twenties, and women with higher bone mass in early adulthood may be able to resist the effects of age-related bone loss (Lappe, 1994). Anorexia and exercise to the point of amenorrhea may be hazardous to women's bones. Athletic women should be counseled about preserving bone density. Nursing interventions for adult women include gathering a careful family, social, and dietary history and teaching preventive behaviors. Bone mass can be measured by various methods, including single-photon and dual-photon absorptiometry, dual-energy x-ray absorptiometry, and computed tomography. However, bone density measures are not recommended for osteoporosis screening in the general population. Much more research and development are needed before affordable sensitive screening tests are available (Polan, 1994).

For postmenopausal women, nurses should obtain yearly height measures and observe for clinical features of osteoporosis (kyphosis). Nurses can also teach women how to prevent or slow the progression of osteoporosis. In one nursing study (Ali and Twibell, 1994), women over age 50 years consumed less than half the recommended daily calcium intake from milk and yogurt. A number of barriers to prevent osteoporosis were found. These included lack of knowledge about the importance of calcium, exercise, and estrogen replacement therapy to prevent osteoporosis. Moreover, for many women, a low income created an economic barrier to obtaining adequate calcium.

Urinary Incontinence

Urinary incontinence (UI) is a major women's health issue. Most literature uses the definition of incontinence specified by the International Continence Society, a condition in which involuntary loss of urine is a social or hygienic problem and is objectively demonstrable (Bo et al., 1994). It has been estimated that at least 10 million adults in the United States have UI. Women have twice the rates of UI as men.

Between 15 and 64 years of age, up to 25% of women report experiencing UI, and 14% perceive it as a social or hygienic problem. It is believed that the incidence of UI is greatly underreported, since many women believe that losing continence is just the normal result of childbearing or growing older. Urine loss may vary from small infrequent amounts to large frequent amounts.

The consequences of UI can be devastating. UI creates an economic burden on individuals. Individuals typically experience a loss in self-esteem, a sense of guilt, and isolation. UI in elderly persons is the major factor contributing to the family's decision to seek institutional care. In elderly persons, skin breakdown can contribute to the development of pressure ulcers.

As evidenced by the advertising and brisk sales of perineal pads or diapers, many women attempt to manage the problem without seeking professional help. Some studies have estimated that fewer than 50% of individuals with severe incontinence seek professional help. Individuals may wait between 7 and 9 years to seek help (Wallace, 1994). The vast majority of women are never asked questions about UI during a routine physical examination. An objective of *Healthy People 2000* is to increase to at least 60% the proportion of providers of primary care for older adults who routinely evaluate people aged 65 years and older for UI. UI is not restricted, however, just to the older population. Evidence is mounting that young, healthy, nulliparous females often experience UI, especially during exercise. Activities that provoke the highest degree of UI involve jumping, high-impact landings, and running. Women who participate in gymnastics, basketball, and running typically experience UI.

Because so many women will not initiate discussion about problems with UI, introducing the topic and taking a urinary history to determine if a woman has urinary control difficulties are important. Simple questions may invite a woman to begin sharing. "Are you having any problems with urination or bladder control?" "Do you ever unintentionally lose urine?"

Studies have documented that women initiate a variety of self-discovered methods to prevent, minimize, and hide UI (Skoner and Haylor, 1993). Strategies frequently employed include wearing protective pads, avoiding activities that cause urine loss, urinating frequently, limiting fluid intake, performing pelvic muscle exercises, and avoiding or limiting caffeinated beverages.

Community health nurses can encourage a number of behavioral activities that can prevent or minimize UI. Women should be encouraged to maintain adequate hydration (2000 to 3000 ml a day). Women often restrict fluids because of urge incontinence. Restricting fluids may actually worsen incontinence because the bladder does not fill to its normal capacity. Fluids help to distend the bladder to its normal capacity. Decreased fluid intake can also lead to dehydration, cystitis, and constipation. Highly concentrated urine can irritate the bladder mucosa and increase the urge to urinate. Constipation can exacerbate incontinence by putting pressure on the bladder and obstructing the urethra. Some fluids increase the urge to urinate; caffeine beverages and citrus juices should be avoided. Obesity can contribute to incontinence; therefore, weight reduction may reduce UI. Low estrogen levels can lead to flaccid muscle tissue, causing stress incontinence. Perimenopausal and postmenopausal women can be counseled about HRT. Strengthening the sphincter and supporting structures of the bladder (Kegel exercises) should be promoted. Pelvic muscle assessment should become as much a part of preventive health care of women as annual Pap tests and regular mammography. Although several surgical interventions exist for UI, the success rate varies greatly. Comprehensive behavioral and medical management of UI is recommended before referral for surgery (AHCPR, 1992).

Depression

Mental illness patterns vary for women and men. Findings from epidemiological community-based surveys indicate that women are more likely to experience major depression and phobias. Men have higher rates of antisocial personality disorder and alcohol abuse.

Women have twice the rates of depression as men. These rates persist even when income level, education, and occupation are controlled. Women ages 18 to 44 years have the highest rates of depression. Depressive symptoms may range from feelings of sadness to thoughts of death.

A number of factors that may contribute to the development of depression in women have been identified, including unhappy intimate relationships, history of sexual and physical abuse, reproductive events, multiple roles, ethnic minority status, low self-esteem, poverty, and unemployment. Nursing research has also documented the importance of women's social networks in protecting them from depression and enhancing their self-esteem (Woods et al., 1994). Women may derive great satisfaction from interpersonal relationships, but they are also at greater risk for depression when conflict in these relationships occur. When women report unhappiness in their marriages, they are three times as likely as men to be depressed (Wollersheim, 1993).

Research is beginning to document that older women are a high-risk group for depression. Estimates of depression in older women vary greatly across studies (from 2% to 50%). Causes of depression in older women are loss of physical health, loss of a spouse from death or divorce, and financial problems.

Community health nurses should be aware of the signs and symptoms of depression. Depression may be identified in the workplace, adversely affecting the woman's work satisfaction and performance. Prompt referral for professional mental health services should be made if depression is suspected. Women may also benefit from group support focusing on developing coping skills for dealing with difficult relationships and role conflict/overload.

REPRODUCTIVE HEALTH

Women often enter the health care system because of reproductive issues or problems. It is not surprising that community health nurses provide a range of services in the area of reproductive health. *Healthy People 2000* identifies several objectives for improving maternal and infant health during the childbearing years, including increasing prenatal care, reducing complications of pregnancy, and decreasing low birth weight and infant mortality. In addition, improvement in preconceptional counseling and prenatal and newborn screening is sought. A number of initiatives have been recommended to improve maternal and infant health (see box on p. 555). Some progress has been made, but more work is needed.

Family Planning

U.S. women have a wide array of effective contraceptives from which to choose. Unfortunately, more than half of the 6 million annual pregnancies in the United States are unplanned, and about half end in abortion (Pasquale, 1994). Community health nurses need to take an active role in discussing contraception use with all women of childbearing age. Much of the literature focuses on the problem of unintended pregnancy among adolescents. Little attention has been paid to the contraceptive concerns of adult women. Health care providers erroneously assume that adult women are fully informed about contraception, use their method correctly and con-

Initiatives to Improve Maternal and Infant Health

Providing family planning services for all women who want to use them.

Providing preconceptional and interconceptional counseling.

Providing maternity benefits for all pregnant women.

Improving accessibility of health care services for pregnant women by the provision of an adequate number of strategically located clinics, transportation, and child care facilities.

Removing barriers to prenatal care, including negative provider attitudes, lack of continuity in care, and unnecessary waiting for care.

Protecting childbearing women from occupational hazards.

Extending the Special Supplemental Food Program for Women, Infants, and Children (WIC) to all pregnant and breast-feeding women.

Implementing programs to help pregnant women decrease smoking and use of drugs and alcohol.

Providing special follow-up of all high-risk women after delivery.

Granting parental leave for employed parents.

---

sistently, and are highly satisfied (Pasquale, 1994).

Effective contraceptive counseling not only requires accurate knowledge of current contraceptive choices but also a nonjudgmental approach. Women should be encouraged to talk about intimate family and individual issues. The goal of contraceptive counseling is to ensure that women receive appropriate instruction to take charge of their own reproductive choices.

Assessment should include questions about sexual behavior; medical history; health habits, including smoking; past contraceptive failures; and motivation. Choice of method depends on compliance motivation. Is the woman able to take daily pills or insert a diaphragm before each act of intercourse? Does the woman want to practice minimal compliance required by the intrauterine device (IUD), Norplant, or Depo-Provera?

Contraception instruction should include discussion of all the options available. Women may put themselves at risk for unintended pregnancy through their method choices and changes. Many women seek contraceptive services with a specific contraception chosen. Research has documented, however, that many women have much wrong information regarding the relative risks of methods. For example, women often overestimate the cancer risks of oral contraceptives. A comprehensive presentation of contraception options is also important because women use many different methods and change methods often. Many times they never fill a prescription or purchase the over-the-counter method. Sometimes, women change contraception methods between health care visits. Women who had previously selected a highly effective pregnancy prevention option (e.g., oral contraceptives) may switch to a method that is much less effective (e.g., condoms or withdrawal) (Matteson and

Hawkins, 1993). Careful discussion may prevent some of these problems.

Preconceptional Counseling

In recent years a movement to expand the concept of prenatal care to include preconceptional counseling has gained momentum (Moos, 1994). **Preconceptional counseling** includes education, assessment, diagnosis, and interventions to address risks before conception (Frede, 1992). The goal of preconceptional care is to reduce or eliminate risks for both the woman and the infant. Enthusiasm for preconceptional care has increased as the rates for low birth weight, infant mortality, and congenital malformations have remained stagnant. Increasingly, it is recognized that many risks can be identified and corrected before conception. For example, research has linked inadequate intake of folic acid with the development of neural tube defects. Additional folic acid during the first 6 weeks of pregnancy may protect against neural tube defects. Thus, the U.S. Public Health Service recommends that all women of childbearing age who are capable of becoming pregnant should consume 0.4 mg of folic acid per day.

Preconception assessment should include discussion of a woman's family, medical, reproductive, nutritional, and social history. During assessment, areas deserving attention can be uncovered. For example, exposure to tobacco and alcohol may be detected. Education about the effects of these on the fetus can be explored, and efforts aimed at decreasing exposure can be taken.

Prenatal Care

Prenatal care is a variable strongly associated with improved birth outcomes. A number of barriers exist, however, in women seeking prenatal care. Many times, women are hesitant to seek early prenatal care because of the cost. Twenty-five percent of women of childbearing age are without public or private health insurance (Stevens and O'Connell, 1992). Of the women who have health insurance, 25% do not have maternity insurance coverage. Many women lack transportation and must travel great distances to seek care. Women may face a bureaucratic system that is understaffed and underfinanced. Some physicians will not treat Medicaid patients or those with little insurance (Lucas-Holt, 1994). Often, clinics are crowded; the waiting time is long. Moreover, most clinics do not offer child care services.

Pregnant women cite a number of factors that increase their motivation to seek prenatal care, including transportation assistance, telephone or mailed reminders, child care, cash payments, layette gifts, and posters (Stevens and O'Connell, 1992).

U.S. social policy dictates few supports for childbearing families. This in direct contrast to most other

Research Brief

Freda MC, Fogarassy MMA, Davini D, DeVore NE, Damus K, Merkatz IR: Are they watching? Are they learning? Prenatal video education in the waiting room, J *Perinatal Educ* 3(1):20-28, 1994.

One method of educating pregnant women has become common practice in prenatal clinics; education videotapes are shown continually in the waiting rooms. The expectation is that women will watch them and learn important information about prenatal care and infant care. This study was conducted to determine whether women learned from these videotapes. Videos were shown in the prenatal waiting room on alternating weeks in an inner-city prenatal clinic. The experimental group included women having their first prenatal visit on a week when videos were shown. The control group included women having their first prenatal visit when videos were not shown. Test scores were significantly higher for the group exposed to the videotapes. However, women had little knowledge about the videotape topics whether or not they were exposed to videotapes. Although some women learned from the videos, passive waiting room education should be considered only as a supplementary educational technique. It should not be used as a single strategy for teaching women important information during pregnancy.

industrialized countries. European countries, with infant mortality rates less than the U.S. rate, provide all mothers with early adequate prenatal care. Many countries offer additional support for pregnant women. Pregnant Japanese women can ride free on city buses. In England, health visitors visit all new mothers. France has developed an elaborate cash payment program for women engaged in prenatal care.

Most industrialized countries have established policies that protect not only the mother and infant, but the family as well. Among these countries, only the United States and South Africa do not have a charter that states that the health and well-being of families is a national priority (Grad, 1989). The United States is also one of the few industrialized countries without a central administrative office to coordinate policies and initiatives for maternal-child health.

In addition to lack of prenatal care, life-style problems such as inadequate nutrition, smoking, substance use, poor maternal health, psychological distress, and violence are important contributors to high infant mortality (Stevens and O'Connell, 1992). Promoting healthy life-style behaviors and reducing risk factors should provide the core of prenatal care. In addition to assessing development of the fetus and the general health of the woman, community health nurses should address areas such as eating proper foods, taking vitamin or mineral supplements, stress management, smoking cessation, alcohol/drug treat-

ment, gaining an appropriate amount of weight, seeking social support, and parent education. A U.S. Public Health Service Expert Panel has recommended a set of basic screening, education, and counseling components that all women should receive during prenatal care. Many women do not receive this prenatal content (Kogan et al., 1994). Improvements in the delivery of prenatal care are needed.

A community nursing model of innovative prenatal care developed for women in Hawaii uses themes to guide nurses in monitoring the woman's pregnancy-postpartum adaptation (Affonso et al., 1992). These themes communicate the goals for prenatal care to women. Themes for the first trimester include "Am I really pregnant?" "What does it mean to be pregnant?" "What's happening to me and my baby?" and "Having status as a pregnant woman." Second-trimester themes include "Staying healthy through self-care" and "Is my baby okay?" Third-trimester themes include "Preparing for labor and birth," "Expectations for my baby and myself," and "Lady in waiting." Within this model of care, essential prenatal screening, education, and counseling can take place while incorporating understanding of women's needs within their social environment and cultural lifestyles. This model provides an exciting nursing alternative to the traditional medical model of prenatal care.

WOMEN AT MIDLIFE

Ages 35 to 65 years are commonly referred to as midlife. This transition time represents the more mature years after young adulthood but before the senior years. During this time, women typically experience many physiological, psychological, and social changes.

The average life expectancy for a woman born 100 years ago was about 49 years; many women did not live beyond menopause. Today it is expected that a woman will live one-third of her life past menopause. Thus, interest in midlife women's health has grown.

Menopause is a biological transition in women's lives that has personal, social, and cultural significance (Woods, 1994a). Society is beginning to replace the image of menopause as a time of great emotional imbalance and the beginning of the end of a woman's life with the positive image of menopause as a time of individual growth, vitality, and aging with dignity. Although menopause is a universal life transition for women during midlife, women are poorly prepared for what to expect during this stage. Natural menopause is a gradual process with progressive changes in anovulatory cycles and eventual cessation of menses. In the 8 to 10 years preceding menopause, hormonal changes occur that eventually lead to amenorrhea.

During the **perimenopausal** period, women may note a number of changes in their menstrual periods. They may experience longer periods, with 2 to 3 days of spotting, followed by several days of heavy bleeding. They may also have regular menses followed by several days of spotting.

Reduced production of estrogen results in many physiological changes. Some of these changes are apparent (hot flashes), but others are silent (cardiovascular and bone changes), having no immediate signs or symptoms. One menopause center reported that of the women who sought help, 79% reported physical symptoms and 63% reported emotional symptoms (Rebar, 1994). The most common physical symptoms were hot flashes, muscle and joint pains, headaches, and weight gain. The most common emotional symptoms included irritability, fatigue, tension, nervousness, depression, and inability to concentrate. When women identified emotional symptoms, these tended to be more vague than the physical symptoms.

Hot flashes are a significant problem, affecting the daily functioning and quality of life for many perimenopausal and postmenopausal women (Kronenberg, 1994). Hot flashes may disrupt sleep, leading to fatigue and irritability during the day. Hot flashes may cause profuse sweating and result in embarrassment, particularly in the workplace. While HRT can relieve hot flashes, the exact mechanism by which this works is not well understood. A number of self-management remedies may also be helpful for women who do not want or cannot take HRT. Many women have a particular pattern to their hot flashes. Tracking hot flashes over several days may increase a woman's awareness of the pattern as well as any precipitating factors, such as particular foods to avoid. Many women find that their hot flashes are worse when environmental temperatures are highest. Women may be able to reduce nighttime awakenings by sleeping in a cool bedroom. Particular foods may trigger hot flashes, and spicy foods, alcohol, and caffeine may increase hot flashes. Some research indicates that regular exercise may reduce the severity of hot flashes. Smoking reduces estrogen levels and may increase the risk of hot flashes.

HRT is the most frequently prescribed therapy for symptoms related to menopause. In addition to reducing hot flashes, HRT appears to retard the development of osteoporosis, reduce urinary incontinence and vaginal dryness, prevent thinning of the skin, reduce the risk of heart disease, reduce the risk of Alzheimer's disease, and positively affect mood. Despite the number of health benefits that can be documented for HRT, great controversy still surrounds this form of therapy. Some women do not like the side effects of HRT, such as headaches, nausea and vomiting, bloating, weight gain, and irritation with contact lenses. Moreover, HRT may increase the likelihood of development of gallbladder disease and endometrial and breast cancer.

Many women do not have an understanding of the long-term health-related consequences of menopause. Nurses should emphasize the importance of health maintenance for all midlife women. During the midlife, women can be encouraged to make additional

 Possible Components of a Comprehensive Midlife Women's Health Program

Blood chemistry profile
Complete blood count
Lipid profile
Complete history
Comprehensive physical examination
Pap test
Endometrial biopsy
Mammography
Bone density screening
Health risk appraisal
Dietary profile
Flexibility/exercise screening
Hemoccult screening
Education programs on osteoporosis, mammography, breast self-examination, menopause, and hysterectomy
Individualized educational components on incontinence, heart disease, smoking cessation, skin cancer, and fibrocystic breast disease

Modified from Garner CH: *NAACOG Clin Issues* 2(4):480, 1991.

life-style changes to avoid ill health during later years. Some potential life-style changes include (1) stop smoking, (2) reduce obesity, (3) reduce dietary fat, (4) increase dietary fiber, (5) adopt a sensible exercise regimen, (6) minimize sun exposure, (7) decrease alcohol and caffeine, (8) avoid abuse of medications, (9) seek screening examinations, and (10) adopt a stress management program (Frank, 1991). Possible components of a comprehensive midlife women's health program are identified in the box above.

Increasingly, women want to be actively involved in selecting therapies for managing the effects of symptoms that occur during midlife, such as hot flashes. Many women choose self-management approaches, including self-help groups, relaxation techniques, biofeedback, imagery, exercise, and herb and vitamin therapy.

TRANSITIONS IN AGING

For many women, the years past retirement are a time of enrichment and personal growth. After years of working and caring for their families, they finally have time for themselves. Some women discover a creativity within themselves that they were not aware existed or previously did not have time to foster. Some become writers and artists for the first time at 60 or 70 years old. Women also enjoy their older years traveling, reading, studying, gardening, and spending time with family. Unfortunately, for some of these women and many others, growing older also means facing a series of hardships and losses (Szwabo, 1993).

Older adults, of which women are the majority, are the fastest-growing segment of the population. Predictions are that by the end of the twenty-first century, the number of older people will double (Olshansky et al., 1990). In the 65- to 74-year-old age group, 6.5% are men and 7.9% are women. In the 65- to 69-year-old age group, there are 84 men to every 100 women. However, among the oldest elderly, the number of men over 85 years old drops to 39 men for every 100 women. For those women who live beyond 85 years old, there are often no loved ones to care for them. They may die alone, often abused and neglected.

Caregiving has defined the lives of many women. This continues as women age and care for ill husbands. The demands of spousal caregiving are often the most difficult for women because of their own age, fading health, and lack of resources.

Women are more likely than men to be widowed. The average age of widowhood is 56 years, and the average woman can expect to live another 30 years. Many widowed women are at increased risk for social isolation, depression, poverty, and substance abuse (Szwabo, 1993). Widowed women incur more health care costs than married women. Although Medicare pays 44% of an elderly couple's health care costs, only 33% of a single woman's health care costs are covered (Arendell and Estes, 1991). As the need for health care services increases with age, many elderly women are propelled further into poverty.

Because women have a greater life expectancy than men, they are more susceptible to disabilities associated with aging. It is estimated that half the additional life expectancy of women is spent in a state of disability. The cost of these years of disability further depletes the already limited resources of elderly women.

Older minority women are most likely to live in poverty. While 15% of women over age 65 live in poverty, that number increases to 25% among Hispanic women and 33% among African-American women (Szwabo, 1993). The consequences of older minority women with a history of poor health living their lives in poverty place them at the greatest risk for health problems (Hopper, 1993).

When elderly women require care, it is frequently middle-aged daughters that assume responsibility for their mothers. Thus, the cycle of caregiving is complete for one woman and continues for another.

WOMEN'S USE OF HEALTH SERVICES

Caregiving is a major role of women throughout their lifespan. For many women, caring for family members is informal care that they provide in addition to paid employment outside the home. Mothers assume the primary responsibility for the health and illness of their young families, wives often care for their aging and ill husbands, and daughters and daughters-in-law care for aging parents or in-laws. Unfortunately, in today's society the role of caregiver is devalued. Most women today are juggling the roles of wife, employee, and caregiver to children, parents, and in-laws with

little assistance from spouses, employers, and government.

The wages lost by women to fulfill their role as caretaker of the family's health are immeasurable. It has been estimated that employed mothers spend 15 hours a week more than men fulfilling their caregiver responsibilities; over a year's time, this "second shift" work totals an extra month of 24-hour days (Hochschild, 1989). Midlife women with children in the home who are caring for an elderly family member spend an additional 20 to 28 hours a week (Russo, 1990). The added responsibility and financial strain of the caregiver role can lead to **caregiver burden** and increased stress. When a young mother must take time off of work to keep a health care provider appointment or to care for a sick child, she loses wages. When a daughter who is caring for an elderly relative at home is forced to quit her job or work part time, the interruption in employment can mean a decline in family income and loss of insurance coverage and retirement contributions (Russo, 1990).

Access to medical care is inextricably linked to health insurance. Women lack health insurance for various reasons. Many women work part time or are employed in low-paying jobs that do not provide insurance coverage. For example, of the 1.5 million women who work in nursing homes and home health agencies, 75% earn under $10,000 per year and few have employer-provided health insurance (Older Women's League, 1992). Also, 94% of the 2 to 3 million child care workers earn incomes below poverty level, and few have health insurance (McGovern et al., 1992).

Many women have health insurance through their husband's employer. If the marriage ends in divorce, a women's coverage is dropped. With 50% of all marriages ending in divorce, the number of women without the benefit of their spouse's health insurance is swelling.

The health behaviors of women are influenced by their access to health care, and in turn, their access to health care is influenced by their level of education and income. Well-educated women with sufficient financial means are more likely to eat healthy, drink less alcohol, and smoke less (Woods et al., 1993).

Poverty and lack of education increase the incidence of stress, depression, and health-damaging behavior. Moreover, women of color are overrepresented in the category of the poorly educated, unemployed, and divorced. Not surprisingly, therefore, they also have the poorest physical health of any social group (Cummings et al., 1993).

The impact of paid employment on the health of women may vary (Facione, 1994; Rankin, 1993). For some women, the financial and emotional benefit of paid employment is associated with an increased sense of well-being. For others, the multiple, often conflicting, roles can lead to stress and self-neglect. Community health nurses can teach women time and stress management, particularly how to share the work at home with other family members (Rankin, 1993).

Paradoxically, despite women's pivotal role in providing care, very few women participate in public decisions regarding health care. A powerful minority of male physicians, legislators, and health care administrators control decisions regarding research, public policy, and health care (Quimby, 1994). In recent years, this has begun to change. Women are now entering traditionally male-dominated fields of medicine, research, and health care administration. There are now more women in Congress than at any other time in U.S. history. As more women participate in the decision-making process, more women's health issues will be addressed. Community coalition building is one way that nurses can increase community awareness of women's issues.

PROGRAMS FOR WOMEN'S HEALTH SERVICES

An encounter with a health provider can be an opportunity for women to share issues of concern in their lives and glean information to make informed decisions about their family's health. Instead, many women dread this experience. Too many health care providers view their own time as more valuable than that of their clients. Women, whose time is viewed as less valuable, are expected to endure frequent long waits to see a health care professional. Because of their role as family caregiver, women experience this much more than men. The treatment experienced by women who receive public health care is even worse. They often wait several hours for treatment, only to be rushed through their examination, provided little information, and discouraged from asking questions. Health care providers must take the time to interact with their female patients, and women must be provided with the information that they need to make informed decisions (Gauthier and Krassen-Maxwell, 1991).

Programs for women's health should offer comprehensive screening and education for women in one convenient setting. Clustering of services and collaboration with other disciplines and medical specialties are important. A team approach might include a nurse who coordinates services. Nurses can interview women before they see their primary provider and assemble patient education materials.

One suggested model involves a 1-day or two-part program. One visit would consist of testing and the second for interpretation of results and education/counseling. Some education and counseling can be provided in groups, but attention to individual women still requires quality provider time. Although women may spend some time waiting for some services, this time can be valuable for patient education.

SPECIAL POPULATIONS

Three groups of women warrant special consideration because of the uniqueness of their lives. In this section, lesbians, women in prison, and single mothers are discussed. Adolescent pregnancy is discussed in Chapter 34.

Lesbians

It is difficult to determine the actual number of lesbians because they are a hidden population. Estimates range from 2% to 10% of the female population. There are lesbian women in all races, classes, and ethnic groups. Lesbians are both similar to and different from heterosexual women.

Many lesbian women hide their sexual preference from neighbors, family, co-workers, and health care providers out of fear of discrimination and reprisal. Although the American Psychiatric Association recognized lesbianism as a normal sexual choice in 1972, **heterosexism** and **homophobia** contribute to the prejudice, fear, and discrimination that lesbian women endure. Many lesbians are denied jobs, housing, and custody of their children on the basis of their sexual orientation. Sometimes, prejudice and fear are acted out in the form of violence against lesbian women.

The decision to live openly as a lesbian is a difficult one. The term "coming out" refers to the decision to disclose one's sexual identity rather than hiding it. Many women report knowing as teenagers that they were attracted to females but denying their feelings out of fear. Many marry, have children, and only later in life acknowledge their sexual preference. Divorced lesbians with children are often denied custody of their children on the basis of their sexual preference.

The 1980s are known as the "lesbian baby boom." The number of lesbian couples who have children increased significantly. Some women choose to conceive a child through artificial insemination or heterosexual intercourse, whereas others opt to adopt or become foster parents (Zeidenstein, 1990).

Although many of the health care needs of lesbian women are the same as those of heterosexual women, some special considerations exist. Lesbians are at low risk for vaginal infections, STDs, and HIV. A lesbian woman's risk of HIV may increase because of previous and current contact with HIV-infected semen, IV drug use, or sexual partners with unknown sexual history. The community health nurse can teach lesbian women to have regular pelvic examinations and avoid unprotected oral sex by using latex barriers, such as a dental dam (Zeidenstein, 1990).

Many lesbian women neglect their health care needs. One nurse researcher found that 50% of the respondents reported receiving gynecological examinations every 3 to 5 years to not at all. Even more shocking is that most respondents were highly educated professional women with access to health care. The majority of the women believed that they were at less risk than heterosexual women for an abnormal Pap test. Lesbian women who have had heterosexual intercourse are at risk for cervical cancer (Zeidenstein, 1990). The adverse effects of a lack of regular gynecological screening and breast examination is well documented in this chapter.

Many lesbians delay health care to avoid an encounter with a health care provider. Lesbian women complain of health care providers assuming their heterosexuality with questions such as "What method of birth control do you use?" If a woman can feel comfortable enough to disclose her lesbianism, the quality of health care that she receives is improved. Nurses can create a nonthreatening environment by asking questions such as "What is your sexual status (heterosexual, homosexual, bisexual)?" (Zeidenstein, 1990). Lesbian women are more likely to reveal their true selves to nurses who are open and nonjudgmental.

Many lesbian women experience increased stress and depression because of social isolation, prejudice, and discrimination. Substance abuse is also a major problem for 30% of all lesbian women (Deevey and Wall, 1992). Many cities have special Alcoholics Anonymous meetings for lesbian women. Mental health counseling, particularly by therapists trained for dealing with this special population, is recommended for depression. Many communities have active lesbian women's support groups.

Women in Prison

Although women represent only a small percentage (5.5%) of the total state prison population, this number is drastically increasing (Bureau of Justice Statistics, 1991). In the past decade, the number of African-American women in prison has quadrupled (French, 1991). The upsurge in the female prison population is directly attributed to drugs and drug-related crimes. Many women in prison are poor, minority, single mothers.

The problems of incarcerated women are not unlike those of women everywhere. For example, they are in need of routine gynecological and breast examinations. Also, many have children; making child care arrangements while they are in prison is worrisome. Many women inmates have a history of drug use, but there are few drug treatment programs for incarcerated women.

Many inmates enter prison pregnant and are more likely than women in the general population to be chemically dependent and enter prenatal care late (Fogel, 1993). The stress of being in prison is compounded by being pregnant. Community health nursing interventions must be aimed at intensive health education related to childbirth and child care. Inmates should be encouraged to discuss their concerns in self-help groups. Also, group counseling sessions for inmates and their families are suggested, as well as

instruction in stress management and self-esteem enhancement (Fogel, 1993).

Single Mothers

In the past two decades, the traditional two-parent family has gained minority status. Only 35% of family households in the United States have two parents. Single parents now maintain one third of all households. Divorce accounts for 37% of single-parent households, while 35% are maintained by a parent who had never married. Single mothers are six times as likely as single fathers to be raising children (Bureau of Census, 1993).

The poverty rate for families supported by single women is six times as high as for married couple families. In 1992, women maintained 52% of all poor families. Among white and Hispanic families, 43% were maintained by women, and 75% of African-American families living in poverty were supported by women (U.S. Department of Labor, 1992).

Divorced women often live in poverty. Nonpayment of child support is a major factor that contributes to the economic decline of many female-headed families. In 1989, of the 5 million women due to receive child support payments, only 50% received the full amount awarded by the courts. The average amount of child support received in 1989 was $2995 dollars (Scarr, 1994).

Some women are single mothers by choice. Many of these women have had a previous pregnancy that ended in abortion or adoption. Some adopt, and others become pregnant through artificial insemination or intercourse. Some plan their pregnancy, and others choose to become mothers when they learn they are pregnant. The profile of single mothers by choice is changing. A growing population of single mothers by choice is characterized by a woman who is older, well educated, and financially able (Pakizegi, 1990).

Most single mothers do the work of two with resources for one. The synergistic effect of the multiple responsibilities of home and a job can lead to depression and stress. Single mothers often feel lonely and isolated. A sound social network of family and friends can contribute to the well-being and satisfaction of single mothers.

HEALTH POLICY

With the exception of reproductive health, policy makers have paid little attention to the needs of women. Until the 1990s, women's health issues were absent in public policy and medical research (Quimby, 1994). With the passages of two pieces of legislation, the Family and Medical Leave Act of 1993 (FMLA) and the Women's Health Equity Act (WHEA) of 1990, many of the needs specific to women will finally be addressed.

The FMLA provides job protection and continuous health benefits (if applicable) to eligible employees

What Do You Think?

Women are underrepresented at every level of health policy decision making.

who need extended unpaid leave. Eligible employees can take 12 weeks annually for serious personal or family health conditions or for the birth or adoption of a child. Family is defined as the employee's child, spouse, or parents (Zuffoletto, 1994). The FLMA is particularly beneficial to women who work outside of the home and are family caregivers. Before this legislation, many women had to quit or were terminated from their jobs in order to care for a newborn or an ill family member. The loss of employment benefits created financial hardship for many women and served to punish women caregivers. The FLMA may be of little benefit for low-income women, since 12 weeks without pay is financially ruinous.

In response to the gross inequities in research between men and women's health issues, the WHEA was passed in 1990. As a result of WHEA, women's health has emerged as a field of discussion, study, and research in many schools of nursing and medicine (Quimby, 1994).

In 1990 the Office of Research in Women's Health was created within the National Institutes of Health (NIH). Shortly thereafter, the Women's Health Initiative, a $625-million, 14-year study of diseases in women, began in 1993. It is the largest study of diseases in women ever conducted (Sharp, 1993). This initiative will begin to identify the uniqueness of women's health.

Although women's issues are at the forefront of public policy today, much work still needs to be done. Those most vulnerable populations in a society are the very young and the very old. Because women are the primary family caregivers at both ends of the age continuum, a national child care policy and a policy on aging is of particular concern.

The United States is the only country in the industrialized world that does not have a national child care policy. In Europe, parents pay much less for child care that is rated better than that in the United States. Whereas parents in Europe typically pay 5% to 15% of the cost of their children's childcare, their U.S. counterparts pay more than 90%. It is estimated that the average parent pays $2600 for child care annually. It is further estimated that in order to provide good child care, the cost would be $5000 annually. In Europe the cost is $7000 to $10,000 per child per year. The added cost goes to fund the salary and benefits of European child care workers. A national policy on child care similar to that in European countries would not only provide assistance to parents, but would also lift millions of child care workers out of poverty (Scarr et al., 1993).

Although the FLMA has provided much needed assistance to families caring for aging family members, much work still needs to be done. Currently, the law requires elderly married couples to spend much of their assets in order for Medicare to pay for the cost of nursing home care. Because wives are typically younger than their husbands, it is often the wife who must place her husband in a nursing home and as a consequence live in poverty.

The community health nurse must advocate for legislation of public policies that support issues important to the lives of women and their families. It is also important that the community health nurse promote self-advocacy among women.

 ## Clinical Application

The following situation involves the needs and health problems of a middle-aged woman and her family. A student can apply knowledge of the nursing process, women's health, and community health nursing to make clinical decisions.

Mrs. Johnson is a 50-year-old black woman who works as a nursing assistant at a long-term care facility for elderly persons. She is a widow with two adult children. Her third child, Michael, was murdered 2 years ago while walking home one night. He was 18 years old. Her daughters Vicky, age 32, and Jackie, age 30, live in the neighborhood. She has five grandchildren: Jamil, age 14; Shandra, age 12; Chrystal, age 8; and Shaquil, age 6. Mrs. Johnson's 70-year-old mother, Mrs. Smith, now lives with her since she suffered a mild stroke 2 months ago and can no longer manage alone. The community health nurse

visits three times a week to monitor Mrs. Smith's blood pressure and cardiovascular status.

Mrs. Johnson rises early to prepare breakfast for her mother and assist her to dress. She also prepares her mother's lunch before she leaves for work. Mrs. Smith can ambulate around the house with the aid of a walker and is independent in most of her activities of daily living.

When Mrs. Johnson returns home in the evening, she prepares dinner and assists her mother to prepare for bed. She shops, cleans her house, and does laundry on Saturdays. She relies on public transportation. Vicky and Jackie provide assistance when they can, although both women work full time and have children.

Since her son's death, Mrs. Johnson has become active in community organizing efforts to stop the vi-

Continued.

Clinical Application—cont'd

olence in her neighborhood. She attends weekly meetings at her church. The neighborhood has changed in the 30 years that she has lived there. It is now a dangerous place to live. She knows that there is drug dealing, and sometimes at night she hears the sound of gunfire. She worries about the safety of her grandchildren, especially Jamil. On Sundays she attends church and cooks dinner. Her daughters and grandchildren often come for Sunday dinner.

One day when the nurse visits Mrs. Smith, Mrs. Johnson is home. Mrs. Johnson mentions to the nurse that she has a history of hypertension that is controlled with medication and diet. However, she has not taken her Aldomet for 2 days. She will not be able to fill her prescription until Friday when she is paid. The nurse takes her blood pressure, which is 190/100.

The nurse recommends that Mrs. Johnson go to the public health clinic and see the nurse practitioner. At the clinic the nurse completes a health history and learns that Mrs. Johnson has smoked 15 to 20 cigarettes a day for the past 30 years. She has not had a

Pap test in 5 years. She has no health insurance and no sick leave. A 24-hour dietary recall reveals that Mrs. Johnson had eggs, bacon, and juice for breakfast; hamburger and french fries for lunch; and red beans with sausage for dinner. She had potato chips and a coke for an afternoon snack and cookies and milk at bedtime. Her blood pressure remains high at 190/96.

- ◆ What additional information should be collected about Mrs. Johnson?
- ◆ What are the nursing diagnoses?
- ◆ What factors must be considered when developing a plan of care?
- ◆ Develop a plan of care for Mrs. Johnson.
- ◆ What are the criteria to evaluate the plan of care?
- ◆ Identify the teaching and learning needs of Mrs. Johnson.
- ◆ What are the continued health risks for Mrs. Johnson and her family?
- ◆ Identify women's health issues from the chapter that apply to Mrs. Johnson's life.
- ◆ Identify community resources that might be of assistance to Mrs. Johnson and her mother.

Key Concepts

- ◆ Relationships are pivotal in the development of female identity.
- ◆ Women have a longer life expectancy than men. However, women are more likely to have acute and chronic conditions that require them to use health services more than men.
- ◆ The three major causes of mortality in women are heart disease, cancer, and cerebrovascular disease. The three major chronic conditions women experience are heart conditions, arthritis, and hypertension.
- ◆ The failure to include women in medical research has resulted in a lack of understanding about the distinctive issues surrounding the diagnosis and treatment of the major diseases for women.

- ◆ Smoking is a risk factor for a number of major health problems: lung cancer, heart disease, osteoporosis, and poor reproductive outcomes.
- ◆ Women assume the primary responsibility for the health of their family members.
- ◆ Women of color are more likely to have poor health outcomes because of a poor understanding of health, lack of access to health care, and life-style practices.
- ◆ There are very few early warning signs for a number of potential health problems for mid-life women, such as osteoporosis and heart disease. Women can engage in various preventive health care practices to avoid ill health.

Critical Thinking Activities

1. Design a teaching plan for a middle-age woman that reflects a maximum level of health promotion.
2. Analyze mortality and morbidity data in your county and rank the order of the 10 most prevalent health problems for women. Compare these to men's health problems.

3. Interview three women (young, middle age, and older). Compare and contrast their major health concerns.
4. Using a telephone book or community resources directory, list and evaluate health promotion and prevention services available for women. Include fees, location, and range of services.

Bibliography

Affonso DD, Mayberry LJ, Graham K, Shibuya J, Kunimoto J, Kuramoto M: Adaptation themes for prenatal care delivered by public health nurses, *Public Health Nurs* 9:172-176, 1992.

Agency for Health Care Policy and Research: *Urinary incontinence in adults*, Rockville, Md, 1992, US Department of Health and Human Services.

Agency for Health Care Policy and Research: *Quality determinants of mammography*, Rockville, Md, 1994, US Department of Health and Human Services.

Ali N, Twibell R: Barriers to osteoporosis prevention in perimenopausal and elderly women, *Geriatr Nurs* 15(4):201-205, 1994.

American Cancer Society: *Cancer facts and figures—1994*, Atlanta, 1994, The Society.

American College of Obstetricians and Gynecologists: *Routine cancer screening*, ACOG Committee Opinion No 128, Washington, DC, 1993, Committee on Gynecologic Practice.

American Heart Association: *Heart and stroke facts*, Dallas, 1994, The Association.

Arendell T, Estes CL: Older women in the post-Reagan era. In Minkler M, Estes CL, editors: *Critical perspectives on aging: the political and moral economy of growing old*, Amityville, NY, 1991, Baywood.

Arras JD: AIDS and reproductive decisions: having children in fear and trembling, *Milbank Q* 68(3):353-382, 1990.

Averette H, Steren A, Nguyen HN: Screening in gynecologic cancers, *Cancer (Suppl)* 72:1043-1049, 1993.

Barrett-Conner E, Bush TL: Estrogen and coronary heart disease in women, *JAMA* 265:1861-1867, 1991.

Birenbaum A: Courtesy stigma revisited, *Ment Retard* 30:265-268, 1992.

Birge, SJ: Osteoporosis and hip fracture, *Clin Geriatr Med* 9(1):69-86, 1993.

Bo K, Stien R, Kulseng-Hanssen S, Kristofferson M: Clinical and urodynamic assessment of nulliparous young women with and without stress incontinence symptoms: a case-control study, *Obstet Gynecol* 84:1028-1032, 1994.

Breen N, Kessler L: Changes in the use of screening mammography: evidence from the 1987 and 1990 National Health Interview Surveys, *Am J Public Health* 84:62-67, 1994.

Buckley LM, Vacek P, and Cooper SM: Educational and psychosocial needs of patients with chronic disease: a survey of preferences of patients with rheumatoid arthritis, *Arthritis Care Res* 3(1):5-10, 1990.

Bureau of Census: *Families in the US*, Washington, DC, 1993, US Department of Commerce.

Bureau of Census: *Statistical abstract of the United States*, Washington, DC, 1994, US Department of Commerce.

Bureau of Justice Statistics: Survey of state prison inmates. In *Statistical abstract of the United States*, Washington, DC, 1991.

Champion VL: Relationship of age to factors influencing breast self-examination practice, *Health Care Women Int* 13:1-9, 1992.

Chodorow N: *The reproduction of mothering*, Berkeley, 1978, University of California Press.

Cohen FL: Clinical manifestations and treatment of HIV infection and AIDS in women. In Cohen FL, Durham JD, editors: *Women, children, and HIV/AIDS*, New York, 1993, Springer.

Cohen SS: Overview of maternal-child health policies. In Natapoff JN, Wieczorek RR, editors: *Maternal-child health policy: a nursing perspective*, New York, 1990, Springer.

Croft P, Hannaford PC: Risk factors for acute myocardial infarction in women: evidence from Royal College of General Practitioners' Oral Contraception Study, *Br Med J* 298:165-168, 1989.

Cummings CM, Robinson AM, Lopez GE: Perceptions of discrimination, psycho-social functioning, and physical symptoms of African-American women. In Bair B, Cayleff SE, editors: *Wings of gauze: women of color and the experience of health and illness*, Detroit, 1993, Wayne State University Press.

Dan AJ, editor: *Reframing women's health: multidisciplinary research and practice*, Thousand Oaks, Calif, 1994, Sage.

Das BN, Banka VS: Coronary artery disease in women: how it is—and isn't—unique, *Postgrad Med* 91(4):197-206, 1992.

Deevey S, Wall LJ: How do lesbian women develop serenity, *Health Care Women Int* 13(2):199-208, 1992.

Dodd GD: Screening for breast cancer, *Cancer (Suppl)* 72:1038-1042, 1993.

Facione NC: Role overload and health: the married mother in the waged labor force, *Health Care Women Int* 15:157-167, 1994.

Fogel CI: Pregnant inmates: risk factors and pregnancy outcome, *J Obstet Gynecol Neonatal Nurs* 22(1):33-39, 1993.

Frank MEV: Transition into midlife, *NAACOG Clin Issues* 2(4):421-428, 1991.

Freda MC, Fogarassy MMA, Davini D, DeVore NE, Damus K, Merkatz IR: Are they watching? Are they learning? Prenatal video education in the waiting room, *J Perinatal Educ* 3(1):20-28, 1994.

Frede DJ: The state of preconceptional health education, *J Perinatal Educ* 1(2):19-26, 1992.

French L: A profile of the incarcerated black female offender, *Prison J*, 1991, pp 80-87.

Garfinkel L: Current trends in breast cancer, *CA Cancer J Clin* 43(1):5-6, 1993.

Garner C: Midlife women's health, *NAACOG Clin Issues* 2(4):473-481, 1991.

Gauthier CC, Krassen-Maxwell E: Time demands and medical ethics in women's health care, *Health Care Women Int* 12:153-165, 1991.

Gilligan C: Woman's place in a man's life cycle, *Harvard Educ Rev* 49:431-446, 1979.

Gilligan C: *In a different voice*, Cambridge, Mass, 1982, Harvard University Press.

Grad RK: National commission acts on behalf of children, *Matern Child Nurs J* 14:237-242, 1989.

Gray M: Assessment of patients with urinary incontinence. In Dougherty DB, editor: *Urinary and fecal incontinence: nursing management*, St Louis, 1991, Mosby.

Hanson MJS: Modifiable risk factors for coronary heart disease in women, *Am J Crit Care* 3(3):177-184, 1994.

Hawthorne M: Gender differences in recovery after coronary artery surgery, *Image J Nurs Scholarship* 26(1):75-80, 1994.

Hochschild A: *The second shift*, New York, 1989, Avon.

Holm K, Penckofer S, Keresztes P, Biordi D, Chandler P: Coronary artery disease in women: assessment, diagnosis, intervention, and strategies for life style change, *AWHONN Clin Issues* 4(2):272-285, 1993.

Hopper SV: The influence of ethnicity on the health of older women, *Clin Geriatr Med* 9(1):231-259, 1993.

Hueston WJ, Stiles MA: The Papanicolaou smear as a sentinel screening test for health screening in women, *Arch Intern Med* 154:1473-1477, 1994.

Ickovics JR, Rodin J: Women and AIDS in the United States: epidemiology, natural history, and mediating mechanisms, *Health Psychol* 11(1):1-16, 1992.

Jones DA: HIV-seropositive childbearing women: nursing management, *J Obstet Gynecol Neonatal Nurs* 20(6):446-452, 1991.

Kaluzny AD, Rimer B, Harris R: The National Cancer Institute and guideline development: lessons from the breast cancer screening controversy, *J Natl Cancer Inst* 86(12):901-905, 1994.

Kelley KF, Galbraith MA, Vermund SH: Genital human papillomavirus infection in women, JOGGN; *J Obstet Gynecol*, Neonatal Nursing 21(6):503-515, 1992.

Knobf MT, Morra ME: Women and cancer, *AWHONN Clin Issues* 4(2):287-301, 1993.

Kogan MD, Alexander GR, Kotelchuck M, Nagey DA, Jack BW: Comparing mothers' reports on the content of prenatal care received with recommended National Guidelines for Care, *Public Health Rep* 109:637-646, 1994.

Kronenberg F: Hot flashes: phenomenology, quality of life, and search for treatment options, *Exp Gerontol* 29(3/4):319-336, 1994.

Lacey LP, Manfredi C, Balch G, Warnecke RB, Allen K, Edwards C: Social support in smoking cessation among black women in Chicago public housing, *Public Health Rep* 108(3):387-394, 1993.

Lambert JS: Maternal and perinatal issues regarding HIV infection, *Pediatr Ann* 19(8):468-472, 1990.

Lappe JM: Bone fragility: assessment of risk and strategies for prevention, *J Obstet Gynecol Neonatal Nurs* 23:260-268, 1994.

Leaf DA: Women and coronary artery disease: gender confers no immunity, *Postgrad Med* 87(7):55-60, 1990.

Lucas-Holt JC: The effectiveness of incentive programs for prenatal care, *J Perinatal Educ* 3(1):29-39, 1994.

Matteson PS, Hawkins JW: What family planning methods women use and why they change them, *Health Care Women Int* 14:539-548, 1993.

McGovern P, Gjerdingen DK, Froberg D: The parental leave debate: implications for policy relevant research, *Women Health* 18:97-118, 1992.

Miller B, Feuer EJ, Hankey BF: Recent incidence trends for breast cancer in women and the relevance of early detection: an update, *CA Cancer J Clin* 43(1):27-41, 1993.

Moos MK: Preconception health, *Adv Nurse Pract* 2(6):8-10, 1994.

National Center for Health Statistics: *Health promotion and disease prevention: United States, 1990,* Series 10, No 163, DHHS Pub No 185, Hyattsville, Md, 1993a, US Department of Health and Human Services.

National Center for Health Statistics: *Vital statistics of the United States,* Washington, DC, 1993b, US Government Printing Office.

National Research Council: *AIDS: the second decade,* Washington, DC, 1990, National Academy Press.

Oakley A: Who cares for health? Social relations, gender and the public health, *J Epidemiol Community Health* 48:427-434, 1994.

Older Women's League: *Critical condition: midlife and older women in America's health care system,* Washington, DC, 1992, The League.

Olshansky SJ, Carnes BA, Cassel C: In search of Methuselah: estimating the upper limits of human longevity, *Science* 250:634, 1990.

Pakizegi B: Emerging family forms: single mothers by choice—demographic and psychosocial variables, *Matern Child Nurs J* 19(1):1-19, 1990.

Pasquale SA: Helping patients make informed contraceptive decisions, *Contemp OB/GYN* 39(Special Issue):9-10, 12, 21-22, 1994.

Pittman DA, Kirkpatrick M: Women's health and the acute myocardial infarction, *Nurs Outlook* 42:207-209, 1994.

Pizzi M: Women, HIV infection, and AIDS: tapestries of life, death, and empowerment, *Am J Occup Ther* 46(11):1021-1027, 1992.

Polan ML: Value of early screening for osteoporosis, *Contemp OB/GYN* 39(Special Issue):63-67, 1994.

Price JH: Economically disadvantaged females' perceptions of breast cancer and breast cancer screening, *J Natl Med Assoc* 86(12):899-906, 1994.

Quimby CH: Women and the family of the future, *J Obstet Gynecol Neonatal Nurs* 23(2):113-123, 1994.

Ragsdale D, Morrow JR: Quality of life as a function of HIV classification, *Nurs Res* 39(6):355-359, 1990.

Rankin EAD: Stresses and rewards experienced by employed mothers, *Health Care Women Int* 14:527-537, 1993.

Rebar RW: Unanswered questions in hormonal replacement therapy, *Exp Gerontol* 29(3/4):447-461, 1994.

Russo NF: Forging research priorities for women's mental health, *Am Psychol* 45:368-372, 1990.

Scarr HA: A typical American as seen through the eyes of the Census Bureau. In *Almanac and book of facts,* Mahwah, NJ, 1994, Funk and Wagnalls.

Scarr S, Phillips D, McCartney K, Abbott-Shim M: Quality of child care as an aspect of family and child care policy in the United States, *Pediatrics* 91(1):182-188, 1993.

Sharp N: Women's Health Equity Act of 1990, *Nurs Manage* 21(12):23-24, 1990.

Sharp N: Women's health: A powerful public issue, *Nurs Manage* 24(6):17-19, 1993.

Shaul MP: Rheumatoid arthritis and older women: economics tell only part of the story, *Health Care Women Int* 15:377-383, 1994.

Sherr L: *HIV and AIDS in mothers and babies,* London, 1991, Blackwell.

Shervington DO: Attitudes and practices of African-American women regarding cigarette smoking: implications for interventions, *J Natl Med Assoc* 86(5):337-343, 1994.

Sidel R: Putting women and children first: priorities for the future of America, *J Public Health Policy* 12(1):37-49, 1991.

Sipes C: Guidelines for assessing HIV in women, *Matern Child Nurs J* 20:29-33, 1995.

Skoner MM, Haylor MJ: Managing incontinence: women's normalizing strategies, *Health Care Women Int* 14:549-560, 1993.

Smeltzer SC, Whipple B: Women and HIV infection, *Image J Nurs Scholarship* 23(4):249-256, 1991.

Sotosky JR, McGrory CH, Metzger DS, DeHoratius RJ: Arthritis problem indicator: preliminary report on a new tool for use in the primary care setting, *Arthritis Care Res* 5(3):157-162, 1992.

Stevens KA, O'Connell ML: The problem of access: meeting needs of pregnant women, *J Perinatal Educ* 1(2):1-11, 1992.

Stratton P, Mofenson LM, Willoughby AD: Human immunodeficiency virus infection in pregnant women under care at AIDS clinical trials centers in the United States, *Obstet Gynecol* 79(3):364-368, 1992.

Szwabo PA: Substance abuse in older women, *Clin Geriatr Med* 9(1):197-208, 1993.

US Department of Labor: *Facts on working women,* Washington, DC, 1992, US Government Printing Office.

US Preventive Services Task Force: *Guide to clinical preventive services: report of the US Preventive Services Task Force,* Washington, DC, 1989, US Department of Health and Human Services.

Vickers MJ: Understanding obesity in women, *J Obstet Gynecol Neonatal Nurs* 22(1):17-23, 1993.

Wallace K: Female pelvic floor functions, dysfunctions, and behavioral approaches to treatment, *Clin Sports Med* 13:459-481, 1994.

Williams AB: Reproductive concerns of women at risk for HIV infection, *J Nurse Midwifery* 35(5):292-298, 1990.

Wollersheim JP: Depression, women, and the workplace, *Occup Med* 8(4):787-795, 1993.

Woods NF: Menopause—challenges for future research, *Exp Gerontol* 29(3/4):237-243, 1994a.

Woods NF: Women and their health. In Fogel CI, Woods NF, editors: *Women's health care: a comprehensive handbook,* Thousand Oaks, Calif, 1994b, Sage.

Woods NF, Lentz M, Mitchell E: The new woman: health-promoting and health damaging behavior, *Health Care Women Int* 14:389-405, 1993.

Woods NF, Lentz M, Mitchell E, Oakley LD: Depressed mood and self-esteem in young Asian, black and white women in America, *Health Care Women Int* 15:243-262, 1994.

Wuest J: Institutionalizing women's oppression: the inherent risk in health policy that fosters community participation, *Health Care Women Int* 14(5):407-417, 1993.

Zeidenstein L: Gynecological and childbearing needs of lesbians, *J Nurse Midwifery* 35(1):10-18, 1990.

Zuffoletto JM: The federal family and medical leave act, *AORN J* 60(1):91-93, 1994.

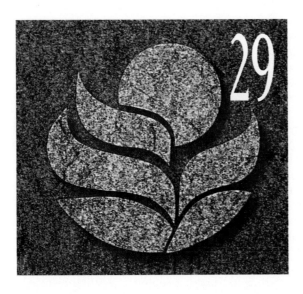

29 Men's Health

Thomas Kippenbrock*

Objectives ▼

After reading this chapter, the student should be able to do the following:

◆ Explain the unique aspects of developmental stages and tasks that affect young and middle-aged men.
◆ Discuss risk factors and their consequences on men's health.
◆ Understand how the life-styles men lead affect their health.
◆ Identify legislation affecting men's health.
◆ Describe the community health nurse's role in maintaining and promoting men's health.
◆ Describe the advanced practice nursing role in men's health.

Key Terms ▼

body maintenance
development
digital rectal examination
generativity versus stagnation
intimacy versus isolation
men's health nurse practitioner (MHNP)
men/women death ratio
moral development
prostate cancer
psychosocial development
testicular cancer
testicular self-examination (TSE)

Outline ▼

*The author acknowledges the contribution of Paul Gordier, BSN and David E. Hiatt, BSN

Men's health, as a separate and distinct practice of care, is at an early developmental level. Men's health goes beyond care of the prostate, genitalia, sexual dysfunction, and associated diseases. Today's focus is on the entire person, requiring a holistic approach.

The data are quite convincing: men are physiologically the more vulnerable gender. More male infants die at birth. More men die of cardiovascular, liver, and chronic pulmonary diseases, as well as cancers and suicide. Further, a man has a shorter predicted lifespan. Many explanations exist for such differences in gender health outcomes: genetics, risk-taking behaviors, stressors, ignoring warning signs, and many others. This chapter discusses men's health by reviewing developmental stages of men, identifying men's health problems and needs, and exploring the nurse's role in maintaining and promoting men's health in the community.

This chapter also addresses the goals of *Healthy People 2000* (1991) of increasing the healthy lifespan of Americans, reducing health disparities among Americans, and helping people achieve access to preventive services by focusing on the unique health needs of men. Health promotion strategies are described to help men deal effectively with the leading causes of death affecting them. In addition, nursing interventions are discussed that are designed to assist men to take advantage of preven-tive services that they tend to overlook to a greater extent than do women. The strategies described in this chapter illustrate the many ways in which the *Healthy People 2000* goals and objectives can be applied to men.

HOW MEN DEFINE HEALTH

Although men and women have similar ideas about health, there are some distinct differences. Most people view health as being closely associated with well-being. Both men and women define health comprehensively and refer to it as a state or condition of being, and they often relate this condition to capacity, performance, and function.

Further, health is grounded in a sense of self and the physical body, and both are tied to conceptions of past and future actions. When men are asked about health, they look at physical, mental, and emotional well-being. Also, they believe the state of self has the potential to affect the state of others. Many men believe health is individualized. This means one person's idea of health and well-being may differ from another's thoughts of being healthy. Men frequently refer to healthiness as "keeping" or "being in control" and "minding" one's body. Men seem to imagine themselves as having "power over" the relationship to their bodies. Men speak about their bodies as though they "belong" to them in the same way an object belongs to them (Saltonstall, 1993).

The times are changing from focusing on diseases with their associated treatments to a new health care focus on identifying needs and prevention concerns. This preventive focus is a wise one: men have been identified as an unmistakably high-risk group. They frequently engage in compensatory, aggressive, and risk-taking behavior predisposing them to illness, injury, and even death (Forrester, 1986).

Abel et al. (1989) analyzed men's life-styles and self-direction in employment and found that men are changing their ideas about health. Nonsmoking males regularly participate more in sports and various exercises, undertake regular physical examinations, and perceive themselves to be in good health. Further, men earning high incomes perceived themselves as being healthier than did their less affluent counterparts; however, socioeconomic status was not a strong predictor of healthy life-styles.

Men tend to avoid medical help as long as possible, leading to serious health problems. With the exception of orthopedics and pediatrics, females use medical specialties more often than men. Naphon stated, "Many men simply don't seek medical advice, or take action in preventive health care, unless it's absolutely necessary" (Rafuse, 1993 p. 329).

Men need to openly express their health care concerns. Health care professionals can help men examine their concerns by encouraging them to discuss nonhealth problems, as well as health care problems, and by promoting preventive health care. Although some men are apprehensive about intimate interaction with professionals, strategies can be employed to reduce men's anxiety. Nurses should remove physical barriers separating themselves from the patient, use handouts and other written information to support oral instructions, and show a genuine interest in men's needs.

MALE DEVELOPMENT

Development is a process by which humans change in structure, thoughts, or behaviors as a consequence of biological or enviromental factors. Usually these changes are progressive and cumulative; they are not as rapid in adults as they are in children. Because adult men and women follow similar developmental patterns, developmental theorists have not typically separated the genders.

Psychosocial

Erikson (1968) explained the **psychosocial development** of adults as stages in which a person's capacities or experiences dictate major life adjustments in his or her social environment or self. The following is an overview of psychosocial development focusing on men during their young and middle adulthood.

Young Adulthood (20 to 45 years)

Erickson labels this stage **intimacy versus isolation.** Each person must establish a secure personal identity. Once this task is accomplished, the person is able to

Tasks of the Young Adult Male

1. Develops an intimate relationship with another
2. Chooses a mate
3. Establishes a husband or father role or both
4. Manages a household independent of his parents' home and care
5. Develops a career or vocation
6. Continues development of a social structure
7. Develops a community role focusing on citizenship
8. Develops a life-style suitable to his philosophy on life

form intimate and loving relationships. The young adult male begins to focus on developing close relationships with others and eventually choosing a mate (see box above for a summary of tasks). These relationships lead to forming his own family and pursuing a career. Around 30 years of age and again at 40 years, there is a time of reevaluation during which the person closely examines himself regarding goals and accomplishments. This may be a crisis period for men, and they may decide to make changes in their lives.

Middle Adulthood (40 to 65 years)

Erickson labels middle adulthood as **generativity versus stagnation.** This stage focuses on contributions to the next generation. Men are involved in sharing, nurturing, and contributing to the growth of others (see box below, left, for a summary of tasks). Middle adulthood has been typically defined as being a period of stability; yet many men undergo a transition period equal to or greater than the one they experienced in adolescence. Jung (1933) noted a gradual personality change in which men search their inner selves for a greater meaning in their lives. At this time, men may begin to acknowledge "tender feelings" and are more expressive. Marriage and the spousal relationship are the best predictors of male midlife satisfaction and perceived stress reduction. Thus a redefinition of husband and father roles may occur. Men also must cope with the physical changes that occur during this time.

Tasks of the Middle Adult Male

1. Promotes a deep relationship with the spouse
2. Nurtures and shares in the growth of children and the next generation
3. Adjusts to physical changes
4. Reassesses self and career goals
5. Achieves desired goals in life and career
6. Builds acceptable leisure activities
7. Copes with the empty nest syndrome

Moral

Over time, society has changed from hunting and gathering to farming, manufacturing, and service. In prehistoric time, human's need to hunt and kill game was essential for survival; however, with the discovery of machines, energy, and agriculture, the need to kill should cease. Yet humans continue to kill and commit crimes against humanity. Questions about human **moral development** can be explained by reviewing related theory. This chapter further explores why some men resort to violence.

Kohlberg (1984) focused on the moral development of the individual. As a person reasons and thinks about moral issues and problems, the individual should become motivated to develop new and broader viewpoints. People do not lose the insight they have gained earlier but instead build on it. Kohlberg divided moral development into stages or levels of reasoning (see the box below, right, for a summary of the stages). The stages are hierarchical. Progression usually occurs with advancement from one stage to the next; however, individuals may regress to a previous stage. Stage advancement does not depend on physical maturity. The typical movement through stages is an orderly process from a focus on self to the larger society and universal principles.

MEN'S HEALTH AND MORTALITY

In the United States, men's life expectancy for all ages is one of the lowest in developed countries. At birth a male born in the United States can expect to live until 72 years of age, compared with Japan (76.17 years), France (73.37 years), Canada (73.81 years), and the Netherlands (74.17 years). Further, international data reveal similar shorter life expectancies at

Stages of Morality

STAGE I: PRECONVENTIONAL MORALITY

The individual is guided by rules dictating good or bad, right or wrong. The individual translates these rules into physical or hedonistic consequences of action such as rewards, favors, and physical power over others.

STAGE II: CONVENTIONAL MORALITY

Usually in the teens, the individual shifts from unquestioning obedience to a concern for "good" motives. Assumptions about family, groups, and society as valuable in their own entity occur in this stage. Conforming to personal and social expectations as well as loyalty, support, maintenance, and championing order results in this stage.

STAGE III: UNIVERSAL PRINCIPLES

The individual is concerned with individuals' rights and social contracts apart from his or the group's needs. The individual is concerned with consistent, comprehensive ethical principles.

15, 45, and 65 years of age. The only exception is at 80 years, at which time American men are in the middle ranking of developed countries with a continued life expectancy of 9 years.

For American adolescents (15 to 24 years) and early adult men (25 to 34 years), death rates are more than twice those of men in Japan and the Netherlands. In addition, American men ages 45 to 54 years rank second highest in death rates among the 13 developed countries; but interestingly enough, mortality has significantly declined for American men ages 45 to 54 years. The least progress toward mortality decline is in the men's age group of 25 to 34 years. Accidents, homicides and other violence, cancers, circulatory system diseases, and infectious and parasitic diseases account for most deaths in developed countries. American men rank high in all areas except the latter. The good news is that there has been a decline in men's ischemic heart disease in the United States; however, American men's and women's heart disease mortalities are still among the highest in the world (U.S. Congress, Office of Technology Assessment, 1993).

GENDER DIFFERENCES

Men have a shorter life expectancy than women. Government data revealed that the U.S. life expectancy for men at birth is 72.0 years, compared with 78.9 years for women ("Advance Report of Final Mortality Statistics, 1991," 1993). In 1991 the age-adjusted death rate for men of all races was 1.7 times that of women. The **men/women death ratio** has fluctuated somewhat over the past years. The recent low was 1.5 in 1950 compared with 1.8 in 1970.

Men do engage in more risk-taking behaviors than women. This is particularly true with behaviors involving physical challenges or illegal behavior. Men drink more alcohol than women, which may explain men's higher mortalities from accidents, liver cirrhosis, and some types of cancer. Men's jobs are more hazardous, resulting in more job-related accidents. Men are also exposed to more industrial carcinogens. Other areas contributing to gender differences in morbidity or mortality may include stress responses, genetics, physiological differences, environmental factors, and preventive behavior. Often, differences are related to several combined factors.

Similarities and differences exist as to the leading causes of death among men and women (Table 29-1). Heart disease and cancer are by far the leading causes of men's mortality; however, women have similar death rates. The most prominent gender death rate differences are for accidents, pulmonary diseases, human immune viruses (HIV), suicides, homicides, and alcoholism-related liver diseases. For example, HIV deaths are almost eight times higher in men than in women; suicides are more than four times higher; homicides are more than three times higher; and accidents are more than two times higher. Even though cerebrovascular disease, pneumonia and influenza,

Table 29-1 Leading Causes of Death among Men (as Compared to Those among Women)

Disease	Death rate — Males	Death rate — Females	Death ratio
Heart	292.6	279.5	1.05
Cancer	221.5	187.5	1.18
Accidents	48.6	22.9	2.13
Motor vehicles	24.4	10.5	2.30
Others	24.2	12.4	1.95
Cerebrovascular disease	46.1	67.2	0.68
Chronic obstructive pulmonary disease	41.1	31.2	1.33
Pneumonia	29.4	32.2	0.90
HIV	21.2	2.7	7.85
Suicide	20.1	4.7	4.27
Diabetes	17.2	21.6	0.79
Homicide	16.9	4.4	3.80
Chronic liver	13.2	7.1	1.86

Advance report of final mortality statistics, 1991, *Monthly Vital Statistics Rep* 42 (2; suppl), 1993.

and diabetes mellitus are leading causes of men's death, they are not discussed because women have even higher death rates.

LEADING CAUSES OF MEN'S DEATHS
Heart and Cardiovascular Diseases

For men, heart disease is the leading cause of death. The men's death rate in 1991 was 912 per 100,000 population, accounting for 32% of all men's mortalities. This health statistic is unquestionably significant in young and middle-aged men. For young men (25 to 44 years), heart disease is 2.7 times higher than for females; for middle-aged men (45 to 64 years), it is 2.57 times higher (Table 29-2) ("Advance Report of Final Mortality Statistics, 1991," 1993).

Several physiological changes occur as a person ages, including an increase in the size of the heart. The biggest changes take place on the left side of the heart, or the pumping side. Heart mass increases 1 to 1.5 g/yr between ages 30 and 90 years (Holm and Penckofer, 1990). However, the heart may atrophy if the person has extended illness. Aging results in valve and vascular changes and systolic blood pressure rises because of less compliant blood vessels.

Smoking, sedentary life-styles, improper diet, and obesity are risk factors associated with heart diseases. Although the number of U.S. men who smoke has declined in recent years, young people continue to start smoking. The positive news is that the adverse effects of smoking may be reversed by cessation at any age

Table 29-2 Heart and Vascular Disease Death Rates and Death Ratios of Young and Middle-Aged Men and Women

| | Age 25-44 years | | | Age 45-64 years | | |
| | Death Rate | | | Death Rate | | |
	Men	Women	Death ratio	Men	Women	Death ratio
Heart	28.1	10.5	2.70	330.1	128.3	2.57
Cerebrovascular disease	4.3	3.8	1.13	34.6	27.5	1.26

Advance report of final mortality statistics, 1991, *Monthly Vital Statistics Rep* 42(2; suppl), 1993.

(Higgins, et al., 1993). Exercise and physical activity clearly have a positive effect on the cardiovascular system. With jobs becoming less physical, attention is being focused on leisure activities. Bittner and Oberman (1993) reported low levels of exercise such as jogging, walking, and swimming on a regular basis have cardiovascular benefits. In fact, Pate et al. (1995) found people can benefit from minor brief stints of exercise. Reduction of cardiovascular risk occurs with exercises such as climbing stairs and gardening. The key is to make the activity intense, such as a brisk walk.

Diet is an important determinant of health. The typical American diet is high in calories, saturated fats, cholesterol, and sodium. For example, one of the most popular fast food sandwich and french fries combinations has 1131 calories, 21 g of saturated fat, 66 g of total fat, 115 mg of cholesterol, and 1.5 g of sodium chloride. The issue of high cholesterol has come to the forefront in recent years. Although cholesterol-lowering drugs are available, diet is one of the key factors in determining cholesterol levels.

In earlier years, patients who had suffered a myocardial infarction were kept on strict bed rest. Now, however, the benefits of physical activity are reported in rehabilitation programs. Bittner and Oberman (1993) demonstrated exercise used in rehabilitation programs consistently decreased cardiovascular mortality after a myocardial infarction.

Cancer

Malignant neoplasms are the second leading cause of death for men of all ages. The death rate is 221 per 100,000 population, accounting for 24% of all men's deaths in the United States ("Advanced Report on Final Mortality Statistics, 1991," 1993). A discussion of the most significant cancers affecting men will be addressed: prostate, testicular, and skin.

Prostate Cancer

The most common cancer among U.S. men, with a reported incidence of 89 per 1000 men, is **prostate cancer** (*Vital and Health Statistics*, 1994). The risk for prostate cancer increases with each decade after 50 years of age. Overall, black men have a 45% higher incidence rate than white men. The lowest incidence rates are found in Asian populations, whereas Scandinavian, northern European, and North American countries have the highest rates (Pack, 1993).

The exact cause of prostatic cancer is unknown. Genetics, hormones, diet, environment, and viruses have all been implicated as risk factors. Early diagnosis is essential because treatment is usually unsuccessful unless it is done in the early stages of the disease. One diagnostic problem is the lack of symptoms; thus the cancer may be advanced before detection.

An annual **digital rectal examination** is recommended for men over 40 years of age. Other forms of testing have been developed such as transrectal ultrasound, screening for tumor markers such as serum acid phosphatase and prostate-specific antigen (PSA), x-ray assessment, and biopsy. More frequent examinations are recommended for men who are considered at risk. Two factors considered to indicate risk are (1) men with continuing urinary symptoms and a history of blood relatives with prostatic cancer and (2) men with benign prostatic hypertrophy or a partial prostatectomy.

Treatment may include one or a combination of the following: radiation therapy, pharmacological management, or surgical management. Even though survival rates have improved, it is still necessary to continue to educate men concerning the risks and the need for regular examinations.

Closely related and a precursor to prostate cancer is benign prostatic hyperplasia (BPH). Aging is the major risk factor for BPH. By 60 years of age, more than 50% of men will experience BPH. This rate increases to 90% by 85 years of age. In fact, one in four U.S. men will require treatment of symptomatic BPH by 80 years (*Treating Your Enlarged Prostate*, 1994). Symptoms may include frequency of urination, nocturia, urgency, straining to urinate, hesitancy in urination, weak or intermittent stream, and a sensation of incomplete emptying. Prostate enlargement does not necessarily correlate with the severity of the symptoms or the amount of restriction to urine flow. Complications may include urinary retention, renal insufficiency, urinary tract infections, hematuria, or bladder stones.

Symptom assessment may be done using a self-administered questionnaire called the International Prostate Symptom Scores (I-PSS). This questionnaire consists of six symptom-related questions and one quality of life question. The symptoms include most of those discussed above: incomplete emptying, fre-

Step-by-step Guide to Monthly TSE

1. Perform the TSE during a warm bath or shower.
2. Roll each testicle between your thumb and fingers using warm hands. Testicles should be egg shaped, 4 cm oblong, and similar in size and have a rubbery texture; the left dangles lower than the right.
3. Check the epididymis for softness and slight tenderness.
4. Check the spermatic cord for firm smooth tubular structure.

quency, intermittency, urgency, weak stream, and straining. Symptoms are scored from 0 (not at all) to 5 (almost always). The total score can range from 0 (asymptomatic) to 35 (symptomatic). The quality of life question has six possible responses ranging from delighted to terrible. Additional diagnostic tests are also used to reach a diagnosis. These include uroflometry, postvoid residual urine, pressure flow studies, and urethrocystoscopy.

Treatment consists of several options ranging from medications to surgery. New technologies are emerging, including laser prostatectomy.

Testicular Cancer

Testicular cancer is the most commonly found solid tumor malignancy in men 15 to 35 years of age, representing 20% of the cancers in this age group. In 1993, 6600 new cases were reported and 350 men died (Boring et al., 1993). The etiology of this cancer, testicular germ cell, is unknown. Many possible explanations exist, such as age, endocrine and genetic disorders, or socioeconomic and occupational factors.

The most common presenting symptom is a painless, firm scrotal mass or swelling accidentally discovered. Low back pain may result with retroperitoneal lymph node involvement. It is unfortunate that most men do not practice risk appraisal strategies to detect this cancer. Walker (1993) found 83% of men do not perform **testicular self-examination (TSE).**

Modeling and guided practice should be components of a comprehensive testicular educational program (see box above for a step-by-step guide to TSE). A program may consist of audiovisual aids and pamphlets followed by step-by-step procedures and return demonstrations. These approaches lead to increased frequency of TSE and enhanced comfort levels of the men performing the procedure (Walker, 1993). If tumors are found, the most common form of management is retroperitoneal lymph node dissection and chemotherapy for metastases larger than 3 cm.

Skin Cancer

This cancer is the most common of all cancers. About 600,000 new cases are diagnosed annually (Preston and Stern, 1992). Men's death rate (3.3/100,000 population) is much higher than women's death rate (1.9/100,000 population) ("Advance Report of Final

Mortality Statistics, 1991," 1993). The three main types of skin cancers are basal and squamous cell carcinoma and malignant melanomas. More than 90% of all skin cancers are either basal cell carcinoma or squamous cell carcinoma with a 95% cure rate or more (Black et al., 1993).

Prolonged sun exposure and high ultraviolet B cause skin cancer. Red-, blond-, or light brown–haired men with light complexions or freckles are the most susceptible. Also, men with a history of long-term occupational or recreational sun exposure such as farmers, construction workers, sailors, swimmers, surfers, and sunbathers are at high risk.

Malignant melanoma is the deadliest form of skin cancer, and the incidence is rising worldwide. Of the 272,380 U.S. cancer deaths in 1991, there were 4017 melanoma deaths in men, or a rate of 3.3 per 100,000 population with malignant melanoma ("Advance Report of Final Mortality Statistics, 1991," 1993). This cancer can metastasize to the brain, lungs, bones, liver, and other areas of the skin with generally fatal results.

Prevention includes decreasing exposure to direct sunlight, especially between the peak hours of 10 AM and 3 PM. Men should wear protective clothing and use a sunblock of at least SPF 15 or higher rating when outside. Regular skin inspection and assessment are also important. Early diagnosis and treatment enhance the chances of recovery.

Accidents

The third leading cause of men's death for all ages, accounting for 48 deaths per 100,000 population, is accidental death. The death rate data are highly significant in men 15 to 24 years old (62 per 100,000 population) and 25 to 44 years old (50 per 100,000 population) ("Advance Report of Final Mortality Statistics, 1991," 1993).

Fatal Accidents

Men are at higher risk for fatal occupational injuries than women. In 1992 men accounted for about 90% of all fatally injured workers. This is high, since men accounted for approximately 55% of the workforce. A breakdown of occupational fatalities by gender is listed in Table 29-3.

The most recent data reveal that transportation and assault/violent acts were the two leading fatal occupational injuries, accounting for 58% of men's deaths in this category. Other leading fatal injuries were contact with objects and equipment, falls, exposure to harmful substances or environment, and fires. The men/women occupational death ratios differed immensely. For example, the men's death rate resulting from contact with objects and equipment was 46 times greater than in women, 42 times greater for fire and exposure, 33 times greater for harmful substances and environmental exposure, 19 times greater for falls, 14 times greater for transportation, and 6 times greater for assaults and violent acts (Toscango and Windau, 1994).

Table 29-3 Number and Percent Distribution of Fatal Occupational Injuries By Gender

	Men (n = 5657)		Women (n = 426)	
	Number	Percent	Number	Percent
Transportation	2263	40	162	38
Assaults and violent acts	1018	18	183	43
Contact with objects and equipment	962	17	21	5
Falls	566	10	30	7
Exposure to harmful substances or environment	566	10	17	4
Fire and exposure	170	3	4	1

From Toscano G, Windau J: *Fatal work injuries: results from* 1992 *national census.* Report 870, Washington, DC, 1994, US Department of Labor, Bureau of Labor Statistics.

Nonfatal Accidents

Sprains and strains accounted for approximately 1 million of the total 2.3 million work-related injuries in 1992. About one-fifth of the nonfatal injuries occurred to the back, caused by overexertion from lifting, pulling, or pushing objects or persons. Again, men accounted for nearly two-thirds of these cases. Occupations with the highest back injuries were nonconstruction laborers, truck drivers, and nursing aides or orderlies (U.S. Department of Labor, 1994).

Pulmonary Diseases

Chronic obstructive pulmonary disease is the fifth leading cause of death among men. Men have a 1.33-fold greater chance of dying from chronic pulmonary problems than women (Advance Report of Final Mortality Statistics, 1991, 1993). It should be noted that the incidence of emphysema is more than twice as high in men as in women (48.9 for men and 24 for women per 1000 population). Further, respiratory system cancer death rates are 1.8 times higher in men than in women *(Vital and Health Statistics,* 1994).

Smoking is a definite pulmonary disease risk factor. Traditionally, men have used tobacco more than women; however, this trend is changing. Early studies found that men were more likely than women to become regular smokers. More recent data indicate women are more likely than men to have tried smoking. In recent decades the public, and especially men, have received education concerning the dangers of smoking. This has resulted in a decrease in the prevalence of smoking, chiefly in men. Evidence indicates men's cessation rates were higher than women's in

middle-aged and older smokers during the 1960s and 1970s (Waldron et al., 1991).

In the United States, education is an important factor concerning gender differences in smoking. Men in two categories—ages 19 to 24 years old, and those who had attended college—are less likely than females to become smokers (Waldron et al., 1991). A study done by Higgins et al. (1993) on smoking and lung function in elderly persons showed smokers who quit before age 40 had pulmonary functions similar to people who never smoked. The same study showed that termination of smoking between ages 40 and 60 years resulted in a 7% decrease and a 14% decrease after quitting at 60 years old or older.

What Do You Think?

It is clear that tobacco use in any form has detrimental effects on personal health. Current legislation has limited or banned smoking in public places. These policies have been criticized by smokers who cite the "common courtesy approach" as being effective.

Human Immune Virus and Acquired Immunodeficiency Syndrome

Acquired immunodeficiency syndrome (AIDS) has become a major health concern in the world and in the United States. AIDS is the second leading cause of death in the United States for men ages 25 to 44 years, and it is the seventh leading cause of death for men of all age groups. There is a wide difference in death rates between men and women. For all ages and all races, the men's death rate is 21.2 per 100,000 population compared with women's 2.7 per 100,000 population. White male death rates are even higher at 16.7, compared with 1.3 for females ("Advance Report of Final Mortality Statistics, 1991," 1993).

AIDS was first reported in 1981. Since that time the occurrence of AIDS has steadily increased. The human immune virus (HIV) is the precursor to AIDS. The World Health Organization (WHO) reported in 1995 that worldwide cumulative AIDS infections stood at 20 million people (Global AIDS news, 1995). AIDS is of special concern for men, considering that the highest infection rates have occurred in homosexual and bisexual men.

This trend is changing: the fastest growing affected population is now heterosexuals who abuse drugs. The WHO reported 60% of HIV transmission is heterosexual (Pozgar and Pozgar, 1993). The estimated occurrence of heterosexual transmission is expected to increase to 75% to 80% by the turn of the century. The incidence of infection is increasing in minorities, especially blacks and Hispanics.

AIDS spreads by direct contact with infected blood or body fluids, including vaginal secretions, semen, and breast milk. High-risk groups include sexually active men with multiple partners and intravenous drug users. The risk of HIV and AIDS being introduced through blood and blood products has been greatly reduced. All blood donated in the United States has been tested for the HIV antibody since 1985. Individuals who donate are also screened as to health history and risk behaviors.

The signs and symptoms of AIDS vary from person to person but may include diarrhea, night sweats, fever, weight loss, fatigue, persistent cough, and memory problems. A person may be asymptomatic or have any one or a combination of symptoms. Treatment is directed at symptom relief, and two drugs are used to slow the progression of the disease: azidothymidine (AZT) and dideoxyinosine (ddI).

The occurrence of this disease has created both ethical and financial questions. The cost for care and treatment of AIDS continues to grow, and many male AIDS patients find insurance companies refusing to pay as costs soar. Men have been fired from their jobs, refused medical treatment, and driven out of their communities. Although such discrimination is against the law, it still occurs. Ethical standards of confidentiality, privacy, and treatment have been challenged. The result is that men with HIV and AIDS remain silent about their disease. Many people in high-risk groups decline to be tested out of fear of potential results. Healthcare workers both in acute care and community health must maintain confidentiality and demonstrate high ethical standards.

Did You Know?

If a person with HIV or AIDS knowingly infects another person, it may be considered a criminal offense.

Suicide

Some of the most significant gender health differences occur in the mental health domain. The suicide rate in men is 20.1 per 100,000 population compared with 4.7 for women, representing a greater than fourfold gender difference. In addition, suicide is the eighth leading cause of death overall for men; high-risk groups are men 15 to 24 years old (the second leading cause) and men 25 to 44 years old (the fifth leading cause) ("Advanced Report of Final Mortality Statistics, 1991," 1993).

Suicide is a significant problem in men, since they are more likely to make a serious attempt to kill themselves rather than to use a suicide attempt as a cry for help (Mellick et al., 1992). Elderly persons are more

Table 29-4 Suicidal Risk Factors

Factors	Conditions
Gender	Men use more violent means and have a higher completed suicide rate.
Marital status	Unmarried men have a greater risk than married men.
Employment	Unemployed men are at a higher risk.
Previous attempts	Men with more than one attempt have a much higher chance of attempting it again. One-quarter to one-half of deaths are by people who have made previous attempts.
Family history	A positive family history increases the risk of suicides.
Medical illness	Men suffering from terminal illness or other medical conditions are at high risk.

likely to use violent and lethal means, and they communicate their intentions less frequently.

Suicide is tragic, since it can often be prevented and such a loss causes grief for family members and friends. Nurses in community health often can identify men at risk for suicide. Table 29-4 shows the suicidal risk factors identified by Barklage (1991).

Despite the widespread use of telephone crisis lines, school-based intervention programs, and antidepressive medications, high rates of suicide continue. All suicide attempts should be taken seriously. The nursing goal is to detect risk factors, promote safety, prevent self-harm, make appropriate referrals, and assist people back to health.

Homicide

Men are also prone to engage in dangerous and risky behavior, such as carrying weapons and fighting. The homicide death rate for men is 16.9 per 100,000 population, compared with 4.4 for women. Homicides are the tenth leading cause of death in men of all ages. More significantly, for 15- to 24-year-old men, the death rate is 37.2 per 100,000 population and the third leading cause of death ("Advance Report of Final Mortality Statistics, 1991," 1993).

Assaultive violence is defined as "nonfatal and fatal interpersonal violence where physical force or other means is used by a person with intent of causing harm, injury, or death to another" (Rosenberg and Mercy, 1991, p. 14). Specifically, a national poll found that 34% of U.S. adults have witnessed a man beating his wife or girlfriend. Also, the violent nature of men is exemplified by research that found that 14% of all women have had a violent action committed against them by a man at some time (EDK Associates, 1993).

Multiple etiologies are attributed to violent behavior. For example, brain dysfunction is associated with irregularities in the limbic system, the part of the brain that regulates emotions and motivation and is associated with violence. Other causes of dysfunction include organic brain disease, psychosis, depression, mental retardation, and brain tumors.

Violence is associated with social, economic, cultural, and environmental factors that especially contribute to assaults among black youth (Hammond and Yung, 1993). Poverty and inner city residency also have been shown to be strongly associated with violent victimization among all adolescents (Fingerhut et al., 1992). For black males 15 to 24 years, homicide is the leading cause of death at 158.9 per 100,000 population. Further, for black males 25 to 44 years, the death rate is 103.9 per 100,000 population, making it the second leading death cause in their age bracket ("Advance Report of Final Mortality Statistics, 1991," 1993).

According to the National Rifle Association (1990), approximately 200 million firearms are owned by private U.S. citizens. One example of health-related problems of gun ownership is workplace homicides. Gunshot wounds account for more than 80% of workplace homicides, and male workers comprise 83% of the victims (Windau and Toscano, 1994).

Little is known about the long-term effects men experience following sexual assaults. Nurses need to understand violent crimes and develop prevention and educational programs for assisting the male victim. For now nurses must continue to support and provide counseling for the male victim who demonstrates emotional distress.

Violence is a public health emergency. Solutions are complex but are believed to be reachable. First, nurses need to identify signs and symptoms of violent behavior. The practitioner should be concerned about a man who is excessively restless and agitated; he may pace up and down or start pounding on walls, doors, furniture, and other objects. He may appear angry and tense by clenching his teeth, jaw, and fists. His voice may become loud, and he may use profanity. He may become argumentative by refusing to follow directions and making threats. Another sign to watch for includes impulsive behaviors. Alcohol and drug abuse and psychiatric disorders are highly associated with violent behavior. Finally, the most predictive indicator of violence is a history of aggressive behavior and family violence (Blomhoff et al., 1990).

Alcohol-induced Disorders

In 1991 the National Council on Alcoholism and Drug Dependence (1991) estimated 10.5 million U.S. adults showed symptoms of alcoholism. In addition, 7.2 million showed continued heavy drinking patterns with impaired health or social functioning. An evaluation of gender differences reveals the men's death rate for alcohol-induced causes is 10.9 per 100,000 population compared with 3.2 for women.

Chronic liver disease and cirrhosis represent a health hazard associated with alcohol abuse. Gender death rates from alcohol abuse demonstrate striking differences: 11.7 for men compared with women's 5.2 per 100,000. Further, black men have an even higher death rate of 17.4. Age-related data demonstrate some interesting comparisons. The death rate for men 25 to 44 years old was 7.7 per 100,000 population, making it the seventh leading cause of death, and for men ages 45 to 64 years it was 32.5, making it the fifth leading cause of death ("Advance Report of Final Mortality Statistics, 1991," 1993).

Patterns of alcohol, tobacco, and drug usage established during the teen years often persist into adulthood, contributing to a leading cause of mortality and morbidity. Alcohol is closely associated with several negative aspects of society: suicide, violent crime, birth defects, and domestic and sexual abuse (Englemann, 1991).

Alcohol is the major cause of all fatal and nonfatal motor vehicle accidents among teenage drivers. Bachman et al. (1991) described the highest drinking rates in teens among white, American-Indian, and Mexican-American males in their senior year of high school. Among high school seniors, males drink more (binge drinking) than females in all ethnic groups. In addition to alcohol-related injuries, illnesses, and deaths, drinking can have negative consequences on family, friends, and employment.

Alcohol leads to dependence associated with one's inability to cut down on drinking, morning drinking, memory losses, and other related medical problems. Almost 50% of separated and divorced men under 45 years of age have been exposed to alcoholism in the family. Also, separated and divorced men are three times more likely than married men to say they have

Research Brief

Lipscomb G, Muram D, Speck P, Mercer B: Male victims of sexual assault, JAMA 267:3064-3066, 1992.

Men are both the assailants and the victims of violence. For example, a study involving 99 sexually assaulted men in a prison or the community were evaluated over a 3-year period. Victims were usually assaulted by multiple male assailants. A majority of the assailants and victims were black. None of the victims sustained injuries serious enough to require medical attention; however, the reported injuries did not just involve the perineal area but were the result of beatings that occurred over the body. Weapons were used in most of the community assaults and in one-third of the prison crimes.

been married to an alcoholic or problem drinker (National Council on Alcoholism and Drug Dependence, 1991).

Society must remember that alcohol consumption is a major drug problem. Nurses must start educating the younger population about the effects of alcohol. One focal point is the message to "stop underage drinking." Even though alcohol use under 21 years of age is illegal in most states, alcohol is easily accessible. Education is the best prevention at this time.

MEN'S HEALTH PRACTICES IN EVERYDAY LIFE

Men and women both have unquestionable biological and physiological needs for rest, exercise, and food consumption to maintain health. When asked, men and women differ on the most important needs to maintain health. Women listed food first, then exercise, and then rest. Men rate exercise first, then sleep, and food last. Men emphasized the nutrient quality of food; women focused on the food's calories rather than its nutrient quality. Men perceived body maintenance activities as essential to producing health for oneself and emphasized sports and outdoor activities as influencing better body maintenance. Further, men viewed the body as a medium of action; function and capacity were of paramount importance (Saltonstall, 1993).

The concept of **body maintenance** images has two components: inner and outer. Inner refers to optimal functioning, performance, and capacity to do things. Outer refers to appearance, movement within social space, and having the potential to be heard and touched. Men discern the inner phenomenon as a function and capacity more than the outer body phenomenon of appearance. Men would rather look at how they went through the day, what they accomplished, and what kind of physical shape they are in so they can perform. Less attention is given to having good color and skin tones.

Bird and Fremont (1991) compared men's and women's social roles related to time use and health. Even though men reported poorer health than women, men spend more time in paid work hours with higher wages associated with better health. Women, on the other hand, spend more time doing housework, have a slightly lower educational level, and have less paid work hours and lower wages, all of which are associated with poorer health. Neither gender was shown to spend much time helping others, which has been shown to improve health. Gender differences favor men's health and their perception of health. Men do benefit from the role of being the family's primary breadwinner.

Men need to take an individual conscious look at themselves and develop a plan to stay healthy and free of illness by becoming knowledgeable about health and their own individual bodies. Along with knowledge comes desire to be healthy. In addition,

men need to set health-related goals and develop an action plan. With the support of the nursing profession, men can take responsibility in changing and maintaining healthier life-styles. Table 29-5 summarizes men's biological and psychosocial health care needs.

LEGISLATION AFFECTING MEN'S HEALTH

As described in Chapter 3, the 1990s have seen considerable attention focused on health reform with economics playing a key role. Both men and women will be affected by changes in health care. Review of past health care legislation affecting men may provide clues to where future legislation is headed. Rules and regulations on elder care, work-related injuries, and veterans' services have affected particularly men's health.

Most Americans turning 65 years old are eligible for Medicare, Part A, consisting of hospital insurance, skilled nursing facilities, home health care, and hospice care. Disabled men are also eligible for these benefits. Currently, millions of men participate in this government-operated insurance plan. Medicare, Part B, which requires subscribers to pay a monthly fee, provides 80% coverage on other medical-related expenses such as physician costs.

As described in Chapter 5, to hold down the spiraling cost of Medicare, a prospective payment system was established based on 467 diagnostic-related groups (DRGs). These laws allow pretreatment diagnosis billing categories for almost all U.S. hospitals reimbursed by Medicare.

The Worker's Compensation Act (WCA) and Americans with Disabilities Act (ADA) are two significant laws affecting men's health because of the high occupational accident rate. The WCA required all industrial employers to carry worker's compensation for their employees in case of job-related injuries; however, some nonprofit organizations are exempt. Worker's compensation insurance pays for an employee's partial lost wages and medical costs encountered. If the employee is permanently disabled, the worker is entitled to additional compensation.

ADA was designed to protect people from being discriminated against in the workplace; this means employers are prohibited from discriminating against qualified disabled individuals in hiring, promotion, job assignment, discharge, compensation, and all other "terms, conditions, and privileges" of employment. An ADA-qualified individual is defined as a person with a disability who meets the skill, experience, education, and other job-related requirements of a position held or desired and who, with or without a reasonable accommodation, can perform the essential functions of a job. If a person is injured on the job, the employer has to look at all circumstances and evaluate how the employee may be taken care of after the injury.

With more men assuming parenting and elder caregiver roles, the Family and Medical Leave Act offers

Table 29-5   Men's Health Care Needs

	Biological	Psychosocial	Combination
Expression		Desire to communicate to others about health care concerns	
Support		Support from others about certain sex roles and life-styles that influence their physical and mental health	
Respect and dignity			Attention from professionals regarding factors that may cause illness or impact a man's expression of illness, including occupational factors, leisure patterns, and interpersonal relationships
Health-seeking knowledge and behaviors	Information about their bodies' functions, what is normal and abnormal, what action to take, and the contributions of proper nutrition and exercise Self-care instruction including testicular and genital self examinations Physical examination and history taking that include sexual and reproductive health and illness across the lifespan		
Holistic medical care and availability		Adjustment of health care system to men's occupational constraints regarding time and location of source of health care	Treatment for problems of couples, including interpersonal problems, infertility, family planning, sexual concerns, and sexually transmitted diseases
Parental guidance		Help with fathering (i.e., being included as a parent in care of children) Help with fathering as a single parent, in particular, with a child of the opposite sex, in addressing child's sexual development and concerns	
Coping		Recognition that feelings of confusion and uncertainty in a time of rapid social change are normal and may mark onset of healthy adaptation to change	
Fiduciary		Financial ways to obtain the above	

opportunities to meet family responsibilities. An eligible employee is entitled to a maximum of 12 weeks for the birth of a child, to care for an ill child or spouse, to adopt or accept a foster or an adoptive child, and last, for his recovery from a serious health condition. When the person's leave is over, he is entitled to return to work in the same or an equivalent position with the same or equivalent pay scale and benefits. During the leave, the employer is not required to pay the employee, although vacation time, personal time off (PTO), or sick leave can be used. Other benefits such as life insurance and health insurance will continue; however, the employer is only required to pay for the employee.

The effects of war have influenced men's health care legislation. Until the Vietnam era, most American veterans were men. Since the mid-1970s women have entered the armed forces and are eligible for veterans' benefits. Nevertheless, the majority of veterans are men. Health-related veterans' benefits include hospital and nursing home care, counseling for sexual trauma, alcohol and drug treatments, prosthetic services, outpatient pharmacy services, and dental services. Other entitlements include a pension program.

COMMUNITY HEALTH NURSE'S ROLE IN MEN'S HEALTH

Community health nurses have knowledge and skills enabling them to assess, diagnose, plan, implement, and evaluate the care of men. Nurses using a range of skills and in a variety of roles work with men in diverse communities ranging from isolated agricultural regions to densely populated cities. The roles of educator, patient advocate, case manager, and men's health nurse practitioner are discussed.

Educator

The goal of patient education is to provide knowledge and skills for learning new behaviors or changes affecting health-related behaviors. The educator's goal is to improve or maintain the health status of men. When the community health nurse encounters men in the clinics, health departments, or their homes, a teaching opportunity exists. The myth about men not being receptive to health information is not substantiated. Glasser (1990) reported men were willing to use health departments to receive health care information and products. Survey findings indicated men used family planning services at a midwestern county public health department. The authors reported that men not only accompanied their female partners in the family planning process and provided emotional support to their partners, but also took an active part in the family planning process. Also, other men received birth control products distributed by the department.

Patient Advocate

The goal of patient advocacy is to ensure that men's long-term health care needs are met. The goal for the advocacy role is to inform and support men in their health care decisions. The nurse needs to become knowledgeable about the health care options and to support the patient in his decisions. For example, a male patient who had post–myocardial infarction needs to be informed about his treatment options, (i.e., diet, exercise, drugs, therapy, stress reduction, and surgical interventions). The nurse should assist the man in making his decisions in the most effective and cost-conscious manner.

Case Manager

Being a case manager of men's health means more than just coordinating patient services. The role involves problem solving and managing men's health care services in a supportive, effective, and efficient manner. The American Nurses Association (1988) described the nursing care manager's role as "a health care delivery process whose goals are to provide quality health care, decrease fragmentation, enhance the client's quality of life, and contain cost." The actual role of the case manager is structured to the patient's needs.

Men's Health Nurse Practitioner

Bozett and Forrester (1989) argued that mens' health care needs were not being met by physicians. Typically, men choose not to communicate their health concerns to physicians. In the office and clinics, pleasantries and shallow comments are exchanged, with critical health care concerns avoided. Physicians rarely give their male patients adequate time for reflective discussion and thoughtful communications about their health needs. Further, physicians focus on pathologic findings and "cure" treatments. Prevention and health promotion activities are not high priorities.

A **men's health nurse practitioner (MHNP)** would alleviate some of these concerns. This advance practice role would deliver comprehensive men's health care. The provider would assess and manage minor health problems, as well as manage acute and chronic conditions. Conducting histories and physical examinations, ordering and interpreting diagnostic studies, prescribing medications and treatments, providing health maintenance care, promoting positive health behaviors and self-care, and collaborating with physicians and other health professionals are some of the MHNP's functions and roles. Effective interpersonal skills and empathetic listening are important communication skills the nurse practitioner would use to facilitate men discussing their health concerns.

Clinical Application

Using the concepts in this chapter, analyze the following case. Focus on the issues of how men define health, developmental patterns, the health practices of men, and a nursing care plan.

John, a 29-year-old caucasian man with a wife and three children, was employed as a sales representative in a small, rural community. John's health was excellent except for injuries sustained in a car accident several years ago that required three blood transfusions. After the accident, John returned to work, thinking he was fully recovered. His business success continued, and he was well respected by employers, coworkers, and community leaders.

Years after the accident, John became ill with pneumonia requiring hospitalization. While he was hospitalized, a blood test discovered HIV. A series of devastating events followed. John and his family decided to keep his condition confidential so he could live the rest of his life as normally as possible.

When John returned to work from the hospital, his coworkers seemed distant and they avoided him. He began to receive threatening telephone calls telling him to leave town, and his car was spray painted with derogatory words. Clearly, there had been a breach of confidentiality. John later discovered his hopsital file was marked "AIDS" in large red letters. Further, he learned nurses refused to care for him while he was hospitalized and he was the dinner conversation focus throughout the hospital.

John's circumstances worsened, and he felt isolated and rejected. He eventually was fired from work, thereby losing health insurance for himself and his family. His wife divorced him. All his accumulated wealth was depleted. He could not pay his hospital bills; his financial state was compounded by filing for bankruptcy. John was now homeless. His symptoms gradually progressed. He had a fever, tachypnea, lymphadenopathy, night sweats, and diarrhea. A friend suggested he visit the clinic.

Imagine you are the nurse in the public health clinic. What information do you want to collect? What nursing diagnoses are relevant based on the collected data? What short-term goals are appropriate for the first clinic visit? What long-term goal do you want to plan with John? What social and health agencies would you consult in planning for John's care?

John is reluctant to speak about his disease. He is extremely fatigued and whispers softly. Further, he refuses any governmental services; however, you are able to convince him to enter the homeless shelter across the street for the night. You ask him to return to the clinic in the morning. What outcome criteria should you use to evaluate the effectiveness of your plans and interventions?

Key Concepts

- Men are physiologically the more vulnerable gender, demonstrated by shorter lifespans and a higher infant mortality.
- Men's psychosocial and moral development continues through young and middle adulthood.
- Life expectancy of men in the United States is one of the lowest in developed countries.
- Men engage in more risk-taking behaviors such as physical challenges and illegal behaviors than do women.
- The most significant death rate differences between men and women are AIDS, suicides, homicides, and accidents.

- Men tend to avoid diagnosis and treatment of illnesses that may result in serious health problems.
- Legislation has been enacted that is helpful to men in the areas of elder care, worker's compensation, Americans with disabilities, family and medical leaves, and veterans.
- The men's health nurse practitioner is an advance practice role focusing on the comprehensive health needs of men.

Critical Thinking Activities

1. Interview six men ranging in age from 21 to 70 years and ask them to list what they believe are health risk factors for them, what activities they regularly engage in that promote health, and what changes they believe they should make to promote their own health and reduce any existing risk factors.

2. Using the information gathered in activity 1, design a plan for health promotion for each man who is interviewed using the man's life-style, occupation, interest in social and recreational activities, income level, health risks, limitations in activities, and medical conditions. Review this plan with the man and determine how effectively the plan fits his perception of what he might do to ensure a healthier state.

3. Using the information gathered from the interviews and from the design of the health plan, determine at which developmental level the man is functioning. Is the level consistent with the age of the man?

4. Because morbidity and mortality data indicate that women live longer than men in the United States, interview 10 women ranging in age from 21 to 70 years and compare their health status, health risks, and participation in health-promoting behaviors with those of the 10 men who were interviewed to see what differences exist that might explain this differing life expectancy.

5. Using the leading causes of death described in this chapter that affect men, design a diet for men from two different cultural groups in the United States that would promote health and reduce the risks from the leading causes of death among men.

6. Because violence, suicide, and accidents are major causes of mortality for men in the United States, look at your community and describe the leading risk factors for violence, suicide, and accidents. Do each category separately. Use statistical data to document incidence. What agencies exist in the community to help prevent death or disability from these three risk factors?

Bibliography

Abel T, Cockerman W, Lueschen G, Kunz G: Health lifestyles and self-direction in employment among American men: a test of the spillover effect, *Soc Sci Med* 28:1269-1274, 1989.

Advance report of final mortality statistics, 1991, DHHS Pub No (PHS) 93-1120 *Monthly Vital Statistics Rep* 42, 2;(Suppl), 1993.

American Nurses Association: *Nursing care management,* Kansas City, 1980 American Nurses Association.

Bachman JG, Wallace JM, O'Malley PA, et al: Racial/ethnic differences in smoking, drinking, and illicit drug use among American high school seniors, *Am J Pub Health* 81(3):372-377.

Barklage N: Evaluation and management of the suicidal patient, *Emergency Care Q* 7:9-17, 1991.

Bird C, Fremont A: Gender, time use, and health, *J Health Soc Behav* 32:114-129, 1991.

Bittner V, Oberman A: Efficacy studies in coronary rehabilitation, *Cardiol Clinics* 11(2):333-347, 1993.

Black J, Matassarin-Jacobs E, Luckman J: *Luckman and Sorensen's medical-surgical nursing: a psychophysiologic approach,* Philadelphia, 1993, WB Saunders.

Blomhoff S, Seim S, Friis S: Can prediction of violence among psychiatric inpatients be improved? *Hosp Commun Psychiatry* 41:771-775, 1990.

Boring C, Squires T, Tong T: Cancer statistic, *CA Cancer J Clinicians* 43:7-26, 1993.

Bozett FW, Forrester DA: A proposal for men's health nurse practitioner, *Image J Nurs Schol* 21:158-161, 1989.

Davis R, Boyd G, Schoenborn C: Common courtesy and elimination of passive smoking, *JAMA* 26:2208-2210, 1990.

DeHoff JB, Forest K: Men's health. In Swanson J, Forest K, editors: *Men's reproductive health,* New York, 1984, Springer.

EDK Associates: *Men beating women: ending domestic violence—a qualitative and quantitive study of public attitudes on violence against women,* New York, 1993, EDK Associates.

Engelmann J: America ignores its number one drug problem—alcohol, *Hazelden News Professional Update,* pp 1-2, May 1991.

Erikson E: *Identity: youth and crisis,* New York, 1968, WW Norton.

Fingerhut L, Ingram D, Feldman J: Firearm and nonfirearm homicide among persons 15 through 19 years of age, *JAMA* 276:3048-3053, 1992.

Forrester D: Myths of masculinity: impact upon men's health, *Nurs Clin North Am* 21:15-23, 1986.

Glasser M: Males use of public health departments' family planning services, *Am J Pub H* 80:611-612, 1990.

Global AIDS News: Cumulative infections approach 20 million, *The Newsletter of the World Health Organization* Global Programs on AIDS 1:5, 1995.

Hammond W, Yung B: Psychology's role in public health response to assaultive violence among young African-American men, *Am Psychologist* 48:142-154, 1993.

Healthy People 2000: national health promotion and disease prevention objectives, Washington, DC, 1991, USDHHS, Public Health Service.

Higgins M, Enright P, Kronmal R: Smoking and lung function in elderly men and women: the cardiovascular study, *JAMA* 269:2741-2748, 1993.

Holm K, Penckofer S: Coronary heart disease: requisite knowledge for developing prevention strategies for the aging adult, *Prog Cardiovasc Nurs* 5:118-125, 1990.

Julian T, McKenry P, McKelvey M: Components of men's well being at mid-life, *Issues Mental Health Nurs* 13:285-299, 1992.

Jung CG: *Modern man in search of a soul,* New York, 1933, Harcourt Brace Jovanovich.

Kohlberg L: *Psychology of moral development: the nature and validity of moral stages,* San Francisco, 1984, Harper.

Lipscomb G, Muram D, Speck P, Mercer B: Male victims of sexual assault, *JAMA* 267:3064-3066, 1992.

Mellick E, Buckwalter K, Stolley J: Suicide among elderly white men: development of a profile, *J Psychosoc Nurs* 30:29-34, 1992.

National Council on Alcoholism and Drug Dependence, Inc: *Alcoholism in the family,* Hyattsville, Md, 1991, National Center for Health Statistics.

National Rifle Association: *1990: Firearms Fact Card,* Washington, DC, NRA Institute for Legislative Action.

Pack R: Descriptive epidemiology of genitourinary cancers, *Semin Oncol Nurs* 9:218-223, 1993.

Parks J: Violence. In Hillard JR, et al, editors: *Manual of clinical emergency psychiatry,* Washington, DC, 1990. American Psychiatric Press.

Pate RR, Pratt M, Blair SN, et al: *Physical activity and public health: a recommendation from the Center of Disease Control and Prevention and the American College of Sports Medicine,* *JAMA* 273(5):402-407, 1995.

Pozgar G, Pozgar N: *Legal aspects of healthcare administration,* ed 5, Gaithersburg, Md, 1993, Aspen Publishers.

Preston DS, Stern RS: Nonmelanoma cancers of the skin, *N Engl J Med* 327:1649-1659, 1992.

Rafuse J: Men's attitudes about seeking healthcare may put them at risk, conference told, *J Can Med Assoc* 149:329-330, 1993.

Rosenberg M, Mercy J: Assaultive violence. In Rosenberg M, Mercy J, editors: *Violence in America: a public health approach,* New York, 1991, Oxford University Press.

Saltonstall R: Healthy bodies, social bodies: men's and women's concepts and practices of health in everyday life, *Soc Sci Med* 36:7-14, 1993.

Toscano G, Windau J: *Fatal work injuries: results from 1992 national census,* Report 870, Washington, DC, 1994, US Department of Labor, Bureau of Labor Statistics.

Treating your enlarged prostate, AHCPR Pub No 94-0583, Rockville, Md, 1994, Public Health Service, Agency for Health Care Policy and Research.

US Congress, Office of Technology Assessment: *International health statistics: what the numbers mean for the United States—Background paper,* Pub No OTA-BP-H-116, Washington, DC, 1993, US Government Printing Office.

US Department of Labor: *Work injuries and illnesses by selected characteristics,* Pub No USDL-94-213, Washington, DC, 1994, Bureau of Labor Statistics.

Vital and health statistics: current estimates from the National Health Interview Survey, 1992, DHHS Pub No (PHS) 94-1517, Hyattsville, Md, 1994, Public Health Services, Centers for Disease Control and Prevention.

Waldron I, Lye D, Brandon A: Gender differences in teenage smoking, *Women and Health* 17:65-90, 1991.

Walker R: Modeling and guided practice as components within a comprehensive testicular self-examination educational program for high school males, *J Health Educ* 24:162-168, 1993.

Windau J, Toscano G: *Workplace homicides in 1992,* Report 870, Washington DC, 1994, US Department of Labor, Bureau of Labor Statistics.

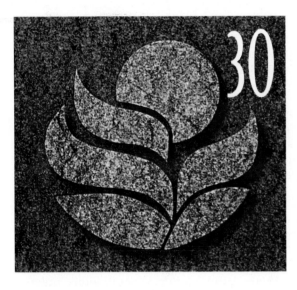

30

Elder Health

Patricia C. Birchfield*

Objectives ▼

After reading this chapter, the student should be able to do the following:

◆ Identify at least three demographic facts about elders.
◆ Define ageism and how it affects society's bias about elders.
◆ Discuss at least two theories of aging.
◆ List the major health problems of elders.
◆ Identify the components of a comprehensive assessment of elders.
◆ Discuss the role of the community health nurse in the delivery of care to elders.

Key Terms ▼

activities of daily living
advance directives
ageism
Alzheimer's type of dementia
assisted living
confusion
delirium
dementia
depression
developmental tasks
elder abuse
extended care facilities
home care
instrumental activities of daily living
life review
long-term care
malnutrition
multi-infarct dementia
respite care
return migration
social network

*The author acknowledges the contribution of Dr. Delois Skipwith for the chapter in previous editions of this book, from which this chapter is revised.

The population of the United States in the age group 65 years of age and older, or elders, is increasing at a more rapid pace than the population as a whole. This "graying" of America is a phenomenon of the twentieth century that is without precedence. Increased numbers of persons 65 years of age and older are often accompanied by an increase in chronic conditions and a greater demand for services. These services can be costly and may not be accessible to all elders. This chapter describes elders, including theories and myths of aging, developmental tasks of aging, health problems and health assessment of elders, the role of the community health nurse, and health care delivery issues that may affect the delivery of service to elders.

DEMOGRAPHY

At the turn of the twentieth century, the average life expectancy in the United States was 47 years; in 1987 it was almost 75 years, an increase of almost 28 years (U.S. Department of Health and Human Services [DHHS], 1990). It is estimated that by the year 2030, because of the graying of the "baby boom" generation, 21.8% of the population will be 65 years of age or older. By 2050, 80 million persons in the United States will be 65 years of age or older (Figure 30-1).

For the first decade since 1910, males in the United

States showed a greater increase than females in the population, but women continue to have a longer life expectancy than men: 78.3 years for women and 71.5 years for men (Hollmann, 1992). Even with the improvement of male life expectancy, women outnumber the men in the later years of life (Figure 30-2).

Aging of the U.S. population has resulted from the steady decline in birth rates that began in the late 1950s and a combination of the discovery of antibiotics, increased life expectancy, declining fertility, and immigration (Olson, 1994). Health care beliefs and practices differ across ethnic populations, and community health nurses must be prepared to adapt in response to ethnic differences. African-Americans are the largest minority in the United States, accounting for 8.2% of elders, and Hispanics comprise 3% of elders (American Association of Retired Persons [AARP], 1990). Minority elderly populations undergo not only the infirmities of age, but also the problems of discrimination, stress, lack of education, and poverty (Greene et al., 1992).

Geography and Elders

An erroneous perception exists that elders are geographically concentrated in the Sunbelt states. Geographical distribution patterns reveal that this is not true. In 1987, states with the highest proportion of elderly residents were those states in the Midwest and Plains (Iowa, Arkansas, Wisconsin, South Dakota, Ne-

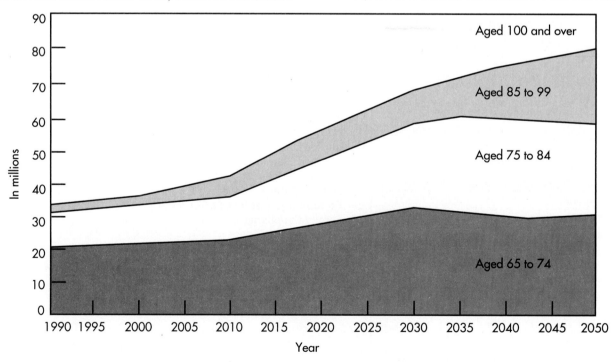

FIGURE 30-1

Population of persons aged 65 and over: 1990 to 2050. (From US Senate Subcommittee on Aging, American Association of Retired Persons, Federal Council on Aging, US Administration on Aging: *Aging America: trends and projections*, DHHS Pub No (FCOA) 91-28001, Washington, DC, 1991, US Department of Health and Human Services.)

braska, Missouri, Kansas), the Northeast (Pennsylvania, Rhode Island, Massachusetts, Maine, Connecticut, New Jersey, New York), as well as West Virginia and Oregon. One notable exception is Florida, where 17.8% of the population was over age 65 (U.S. Senate Subcommittee, 1990).

One geographic pattern that has been recognized recently is that of return migration. **Return migration** occurs when elders return to their home town communities after having spent their working life elsewhere. This pattern is more common in the rural South, where retirees return to their roots to pursue retired life. Rural communities often have a lower cost of living, and the retirement income goes further (Greene et al., 1992).

Living Arrangements and Elders

Most elders live independently, either alone or with their spouses; only about 5% of elders are living in an institution (Greene et al., 1992). More men than women age 85 and older are still married; as a consequence, more women live alone in later life than men (Barer, 1994). Almost 65% of impaired elders live with someone else because of their health problems, while the remaining 35% live alone (Greene et al., 1992).

Economics and Elders

Despite important gains, elders as a group experience more economic insecurity than do younger persons.

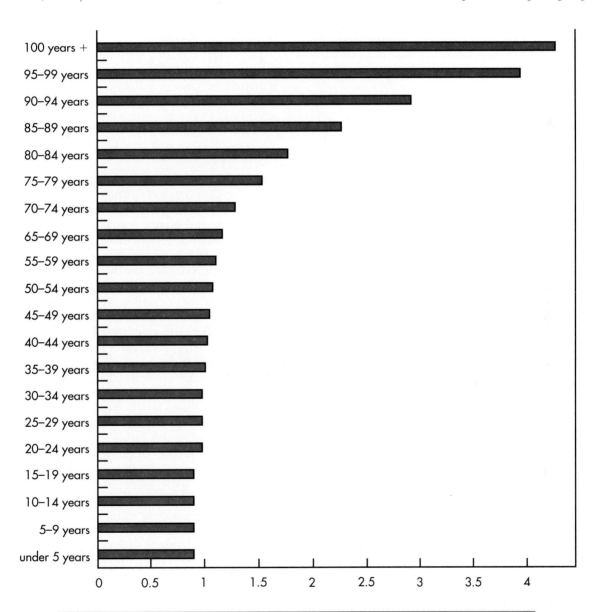

FIGURE 30-2

Ratio of women to men by age in 1990. (From US Bureau of the Census, US Department of Commerce: Projections of the population of the US by age, sex, and race, 1988-2050. In *Current Population Reports, Population Estimates, and Projections*, series p-25, No 118, Washington, DC, 1991, US Government Printing Office.)

In 1966, 28.5% of elders were living in poverty; in 1988, 12.2% of the elderly had incomes below the poverty level. Elderly women are especially vulnerable; women age 85 and older are more likely to live at the poverty level. This group of women either did not work outside the home or had work patterns that were interrupted, resulting in exclusion from pensions and other retirement benefits (Barer, 1994). Even with significant improvement, 15.2% of elders had incomes no more than 1.5 times the poverty level in 1987; elders with incomes in this range are more vulnerable economically, especially if they find themselves in a situation where they must pay high out-of-pocket health care expenses (Greene et al., 1992).

Educational Level and Elders

The elder population is much less educated than the younger population; however, the gap is narrowing and is expected to decline even further by the end of this decade. It is predicted that by the year 2000, the median number of school years completed for elders will be 12.4 compared with 12.8 years for those persons aged 25 and older. Racial and ethnic differences are pronounced; whites comprised 70% of those graduating from high school, while 40% of African-Americans and 32% of Hispanics were high-school graduates (U.S. Senate Subcommittee, 1990).

MYTHS AND THEORIES OF AGING
Myths

Aging is a normal process that is not well understood, and over the years, myths associated with aging have evolved. Some of the common myths involve the perception that all elders are infirm, senile, hard of hearing, cannot adapt to change, love to sit and rock in their rocking chairs, are bad drivers, are not interested in or capable of sexual activity, cannot learn, and are all alike (Skipwith, 1992; Swanson and Albrecht, 1993). These myths are grossly unfair to elders and characterize them in a way that is neither correct nor humane. If Americans would observe the activities of some elders, they would see them engaged in gardening, performing church and volunteer work, involved with family members, attending classes, and being productive and vibrant members of society.

Many myths surrounding aging foster ageism. **Ageism** is the term for prejudice about older people; it is similar in many ways to racism and sexism and is just as harmful. Ageism fosters a stereotype of elders that does not allow them to be viewed realistically. Ageism can result in social isolation of elders and perpetuates the fear of growing old that resides in all of us (Berger, 1994).

Theories

Even though the process of aging is not well understood, several theories have been proposed as a way to explain the aging process. Not all have been accepted either when first published or at present.

Biological Theories

Several biological theories have been developed to explain the process of aging. The *cellular interaction theory* suggests that an organism's individual cells are influenced by other cells. Unless the cells are functioning in harmony, the feedback mechanisms will fail and the cells will degenerate (Berger, 1994).

The *somatic mutagenesis theory* states that as cells divide, they develop spontaneous mutations. These mutations eventually lead to death (Kane et al., 1994).

The *error catastrophe theory* proposes that errors occur in deoxyribonucleic acid (DNA), ribonucleic acid (RNA), and protein synthesis. Each error augments the other and culminates in an error catastrophe (Kane et al., 1994).

The oldest and most general biological theory of aging is the *wear-and-tear theory*. This theory maintains that just as parts of machines wear out, parts of the human body also deteriorate with each year of use. According to this theory, we wear out our bodies just by living (Berger, 1994).

Psychosocial Theories

The first theoretical approach in gerontology came from the University of Chicago and resulted in the *disengagement theory*. In brief, the disengagement theory (Cumming and Henry, 1961) maintains that society and individuals disengage in a mutual withdrawal, allowing the individual to invest in more self-focused activities and establish balance at this stage of life.

Many critics of the disengagement theory embraced an opposing theory called the *activity theory*. Activity theory states that older persons need and want to become involved with a variety of activities. The new involvements substitute for changes that come with growing older and the roles that were lost with retirement (Berger, 1994; Gelfand, 1994).

With *continuity theory*, each person copes with the later years of life in much the same way as they coped with the earlier period. In this sense, aging is seen as a continuation of the earlier life rather than as a separate period (Berger, 1994; Gelfand, 1994).

Exchange theory views elders with great esteem as a result of their experience and greater knowledge of lore and history. The elder "exchanges" this knowledge for a position of deferment and respect from younger individuals (Gelfand, 1994).

Humanistic theorists, such as Abraham Maslow and Carl Rogers, have taken a more holistic view of development and have tried to account for diverse human experiences. *Humanistic theory* views people as unique, self-determined, worthy of respect, and guided by a variety of basic human needs (Berger, 1994).

According to Maslow, an individual's behavior is motivated by universal needs that range from the most basic (food, sleep, safety) to the highest need of self-actualization. If the basic needs are not met, self-actualization cannot be attained (Maslow, 1968). Rogers believed that the process of becoming a fully functioning adult is aided throughout life by those who are important to us when they provide unconditional positive regard, allowing the perception of being loved no matter what we do (Berger, 1994).

Harry Stack Sullivan's *interpersonal theory* (1956) involves developing satisfactory interpersonal relationships as a sign of maturity. As these relationships are lost, the individual may also experience a loss of interpersonal security.

Theories of aging may provide a useful framework for practice for community health nurses. One or several theories may be appropriate, but if the community health nurse selects a theoretical framework, it must match the elder to whom it is applied.

DEVELOPMENTAL TASKS OF AGING

Despite wide acceptance of the heterogeneity of the elder population, most references to developmental tasks of elders view this period of life as one stage of life, or two at most. **Developmental tasks** refer to age-appropriate skills that need to be accomplished. One approach to elders is to designate stages of older adulthood arbitrarily based on chronological age, such as dividing the population into young-old, old-old, or frail elderly. This approach seems inadequate, since chronological age is an inappropriate basis on which to identify differences among elders (Fisher, 1993).

Erik Erikson's stages of development (1950) are widely cited as a way of viewing development across the lifespan (see box below). Erikson's eighth stage, integrity versus despair, is frequently cited in describing older adulthood. Erikson, now an octogenarian, admitted to being surprised at the creativity and generativity of older adults. With increased life expectancy, Erikson suggested that the entire life cycle

should be reexamined rather than adding another stage toward the end (Erikson et al., 1986).

Havighurst (1952) also described older adulthood as one stage beginning at age 55, which was termed *later maturity*. Later maturity was seen as a time during which the older adult was faced with adjusting to retirement and reduced income, adjusting to decreased physical strength, adjusting to the death of a spouse, establishing alliances with others of the same age, and adapting to changing social roles.

Butler (1963) proposed the process of **life review,** which involves integrating past life experiences in an attempt to believe that life has had meaning. Life review was characterized as a universal process that occurs at any point in life when a person is forced to confront his or her mortality. Perceiving that life has had meaning enables the individual to prepare for death without fear.

With a better understanding of elders, it is easier for health care providers to plan appropriate care for them. Understanding the anticipated demographic changes, theories of aging, and expected developmental tasks assists the community health nurse in preparing for comprehensive delivery of service to elders.

MAJOR HEALTH PROBLEMS OF ELDERS

Not all elders are afflicted with health problems, but elders as a group show a significant incidence of chronic conditions. Table 30-1 demonstrates these, as well as measures that elders can take, or the community health nurse can teach, to prevent or reduce the

Erikson's Stages of Psychosocial Development

Stage 1	Trust versus mistrust: focuses on developing a sense of self and others
Stage 2	Autonomy versus shame and doubt: focuses on ability to express oneself and cooperate with others
Stage 3	Initiative versus guilt: focuses on purposeful behavior and evaluation of that behavior
Stage 4	Industry versus inferiority: focuses on developing confidence in one's abilities
Stage 5	Identity versus role confusion: focuses on developing a clear sense of self
Stage 6	Intimacy versus isolation: focuses on developing one's capacity for reciprocal love
Stage 7	Generativity versus stagnation: focuses on creativity, productivity, and developing the capacity to care for others
Stage 8	Integrity versus despair: focuses on acceptance of one's life as having had meaning

Table 30-1 Most Common Chronic Conditions in Adults Ages 65 Years and Older

Problem	% Affected	Measures available to prevent onset or reduce disability
Arthritis	46	Weight control, exercise
Hypertension	38	Salt restriction, weight control, antihypertensive medication
Hearing loss	28	Avoid exposure to loud noises or wear hearing protection
Heart conditions	28	Diet, control of hypertension, nonsmoking, low-fat diet
Chronic sinus problems	18	Nonsmoking
Visual loss	14	Wear sunglasses in bright light
Bone problems	13	Adequate calcium intake, exercise, avoid smoking and excessive alcohol use

From Ham RI, Sloane PD, editors: *Primary care geriatrics: a case-based approach,* St Louis, 1992, Mosby. Reprinted with permission.

Table 30-2 Changes in Most Common Causes of Death, 1900 and 1985, All Ages and For Those 65 +

| | All Ages | | | | 65 + | |
| | 1900 | | 1985 | | 1985 | |
Cause	Rate*	Rank	Rate	Rank	Rate	Rank
Diseases of heart	13.8	4	32.3	1	217.3	1
Malignant neoplasms	6.4	8	19.3	2	104.7	2
Cerebrovascular disease	10.7	5	6.4	3	46.4	3
Accidents	7.2	7	3.9	4	8.7	6
Influenza and pneumonia	22.9	1	2.8	5	20.6	4
Diabetes mellitus	1.1		1.5	6	9.6	5
Suicide	1.0		1.2	7	2.0	11
Cirrhosis of liver	1.2		1.1	8	3.4	10
Atherosclerosis	NR		1.0	9	8.0	7
Bronchitis, emphysema, asthma	4.5	9	0.9	10	5.7	8
Nephritis and nephrosis	8.9	6	0.9	10	5.7	8
Homicide	0.1		0.8	12	0.4	12
Tuberculosis	19.4	2	0.07		0.4	12
Diarrhea and enteritis	14.3	3	NR			
Diphtheria	4.0	11	NR			
Typhoid fever	3.1	12	NR			
Senility	5.0	10	NR			

From Kane RL, Ouslander JG, Abrass IB: *Essentials of clinical geriatrics*, ed 3, New York, 1994, McGraw-Hill. Used with permission.
NR, Not reported.
*Rate per 10,000 population.

disability associated with the chronic conditions (Sloane, 1992).

Ischemic heart disease continues to be the most common cause of death for elders, followed by malignant neoplasms, cerebrovascular disease, and diabetes mellitus. Table 30-2 outlines the causes of death for elders and all ages.

The most common acute condition experienced by elders is an infection of the respiratory tract. Other common acute conditions for elders include eye and ear conditions, urinary tract infections, skin conditions, and a variety of musculoskeletal conditions (Mermelstein et al., 1993). With both acute and chronic conditions, elders use a disproportionate share of health care services (Figure 30-3) (Furner, 1993).

Several other conditions affect elders and are most common in elders over 80 years of age. These conditions are often referred to as the "five I's" (Tierney et al., 1994): (1) intellectual impairment, (2) immobility, (3) instability, (4) incontinence, and (5) iatrogenic drug reactions.

Progressive intellectual impairment, dementia, is manifested as a gradually progressive course, usually over the course of months to years. Dementia is the most feared condition among the aging population, even though it is not inevitable. Aging itself does not cause dementia, but aging is associated with changes in the central nervous system and detectable changes in memory called "benign senescent forgetfulness" (Kane et al., 1994).

Depression is a fairly common cause of intellectual impairment but one that is often overlooked. Depression occurs in 5% to 10% of elders living in the community. Depression requires the presence of a depressed mood for at least 2 weeks plus at least four of eight vegetative signs, including sleep disturbance, lack of interest, feelings of guilt, lack of energy, decreased concentration and appetite, psychomotor agitation, and suicidal ideation (Kane et al., 1994; Tierney et al., 1994).

Immobility in elders is caused by pain, stiffness, imbalance, and psychological problems. Fear of falling is a major cause of immobility. The most important step in the area of immobility is prevention. Adequate nutrition should be ensured, appropriate exercise should be encouraged, and assistive aids should be installed if necessary (Tierney et al., 1994).

Instability and the resulting falls are a problem for

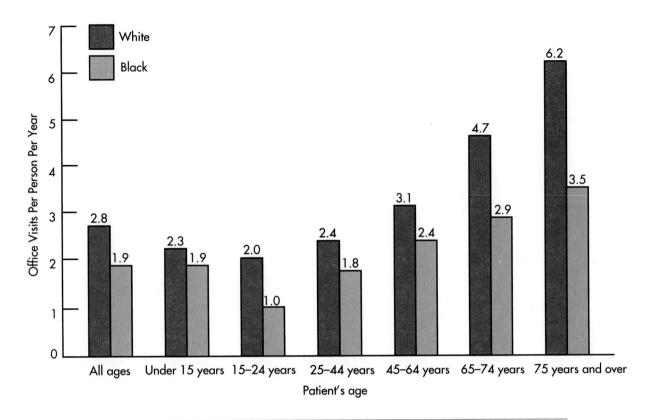

FIGURE 30-3

Annual rate of visits to office-based physicians by patient's age and race: United States, 1991. (From US Department of Health and Human Services, Public Health Service: *National Ambulatory Medical Care Survey*: 1991 *summary*, DHHS Pub No (PHS) 94-1777, Washington, DC, 1994, US Government Printing Office.)

elders, especially women. Thirty percent of elders fall each year, and one of four of those who fall sustain serious injuries, including fractures. Many environmental factors affect the likelihood of a fall occurring. These factors can be modified, as outlined in Table 30-3. Falls are a leading cause of death and are a contributing factor in 40% of the admissions to nursing homes. One in 40 of those who sustain a fall requires hospitalization, and only one half of elders hospitalized as a result of a fall are alive 1 year later. Even in light of these statistics, falls should not be considered as inevitable (Kane et al., 1994; Tierney et al., 1994).

Urinary incontinence often contributes to institutionalization. Incontinence can also lead to psychological problems and self-imposed social isolation. There are medical causes that are correctable; surgical procedures can also correct some causes of urinary incontinence. Pelvic muscle exercises are easily accomplished, and underwear liners are available for both men and women (Tierney et al., 1994).

Iatrogenic drug reactions are more common in elders for several physiological reasons, including changes in absorption, decreased renal flow, decreased blood flow to the liver, and altered responses to drugs. Many elders take several medications, both prescribed and over the counter, increasing the chance of drug reactions (Tierney et al., 1994). It has been estimated

Table 30-3 Environmental Factors Affecting Risks of Falling in the Home

Environmental area or factor	Objective and recommendations
All areas: lighting	Absence of glare and shadows; accessible switches at room entrance; night light in bedroom, hall bathroom
Floors	Nonskid backing for throw rugs; carpet edges tacked down; carpets with shallow pile; nonskid wax on floors; cords out of walking path; small objects (e.g., clothes, shoes off floor)
Stairs	Lighting sufficient, with switches at top and bottom of stairs; securely fastened bilateral handrails that stand out from wall; top and bottom steps marked with bright, contrasting tape; stair rises of no more than 6 inches; steps in good repair; no objects stored on steps
Kitchen	Items stored so that reaching up and bending over are not necessary; secure step stool available if climbing is necessary; firm, nonmovable table

Continued.

Table 30-3   Environmental Factors Affecting Risks of Falling in the Home—cont'd

Environmental area or factor	Objective and recommendations
Bathroom	Grab bars for tub, shower, toilet; nonskid decals or rubber mat in tub or shower; shower chair with hand-held shower; nonskid rugs; raised toilet seat; door locks removed to ensure access in an emergency
Yard and entrances	Repair of cracks in pavement, holes in lawn; removal of rocks, tools, other tripping hazards; well-lit walkways, free of ice and wet leaves; stairs and steps as above
Institutions	All the above; bed at proper height (not too high or low); spills on floor cleaned up promptly; appropriate use of walking aids and wheelchairs
Footwear	Shoes with firm, nonskid, nonfriction soles; low heels (unless person is accustomed to high heels); avoidance of walking in stocking feet or loose slippers

From Tinetti ME, Speechley M: N Engl J Med 320:1055-1059, 1989. Reprinted with permission.

that adverse drug reactions account for 10% to 30% of all hospital admissions for elders and that 1 in 1000 hospitalized elders die as a result of side effects of medications (Kotthoff-Burrell, 1992).

ROLE OF THE COMMUNITY HEALTH NURSE

Community health nurses focus on the prevention of disease and the promotion and maintenance of health. To achieve these goals, community health nurses are involved in client and community education, counseling, advocacy, and management of care (Table 30-4). The overall goal is improvement of the individual's and the community's health through collaborative practice with other members of the health care team (Lancaster et al., 1992). Achieving this goal involves the community health nurse in all three levels of prevention: primary, secondary, and tertiary, with an emphasis on primary prevention. The community health nurse should be familiar with the guidelines for screening preventive services for individuals 65 years of age and older (Appendix A) recommended by the U.S. Guide to Clinical Preventive Services. Awareness of the guidelines facilitates counseling of elders to obtain the recommended screening tests.

Health promotion includes many activities such as exercise, nutrition, screening, self-care, relaxation, stress management, and accident prevention. Health promotion and prevention of disease are infrequently associated with elders because of the image of aging

 Summary of Selected National Health Objectives Related to Elders

1. Reduce suicides among white men aged 65 and older to no more than 39.2:100,000.
2. Reduce deaths from falls and fall-related injuries to no more than 14.4:100,000.
3. Reduce to no more than 90:1000 who have difficulty performing two or more personal care acts.
4. Reduce hip fractures among those 65 and older so that hospitalizations are no more than 607:100,000.
5. Reduce significant hearing impairment among people 45 and older to no more than 180:1000.
6. Reduce significant visual impairment among people 65 and older to no more than 70:1000.
7. Increase pneumococcal and influenza immunizations in institutionalized elders to at least 80%.
8. Increase length of healthy life to at least 65 years.
9. Increase to at least 30% the proportion of those 65 and older who engage regularly in light to moderate physical activity.
10. Reduce to no more than 20% those elders who have lost all their natural teeth.

being associated with pathology. This view must be challenged by nurses' practice and by the way in which nurses are educated. Health promotion for elders should place health in its widest context and should include social and political action as well as advocating for life-style changes (Lauder, 1993).

Prevention may improve the quality of life and may lead to preserved or improved physical and mental health, functional status, and role function (Klinkman et al., 1992; Kotthoff-Burrell, 1992). Contrary to the myths, *all* elders can gain from health promotion and disease prevention, not just elders residing in the community.

The federal government, with its increased support for health promotion, has published *Healthy People 2000: National Health Promotion and Disease Prevention Objectives* (1991), which includes health promotion priorities and strategies for older adults (see box above). It is essential for the nursing profession to include the older population in planning for health promotion activities and strategies. Not only should consideration be made for those elders still living in the community, but also for those who reside in an institution. Institutionalized elders benefit from humanistic approaches and an enhanced life-style (Robertson, 1991).

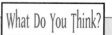 What Do You Think?

Health promotion activities should only be included in the care of elders residing in the community.

Table 30-4   Major Health Problems in Elders and Community Health Nursing Roles

Problem	Community health nursing roles
Hypertension	Monitor blood pressure and weight; educate about nutrition and antihypertensive drugs; teach stress management techniques; promote an optimal balance between rest and activity; establish blood pressure screening programs; assess client's current life-style and promote life-style changes; promote dietary modifications by using techniques such as a diet diary.
Cancer	Obtain health history; promote monthly breast self-examinations and yearly Pap smears and mammograms for older women; promote regular physical examinations; encourage smokers to stop smoking; correct misconceptions about processes of aging; provide emotional support and quality care during diagnostic and treatment procedures.
Arthritis	Help adult avoid the false hope and expense of arthritis quackery; educate adult about management of activities, correct body mechanics, availability of mechanical appliances, and adequate rest; promote stress management; counsel and assist the family to improve communication, role negotiation, and use of community resources.
Visual impairment (e.g., loss of visual acuity, eyelid disorders, opacity of the lens)	Provide support in a well-lighted, glare-free environment; use printed aids with large, well-spaced letters; assist adult with cleaning eyeglasses; help make arrangements for vision examinations and obtain necessary prostheses; teach adult to be cautious of fraudulent advertisements.
Hearing impairment (e.g., presbycusis)	Speak with clarity at a moderate volume and pace and face audience when performing health teaching; help make arrangements for hearing examination and obtain necessary prostheses; teach adult to be cautious of fraudulent advertisements.
Confusional states	Provide complete assessment; correct underlying causes of disease (if possible); provide for a protective environment; promote activities that reinforce reality; assist with adequate personal hygiene, nutrition, and hydration; provide emotional support to the family; recommend applicable community resources such as adult day care, home health aides, and homemaker services.
Alzheimer's disease	Maintain optimal functioning, protection, and safety; foster human dignity; demonstrate to the primary family caregiver techniques to dress, feed, and toilet adult; provide frequent encouragement and emotional support to caregiver; act as an advocate for client when dealing with respite care and support groups; ensure that clients's rights are protected; provide support to maintain family members' physical and mental health; maintain family stability; recommend financial services if needed.
Dental problems	Perform oral assessment and refer as necessary; emphasize regular brushing and flossing, proper nutrition, and dental examinations; encourage clients with dentures to wear and take care of them; allay fears about dentist; help provide access to financial services (if necessary) and access to dental care facilities.
Drug use and abuse	Obtain drug history; educate adult about safe storage, risks of drug, drug-drug, and drug-food interactions, and general information about drug (e.g., drug name, purpose, side effects, dosage); instruct adult about presorting technique (using small container with one dose of drug that are labeled with specific administration times).
Substance abuse	Arrange and monitor detoxification if appropriate; counsel adults about substance abuse; promote stress management to avoid need for drugs or alcohol; encourage adult to use self-help groups such as Alcoholics Anonymous and Al-Anon; educate public about dangers of substance abuse.

From Skipwith DH: In Stanhope M, Lancaster J, editors: *Community health nursing: process and practice for promoting health*, ed 3, St Louis, 1992, Mosby.

Reducing susceptibility or exposure to disease for an individual who has no symptoms is *primary prevention.* For elders, this may involve immunizations (influenza, Pneumovax, tetanus), smoking cessation education, chemoprophylaxis (aspirin, hormone replacement therapy), safety factors, dental health, nutrition counseling, sunscreens, exercise, accident prevention, and instruction in the appropriate use of medications or herbs (Kotthoff-Burrell, 1992).

Secondary prevention for elders includes screening for early detection, diagnosis, and treatment of disease in asymptomatic persons. The goal is to decrease pathology and disability through early detection. Secondary measures include screening for hypertension; breast, colorectal, cervical, ovarian, skin, and prostate cancer; visual and hearing impairments; diabetes mellitus; hyperlipidemia; cardiovascular disease (bruits, pulses); tuberculosis; depression and dementia; urinary incontinence; abuse and neglect; and thyroid disease (Kotthoff-Burrell, 1992). It has been estimated that as many as 94% of elders screened revealed a positive finding. Advocates maintain that preventive programs can result in healthier elders, which would result in reducing health care costs (Beers et al., 1991).

Tertiary prevention involves maximizing independent functioning in those persons in whom disease is diagnosed. Activities include those aimed at maximizing function in persons with incontinence, early dementia, suicidal ideation, and depression. The nature and extent of the interventions should be guided by the wishes of the individual and the family (Kotthoff-Burrell, 1992).

Federal regulations require that elders be advised of their rights to self-determination when they are admitted to either an acute or long-term care institution. Living will (Appendix C.2) and surrogate decision making legislation exists in many states (Kotthoff-Burrell, 1992). A routine discussion of **advance directives** may be facilitated by the community health nurse in an open discussion with both elders and family members.

Health Assessment of Elders

Effective care of elders by a community health nurse requires an accurate assessment of their health status. The goal of care for elders is to optimize their general health and functioning capabilities. At the core of this goal is enabling elders to remain in their homes, which helps reduce health care costs, improves quality of life, and preserves functional status (Ramsdell, 1991).

Comprehensive assessment of elders by community health nurses includes identifying health, nutritional, functional, psychosocial, and other problems that elders encounter. This comprehensive assessment allows the community health nurse to devise an individualized management plan that will optimize the elder's functional level (Ramsdell, 1991).

Health History

It is vital that health care providers have accurate and current health information for the elders they serve. A comprehensive assessment that includes the health history may be one that has evolved over time and includes the individual's perception of his or her health. The history should be the basis for recommended screening measures, preventive and health-promoting plans, and practical plans for implementing comprehensive and continuing future care of elders (Ham, 1992). Tools are available for comprehensive assessment, including the Comprehensive Older Persons' Evaluation (COPE) (Appendix J.3).

Most elders are able to give an accurate health history to the community health nurse, but obtaining a history from elders can potentially present communication difficulties. Impaired hearing and vision may interfere with communication; impaired intellectual functioning may render the attempt at obtaining a history from the elder useless, indicating that other sources must be sought; the multiplicity of complaints may frustrate the interviewer; and symptoms may be vague or underreported (Kane et al., 1994; Tierney et al., 1994).

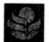 **Research Brief**

Schoenfeld DE, Malmrose LC, Blazer DG, Gold DT, Seeman TE: Self-rated health and mortality in the high-functioning elderly—a closer look at healthy individuals: MacArthur Field Study of Successful Aging, *J Gerontol Med Sci* 49(3):M109-M115, 1994.

A study, focusing on high-functioning elderly, tested the predictive value of self-rated health on mortality. Data from the MacArthur Field Study of Successful Aging were utilized. The subjects were aged 70 to 79 years at baseline, and in-home interviews were conducted in 1988 and 1991. Logistic regression was performed to create odds ratios for age, sex, marital status, education, alcohol consumption, cigarette smoking, chronic disease, past hospitalization, and cognitive functions.

Mortality and survival chances appear to be directly linked to perceptions of health, with the greatest influence seen in healthy individuals. Elders' perceptions of their health may differ from what might be expected on the basis of their health history, their diagnoses, and the physical examination findings. Self-rated health may be more meaningful in healthy individuals and should be utilized to identify those healthy elders at risk. After identification of those at risk, the health care provider can explore the factors that caused elders to rate their health as poor. Clinical use of self-rated health may be a step toward early identification and treatment of health problems, resulting in reduced costs.

Did You Know?

A multidisciplinary visit assessing all aspects of elders is the best way to achieve a comprehensive geriatric assessment, enabling prioritization of problems, implementation, and ongoing management of an elder's situation.

An elder's past health history is important in understanding the elder's health and helps to put the current problems with health status into perspective. A detailed medication history is critical, since elders may not be complying with a prescribed medical regimen, may be self-medicating, or may be having adverse effects from medications (Kane et al., 1994).

A systems review, with an emphasis on potentially important symptoms in the elderly can assist in completing the health picture of elders (Table 30-5). Because symptoms are not as keenly experienced by elders, this part of the history may be time consuming and difficult to interpret (Kane et al., 1994).

Nutrition Assessment

Community health nurses, in performing a comprehensive assessment on elders, must be aware of the possibility of inadequate nutrition in elders. The prevalence of malnutrition among elders is high; some studies reveal that as many as 10% to 50% of community-residing elders have inadequate nutrition. Malnutrition is a major risk for morbidity and mortality among institutionalized elders. Despite prevalence rates, nutrition assessment is frequently overlooked (Mion, McDowell, and Heanet, 1994).

Malnutrition is a multifactorial problem that involves physical, psychosocial, and economic factors. Elders who live alone eat less; this finding may be greater for men. Cognitive and mood disturbances can also result in altered nutritional intake. In addition, approximately 10% of elders misuse or abuse alcohol, which is often overlooked by health care professionals. Problems with alcohol may present as new urinary incontinence or decreased appetite (Kane et al., 1994).

The diet history is used to determine nutritional status; the diet history includes not only recent food intake but meal preparation and frequency, location and sharing of meals, weight history, and use of nutritional supplements. Two methods frequently utilized are the 24-hour dietary recall and the 3-day written record. The 24-hour recall relies on the elder's memory but is quick and simple if the information can be considered accurate. The 3-day written record is more accurate but requires another visit. Interviewing others who have information about the elder's eating patterns can add validity to the information (Mion et al., 1994).

Psychosocial Assessment

Assessing an elder's mental and emotional status is critical for a comprehensive assessment. The community health nurse should present this to the elder as part of a routine assessment. Disoriented elders can mask their status in such a pleasant and lucid-appearing manner that others may not suspect deficits in their mental status functioning (Beck, Freedman, and Warshaw, 1994; Kane et al., 1994).

An important aspect of determining an elder's ability to function independently in the community is the

Table 30-5 Important Aspects of Systems Review in Elders

System	Key symptoms
Respiratory	Increasing dyspnea
	Persistent cough
Cardiovascular	Orthopnea
	Edema
	Angina
	Claudication
	Palpitations
	Dizziness
	Syncope
Gastrointestinal	Difficulty chewing
	Dysphagia
	Abdominal pain
	Change in bowel habit
Genitourinary	Frequency
	Urgency
	Nocturia
	Hesitancy, intermittent stream, straining to void
	Incontinence
	Hematuria
	Vaginal bleeding
Musculoskeletal	Focal or diffuse pain
	Focal or diffuse weakness
Neurological	Visual disturbances (transient or progressive)
	Progressive hearing loss
	Unsteadiness or falls
	Transient focal symptoms
Psychological	Depression
	Anxiety or agitation
	Paranoia
	Forgetfulness or confusion

From Kane RL, Ouslander JG, Abrass IB: *Essentials of clinical geriatrics*, ed 3, New York, 1994, McGraw-Hill. Used with permission.

extent of their social network. **Social network** can be defined as those individuals with whom elders have contact because of proximity or reciprocity, some of whom may be involved in their care. Most care given to elders is provided by family members; even formalized community support services rely heavily on family and friends to see that adequate care is given to maintain elders in the community (Kane et al., 1994; Olson, 1994). The community health nurse must be aware of formal and informal members of elders' social network when planning care.

Women, wives, daughters, daughters-in-law, sisters, or other female relatives represent more than 70% of all caregivers. Elderly men are generally cared for by their wives, whereas elder women rely on their adult children. Family members in general prefer to provide care rather than to institutionalize their relatives (Olson, 1994).

The community health nurse should assess interaction among elders and their caregivers to observe for actual or potential neglect, exploitation, and abuse. **Elder abuse** is typically defined as an act of commission or omission that leads to harm or threatened harm to the welfare of an elder (O'Brien, 1992; Ramsdell, 1991).

Older demented or dependent women and elders who exhibit difficult behaviors are the typical victims of elder abuse. Elder abuse is underreported, and the community health nurse should become proactive and consider the possibility of abuse more frequently. When abuse is suspected, elders should be questioned directly about being harmed, confined against their will, or being victims of theft; their response should also be noted. In many states, nurses are mandated to report abuse or suspected abuse. The primary goal is to ensure the victim's safety and to intervene in a way that is the least disruptive for the elder and the family (O'Brien, 1992).

Many elders are also fearful of being the victims of crime. Door and window locks should be assessed for security and fixed if not in good repair. Although costly, security systems may provide a feeling of security for those who can afford them. Elders may also be victims of crime against person and property (Skipwith, 1992). Community health nurses, as well as family members, should caution elders about being fooled by home repair schemes, letting strangers into their homes, giving out credit card numbers over the phone, having large amounts of cash in the house, being outside alone at night, or paying cash before receiving goods.

The aging process is characterized by various losses, including loss of job, income, friends, or family through death or moving; declining health; death or disability of their spouse; and loss of roles that accompany other losses (Gelfand, 1994; Miceli, 1993; Sloane, 1992). These multiple losses have been suggested by Kastenbaum (1969) as a way of explaining negative behavior patterns often associated with aging. The result is termed "bereavement overload." The loss or absence of a confidante places elders at risk. A tie with another person can make the critical difference between satisfaction and unhappiness (Solomon and Peterson, 1994).

The loss of a spouse is one of the most profound losses that one can suffer. Adjusting to and eventually accepting the reality of the death is a long, slow, and painful healing process. Successful mastery of this major transition is an important feature of the aging experience (Wortman and Silver, 1990). Women can expect to spend some time in later life as widows, but few are ready for the devastation that the death of a spouse brings. Community health nurses should allow bereaved spouses to talk about their spouse and their life together. Bereaved spouses are not prepared for the new roles thrust on them, and the nurse must be

there to assist with this process. Implicit in assisting is recognizing when assistance is needed, since this is not always apparent. Nurses must provide a climate that is nonjudgmental and conducive for self-disclosure to enable bereaved individuals to mourn and share their feelings.

Signs and symptoms of **depression** are common in elders; 10% to 20% of elders in the community may express sadness or have a clinically diagnosable depression. Depression may go unrecognized unless specific questions are asked. The Geriatric Depression Scale (GDS) is often used for this purpose (Appendix J.4).

Suicide is the most serious and most preventable consequence of depression. Given the many factors that predispose elders to depression, it is not surprising that male elders have the highest rate of suicide (Kane et al., 1994). The community health nurse and caregivers of elders should be alert for the signs and symptoms that an elder is depressed; however, these should be interpreted cautiously, since many age-related or disease-related changes can mimic depression. Awareness of potential depression by the community health nurse aids in identifying those elders at risk and in avoiding both the underreporting and the overreporting of depression in elders.

The term confusion is often misused, and its misapplication to an elder can have long-lasting effects. **Confusion** has been defined, imprecisely, as a mental state in which inappropriate reactions to various stimuli are observed. It is more accurate to report *cognitive impairment* with documentation of what defined the impairment. In the community, about 5% of those older than 65 and almost 20% of those older than 75 have some degree of clinically detectable impairment of cognitive function. As more elders live into the tenth decade of life, the incidence of cognitive impairment will rise (Kane et al., 1994).

Delirium is characterized by an acute onset and disordered attention and changes in cognition, psychomotor behavior, and the sleep-wake cycle (Lusis, et al., 1993). Delirium is often associated with an acute illness or a drug reaction. It may represent a significant change in functioning for the individual.

Dementia is another cause of confusion that must be considered. Dementia is a slow, progressive loss of cognitive function and memory without loss of alertness (Kane et al., 1994). Approximately 60% to 70% of dementia cases are of the Alzheimer's type, and 15% to 20% are caused by multiinfarct dementia (Tierney et al., 1994).

The most frequent form of dementia is **Alzheimer's type of dementia,** or primary degenerative dementia of the Alzheimer's type (Ham, 1992; Kane et al., 1994). Alzheimer's type of dementia is a gradually progressive dementia that affects more women than men, especially if over age 75. Dementia is characterized by short-term memory loss, gradual loss of expressive and comprehensive language, visual-perceptual defects, decreased olfactory sense, and problem-solving difficulties. Personality changes include thought disorder and increased irritability. There is enormous diversity, both in symptomatology and progression of the dementia (Tierney et al., 1994).

Multi-infarct dementia results when persons have either sustained or recurrent cortical or subcortical cerebrovascular accidents (CVAs, strokes). Many CVAs are too small to cause residual neurological deficits. Differentiation between Alzheimer's and multiinfarct dementia may be difficult, and many persons may have evidence of both (Kane et al., 1994).

Several screening instruments provide immediate information as to the level of cognitive functioning. The easiest to administer is the *Short Portable Mental Status Questionnaire* (SPMSQ) (see box below), but the *mini-mental status examination* (Appendix J.5) is also often used (Folstein, Folstein, and McHugh, 1975). Another screening procedure involves naming three objects and asking the individual to repeat them 1 minute later. The Draw-a-Clock test is a rapid way to assess cognitive functioning. The nurse simply hands clients a piece of paper with a circle on it and asks them to fill in all the numbers on a clock and then draw the hands to show 2:45 (Schneiderman, 1993).

Functional Assessment

Elders' functional status is typically defined in terms of the individual's ability to perform **activities of daily living** (ADLs) and **instrumental activities of daily living** (IADLs). ADLs include seven personal care activities: (1) eating, (2) toileting, (3) dressing, (4) bathing, (5) transferring, (6) walking, and (7) getting outside. IADLs refer to six home management activities: (1) meal preparation, (2) money management, (3) shopping, (4) telephone use, (5) light housework, and (6) heavy housework (Prohaska et al., 1993).

Katz et al. (1970) devised a frequently used measure of functional status, the index of ADLs (see box on p. 594). Data come from the individual or a caregiver who has had sufficient opportunity to observe the individual. The Katz ADL scale is a simple way to summarize the individual's ability to carry out the basic tasks needed for self-care. Experience with the scale suggests that functional losses tend to occur in an order from bathing to feeding. Results of the ADL scale also allow monitoring of change in an individual's basic functioning.

The ADL scale does not evaluate higher levels of functioning that require both physical and cognitive functioning. The IADLs may be assessed either by report or direct observation. Conflicting information may be obtained for both ADLs and IADLs, but the discrepancies provide important insights as to the individual's and caregiver's perceptions of ability (Kane et al., 1994).

Physical Examination

A comprehensive physical examination with laboratory evaluation is essential to further develop the health care picture of elders. The nurse typically finds multiple pathological physical findings as well as age-related physical changes. The community health nurse, in providing care to elders, should be aware of normal age-related physical changes (Table 30-6) and also should make elders aware that periodic physical examinations are necessary and assist in making the arrangements.

Intervention Strategies

The comprehensive assessment of elders performed by the community health nurse may reveal health or safety concerns. Based on the data obtained from the assessment, the nurse may find it necessary to make appropriate referrals to other health care providers, such as physicians or physical therapists, or community agencies such as Meals-on-Wheels. Community health nurses, with their knowledge of available resources in the community, state, and nation, are well qualified to make appropriate referrals and act as case managers for an elder's care.

In planning strategies to meet the health care needs of elders served, community health nurses should plan *with* rather than for the elders. Planning with elders assists in the elder maintaining independence and promotes investment in the management plan. Investment in the plan is more likely to result in compliance with the recommendations derived through

---

Short Portable Mental Status Questionnaire

1. What is the date today (month/day/year)? (All three correct needed to score.)
2. What day of the week is it?
3. What is the name of this place? (Any correct description needed to score.)
4. What is your telephone number? If you do not have a telephone, what is your street address?
5. How old are you?
6. When were you born (month/day/year)? (All three correct needed to score.)
7. Who is president of the United States now?
8. Who was president just before him?
9. What was your mother's maiden name?
10. Subtract 3 from 20 and keep subtracting 3 from each new number all the way down. (Whole series corrected needed to score.)

Error score (out of 10): Add one if patient is educated beyond high school; subtract one if patient is not educated beyond grade school.

Scoring: 0 to 2 errors—intact intellectual function
        3 to 4 errors—mild intellectual impairment
        5 to 7 errors—moderate intellectual impairment
        8 to 10 errors—severe intellectual impairment

From Pfeiffer E: *Am Geriatr Soc* 23(10):433-441, 1975. Reprinted with permission of the American Geriatric Society.

Index of Independence in Activities of Daily Living

The Index of Independence in Activities of Daily Living is based on an evaluation of clients' functional independence or dependence in bathing, dressing, toileting, transferring, continence, and feeding. Specific definitions of functional independence and dependence are provided.

A   Independent in feeding, continence, transferring, toileting, dressing, and bathing
B   Independent in all but one of these functions
C   Independent in all but bathing and one additional function
D   Independent in all but bathing, dressing, and one additional function
E   Independent in all but bathing, dressing, toileting, and one additional function
F   Independent in all but bathing, dressing, toileting, transferring, and one additional function
G   Dependent in all six functions

Other: dependent in at least two functions not classifiable as C, D, E, or F

Independence refers to clients' ability to function without supervision, direction, or active personal assistance except as specifically noted in the definitions. This is based on actual status and not ability. Clients who refuse to perform a function are considered not able to perform the function even though they are deemed able.

BATHING (sponge, shower, or tub)

Independent: assistance only in bathing a single part (e.g., back, disabled extremity) or bathes self completely
Dependent: assistance in bathing more than one body part, assistance in getting in or out of the tub or does not bathe self

DRESSING

Independent: gets clothes from closet and drawers; puts on clothes, outer garments; manages fasteners; act of tying shoes excluded
Dependent: does not dress self or remains partly undressed

TOILETING

Independent: gets to toilet; gets on and off toilet; arranges clothes; cleans organs of excretion (may manage own bedpan used only at night and may use mechanical supports)
Dependent: uses bedpan or commode or receives assistance in getting to toilet and using it

TRANSFERRING

Independent: moves in and out of bed independently; moves in and out of chair independently (may use mechanical supports)
Dependent: assistance in moving in or out of bed and chair; does not perform one or more transfers

CONTINENCE

Independent: urination and defecation entirely self-controlled
Dependent: partial or total incontinence in urination or defecation; partial or total control by enemas or catheters or regulated use of urinals and bedpans

FEEDING

Independent: gets food from plate or its equivalent into mouth (precutting of meat and preparation of food, e.g., buttering bread, are excluded from evaluation)
Dependent: assistance needed in act of feeding; does not eat at all or uses parenteral feeding

From Katz S, Downs TD, Cash HR, Grotz RC: *Gerontologist* 10(1):20-30, 1970. Reprinted with permission. Copyright by The Gerontological Society of America.

mutual consent. Planning care with elders should take into consideration the elder's available resources. Resources available can be considered as financial, social, and other means (e.g., transportation) to achieve goals.

One area that is often missed in the care of elders involves preparation for death. Community health nurses can allow elders to reflect on their life, make legal referrals for wills and advance directives, assist in funeral planning, and support them in arranging for discussing this topic with friends and family.

An important aspect of caring for elders is advocacy. *Advocacy* may involve educating friends and family about an elder's condition or care, intervening in

abuse situations, not participating in or allowing age-related jokes to be told, or just being supportive of elders. Advocacy may also involve political activism. Policymakers need factual information from informed sources; the information can come from private discussions with policymakers on behalf of elders, letter writing, editorials in the local newspaper, and speaking to local clubs and churches. The community health nurse, in acting to dispel ageism, is acting as an advocate for the elder population.

Community health nurses are in ideal positions to assist in meeting the present and future health needs of elders because of their knowledge of disease prevention and health promotion. In addition, commu-

Table 30-6 Selected Age-Related Physical Changes in Elders

System	Physical findings
Integumentary	Loss of subcutaneous fat Dry and thin skin with increased vulnerability to trauma and irritation with decreased healing
Eyes	Arcus senilis Decreased visual acuity
Ears	Decreased hearing acuity with potential for speech discrimination difficulty
Cardiopulmonary	Decreased cardiac output and elasticity of heart and arteries Presence of fourth heart sound (S4) or systolic ejection murmur Decreased forced vital capacity, forced expiratory volume, and elastic recoil of lungs Basilar rales may be found in absence of disease
Musculoskeletal	Skeletal mass loss, greater in women than men Size and number of muscle and fibers decreased Lean body mass replaced with fat with accompanying loss of body water
Gastrointestinal	Decreased intestinal mobility, absorption, taste, and saliva production
Neurological	Decreased vibratory sensation, arm swings Increased waddling and narrow-based gait for women; men have wider-based and small-stepped gait Potential for changes in mental status

nity health nurses have a long history of service in the home and in the community, have experience with multidisciplinary teams as case managers, can perform comprehensive assessments, and are expert health educators. An emphasis on cost containment, coupled with an increased demand for services to elders, prepares the community health nurse to deliver the services needed.

LONG-TERM CARE FOR ELDERS

Long-term care refers to care that is delivered to individuals who are dependent on others for assistance with basic tasks over a sustained period. Long-term care can be delivered in an institutional setting, such as a nursing home, or it can be delivered in the community with the assistance of a caregiver (Furner, 1993). Long-term care for elders has become an in-

creasingly significant portion of the health care system in the United States. With increased age and chronicity, the demand for and use of health care services has increased.

Federal Programs

The Social Security Act, passed in 1935, provided retirement benefits based on work history and age. It also provided for survivor, disability, and health benefits (Skipwith, 1992). Title 18 (Medicare) of the Older Americans Act was passed in 1965, and since that time it has become a major component of the health care system. Out-of-pocket costs for health care services that are not covered by Medicare, referred to as Medigap, average about 15% of elder's incomes (DHHS, 1994). Its benefits include institutional services but exclude custodial and nonresidential services for elders. Medicaid is a federally regulated program for the poor, under which states offer basic health care services, including the cost of long-term care, to eligible low-income individuals (Alber, 1992).

Nursing Homes

The nursing home industry has exploded in recent years and has resulted in stretching the Medicaid budget to its limits. In 1987 the Omnibus Budget Reconciliation Act (OBRA) was passed and contained a major nursing home reform package aimed at the improvement of health care (Olson, 1994). Nursing home care was previously divided into at least two levels of care based on the amount of nursing care available. The OBRA 1987 regulations have eliminated these distinctions and call for a single level of nursing facility, although there has been a trend to place cognitively impaired elders in special care units (SCUs) within the nursing home (Kane et al., 1994).

Residential care in nursing homes is largely financed from private out-of-pocket resources and the state-administered Medicaid program. A large percentage of institutionalized elders funded by Medicaid enter as private-paying patients and convert to Medicaid after nursing home costs have impoverished them and their spouses as well (Olson, 1994). Medicaid was never intended to provide large amounts of money for long term-care for elders. In 1990, however, elders represented approximately 20% of the 26 million Medicaid recipients and about 40% of its total expenditures of $70 billion (Pepper Commission, 1990).

The American nursing home tends to be organized around the medical model, fostering a hospital-like environment. The major focus is on custodial care rather than meaningful social activities, psychological care, or rehabilitative services. Most elders, even those with disabilities, live in their own home or with a family member; only 5% of elders reside in nursing homes (Olson, 1994). However, approximately 36% to 45% of elders will spend some time in a nursing home, and 20% will die in a nursing home (Pepper Commission, 1990).

Extended care facilities (ECFs) are available in some areas. These facilities may be free-standing or may be associated with a hospital. ECFs are designed to ease the transition from hospitalization to returning home and serve as an alternative to short-term nursing home stays. Services are offered to assist individuals to return to independent living.

Quality of care in nursing homes has become a national concern. Most problems are directly related to situations in which good nursing care could make a difference. In addition to clinical issues in nursing homes, there is the problem of image within nursing; nurses who choose to work in nursing homes are often looked on as less capable than other nurses (DHHS, 1994).

Community-Based Long-Term Care

Home care refers to health care and social services provided to individuals in their homes or in community and homelike settings. Home care may include nursing, rehabilitation, social work, home health, and other long-term services (DHHS, 1994). Home care can enable elders to remain in their own homes for as long as possible, relieve the burden on hospitals, and improve the quality of life for the elder and the caregiver (Jamieson, 1992).

Neither Medicare nor Medicaid provides significant funding for home care services; a large percentage of elders with limited incomes are not able to obtain home-based care at all. The type and quality of care available and received in the United States depend mostly on costs, who pays for them, and other factors unrelated to the actual service needs of elders. Home care services have not significantly replaced nursing homes in the United States primarily because it has not been proved that home care services save money (Olson, 1994). Patterns of care are influenced by government funding sources that favor acute care or institutionalization. Without government funding of community health services, elders residing in the community, but not in need of skilled care services, are not in a position to access needed health care services.

Increasing proportions of elders in the rural areas, along with the out-migration of the younger workforce, heighten the possibility that rural communities will experience the loss of financial resources needed for the delivery of services (McCulloch and Lynch, 1993). Elders may be at increased risk of health impairment not only because of their geographical location, but also because of the loss of formal services that can aid in maintaining their quality of life (Coward et al., 1993).

Community health nurses, in collaboration with elders and their families, are involved in making referrals of elders who have been identified as needing

home care. In addition, nurses should collaborate with the home care agency in planning for elders' present and future care.

Assisted living is a form of care that has emerged and is designed to provide services in an environment that more closely resembles a home. Residents may choose to use common facilities, such as a dining room. This approach is aimed at maximizing the resident's sense of self, privacy, and independence as much as possible (Kane et al., 1994). Community health nurses are often involved in the delivery of population-focused care to residents in these facilities. In addition to case management, the care delivered may include counseling on ways to maximize health status, screening measures, education, and advocacy for residents' rights. In case management the community health nurse is involved in coordinating and monitoring the full range of geriatric services available.

Other community services available include **respite care** or day care, which targets individuals with limited functional ability and combines recreational and restorative activities. The aim is to return the elder to a refreshed caregiver (Kane et al., 1994; Skipwith, 1992). Hospice is available for terminally ill elders, and elders in the community may rely on the community health nurse for a referral to a hospice.

Family Caregiving

In the past two decades, the role of informal caregivers in providing care to elders has undergone change as a result of sociopolitical trends. Since many institutions have been unwilling to accept government fee levels and the costs are beyond what most families can afford, more caregiving for elders has become the family's responsibility (Olson, 1994). Consequently, informal caregivers are viewed as nurse extenders (DHHS, 1994). Approximately 80% of community-based long-term care comes from informal networks of family and friends, most of whom are women (Furner, 1993). Both elders and family members strongly resist nursing home placement and view institutionalization as a personal failure (Olson, 1994).

Family caregiving places enormous demands on the individual and their families. Many undergo psychological, physical, and financial stresses. Women caregivers may find themselves in a position of having to sacrifice their employment and economic future.

The four-generation family is now commonplace, increasing the potential of more elders needing care. Lower fertility rates mean a decrease in family size, with fewer children to share the responsibility of caregiving. Many women find themselves thrust into a caregiver role just as their youngest child is leaving home. Caregivers usually do not have a choice about assuming care, since the costs for their family member's care is often too high for the financial resources available (Olson, 1994).

Resources for Elders

Numerous organizations and services are available to assist elders and their families. Agencies may be concerned with advocacy, special populations, and volunteer services in which elders can become involved. Appendix G lists selected examples of organizations.

HEALTH CARE DELIVERY ISSUES

In the context of today's health care system, quality and cost have become issues of great concern. Some health care providers' sense of responsibility to meet humanitarian needs is largely gone; the focus has shifted to reimbursement. These factors have given rise to delayed or neglected access to appropriate care or both (Benson and McDevitt, 1994).

Many groups have called for reform in financing care needed by elders. The Pepper Commission (1990) has proposed long-term care financing that would include a limited social mechanism that guarantees subsidized home care services, 3 months of nursing home care, a public program for longer nursing home stays that protects clients against impoverishment, and measures to promote private long-term care insurance. Many obviously resist reform that requires new social programs. Proposals that include new taxes to pay for services for elders to not appear feasible in a climate of economic restraint, especially when some believe that elders have already received more than their fair share of services. Also, new programs would benefit middle-class and upper-class elders, since Medicaid already covers a large share of the poor elders (Zedlewski and McBride, 1992).

There is a rapidly growing market of private long-term care insurance. However, it is not clear whether this can improve the financing portion of long-term care costs. Few elders can afford today's long-term care insurance premiums. Elders' ability to pay for long-term care will depend on their economic status from 1990 to 2030, the future cost of long-term health care, and the mechanism to finance care (Zedlewski and McBride, 1992).

Controlling national health care expenditures is a major issue in health care reform; however, it appears that the rapidly growing managed care networks will be crucial. Most agree that managed care can cut costs, but by how much and where the savings will come from are less clear. Often, practice is underprovided in order to cut costs and increase salaries. Typically, those persons with no health care problems are attracted to managed care programs, whereas those with health problems, which include a large percentage of elders, prefer the traditional fee-for-service insurance programs (Warren, 1994).

Policymakers must recognize the social, economic, and health needs of all the U.S. population. By focusing only on elders, policymakers foster intergenerational conflict; the reality is that the well-being of all generations are interlocked (Olson, 1994). New systems of coverage should incorporate the values and beliefs of the elders being served and provide acceptable alternatives for care.

Since elders already account for 31% of the U.S. health care expenditures, the changes in demographics will have an enormous economic influence on health care. Meeting the needs of the elderly will require emphasis on primary and preventive care, multidisciplinary teams, service in the home, long-term care, and education in the field of gerontology (Lindbloom, 1993).

The community health nurse may be the provider that elders turn to for advice and counseling about the array of available health care services. The nurse can help elders understand the services and how they differ, determine whether they are eligible for a particular service, and assist in accessing the appropriate service.

 ## Clinical Application

Mrs. Eldridge, a 79-year-old widow, was reported by neighbors and the administrator of the senior high rise where she lived to the community health nurse who visited residents of the high rise. Mrs. Eldridge lives alone, and no one had been observed coming or going from her apartment recently. When Mrs. Eldridge has been seen by her neighbors, she appears self-neglected and does not appear to recognize her neighbors.

The community health nurse made a visit to Mrs. Eldridge's apartment and validated the unkempt appearance of both. Mrs. Eldridge answered the door and was pleasant but unkempt with an odor of stale urine. Even though Mrs. Eldridge was hesitant and unsure in her answers, the history revealed medical problems. A son and daughter-in-law lived in the next county and phoned at least once a week; their number was taped to the table by the phone. Several pill bottles were observed on the kitchen counter with the name of a local physician and pharmacist.

The medications, an antihypertensive and a diuretic, were verified with the physician and the pharmacist. One pill bottle did not have a label, and the pharmacist said that the unknown medication was probably a sleeping pill because its description fit one that had been prescribed. The pharmacist said that the sleeping pill was an old prescription and had not been refilled in some time.

Continued.

Clinical Application—cont'd

The community health nurse, while at Mrs. Eldridge's home, noted that both she and her clothes were dirty and that she moved without aids and appeared steady on her feet. The kitchen was littered with unwashed dishes and empty frozen-food boxes, which Mrs. Eldridge could not recall being bought or delivered. An open billfold with several bills was lying open on the kitchen counter, as well as an uncashed Social Security check.

The community health nurse administered the SPMSQ and found that Mrs. Eldridge had eight errors. A meeting was arranged with the son at the health department after a neighbor agreed to stay with Mrs. Eldridge. After revealing what had been observed, the son was both shocked and saddened. He went on to say that he had an uneasy feeling about his mother for the past couple of weeks but that he "just couldn't put a finger on what was going on." Because of Mrs. Eldridge's obvious cognitive impairment, the nurse asked for validation of what information she had been able to obtain. She learned that Mrs. Eldridge had been hypertensive for several years and had always been faithful about taking her medications, keeping appointments, and eating a healthy diet. He revealed that the 1-year anniversary of his father's death had been a month ago and that his mother had seemed to dread facing that particular day. He went on to say that he had been dreading the day when he would have to look for a nursing home for his mother for an extended stay.

Mrs. Eldridge's son and community health nurse met again 2 weeks later at Mrs. Eldridge's home. The home and Mrs. Eldridge were clean, and Mrs. Eldridge apologized for not remembering the first meeting. It appeared that the sleeping pill, which she had taken to help with the sad feeling and insomnia that accompanied the anniversary of her husband's death, had caused Mrs. Eldridge's intellectual impairment. Mrs. Eldridge and her son had a frank discussion about her living arrangements, and both agreed she would stay in her apartment. Mrs. Eldridge also wished that should her health deteriorate to a point that all hope for recovery was lost, she be allowed to die a peaceful death. The nurse suggested that both mother and son discuss this issue and come to an agreement on an advance directive measure; both agreed. The son admitted that he had learned a lesson about assuming that all older people would end up confused and needing nursing home care.

The community health nurse admitted that she too had learned from this experience and was planning a class for the residents of the senior high rise about the dangers of self-medicating. In addition, she had consulted with the administrator of the high rise and discovered that several men and women had experienced the death of their spouses in the last 2 or 3 years. Because of the number of widows and widowers, the community health nurse had begun organizing sessions, in collaboration with a grief counselor, that allowed for an open discussion about bereavement for any elders interested in attending.

Key Concepts

- A "graying" of America is occurring that is accompanied by an increase in chronic conditions and a greater demand for services.
- The increase in demand for services has resulted in budgets being stretched to their limits.
- More and more elders are not able to access health care services, and their family members are being called on to provide for them.
- Only 5% of elders are institutionalized; the rest either live alone or with family members.
- Community health nurses work to improve the health of elders through collaborative

practice with other members of the health care team.
- The delivery of nursing care to elders involves all three levels of prevention, with the goal to optimize elders' general health and functioning capabilities.
- Community health nurses assist elders to remain in their homes to improve the quality of their lives, preserve their functional status, and reduce their health care costs.

Critical Thinking Activities

1. Describe your impression of a typical elder and compare it with the demographic information on elders given in this chapter.
2. From the previous clinical application, identify an example of a theory of aging, an example of ageism, and write at least two nursing diagnoses.
3. From television portrayals, identify both positive and negative ways in which elders are portrayed.
4. Interview an elder within your family, and ask him or her to list any health problems, how your relative would rate his or her health on a scale of 1 to 10 (with 10 being the highest), and what is included in a typical day's activities. Also, ask the elder to keep a 24-hour dietary recall.
5. From the information in activity 4:
   a. Devise screening recommendations for your relative.
   b. Derive at least one nursing diagnosis.
   c. What theory of aging best fits your relative?
6. Interview a peer to determine what myths of aging they perceive about elders.
7. Describe what you can do to aid in overcoming the myths and examples of ageism that are pervasive in society.
8. Discuss the perceptions of nurses who work in long-term care institutions.

Bibliography

Alber J: Residential care for the elderly, *J Health Polit Policy Law* 17(4):929-957, 1992.

American Association of Retired Persons (AARP), Administration on Aging, US Department of Health and Human Services: *A profile of older Americans*, Pub No PF 3049 (1289), D996, Washington, DC, 1990, AARP.

Barer BM: Men and women aging differently, *Int J Aging Hum Dev* 38(1):29-40, 1994.

Beck JC, Freedman ML, Warshaw GA: Geriatric assessment: focus on function, *Patient Care*, Feb 28, 1994.

Beers MH, Fink A, Beck JC: Screening recommendations for the elderly, *Am J Public Health* 81(9):1131-1140, 1991.

Benson ER, McDevitt JQ: When third party payment determines service: the elderly at risk, *Holistic Nurs Pract* 8(2):28-35, 1994.

Berger KS: *The developing person through the lifespan*, ed 3, New York, 1994, Worth.

Butler RN: The life review: an interpretation of reminiscence in the aged, *Psychiatry* 26:65-76, 1963.

Coward RT, Duncan RP, Netzer JK: The availability of health care resources for elders living in nonmetropolitan persistent low-income counties in the south, *J Appl Gerontol* 12(3):368-387, 1993.

Cumming E, Henry W: *Growing old: the process of disengagement*, New York, 1961, Basic Books.

Erikson EH: *Childhood and society*, New York, 1950, Norton.

Erikson EH, Erikson JM, Knivick HQ: *Vital involvement in old age*, New York, 1986, Norton.

Fisher JC: A framework for describing developmental change among older adults, *Adult Educ Q* 43(2):76-89, 1993.

Folstein MF, Folstein SE, McHugh PR: Mini-mental state: a practical method for grading the cognitive state of patients for the clinician, *J Psychiatr Res* 12:189-198, 1975.

Furner SE: Chartbook on health data on older Americans: United States, 1991, *Vital Health Stat* 29:21-36, 1993.

Gelfand DE: *Aging and ethnicity*, New York, 1994, Springer.

Greene VL, Monahan D, Coleman PD: Demographics. In Ham RJ, Sloane PD, editors: *Primary care geriatrics: a case-based approach*, St Louis, 1992, Mosby.

Ham RJ: Assessment. In Ham RJ, Sloane PD, editors: *Primary care geriatrics: a case-based approach*, St Louis, 1992, Mosby.

Ham RJ: Characteristics of the ill elderly patient. In Ham RJ, Sloane PD, editors: *Primary care geriatrics: a case-based approach*, St Louis, 1992, Mosby.

Havighurst RJ: *Developmental tasks and education*, ed 2, New York, 1992, David McKay.

Healthy People 2000: national health promotion and disease prevention objectives, Washington, DC, 1991, USDHHS, Public Health Service.

Hollmann FW: *National population trends*. Series P-23, No. 175, US Department of Commerce, Bureau of the Census, Washington, DC, 1992, US Government Printing Office.

Jamieson A: Home care in old age: a lost cause? *J Health Polit Policy Law* 17(4):879-898, 1992.

Kane RL, Ouslander JG, Abrass IB: *Essentials of clinical geriatrics*, ed 3, New York, 1994, McGraw-Hill.

Kastenbaum R: Death and bereavement in later life. In Kirtschner A, editor: *Death and bereavement*, Springfield, Ill, 1969, Charles C Thomas.

Katz S, Downs TD, Cash HR, Grotz RC: Progress in the development of the index of ADL, *Gerontologist* 10(1):20-30, 1970.

Klinkman MS, Zazove P, Mehr DR, Ruffin MT: A criterion-based review of preventive health care in the elderly, *J Fam Pract* 43(2):205-224, 1992.

Kotthoff-Burrell E: Health promotion and disease prevention for the older adult: an overview of the current recommendations and a practical application, *Nurse Pract Forum* 3(4):195-209, 1992.

Lancaster J, Lowry L, Lee G: Conceptual models for community health nursing. In Stanhope M, Lancaster J, editors: *Community health nursing: process and practice for promoting health*, ed 3, St Louis, 1992, Mosby.

Lauder W: Health promotion in the elderly, *Br J Nurs* 2(8):401-404, 1993.

Lindbloom E: America's aging population: changing the face of health care, *JAMA* 269(5):674-679, 1993.

Lusis SA, Hydo B, Clark L: Nursing assessment of mental status in the elderly, *Geriatr Nurs* 14(5):255-258, 1993.

Maslow A: *Toward a psychology of being*, ed 2, Princeton, NJ, 1968, Van Nostrand.

McCulloch BJ, Lynch MS: Barriers to solutions: service delivery and public policy in rural areas, *J Appl Gerontol* 12(3):388-403, 1993.

Mermelstein R, Miller B, Prohaska T: Health data on older Americans: 1991, *Vital Health Stat* 27:9-21, 1993.

Miceli DG: Evaluating the older patient's ability to function, *J Am Acad Nurs Pract* 5(4):167-174, 1993.

Mion LC, McDowell JA, Heanet LK: Nutritional assessment in the ambulatory care setting, *Nurse Pract Forum* 5(1):46-51, 1994.

O'Brien JG: Elder abuse. In Ham RJ, Sloane PD, editors: *Primary care geriatrics: a case-based approach*, St Louis, 1992, Mosby.

Olson LK: *The graying of the world: who will care for the frail elderly?* New York, 1994, Haworth Press.

Pearlman R: Development of a functional assessment questionnaire for geriatric patients: the Comprehensive Older Persons Evaluation (COPE), *J Chronic Dis* 40:85S-94S, 1987.

Pepper Commission, US Bipartisan Commission on Comprehensive Health Care: *A call for action: final report*, Washington, DC, 1990, US Government Printing Office.

Pfeiffer EJ: A short portable mental status questionnaire for the assessment of organic brain deficit in elderly patients, *J Am Geriatr Soc* 23(10):433-441, 1975.

Prohaska T, Mermelstein R, Miller B: Health data on older Americans: United States, 1991, *Vital Health Stat* 3, Anal Epidemiol Stud 27:23-39, 1993.

Ramsdell JW: Geriatric assessment in the home, *Clin Geriatr Med* 7(4):677-693, 1991.

Robertson JR: Promoting health among the institutionalized elderly, *J Gerontol Nurs* 17(6):15-19, 1991.

Roen OT: Senior health. In Swanson JM, Albrecht MA, editors: *Community health nursing: promoting the health of aggregates,* Philadelphia, 1993, WB Saunders, Co.

Schneiderman H: Physical examination of the aged patient, *Conn Med* 57(5):317-324, 1993.

Schoenfeld DE, Malmrose LC, Blazer DG, Gold DT, Seeman TE: Self-rated health and mortality in the high-functioning elderly—a closer look at healthy individuals: MacArthur Field Study of Successful Aging, *J Gerontol Med Sci* 49(3):M109-M115, 1994.

Skipwith DH: The older adult. In Stanhope M, Lancaster J, editors: *Community health nursing: process and practice for promoting health,* ed 3, St Louis, 1992, Mosby.

Sloane P: Normal aging. In Ham RJ, Sloane PD, editors: *Primary care geriatrics: a case-base approach,* St Louis, 1992, Mosby.

Solomon R, Peterson M: Successful aging: how to help your patients cope with change, *Geriatrics* 49(4):41-47, 1994.

Sullivan HS: The dynamics of emotion. In Sullivan HS, editor: *Clinical studies in psychiatry,* New York, 1956, Norton.

Tierney LM, McPhee SJ, Papadakis MA: *Current medical diagnosis and treatment,* East Norwalk, Conn, 1994, Appleton & Lange.

Tinneti ME, Speechley M: Prevention of falls among the elderly, *N Engl J Med* 320:1055-1059, 1989.

US Bureau of the Census, US Department of Commerce: Projections of the population of the US by age, sex, and race, 1988-2050. In *Current Population Reports, Population Estimates, and Projections,* series p-25, No 118, Washington, DC, 1991, US Government Printing Office.

US Department of Health and Human Services, Public Health Resources and Services Administration: *Seventh report to the President and the Congress on the status of health personnel in the United States,* DHHS Pub No HRS-POD-90-1, Washington, DC, 1990, US Government Printing Office.

US Department of Health and Human Services, Public Health Service: *National Ambulatory Medical Care Survey: 1991 summary,* DHHS Pub No (PHS) 94-1777, Washington, DC, 1994, US Government Printing Office.

US Department of Health and Human Services, Public Health Service, National Institutes of Health: *Long term care for older adults,* NIH Pub No 94-2418, Washington, DC, 1994, US Government Printing Office.

US Preventive Services Task Force: *Guide to clinical preventive services,* Baltimore, 1989, Williams & Wilkins.

US Senate Subcommittee on Aging, American Association of Retired Persons, Federal Council on Aging, US Administration on Aging: *Aging America: trends and projections,* DHHS Pub No (FCOA) 91-28001, Washington, DC, 1990, US Government Printing Office.

Warren J: Latest Medicaid dispute pushes Kentucky doctors over the edge, *Lexington-Herald Leader,* Sept 6, 1994, pp A1, A4.

Wortman CB, Silver RC: Successful mastery of bereavement and widowhood: a life course. In Baltes P, Baltes M, editors: *Successful aging: perspectives from the behavioral sciences,* Cambridge, England, 1990, Cambridge University Press.

Yesavge HA, Brink TL, Rose T: Development and validation of a geriatric depression scale: a preliminary report, *J Psychiatr Res* 17:39-49, 1983.

Zedlewski S, McBride TD: The changing profile of the elderly: effects of future long-term care needs and financing, *Milbank Q* 70(2):246-275, 1992.

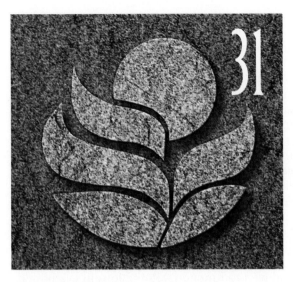

31 The Physically Compromised

Mary Ann McClellan

Objectives ▼

After reading this chapter, the student should be able to do the following:

◆ Define selected terms related to the concept of physically compromised.
◆ Discuss implications of definitions of developmentally disabled, handicapped, disabled, impaired, and chronically ill.
◆ List six types of conditions which may cause a person to become physically compromised.
◆ Compare the effects of being physically compromised on the individual, the family, and the community.
◆ Describe implications of being physically compromised for selected populations (rural, low income, work site populations).
◆ Examine selected issues for those who are physically compromised (abuse, health promotion).
◆ Discuss relationships between being physically compromised and the objectives of both *Healthy People 2000* and *Healthy Communities 2000*.
◆ Examine the community health nurses' role in caring for people who are physically compromised.

Key Terms ▼

Americans with Disabilities Act
chronic disease
congenital disability
developmental disability
disability
functional limitation
handicap
impairment
learning disability
medically fragile
physically compromised
work disability

Early public health nursing emphasized home care of the sick and the poor, prevention of communicable diseases, and efforts toward hygienic conditions in the home and the community. Federal funding in the 1960s allowed for state and local health departments to expand services to include the following: secondary prevention through early detection of selected chronic diseases (e.g., cancer, glaucoma) family planning services to improve the health of mothers and newborns, and expanded community health nursing services to those who were mentally retarded. Home health care through the Medicare program increased at about the same time. These changes, along with legislation affecting handicapped and developmentally disabled people and many of the objectives of *Healthy People 2000* and the Healthy Cities movement, have led to more opportunities for community health nurses to work with families and other community groups that have members who are physically compromised in some manner.

This chapter defines several terms related to being physically compromised, discusses the scope of the problem, and describes the effects on individuals, families, and communites, as well as the relationships between these problems and *Healthy People 2000* and *Healthy Communities 2000* specific objectives and the concepts of Healthy Cities. Of special importance is the community health nurse's role and interventions with individuals, families, and communities in dealing with or preventing these health problems.

DEFINITIONS AND CONCEPTS

This chapter's topic, community members who, at some point across the lifespan are physically compromised, is so broad that definitions of several related terms are necessary.

The term **developmental disability** is a functional one as a result of the Rehabilitation, Comprehensive Services, and Developmental Disabilities Amendments of 1978 (P.L. 95-602):

A severe, chronic disability of a person which (A) is attributable to a mental or physical impairment or combination of mental and physical impairments; (B) is manifested before the person attains the age twenty-two; (C) is likely to continue indefinitely; (D) results in substantial functional limitations in three or more of the following areas of major life activity; (1) self-care, (2) receptive and expressive language, (3) learning, (4) mobility, (5) self-direction, (6) capacity for independent living, and (7) economic sufficiency; and (E) reflects the person's need for a combination and sequence of special interdisciplinary, or generic care, treatment, or other services which are of life-long or extended duration and are individually planned and coordinated (Rubin and Crocker, 1989).

A **disability** ". . . is any restriction or lack (resulting from an impairment) of ability to perform an activity in the manner or within the range considered normal for a human being" (Badley, 1993) "at that chronological age." (Heerkens et al., 1994) "Disability is char-

acterized by excesses or deficiencies of customarily expected activity, performance, and behavior, and these may be temporary or permanent, reversible or irreversible, and progressive or regressive" (Badley, 1993, p. 163).

An **impairment** ". . . is any loss or abnormality of psychological, physiological or anatomical structure or function. 'Impairment' is more inclusive than 'disorder' in that it covers losses—e.g., the loss of a leg is an impairment, but not a disorder" (Badley, 1993, p. 162).

Functional limitations are essentially descriptions of ". . . functions such as hearing, seeing, grasping, moving, climbing, reading and so on. Emphasis is placed on the level of function rather than the purpose of the activity so that functional limitation can be associated with consequent disability. For example, an impairment in the strength or range of motion of the arm could lead to functional limitations in grasping or reaching. These in turn could give rise to disabilities—for example, in reaching up to high shelves, getting dressed, hair care or cooking" (Badley, 1993, p. 165).

Handicap refers to social implications for a person who is impaired or disabled. "A handicap is a disadvantage for a given individual resulting from an impairment or a disability that limits or prevents the fulfillment of a role that is normal (depending on age, sex, and social and cultural factors) for that individual.

"Handicap is concerned with the value attached to an individual's situation or experience when it departs from the norm. It is characterized by a discordance between the individual's performance or status and the expectations of the individual himself or of the particular group of which he is a member" (Badley, 1993, p. 163).

Chronic disease, or illness, refers to any condition or illness lasting 3 or more months and requiring at least 1 month of hospitalization (Perrin and MacLean, 1988). With today's emphasis on short-term hospital stay and home care, the second part of that definition may need revision. Chronic illness may indicate a disease process (e.g., diabetes mellitus, cancer, tuberculosis) or a congenital or acquired condition (e.g., Down syndrome, severe burns, amputation of a limb). Therefore, concepts related to disabilities, handicaps, impairments, and functional limitations may apply to individuals with a chronic disease or condition.

For nurses working with those with a chronic disease, the onset, course, outcome, and degree of incapacitation are important factors to assess in considering the significance of the disease to individual clients. Moreover, recognition of the clients' and families'

Did You Know?

Diabetes mellitus is a significant chronic disabling condition with estimated annual costs of treatment in the U.S. alone being $92 billion (American Diabetes Association, 1993).

stages in the disease process as crisis (onset and diagnosis), chronic, or terminal is crucial to the effectiveness of nursing care (Collier, 1990).

A person who is **physically compromised** may have any or all of the above-listed conditions. Thus, there are nursing implications for individuals who are physically compromised, for their families, as well as for the populations and subpopulations which they constitute and the communities in which they live. The community health nurse must remember that some clients prefer to be regarded as being physically challenged or physically compromised while others may think such terminology trivializes the needs and problems of people who are disabled. See Appendixes H.3, I.6, and J.6 for a thorough review of assessment tools for use with people who are physically compromised.

SCOPE OF THE PROBLEM

People may be physically compromised from many different causes. Three major categories of such causes summarized in Figure 31-1 are injuries, developmental disabilities, and chronic diseases. As Figure 31-1 demonstrates, some of these conditions may occur or may become manifest at different ages and stages of development of the individual. Therfore, the effects in the person's life are influenced by the timing as well as the severity of the condition. According to Marge (1988), several specific individual conditions and hereditary problems can result in disability. These include genetic disorders, acute and chronic illnesses, violence, tobacco use, lack of access to health care, or, finally, failure to either eat correctly, exercise regularly, or manage stress effectively. Other causes include perinatal complications, injuries, substance abuse, environmental quality problems, and unsanitary living conditions. Appendix B.1 lists selected national organizations related to disabilities.

By definition, the onset of developmental disabilities occurs before age 22 and continues throughout the person's lifetime. While there are no specific statistics available on total numbers of children's developmental disabilities in this country, approximately 10% to 15% of children in the United States will have some type of special health care needs. About 1% to 2% of the entire child population have conditions severe enough to limit daily functioning (Francis, 1995). Nearly 6.2% of adolescents (almost 2 million) ages 10 to 18 years, live with some degree of limitations on their activities due to chronic conditions (Newacheck, 1989).

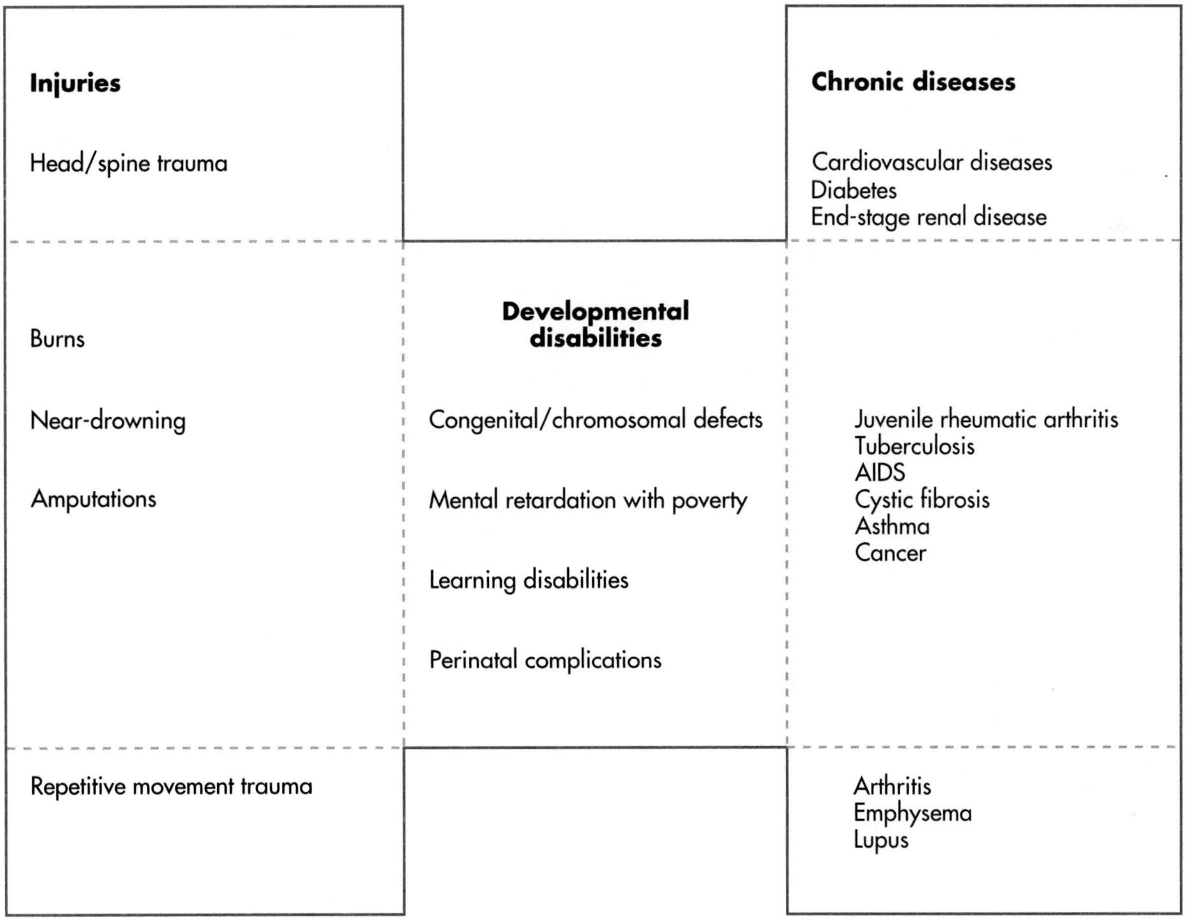

Injuries

Head/spine trauma

Burns

Near-drowning

Amputations

Repetitive movement trauma

Developmental disabilities

Congenital/chromosomal defects

Mental retardation with poverty

Learning disabilities

Perinatal complications

Chronic diseases

Cardiovascular diseases
Diabetes
End-stage renal disease

Juvenile rheumatic arthritis
Tuberculosis
AIDS
Cystic fibrosis
Asthma
Cancer

Arthritis
Emphysema
Lupus

FIGURE 31-1

Examples of conditions related to being physically compromised.

Conditions Related to Disability in Persons 15 Years Old or Older

AIDS or AIDS-related condition
Alcohol- or drug-related problem or disorder
Arthritis or rheumatism
Back or spine problems (including chronic stiffness or deformity of the back or spine)
Blindness or other visual impairment (difficulty seeing well enough, even with glasses, to read a newspaper)
Broken bone/fracture
Cancer
Cerebral palsy
Deafness or serious trouble hearing
Diabetes
Epilepsy
Head or spinal cord injury
Heart trouble (including coronary heart disease and arteriosclerosis)
Hernia or rupture
High blood pressure (hypertension)
Kidney stones or chronic kidney trouble
Learning disability
Lung or respiratory trouble (asthma, bronchitis, emphysema, respiratory allergies, tuberculosis, or other lung trouble)
Mental retardation
Missing legs, feet, arms, hands, or fingers
Paralysis of any kind
Senility/Dementia/Alzheimer disease
Speech disorder
Stiffness or deformity of the foot, leg, arm, or hand
Stomach trouble (including ulcers, gall bladder, or liver conditions)
Stroke
Thyroid trouble or goiter
Tumor, cyst, or growth
Other

From Centers for Disease Control, Prevalence of Disabilities and Associated Health Conditions, United States, 1991-1992. *MMRW* 43(40):730-731, 737-739.

 Potential Effects of Being Physically Compromised Related to Individuals, Families, and Communities

PERSON

Related health problems (e.g., nutrition, oral health, hygiene, limited activity and stamina)
↓ Self-concept/self esteem
↓ Life expectancy and ↑ risk for infection and secondary injury
Developmental tasks; change in role expectations

FAMILY

Stress on family unit
Need for ↑ use of external resources in role expectations
↓ options in use of any discretionary income
Social stigma

COMMUNITY

Need/demand to reallocate resources
Discomfort or fear due to lack of knowledge of disability
Need to comply with legislation
Services provided by health department, health care providers
↑ need for other services beyond medical diagnosis (e.g., transportation, etc.)

Data about disabilities among adults is also inadequate. One recent report—"Prevalence of Disabilities and Associated Health Conditions: United States, 1991-1992,"—discussed results of the Survey of Income and Program Participation (SIPP) subsample of the 1990 U.S. census (CDC, 1994). Respondents ages 15 years or older were asked about any existing disabilities; the result was that almost one-fifth of the U.S. population had some type of disability. Conditions reported in the SIPP are listed in the box above, left, and include chronic diseases, injuries, and some conditions that are **congenital** (CDC, 1994).

Work disability, the inability to perform work for 6 months or more due to a mental, physical, or other health condition (CDC, 1993), costs about $111.6 billion each year in lost wages and direct and indirect medical costs in this country (Ycas, 1991). In 1990 an estimated 12.8 million people ages 16 to 64 years were believed to have a work disability, about half of which were severe and half not severe. Prevalence rates were highest in the following states: West Virginia, Kentucky, Arkansas, Louisiana, and Mississippi (CDC, 1993). As the average age of a population increases, there is usually an increase in work disability (Wolfe and Haveman, 1990).

EFFECTS OF BEING PHYSICALLY COMPROMISED

The extent to which the physically compromised individual may need extra support, care, and services from the family unit and the community is reflected in the box above, right. A comprehensive understanding of the interrelationships of these three is best grasped by starting with the stresses placed on the individual.

Effects on the Individual

Health care tends to be organized around medical diagnoses rather than an individual's degree and kind of functional strengths and limitations. The problem is, the effects of being physically compromised vary according to the cause of the disability, the person's resiliency, the severity of limitations, and other considerations (Keith, 1994; Turner-Henson and Holaday, 1995). Since it is not possible to discuss here every potential cause of being physically compromised, their effects will be discussed, instead, from a lifespan perspective.

Children: Infancy Through Adolescence

Perhaps the wide variability of effects, as they are related to cause, is best demonstrated by looking at several specific examples. For instance, children with significant sensory deficits (e.g., hearing or vision impairments) are at risk for social isolation, congnitive and neuropsychological impairment, and developmental delays (Kravitz and Selekman, 1992; Tröster and Brambring, 1992; Schilling and DeJesus, 1993). Second, many children with leukemia may require special education services following successful central nervous system (CNS) irradiation or intrathecal chemotherapy (Brown and Madan-Swain, 1993). In a third example, a pilot study found that children with elevated lead levels were significantly slower in a reaction-time test and in flexibility in changing their focus of attention (Minder et al., 1994).

Social implications for children who are chronically ill are significant. For example, school-age children who are chronically ill may be discriminated against in their school systems, peer groups, communities, and government institutions. Such discrimination can interfere with children's development by limiting their opportunities to take part in customary roles and functions (Turner-Henson et al., 1994).

Finally, the effects on adolescents' development may vary with the time of onset of the physical problem. The impact seems to be less when the onset occurs in early adolescence rather than in middle or late adolescence. Children with previously diagnosed chronic diseases may be viewed as regressing in development during adolescence. However, their behavior may simply indicte a change in already achieved tasks that permit chronically ill adolescents to express themselves in new ways (Weekes, 1995). This is not unlike adolescents who are not physically compromised—it is important to keep in mind that adolescence is frequently a time when behaviors seem to regress.

Adults

Chronic diseases may have profound effects on adults. For instance, older adults with diabetes mellitus live with substantial comorbidity, including greater likelihood of having myocardial infarction, stroke, vision problems, incontinence, physical disability, and nursing home stays compared with those without diabetes (Moritz et al., 1994). For those who have suffered a stroke, the resulting condition affects activities of daily living, depression, socialization, and reintegration (Bronstein, 1991).

But in adults, chronic disease effects go far beyond the expected physical and safety issues to include emotional and social functioning. For instance, adults with severe asthma are often at increased risk for emotional problems; although these may be separate from the disease, depression in these patients is often related to dealing with the asthma itself or with the effects of corticosteroids (Rubin, 1993). Self-care stresses, perceived life stress, nocturnal symptoms, and the degree of distress occurring in asthma episodes have been identified as predictors of depression (Janson-Bjerkle et al., 1993). Asthma is certainly not the only chronic disease affecting the emotions; as many as one-third of adults may report emotional distress several years after being

hospitalized for coronary heart disease (Nickel et al., 1990). Finally, in any chronic disorder, there is evidence that a combination of physical disability and depressive symptoms can trigger a downward spiral in emotional and physical health (Bruce et al., 1994).

In addition to chronic disorders, sensory loss in adults can be devastating, and these, too, can affect emotional well-being. For instance, vision loss involves a wide variety of issues including loss of a body part, mobility, self-sufficiency, possible economic security, and some contact with reality (Vader, 1992). Also, the effects of hearing loss on older adults vary with the extent of the individual's isolation, maladjustment, anxiety, depression, loneliness, and frustration (Chen, 1994).

Outside factors that influence the effects of chronic illness on adults include previous problem-solving skills and management of tasks related to their conditions and to development. For example, in one study, women with congenital heart disease experienced these problems: lack of information about their health status and reproductive options, overinvolvement of their mothers and of health care professionals on their bodies, leaving them with a limited sense of ownership of their own bodies, and poor self-esteem, self-concept, and body image (Gantt, 1992). Effects on sexual functioning are often related to clients' lack of information as it relates to the specific disorder (Katzin, 1990).

Finally, adults with long-term illnesses may be at special risk for unsuccessful completion of transition points. These may include establishing a life outside the family of origin, employment or a career, parenting responsibilities, setting and reassessing life goals (Catanzaro, 1990).

Effects on the Family

Most people who are physically compromised are cared for at home by one or more family members. Figure 31-2 depicts some of the issues and concerns that occur when a family member is disabled and the impact of the disability on the family unit. Clearly, the entire family system is affected in families with members who are disabled (Garlow and Turnbull, 1993).

Children

Many children with chronic illnesses or defects are surviving conditions that would have been fatal 20 years ago (Diamond, 1994). Upon receiving the diagnosis, parents may experience a range of normal emotions including denial and grief, as well as reactions to any developmental crisis that the child may be experiencing (Johnston and Marder, 1994). The way in which families respond to the diagnosis of developmental disorders in older children seems to be influenced by the quality of the information provided to them. This includes information about directions to the clinic where the children are assessed as well as information about the disorder itself (Piper, 1992). Other critical times for

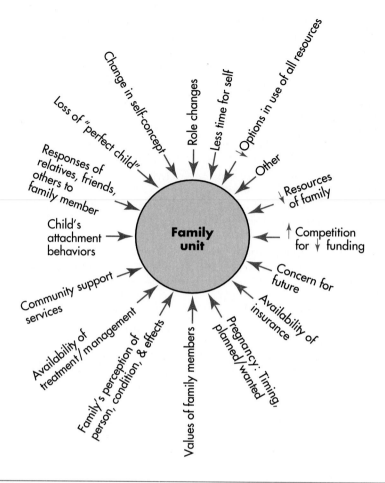

FIGURE 31-2

Factors influencing a family unit when a member is physically compromised.

the family of a child with a chronic condition result from change in the family's support or an increase in any individual's needs. These include worsening of physical symptoms, relocating the child, as in rehospitalization, parental absence, or developmental changes of any family member (Clements et al., 1990).

Adolescence may be a particularly difficult developmental stage for the families of children with **learning disabilities.** Adolescents may misinterpret parents' decisions to let them deal with the consequences of their behavior as indifference. Parents may have increasing stress in realizing that their caregiving roles for these children may have to continue into adulthood (Dane, 1993).

Families with **medically fragile** children, those requiring skilled nursing care with or without medical equipment for support of vital functions, may experience greater stress with increased demands for the affected child and reduction in their resources (Youngblut et al., 1994). For example, for children on apnea monitors, family adjustment and responses may change over time. Studies have shown variations in persistence of stress and anxiety and occurrence of depression and higher risk to the health of mothers (Ahmann, 1992).

Siblings may have special needs and problems in relation to children in their families who are physically compromised, including increased rivalry, anger, and hostility between ill and healthy children. By the same token, other studies have shown well siblings of chronically ill or disabled children to be protective of and sensitive towards them (Faux, 1991). Also, several studies have indicated that well siblings of chronically ill children are not at greater risk for psychosocial adjustment problems than are siblings of well children (Thompson et al., 1994). Well siblings may recognize that chronically ill children in their families may be stigmatized by their health problems. Well siblings may go to great lengths to emphasize the normal characteristics of these children and to reveal information about their health problems selectively (Gallo et al., 1991). In the case of childhood cancer, well siblings' reactions to their ill brothers or sisters may be mediated by the siblings' knowledge of the disease and treatment and their social competence (Evans et al., 1992).

Adults

Adults who are physically compromised may also have a variety of effects on their family units. For example, the financial impact of having a disabled family member may be significantly worsened if that person has been the primary source of family income. In other families, the wage earners may take lower paying jobs, reduce work hours, or take unpaid leave in order to accommodate the needs of the disabled person (Paterson, 1993; Stone and Short, 1990).

Another way in which adults with disabilities can affect families is in their parenting roles. There are conflicting results from studies evaluating parenting skills of adults who are mentally retarded. While some researchers believe such parents provide adequate care, others describe limited parenting abiliites. There is an increased prevalence of mental retardation among children whose parents are retarded. With one parent who is retarded, it is 15%. If both parents are retarded, it is as high as 40% (Dowdney and Skuse, 1993). Some researchers believe that children of parents who are mentally retarded are more likely to be abused than are children of nonretarded parents. In some conditions children may be guided or coerced into parenting their own parents, may fear being abandoned (e.g., through death of the disabled parents), or may fear that they will acquire or "catch" the parent's conditions (Lannon, 1992).

Other concerns for children living in a home with one or more disabled family members are their risks for accidental injuries and their potential for behavioral problems. The average number of common and serious behavioral problems were significantly greater when a disabled family member was in the home. The presence of more than one disabled family member in the homes increased children's risks for accidents, injuries, or poisonings (LeClere and Kowalewski, 1994).

With maternal chronic diseases or disabilities, families may also differ in the mothers' and families' adaptation. The major objective factor seems to be income, while the major subjective factors are the mothers' perceptions of the marital relationships and of the amount and quality of social support that they receive. Low income women are significantly more likely to perceive more stress and strain and less effective support. These perceptions negatively affect their own and their families' adaptations to the mothers' chronic health problems (Florian and Dangoor, 1994; Hough et al., 1991). In a study of 103 middle to upper-middle class families, Stetz and associates (1994) found that family system goals do not differ by type of disease, either breast cancer, diabetes mellitus, or fibrocystic breast disease. Also, family system goals seem to be consistent over time and are not easily influenced by health status nor illness in the mothers.

Family members who are caregivers for physically compromised adults are most likely to be spouses or daughters of the affected individuals. Between spouses, issues of strain upon the marital relationships, sexual functioning, concerns in case the caregivers become incapacitated, and isolation are important (DesRosier et al., 1992; Fisher and Lieberman, 1994; Garwick et al., 1994; Griffiths and Unger, 1994). For daughters and other caregivers, conflicting demands of their own families and their employment are areas of concern (Stone and Short, 1990). Moreover, female offspring and inlaw caregivers have reported more anxiety or depression than males have (Fisher and Liberman, 1994). Others have shown strong correlations of the burden of caregiving with patients' deviant behaviors and depression in the care providers (Gerritsen and van der Ende, 1994). All caregivers may deal with issues of fatigue, resentment at the demands of patients, limitations of available resources, demands of other family members, ambiguity of outcomes and crises with a chronic disease or disability, and guilt if the caregivers take advantage of respite care (Homer and Gilleard, 1994). However, effective caregiving can make the difference in a technologically dependent adult's recovering and returning to work, as well as normalizing family life (Davis and Grant, 1994).

 ## Research Brief

Fisher L, Lieberman MA: Alzheimer disease: The impact of the family on spouses, offspring, and inlaws, *Fam Proc* 33:305-325, 1994.

Ninety-seven multigeneration families of clients having Alzheimer disease participated in this study by completing a questionnaire, and appraisals of three major domains of a family's life (Emotion Management, World Views, and Structure/Organization), and three well-being indices (Well-being, Anxiety Depression, and Somatic Symptoms) through a telephone interview. Family members involved in this study included spouses, offspring and their spouses, or "inlaws."

There was no significant correlation between a family member's health and well-being and the severity of the client's disease. There was poorer health and well-being reported among female family members than among male family members. Strain for the primary caregiver was associated negatively with the health and well-being of the family member in this role. Some qualities of families have a negative influence on family members, (e.g., life engagement and organized cohesiveness), while others may have a protective function.

Implications for community health nursing practice are as follows:
1. Assessment and interventions for clients with Alzheimer and other chronic conditions need to focus on the multigenerational family instead of solely on the primary caregiver.
2. Family members who are geographically distant may still be closely involved in decision-making and should be included in the community health nurse's plans.

Effects on the Community

The presence of physically compromised people and their families in a community may have far-reaching effects on all aspects of community life. The community may be called upon to respond in new ways to these citizens, especially as a result of federal laws affecting those who are disabled.

Children

In Iowa the legislature created the Iowa Council on Chemically exposed Infants to study the scope of the problem, identify resources for these children, and look at the educational needs of those serving these children. Their study resulted in such recommendations as educating health care professionals in maternal-child health clinics about ways to identify and intervene with these children (Saunders et al., 1994). These same recommendations could be applied not only to the broader population of physically compromised children, but also to *non*health care community members, particularly members of the educational community. For instance, technology-dependent children from birth to 6 years old are reportedly welcome by directors of day care centers. However, enrollment in day care centers is low due to lack of funding and inadequately trained staff. Some communities have used resources to make prescribed child care centers, or medically fragile day care centers, available for children who use a specific device daily and need ongoing care or monitoring by trained personnel (Stutts, 1994).

Transition points in children's lives may require the investment of additional community resources. Successful transition of children with disabilities from preschool to kindergarten requires time and funding to coordinate parents' participation in plans and program and to coordinate arrangements between schools (Fowler et al., 1991). Children who are chronically ill or disabled and who enter school for mainstream education also need more support from the community. Assessment of the children's needs and abilities, preparation of school personnel and peer groups, adaptation of school buildings, provision of transportation, and training of parents in advocacy and negotiations skills and knowledge of services available are all important activities that may affect communities' resources to deal with them (Rabin, 1994). Other transitions to which communities need to respond are preparation of children in independent living skills and advice and guidance in education, training and employment, and career guidance and counseling (Gordon, 1992).

Incongruent perceptions or goals are also potential issues between families and school personnel in providing education for chronically ill children. In one study, school systems identified inadequate funding and lack of public and staff awareness as major barriers to children's success in school. Parents thought that teachers' misunderstanding of children's needs and inaccurate information about their illnesses were the major stumbling blocks (Lynch et al., 1993).

The use of the medical model which defines disabilities as problems or defects of indiviudals that must be repaired minimizes the importance of the environment and thus affects the way in which the person interacts with the community. Law and Dunn (1993) say that disability should be defined with a sociopolitical model stressing social policies that change the environment. The goal is for people with and without disabilities in communities to cooperatively change environments to increase children's involvement in community activities.

Adults

One of the most visible ways in which those with disabiliites affect their communities is through changes to accommodate mandated architectural accessibility to buildings. However, in spite of federal legislation, access to public buildings is still a significant problem in many communities (Ahn et al., 1994; McClain and Todd, 1990). A study of wheelchair accessibility in restaurants found no differences between rural and urban restaurants or between fast food and conventional restaurants (McClain et al., 1993). Up to 60% of restaurants studied had problems with parking and accessible restrooms for those who were disabled.

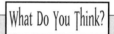

What Do You Think?

The expense of making all buildings on a college campus accessible to the physically compromised person is prohibitive; therefore, a few buildings should be made accessible and classes scheduled so that all those with physical limitations will be able to take their classes in the designated buildings.

Another issue that has implications for communites is that of independent living arrangements for adults who are disabled. One study found that men with multiple disabling conditions were more likely to live with adult relatives than were nondisabled men or those with only one disabling condition (Stinner et al., 1990). This finding has implications for community planning for caregiver support. Generally, the community needs to be concerned with ensuring adequate, appropriate housing for those who are physically compromised without stigmatizing them (Lowry, 1990). Disabled adults who live independently in apartments value control, safety and security, accessibility and mobility, function, flexibility, and privacy (Cooper and Hasselkus, 1992). Communities must try to balance resources for housing with the varying needs of those who are disabled. Some of the effects on communities are less obvious. For instance, some chronic conditions, such as AIDS and tuberculosis, can elicit fear from communities. People with epilepsy and other seizure disorders may also be feared by others in their communities or may be seen as unpredictable and lacking in self-control, which frequently results in their being stigmatized (Hartshorn and Byers, 1992).

Some communities have developed flexible care services to allow those who are physically compromised to remain at home. Such services can include in-home respite care for family members who are care providers (Sahai, 1992). Others have responded to specific needs by becoming involved with nationally developed, locally implemented programs. The Bone Up on Arthritis (BUOA) program has been shown to improve clients' knowledge of arthritis, self-care behaviors, learned helplessness, and pain (Oppewal, 1992). Community-based rehabilitation is the provision of primary care and rehabilitative assistance to those who are disabled by using resources available in their respective communities. Communities in which this approach is taken have been shown to develop more favorable attitudes toward people who are physically compromised (Mitchell et al., 1993).

Communities are also affected both by employment expectations of those who are disabled and by legislative mandates for employers. Those who are disabled may be employed in various sheltered workshops. However, more adults anticipate employment in positions and settings which use their strengths and can reasonably accommodate their needs. A study by

Craig and Boyd (1990) showed that more disabled people are hired by public administration, transportation, and service industries than by private businesses.

SPECIAL POPULATIONS
Rural Populations

As mentioned in Chapter 16, rural dwellers may be at greater risk for disability than urbanites, in particular from agricultural-related injuries and chronic illness (Bigbee, 1993; Coghill et al., 1991; Hohman, 1994; Townley and McKnight, 1994; Zejda et al., 1993). Table 31-1 summarizes some of the hazards and their potentially disabling effects. In addition to health problems peculiar to their lifestyle, people who live in rural areas can also have some of the same health problems as urban dwellers and with fewer options for dealing with these problems, both for informal and formal sources of care and support (Dana et al., 1990; Eaton et al., 1994; Henderson, 1992; Labuhn et al., 1993; Long and Weinert, 1992; Parker et al., 1992; Schroeder and Wilkerson, 1993). For example, children screened for blood lead levels in clinics in rural North Carolina were found to have a surprisingly high prevalence of elevated blood lead (Norman et al., 1994). After all, rural areas have a higher percentage of children in poverty and a higher percentage of older houses with lead paint.

Even though health care, particularly for specialized care, is limited in rural areas, there are several examples available showing how different groups have worked to provide services to those in rural areas who are disabled. Community health nurses have been in-

Table 31-1 Agricultural Industry and Disabling Conditions

Organ system or disorder	Principal exposures	Possible disability manifestations
Lungs	Organic dust, microbes, molds, fungi, endotoxins, allergens	Chronic bronchitis, asthma, hypersensitivity pneumonitis, organic dust, toxic syndrome
Cancer	Herbicides, insecticides, fungicides, fumes, sunlight, diet, unknown	Non-Hodgkin lymphoma; Hodgkin disease, multiple myeloma, soft-tissue sarcoma, leukemias, skin cancer, prostate cancer, stomach, pancreas, testicle, glioma
Neurologic disorders	Herbicides, insecticides, fungicides, solvents, fumigants	Acute intoxication, Parkinson disease, peripheral neuritis, Alzheimer disease, acute and chronic encephalopathy
Accidents	Tractor rollovers, machine injuries, animal injuries, farmyard injuries	Suffocation, crushing, amputations, eye injuries
Hearing loss	Motor noise, animal noise	Deafness
Skin	Pesticides, fuels, fungi, sun	Dermatitis, cancer
Stress and well-being	Isolation, intergenerational problems, violence, substance abuse, incest	Depression, suicide, poor coping, physical disability resulting from inadequate attention to health.

From Zejda TE, McDuffie HH, Dosman JA: *West J Med* 158(1):56-63, 1993.

volved with these projects as participants or as referral sources. These projects include efforts to reduce disability in North Carolina from such diseases as strokes, diabetes, several forms of cancer and others (Stoodt and Lengerich, 1993). The Rural Efforts to Assist Children at Home (R.E.A.C.H.) project in north central Florida and a case management program described in a Tennessee genetics program both involve provision of services to children who are developmentally disabled (Cook et al., 1986; Fiene and Taylor, 1991). Other states provide such services as a transdisciplinary mobile intervention program in rural areas of New York state for young children with developmental disabilities (Magrun and Tiggs, 1982). In Missouri, the Elks Mobile Dental Program provides cost-effective dental services to those who are developmentally disabled and live in rural areas of the state (Dane, 1990). All these examples of projects that may provide a variety of services to those who are physically compromised demonstrate the importance of the community health nurse's maintaining current knowledge about services available at the local, county, and state levels. Some demonstration projects, for example, may be funded for a limited number of years and may not be supported by other sources when initial funding is terminated.

Low Income Populations

Physically compromised individuals often experience poverty (Chubon, et al., 1994; Najman, 1993; Pope and Tarlov, 1991). However, the groups most likely to experience poverty are the following: single parents and their children, the aged, the unemployed, members of racial and ethnic minorities, and the disabled (Najman, 1993). People with low incomes have less access to health care throughout their lives and are less likely to participate in all levels of prevention (Aday et al., 1993; Bosco et al., 1993; Leveille et al., 1992; Martin, 1992). Therefore, they are at greater risk for the onset of disabling conditions and for more rapid progression of disease processes. Those in poverty are also at greater risk for disabling conditions resulting from lifestyle, such as injuries, tobacco abuse, and inadequate nutrition (Najman, 1993; Pope and Tarlov, 1991; Price and Everett, 1994). Those who are disabled and in poverty are less likely to be able to provide for their special needs from their own resources. Also, those who are physically compromised are often unemployed, including those who are able to work and who seek jobs. Employers may be reluctant to hire personnel whose conditions may increase insurance costs. Therefore, lack of insurance through the work setting further limits access to health care by those who are physically compromised. Other factors that affect low-income, physically-compromised clients' access to needed services are inadequate transportation, lack of coordination of care, and limited locally available services for those who cannot pay for them (Pope and Tarlov, 1991). See Figure 31-3 for an

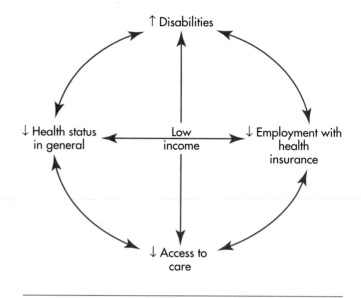

FIGURE 31-3

Relationships of poverty and disability.

illustration of the relationships between poverty and disabilities.

Occupation and Worksite

Several issues related to occupation and disability are of concern to the community health nurse. Many chronic diseases can result from or be exacerbated by worksite hazards (Behrens et al., 1994; Borkgren and Gronkiewicz, 1995; Bowden and McDiarmid, 1994; Kraut, 1994; Stellman, 1994). In addition, work-related injuries are believed to be seriously under-reported. Data about the severity and length of disability are also limited (Oleinick et al., 1994; Parker et al., 1994). Consequently, plans for population-level nursing interventions are hampered. Another concern is the correlation of other family members' disability status and causative worksite conditions (Bowden and McDiarmid, 1994). For example, a positive association has been identified between mental retardation in 10-year-old children and their mothers' employment in textile and garment industries (Decouflé et al., 1993).

Of special interest to the community health nurse is the need and opportunity for health promotion at the work site (Goetzel et al., 1994; Nelson et al., 1994). (See Chapter 45 for a more indepth discussion of this topic.) The Americans with Disabilities Act of 1990 includes provisions for certain employers to make "reasonable accommodations" in the work environment in order to facilitate employment of those who are physically compromised. However, there are many continuing questions in interpreting and carrying out the requirements of the law. For example, an elevator may have a control panel with Braille printing, maybe at wheelchair level, and may have "buttons" to press that are sensitive to warmth for those with inadequate strength to press them. What is the employer's responsibility to an employee who has bilateral amputation of both arms below the shoulder and whose prostheses includes a type of hook that prevents his readily pressing elevator "buttons? Also, under the Rehabilitation Act of 1973 and 1994, is obesity a "handicap"?

SELECTED ISSUES
Abuse

Most of the literature on abuse of those who are physically disabled concerns children and the elderly. However, community health nurses must be knowledgeable about state laws related to reporting suspected abuse of those of any age who are disabled. The particular law's definition of the characteristics defining "disabled" is especially important in view of the definition of the term in the 1990 Americans with Disabilities Act (Barton, 1993; Sheff, 1993).

For adults, abuse associated with physical disability has been identified as following disablement. In children, physical disability may result from abuse or neglect; or abuse may occur after the onset of disability (Cohen and Warren, 1990; West et al., 1992). A form of child abuse, Munchausen syndrome by proxy, may present as a developmental disability or with neurological symptoms, especially seizure activity (Baldwin, 1994; Stevenson and Alexander, 1990). Several studies have shown that adults and children who are mentally retarded are at higher risk for sexual abuse than is the general public (Ammerman et al., 1994; Cohen and Warren, 1990; Elvik et al., 1990; Tharinger et al., 1990; Westcott, 1991). Furthermore, girls who have been sexually abused and who are mentally retarded may be held responsible by adults for the abuse if the girls' behavior is considered encouraging (Podell et al., 1994).

Much has been written about characteristics of abusers and the children and elderly adults who are abused (Lachs et al., 1994). However, other authors think that the interaction among the environment, the victim, and the abuser is most important (Ammerman, 1991; Benedict et al., 1990; Benedict et al., 1992). Figure 31-4 includes several factors to consider in each component. For example, those who are physically compromised and who are in group residences or who must travel long distances in buses may be at risk for abuse from a variety of possible perpetrators. Such potential victims seem to be especially at risk if they are

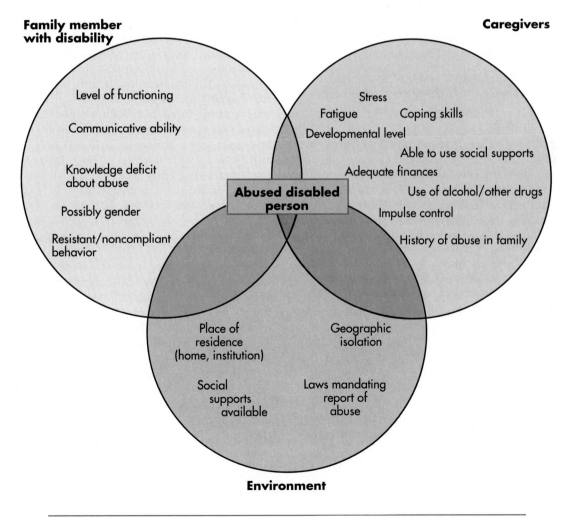

FIGURE 31-4

Factors influencing the abuse of those who are physically compromised.

Table 31-2   Impediments to Primary Health Care of the Physically Compromised

Issues	Examples
1. Transportation	1. May not be able to drive; limited flexibility in public/private transporation; may need specially equipped van
2. Access to clinic/office	2. Entrances, halls, restrooms may all be inadequate. Exam tables, scales, life equipment unavailable or inappropriate. Increased time needed for disabled client's visit.
3. Inadequate care from primary care providers	3. Limited or no training in primary care needs/health promotion of those with disabilities; lack of understanding reasons that those with disabilities often delay treatment until at crisis levels; limited ability to distinguish between progress in a disability and different, new health problems.
4. Information given to clients	4. Often unavailable or available only to few specialists; may not have been given basic health information in school; most have never received comprehensive rehabilitation.
5. Finances	5. Health maintenance/health promotion costly: good food, someone to obtain and prepare it; exercise: transporation, fees of facilities and assistant with exercise.
6. Personal assistance	6. Needed by some with disabilities for most basic health activities, hygiene, laundry, etc.

Data from Gans BM: *Arch Phys Med Rehabil* 74 (12-S): S-15-S-19; Nosek MA: J *Womens Health* 1(4).

communicatively handicapped (Porter et al., 1995). Research about interactions and mediations leading to abuse of those who are physically compromised is not currently well developed. Nevertheless, the community health nurse's comprehensive approach to health problems promotes his or her ability to consider multiple factors in these situations.

Health Promotion

Health promotion usually focuses on primary prevention of conditions in healthy people that may lead to disability (e.g., smoking cessation to prevent lung cancer). However, physically compromised clients also need information and counseling for health promoting behavior since such behavior may slow the progression of a condition or prevent added pathology (Pope and Tarlov, 1991). For example, a child with a serious congenital heart defect does not need the added insult of increased respiratory infections from exposure to second-hand cigarette smoke.

Many health promotion and disease prevention needs are similar across the lifespan; these include exercise, diet, avoidance of excess substance use, and injury prevention. However, specific problems and interventions to deal with these needs may vary with the person's age, specific disabling condition, and developmental status, among other factors. For example, nutritional needs of premature infants may focus on adequate energy, protein, fat, vitamins and minerals. Mechanical difficulties in chewing and swallowing may be the major obstacles to adequate nutrition for a child with Down syndrome, while a young adult confined to a wheelchair and with low energy expenditure may become overweight. An older adult with Type II diabetes mellitus may be concerned primarily with reducing his risk of experiencing a myocardial in-

farction. All these different needs are related to promotion of health through appropriate nutrition.

It is especially important to establish life-long, health-promoting behaviors in children who are disabled. Unfortunately, parents may be so overwhelmed by care for such children that this aspect of care is not considered. Furthermore, health promotion and disease protection for those who are physically compromised often have not been emphasized in primary care or in rehabilitation (Becker et al., 1991; Bruder and Cole, 1991; Hulseman and Normah, 1992; Parker and Beales, 1993; Rodgers, 1994). Table 31-2 summarizes issues that limit access to health care and health promotion for those who are physically compromised (Gans et al., 1993; Nosek, 1992).

HEALTHY PEOPLE 2000 OBJECTIVES

Appendix A.1 summarizes the *Healthy People 2000* objectives. Clearly many of the national health goals that apply to people without disabling conditions also apply to people who are physically compromised. For example, Objective 17 of the *Healthy People 2000* objectives deals with diabetes mellitus and the resulting disabling complications. Other objectives with clear relevance to the disabled person include those that deal with physical activity and fitness, nutrition, educational and community-based programs, unintentional injuries, occupational safety and health, environmental health, oral health, maternal and infant health, immunization and infectious diseases, and clinical preventive services. Objective 22, surveillance and data systems, is also pertinent.

Sexually transmitted diseases, Objective 19, may also be seen to be potentially disabling for the infants who are congenitally infected (Healthy People 2000, 1991). Consequently, it is evident that most of the

Healthy People 2000 objectives are related directly or indirectly to conditions that result in people being physically compromised. It is beyond the scope of this chapter to deal with all potential relationships. However, some examples of health problems that may be disabling but which do not relate to a specific major *Healthy People 2000* objective are included in this chapter.

HEALTHY CITIES

Healthy Communities 2000 (1991) gives communities a way to establish local goals to achieve the objectives of *Healthy People 2000*. This approach emphasizes the belief that an entire community is responsible for its health, and all subsystems of the community must contribute to the improvement and maintenance of that health status (Allukian, 1993; Milio, 1990). One of the subsystems within a community that is identified as a committtee is Population Groups (Flynn et al., 1991). These committees should include, in addition to "able-bodied people," those who are physically compromised or their representatives if they are unable to particpate. It would also be useful if those who are physically compromised could participate on other committees (e.g., Education, Employment, Planning and Housing) (Flynn et al., 1991). Such involvement can aid people with disabilities to enhance their leader-ship skills, specifically interpersonal and decision-making skills. These improved skills can lead to empowerment of those in this population (Walker and Doherty, 1994).

One of the major elements of the Healthy Cities Project as described in Chapter 17 is the understanding that the health of communities and people who live in them are dependent upon the environment (Ashton, 1991; Chamberlin, 1992; Flynn, 1993; Hancock, 1988; Hudson-Rodd, 1994; LaBonté, 1993; Milburn, 1993; Sabourad, 1992). This concept has several implications in terms of becoming or being physically compromised in relation to *Healthy People 2000* (1991). Environment health objectives include those for control of asthma and lead poisoning from environmental conditions. Asthma is a relatively common cause of being physically compromised, and lead poisoning may result in the developmental disability of being learning disabled. Tobacco use may also be regarded as having significance for the environmental effects on health. Objective 3.5 deals with reducing the beginning of smoking by children and youth, which is influenced by imitation of others and by advertisement. Also, Objective 3.5 recognizes the importance of second-hand smoke for children's health.

In order to prevent disabilities and to promote optimal health of those who are physically compromised, Objectives 8 to 14 must be addressed. It asserts: "Increase to at least 90 percent the proportion of people who are served by a local health department that is effectively carrying out the core functions of public health" (Healthy People 2000, 1991).

In *Disability in America,* Pope and Tarlov (1988) recommend, among other actions, improved access to care and preventive services to prevent disabilities and to provide health promotion for those who are disabled. This approach specifically includes local capacity building. Consequently, their National Agenda for the Prevention of Disability recommendations are a useful guide to integrating the Healthy Cities approach and selected objectives from *Healthy People 2000* for the community health nurse working with individuals or populations who are physically compromised.

THE ROLE OF THE COMMUNITY HEALTH NURSE

There are many factors that influence the role of the community health nurse who works with those who are physically compromised. These factors will include, of course, the community's awareness of those who are disabled and its commitment to their health needs. But of particular influence is the agency in which the nurse works. The structure and priorities of an agency determine whether a nurse will carry a general caseload or focus on service to a special population. If funding sources are dedicated to particular programs (e.g., tuberculosis control, maternal-child health services), care for those who are physically compromised may be dispersed throughout several program areas and may be difficult to identify.

In dealing with those who are physically compromised, the community health nurse's role may further change as the focus varies from the levels of individuals, families, groups, or entire communities. For instance, the nurse may be a caregiver and apply the nursing process and principles of epidemiology at any of the above listed levels. This may include, among other things, assessing, implementing, and evaluating technical care for a ventilator-dependent client at home.

A second role long associated with community health nurses is that of educator, that is, one who provides clients at any level with sufficient knowledge to enable them to decide on the most appropriate behavior for their own needs (Clark, 1992). The community health nurse may provide an entire community with information about reducing disability by decreasing a specific cause, such as spinal cord injury. The closely-related counseling role of the community health nurse is of value in that clients learn to improve their problem-solving skills as the community health nurse guides them.

The community health nurse's role as an advocate for individuals and families or groups of those who are physically compromised is especially important. An advocate is someone who speaks on behalf of others who are unable to speak for themselves (Clark, 1992). One of the potential problems with this role is that the community health nurse may unintentionally foster excessive dependence by individuals, families, or other groups. The community health nurse focuses on using advocacy to support those who need this service. At the same time, the chance to observe the community health nurse's data collecting and negotiating skills can be of use as a model for clients who are capable of using such knowedge.

For example, the community health nurse might advocate a school environment that is adapted to the specific needs of children who are wheelchair mobile, but who do not necessarily have to be limited to their chairs, without explicitly telling the children what they should do about the use of their wheelchairs. The community health nurse may assist a family caregiver of a disabled individual by validating that the caregiver's own basic needs are being sacrificed and by identifying ways that this problem can be moderated.

As a referral agent, the community health nurse maintains current information about agencies whose services are of potential use to those who are disabled. Referral, one of the most important functions of the community health nurse, is the process of directing clients to the resources that can meet their needs (Clark, 1992). For self-directing clients and families, information about an agency's services, phone number, and address may be adequate. For a family with little understanding of how systems work and a developmentally delayed child, more specific guidance and case conferences with the local school may be necessary to coordinate the child's health-related and educational needs.

As a primary care provider, one who gives essential care universally accessible to all, the community health nurse may be the most logical person to ensure that primary prevention for other health problems (e.g., communicable diseases), and information about health promotion are made available to clients who are physically compromised. On a more individualized basis, the case manager role means meeting the needs of clients by developing a plan of care to reach that goal. The nurse may also see that others carry out the plan (Clark, 1992) and is responsible for evaluating the plan's effectiveness. For example, a client who has been disabled through complications of diabetes mellitus may have several complex needs related to dealing with immediate problems such as adjusting to the amputation of one or more limbs, learning strategies for better management and compliance to slow progression of other complications. The community health nurse or case manager will, with the client and family, develop a plan to meet those needs and establish a time frame to evaluate specific outcomes.

In the quite different role of coordinator, the community health nurse is not responsible for developing the overall plan of client care. Instead, responsibilities include assisting clients and families by organizing and integrating the resources of other agencies or care providers to meet clients' needs most efficiently (Clark, 1992). For example, with the family's agreement, the community health nurse may arrange for a family to see a social worker on the same day that they bring their child to be followed up in a pediatric cardiology clinic.

The community health nurse performs the functions of a collaborator by taking part in joint decision making with clients, families, groups, and communities. Collaboration may, of course, be part of the community health nurse's role with other care providers, too. This role is of particular importance as the community health nurse seeks to involve those who are physically disabled in community-level decisions that affect their lives. An example is working with agencies or groups who make decisions about community housing for those who are physically compromised.

The role of the community health nurse as casefinder is historically a basic part of public health nursing. Nurses identify individuals with disabilities who need services they are not currently receiving. Developmental, vision, and hearing screening of young children by the community health nurse are examples of ways in which this role is carried out. It is important to bear in mind that, although the nurse's efforts are for a particular client, the focus of casefinding is on monitoring the health status of entire groups or communities (Clark, 1992). Casefinding in tuberculosis may indicate the increase in a population of this chronic disease, which is also a communicable disease. The community health nurse may also identify those who are members of vulnerable populations and who are not yet physically compromised. Such people may have limited or no access to health promotion or disease prevention services or may be unaware of those for which they are eligible.

The community health nurse may function as a change agent at all levels, including the health care delivery system. A change agent is one who originates and creates change. This process includes identifying a need for change, enlightening and motivating others as to this need, and starting and directing the proposed change (Clark, 1992). The nurse may function in the role by helping to obtain more appropriate health care services for those who are physically compromised.

These are some of the major roles in which community health nurses function to meet the complex needs of people who are physically compromised, their families, groups, and their communities.

Legislation

A community health nurse who works with clients who are physically compromised may have a general caseload of clients of all ages while another, such as a school nurse, may see clients in a specific age group. A community health nurse's need to know about laws related to specific groups will vary with the population that is the nurse's focus of care. The box on p. 615 summarizes categories of historically significant federal legislation designed to benefit those who are disabled. For indepth information about federal laws in each category since 1914, consult the National Information Center for Children and Youth with Disabilities (1991) and the Reed reference (1992).

Categories of Federal Legislation for those with Disabilities

EDUCATION

Early childhood special education
Elementary and Secondary Education Act and Amendments
Vocational education for those who are disabled

REHABILITATION

Vocational
Medical, including Medicare and Medicaid
Rehabilitation

SERVICES

Economic assistance
Facility construction and architectural design
Deinstitutionalization and independent living

CIVIL RIGHTS AND ADVOCACY

Data from National Information Center for Children and Youth with Disabilities: *NICHCY* News Digest 1(1):12-13, 1991.

Rehabilitation services were originally developed through legislation for veterans of World War I. In time, others who were physically compromised were regarded less as sources of embarrassment to their families and more as citizens who should participate as fully as possible in all aspects of society. This change in attitudes is reflected in such major laws as P.L. 93-112, 94-142 and the subsequent amendments of each. Most recently, the **Americans with Disabilities Act** of 1990, P.L. 101-336, has had far reaching effects on the civil rights of those in the community who are physically compromised. Significantly, this act includes any one of the following:

1. Persons who have a physical or mental impairment that substantially limits one or more of the major life activities of such an individual;
2. Persons who have a record of such an impairment;
3. Persons who are perceived or regarded as having a disability.

Examples include someone with a condition that is not presently disabling, (e.g., hypertension, mild congenital special deformity, or a badly scarred burn survivor) (Gammon and Abrams, 1993).

Both federal and state legislation and rules and regulations have implications for the community health nurse working with those who are disabled. The community health nurse must also remember that other state and federal laws and rules and regulations are applicable for all citizens. For example, some states have "wrongful death" laws which specify who must be consulted and who can make decisions about the type of resuscitation to be used and under what circumstances when any patient has died.

Clinical Application

A referral was made to a public health department from a nearby regional level III neonatal intensive care unit (NICU) regarding discharge plans for a developmentally delayed infant. The infant, Joel, was born at 27 weeks of gestation and had remained in intensive care for 7 months. His hospital course was complicated by hyaline membrane disease, bronchopulmonary dysplasia, and intraventricular hemorrhage. At the time of discharge, Joel was receiving neither supplemental oxygen nor medications and was taking all of his feedings orally. There were strong indications of spastic diplegia, and he was diagnosed as having severe retinopathy of prematurity with the expectation of eventual blindness. Family financial resources were extremely limited. Although Medicaid coverage was available for subsequent needs, the family owed over $100,000 to the hospital. Joel's 17-year-old mother Mary was unmarried. Joel's grandmother would babysit while Mary finished high school. Joel's father, who was also 17 years old and unemployed, had not been active with Mary and her mother in the hospital discharge planning program. His involvement with Mary and Joel was expected to be minimal. The hospital was seeking a home evaluation before discharge.

The community health nurse planned to evaluate the safety of the home environment and to begin her assessment of the family's understanding of the situation and their concerns. She found that Joel's mother and grandmother were optimistic about the future and delighted to bring him home after such a long hospitalization. They recognized that he would probably suffer motor and visual impairments, yet they wanted to participate in a program to help him develop to his best potential.

The nurse also assessed knowledge of infant care and availability of infant care items. The nurse recommended the purchase of a cool mist humidifier. Because the family had been so involved in providing Joel's daily care in the nursery, they had become skilled in this area and no knowledge deficits were identified.

In planning for early intervention services, several factors were considered. Joel's family expressed a desire for developmental services. Joel's chronic lung disease made him susceptible to complications of respiratory tract infections, making it unwise to expose him to groups of young children. Lack of financial resources limited access to services. Available community resources were center-based, offered no provision for home programs, and primarily served children ages 3 to 6 years. NICU follow-up clinic was a multidisciplinary program that could offer periodic evaluations and recommendations for developmental intervention. The health department staff—the nutritionist, physical therapist, and nurse—would receive recommendations from the hospital and follow-up program staff to develop a home program for Joel.

Continued.

Clinical Application—cont'd

Later the community development center would serve as the main program.

During the week following Joel's discharge from the hospital, he was seen at the health department by the pediatrician and nurse to establish a baseline health appraisal. The DDT Denver II was administered using Joel's corrected age (birth age in weeks minus number of weeks premature). Results showed delays in all areas. Nutritional assessment showed that weight gain was only minimally acceptable but consistent with the growth demonstrated in the hospital. Feeding practices were assessed; Joel continued to take a high-calorie formula and rice cereal with a spoon. He tired easily with feedings and was fed small amounts on a frequent schedule. Joel's immunization status was also reviewed. He had received a DPT vaccine in the nursery at 5 months of age but had not been given oral polio vaccine (OPV). An immunization schedule was established. Mary and her mother had concerns about his irregular sleeping habits and irritability. The nurse counseled them regarding behavioral and environmental interventions to promote a more organized sleeping pattern. Before the family left the clinic, the nurse checked Joel's position in his carseat and made recommendations about support for correct posture.

The physical therapist and nurse made a home visit in the following week to assess the family's success with interventions begun in the nursery and their readiness to continue the program. Mary and her mother demonstrated the exercises the hospital physical therapist had taught them. They expressed a desire to set goals, including fostering appropriate parenting skills, developing Joel's awareness of sensory stimuli, and facilitating optimal motor functioning. Examples of interventions for promoting development included recognizing Joel's behavior cues (for hunger, sleepiness, overstimulation, and boredom), offering auditory and tactile stimulation in addition to visual stimulation, and demonstrating handling techniques that promote appropriate muscle tone. Joel's mother, father, and grandmother were taught how to incorporate the interventions into Joel's playtimes and daily care. Assessment of the family's coping abilities continued to indicate that the family was adjusting to the complexity of Joel's care and his physical and sensory limitations.

The nurse planned to continue biweekly home visits with the physical therapist to develop further intervention techniques and establish goals in self-help, social, emotional, cognitive, and language skills. Periodic evaluations were performed by the multidisciplinary staff at the follow-up clinic. In collaboration with the physician and nutritionist, the nurse also planned a schedule of health appraisal, nutritional assessments, and family assessments to identify health problems and to guide well-child care.

At Joel's 1-year health assessment (9¾ months corrected age), Mary was upset about Joel's delays. The nurse encouraged her to discuss her frustrations and pointed out the progress Joel had made. Mary expressed anger and guilt and was unable to handle the constant demands placed on her. She was having difficulty understanding her own feelings because she usually seemed able to adjust to everything. The nurse supported her in her grief responses and helped her recognize that the was experiencing natural emotions that other parents had also described. The nurse helped her to realize that, although she accepted Joel's limitations, she might experience times of intense pain and grief. The nurse recommended that Mary and other family members attend parent support-group meetings through the community's developmental program.

Key Concepts

♦ The community health nurse has numerous opportunities to influence the development of disabling conditions through health promotion, especially health education for parents who might be high risks for having a disabled child, for children at risk for accidents and injuries, and for adults with chronic illnesses who might prevent disability through careful health practices.

♦ The majority of the objectives identified in *Healthy People 2000* apply to physically compromised individuals, their families, and communities.

♦ Physically compromised people need to participate in health promotion to prevent the onset of a new health disruption, to strengthen their well-functioning aspects and to prevent further deterioration of their health problem.

♦ Nursing interventions for physically compromised clients requires attention to their health as well as the environment in which they live.

♦ Community health nurses influence policy decisions that effect the health and well-being of physically compromised individuals.

♦ Community health nurses must know both federal and state laws pertaining to disabilities in order to most effectively assist clients and their families.

Critical Thinking Activities

1. Divide either the class or clinical group into two teams and debate: Children with developmental disabilities should (should not) be mainstreamed into classrooms with nondisabled children.

2. During a home visit to an adult (and then to a child) who has a chronic illness that leaves them physically compromised, answer the following questions: 1) Could this disability have been prevented? If so, what steps might the community health nurse have taken to provide health promotion activities to prevent the occurrence of the disabling condition. 2) What role, if any, does the environment play in the onset of this compromising health condition? 3) What preventive activities are currently needed to assure the highest possible quality of life for this person?

3. For the next week look at each building that you enter and keep a log with two parts: 1) What accommodations have been made to allow physically compromised people to enter this building? 2) What accommodations should still be made? 3) Who should pay for these architectural accommodations?

4. Spend one day following your usual schedule, either using crutches or in a wheelchair, so you can understand better what it means to be physically compromised.

5. Using a telephone book or community resource directory for your town, identify all agencies whose scope of work would be devoted to assisting physically compromised individuals and their families.

Bibliography

Aday LA, Lee ES, Spears B, Chung CW, Youssef A, Bloom B: Health insurance and utilization of medical care for children with special health care needs, *Medical Care* 31(11):1013-1026, 1993.

Ahmann E: Family impact of home apnea monitoring: an overview of research and its clinical implications, *Pediatr Nurs* 18(6):611-616, 1992.

Ahn HC, McGovern EE, Walk EE, Edlich RF: Architectural barriers to persons with disabilities in businesses in an urban community, *J Burn Care and Rehabil* 15(2):176-180, 1994.

Allukian M: Forging the future: the public health imperative, *Am J Public Health* 83(5):655-660, 1993.

American Diabetes Association: *Direct and indirect costs of diabetes in the United States in 1992,* Alexandria, Va, 1993, American Diabetes Association.

Ammerman RT: The role of the child in physical abuse: A reappraisal, *Violence Vic* 6(2):87-101, 1991.

Ammerman RT, Hensen M, Van Hasselt VB, Lubetsky MJ, Sieck WR: Maltreatment in psychiatrically hospitalized children and adolescents with developmental disabilities: prevalance and correlates, *J Am Acad Child Adolesc Psychiatry* 33(4):567-576, 1994.

Appleton PL, Minchon PE, Ellis NC, Elliott CE, Boll V, Jones P: The self-concept of young people with spina bifida: a population-based study, *Dev Med Child Neruol* 36(3):198-215, 1994.

Ashton J: The Health cities project: a challenge for health education, *Health Educ Q* 18(1):49-58, 1991.

Badley EM: An introduction to the concepts and classifications of the international classification of impairments, disabilities, and handicaps, *Disabil Rehabil* 15(4):161-178, 1993.

Baldwin MA: Munchausen syndrome by proxy: neurological manifestations, *J Neurosci Nurs* 26(1):18-23, 1994.

Barton HM: Failure to report child, elder abuse is criminal offense in Texas, *Tex Med* 89(2):22-24, 1993.

Becker H, Stuifbergen AK, Sands D: Development of a scale to measure barriers to health promotion activities among persons with disabilities, *Am J Health Promot* 5(6):449-454, 1991.

Behrens V, Seligman P, Cameron L, Mathias CGT, Fine L: The prevalence of back pain, hand discomfort, and dermatitis, *Am J Public Health* 84(11):1780-1785, 1994.

Benedict MI, Wulff LM, White TB: Current parental stress in maltreating and normaltreating families of children with multiple disabilities, *Child Abuse Negl* 16(2):155-163, 1992.

Benedict MI, White RB, Wulff LM, Hall BJ: Reported maltreatment in children with multiple disabilities, *Child Abuse Negl* 14(2):207-217, 1990.

Bernbaum JC, Friedman S, Hoffman-Williamson M, D'Agostino J, Farran A: Preterm infant care after hospital discharge, *Pediatr Rev* 10(7):195-206, 1989.

Bigbee JL: The uniqueness of rural nursing, *Nurs Clin North Am* 28(1):132-144, 1993.

Borkgren MW, Gronkicwicz CA: Update your asthma care, *Am J of Nurs* 95(1):26-34, 1995.

Bosco LA, Gerstman BB, Tomita DK: Variations in the use of medication for the treatment of childhood asthma in the Michigan Medicaid population (1980-1986), *Chest* 104(6):1727-1732, 1993.

Bowden KM, McDiarmid MA: Occupationally acquired tuberculosis: what's known, *J Occup Med* 36(3):320-325, 1994.

Bronstein KS: Psychosocial components in stroke, *Nurs Clin North Am* 26(4):1007-1017, 1991.

Brookins GK: Culture, ethnicity, and bicultural competence: implications for children with chronic illness and disability, *Pediatrics* 91(5):Part 2, 1056-1062, 1993.

Brown RT, Madan-Swain A: Cognitive, neuropsychological, and academic sequelae in children with leukemia, *J Learning Disabil* 26(2):74-90, 1993.

Bruce ML, Seeman TE, Merrill SS, Blazer DG: The impact of depressive symptomatology on physical disability: MacArthur studies of successful aging, *Am J Public Health* 84(11):1796-1799, 1994.

Bruder MB, Cole M: Critical elements of transition from NICU to home and follow-up, *Child Health Care* 20(1):40-49, 1991.

Catanzaro M: Transitions in midlife adults with long-term illness, *Holistic Nurs Pract* 4(3):65-73, 1990.

Centers for Disease Control: Prevalence of selected risk factors for chronic disease by education level in racial/ethnic populations—United States, 1991-1992, *MMWR* 43(48):894-899, 1994.

Centers for Disease Control: Prevalence of work disability—United States, 1990, *MMWR* 42(39):757-759, 1993.

Centers for Disease Control: Prevalence of disabilities and associated health conditions, United States, 1991-92, *MMWR* 43(40):730-731, 737-739, 1994.

Chamberlin RW: Think globally act locally: the WHO Healthy Cities Project, *Dev Behav Pediatrics* 13(5):366-367, 1992.

Chen HL: Hearing in the elderly: relation of hearing loss, loneliness, and self-esteem, *J Gerontol Nurs* 20(6):22-28, 1994.

Chubon SJ, Schulz RM, Lingle EW, Coster-Schulz MA: Too many medications, too little money: how do patients cope? *Public Health Nurs* 11(6):412-415, 1994.

Clark MA: *Nursing in the community*, Norwalk, Conn, 1992, Appleton and Lange.

Clements DB, Copeland LG, Loftus M: Critical times for families with a chronically ill child, *Pediatr Nurs* 16(2):157-161, 224, 1990.

Coghill TH, Steenlage ES, Lander-Casper J, Strutt PJ: Death and disability from agricultural injuries in Wisconsin: a 12-year experience with 739 patients, *J Trauma* 31(12):1632-1637, 1991.

Cohen S, Warren RD: The intersection of disability and child abuse in England and the United States, *Child Welfare* LXIX (3):253-262, 1990.

Collier JAH: Developmental and systems perspectives on chronic illness, *Holistic Nurs Prac* 5(1):1-9, 1990.

Cook BA, Krischer JP, Kraft P: Health care provider and family acceptance of a rural community-based nursing service for chronically ill children, *J Comm Health* 11(2):98-110, 1986.

Cooper BA, Hasselkus BR: Independent living and the physical environment: aspects that matter to residents, *Can J Occup Ther* 59(1):6-15, 1992.

Craig DE, Boyd WE: Characteristics of employers of handicapped individuals, *Am J Ment Retard* 95(1):40-43, 1990.

Dana MR, Tielsch JM, Enger C, Joyce E, Santoli JM, Taylor HR: Visual impairment in a rural Applachian community, *J Am Med Assoc* 264(18):2400-2408, 1990.

Dane E: Family fantasies and adolescent aspirations: a social work perspective on a critical transition, *Fam Community Health* 16(3):34-45, 1993.

Dane JN: The Missouri Elks Mobile Dental Program: dental care for developmentally disabled persons, *J Public Health Dent* 50(1):42-47, 1990.

Davis LL, Grant JS: Constructing the reality of recovery: family home care management strategies, *Adv Nurs Sci* 17(2):66-76, 1994.

Decouflé P, Murphy CC, Drews CD, Yeargin-Allsopp M: Mental retardation in ten-year-old children in relation to their mothers' employment during pregnancy, *Am J Ind Med* 24(5):567-586, 1993.

DesRosier MB, Catanzaro M, Piller T: Living with chronic illness: social support and the well spouse perspective, *Rehabil Nurs* 17(2):87-91, 1992.

Diamond J: Family-centered care for children with chronic illnesses, *J Pediatr Health Care* 8(4):196-197, 1994.

Dowdney L, Skuse D: Parenting provided by adults with mental retardation, *J Child Psychol Psychiatry* 34(1):25-47, 1993.

Eaton CB, Nafziger AN, Strogatz DS, Pearson TA: Self-reported physical activity in a rural county: a New York county health census, *Am J Public Health* 84(1):29-32, 1994.

Elvik SL, Berkowitz CD, Nicholas E, Lipman JL, Inkefis SH: Sexual abuse in the developmentally disabled: dilemmas of diagnosis, *Child Abuse Negl* 14(4):497-502, 1990.

Evans CA, Stevens M, Cushway D, Houghton J: Sibling response to childhood cancer: a new approach, *Child Care Dev* 18(4):229-244, 1994.

Faux SA: Sibling relationships in families with congenitally impaired children, *J Pediatr Nurs* 6(3):175-184, 1991.

Fiene JA, Taylor PA: Serving rural families of developmentally disabled children: a case management model, *Soc Work* 36(4):323-327, 1991.

Fisher L, Lieberman MA: Alzheimer's disease: the impact of the family on spouses, off-spring, and inlaws, *Fam Process* 33:305-325, 1994.

Florian V, Dangoor N: Personal and familial adaptation of women with severe phsyical disabilities: a further validation of the double ABCX model, *J Marriage Fam* 56(3):735-746, 1994.

Flynn BC: Healthy cities: the future of public health, *Health Trends Transit* 4(3):12-16, 18, 80, 1993.

Flynn BC, Rider M, Ray DW: Healthy Cities: the Indiana model of community development in public health, *Health Educ Q* 18(3):331-347, 1991.

Fowler SA, Schwartz I, Atwater J: Perspectives on the transition from preschool to kindergarten for children with disabilities and their families, *Exceptional Children* 58(2):136-145, 1991.

Francis S: Disability and chronic illness. In Johnson BS: *Child, adolescent and family psychiatric nursing*, Philadelphia, 1995, JB Lippincott.

Gallo AM, Breitmayer BJ, Knafl KA, Zoeller LH; Stigma in chronic illness: a well sibling perspective, *Pediatr Nurs* 17(1):21-25, 1991.

Gammon EA, Abrams TE: Burn survivors and the Americans with Disabilities Act, *Burns* 19(6):531-534, 1993.

Gans BM, Mann NR, Becker BE: Delivery of primary care to the physically challenged, *Arch Phys Med Rehabil* 74 (12-S): S-15-S-19, 1993.

Gantt LT: Growing up heart-sick: the experiences of young women with congenital heart disease, *Health Care Women Int* 13(3):241-248, 1992.

Garlow JE, Turnbull HR III: Families and Disability, *Vision 2010* 1(1):26-27, 1993.

Garwick AW, Detzner D, Boss P: Family perceptions of living with Alzheimer's disease, *Fam Process* 33:327-340, 1994.

Gerritsen JC, van der Ende PC: The development of a care-giving Burden Scale, *Age Ageing* 23(6):483-491, 1994.

Goetzel R, Sepulveda M, Knight K, Eisen M, Wade S, Won J, Fielding J: Association of IBM's 'A Plan for Life' health promotion program with changes in employees' health risk status, *J Occup Med* 36(9):1005-1009, 1994.

Gordon N: Independence for the physically disabled, *Child Care Dev* 18(2):97-105, 1992.

Griffiths DL, Unger DG: Views about planning for the future among parents and siblings of adults with mental retardation, *Family Relations* 43(2):221-227, 1994.

Hancock T: The future of public health in Canada: developing healthy communities, *Can J Public Health* 79(6):416-419, 1988.

Hartshorn JC, Byers VL: Impact of epilepsy on quality of life, *J Neurosci Nurs* 24(1):24-29, 1992.

Healthy Communities 2000: model standards, 3rd ed, Washington, DC, American Public Health Association, 1991.

Healthy People 2000: national health promotion and disease prevention objectives, Washington, DC, 1991, USDHHS, Public Health Service.

Heerkens YF, Brandsma JW, Lakerveld-Heyl K, van Ravensberg CD: Impairments and disabilities—the difference: proposal for adjustment of the international classification of impairments, disabilities, and handicaps, *Phys Ther* 74(5):430-442, 1994.

Henderson MC: Families in transition: caring for the rural elderly, *Fam Community Health* 14(4):61-70, 1992.

Hohman S: Farm safety: a missing topic in comprehensive school health education, *Wellness Perspectives: Research, Theory and Practice* 10(3):26-36, 1994.

Homer AC, Gilleard C: Abuse of elderly people by their carers, *Br Med J* 301(6765):1359-1362, 1990.

Homer AC, Gilleard CJ: The effect of impatient respite care on elderly patients and their carers, *Age Ageing* 23(4):274-276, 1994.

Hough EE, Lewis FM, Woods FG: Family response to mothers' chronic illness, *Western J Nurs Research* 13(5):568-596, 1991.

Hudson-Rodd N: Public health: people participating in the creation of healthy places, *Public Health Nurs* 11(2):119-126, 1994.

Hulseman ML, Normah LA: The neonatal ICU graduate: Part I, Common problems, *Am Fam Physician* 45(3):1301-1305, 1991.

Hulseman ML, Normah LA: The neonatal ICU graduate: Part II, Fundamentals of outpatient care, *Am Fam Physician* 45(4):1696-1702, 1992.

Is obesity a handicap under the Rehabilitation Act: The Regan Report on Hospital Law 34(8):1, 1994.

Jackson CB: Primary health care for deaf children, Part I, *J Pediatr Health Care* 3(6):316-318, 1989.

Jackson CB: Primary health care for deaf children, Part II, *J Pediatr Health Care* 4(1):39-41, 1990.

Jackson PL: Primary health care needs of children with hydrocephalus, *J Pediatr Health Care* 4(2):59-71, 1990.

Janson-Bjerkle S, Ferketich S, Benner P: Predicting the outcomes of living with asthma, *Res Nurs Health* 16(4):241-250, 1993.

Johnston CE, Marder LR: Parenting the child with a chronic condition: an emotional experience, *Pediatr Nurs* 20(6):611-614, 1994.

Katzin L: Chronic illness and sexuality, *Am J Nurs* 90(1):56-59, 1990.

Keith RA: Functional status and health status, *Arch Phys Med Rehabil* 75(4):478-483, 1994.

Kraut A: Estimates of the extent of morbidity and mortality due to occupational diseases in Canada, *Am J Ind Med* 25(2):267-278, 1994.

Kravitz L, Selekman J: Understanding hearing loss in children, *Pediatr Nurs* 18(6):591-594, 1992.

Labonté R: A holosphere of healthy and sustainable communities, *Aust J Public Health* 17(1):4-12, 1993.

Labuhn K, Lewis C, Koon K, Mullooly JP: Smoking cessation experiences of chronic lung disease patients living in rural and urban areas of Virginia, *J Rural Health* 9(4):305-313, 1993.

Lachs MS, Berkman L, Fulmer T, Horwitz RI: A prospective community-based pilot study of risk factors for the investigation of elder mistreatment, *J Am Geriatr Soc* 42(2):169-173, 1994.

Lannon SL: Meeting the needs of children whose parents have epilepsy, *J Neurosci Nurs* 24(1):14-18, 1992.

Law M, Dunn W: Perspectives on understanding and changing the environments of children with disabilities, *Phys Occup Ther Pediatr* 13(3):3-24, 1993.

LeClere FB, Kowalewski BM: Disability in the family: the effects on children's well-being, *J Marriage Fam* 56(5):457-468, 1994.

Leveille SG, LaCroix AZ, Hecht JA, Grothaus LC, Wagner EH: The cost of disability in older women and opportunities for prevention, *J Womens Health* 1(1):53-61, 1992.

Long KA, Weinert C: Descriptions and perceptions of health among rural and urban adults with multiple sclerosis, *Res Nurs Health* 15(5):335-342, 1992.

Lowry S: Housing for people with special needs, *Br Med J* 300(6720):321-323, 1990.

Lynch EW, Lewis RB, Murphy DS: Educational services for children: perspectives of educators and families, *Exceptional Children* 59(3):210-220, 1993.

Magrun WM, Tiggs KN: A transdisciplinary mobile intervention program for rural areas, *Am J Occup Ther* 36(2):90-94, 1982.

Marge M: Health promotion for persons with disabilities: moving beyond rehabilitation, *Am J Health Promot* 2(4):29-35, 44, 1988.

Martin DA: Children in peril: a mandate for change in health care policies for low-income children, *Fam Community Health* 15(1):75-90, 1992.

McClain L, Beringer D, Kuhnert H, Priest J, Wilkes E, Wilkinson S, Wyrick L: Restaurant wheelchair accessibility, *Am J Occup Ther* 47(7):619-623, 1993.

McClain L, Todd D: Food store accessibility, *Am J Occup Ther* 44(6):487-491, 1990.

McIntyre L: The evolution of health promotion, *Can Dent Hyg/Probe* 26(1):15-22, 1992.

Milburn LT: Partnerships for healthy communities: Part I, Lessons from the Texas Cancer Network, *Healthc Trends Transit* 5(2):10-14, 1993.

Milio N: Healthy cities: the new public health and supportive research, *Health Promot Int* 5(4):291-297, 1990.

Minder B, Das-Smaal EA, Brand EFJM, Orlebeke JF: Exposure to lead and specific attention problems in schoolchildren, *J Learning Disabil* 27(6):393-399, 1994.

Mitchell RA, Zhou D, Lu Y, Watts G: Community-based rehabilitation: does it change community attitudes towards people with disability? *Disabil Rehabil* 15(4):179-183, 1993.

Moritz DJ, Ostfeld AM, Blazer D, Curb D, Taylor JO, Wallace RB: The health burden of diabetes for the elderly in four communities, *Public Health Rep* 109(6):782-790, 1994.

Najman JM: Health and poverty: past, present, and prospects for the future, *Soc Sci Med* 36(2):157-166, 1993.

National Information Center for Children and Youth with Disabilities: Selected, key federal statutes affecting the education and civil rights of children and youth with disabilities, *NICHCY News Digest* 1(1):12-13, 1991.

Nelson DE, Emont SL, Brackbill RM, Cameron LL, Peddicord J, Fiore MC: Cigarette smoking prevalence by occupation in the United States, *J Occup Med* 36(5):516-525, 1994.

Newacheck PW: Adolescents with special health needs: prevalence, severity, and access to health service, *Pediatrics* 84:872-81, 1989.

Nickel JT, Brown KJ, Smith BA: Depression and anxiety among chronically ill heart patients: age differences in risk and predictors, *Res Nurs Health* 13(2):87-97, 1990.

Norman EH, Bordley WC, Hertz-Picciotto I, Newton DA: Rural-urban blood lead differences in North Carolina children, *Pediatrics* 94(1):59-64, 1994.

Nosek MA: Primary care issues for women with severe disabilities, *J Womens Health* 1(4):245-248, 1992.

Oleinick A, Guire KE, Hawthorne VM, Schork MA, Gluck JV, Lee B, La S: Current methods of estimating severity for occupational injuries and illnesses: data from the 1986 Michigan comprehensive compensable injury and illness database, *Am J Ind Med* 23(2):231-252, 1993.

Oppewal SR: Implementing a community-based innovation: organizational challenges and strategies, *Fam Community Health* 15(3):70-79, 1992.

Parker DL, Carl WR, French LR, Martin FB: Characteristics of adolescent work injuries reported to the Minnesota Department of Labor and Industry, *Am J Public Health* 84(4):606-611, 1994.

Parker G, Beales D: Provision to reflect real needs, *Prof Nurs* 8(12):820-825, 1993.

Parker M, Quinn J, Viehl M, et al: Issues in rural case management, *Fam Community Health* 14(4):40-60, 1992.

Paterson MA: The financial impact of disability on the family: issues and interventions, *Fam Community Health* 16(3):46-55, 1993.

Perrin JM, MacLean WE: Children with chronic illness: the prevention of dysfunction, *Pediatr Clin North Am* 35(6):1325-1337, 1988.

Piper E: Assessing and diagnosing developmental disorders that are not evident at birth: parental evaluations of intake procedures, *Child Care Health, Dev* 18(1):35-55, 1992.

Podell DM, Kastner J, Kastner S: Mental retardation and adult women's perceptions of adolescent sexual abuse, *Child Abuse Negl* 18(10):809-819, 1994.

Pope AM, Tarlov AR, eds: *Disability in America*, Washington, DC, 1991, National Academy Press.

Porter S, Yuille JC, Bent A: A comparison of the eyewitness accounts of deaf and hearing children, *Child Abuse Negl* 19(1):51-61, 1995.

Price JH, Everett SA: Perceptions of lung cancer and smoking in an economically disadvantaged population, *J Community Health* 19(5):361-375, 1994.

Rabin NB: School re-entry and the child with a chronic illness: the role of the pediatric nurse practitioner, *J Pediatr Health Care* 8(5):227-232, 1994.

Reed KL: History of federal legislation for persons with disabilities, *Am J Occup Ther* 46(5):397-408, 1992.

Rodgers J: Primary health care provision for people with learning difficulties, *Health Soc Care Community* 2(1):11-17, 1994.

Rubin IL, Crocker AC: *Developmental disabilities*, Philadelphia, 1989, Lea and Febiger.

Rubin NJ: Severe asthma and depression, *Arch Fam Med* 2(4):433-440, 1993.

Sabourad A: A better prospect for city life, *World Health Forum* 13:2-3, 232-236, 1992.

Sahai ICM: Setting an example to improve quality of life, *Prof Nurse* 8(1):62-64, 1992.

Saunders JA, Saunders EJ, Butler MA: Serving chemically exposed infants: a survey of Iowa's maternal and child health clinics, *Fam Community Health* 16(4):39-48, 1994.

Schilling LS, DeJesus E: Developmental issues in deaf children, *J Pediatr Health Care* 7(4):161-166, 1993.

Schroeder CA, Wilkerson NN: A multidisciplinary model for perinatal substance abuse prevention in rural Wyoming, *Fam Community Health* 16(2):20-29, 1993.

Sheff M: Abuse of disabled persons, *Journal of the Massachusetts Dental Society* 42(1):40, 1993.

Stellman JM: Where women work and the hazards they may face on the job, *J Occup Health* 36(8):814-825, 1994.

Stetz KM, Lewis FM, Houck GM: Family goals as indicants of adaptation during chronic illness, *Public Health Nurs* 11(6):385-391, 1994.

Stevenson RD, Alexander R: Munchausen syndrome by proxy presenting as a developmental disability, *J Dev Behav Pediatr* 11(5):262-264, 1990.

Stinner WF, Byun Y, Paita L: Disability and living arrangements among elderly American men, *Res Aging* 12(3):339-363, 1990.

Stone RI, Short PF: The competing demands of employment and informal caregiving to disabled elders, *Med Care* 28(6):513-526, 1990.

Stoodt G, Lengerich EJ: Reducing the burden of chronic disease in rural North Carolina, *NC Med J* 54(10);532-535, 1993.

Stutts AL: Selected outcomes of technology dependent children receiving home care and prescribed child care services, *Pediatr Nurs* 20(5):501-507, 1994.

Sullivan RM, Brookhouser PE, Knutson JF, Scanlon JM, Schulte LE: Patterns of physical and sexual abuse of communicatively handicapped children, *Ann Otol Rhinol and Laryngol* 100(3):188-194, 1991.

Tharingor D, Horton GB, Millea S: Sexual abuse and exploitation of children and adults with mental retardation and other handicaps, *Child Abuse Negl* 14(3):301-312, 1990.

Thompson AB, Curtner ME, O'Rear MR: The psychosocial adjustment of well siblings of chronically ill children, *Child Health Care* 23(3):211-226, 1994.

Townley KF, McKnight RH: Developmentally inappropriate play areas in rural day care: is it safe to go outside? *Pediatrics* 94(6):Part 2 of 2, 1050, 1994.

Trachtenbarg DE, Miller EC: Office care of the premature infant, *Am Fam Physician* 33(5):119-127, 1986.

Tröster H, Brambring M: Early social-emotional development in blind infants, *Child Care Dev* 18(4):207-227, 1992.

Turner-Henson A, Holaday B: Daily life experiences for the chronically ill: a life-span perspective, *Fam Community Health* 17(4):1-11, 1995.

Turner-Henson A, Holaday B, Corser N, Ogletree G, Swan JH: The experiences of discrimination: challenges for chronically ill children, *Pediatr Nurs* 26(6):571-577, 1994.

Turnock BJ, Handler A, Hall W, Potsic S, Nalluri R, Vaughn EH: Local health department effectiveness in addressing the core functions of public health, *Public Health Rep* 109(5):653-658, 1994.

US Office of Special Education and Rehabilitation Services: *Fifth annual report to Congress on the implementation of P.L. 94-142.* Washington, DC, 1983, US Government Printing Office.

Vader LA: Vision and vision loss, *Ophthalmic Nurs* 27(3):705-714, 1992.

Walker MB, Doherty AA: Healthy cities: empowering vulnerable populations for health through partnerships, *Fam Community Health* 17(2):77-79, 1994.

Weekes DP. Adolescents growing up chronically ill: a life-span developmental view, *Fam Community Health* 17(4):22-34, 1995.

West MA, Richardson M, LeConte J, Crimi C, Stuart S: Identification of developmental disabilities and health problems among individuals under child protective services, *Ment Retard* 30(4):221-225, 1992.

Westcott H: The abuse of disabled children: a review of the literature, *Child Care Dev* 17(4):243-258, 1991.

Wolfe BL, Haveman R: Trends in the prevalence of work disability from 1962 to 1984 and their correlates, *Milbank Q* 68:53-80, 1990.

Ycas MA: Trends in the incidence and prevalence of work disability. In Thompson-Hoffman S, Storek IF, editors: *Disability in the United States: a portrait from national data,* New York, 1991, Springer.

Youngblut JM, Brennan PF, Swegart LA: Families with medical fragile children: an exploratory study, *Pediatr Nurs* 20(5):463-468, 1994.

Zejda JE, McDuffie HH, Dosman JA: Epidemiology of health and safety risks in agriculture and related industries, *West J Med* 158(1):56-63, 1993.

Part Six

Vulnerability: Predisposing Factors

As the twentieth century draws to an end and the complexity of health and social problems increases, community health problems remain more a societal than an individual problem. Solutions will require an integrated social and health care approach that begins with a commitment to primary health care.

Communities increasingly experience significant problems due to communicable conditions that are often expensive and hard to treat: violence against people and property, unresolved mental health illnesses, abuse of substances among people of all groups, teen pregnancy, and increasing numbers of people disenfranchised from society, whose personal resources and access to health and social services are limited. This section presents a discussion of the most common problems seen in our communities.

Chapter 32 sets the stage for this section by discussing the concept of vulnerability and the implications for communities of the growing number of vulnerable people. Chapter 33 goes on to describe poverty and homelessness as two conditions having profound effects on the health of individuals, families, and communities. Chapter 34 examines the growing community health problems arising from increased rates of teen pregnancy. Chapter 35 looks at the community health implications of the growing migrant populations in cities and rural areas across the country. Mental health issues, substance abuse, and violence and human abuse are discussed in Chapters 36, 37, and 38, respectively. The final two chapters, 39 and 40, discuss communicable diseases and HIV, hepatitis, and sexually transmitted diseases. ▼

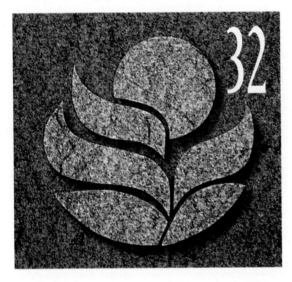

32

Vulnerability and Vulnerable Populations: An Introduction

Juliann G. Sebastian

Objectives

After reading this chapter, the student should be able to do the following:

- ◆ Define what is meant by vulnerability.
- ◆ Describe vulnerable population groups.
- ◆ Analyze trends that have influenced the development of vulnerability among certain population groups and social attitudes toward vulnerability.
- ◆ Analyze the effects of public policies on vulnerable populations.
- ◆ Evaluate the usefulness and validity of a conceptual model of vulnerability.
- ◆ Explain how socioeconomic status, age, health status, and life experiences can predispose people to vulnerability.
- ◆ Describe outcomes of vulnerability from the individual, group, and societal perspectives.
- ◆ Identify assessment issues related to vulnerable population groups.
- ◆ Give examples of the community health nurse's role in planning and implementing care for vulnerable population groups.
- ◆ Explain how to evaluate outcomes of therapeutic nursing interventions with vulnerable population groups.

Key Terms

barriers to access
brokering health services
case finding
case management
chronically homeless
comprehensive services
culturally sensitive strategies
cumulative risks
cycle of vulnerability
differential vulnerability hypothesis
disadvantaged
disenfranchisement
distribution effects
empowerment
enabling
episodically homeless
federal poverty level
health field concept
hidden homeless
homeless
human capital
iterative assessment process
locus of control
market model
medically indigent
near poor
outreach
resilience
risk
self-efficacy
social Darwinism
social isolation
vulnerable population group

Outline

Continued.

Outline—cont'd

This chapter introduces the issue of vulnerability and the roles that community health nurses play in meeting the health needs of vulnerable population groups. Selected vulnerable population groups are described. Public policies that have influenced vulnerable groups and the effects of these policies are explored. The nature of vulnerability is analyzed, and then factors that predispose people to vulnerability are covered. Outcomes of vulnerability and the cycle of vulnerability also are described. Community health nursing interventions are designed to help break the cycle of vulnerability. Numerous interventions are possible at the individual, family, group, and community level. This chapter details the community health nurse's use of the nursing process with vulnerable population groups and presents clinical applications throughout and at the end to clarify these ideas.

PERSPECTIVES ON VULNERABILITY
Definition

Vulnerability is often confused with the concept of risk. **Risk** is based on the natural history of disease model. This model explains how certain aspects of physiology and the environment, including personal habits, social environment, and physical environment, make it more likely that one will develop particular health problems (Valanis, 1992). For example, a smoker is at risk of developing lung cancer because cellular changes occur with smoking. However, not everyone who is at risk develops health problems. Some individuals seem to be more likely than others to develop those health problems for which they are at risk. These people are more vulnerable than others. A **vulnerable population group** is a subgroup of the

population who is more likely to develop health problems as a result of exposure to risk or to have worse outcomes from these health problems than the population as a whole. Members of vulnerable groups frequently have **cumulative risks,** or combinations of risk factors (Nichols et al., 1986) that make them more sensitive to the adverse effects of individual risk factors that others might be able to overcome. Vulnerability, therefore, implies that certain people are more sensitive to risk factors than others (O'Connor, 1994).

Those who are at risk, but who are not as likely to develop the health problem are more resilient than their more vulnerable counterparts. Being at risk for a certain health problem is therefore *necessary* for development of that problem, but it is *not sufficient.* It also seems to be necessary to possess other characteristics that increase one's vulnerability before the health problem actually develops. For example, vulnerable population groups are those who are not only particularly sensitive to risk factors, but also those who possess multiple, cumulative risk factors. This is referred to as the **differential vulnerability hypothesis** (Aday, 1993).

Health care professionals are focusing on the needs of special population groups. Special population groups are defined as low-income groups, minority groups, and people with disabilities in *Healthy People 2000* (1991). Special populations that community health nurses are concerned about include (1) those who are poor or homeless, (2) pregnant adolescents, (3) migrant workers, (4) severely mentally ill individuals, (5) substance abusers, (6) abused individuals, (7) people with communicable diseases and those at high risk for these diseases, and (8) persons who are positive for the human immunodeficiency virus (HIV) or have hepatitis B virus (HBV) or other sexually transmitted diseases (STDs). Vulnerable individuals and

Vulnerable Population Groups of Special Concern to Community Health Nurses

Poor and homeless persons
Pregnant adolescents
Migrant workers
Severely mentally ill individuals
Substance abusers
Abused individuals
Persons with communicable disease and those at risk
Persons who are HIV positive or have hepatitis B virus and sexually transmitted diseases

families often belong to more than one of these groups. For example, community health nurses work with pregnant adolescents who are poor, have been abused, and are substance abusers. Community health nurses also work with substance abusers who are HIV positive and HBV positive as well as those who are severely mentally ill. The box above lists vulnerable population groups.

Community health nurses, other public health professionals, and policy makers are targeting health care interventions toward vulnerable population groups because these groups suffer from disparities in access to care, uneven quality of care, and the poorest health outcomes. Both *Healthy People 2000* and *Healthy Communities 2000* (American Public Health Association [APHA], 1991) highlight vulnerable population groups and illness prevention and health promotion objectives for them. The following discussion points out some of the problems that each of the vulnerable populations just described has with access to care, quality of care, and health outcomes. Chapters 33 to 40 describe these vulnerable populations in more detail.

Description of Vulnerable Population Groups

Poor and Homeless Persons

Economic status is strongly related to health status. People who are poor are more likely to live in hazardous environments, work at high-risk jobs, eat less nutritious diets, and have multiple stressors, since they do not have the extra resources to manage unexpected crises and may not even have adequate resources to manage daily life (Pappas, 1994). In a study of the widening gap in life expectancy between blacks and whites in the United States, researchers concluded that the causes of the differences were related to low socioeconomic status rather than race (Kochanek et al., 1994). The interaction among multiple socioeconomic stressors makes people more susceptible to risks than others with more financial resources might be able to cope with. For example, Felicia Delacorte's situation illustrates how living environment and practical problems such as transporta-

tion and cost interact to make people who are poor particularly vulnerable to health problems.

Felicia Delacorte is a 22-year-old single mother of three children whose primary source of income is Aid to Families with Dependent Children. Felicia recently took all three children with her to the health department because 15-month-old Hector needed immunizations. Felicia was worried about 5-year-old Martina, who had a fever of 100° to 101° F on and off for the past month. Felicia and her friends in the trailer park were worried that some type of hazardous waste from the chemical plant next door to the park was making their children sick. Now that Martina was not feeling well, Felicia was particularly concerned. However, she was told by the health department nurse that they were all booked up for the day and that she would need to bring Martina back to the clinic on the next day. Felicia left discouraged because it was so difficult for her to get all three children ready and on the bus to go to the health department, not to mention the expense. She thought maybe Martina just had a cold and she would wait a little longer before bringing her back.

Homeless people have fewer resources than poor people and must struggle with even more demands as they try to manage daily life. Homeless individuals and families do not have the advantage of shelter and must cope with finding a place to sleep at night and to stay during the day, as well as finding food, before even thinking about health care. In fact, the health care needs of homeless individuals are related to their regular search for shelter and food. For example, homeless individuals often have foot problems from constant walking, hypothermia from exposure to the cold, and exacerbations of chronic health problems because they have no place to store their medications, cannot always find nutritious meals, and cannot maintain a healthy balance of rest and activity because of vagrancy laws that prohibit loitering in one place for a prolonged time (Sebastian, 1985). Ferenchick (1992) compared the medical problems of homeless patients who were seen in a community health clinic with those of patients who had stable housing and those with unstable housing arrangements. He found that homeless patients were significantly more likely to have injuries, fractures, and dental problems than patients with housing. Homeless persons experience problems ranging from violence and trauma associated with life in the streets, to difficulty managing dental care because they have no place to store toothbrushes, toothpaste, and other dental supplies. In a study of homeless shelters for women in Chicago, Barge and Norr (1991) found that the most common health problems of women in their childbearing years were hypertension, mental illness, and injuries, with infections, abuse, and STDs also reported, but less often.

Pregnant Adolescents

Pregnant teenagers are similar to people who are poor because having a baby as a teenager often means that the adolescent mother, her infant, and future children will experience a lower socioeconomic status than they might have otherwise. Most teenage mothers keep and raise their children (Yoos, 1987). This often results in interrupted education for one or both of the parents, limited job opportunities, additional expenses associated with childrearing, and a long-term cycle of economic problems that affect both the parents and their children. The teenage mother often assumes the role of a single parent, with even more economic consequences. The economic problems are worsened by the many health problems associated with adolescent pregnancy.

Adolescent females (especially those under 14 years of age) are more likely to deliver low-birth-weight infants than are women in their twenties and thirties. This is thought to result from the combined interaction of physiological variables (Yoos, 1987) and socioeconomic conditions (Trussell, 1988). Being unable to afford prenatal care, lacking awareness of the importance of prenatal care and how to obtain it, and being likely to initiate prenatal care later in pregnancy than older mothers all contribute to the poor pregnancy outcomes of adolescents. Other health problems that pregnant adolescents experience include toxemia, pregnancy-induced hypertension, and anemia.

Migrant Workers

Migrant workers face a wide variety of risk factors, including occupational risks associated with hazardous work and poor working conditions and socioeconomic risks from poverty and homelessness. The nature of occupational risks varies depending on the type of work. Many are employed on farms, planting and harvesting agricultural products. Others are employed in other types of seasonal labor, such as those who travel the horse racing circuit, working at race tracks and on horse farms (Ireson and Weaver, 1992). In addition to occupational risks, migrant workers are at high risk for tuberculosis (Ciesielski et al., 1994). Crowded living conditions, traveling to work in crowded buses, and malnutrition are risk factors to which migrant workers are exposed.

Migrant workers are **episodically homeless.** "Episodically homeless people are those who frequently go in and out of homelessness" (Institute of Medicine, 1988, p. 23). Because migrant workers obtain shelter in migrant camps while they are working but may not have a reliable place to live at other times, they are among the **hidden homeless.** These distinctions are important to consider when planning health services, since it is easy to forget that migrant workers have many of the same problems as those who are **chronically homeless** (Institute of Medicine, 1988).

Migrant workers also have serious problems with access to health care (Ciesielski et al., 1994). Some, but not all, migrant workers do not have citizenship status. Those who are illegal immigrants may have no legal access to health services, depending on the laws in a particular state.

Severely Mentally Ill Individuals

Severely mentally ill (SMI) individuals, defined as those people with a major psychosis, such as schizophrenia or bipolar disorder, also cope with a combination of health and socioeconomic problems. These disorders often do not manifest themselves until adolescence or young adulthood, at the very time when people are trying to establish themselves financially. Untreated severe mental illness interferes with a person's ability to function on a daily basis and thus makes it difficult to maintain a job. SMI individuals need multiple health and social services, such as antipsychotic medications, counseling and sometimes group therapy, and vocational assistance (Steinwachs et al., 1992).

Throughout the nineteenth and much of the twentieth centuries, SMI individuals in the United States were treated primarily by hospitalizing them for long periods. State mental hospitals were originally developed in the nineteenth century as restful places where a comprehensive, healing environment could be created (Grob, 1973). In fact, the original term, *asylum* was intended to connote this idea of rest and refuge from the stresses of daily living. State mental hospitals were never supposed to become long-term care facilities for SMI individuals. However, the lack of adequate community resources for these people resulted in increasing reliance on them and, eventually, on the abuses and dysfunctions that were documented by Clifford Beers, who had himself been a patient in a state mental hospital (Grob, 1983). Eventually, public concern about mental hospitals led to the passage of the 1963 Community Mental Health Centers Act, which intended to deinstitutionalize the SMI population and create comprehensive services for them in their own communities. Unfortunately, comprehensive service networks did not develop in every community, and many SMI individuals were left with fewer and more fragmented services than they needed to function. In many cases, people who had lived in mental hospitals for many years had no idea how to manage on their own in the community. Community agencies are trying to work together to provide the individualized care that so many SMI people need to help them function and achieve a high quality of life in their communities (Steinwachs et al., 1992).

Substance Abusers

Substance abuse is a growing problem in the United States. It includes abuse of legal and illegal substances, such as alcohol, narcotic pain medications, and street drugs (e.g., cocaine, heroin, marijuana). Substance abuse creates both health and socioeconomic problems. For example, people who use cocaine may have heart problems and develop nasal and sinus pathology. Neurological problems may result from marijuana use. Alcohol abuse damages the liver and is a risk factor for certain forms of cancer. Alcoholic persons who are HIV positive are at a higher risk of developing hepatitis (Anastasi and Rivera, 1994). Substance abusers have serious socioeconomic problems, including financial strain from the cost of the drugs; criminal convictions from illegal activities used to obtain the drugs; communicable diseases from sharing drug paraphernalia, from sexual activity such as prostitution to earn money for drugs, and from decreased inhibitions caused by the drugs themselves; and family breakdown. Substance abusers may be reluctant to seek health care for fear of being "turned in" to criminal authorities.

Abused Individuals

Abuse is a huge problem in the United States, affecting all age groups. Physical, emotional, and sexual abuse are issues, as well as neglect. Adult domestic violence of all types occurs more often than any other crime. Chez (1994, p. 33) says that ". . . the term 'domestic violence' refers to a pattern of regularly occurring abuse and violence, or the threat of violence, in an intimate (though not necessarily cohabitating) relationship." Domestic violence occurs in one of five forms: physical, sexual, psychological, emotional, and economic (Chez, 1994). The incidence of child abuse has risen, with 2.9 million suspected cases reported in 1992 (Devlin and Reynolds, 1994). Child neglect is the most common form of child abuse, followed by physical abuse and then sexual abuse (Finklehor, 1994). Child sexual abuse is a particular problem not only because of its long-term consequences for affected children, including posttraumatic symptoms, emotional problems, and addictive behaviors (Briere and Elliott, 1994), but also because the reported cases of child sexual abuse are rising faster than those for neglect and physical abuse (Finklehor, 1994). Abusive behavior seems to be related to a combination of problems, including mental health problems, substance abuse, and socioeconomic stressors such as dysfunctional families and financial strain. Stressed families and those practicing substance abuse are at high risk for child abuse (Devlin and Reynolds, 1994).

People with Communicable Diseases and Those at Risk

Vulnerable populations are at a particularly high risk of contracting communicable diseases. The incidence of communicable and infectious diseases is increasing in the United States, partly because not all children are fully immunized, so the level of "herd immunity" for childhood diseases has dropped in some communities. Also, as more strains of drug-resistant bacteria develop, the incidence of communicable diseases increases. The measles outbreak in the United States in

Research Brief

Kelleher K, Chaffin M, Hollenberg J, Fischer E: Alcohol and drug disorders among physically abusive and neglectful parents in a community-based sample, *Am J Public Health* 84(10):1586-1590, 1994.

Researchers compared the frequency of substance abuse between people who reported that they physically abused or neglected a child and those who did not abuse or neglect children. They interviewed 169 adults who said they had physically abused a child and 209 adults who said they had neglected a child and compared the results of those interviews with interviews from the same numbers of adults who reported no abuse or neglect of a child. The researchers found that ". . . adults with alcohol or drug disorders were 2.7 times more likely to have reported abusive behavior toward children and 4.2 times more likely to have reported neglectful behavior toward children than were their matched control subjects. Adults living in larger households or with a history of depression were also significantly more likely to have acted abusively toward children than their matched control subjects. A history of antisocial personality disorder remained a significant predictor of child neglect" (pp. 1588-1589). The results of this study demonstrate that abusive behavior, substance abuse, and mental health problems may coexist. These results suggest that abusive parents should be screened for substance abuse and mental health problems and should be provided treatment for these problems if necessary.

the early 1990s is one example of increased incidence from inadequate levels of herd immunity. Increases in numbers of people infected with dangerous strains of drug-resistant *Staphylococcus aureus* have been seen in recent years (Shovein and Young, 1992). The incidence of tuberculosis (TB) increased throughout the 1980s and 1990s, partly because of the decreased resistance of HIV-infected people to opportunistic infections (O'Brien and Bartlett, 1992). People who live or work in homeless shelters or drug treatment centers and substance abusers have a higher risk of becoming infected with TB than the rest of the population (Avey, 1993). New infectious syndromes are occurring, such as *Mycobacterium avium* complex (MAC) (Anastasi and Rivera, 1994; Benenson, 1990), which affects people who are HIV positive. Crack cocaine users risk TB infection, partly because of the crowding and high traffic in crack houses and because of the coughing caused by smoking cocaine (Leonhardt et al., 1994).

Concerns have been raised in recent years about the safety of food and water supplies. For example, epidemics of staphylococcal food poisoning have occurred in the United States related to both political and economic problems. These outbreaks were traced to a chain of fast-food hamburger restaurants. Investigation revealed that standards for detecting potentially harmful levels of bacterial contaminants in raw meat were inadequate. Public health officials advised restaurants to cook meat to a high enough temperature to kill the bacteria, but this was not always done. As a result, large numbers of people became ill and two young children died. People who are the most vulnerable to communicable and infectious diseases are those with compromised immune systems, such as people with HIV, acquired immunodeficiency syndrome (AIDS), and cancer, as well as very young and very old persons. Communicable disease prevalence can influence the social and economic health of a community because the greater the number of people who are sick, the fewer people who are available to do the work necessary to sustain other community functions.

Persons Who Are HIV Positive or Have Hepatitis and other Sexually Transmitted Diseases

Persons who are HIV positive or have HBV and other STDs are susceptible to further health and socioeconomic risks. They are more likely to develop other infectious diseases and certain forms of cancer. For example, people who are HIV positive risk developing opportunistic infections such as TB and cancers such as Kaposi's sarcoma. People who have certain STDs, such as herpes simplex virus 2 infection, also risk cancer. Socioeconomic problems result from interferences with work, family, and life-style disruptions. These problems are compounded if the individual loses his or her insurance. This can happen as a result of changing jobs and being refused coverage because of a preexisting condition, because the insurance rates for someone with a preexisting condition were high, or because the insurance company dropped that person's coverage altogether. Social, psychological, and emotional problems associated with these illnesses can be the most disruptive aspects.

Trends in Health Care

During colonial times, people with chronic physical or mental conditions were cared for in their own communities. Later, the social reforms of the nineteenth century led to institutional care for many of these individuals. In the latter part of the twentieth century, there is a renewed emphasis on caring for vulnerable population groups in the community. Many of the vulnerable population groups described in this chapter and Chapters 33 to 40 have less access to health services than other groups. The trend is toward more outreach and case finding to make access easier and more culturally competent (AAN, 1992). There is also a trend toward providing more comprehensive, family-centered services when treating vulnerable population groups. Felicia Delacorte's situation, described

previously, is a good example of the importance of providing comprehensive, family-centered, "one-stop" services. If Felicia had been able to have Martina checked while she was in for Hector's immunizations, Martina's health problem would have been treated at an earlier stage. Finally, the trend is toward providing more of these comprehensive services in locations where people live and work, including schools, churches, neighborhoods, and workplaces. Nurses are beginning to develop mobile outreach clinics and take them to migrant camps, schools, and local communities. The shift away from hospital-based care includes a renewed commitment to the public health services that vulnerable populations need to prevent illness and promote health (Baker et al., 1994; Fielding and Halfon, 1994), such as reduction of environmental hazards and violence and assurance of safe food and water.

PUBLIC POLICIES AFFECTING VULNERABLE POPULATIONS
Landmark Legislation

Public policy is shaped by legislation that specifies the general directions for government bodies to take. Even though laws may only relate to a certain proportion of the population, they tend to have a ripple effect and result in other groups following the general intent of the law. Various pieces of landmark legislation have affected vulnerable population groups throughout the twentieth century (see box below).

Two of these pieces of legislation *provided for direct and indirect financial subsidies to certain vulnerable groups.* The Social Security Act created the largest federal support program for elderly and poor Americans in history. This act was intended to ensure a minimal level of support for people who otherwise had a level of

---

 Legislation That Has Affected Vulnerable Population Groups in the United States

LEGISLATION THAT PROVIDED FOR DIRECT AND INDIRECT FINANCIAL SUBSIDIES TO CERTAIN VULNERABLE POPULATION GROUPS

Social Security Act of 1935
Medicare and Medicaid Social Security Act amendments of 1965

LEGISLATION THAT PROVIDED FINANCIAL SUPPORT FOR BUILDING HEALTH CARE FACILITIES

Hill-Burton Act of 1946
Community Mental Health Centers Act of 1963
Stewart B. McKinney Homeless Assistance Act of 1988

LEGISLATION THAT AFFECTED HOW HEALTH CARE RESOURCES WERE USED

National Health Planning and Resources Development Act of 1974
Tax Equity and Fiscal Responsibility Act of 1982

vulnerability to problems resulting from inadequate financial resources. This was accomplished by direct payments to eligible individuals. Later, the Medicare and Medicaid amendments to the Social Security Act of 1965 were intended to provide for the health care needs of elderly, poor, and disabled people who might be vulnerable to impoverishment resulting from high medical bills or to poor health status from inadequate access to health care. These acts created third-party payers at the federal and state levels who provided financial assistance by paying for health services.

Three of the other laws created *financial support for building health facilities,* thereby improving access to health services for vulnerable groups. The Hill-Burton Act of 1946 provided financial support to build hospitals that would provide care to indigent people. The Community Mental Health Centers Act of 1963 made money available to construct community mental health centers and train mental health professionals who would provide community-based care for the severely mentally ill individuals who were discharged from state mental hospitals. This overall policy of deinstitutionalization from mental hospitals was also included in the act and is similar to the current trend to treat more people in their communities and homes rather than in institutions. A policy that encourages more community-based care also requires that the community-based services that people need are developed and implemented. Finally, the Stewart B. McKinney Homeless Assistance Act of 1988 resulted in money for clinics and a wide variety of educational and social services for homeless individuals and families.

The other two pieces of legislation, the National Health Planning and Resource Development Act of 1974 and the Tax Equity and Fiscal Responsibility Act of 1982, *influenced the use of resources* for providing health services. The National Health Planning and Resource Development Act was intended to provide local mechanisms for planning which types of health services and facilities were really needed so that duplication of expensive facilities and services would be avoided. The goal was to reduce the increasing cost of health services; this would indirectly influence access for vulnerable population groups by making health services more affordable. Also, part of the planning process included community health needs assessment, with the goal of providing balanced services so all would have access to the care they needed. The Tax Equity and Fiscal Responsibility Act of 1982 also focused on the cost of health services but did so in a very different way. This act was also designed to limit the rapid increase in health care costs, but it did not focus on community planning. Instead, this act mandated that payment for hospital services for all Medicare patients would no longer be done on a retrospective cost basis; that is, the Health Care Financing Administration (HCFA) would no longer simply pay the bills that were submitted to them for Medicare enrollees. Now,

the HCFA would pay for services on a prospective basis. The agency did so by developing a list of common medical diagnoses (diagnosis-related groups, or DRGs) and determining what they would pay for caring for people with these diagnoses. If hospitals provided services that cost more than the amount indicated on the list, those hospitals lost money. The effect was an increased emphasis on shorter hospital stays, more emphasis on identifying cost-effective treatments, and more emphasis on community-based care and care in the home. This was difficult for certain vulnerable groups, such as the homeless, who did not have the same level of resources and support to continue with the care necessary after discharge.

Implementation Issues

Once a law is passed, it must be put into place before it will have a substantial effect on the public. Often, unanticipated problems occur during the implementation phase. These problems sometimes mean that the "letter of the law" is followed but that the intentions of the law are not met. For example, the Community Mental Health Centers Act intended to move treatment of severely mentally ill people into the communities so they would have better outcomes. However, the community supports necessary to help this population were not always adequate, so many eventually lost contact with families and jobs and became homeless (Institute of Medicine, 1988). Implementation problems also occur because the law has unintended effects on other groups that lawmakers do not anticipate. These are called **distribution effects.** Distribution effects are exemplified by the criticisms that mental hospitals did not discharge people quickly because the administrators and staff had much to lose. Staff lost jobs and administrators lost perquisites such as homes and their own personal staff as censuses dropped (Torrey et al., 1990).

Even though laws such as Medicaid and the McKinney Act were passed to help provide money to care for vulnerable groups, some vulnerable individuals and families still do not have adequate access to care. Friedman (1994) argues that nonfinancial **barriers to access** include subtle and often unintentional discrimination. Subconscious discrimination can result in an inadequate number of providers who are willing to treat certain racial groups and people with certain diagnoses, such as HIV. Discrimination against certain diagnoses can influence which conditions insurers are willing to pay for. Other nonfinancial barriers include inadequate providers in rural areas and certain sections in urban areas, as well as cultural barriers such as the inability of many vulnerable groups to manage the health care system (Friedman, 1994). Thus, even though laws have been passed to increase access to health services by vulnerable groups, inequities still exist for these populations because of attitudes.

Health Care Reform

Health care reform efforts are focusing both on reducing the cost of care and on covering the cost of caring for vulnerable groups. Universal health insurance coverage is a major issue in these discussions. Many predict that universal health insurance coverage will mean that public health agencies will be much less likely to provide personal health services for individuals (e.g., primary care clinics in health departments) (Aiken and Salmon, 1994). It will be more attractive to private clinics and physicians' offices to provide the personal care services that some public health departments now provide because they can obtain payment for these services. Public health departments may find it less costly to eliminate these services and focus on providing population-focused services only, such as communicable disease control, environmental services, and managing public food and water supplies.

However, if public health no longer provides personal health services to vulnerable populations, private health agencies may not want to provide them with services, and disparities in health care access and outcomes could grow even greater. Aiken and Salmon (1994) explain that vulnerable populations are more expensive to treat, since they possess multiple, cumulative risks and require special service delivery considerations (e.g., to help overcome transportation problems or provide culturally competent care). For example, managed care organizations possess strong incentives to control costs by keeping their enrollees healthy. These groups may prefer to care for the healthiest people rather than those who are most vulnerable.

Many argue that fundamental changes are needed in the way that health services are delivered (Baker et al., 1994). The American Nurses Association's proposal for reform (ANA, 1991) specifically focuses on the need for special programs for vulnerable groups. This document proposes that special programs and outreach activities be developed for these groups. It also notes that improved health care is not solely a result of health services, but also results from improvements in the broader environment. Nursing's plan for health care reform is unique in its emphasis on both health services and broader social change. "National health reform must also consider the interrelationships between health and such factors as education, behavior, income, housing and sanitation, social support networks, and attitudes about health. Better health cannot be the nation's only goal when hunger, crime, drugs, and other social problems remain" (ANA, 1991, p. 14). This approach to reform is much broader than an emphasis on costs alone and is particularly responsive to the multidimensional nature of vulnerability.

CONCEPTUAL BASES OF VULNERABILITY

Vulnerability is *multidimensional;* that is, multiple concepts are needed to understand what vulnerability means to those who experience it. Limited control, victimization, disadvantaged status, disenfranchisement, powerlessness, and health risks are the dimensions emphasized in this chapter. Figure 32-1 illustrates the dynamic interactions among these dimensions.

Limited Control

The **health field concept** explains how limited control over one's own health is part of vulnerability. This concept was developed by LaFramboise (1973, cited in Dever et al., 1988, p. 26) and expanded by Lalonde (1974, cited in Dever et al., 1988, p. 26). Individual control of health is only one factor in a comprehensive model of health in which biology, environment, and the health care system make up the remaining three foci. According to the health field concept, individuals share *control and responsibility* for their health status with society as a whole.

Individuals largely determine the behaviors they engage in that are health promoting or potentially health damaging. Although individuals do not control their biological heritage, they share some responsibility for the heritage they pass on to their offspring (e.g., through the effect that prenatal health and maternal life-style have on infant health). Society determines the types of health services and the types of reimbursement mechanisms available. Also, society is responsible for many environmental hazards. Thus the health field concept explains how health status is affected by both individual factors (individual and biology) and broader societal factors (environment and health care system). The ongoing health of the women with AIDS described in the case of Pam Swift is affected not only by their own health behaviors, but by the fact that they may lose access to medications and laboratory tests when their insurance is cancelled.

In many cases, aspects of the physical and social environment that adversely affect the health status of vulnerable populations are beyond their control and

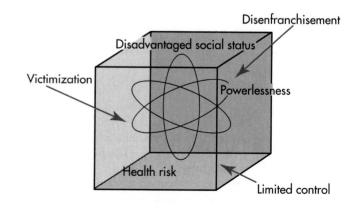

FIGURE 32-1

Dimensions of vulnerability.

are the responsibility of society. For example, communities sometimes find it difficult to locate group homes for severely mentally ill clients in residential neighborhoods despite the emphasis on providing care for these individuals in more normal environments. Neighbors may fear mentally ill people, or they may worry that their property values will drop. If group homes are located in poor neighborhoods, residents are more likely to be victims of crime, to be exposed to environmental hazards such as air pollutants, and to feel ostracized.

Victimization

Limited individual control over behavior is not the only issue related to health status and vulnerability. Dever et al. (1988) express concern that the current emphasis on individual control of health through lifestyle choices may result in blaming the victim for areas outside individual control. In the extreme, victim blaming relieves society from assuming responsibility for environmental issues and health service delivery issues.

Rosner (1982) concluded that victim blaming has become part of the outlook on care for the poor in American society. In the early days of the United States, the public believed that poverty was temporary and could be overcome. People felt a sense of responsibility to help the "truly needy" and believed that poor people were worthy of help. The thought that poverty might be permanent was in opposition to the developing American ideas of self-sufficiency and individual achievement.

Later, during the Industrial Revolution and the early part of the twentieth century, social attitudes shifted, and people thought that poor and dependent members of society somehow deserved their situations. This attitude justified limitations on social welfare that were actually caused by financial constraints on service availability. Ultimately, affluence was seen as a sign of morality, as the just reward for clever and hard-working members of society, and poverty was viewed as the outcome of immorality and slothfulness. Americans eventually adopted an attitude of ambivalence toward poor and dependent persons; those who were seen as temporarily poor were considered worthy of help, and those for whom poverty was considered a permanent state were not considered worthy of help (Rosner, 1982). Ambivalent attitudes toward vulnerable populations are common; for example, the public sometimes objects to spending tax dollars for treatment of HIV and substance abuse because some still think that people create these problems for themselves.

Such ambivalence seems to have increased in the last decade. Strict eligibility criteria are becoming more common for health and social services. Policy makers are concerned about welfare reform. Public sentiment seems to favor not providing financial entitlements for those who do not want to help themselves. Also, ambivalence toward the poor may have resulted partly from professional opinions regarding enabling behavior. The concept **enabling** comes from the literature on addictions and refers to the behavior of people in the dependent person's environment that makes it possible for the addiction to continue, such as covering up and "making things right." Some think that the presence of loose eligibility criteria for health and social services enables individuals to maintain patterns of dependency. Rosner (1982) argued that attitudes favoring strict eligibility criteria are more likely during times of severely limited economic resources and that certain functions are served by blaming the victims of poverty and dependency.

These functions include the maintenance of a class system and the opportunity for middle-class and upper-class groups to practice charity and benevolence toward poor and dependent persons (Rosner, 1982). Curtin (1986) pointed out that contributing to these persons' needs gives people an opportunity for tax deductions and feelings of self-satisfaction from helping the less fortunate. The functions served by having lower-class groups in society are therefore both financial and psychological. Further division of the health care system into a two-tiered system of care based inherently on victim blaming of those at the lower level has resulted in part from a shift in the focus of health care from patient care to a consumer commodity (Curtin, 1986). The emphasis on cost containment resulted in policies designed to limit those eligible for free or government-financed care, as opposed to earlier efforts to expand accessibility of services (Grau, 1987; Rosner, 1982), although health system reform may reverse this.

Disenfranchisement

Disenfranchisement refers to a feeling of separation from mainstream society in which the individual does not have an emotional connection with any group in particular or the larger social fabric in general. In addition to perceived disenfranchisement, certain groups such as the poor, the homeless, and migrant workers may essentially be "invisible" to society as a whole and forgotten in health and social planning. Disenfranchisement *suggests* that vulnerable groups do not have the social supports necessary to manage effectively an emotionally and physically healthy life-style. Many vulnerable individuals have limited formal support networks because they do not have well-established linkages with formal organizations in their communities, such as churches and schools. They may also have few informal sources of support, such as family, friends, and neighbors. For example, homeless individuals are often isolated and have few people that they can call on for assistance. It is not true, however, that all vulnerable groups have no sources of social support. Community health nurses should remember that although disenfranchisement is part of being vulnerable for many, strong support from churches, family, and neighbors may be advantages that some vulnerable individuals can draw on, even though they may feel disenfranchised from society as a whole. Pam Swift, the nurse mentioned earlier, is helping women with AIDS overcome feelings of disenfranchisement through her health education efforts in the schools and through the support group she is establishing.

Disadvantaged Status

Thus, in many ways, vulnerable groups have limited control over potential and actual health needs. Since these groups are in the minority, they are more **disadvantaged** than others because typical health planning focuses on the majority. Ironically, traditional public health emphasis on the utilitarian value of "the greatest good for the greatest number" places vulnerable populations at a disadvantage. Disadvantage also results from lack of resources that others may take for granted. Vulnerable population groups have limited social and economic resources with which to manage their health care. The Family Resiliency Model predicts that families who have access to adequate resources are better able to withstand stressors effectively (McCubbin and McCubbin, 1991). For example, women sometimes choose to tolerate domestic violence rather than risk losing a place for themselves and their children to live. Women who are among the working poor are more likely to become homeless when they leave an abusive partner. They may not have adequate financial resources to pay for a place to live when they lose their partners' income. In their epidemiological study of the effects of undesirable life events, McLeod and Kessler (1990) found that lower socioeconomic status resulted in ". . . pervasive disadvantages inherent in the lives of persons who occupy lower-status positions" (p. 169). These disadvantages resulted not only from inadequate financial resources, but also from poor coping skills, low self-esteem, and a sense of powerlessness.

Powerlessness

Moccia and Mason (1986) stated that poverty is a power issue because it involves a lack of control over critical resources needed to function effectively in society. In contemporary American society, money is one of the most critical resources; insufficient financial means put individuals in dependent positions and further removes control over choices between available options. In addition, insufficient financial resources limit the degree of participation they may have in making decisions that will affect them, thus limiting their potential to influence even the kinds of options available to them. In the past, community health planning efforts were often unintentionally patriarchal. Health professionals thought they knew better than lay people which health needs were most im-

portant and the best ways to provide services to meet those needs. This belief is changing because community health professionals emphasize empowering vulnerable groups and working as partners with them.

Health Risk

Vulnerable populations not only experience multiple, cumulative risks, but they seem to be particularly sensitive to the effects of those risks. Risks may originate in environmental hazards (e.g., lead exposure from peeling, lead-based paint) or social hazards (e.g., crime and violence), in personal behavior (e.g., diet and exercise habits), or from biological or genetic makeup (e.g., congenital addiction or compromised immune status). Members of vulnerable populations often have comorbidities, or multiple illnesses, with each affecting the other. These elements of multiple risk factors, cumulative effects of risk factors, and low thresholds for risk must be addressed when assessing the needs of vulnerable populations and designing services for them.

PREDISPOSING FACTORS
Socioeconomic Status

Social and economic factors predispose people to vulnerability. Economically, poverty is a primary cause of vulnerability and is a growing problem in the United States (Pesznecker, 1984). Poverty is a relative state. The federal definition of poverty is used to develop eligibility criteria for entitlement and other programs. According to *Healthy People 2000* (1991, p. 29) "Nearly 1 of every 8 Americans lives in a family with an income below the Federal poverty level." In 1994, the **Federal poverty level** for a family of four was $14,800 for all states except Hawaii, Alaska, and the District of Columbia (Superintendent of Documents, 1994). However, many people who earn just a little more than the federal poverty level are not able to manage their living expenses and are not eligible for assistance programs. Poverty causes vulnerability by making it more difficult for people to function in society. It is often difficult for a young family with an employed father in the home to obtain financial support from social services, even if the father is earning less money than the family needs. A family such as this is considered **near poor;** sometimes in these situations, families decide they would be better off financially if the fathers were absent because they become eligible for welfare. Vulnerability results from families' efforts to do what is necessary to manage, even though it is disruptive to the family system.

People who do not have the financial resources to pay for medical care are considered **medically indigent.** They may be self-employed or work in small businesses and are unable to afford health benefits. Some people have inadequate health insurance coverage. This may be because either their deductibles and copayments are so high they have to pay for most expenses out-of-pocket or because few conditions or services are covered. In these situations, poverty in its relative sense causes vulnerability because uninsured and underinsured people are less likely to seek preventive health services because of the expense and are more likely to suffer the consequences of preventable illnesses.

Currently, the structure of health care reimbursement policies (and the mood of the United States in general) is based more on a **market model** than on a human service model. This type of model perpetuates inequities in service availability and accessibility. The market model assumes that people who have the resources to purchase services are the ones entitled to those services. Individuals unable to purchase services must somehow not be "fit" to receive services. Moccia and Mason (1986) observed that Social Darwinism is a subtle social value in the United States. **Social Darwinism** refers to the idea of survival of the fittest in relation to the ability to purchase goods and services. Social Darwinism conflicts with the belief that at least some basic level of health care is a right and should be provided regardless of ability to pay. The two perspectives reflect the controversy in health care reform over how involved the government should be in providing health and social services to vulnerable groups.

One of the problems that results from this idea, whether intentional or not, is that policies that reflect this posture reinforce a cycle that may be almost impossible for disenfranchised individuals and groups to break out of (Curtin, 1986). For example, groups who are unable to afford adequate preventive services are likely to develop more chronic diseases, which further deplete the human potential in those groups. This is referred to as a drain on **human capital,** where human capital means that the potential of all people in the community is a valuable resource. Depletion of health status results in decreased human capital and limits the abilities of group members to obtain employment, seek advanced education, or do the things leading to improvement of their situations in society. Not only does poor health lead to reduced human capital, but also reduction in human capital leads to higher overall levels of health risks (Aday, 1993). Ultimately the whole community suffers if the potential of its members is limited.

In addition to economic status, **social isolation** is strongly related to vulnerability. In one study of gay men with AIDS (Rabkin et al., 1993), the researchers found that the men were optimistic, although they did not deny the severity of their illnesses, and displayed high levels of psychological **resilience.** The researchers attributed this to the fact that almost all the men reported having confidants, or "someone who was 'there' for them" (p. 167). Similarly, Hogan and DeSantis (1994) reported that adolescents who had experienced the death of a sibling were helped when they felt that their friends were "there for them."

Age-related Causes

Vulnerable groups may share certain physiological and developmental characteristics that predispose them to unique risks. Among these, *age* is probably the most central variable. It has long been known that clients at the extreme ends of the age continuum are less able physiologically to adapt to stressors. For example, infants of substance-abusing mothers risk being born addicted and having severe physiolog-ical problems and developmental delays. Elderly individuals are more likely to develop active infections from communicable diseases such as TB and generally have more difficulty recovering from infectious processes than younger people because of their less effective immune systems. Chapter 37 discusses substance abuse, and Chapter 39 describes communicable disease risk.

It seems that certain individuals are vulnerable at particular ages because of the interaction between crucial developmental characteristics and socioeconomic tensions. For example, adolescent females (especially those under age 14 years) are more likely to deliver low-birth-weight infants than women in their twenties, probably because of physiological variables (Yoos, 1987), although socioeconomic conditions may play an equally important role (Trussell, 1988). An inability to afford prenatal care, lack of awareness of the existence of or importance of prenatal care, and a tendency to seek such care later in pregnancy than older mothers also contribute to poor pregnancy outcomes of adolescent females. Chapter 34 describes adolescent pregnancy in more detail.

Health-related Causes

Alteration in normal physiological status predisposes individuals to vulnerability. This may result from disease processes, such as in someone with single or multiple concomitant chronic diseases. Infection with HIV is a good example of a pathophysiological situation that increases vulnerability to opportunistic infections such as MAC because of immunodeficiency. Chapter 40 describes HIV, hepatitis, and STDs in detail. Physiological alterations may also result from accidents, injuries, or congenital problems leading to mental or physiological disability. Elderly individuals often exhibit vulnerability resulting both from age and from multiple chronic illnesses. Isaac Rood exemplifies this combination of vulnerability caused by age and chronic illness. Both factors result in limitations in functional status for many elderly persons, thereby leading to vulnerability to safety hazards and to loss of independence. Chapter 30 discusses elder health. Physically compromised individuals are another example of a vulnerable group, as discussed in Chapter 31.

Life Experiences

One's life experiences, especially experiences early in life, influence development of psychological vulnerability or resilience. For example, children who survive disasters may experience difficulties in later life if they do not receive adequate counseling (Yule, 1992). Internal locus of control appears to protect children (particularly adolescents) from the negative effects of disaster (Kimchi and Schaffner, 1990; Yule, 1992). Vulnerable population groups often develop an external locus of control. They may believe that events are outside their control and result from bad luck or fate. An external locus of control makes it more difficult for people to initiate action or to seek care for health problems. Such a point of view may make a person believe that health promotion and illness prevention activities are unimportant or ineffective because they do not believe they have much personal control over their own health status. Extroversion and flexibility are other personality characteristics that appear to be protective factors against early adversity (Yule, 1992). People who have been abused or those who have experienced chronic stressors throughout life may have depleted the reserves that others would normally have for coping with new stressors (Nurius et al., 1992).

OUTCOMES OF VULNERABILITY

Outcomes of vulnerability may be negative, such as lower health status than the rest of the population, or they may be positive with effective interventions. For example, culturally competent, family-focused community health nursing interventions may improve vulnerable populations' health status and empower such groups to promote their own health. Figure 32-2 illustrates the relationship between predisposing factors for vulnerability and outcomes of vulnerability.

Poor Health Outcomes

Vulnerable populations typically have worse health outcomes than others in terms of morbidity and mortality. These groups have high prevalence of chronic illnesses, such as hypertension, and high levels of communicable diseases, such as TB, HBV, STDs, and upper respiratory illnesses, including influenza. They have high mortality rates from crime and violence, including domestic violence. It is not clear whether their mortality rates from other chronic and acute health problems are higher than in the population as a whole; this is an area that would be useful for community health nurses to research. Other types of health outcomes that deserve further study include functional status, overall perception of physical and emotional well-being, quality of life, and satisfaction with health services.

Chronic Stress

Poor health creates stress as individuals and families try to manage health problems with inadequate resources. For example, if someone with AIDS develops one or more opportunistic infections and is either uninsured or underinsured, that person and the family and caregivers will have more difficulty managing than if that person had adequate insurance. Vulnerable populations typically cope with multiple stressors, so managing multiple stressors creates a sort of "domino effect," with chronic stress likely to result. This can lead to feelings of hopelessness. Evelyn, in the case of Isaac Rood described earlier, may very well feel hopeless in her situation.

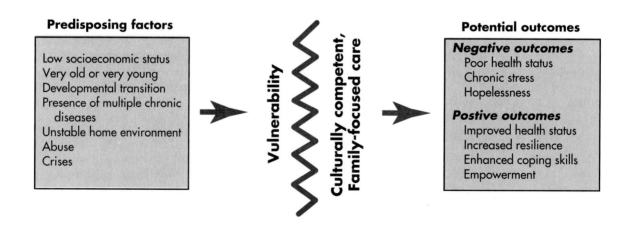

FIGURE 32-2

Predisposing factors for vulnerability and potential outcomes of vulnerability.

Hopelessness

Hopelessness results from an overwhelming sense of powerlessness and social isolation. For example, substance abusers who feel powerless over their addiction and who have isolated themselves from the people they care about may believe that no way exists to change their situation. Feelings of hopelessness contribute to a continuing cycle of vulnerability.

Cycle of Vulnerability

The factors that predispose people to vulnerability and the outcomes of vulnerability create a cycle in which the outcomes reinforce the predisposing factors, leading to even more negative outcomes. Figure 32-3 depicts this **cycle of vulnerability.** Unless the cycle is broken, it is difficult for vulnerable populations to change their health status. Community health nurses identify areas where they can work with vulnerable populations to break the cycle. The nursing process guides community health nurses in *assessing* vulnerable individuals, families, groups, and communities; developing *nursing diagnoses* of their strengths and needs; *planning* and *implementing* appropriate therapeutic nursing interventions in partnership with vulnerable clients; and *evaluating* the effectiveness of interventions.

ASSESSMENT ISSUES

The box on p. 636 lists guidelines for assessing members of vulnerable population groups, whether individual or families. The following discussion expands on the points listed in that box.

Nursing Conceptual Approaches

Nursing assessment of vulnerable populations may be organized around any nursing conceptual framework that takes into account the multiple stressors experienced by these groups and the particular difficulties they have managing their health. Neuman, Roy, and Orem are particularly appropriate to use with vulnerable populations. Neuman's focus on identifying stressors and lines of resistance is a useful framework for organizing a nursing assessment because vulnerable populations experience multiple, overlapping stressors. Roy's emphasis on health-promoting modes of adaptation helps the nurse emphasize client strengths that are resources for coping with stressors. Orem's self-care approach directs the nurse to assess the client's self-care needs and abilities so therapeutic nursing interventions can target self-care deficits. These three nursing models are consistent with Pesznecker's (1984) *adaptational model of poverty,* which states that poor persons possess both individual and group factors, past experiences, and coping skills that, when combined with environmental factors such as stressors and stigma, lead to either healthy or unhealthy adaptive responses. Mediating factors such as public policy and social support can influence whether health-promoting or health-damaging adaptive responses are more likely. Pesznecker's model is particularly relevant to vulnerable populations, so commu-

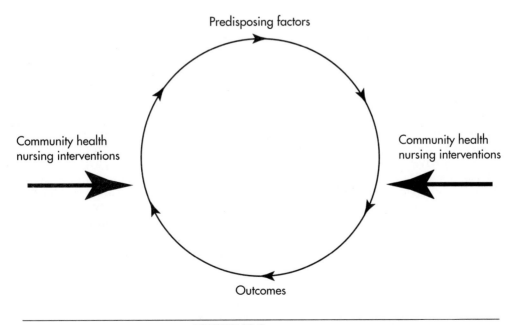

FIGURE 32-3
The cycle of vulnerability.

Guidelines for Assessing Members of Vulnerable Population Groups

SETTING THE STAGE

◆ Create a comfortable, nonthreatening environment.

◆ Learn as much as you can about the culture of the clients you work with so that you will understand cultural practices and values that may influence their health care practices.

◆ Provide culturally competent assessment by understanding the meaning of language and nonverbal behavior in the client's culture.

◆ Be sensitive to the fact that the individual or family you are assessing may have other priorities that are more important to them. These might include financial or legal problems. You may need to give them some tangible help with their most pressing priority before you will be able to address issues that are more traditionally thought of as health concerns.

◆ Collaborate with others as appropriate; you should not provide financial or legal advice. However, you should make sure to connect your client with someone who can and will help them.

NURSING HISTORY OF AN INDIVIDUAL OR FAMILY

◆ You may have only one opportunity to work with a vulnerable person or family. Try to complete a history that will provide all the essential information you need to help the individual or family on that day. This means that you will have to organize in your mind exactly what you need to ask, and no more, and why the data are necessary.

◆ It will help to use a comprehensive assessment form that has been modified to focus on the special needs of the vulnerable population group with whom you work (Fogel, 1995). However, be flexible. With some clients, it will be both impractical and unethical to cover all questions on a comprehensive form. If you

know that you are likely to see the client again, ask the less pressing questions at the next visit.

◆ Be sure to include questions about social support, economic status, resources for health care, developmental issues, current health problems, medications, and how the person or family manages their health status. Your goal is to obtain information that will enable you to provide family-centered care.

◆ Does the individual have any condition that compromises his or her immune status, such as AIDS, or is the individual undergoing therapy that would result in immunodeficiency, such as cancer chemotherapy?

PHYSICAL EXAMINATION OR HOME ASSESSMENT

◆ Again, complete as thorough a physical examination (on an individual) or home assessment as you can. Keep in mind that you should only collect data for which you have a use.

◆ Be alert for indications of physical abuse, substance use (e.g., needle marks, nasal abnormalities), or neglect (e.g., underweight, being inadequately clothed).

◆ You can assess a family's living environment using good observational skills. Does the family live in an insect- or rat-infested environment? Do they have running water, functioning plumbing, electricity, and a telephone? Is perishable food (e.g., mayonnaise) left sitting out on tables and countertops? Are bed linens reasonably clean? Is paint peeling on the walls and ceilings? Is ventilation adequate? Is the temperature of the home adequate? Is the family exposed to raw sewage or animal waste? Is the home adjacent to a busy highway, possibly exposing the family to high noise levels and automobile exhaust?

---

nity health nurses should consider using nursing conceptual frameworks that expand on Pesznecker's model as the basis for client assessment.

Because members of vulnerable populations often experience multiple stressors, nursing assessment must balance the need to be comprehensive and yet focus only on information that the nurse has a need for and that the client is willing to provide. The discussion that follows focuses on assessment of individual clients and families and on assessment of entire vulnerable population groups. With individuals and families, assessment can be intrusive and tiring, so it is important that the nurse have a reason for obtaining the data before asking the client. This means that assessing becomes an **iterative assessment process,** involving progressively more depth as the nurse refines his or her hypotheses about the nursing diagnoses.

Socioeconomic Considerations

One of the distinguishing features of vulnerable populations is their limited socioeconomic resources. Nursing assessment should include questions about the client's perceptions of his or her socioeconomic resources, including identifying people who can provide

support and financial resources. Support from other people may include information, caregiving, emotional support, and help with instrumental activities of daily living, such as transportation, shopping, and babysitting. Financial resources may include the extent to which the client can pay for health services and medications, as well as questions about eligibility for third-party payment. The nurse should ask the client about the perceived adequacy of both formal and informal support networks.

Physical Health Issues

Often, community health nurses see individual clients in clinic settings. These clients may be concerned about specific problems, which should be the initial priority. However, because vulnerable populations often find it difficult to seek routine health promotion and illness prevention services, community health nurses should take the opportunity to explain to clients the value of preventive assessment. If clients agree, nursing assessment should include evaluation of clients' preventive health needs at that time, including age-appropriate screening tests, such as immunization status, blood pressure, weight, serum cholesterol, Papanicolaou smears, breast examina-tions, mammograms, prostate examinations, glaucoma screening, and dental evaluations. It may be necessary to make referrals to have some of these tests done for clients. Assessment should also include preventive screening for physical health problems for which certain vulnerable groups are at a particularly high risk. For example, people who are HIV positive should be evaluated regularly for their T4 cell counts and for common opportunistic infections, including TB and pneumonia. Intravenous (IV) drug users should be evaluated for HBV, including liver palpation and serum antigen tests as necessary. Alcoholic clients should also be asked about symptoms of liver disease and should be evaluated for jaundice and liver enlargement. Severely mentally ill clients should be assessed for the presence of tardive dyskinesia, indicating possible toxicity from their antipsychotic medications. Chapters 33 to 40 provide more specific details about physical health assessment for vulnerable groups.

Biological Issues

Vulnerable populations should be assessed for congenital and genetic predisposition to illness and either receive education and counseling as appropriate or be referred to other health professionals as necessary. For example, pregnant adolescents who are substance abusers should be referred to programs to help them quit using addictive substances during their pregnancies and ideally after delivery of their infants as well. Pregnant women over age 35 should receive amniocentesis testing to determine if genetic abnormalities exist in the fetus. Specialized counseling about treatment and anticipatory guidance regarding the infant's needs may need to be provided by an advanced practice nurse or physician.

Psychological Issues

Vulnerable family groups should be assessed for the extent of stress the family may be experiencing and the presence of healthy or dysfunctional family dynamics. The community health nurse should also evaluate these families for effective communication patterns, caregiving capabilities, and the extent to which family developmental tasks are being met. Vulnerable individuals should be assessed for the presence of stressors, their usual coping styles, levels of **self-efficacy** (or the belief that one is capable of meeting life's challenges), their overall sense of well-being and level of self-esteem, and the presence of depression and anxiety (Berne et al., 1991; Pesznecker, 1984).

Life-style Issues

Community health nurses should assess life-style factors of vulnerable individuals, families, and groups that may predispose them to further health problems. Life-style factors include usual dietary patterns, exercise, rest, and the use of drugs, alcohol, and caffeine.

For example, many homeless individuals eat their meals either at shelters or at fast-food restaurants. Because of the unpredictability of meals and food availability, it is often difficult for them to eat a diet that is low in fat, cholesterol, and sodium, and it is particularly difficult to eat the recommended five servings of fruit and vegetables per day. Cultural preferences may also influence life-style.

Environmental Issues

Vulnerable groups are more likely to be exposed to environmental hazards than other groups. Community health nurses should assess the living environment and neighborhood surroundings of vulnerable families and groups for environmental hazards such as lead-based paint, asbestos, water and air quality, industrial wastes, and the incidence of crime. Community health nurses must often establish partnerships with vulnerable groups to put changes into place, such as persuading a local industry to reduce the levels of effluents from their plants or working with local government and law enforcement to develop crime prevention programs.

PLANNING AND IMPLEMENTING CARE FOR VULNERABLE POPULATIONS

Planning and implementing care for members of vulnerable populations involves partnership between nurse and client. If the community health nurse directs and controls the client's care, the nurse will not be able to establish a trusting relationship and may inadvertently foster a cycle of dependency and lack of personal health control. In fact, the most important initial step is for the nurse to establish that he or she is trustworthy and that the client can depend on the nurse. For example, if the nurse works in a community clinic for substance abusers, he or she must overcome any suspicion that clients may have of the nurse and eliminate any fears that the nurse will manipulate them with "games."

 Community Health Nursing Roles When Working With Vulnerable Population Groups

Case finder
Health teacher
Counselor
Direct care provider
Monitor and evaluator of care
Case manager
Advocate
Health program planner
Participant in developing health policies

Community Health Nursing Roles

Community health nurses working with vulnerable populations may fill numerous roles, including those listed in the box on p. 637. Community health nurses identify vulnerable individuals and families through **outreach** and **case finding.** They encourage vulnerable groups to obtain health services and develop programs that respond to their needs. Community health nurses *teach* vulnerable individuals, families, and groups strategies to prevent illness and promote health. They *counsel* clients about ways to increase their sense of personal power and help them identify strengths and resources (Chez, 1994). They provide *direct care* to clients and families in a variety of settings, including storefront clinics (Aiken and Salmon, 1994), mobile clinics, homes, work sites, churches, and schools. For example, a nurse in a mobile migrant clinic might administer a tetanus booster to a client who has been injured by a piece of farm machinery and may also check that client's blood pressure and cholesterol level during the same visit. A home health nurse seeing a family referred by the courts for child abuse may weigh the child, conduct a nutritional assessment, and assist the family in learning how to manage anger and disciplinary problems. A nurse working in a school-based clinic may lead a support group for pregnant adolescents and conduct a birthing class on another day during the week for the clients. Nurses working with people being treated for TB *monitor* drug treatment compliance and work with people to ensure that they complete their full course of therapy (Frieden, 1994). Community health nurses often function as *case managers* for vulnerable clients, making referrals and linking them with community services. A critical role for community health nurses is that of *advocate* for vulnerable population groups. The nurse functions as an advocate when referring clients to other agencies, when working with others to develop health programs for vulnerable population groups, and when working to influence legislation and health policies that affect vulnerable populations.

The nature of community health nurses' roles varies depending on whether the client is a single person, a family unit, or a group. For example, a community health nurse might teach an HIV-positive client about the need for prevention of opportunistic infections, or may help a family with an HIV-positive member understand myths about transmission of HIV, or may work with a community group concerned about HIV transmission among students in the schools. In each case, the nurse is teaching how to prevent infectious and communicable diseases, but the size of the client group and the teaching methodologies vary. The box on p. 639 lists principles for intervening with vulnerable populations.

Client Empowerment

Nurses should help all vulnerable groups achieve a greater sense of personal **empowerment,** since one of the core dimensions of vulnerability is a perception of powerlessness that can lead to hopelessness. Clients who feel empowered are more likely to be able to make autonomous decisions about their health care and improve their own health status. Community health nurses empower clients by helping them acquire the skills needed for healthy living and for being an effective health care consumer. For example, one of the first steps in helping abused individuals is to empower them so they can begin to help themselves. Nurses can do this through active listening, by letting clients know that what is happening to them is illegal and that all people have the right to be safe, and by reassuring them that their fears and concerns are normal (Chez, 1994). Chez also suggests assisting the client to make independent decisions and helping clients recognize the strengths they can draw on to change the situation. Some examples of actions that abused women can decide to take include seeking help, seeking shelter, moving out of the house, notifying authorities, and separating or divorcing (Nurius et al., 1992).

One way of helping people feel empowered is to ensure that health-promoting strategies are **culturally sensitive.** For instance, culturally sensitive health education strategies ensure that information is provided in language that is meaningful to the group (semantic approach to cultural sensitivity) and that the cultural context is taken into account (instrumental approach to cultural sensitivity) as the educational program is designed (Bayer, 1994). Culturally sensitive health education strategies are based on respect for cultural diversity and demonstrate that the culture of the participants is respected.

Sometimes, the first step in empowering clients is functioning as an advocate for them, especially in the policy arena, where vulnerable populations may not always be represented. For example, in one commu-

---

What Do You Think?

Bayer (1994) says that public health professionals should not worry about being culturally sensitive when the values of a population subgroup threaten that group's health. According to the principled approach to cultural sensitivity, health professionals should not attempt to change cultural barriers to healthy behaviors because that would amount to imposing the values of the dominant group on the minority group (Bayer, 1994). Is this an example of the dominant culture being paternalistic and not respecting cultural diversity, or is it necessary to ignore cultural barriers to health when the public health at large is likely to be affected?

Principles for Intervening with Vulnerable Populations

GOALS

◆ Set reasonable goals that are based on the baseline data you collected. Remember that many of the U.S. national health goals in *Healthy People* 2000 for special population groups are not set as high as those for the population as a whole to allow for realistic progress. Later, as baseline indicators improve, higher goal thresholds should be set.

◆ Work toward setting manageable goals with the client. Goals that seem unattainable may be discouraging.

◆ Set goals collaboratively with the client as a first step toward client empowerment.

◆ Set family-centered, culturally sensitive goals.

INTERVENTIONS

◆ Set up outreach and case-finding programs to help increase access to health services by vulnerable populations.

◆ Do everything you can to minimize the "hassle factor" connected with the interventions you plan. Vulnerable groups do not have the extra energy, money, or time to cope with unnecessary waits, complicated treatment plans, or confusion. As your client's advocate, you should identify what hassles may occur and develop ways to avoid them. For example, this may include providing comprehensive services during a single encounter, rather than asking the client to return for multiple visits. Multiple visits for

more specialized aspects of the client's needs, whether individual or family group, reinforce a perception that health care is fragmented and organized for the professional's convenience rather than the client's.

◆ Work with clients to ensure that interventions are culturally sensitive and competent.

◆ Focus on teaching clients skills in health promotion and disease prevention. Also, teach them how to be effective health care consumers. For example, role play, asking questions in a physician's office with a client. Help clients learn what to do if they cannot keep an appointment with a health care or social service professional.

EVALUATING OUTCOMES

◆ It is often difficult for vulnerable clients to return for follow-up care. Help your client develop self-care strategies for evaluating outcomes. For example, teach homeless individuals how to read their own TB skin test, and give them a self-addressed, stamped card they can return by mail with the results.

◆ Remember to evaluate outcomes in terms of the goals you have mutually agreed on with the client. For example, one outcome for a homeless person receiving isoniazid therapy for TB might be that the person returned to the clinic daily for direct observation of the compliance with the drug therapy.

---

nity a nursing student learned that a social service agency had restrictive policies toward serving homeless alcoholic men. This was the primary agency that could provide shelter for these men, but their restrictive policies made it difficult for the men to obtain shelter as often as necessary. After advocating for the needs of this vulnerable population and persuading the agency to relax their policies, this nurse participated on the board of the agency to ensure that their policies continued to meet the needs. Providing shelter made it more likely that the men could get adequate rest, bathe, and dress in clean clothes so they could look for jobs, empowering them to become more self-sufficient.

Levels of Prevention

Healthy People 2000 objectives emphasize preventing illness and promoting health. One way to do this is for vulnerable individuals to have a primary care provider who both coordinates health services for them and provides their preventive services. This primary care provider may be an advanced practice nurse or a primary care physician (e.g., a family practice physician). Another approach is for a community health nurse to serve as a case manager for vulnerable clients and, again, coordinate services and provide illness prevention and health promotion services.

One example of *primary prevention* recommended for certain vulnerable groups is that HIV-positive individuals who live in homeless shelters receive prophy-

lactic drug therapy for TB. Anastasi and Rivera (1994) explain that prophylactic drug treatment for people who are HIV positive may be either primary or secondary. The goal of primary drug treatment is to ". . . prevent or delay the onset of symptoms of reactivated as well as newly acquired infections. The goal of secondary prophylaxis is to prevent or delay recurrent episodes of symptomatic infection. Both are intended to reduce the number of episodes of infection over a person's lifetime" (Anastasi and Rivera, 1994, p. 37). Another example of primary prevention is administering influenza vaccinations to vulnerable populations who are immunocompromised unless contraindicated. An example of *secondary prevention* is conducting screening clinics for vulnerable populations. For example, nurses who work in homeless shelters, prisons, migrant camps, and substance abuse treatment facilities should know that these groups are at a high risk for acquiring communicable diseases. Both clients and staff need routine screening for TB (see box on p. 640). An example of *tertiary prevention* is conducting a therapy group with the residents of a group home for severely mentally ill adults. Community health nurses who work with abused women to help them enhance their levels of self-esteem are also providing tertiary preventive activities.

Strategies for Promoting Healthy Life-styles

Helping members of vulnerable populations develop healthy life-style behaviors requires great sensitivity

Primary and Secondary Prevention for Populations at Risk for Communicable Diseases

People who spend time in homeless shelters, substance abuse treatment facilities, and prisons risk acquiring communicable diseases such as influenza and TB. Nurses who work in these facilities should plan regular influenza vaccination clinics and TB screening clinics. When planning these clinics, community health nurses should work with local physicians to develop signed protocols and should plan ahead for problems related to the transient nature of the population. For example, nurses should develop a way for homeless individuals to read their TB skin tests if necessary and transfer the results back to the facility where the skin test was administered. It is helpful to develop a portable immunization chart, such as a wallet card, that mobile population groups such as the homeless and migrant workers can carry with them.

by community health nurses. Community health nurses should focus on identifying clients' priorities and helping them meet these priorities. For example, discussing exercise with a homeless person requires empathy and creativity. Often, vulnerable individuals and families are coping with crises, so the nurse must begin by using crisis intervention strategies. After the crisis has been managed, a trusting relationship is likely to exist between the nurse and client, so this interpersonal relationship forms the basis for health promotion interventions. Community health nurses must be sensitive to the life-styles of their vulnerable clients and must develop methods of health promotion that recognize these life-style factors. For instance, Brennan's ComputerLink program for people with AIDS provides personal computers in the homes of people with AIDS and enables them to obtain information about ways to maintain a high quality of life in the privacy of their homes (Brennan and Ripich, 1994). Another example is a program that was designed to encourage inner-city Latino families to increase their intake of low-fat milk (Wechsler and Wernick, 1992). This successful program included providing money-off coupons for low-fat milk, making it less costly for families to purchase the milk.

Healthy People 2000 Objectives and *Healthy Communities* 2000 Standards

The *Healthy People 2000* objectives emphasize illness prevention and health promotion. Objectives have been developed for health promotion, health protection, preventive services, and surveillance and data systems. Objectives that are relevant for vulnerable populations may be found in several areas. Within the health promotion category are objectives related to alcohol and other drugs, mental health and mental disorders, and violent and abusive behavior. Within the preventive services category are objectives targeting maternal and infant health, HIV infection, STDs,

and immunization and infectious diseases. Specific age-related objectives have been developed, as have objectives for special populations. The special population category for low-income persons is directly related to the vulnerable populations described in this chapter. The other special population categories are blacks, Hispanics, Asians and Pacific Islanders, American Indians and Native Americans, and people with disabilities. These categories overlap with many of the vulnerable populations described in this chapter, although it would not be accurate to say that all members of any one of these groups are vulnerable. However, many minority populations are disproportionately represented in vulnerable groups, so community health nurses should focus special attention on the health objectives for the special populations identified in *Healthy People 2000.*

The *Healthy People 2000* objectives include targets for improvement over baseline incidence and prevalence statistics on illness and health problems. Many objectives include unique targets for special population subgroups that have incidence and prevalence statistics that are much higher than for the population as a whole. For example, one of the physical activity objectives for lower-income adults is to "increase to at least 12% the proportion of people who engage in vigorous physical activity that promotes the development and maintenance of cardiorespiratory fitness 3 or more days per week." The target proportion for the population as a whole is 20% and is higher because their baseline level of 12% is higher than the baseline level of 7% for low-income adults. These targets are designed to be realistic improvements over the baseline levels. Communities should determine local incidence and prevalence statistics and establish realistic targets for improvement. For example, it would be unrealistic to establish the same goals for reducing the incidence of HIV infection for IV drug users as for the general population because the baseline rates are so much higher for IV drug users and because their risks are so much greater. Rather, community health nurses should work with local groups to establish goals and objectives that are substantially better than baseline rates but are potentially achievable. Later goals will use the new baselines, and the health status of the vulnerable population group should continuously improve.

A group of public health professionals representing several different agencies, including the American Public Health Association and the Centers for Disease Control and Prevention, developed a guide to help individual communities meet the *Healthy People 2000* national health objectives in their own areas. This guide, entitled *Healthy Communities 2000: Model Standards* (APHA, 1991), describes ways that communities can establish health objectives that are consistent with national health objectives but realistic for local communities. It also suggests activities to achieve local health objectives and ways to determine the capacity of the local health department to implement the activities and emphasizes developing partnerships with other agencies.

Comprehensive Services

In general, more agencies are needed that provide **comprehensive services** with nonrestrictive eligibility requirements. Communities often have many agencies that restrict eligibility for their services to people most likely to benefit from those services, or they limit eligibility to make it possible for more people to receive services. For example, shelters may prohibit people who have been drinking alcohol from staying overnight and sometimes limit the number of sequential nights a person can stay. Food banks usually limit the number of times a person can receive free food. Agencies are frequently very specialized as well. For vulnerable individuals and families, this means that they must go to many agencies to find services for which they qualify and that meet their needs. This is so tiring and discouraging that people are sometimes willing to forego help because it is just too difficult to obtain it. In their study of admission policies in homeless shelters for women in Chicago, Barge and Norr (1991) found that most shelters limited the numbers of pregnant women, women with children, and especially women with teenage boys. It is very difficult to help these clients achieve health promotion and illness prevention objectives if they have difficulty meeting basic needs for shelter.

Resources for Vulnerable Populations

Community health nurses should be thoroughly familiar with community agencies that offer a wide variety of health and social services for vulnerable populations. Nurses should also follow up with the client after the referral if at all possible to ensure that the desired outcomes were achieved. Sometimes, excellent community resources may be available, but are impractical for clients because of transportation or reimbursement problems. Community health nurses should identify if these problems will interfere with clients following through with referrals and work with other team members to make the referral as convenient and realistic as possible. Although clients with social problems such as financial needs should be referred to social workers, community health nurses should understand the close connections between health and social problems and know how to work effectively with other professionals. A list of community resources can often be found in the telephone book, and many communities have publications that list community resources. Examples of agency resources found in most communities are:

◆ Health departments
◆ Community mental health centers
◆ American Red Cross
◆ Food and clothing banks
◆ Missions and shelters
◆ Nurse-managed neighborhood clinics
◆ Social service agencies such as Travelers' Aid and Salvation Army
◆ Church-sponsored health and social service assistance

Did You Know?

Referring clients to community agencies involves much more than simply picking up the phone and making a call or completing a form (Will, 1977). You should be certain that the agency to which you are referring a client is the right one to meet that client's needs. Nurses can do more harm than good by referring a stressed, discouraged client to an agency from which the client is not really eligible to receive services. Be sure to help the client learn how to get the most from the referral.

Two other very important categories of resources for vulnerable populations are their own personal coping skills and social supports (McLeod and Kessler, 1990). These groups must often be quite resourceful and creative to manage in the face of multiple stressors. Community health nurses should work with clients to help them identify their own personal strengths and draw on those strengths when managing their health needs. Also, clients may be able to depend on informal support networks. Even though social isolation is a problem for many vulnerable clients, community health nurses should not assume that clients have no one who can help them.

Case Management

Case management involves linking client with services and providing direct nursing services to clients, such as teaching, counseling, screening, and immunizing (Bower, 1992). Lillian Wald was the first nurse case manager, linking vulnerable families with the wide variety of services needed to help them stay healthy (Buhler-Wilkerson, 1993). Aiken and Salmon (1994, p. 327) explain that ". . . public health nurses represent the interface between personal health services and population-based health promotion." Linking, or **brokering health services,** is accomplished by making appropriate referrals and by following up with clients to ensure that the desired outcomes from the referral were achieved. Nurses have been effective case managers in community nursing clinics, in health departments, and in case management programs where the focus included both community and hospi-

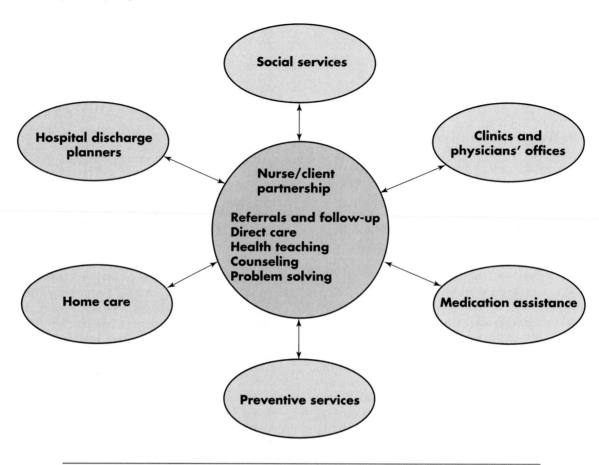

FIGURE 32-4

The community health nurse as case manager for vulnerable populations.

tal care. Community health nurse case managers emphasize health promotion and illness prevention with vulnerable clients and focus on helping them avoid unnecessary hospitalization. Figure 32-4 illustrates the coordination and brokering aspect of the nurse's role as case manager for vulnerable populations.

EVALUATION OF NURSING INTERVENTIONS WITH VULNERABLE POPULATIONS

Evaluation of therapeutic nursing interventions begins with client goals and objectives and *focuses on the extent to which client health outcomes were achieved.* Nurses may evaluate individual client goal achievement, the extent to which a vulnerable family achieved goals developed in partnership with the nurse, or the extent to which a nursing program achieved its objectives. Evaluation takes place while providing care and gives the

nurse a basis for revising therapeutic interventions to make them more effective. Evaluation also takes place when a case is closed or when a program is completed and gives nurses data to use in providing care to similar clients or programs in the future. The types of client outcomes that may be evaluated include improved quality of life, improved indicators of physical health status (e.g., blood pressure, skin integrity, mobility), reduced depression or anxiety, improved functional status, increased levels of knowledge about health behaviors, and satisfaction with care. Nurses use a variety of scales to evaluate these outcome indicators; they sometimes interview clients or administer short questionnaires; and they use laboratory reports and results of health assessments to help evaluate goal achievement with individuals and clients. Incidence and prevalence data, survey data, and service utilization data are used to evaluate health programs for vulnerable populations.

Clinical Application

Use the ideas presented in this chapter to analyze the following situation. Focus on a broad range of issues, including socioeconomic concerns, physical and psychological health issues, and environmental issues. Develop strategies that will help empower this client and break the cycle of vulnerability. Review the nurse's role as a case manager shown in Figure 32-4 to help you identify ideas about therapeutic interventions that may help empower this client.

Imagine you are a nurse in a migrant clinic. Several days ago, Dorothy, a 40-year-old farm worker who is pregnant with her fifth child, came in requesting treatment for swollen ankles. During your *assessment*, Dorothy told you she went to the prenatal clinic at the local health department once a couple of months ago. She was given a couple of sample bottles of vitamins, but she lost them. She is on a waiting list to receive free obstetrical care but does not expect to reach the top of the list before her due date. Her four prior pregnancies were fairly uneventful, although she mentions that she became "toxic" with her last child. She also commented that the middle child, Bobby, had never been "right," but that she guessed he got along okay. Bobby is now 15 years old and in the seventh grade. Dorothy's blood pressure today is 160/90, and she has pitting edema up to her ankles. She said that a physician once told her she should watch her blood pressure, but she has never taken medication for it. She is 5 feet 2 inches tall and weighs 170 pounds.

Dorothy says that she normally takes chlorpromazine hydrochloride (Thorazine), but she ran out of it 3 weeks ago and has not had the money to have the prescription refilled. She did not mention this medication to the nurse practitioner who saw her at the prenatal clinic. She says that she has been in several mental hospitals over the last few years, depending on the state in which she is working. Usually, she becomes increasingly more agitated and has difficulty managing her daily activities, such as caring for her children and keeping house. This is very stressful for her, and as she becomes more and more agitated, she usually begins hearing voices and behaving aggressively.

Dorothy's plans for caring for her infant are vague and include asking her boyfriend for help. He is a race track worker; he and Dorothy usually move from one state to another together. Her other four children range in age from 12 to 23 years. None of them is with her. The two oldest live in another state; the third child lives with the biological father; and the youngest, a son, ran away several months ago.

What other information would you want to help you assess this client's situation? What *nursing diagnoses* are suggested by the brief historical, physical, and socioeconomic data presented here? Which of the potential diagnoses should you focus your efforts on today? Why?

Based on your assessment, you decide it is important to check Dorothy for proteinuria. Her urine specimen is positive for protein (1+) and negative for glucose. Her hands and face seem somewhat swollen, and she has a mild headache. Dorothy has become increasingly agitated as you complete your assessment. She mentions that she is tired and wants to get something to eat. Which *short-term goals* do you think would be most appropriate to focus on today? What *long-term goals* would you want to discuss with Dorothy?

At this point, your *plan* is to contact the health department and make an appointment for her to be seen within the next day or two. She agrees to this but does not seem particularly committed to it. You also suggest that she go to the nearby shelter for a meal and to relax in the lounge area at the shelter. What other plans might help you handle Dorothy's immediate problems? Which therapeutic nursing interventions should you use to manage the long-term problems suggested in this vignette? Give some examples of types of agencies and community resources that might be able to provide services that Dorothy needs. How should you coordinate these services most effectively? How would you function as a case manager in this situation?

Your *interventions* went fairly smoothly. You were able to set up an appointment for Dorothy at the health department later in the afternoon with the same nurse practitioner she had seen earlier. However, because the health department is 5 miles away, you need to help her find transportation. Dorothy went to the shelter and ate lunch, although you learned from the nurse at the shelter that it was high in sodium. Dorothy had a bologna and cheese sandwich, an apple, some carrot sticks and dip, chips, and milk. What *outcome criteria* should you use to evaluate the effectiveness of your interventions so far? How would you evaluate the effectiveness of other therapeutic interventions you may have discussed in class?

Three weeks have passed since you first met Dorothy. A social worker has been working with her to find more stable housing than she has in the migrant camp, especially since it is now October and the camp will close soon. The nurse practitioner at the health department has been monitoring Dorothy carefully and finally referred her to the local hospital, where she was admitted last week with preeclampsia. She is now eligible for free obstetrical care and is happy with her obstetrician. Dorothy met with a therapist at the local community mental health center for counseling and monitoring her psychiatric condition. How would you *evaluate* the effectiveness of your interventions?

Key Concepts

◆ Vulnerable populations are more likely to develop health problems as a result of exposure to risk or to have worse outcomes from those health problems than the population as a whole. Vulnerable populations are more sensitive to risk factors than those who are more resilient and are more often exposed to cumulative risk factors. These populations include poor or homeless persons, pregnant adolescents, migrant workers, severely mentally ill individuals, substance abusers, abused individuals, people with communicable diseases, and people with sexually transmitted diseases, including HIV and HBV.

◆ Health care is increasingly moving into the community. This began with deinstitutionalization of the severely mentally ill population and is continuing today as hospitals reduce inpatient stays. Vulnerable populations need a wide variety of services, and because these are often provided by multiple community agencies, community health nurses coordinate and manage the service needs of vulnerable groups.

◆ Public policies sometimes provide financial assistance for vulnerable populations and sometimes provide money to build health facilities and train professionals to work with vulnerable groups. Unanticipated implementation problems often further disadvantage vulnerable populations. Health care reform policies are focused on controlling costs and may have the unintended effect of limiting services to vulnerable populations.

◆ The health field concept suggests that both individuals and society are responsible for health status. Individuals and groups may be vulnerable to social and health problems both as a result of their own actions and the policies and decisions made at the societal level. There are many dimensions to vulnerability, including limited control over one's own health, victimization, disenfranchisement, disadvantaged status, powerlessness, and cumulative health risks.

◆ Socioeconomic problems, including poverty and social isolation, physiological and developmental aspects of age, poor health status, and highly stressful life experiences, predispose people to vulnerability. Vulnerability can become a cycle, where the predisposing factors lead to poor health outcomes, chronic stress, and hopelessness. These outcomes increase vulnerability.

◆ Community health nurses assess vulnerable individuals, families, and groups to determine which socioeconomic, physical, biological, psychological, and environmental factors are problematic for clients. They work as partners with vulnerable clients to identify client strengths and needs and develop intervention strategies designed to break the cycle of vulnerability.

◆ Community health nursing roles when working with vulnerable populations include health teacher, counselor, direct care provider, case manager, advocate, health program planner, and participant in developing health policies. Nurses focus on empowering clients to prevent illness and promote health, and they work to achieve the *Healthy People 2000* national health objectives with vulnerable populations. Community health nurses link clients with resources in the community and monitor client outcomes to ensure that community referrals are effective.

◆ Evaluation of therapeutic nursing interventions with vulnerable populations occurs both during and after service delivery. Results of evaluations are used to make revisions in nursing care, with the ultimate goal of improving client outcomes.

Critical Thinking Activities

1. Examine health statistics and demographic data in your geographical area to determine which vulnerable groups predominate in your area. Look through your phone book for examples of agencies that you think provide services to these vulnerable groups. Make appointments with key individuals in several of these agencies to discuss the nature of their target population, the types of services provided, and the reimbursement mechanisms for these services. Various class members should visit different agencies and then share their results during class. Based on your findings, identify gaps or overlaps in services provided to vulnerable groups in your community. What might be some ways to manage these gaps and overlaps to help clients receive the services they need?

2. Debate with your class the nature and extent of services that you believe should be made available to the homeless. Defend your position regarding "enabling" and "worthiness."

3. Health care spending accounts for about 14% of the gross domestic product (GDP). Most people do not want to spend any more of the GDP on health care. Assuming then that the amount of money available to spend on health care is fixed at any point in time, explain what proportion of that money you think the federal government should spend on prevention and treatment of AIDS, substance abuse, severe mental illness, and breast cancer. What criteria did you use to arrive at your conclusions?

4. To what extent do you think economic issues and social values play a role in the way that health services are offered to vulnerable population groups? Explain why you think the population as a whole should or should not pay for care for vulnerable groups. Read the article by Grey (1994) in the reference list on the development of health services for migrant workers for an example of this debate.

5. Discuss the types of assistance you might provide to the following clients:
   a. A chronically homeless, pregnant, 33-year-old, mildly mentally retarded woman and her unemployed boyfriend
   b. A 14-year-old runaway girl who is earning money through prostitution and has a drug habit
   c. A 22-year-old woman with four children who is receiving welfare and whose boyfriend smokes crack cocaine
   d. An HIV-positive woman with no family and few friends who is trying to make plans for someone to care for her three children after her death
   e. A 56-year-old alcoholic male migrant farm worker whose TB skin test just came back positive

   What kinds of nursing needs do these clients have in common? Analyze the dimensions of vulnerability described in this chapter in terms of how these clients may possess these characteristics and how you, as a community health nurse, can help them break out of the cycle of vulnerability.

6. Examine the pros and cons of school-based clinics for adolescents. Do you think reproductive services should be included in such clinics? What are the ethical issues involved in providing reproductive information to adolescents, with or without parental consent and involvement?

7. Interview nurses at a health department to identify which personal care services they provide to vulnerable populations and which population-based services they provide. Discuss their opinions about whether personal care services should only be provided by private agencies.

Bibliography

AAN Expert Panel Report: Culturally competent health care, *Nurs Outlook* 40(6):277-283, 1992.

Aday LA: *At risk in America: the health and health care needs of vulnerable populations in the United States,* San Francisco, 1993, Jossey Bass.

Aiken LH, Salmon ME: Health care workforce priorities: what nursing should do now, *Inquiry* 31(3):318-329, 1994.

American Nurses Association: Nursing's agenda for health care reform, Kansas City, Mo, 1991, The Association.

American Public Health Association: *Health communities 2000: model standards,* ed 3, Washington, DC, 1991, The Association.

Anastasi JK, Rivera J: Understanding prophylactic therapy for HIV infections, *Am J Nurs* 94(2):36-41, 1994.

Avey MA: TB skin testing: how to do it right, *Am J Nurs* 93(9):42-44, 1993.

Baker EL, Melton RJ, Stange PV, Fields ML, Koplan JP, Guerra FA,

Satcher D: Health reform and the health of the public: forging community health partnerships, *JAMA* 272(16):1276-1282, 1994.

Barge FC, Norr KF: Homeless shelter policies for women in an urban environment, *Image J Nurs Scholarship* 23(3):145-149, 1991.

Bayer R: AIDS prevention and cultural sensitivity: are they compatible? *Am J Public Health* 84(6):895-898, 1994.

Benenson AS: *Control of communicable diseases in man,* ed 15, Washington, DC, 1990, American Public Health Association.

Berne AS, Dato C, Mason DJ, Rafferty M: A nursing model for addressing the health needs of homeless families, *Image J Nurs Scholarship* 22(1):8-13, 1991.

Bower KA: *Case management by nurses,* Kansas City, Mo, 1992, American Nurses Association.

Brennan PF, Ripich S: Use of a home-care computer network by persons with AIDS, *Int J Technol Assess Health Care* 10(2):258-272, 1994.

Briere JN, Elliott DM: Immediate and long-term impacts of child sexual abuse, *Future Child Sex Abuse Child* 4(2):54-69, 1994.

Buhler-Wilkerson K: Bringing care to the people: Lillian Wald's legacy to public health nursing, *Am J Public Health* 83(12):1778-1786, 1993.

Chez N: Helping the victim of domestic violence, *Am J Nurs* 94(7):32-37, 1994.

Ciesielski S, Esposito D, Protiva J, Piehl M: The incidence of tuberculosis among North Carolina migrant farmworkers, 1991, *Am J Public Health* 84(11):1836-1838, 1994.

Curtin L: Throwaway people? *Nurs Manage* 17(12):7-8, 1986.

Dever GEA, Sciegaj M, Wade TE: Creation of a social vulnerability index for justice in health planning, *Fam Community Health* 10(4):23-32, 1988.

Devlin BK, Reynolds E: Child abuse: how to recognize it, how to intervene, *Am J Nurs* 94(3):26-31, 1994.

Ferenchick GS: The medical problems of homeless clinic patients: a comparative study, *J Gen Intern Med* 7:294-297, 1992.

Fielding J, Halfon N: Where is the health in health system reform? *JAMA* 272(16):1292-1296, 1994.

Finklehor D: Current information on the scope and nature of child sexual abuse, *Future Child Sex Abuse Child* 4(2):31-53, 1994.

Fogel CI: *Measurement issues faced when conducting research with disadvantaged women.* Paper presented at the annual meeting of the Southern Nursing Research Society, Lexington, Ky, 1995.

Frieden TR: Tuberculosis control and social change, *Am J Public Health* 84(11):1721-1723, 1994.

Friedman E: Money isn't everything: nonfinancial barriers to access, *JAMA* 271(19):1535-1538, 1994.

Grau L: Illness-engendered poverty among the elderly, *Women Health* 12(3/4), 1987.

Grey MR: The medical care programs of the Farm Security Administration, 1932 through 1947: a rehearsal for national health insurance? *Am J Public Health* 84(10):1678-1688, 1994.

Grob G: *Mental institutions in America: social policy to 1875,* New York, 1973, Free Press of Glencoe.

Grob G: *Mental illness and American society: 1875-1940,* Princeton, NJ, 1983, Princeton University Press.

Healthy People 2000: national health promotion and disease prevention objectives, Washington, DC, 1991, USDHHS, Public Health Service.

Hogan NS, DeSantis L: Things that help and hinder adolescent sibling bereavement, *West J Nurs Res* 16(2):132-153, 1994.

Institute of Medicine: *Homelessness, health, and human needs,* Washington, DC, 1988, National Academy Press.

Ireson C, Weaver D: Marketing nursing beyond the walls, *J Nurs Adm* 22(1):57-60, 1992.

Kelleher K, Chaffin M, Hollenberg J, Fischer E: Alcohol and drug disorders among physically abusive and neglectful parents in a community-based sample, *Am J Public Health* 84(10):1586-1590, 1994.

Kimchi J, Schaffner B: Childhood protective factors and stress risks. In Arnold LE, editor: *Childhood stress,* New York, 1990, Wiley.

Kochanek KD, Maurer JD, Rosenberg HM: Why did black life expectancy decline from 1984 through 1989 in the United States? *Am J Public Health* 84(6):938-944, 1994.

Leonhardt KK, Gentile F, Gilbert BP, Aiken M: A cluster of tuberculosis among crack house contacts in San Mateo County, California, *Am J Public Health* 84(11):1834-1836, 1994.

McCubbin MA, McCubbin HI: Family stress theory and assessment: the resiliency model of family stress, adjustment, and adaptation. In McCubbin HI, Thompson AI, editors: *Family assessment inventories for research and practice,* Madison, 1991, University of Wisconsin.

McLeod JD, Kessler RC: Socioeconomic status differences in vulnerability to undesirable life events, *J Health Soc Behav* 31:162-172, 1990.

Moccia P, Mason DJ: Poverty trends: implications for nursing, *Nurs Outlook* 34(1):20, 1986.

Nichols J, Wright LK, Murphy JF: A proposal for tracking health care for the homeless, *J Community Health* 11(3):204-209, 1986.

Nurius PS, Furrey J, Berliner L: Coping capacity among women with abusive partners, *Violence Vict* 7(3):229-243, 1992.

O'Brien LM, Bartlett KA: TB Plus HIV spells trouble, *Am J Nurs* 92(5):28-34, 1992.

O'Connor FW: A vulnerability-stress framework for evaluating clinical interventions in schizophrenia, *Image J Nurs Scholarship* 26(3):231-237, 1994.

Pappas G: Elucidating the relationships between race, socioeconomic status, and health, *Am J Public Health* 84(6):892-893, 1994.

Pesznecker B: The poor: a population at risk, *Public Health Nurs* 4(1):237-249, 1984.

Rabkin JG, Remien R, Katoff L, Williams JBW: Resilience in adversity among long-term survivors of AIDS, *Hosp Community Psychiatry* 44(2):162-167, 1993.

Rosner D: Health care for the "truly needy": nineteenth-century origins of the concept, *Milbank Mem Fund Q* 60(3):355-385, 1982.

Sebastian JB: Homelessness: a state of vulnerability, *Fam Community Health* 8(3):11-24, 1985.

Shovein J, Young MS: MRSA: Pandora's box for hospitals, *Am J Nurs* 92(2):48-52, 1992.

Steinwachs DM, Cullum HM, Dorwart RA, et al: Service systems research, *Schizophr Bull* 18:627-668, 1992.

Superintendent of Documents: *Federal Register* 59(28), Washington, DC, 1994, US Government Printing Office.

Torrey EF, Erdman K, Wolfe SM, et al: *Care of the seriously mentally ill: a rating of state programs,* ed 3, Washington, DC, 1990, Public Health Citizen Health Research Group & the National Alliance for the Mentally Ill.

Trussell J: Teenage pregnancy in the United States, *Fam Plann Perspect* 20(6):262-272, 1988.

Valanis B: *Epidemiology in nursing and health care,* ed 2, East Norwalk, Conn, 1992, Appleton & Lange.

Wechsler H, Wernick SM: A social marketing campaign to promote low-fat milk consumption in an inner-city Latino community, *Public Health Rep* 107(2):202-207, 1992.

Will MB: Referral: a process, not a form, *Nursing '77* 7:44-45, 1977.

Yoos L: Perspectives on adolescent parenting: effect of adolescent egocentrism on the maternal-child interaction, *J Pediatr Nurs* 2(3):193-200, 1987.

Yule W: Resilience and vulnerability in child survivors of disasters. In Tizard B, Varma V, editors: *Vulnerability and resilience in human development,* London, 1992, Kingsley.

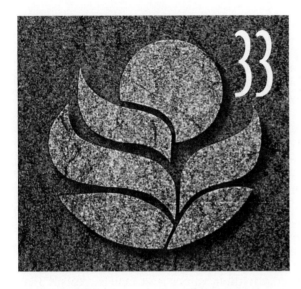

33 Poverty and Homelessness

Teresa Acquaviva ◆ Jeanette Lancaster

Objectives ▼

After reading this chapter, the student should be able to do the following:

◆ Analyze the concept of poverty.
◆ Discuss clients' perceptions about poverty and health.
◆ Describe the social, political, cultural, and environmental factors that influence poverty.
◆ Discuss the effects of poverty on the health and well-being of individuals, families, and communities.
◆ Analyze the concept of homelessness.
◆ Discuss clients' perceptions about homelessness and health.
◆ Describe the social, political, cultural, and environmental factors that influence homelessness.
◆ Discuss the effects of homelessness on the health and well-being of individuals, families, and communities.
◆ Discuss community health nursing interventions for poor and homeless individuals.

Key Terms ▼

Aid to Families with Dependent Children (AFDC)
beliefs
deinstitutionalization
federal poverty guidelines
homelessness
Interagency Council on the Homeless (ICH)
knowledge
near poor
neighborhood poverty
persistent poverty
poverty
poverty guidelines
poverty thresholds
Stewart B. McKinney Assistance Act
underclass poverty
values
Women, Infants, and Children (WIC)

Outline ▼

The concepts of poverty and homelessness are difficult for most Americans to fully understand. For a moment, imagine yourself as a 4-year-old child sleeping on the floor of a condemned apartment building, or as a middle-aged woman with diarrhea walking the street during the day and sleeping in a shelter at night, or as a homeless, aging man with edema looking for a place to rest your feet. Now imagine yourself as the community health nurse looking into the eyes of each of these individuals, knowing that it is your mission to improve their health status and ease their suffering.

Community health nurses seek to provide health care for the poor in their homes as well as on the street and in shelters, schools, churches, clinics, soup kitchens, and nurse-managed centers. To provide quality health care for poor and homeless individuals, nurses must understand the concepts of poverty and homelessness. This understanding begins with a self-examination of personal beliefs, values, and knowledge about poverty and homelessness. Next, from the poor or homeless person's perspective, the nurse must identify health care needs, barriers to care, and essential nursing services. Finally, the community health nurse must be aware of social, political, cultural, and environmental factors that influence poverty and homelessness. It is inadequate for the community health nurse to merely have empathy and compassion for poor and homeless individuals. To provide effective nursing interventions, the nurse also needs to understand the epidemiology, health problems, and risk factors associated with poverty and homelessness (Carney, 1992).

This chapter describes the many ways in which poverty and homelessness affect the health status of individuals, families, and communities. It also outlines strategies for community health nurses to use to promote the health of their poor and homeless clients.

UNDERSTANDING THE CONCEPT OF POVERTY

Understanding the concept of **poverty** necessitates considerable reflection and analysis. The community health nurse's concept of poverty is shaped and influenced by many variables, including personal beliefs, values, and knowledge of poverty; the life stories of those who experience poverty; and social, political, cultural, and environmental factors.

Personal Beliefs, Values, and Knowledge

To be effective, community health nurses must recognize the personal beliefs, values, and knowledge that serve as foundational principles for their practice. Personal **beliefs** are ideas that are thought to be true. Social **values** are ideas of life, customs, and ways of behaving that members of a society regard as desirable. **Knowledge** is an individual's known range of infor-

mation. Community health nurses should ask themselves these questions about poverty and the experience of being poor:

1. What do I believe to be true about being poor?
2. What do I personally know about poverty?
3. How have family and friends influenced my ideas and beliefs about being poor?
4. Have I personally been poor?
5. How has the media shaped my images of poverty?
6. What do I feel when I see a hungry child? A hungry adult?
7. Do I think that people are poor because they just don't try to find work? Or does society have a significant influence on one's becoming poor?
8. What causes poverty?

Although these questions may seem abstract, community health nurses are faced with concrete questions that test their values and beliefs. Nurses may more comprehensively evaluate their beliefs, values, and knowledge regarding poverty by answering the following questions that are based on possible clinical situations:

◆ What would I do if one of my homeless clients asks for change to get bus fare?
◆ What would I do in the home of an elderly client whose kitchen is covered with roaches? Where would I sit if he offers me a chair?
◆ While making a home visit in an especially unclean home, what do I do if the client asks me to eat something?

There are no easy answers to these questions, but community health nurses' responses to these questions influence their relationship with their clients who are poor. A nurse's personal response also comes into play, as illustrated by the poem in Figure 33-1.

In addition to personal beliefs, values, and knowledge, community health nurses should consider the influence that nursing theories and theories from other disciplines have on the care they provide to poor individuals (Carney, 1992). Many nursing theories are based on the assumption that human beings inherently have dignity and worth. Some theories view the human being as a system interacting with the environment. Nursing is based on valuing individuals, health, and the quality of life (Roy and Andrews, 1991). Conflicts in values, beliefs, and perceptions often arise when nurses work with persons from different social, cultural, and economic backgrounds. A lack of agreement between what professionals and clients see as a need can lead to conflict. As a result of this conflict, clients may fail to follow the prescribed treatment protocol (Merton et al., 1983); the nurse may then inaccurately interpret this behavior as resistance, lack of cooperation, or noncompliance.

Nurses should evaluate clients in the context of their environment to develop nursing interventions that meet the needs of individuals, including those who live in poverty. Treating medical problems alone is inadequate. Instead, care must be multidimensional and include biological, psychological, social, environ-

On Hearing the News of a Patient's Death

Morning light glances off the chrome
of a stripped down car in the alley
slices through window panes
along the edges of drawn shades
opens fire on sheets pulled up
to shield the eyes of sleepers.

This summer sun won't light your eyes.
Not even the cries of the baby reach you.
It's too late, for you went early
just as we thought you might
   but not like this
   manacled to a bed
   in the maternity ward
   of D.C. General Hospital.

Hearing the news, I call up your face
a wide-open face with a slow shy smile
as if the shock of life had somehow dazed
you.
You took each day
   each man
   each child
   each welfare check
   each jail cell
   as it came.

It just wasn't in you to ask why or why not
to look ahead or behind.
Since when does someone like you get to
choose?
Since when do poor ignorant women take
charge of their lives?

The world for you was
   your mother's house,
   teeming with kin
   the street
   the welfare office
   hospital and
   jail.
A heroin high was the only place you ever
   had to call your own

and a fix was the only way you knew
   to get there.
the judge decided to keep you in jail
those last few months of your pregnancy-
the best he could do for your unborn child.
Why bring another addict into the world?

Oh, it isn't that you never tried to kick.
You'd come to us in pain
   with abscesses from dirty needles.
You'd come when the drug supply dried up.
You'd come when there was no money to
   buy.
You'd come when you felt too tired to sell.
I can do it alone, you said
   I can kick.
Just give me a few Valiums.
A little help is all I need.

I suppose we'll never know just how you
   died.
It was after the baby was born
after they'd taken you back to the ward.
Some people said they heard calls for help.
When they found you, you were hanging
   over the side of the bed
   dangling by the foot
   they'd shackled to the bedframe.
Your family set up a wail that went on for
   days
   alleged foul play
   hinted at revenge.
There was gunfire at the wake, they say
and eight motherless children destined for
   your mother's house
   the street
   the welfare office
   hospital and
   jail.

The last light you saw in the blank night
   of your life
was your newborn girl.
is that why you named her Star?

Veneta Masson

FIGURE 33-1

Poetry expressing the personal response of a community health nurse to the death of a client who lived in poverty. (From Masson V: *Just who*, Washington, DC, 1993, Crossroad Health Ministry.)

mental, economic, and spiritual factors. As Hilfiker (1994, p. 211) says, "The strictly medical factors are rarely the most crucial to healing. . . . The complex interrelated web of troubles that confront the poor make it impossible to treat the medical portion of their lives in isolation."

Clients' Perceptions About Poverty and Health

Poor people are not a homogeneous group. It is essential to listen closely to clients; their life stories and the words they use can instruct nurses on what it means to be poor. In addition, the fears and misconceptions of health care providers related to poverty can create barriers that prevent them from fully engaging in relationships with those who come from different socioeconomic and cultural backgrounds. By taking the time to know clients by name and to listen to the stories of their lives, community health nurses begin the process of breaking down the barriers of fear, isolation, uncertainty, and the unknown (Figure 33-2).

The following examples provide a glimpse into the lives of some of the clients with whom the author has worked at Community Medical Care, a small nonprofit health clinic that opened its doors in 1978 to provide primary health care to persons in the Shaw neighborhood of Washington, D.C. Most of the families come from the surrounding neighborhood and Wards 7 and 8, which are known for their high infant mortality rate and lack of access to health care. Most of the clients are uninsured or have Medicaid, live on public assistance, and meet the federal government's

definition of poverty. Several clients willingly answered the following questions to provide information about their perceptions about poverty: (1) Do you think of yourself as poor? and (2) What does it mean to be poor?

◆ Demetrius, age 33, is married and the father of four children under age 10. They live in a dark efficiency apartment with a leaking roof and peeling paint in a condemned building. His response to the questions:

Being poor is when you don't have anything at all: no money, no food to put on the table, no house to go home to, no one to love you. I wouldn't trade my life for anything in the world. I have my children and love; that means everything to me.

◆ Linda, age 20, is a single mother of two children. Her life has been one of constant struggle. Her response to the questions:

I'm not poor, I'm surviving. What keeps me from being on the street is my motivation, the good Lord on my side, and my kids. They keep me going. I don't want them to know we're going down. I want them to always know I'm there for them.

◆ Sontia is a 17-year-old mother of one child. She lives with her grandmother. Her response to the questions:

I don't think of myself as poor. To me, being poor don't mean not having money. To be poor means not having no family; no one to talk to.

◆ Sheila, age 38, has recently been diagnosed with systemic lupus erythematous and has been suffer-

---

Why must i . . .
    in the middle of the night
    be awakened by gunshots
    then make sure
    that everything is alright

Why must i . . .
    do everything the good lord
    expects me to do,
    even though other people do
    anything they want to
    get a new pair of shoes

Why must i . . .
    have to get a job to pay
    all the bills, while my
    mother goes back and forth
    to jail for everything
    she steals

Why must i . . .
    put up with these ways
    still trying to be the
    perfect lady no matter
    what my friends say

But in the future, i hope
    everyone will realize that
    poverty is all around us and
    will be until the day we die . . .

    Sontia Lemon

FIGURE 33-2

Poetry by a 17-year-old client at Community Medical Care, Washington, DC, 1994.

ing with severe joint pain. Her response to the questions:

> Yes, I am poor. I can't work. I have so many medical problems, and I can't contribute to the household expenses.

These responses by no means represent all those who come to Community Medical Care, but they provide insight into the perceptions of poor clients. Interestingly, many of the people whom nurses might perceive as poor did not perceive themselves as poor. Also, most of the clients exclude money as a criterion for poverty; however, income level is the criterion used to determine whether someone is poor according to **federal poverty guidelines.** Income is also a qualifying factor for a variety of programs, such as federal housing subsidies; Aid to Families with Dependent Children (AFDC); medical assistance, food stamps; Women, Infants, and Children (WIC); and Head Start.

Social, Political, Cultural, and Environmental Factors

Understanding the meaning of poverty includes looking at one's personal beliefs and values as well as the perspective of those who are poor. Consideration must also be given to the social, political, cultural, and environmental factors that describe the concept of poverty.

Social

Societal definitions of poverty vary depending on what source is consulted. Raspberry (1994) states that one of the difficulties of dealing with poverty and welfare reform is the lack of a common language and a common view. "Poverty refers to having insufficient financial resources to meet basic living expenses. These expenses include costs of food, shelter, clothing, transportation, and medical care" (Sebastian, 1992, p. 369). People who are poor are more likely to live in dangerous environments, to work at high-risk jobs, to eat less nutritious foods, and to have multiple stressors. They often lack the tangible and emotional resources to manage expected crises because for them, managing their daily lives is a serious challenge (Pappas, 1994).

Moccia and Mason (1986) state that poverty is a power issue because it involves a lack of control over critical resources needed to function effectively in society. The federal government uses two terms to discuss poverty: poverty thresholds and poverty guidelines. The **poverty thresholds** are issued by the U.S. Bureau of the Census and are used primarily for statistical purposes. The **poverty guidelines** are issued by the U.S. Department of Health and Human Services (DHHS) and are used to determine whether a person or family is financially eligible for assistance or services under a particular federal program. The poverty guidelines are updated annually to be consistent with the Consumer Price Index. In 1995 the poverty guide-

Table 33-1   1995 Poverty Guidelines for All States and the District of Columbia*

Size of family unit	Poverty guideline ($)
1	7,470
2	10,030
3	12,590
4	15,150
5	17,710
6	20,270
7	22,830
8	25,390

From Annual update of HHS poverty guidelines, *Federal Register* 60(27):7772-7774, 1995.
*Except Alaska and Hawaii.

line for a family of four was $15,150 (*Federal Register*, 1995; Table 33-1). Many people who earn slightly more than the government-defined poverty levels are unable to meet living expenses and are not eligible for government assistance programs. These people are often referred to as the **near poor** (Sebastian, 1992). Poverty has also been defined as a variety of conditions involving differences in home and environment, material possessions, educational and occupational resources, and financial resources (Carney, 1992).

Social science researchers simultaneously discuss different concepts of poverty, such as persistent poverty, neighborhood poverty, and underclass poverty. **Persistent poverty** refers to individuals and families who remain poor for long periods and pass poverty on to their descendants. **Neighborhood poverty** refers to spatially defined areas of high poverty and are characterized by dilapidated housing and high levels of unemployment. **Underclass poverty** is defined as "the display of negative attitudes and behavior that are associated with poverty and indicate deviance from social norms" (Jargowsky and Bane, 1990, pp. 16-17). Raspberry (1994) states that poverty embraces a wide range of conditions: "The poverty of the working poor, for instance, is quite different from the poverty of teenage mothers. The poverty of those idled by plant closings or similar economic events is different from the poverty of those who lack marketable skills and different yet from the poverty of those who can't hold a job or who don't want one" (p. A25). If one asks the clients at Community Medical Care, they will tell you that being poor has less to do with money and more to do with a lack of family, friends, love, and support.

The implication of these societal definitions of poverty for nursing is that although an awareness of these definitions of poverty may be of interest, they are not sufficient. What matters most is the nurse's ability to accept and respect clients and attempt to understand how their life situations influence their health and well-being. Being poor is one variable that must be measured against the presence of other variables that may counteract the negative effects of poverty.

Political

A historical review reveals that poverty in the United States was not recognized as a social problem before the Civil War. The prevalent attitude was that poverty was an individual's problem, and individuals had only themselves to blame if they were poor. Generally, society did not believe it was responsible for alleviating the plight of the poor. However, the post–Civil War industrialized society changed this attitude. "In the face of massive unemployment, poor working conditions, inadequate wages, and inferior housing, preindustrial conceptions of poverty eroded and efforts to combat these problems evolved into major social reforms" (Wilson, 1987, p. 165). A number of laws concerning public health and housing were passed. This social reform movement led to an early interest in urban poverty research (Bremner, 1956; Miller, 1966).

"The early interest in urban poverty research was not sustained, however, despite the heightened public awareness of poverty generated by the depression of the 1930s and the nationwide discussion and debate concerning the New Deal antipoverty programs (e.g., Aid to Dependent Children, unemployment compensation, Social Security, and old-age assistance)" (Wilson, 1987, p. 166). "Aid to Dependent Children (the original title) was enacted in 1935 as part of the Social Security Act to provide financial assistance to needy children under 16 years of age who were deprived of parental support because of death, incapacity or absence of a parent" (Dolgoff and Feldstein, 1984, p. 167). In the 1940s the onset of World War II led to issues other than poverty.

A resurgence of political activity on behalf of disadvantaged groups occurred during the late 1950s and early 1960s. In 1959 the Kerr-Mills Act increased funds for health care for aged persons (Plotnick and Skidmore, 1975). In 1961 President Kennedy approved a pilot food program in response to the hunger he observed on the campaign trail (Price, 1994). In 1963 President Kennedy instructed his administration to develop a major policy effort to combat poverty. After Kennedy's assassination, President Johnson sustained the interest in the antipoverty campaign. "In 1964 the War on Poverty was officially approved by Congress, with emphasis on job-training programs, and community participation and development" (Plotnick and Skidmore, 1975; Wilson, 1987, p. 167). In 1964 the Social Security Administration established the income level of the official poverty line. In 1965 passage of the Medicare amendments to the Social Security Act also occurred. After 1965 a proliferation of research centered on the issue of poverty as it related to education, health, housing, the law, and public welfare (Wilson, 1987).

In the 1970s and 1980s a number of societal and policy changes occurred that still affect poverty. Between 1973 and 1987, median family income increased by less than 1%, much less than the cost of housing increased. Incomes dropped by 11% between 1973 and 1987 for the poorest fifth of the population, thereby pushing more children into poverty. Since the 1970s, housing costs have grown much faster than both general inflation and family incomes, thereby making home ownership impossible for many families (Mihaly, 1991).

Policy changes during the 1980s led to an emphasis on defense spending rather than social programs. Jargowsky and Bane (1990) noted that a series of events in the 1980s, such as the visibility of the homeless in urban areas and the media attention on the "underclass," rekindled public interest in the issues of poverty.

The early 1990s saw an interest in both health care and welfare reform; however, by the middle of the decade, little had been accomplished at the federal level. In contrast, states began making both health care and welfare reform changes, and the public sector, in an effort to control the costs of medical and hospital care, became a major driver of health care reform efforts. In 1994 a record 14.3 million people received welfare benefits, representing a 31% increase since the recession began in 1989 (DeParle, 1994). Welfare reform, with its many political overtones, captured the attention of the media and many powerful groups. Likewise, as the number of underinsured and uninsured people grew and the percentage of the gross national product spent on health care increased, efforts accelerated to try to contain costs. Dealing with underinsured and uninsured persons was tackled as aggressively as was cost.

What Do You Think?

Opinions and beliefs about welfare differ among recipients, taxpayers, politicians, economists, health care providers, and others. Some people believe that welfare benefits are inadequate, whereas others argue that welfare breeds dependency and illegitimacy. Families receiving benefits also have differing views. For some families, it provides temporary support in a time of crisis. For others, it may lead to frustration and isolation. One of the clients at Community Medical Care stated, that in her opinion, "Welfare causes you to accept not expect."

The political debate in the mid-1990s is to abolish versus to reform welfare. What is the relationship between welfare reform and health care reform? What implications does welfare reform have on the community health nurse? How would you redesign the welfare system? (Bane and Ellwood, 1994)

Cultural

Writing about the concept of poverty, Carney (1992) states that the meaning of poverty differs greatly by culture. For example, in India and Japan the poor have been respected because of the political and religious systems that give meaning to their life (Finney, 1969). Anglo cultures, however, tend to view most aspects of poverty in a negative light (Youings, 1984).

Environmental

The causes of poverty are complex and interrelated. In recent decades the number of adult and elderly Americans living in poverty has decreased while the number of women and children living in poverty has increased (Johnson et al., 1991). The following reasons are given for the growing number of poor people in the United States (Velsor-Friedrich, 1992; Wilson, 1987):

- Decreased earnings
- Increased rates of unemployment
- Changes in the labor force
- More female-headed households
- Inadequate education and job skills
- Inadequate antipoverty programs
- Low benefits from Aid to Families with Dependent Children (AFDC)
- Weak child support enforcement
- Dwindling Social Security payments to children
- Increased proportion of births out of wedlock

As the economies in most industrialized nations have changed from an industrialized economy relying on manual labor to a service economy requiring highly skilled employees, job opportunities for people who do not complete at least high school are decreasing. Fewer jobs are available in manufacturing that pay an adequate amount to support a family. Also, many jobs at the lower end of the pay scale do not include health care benefits, which contributes to the growing number of people considered to be poor (Wolch et al., 1988).

POVERTY AND HEALTH: IMPACT ACROSS THE LIFESPAN

Poverty directly affects health and well-being. The poor population has a higher rate of chronic illness, higher infant morbidity and mortality rates, shorter life expectancy, more complex health problems, and greater physical limitations resulting from chronic disease. These health care problems result from barriers that impede access to health care, such as inability to pay for health care, lack of insurance, geographical location, language, maldistribution of providers, transportation difficulties, inconvenient clinic hours, and attitudes of health care providers (Hawkins and Higgins, 1982; Kothoff, 1981).

Researchers in Washington, D.C., found that "residents of low-income communities are hospitalized three times as often as people in high-income communities. They are hospitalized for asthma, diabetes, high blood pressure, and dozens of other medical conditions that can be controlled by getting routine medical care" (Goldstein, 1994, p. A1). The following environmental factors also effect health: lack of heat, inadequate sanitary facilities, inadequate housing, occupational hazards, and presence of vermin, parasites, and rats.

Childbearing Women and Poverty

Poverty, while being a serious obstacle to health across the lifespan, has an especially negative effect on women of childbearing age. Disadvantaged young people, who have not had the opportunity to acquire skills or master knowledge, lack a personal sense of mastery and self-esteem (Schorr and Schorr, 1989). Poor teenagers are four times more likely than nonpoor teens to have below-average academic skills. Poor teenagers, regardless of their race, are nearly three times more likely to drop out of school than nonpoor teenagers. Teenage women who are poor and who have below-average skills, regardless of their race, are 5.5 times more likely to have children than nonpoor teenage women. Poor pregnant women are more likely than other women to receive late or no prenatal care and to deliver low-birth-weight babies, premature babies, or babies with birth defects (Johnson et al., 1991).

Children and Poverty

"Many of the children of the United States are members of the 5H Club. They are hungry, homeless, hugless, hopeless, and without health care" (Elders, 1994). As of 1993, the U.S. Bureau of the Census reported that 15.7 million children (or 22.7%) live in poverty. Child poverty rates remain twice as high as adult rates. One in five American children under age 18 and one in four children under age 6 are poor. Two in three poor children are white, Hispanic, Asian, or Native American. One-third of poor children are black. During the 1980s, Hispanic poverty rates grew the fastest. Children in single-parent homes are twice as likely to be poor as those who live in homes with two parents. The youngest children are most at risk. They are more vulnerable to developmental delays and damage caused by inadequate nutrition or lack of health care (Johnson et al., 1991; Velsor-Friedrich, 1992).

The document *Healthy People 2000* (1991) points out that low income, low educational level, and low occupational level are linked to infant mortality, prematurity, low birth weight, birth defects, and infant deaths (see the box on p. 654). Poverty also increases the likelihood of chronic disease, injuries, traumatic death, developmental delays, poor nutrition, lack of immunizations, iron deficiency anemia, and elevated blood lead levels. Furthermore, children of poverty are more likely than nonpoor children to be hungry and suffer from fatigue, dizziness, irritability, headaches, ear in-

The Effects of Poverty on the Health of Children

Higher rates of prematurity, low birth weight, and birth defects
Higher infant mortality rates
Increased incidence of chronic disease
Increased incidence of traumatic death and injuries
Increased incidence of nutritional deficits
Increased incidence of growth retardation and developmental delays
Increased incidence of iron deficiency anemia
Increased incidence of elevated lead levels
Increased incidence of infections
Increased incidence of delayed immunizations
Increased risk for homelessness
Decreased opportunities for education, income, and occupation

fections, frequent colds, weight loss, inability to concentrate, and increased school absenteeism (Malloy, 1992; Sherman, 1994; Velsor-Friedrich, 1992).

Elderly Persons and Poverty

Elderly persons have been helped by policy changes and the commitment of many people to improve the situation of the older age group. The rate of poverty has decreased for the elderly population in the last 20 years. As of 1993, the U.S. Bureau of the Census reported that 3.8 million Americans aged 65 and over live in poverty. This decrease is primarily a result of improvements in Social Security and the Supplemental Security Income Program. Certain elderly groups, however, continue to be vulnerable to the effects of poverty. For example, "Elderly blacks are three times as likely as whites, and elderly Hispanics are more than twice as likely as whites, to have income below the poverty level" (Wallsten, 1992, p. 21). The poor elderly suffer as well from high rates of chronic illness, higher morbidity rates, shorter life expectancy, and more complex health problems than their more affluent peers. They are more likely to seek acute crisis care rather than preventive health care. Elderly persons are particularly at risk because they may be alone and unable to manage their own affairs. Some elders are eligible for benefits but do not know how to access them.

Did You Know?

It is estimated that 35% of the homeless elderly persons are eligible for Social Security benefits, but only 4% access them (Wallsten, 1992).

The Community and Poverty

Poverty can affect both urban and rural communities. A number of characteristics describe poor communi-

ties. For example, the poorer the neighborhood, the greater is the proportion of residents who are members of minority groups. Family structure is most often a single parent with children. Children of single-parent families are more likely to be poorer in income and other resources. There are higher rates of unemployment and lower wage rates for those who are employed. In addition to the economic deterioration, residents of poor neighborhoods are more likely to be victims of crime, racial discrimination, and police brutality. The rates of crime and substance abuse are higher in poor neighborhoods. Differences in the quality of education in schools and differences in the level of education also exist. Health care is less available in poor neighborhoods. Housing conditions in some areas are deplorable, with families living in run-down shacks or condemned apartment buildings. They are exposed to environmental hazards such as inadequate heating and cooling, exposure to rain and snow, inadequate water and plumbing facilities, and the presence of vermin and pests (Jargowsky and Bane, 1990).

Clearly, being poor affects the health and well-being of people of all ages as well as of families and communities. As Sheila, one of the clients at Community Medical Care, said, "It is easy for the poor to get depressed and despondent; to accept their condition and to have no expectations." Nurses must recognize that poverty exists and influences health and well-being. Poverty is a part of the picture, not the whole picture. Being poor is a health risk factor that should be assessed; however, nurses also need to examine individual and community strengths, resources, and sources of support.

UNDERSTANDING THE CONCEPT OF HOMELESSNESS

Understanding the concept of homelessness similarly necessitates considerable reflection and analysis. The community health nurse's concept of homelessness is influenced by a number of variables. Specifically, these variables include personal beliefs, values, and knowledge of homelessness; the life stories of those who experience homelessness; and social, political, cultural, and environmental factors.

Personal Beliefs, Values, and Knowledge

Poverty can lead to homelessness. **Homelessness,** as with poverty, is a difficult concept to grasp. The following questions may be used by the community health nurse to aid in self-evaluation related to the concept of homelessness:
◆ What does it mean to live on the streets?
◆ What must it be like for a young mother and her children to live in a shelter?
◆ How is it that people are so poor that they have no place to go?
◆ What causes homelessness?

◆ How do you respond to the man on the street asking for change to buy a sandwich?

◆ How do you react to the smell of urine in a stairwell or elevator?

Nurses must explore their personal beliefs, values, and knowledge of homelessness to understand what it means to be homeless.

Clients' Perceptions about Homelessness and Health

Those who live on the street are the poorest of the poor made visible to us. Often, however, they become faceless, nameless, invisible, and inaudible (Cangialosi, 1994). As nurses begin to learn their names and listen to their stories, they can begin to engage in therapeutic relationships. The following are some patient responses to the question, "What is it like to be homeless?"

When you're homeless, nothing is yours anymore. Even the things you carry on your back. Someone will take them if you're not looking.

I'm not here by choice. I used to be married. I lost my wife, my children, my job. I've been out here so long, I don't know my way home.

They gave me a prescription at the emergency room for my baby's infection. But I didn't get it; I didn't have no money. And even if I did, I didn't have no place cold to put it.

Sometimes I wish I had a small room for me and my baby. Some place safe where no one could find us.

They make us leave the shelter at 7 am in the morning. I usually spend the day in the library. They don't let you fall asleep though, otherwise they kick you out.

The homeless long for a place of their own and for stability and relationships. Baumann (1993) studied what the experience of homelessness meant for 15 homeless women with children and found that the following seven themes of homelessness emerged: boundaries, connections, fatigue/despair, lack of self-respect, lack of self-determination, lack of privacy, and mobility.

Who Are the Homeless?

Tragically, "people huddled together asleep under a bus stop shelter, men begging for money, and families digging through dumpsters looking for food are not uncommon sights in many American cities" (Jackson and McSwane, 1992, p. 185). "The federal government defines a homeless person as one who lacks a fixed, regular and adequate address or has a primary nighttime residence in a supervised publicly or privately operated shelter or temporary accommodations including welfare hotels, congregate shelters, and transitional housing for the mentally ill" (Mihaly, 1991, p. 3).

Research Brief

Baumann S: The meaning of being homeless, *Scholarly Inquiry Nurs Pract* 7(1):59-73, 1993.

This study explored the meaning of being homeless as lived by 15 homeless women with dependent children. The significance of being homeless was approached from what is known about the concept of homelessness. The researcher found the emergence of seven themes: boundaries, connections, fatigue/despair, self-respect, self-determination, privacy, and mobility.

◆ Three types of boundaries were significant: physical, social, and symbolic.

◆ The women felt more vulnerable because they lacked physical boundaries.

◆ The women expressed that great energy was needed to maintain connections.

◆ The homeless women experienced fatigue and despair.

◆ Being displaced is a part of the homeless experience that threatened the women's self-respect.

◆ The women experienced frustration with the effort needed to determine the course of their lives.

◆ Privacy emerged as a theme related to individual and family integrity.

◆ Often by circumstance, sometimes by choice, the participants moved regularly.

The homeless population in the United States is estimated to be between 350,000 and 2.5 million people. However, it is very difficult to determine the size of this group of people. There is general consensus that the number of homeless people grew during the 1980s. Link et al. (1994) identified four problems in determining exactly how many people are homeless:

1. Finding people who are homeless at any given time. Simply locating them is difficult because some may sleep in railroad boxcars, on roofs of buildings, in campgrounds, and so on.

2. Once located, homeless respondents may refuse to be interviewed or may deliberately hide the fact of their homelessness.

3. Some homeless people have a short interval of homelessness, or they may have "off and on" episodes, which makes it difficult to find them at a given point in time.

4. It is difficult to generalize from one location to another about homelessness; that is, the numbers and patterns of homelessness may be different in large versus small cities or in urban versus rural areas.

Link et al. (1994) conducted a comprehensive study of homelessness that used a different methodology from most previous studies. His research team found a much higher reported rate of homelessness than other studies. They did telephone household surveys of 1507 residents of the continental United States in a 4-

month period to determine if the respondents had ever been homeless and if they had been homeless in the last 5 years. They found that about 13.5 million adults (or 7.4% of the U.S. population) had been homeless at some time in their lives and that 5.7 million had been homeless in the last 5 years. Because they had such a large number of reported instances of homelessness, the researchers looked at what accounted for these differences. Some of the factors may have been that they did not define homelessness, so people may have interpreted it differently from the usual definition; or people may be more willing to say that they have been homeless if the data are being gathered retrospectively. A third unique factor in their study was that only respondents with telephones at the time of data collection could be included. However, despite the unique features of the methodology used in this study, the data do support the belief that homelessness may be much more widespread than statistics generally indicate.

The study by Link et al. (1994) supports the commonly held belief that the homeless population changed dramatically in the 1990s. Previously, people thought of the homeless as middle-age alcoholic men who lived on the streets. This traditional population is now joined by families, children, single women, recently unemployed persons, substance abusers, adolescent runaways, and mentally ill individuals. Families with children make up one-third of the U.S. homeless population and represent the fastest-growing segment of homeless people (Mihaly, 1991). The typical homeless family has 2.4 children and has exhausted every possible social, economic, and family resource available before they become homeless (Wagner and Menke, 1991).

Many of today's homeless are people who in previous decades had a home and managed to survive on a limited income. Today the homeless population includes people of every age, sex, and ethnic family structure group (Vredevoe et al., 1992). Surprisingly, the single homeless tend to be younger and better educated than stereotypes would suggest; they often represent ethnic minority groups. Many have some history of job success, and they typically are longstanding residents of the area (Vladeck, 1990). The box above summarizes who represents America's homeless.

Homeless people can be found in both rural and urban areas. Many sleep at night in shelters but are asked to vacate the shelters during the day. This means that during the day, they sit or stand on the street, in parks, alleys, shopping centers, libraries, and in places such as trash bins, cardboard boxes, or under loading docks at industrial sites. They may also seek shelter in public buildings, such as train and bus stations. Those who do not sleep in shelters may sleep in single-room occupancy hotels, all-night movie theaters, abandoned buildings, and vehicles, including railroad cars (Vredevoe et al., 1992).

Rural communities, despite their peaceful images, are not immune to homelessness. The extent of the problem is more disguised than in the urban areas be-

Who Are America's Homeless?

Families
Children
Single women
Female heads of household
Adults who are unemployed, earn low wages, or are migrant workers
People who abuse alcohol or other substances
Abandoned children
Adolescent runaways
Elderly people with no place to go and no one to care for them
Persons who are mentally ill
Vietnam-era veterans

cause rural people are more likely to help one another. Family and friends often provide temporary housing to their neighbors who have no place to live (Dahl et al., 1993).

Causes of Homelessness

Most people move into homelessness gradually. Once they give up their own dwelling, they often move in with family or friends. Only when all other options to live in a home are exhausted do people go to shelters or seek refuge on the streets. Numerous factors contribute to the increasing numbers of homeless persons. These factors include an increase in the number of people living in poverty; a decrease in the number of affordable housing units; an emergency demand on income, medical expenses, and loss of equipment or income; gentrification of neighborhoods; alcohol or other drug abuse problems; and a decrease in the number of transitional treatment facilities for deinstitutionalized mentally ill individuals (Interagency Council on the Homeless, 1991).

As discussed earlier, the percentage of people living below the poverty level has increased. Changes in the housing market have also had a profound impact on many people who were marginally meeting their financial obligations. The move to upgrade urban housing, or "gentrification," began with a positive intent that unfortunately led to negative consequences for many of the former residents of urban areas. During the 1980s the supply of low-income housing in the United States dropped by about 2.5 million units; simultaneously, significant growth occurred in the need for such housing. Historically, urban neighborhoods have provided homes for elderly and poor persons. When the neighborhoods were modernized, the former residents were often unable to afford either to use existing housing in the old neighborhoods or to locate new housing elsewhere. In many older neighborhoods, people who are now homeless previously lived in single-room occupancy (SRO) buildings where they rented a room on a long-term basis. Urban renewal eliminated many of the SROs and left a more attractive, better maintained neighborhood that was unaffordable for the former residents.

Deinstitutionalization of chronically mentally ill individuals from public psychiatric hospitals has also led to a growth in the homeless population. The intent of deinstitutionalization was to replace large state psychiatric hospitals with community-based treatment centers. The goal was for clients to have shorter stays in mental health facilities and move into appropriately designed and readily available community-based care. Unfortunately, the hospitals downsized and many closed, but federal and state governments were unable to allocate the needed funds to provide community-based services. Indeed, fewer than 800 of the intended community mental health centers were built (Jackson and McSwane, 1992). According to the Report of the Federal Task Force on Homelessness and Severe Mental Illness (1992), one-third of single homeless adults have a severe mental illness.

HOMELESSNESS: IMPACT ON HEALTH

"Conditions associated with homelessness have a profound effect on an individual's ability to maintain good health, to get treatment when health is compromised, and to recover even after treatment is received" (Jackson and McSwane, 1992, p. 186). Imagine what it is like to be an insulin-dependent diabetic who lives on the street. Even if the person is able to eat one meal a day and sleep in the shelter, the ability to get adequate rest, exercise, take insulin on a schedule, and eat regular, nutrient-controlled meals is virtually impossible. Homeless persons have a higher rate of medical problems and have more difficulty accessing care than the general population. Health care is generally crisis oriented and is often sought from an emergency room when the condition is serious. Once treatment is received, just following the prescribed therapy becomes an obstacle. For example, how does one purchase an antibiotic if no money is available? How is a child treated for scabies and lice when there are no bathing facilities? How does an elderly man with peripheral vascular disease elevate his legs when he must be out of the shelter at 7 AM and on the streets all day? In addition to these challenges, health is a lower priority than food and shelter for many homeless persons. Homeless people spend most of their time trying to survive. Just getting enough money to buy food is a major chore. Some are eligible for entitlement programs, such as AFDC, WIC, or Social Security benefits. Others must beg for money, sell plasma or blood products, steal, deal in drugs, or engage in prostitution.

Some of the specific health problems of the homeless include hypothermia, infestations, peripheral vascular disease, hypertension, respiratory infections, tuberculosis, acquired immunodeficiency syndrome (AIDS), trauma, and mental illness (Jackson and McSwane, 1992). The disorders caused by exposure include hypothermia and heat-related illnesses such as heat-stroke. Compounding the effects of exposure is the prevalence of diabetes, poor skin integrity, chronic diseases, nutritional deficits, trauma, and decreased perceptions secondary to alcohol or substance abuse. The use of psychoactive medications can cause irregularities in thermoregulation (Brickner et al., 1986).

Several factors contribute to the rate of infestation among the homeless. These factors include close physical contact and shared clothing, combs, brushes, and bedding. The most common infestations are scabies and lice. Symptoms of infestation include a rash, itching, and occasionally a low-grade fever. Although several treatment methods are available, once again the lack of water facilities and the inability to treat all clothing and persons prevent adequate eradication (Jackson and McSwane, 1992).

Cardiovascular and respiratory diseases in the homeless population include peripheral vascular disease, hypertension, tuberculosis, pneumonia, and chronic obstructive pulmonary diseases. The homeless spend many hours on their feet and often sleep in upright positions, which compromise their peripheral circulation. Hypertension is exacerbated by the high rates of alcohol abuse and the high sodium content of fast foods and meals available in the shelters. Crowded living conditions put the homeless at risk for exposure to viruses and bacteria that cause pneumonia and tuberculosis. In addition, the homeless have a high rate of tobacco and other substance use, which diminishes immune responses and contributes to chronic obstructive pulmonary disease (Brickner et al., 1986; Jackson and McSwane, 1992).

AIDS is also a growing concern among the homeless population. The seroprevalence of the human immunodeficiency virus (HIV) infection in the homeless is estimated to be at least double that found in the general population. The use of intravenous drugs and sexual assault are additional risk factors. Homeless persons with AIDS tend to develop more virulent forms of infectious diseases, have longer hospitalizations, and are less likely to be able to continue long-term treatment (Fetter and Larson, 1990; Jackson and McSwane, 1992).

Trauma is a significant cause of death and disability in the homeless population. Major trauma includes gunshot wounds, stab wounds, head trauma, suicide attempts, and fractures. Minor trauma includes bruises, abrasions, concussions, sprains, puncture wounds, eye injuries, and cellulitis (Hilfiker, 1994; Jackson and McSwane, 1992).

As discussed earlier, deinstitutionalization has contributed to the growing number of homeless persons. Studies have found that approximately 30% of the homeless have major mental illnesses, including schizophrenia and affective disorders. The prevalence of alcohol and substance abuse compounds the effects of mental illness. Some homeless persons have a history of diagnosed mental illness before becoming homeless, and some homeless persons develop acute mental distress as a result of being homeless. Although treatment modalities may exist, the homeless are often unable to gain access to these services because of several barriers, such as lack of awareness of treatment options, lack of available space in treatment facilities, inability to pay for treatment, lack of transportation, and nonsupportive attitudes of service providers (Hilfiker, 1994; Jackson and McSwane, 1992).

In addition to the physiological effects on health, homelessness also influences psychological, social, and spiritual well-being. Being homeless means more than the loss of a home, a regular place to sleep and eat; it also means losing friends, one's personal possessions, and a neighborhood that is familiar (Wagner and Menke, 1991). Homelessness is an isolating experience that is particularly difficult for children, who are often labeled and ridiculed by other children. Being homeless is an existence filled with chaos, confusion, and fear.

Homelessness and At-Risk Populations

Clearly, being homeless is a significant deterrent to health. Imagine the added implications if you are homeless and pregnant, a homeless child, a homeless adolescent, or a homeless elderly person. Being pregnant and homeless is an especially high-risk condition. Homelessness makes it difficult to maintain adequate nutrition, control hypertension, control gynecological disease, and receive adequate prenatal care (Jackson and McSwane, 1992).

The health problems of homeless children, although similar to those of poor children, may be more severe and numerous. For example, homeless children are at greater risk for inadequate nutrition, which can lead to delayed growth and development, failure to thrive, or obesity. These children also experience high rates of school absenteeism, academic failure, and emotional and behavioral maladjustments. The stress of homelessness can be manifested in behaviors such as withdrawal, depression, anxiety, aggression, regression, or self-mutilating behaviors (Davidhizar and Frank, 1992). The box above lists health problems that occur in higher incidence among homeless children.

Homeless elderly persons are the most vulnerable of the impoverished elderly population. They have lived in longstanding poverty, have fewer supportive relationships, and are likely to become homeless as a result of catastrophic events (Wallsten, 1992). Hilfiker (1994) states "that there is comparatively little geriatric care because so few homeless people live to old age. The life expectancy is about twenty years less than the average middle-class person. Permanent physical deformities are common, often the result of poor or absent medical care: a broken leg not properly set, a congenitally dislocated hip never treated, a leg amputated because of diabetes in a fifty-year old man who had no place to store his insulin and whose needles kept being stolen at the shelter" (pp. 68-69). Homeless elderly persons suffer from untreated chronic health conditions, tuberculosis, hypertension, arthritis, stroke, injuries, malnutrition, and

 Health Problems of Homeless Children

PHYSICAL HEALTH PROBLEMS

Scabies
Lice
Dermatologic infections
Dental problems
Chronic cardiovascular problems
Neurological disorders
Anemia
Asthma
Bronchitis
Incomplete immunization status
Inadequate nutrition

SOCIAL AND DEVELOPMENTAL PROBLEMS

Developmental problems
Behavioral problems
School-related problems
  Erratic attendance
  Failure
Anxiety and depression

hypothermia. They also suffer from acute problems such as frozen appendages or burns from grates. As with the younger homeless population, elderly homeless persons must focus their energy on survival; obtaining food and shelter is a much higher priority than health care (Wallsten, 1992).

Federal Programs for the Homeless

A tremendous need exists for comprehensive, affordable, and accessible care for the homeless population. The federal government officially became involved with meeting the needs of the homeless in 1987 with the passage of the **Stewart B. McKinney Assistance Act** (P.L. 100-77). Title 11 of the McKinney Act provided categorical funding for outpatient health services; however, the financial appropriations have never been large, and many needs go unmet. The act grants homeless children the same access to a "free, appropriate education" as permanently housed children (Title VII, Subtitle B). This act also created the **Interagency Council on the Homeless (ICH)** to coordinate and direct federal homeless activities (Velsor-Friedrich, 1993a, 1993b).

The ICH is made up of the heads of 16 federal agencies that have programs or activities for the homeless. The general goals of the ICH are to improve federal programs for this population through better coordination and linkages, by decreasing the paperwork in securing help, and by reaching the most needy segments of the homeless population. Children are a top priority for the ICH.

Homeless families with children are eligible to receive shelter and nutrition assistance from the U.S. Department of Agriculture program for **Women, Infants, and Children (WIC),** by using food stamps, through school meals, and from special shelters. Also, the **Aid to Families with Dependent Children (AFDC)** program is a key source of income for homeless families.

Unfortunately, health care for the homeless tends to be fragmented and limited in scope (Velsor-Friedrich, 1993a, 1993b). Some of the most useful health care programs for the homeless are begun with grants from the Robert Wood Johnson Foundation and the Pew Memorial Trust. In late 1983, these two foundations, through a call for competitively judged proposals, funded projects in 19 of the 50 largest U.S. cities (Vladeck, 1990). The project guidelines followed sound public health principles by expecting community involvement, public/private partnerships, and a commitment to outreach. Most of the projects relied heavily on nurse practitioners and physician assistants to deliver care in collaboration with physicians, nurses, and social workers. In recent years, several schools of nursing have received funding from the Division of Nursing in the DHHS to establish nurse-managed centers for the homeless. Both faculty and students provide a range of services in these centers. (See Chapter 18 for more details.)

THE ROLE OF THE COMMUNITY HEALTH NURSE

Community health nurses have a critical role in the delivery of care to persons who are poor or homeless. Nurses respect the worth and dignity of the human person and bring to each client they encounter the ability to assess the situation and to intervene in ways that can restore health, maintain health, or promote health (see box below, left). Nurses are prepared to look at the whole picture, that is, the person, the family, or the community interacting with the environment. Working with poor or homeless people involves interventions (see box below, right, and following text).

◆ *Create a trusting environment.* Trust is essential to the development of a therapeutic relationship with poor or homeless persons. Many clients and families have been disappointed by the health care and social systems that are part of their lives. As a result, they may be mistrustful and may not believe that there is hope for any change. Nurses must follow through and do what they say they are going to do.

If the answer to a question is unknown, an appropriate response might be, "I don't know the answer, but I will try to find out. Let me make a few phone calls and I will let you know Friday." The demonstration of trust and reliability builds the foundation for a trusting and therapeutic relationship.

◆ *Show respect, compassion, and concern.* Often, poor and homeless persons think that they are different or less than human. Sheila, a client at Community Medical Care, stated, "The poor get depressed and despondent. Poor people need a lot of support. They need to know that someone cares." It is essential to take the time to listen and ask the questions that probe to the deeper meaning of their life experience. Ask open-ended questions, such as, "Tell me what your day is like" or "Tell me about your experience at the housing department."

When appropriate, use reflective statements that convey your acceptance and understanding of the client's life situation. Tonya, a single mother with AIDS, lives in an apartment with her two children, who are HIV positive, and seven other family members. Tonya does not have transportation and is often unable to keep her children's numerous appointments at the immunology clinic. She calls the clinic often just to talk and share the frustration of her life. A response, such as, "Tonya, it must be difficult to manage day to day. I can see you care deeply for your children," conveys acceptance for Tonya's situation as well as acknowledges her positive caring for her children. An unsolicited telephone call or a visit to a family just to let them know you are thinking about them and wondering how they are doing conveys caring.

◆ *Don't make assumptions.* A comprehensive and holistic assessment is crucial to identifying the underlying need. Tonya, the young mother just mentioned, was to bring her children to the immunology clinic at the city hospital. The staff at the hospital called child protective services to report her failure to keep their appointments. Not showing up for an appointment was falsely interpreted as noncompliance and neglect of the children. A more thorough assessment revealed that Tonya did not have transportation and also was responsible for caring for some of

A Client's Advice to Nurses Caring for the Poor

Treat the poor like everyone else.
Don't be condescending.
Don't make it obvious that someone is poor.
Don't prejudge; ask if someone wants to pay on their bill.
Remember that people can't always pay for their medicine.
Suggest programs that might help, such as food banks, churches, and clothing centers.
Poor people need a lot of support.
Many poor people need to be reeducated on what to eat.

Community Health Nursing Interventions

Creating a trusting environment.
Show respect, compassion, and concern.
Don't make assumptions.
Remember the basics.
Recognize that time isn't measured in hours and days.
Coordinate a network of services and providers.
Advocate for accessible health care services.
Focus on prevention.
Know when to walk beside someone and when to encourage them to walk ahead.
Develop a network of support for yourself.

the other children in the household. The community health nurse made a home visit and then called the immunology clinic to explain the restrictions that Tonya was facing. The nurse obtained taxi vouchers to secure transportation to the clinic, and another family member agreed to watch the other children at home.

Shelley, a young mother of three school-age children, has a part-time job and is ineligible for public assistance or Medicaid. She and her children attend a health clinic that has a sliding scale for uninsured families. Shelley said, "I don't want people to think I'm poor. I don't want them to prejudge me. When someone asks me, 'Can you pay anything on your bill today?' I feel that they trust me; they're treating me like everybody else."

◆ *Remember the basics.* Carla is 17 years old and the mother of 4-month-old Darryl, who has been evaluated for sepsis three times in the emergency room of a children's hospital. One Friday afternoon, Carla called to say, "I'm on my way to the clinic; Darryl is sick again. He hasn't eaten in 2 days and he's just laying around. His eyes are rolling in the back of his head." When Carla and Darryl arrived, a history and physical examination were done by the family nurse practitioner. Darryl had lost 2 pounds since the previous visit and was dehydrated. In addition to assessing Darryl, the nurse practitioner asked to see the baby bottle and discovered that it was coated with dry, spoiled milk, and that the nipple was plugged. The baby bottle was the most likely cause of Darryl's fever and weight loss. Nursing interventions focused on teaching Carla the basics of infant feeding: how to prepare the formula, how to clean the bottles and nipples, how to store the formula, and how to check the nipples for patency. A referral was made for nursing home visits to assess further the home situation and to reinforce parent teaching. The success of the interventions was evident when Darryl began gaining weight and had no other episodes of fevers.

◆ *Recognize that time is not measured in hours and days.* An ongoing pattern occurs at Community Medical Care; the patients rarely arrive on time for their appointments. Frequently, people miss their appointments and walk in when they have an acute illness. For many poor and homeless families, seeking preventive health care is a low priority, and care is often sought only when there is a crisis. Recognizing this fact helps in both scheduling appointments and in deciding when a home visit is indicated. Take into consideration that a family may not be home when a visit is planned; for example, the family may be out paying a utility bill or waiting in the lobby of a housing building to meet with a caseworker.

◆ *Coordinate a network of services and providers.* The multiple and complex needs of poor and homeless people make working with them exceedingly challenging. For example, a school principal might ask the school nurse to evaluate a 7-year-old child with a dry scalp. The nurse would collect the information by interviewing the child and the child's parent(s). In examining the child's head, the nurse might discover a thick, crusted layer of dry skin covering the scalp. The nurse also notes that the child has a strong body odor. The nurse learns that the child has not been bathed in at least a month and lives with her mother in a shelter. A dry scalp, which usually is a relatively simple condition, is now complicated by no available bathing facilities, no soap, no towels, and no clean clothing. The school nurse recognizes personal limits as well as the lack of resources for basic hygiene and contacts agencies that can provide soap, linens, and clothing. The nurse also contacts the shelter director to inquire what kind of bathing arrangements can be made. A referral is made to a social worker to assist the mother in applying for benefits for which she is eligible. A referral is also made to a local food and clothing distribution center to obtain basic supplies for the child and her mother.

Developing a coordinated network of providers involves investigating what federal, state, and local services are available. Where are the food banks? Where can clothing be obtained? What programs are available in the area churches and schools? How do participants gain access to these services? What are the eligibility requirements? How helpful are the people who work at the various agencies? What is the actual level of assistance that is given to individuals and families? Various services and agencies exist, but often the people who could benefit from these services are unaware of them. Both community health nurse and social worker can identify these services and help link families with appropriate resources.

◆ *Advocate for accessible health care services.* Poverty and homelessness create a number of barriers that prevent access to health care services. Nurses can advocate for accessible and convenient locations of health care services. Neighborhood clinics, mobile vans, and home visits are interventions that help bring health care to those who are unable to access care. Coordinating services at one central location improves patient compliance compared with sending patients to multiple agencies and clinics. For example, placing a WIC site in a primary care clinic brings together nutritional and health care services.

◆ *Focus on prevention.* The community health nurse should take advantage of every opportunity to provide preventive care and health teaching, such as immunizing children and ensuring that their immunizations are up to date and providing age-appropriate health screening and health education. It is important to know what other screening and health promotion services are available, such as nutrition programs, employment programs for elderly persons, job training programs, educational programs, housing programs, and legal services in the community. All these services may be needed in the development of a comprehensive plan of care.

◆ *Know when to walk beside someone and when to encourage them to walk ahead.* This intervention is often unclear, with nursing intervention ranging from extensive care activities to minimal support. At times the nursing action will be to encourage, support, and accompany clients through the complicated maze of the health care delivery system while allowing them to do as much for themselves as possible. The role of the community health nurse is to assess for the presence of strengths, problem-solving ability, and the coping ability of the individual or family while providing information on where and how to gain access to services.

For example, in the District of Columbia, several hospitals provide a free mammogram for uninsured women. Many clients at Community Medical Care qualify for this free service, but because they fear breast cancer, they will not take advantage of this opportunity. The nurse is responsible for informing the women of the importance of preventive health care such as breast cancer screening while also assessing and dealing with fear and anxiety. The chal-lenge for the nurse becomes choosing whether to schedule the appointments for the women or provide them with a referral sheet, knowing that most will not follow through. The choice is not clear, but the goal is to make available a needed screening intervention without taking away the woman's right to choose and do for herself.

◆ *Develop a network of support for yourself.* Caring for persons who are poor and homeless can be challenging, rewarding, and at times exhausting. It is important to find a source of personal strength, renewal, and hope. The people you encounter often are looking to you to maintain hope and provide encouragement. Discover for yourself what restores and encourages you. For some nurses it is poetry, music, painting, or weaving. For others it is a walk in a peaceful place, a weekend retreat, or a monthly breakfast meeting with other nurses who are doing the same work. Be attentive to your own needs for healing, and create the time and space to restore your spirit.

Clinical Application

Case management is an intervention strategy that can be used by community health nurses working with families who are poor or homeless (Wagner and Menke, 1992). Community health nurses strive to meet the multiple and complex needs of families by coordinating community resources. Nursing's strengths include the therapeutic use of self, a holistic view of the individual and family, knowledge of health and illness, and the ability to identify variations from normal. The following are specific actions involved in case management:

◆ Determine available services and resources.
◆ Determine missing resources and develop creative solutions for service deficiencies.
◆ Integrate and utilize clinical skills.

◆ Establish long-term therapeutic relationships with families.
◆ Enhance the family's personal coping skills, survival skills, and resourcefulness.
◆ Facilitate service delivery on behalf of the family.
◆ Promote assertive family communication.
◆ Advocate for the individual and family.
◆ Guide the family toward the use of appropriate community resources.
◆ Communicate and collaborate with professionals from multiple service systems.
◆ Advocate for the development of creative solutions.
◆ Participate in policy analysis and political activism.
◆ Manipulate and modify the environment as needed.
◆ Speak to state legislators.

Key Concepts

◆ To understand the concepts of poverty and homelessness, one must consider one's own personal beliefs and attitudes, clients' perceptions of their condition, and the social, political, cultural, and environmental factors that influence the definition of poverty and homelessness.

◆ The definition of poverty varies depending on what source is consulted. The federal government defines poverty based on income, family size, the age of the head of the household, and the number of children under age 18 years. Those who are poor state that poverty has less to do with income and more to do with a lack of family, friends, love, and support.

◆ The factors leading to the growing number of poor people in the United States include decreased earnings, more female-headed households, inadequate education and job skills, low AFDC benefits, weak child support enforcement, and reduced Social Security payments to children.

◆ Poverty has a direct impact on health and well-being across the lifespan. The poor popu-

Continued.

Key Concepts—cont'd

lation has a higher rate of chronic illness, higher infant morbidity and mortality rates, shorter life expectancy, and more complex health problems.

◆ Child poverty rates remain twice as high as for adults. Children in single-parent homes are twice as likely to be poor as those who live in homes with two parents. The younger the child, the more vulnerable the child is to developmental delays and damage caused by inadequate nutrition or lack of health care.

◆ Poverty affects both urban and rural communities. The poorer the neighborhood, the greater is the proportion of residents who are members of minority groups.

◆ The homeless population in the United States is estimated at 350,000 to 2.5 million. Families represent the fastest-growing segment of the homeless population.

◆ At present the following groups often constitute the homeless in both rural and urban areas: families, children, single mothers, single women, recently unemployed persons, substance abusers, adolescent runaways, mentally ill individuals, and single men.

◆ Factors leading to homelessness include an increase in the number of people who live in poverty, decrease in low-cost housing, increased unemployment, substance abuse, lack of available facilities for mentally ill persons, and family conflicts leading to children who run away.

◆ The complex health problems of the homeless population include inability to get adequate rest, exercise, and nutrition; exposure; infectious diseases; acute and chronic illness; infestations; trauma; and mental health problems.

◆ Community health nurses have a critical role in the delivery of care to persons who are poor and homeless. Nurses bring to each client they encounter the ability to assess the whole situation and to intervene in ways that can restore, maintain, or promote health.

Critical Thinking Activities

1. Discuss with your classmates the poem entitled "On Hearing the News of a Patient's Death" (see Figure 33-1). Ask one classmate to read the poem aloud while the others imagine the characters and scenes in the poem. Identify and discuss the persons in the poem. What are your personal reactions to the poem? What emotions does the poem stir in you? How does it make you feel? Explore with your classmates creative outlets for expressing some of the various emotions you experience when working with persons who are homeless or poor.

2. Examine health statistics and demographic data to identify the rate of poverty and homelessness in your geographical area. What resources and agencies are available in your area to support these populations? What services are available through the federal government, the state, and the local community? Identify specific geographical boundaries, and survey the area to identify community resources, soup kitchens, health centers, food banks, and clothing distribution centers. How do persons who need these services access them? Have various class members make appointments with key persons in the community to learn more about avail-

able services, eligibility requirements, and methods of evaluation.

3. Identify nurses in your community who are working with homeless or vulnerable groups. Invite the nurses to a class session. Organize a panel discussion. Ask the nurses to describe their client population and a typical work day. What are the rewards and challenges of working with these high-risk populations? How did these nurses first become involved with their work? How do they deal with the frustrations and challenges of their work? What advice do they have to offer the class?

4. Imagine yourself as a community health nurse working in a homeless shelter or making a home visit to a family that lives in an impoverished neighborhood. What previous experience have you had with these situations? What are you anticipating? Write down your fears, anxieties, and apprehensions as you anticipate this work. Discuss your writings with your classmates.

5. Discuss the issue of welfare reform. What is meant by the welfare system in America? What is your understanding of who is receiving welfare? Who is eligible for welfare? How do people apply for welfare?

Critical Thinking Activities—cont'd

Do you believe in reforming or restructuring the welfare system? Discuss current legislative proposals dealing with welfare reform. What is the financial and personal cost involved in reforming the welfare system? Identify the senators and representatives in your district. Where do they stand on the issue of welfare reform? How do you propose that the welfare system should be restructured?

6. Identify homeless shelters in your area that provide services to families. Ask to visit and meet with the director and staff. Ask what health needs have been identified. Offer to do a teaching session on an identified health need. Once a topic is identified, write an outline, objectives, and a teaching plan that could be used to present health information to homeless families.

Bibliography

Annual update of HHS poverty guidelines, *Federal Register* 60(27): 7772-7774, 1995.

Bane MJ, Ellwood D: *Welfare realities: from rhetoric to reform,* Cambridge, Mass, 1994, Harvard University Press.

Baumann SL: The meaning of being homeless, *Scholarly Inquiry Nurs Pract* 7(1):59-70, 1993.

Bremner RH: *From the depths: the discovery of poverty in the United States,* New York, 1956, University Press.

Brickner PW, Scharer LK, Conanan B, Elvy A, Savarese M: *Health care of homeless people,* New York, 1985, Springer.

Brickner PW, Scanlan BC, Conanan B, Elvy A, McAdam J, Scharer LK, Vicic WJ: Homeless persons and health care, *Ann Intern Med* 104:405-409, 1986.

Cangialosi G: *A kairos winter,* Washington, DC, 1994, Servant Leaderhip School Publication.

Carney P: The concept of poverty, *Public Health Nurs* 9(2):74-80, 1992.

Dahl S, Gustafson C, McCullagh M: Collaborating to develop a community-based health service for rural homeless persons, *J Nurs Adm* 23(4):41-45, 1993.

Davidhizar R and Frank B: Understanding the physical and psychosocial stressors of the child who is homeless, *Pediatr Nurs* 18(6):559-562, 1992.

DeParle J: Welfare as we've known it, *New York Times,* June 19, 1994, p E4.

Dolgoff R, Feldstein D: *Understanding social welfare,* ed 2, White Plains, NY, 1984, Longman.

Elders J: *An urban health crisis.* Keynote address presented at Mothers and Children 1994, Washington, DC, 1994.

Federal Task Force on Homelessness and Severe Mental Illness: *Outcasts on Main Street,* Rockville, Md, 1992, National Institute of Mental Health.

Fetter MS, Larson E: Preventing and treating human immunodeficiency virus infection in the homeless, *Arch Psychiatr Nurs* 4(6):379-383, 1990.

Finney JC, editor: *Culture change, mental health, and poverty,* Lexington, Ky, 1969, University of Kentucky Press.

Fred A, Elman R, editors: *Charles Booth's London,* London, 1969, Hutchinson.

Goldstein A: As patients differ, so do ways of coping, *Washington Post,* Aug 10, 1994, pp A1, A8.

Hawkins JB, Higgins LP: *Nursing and the American health care delivery system,* New York, 1982, Tieresias.

Healthy People 2000: national health promotion and disease prevention objectives, Washington, DC, 1991, USDHHS, Public Health Service.

Hilfiker D: *Not all of us are saints: a doctor's journey with the poor,* New York, 1994, Hill & Wang.

Interagency Council on the Homeless: *The 1990 annual report of the homeless,* Washington, DC, 1991, Department of Health and Human Services.

Jackson MP, McSwane DA: Homelessness as a determinant of health, *Public Health Nurse* 9(3):185-192, 1992.

Jargowsky P, Bane MJ: Ghetto poverty: basic questions. In Lynn LE, McGeary M, editors: *Inner city poverty in the United States,* Washington, DC, 1990, National Academy Press.

Johnson C, Miranda L, Sherman A, Weill J: *Child poverty in America,* Washington, DC, 1991, Children's Defense Fund.

Kothoff ME: Current trends and issues in nursing in the United States: the primary health care nurse practitioner, *Int Nurs Rev* 28(1):24-28, 1981.

Link BG, Susser E, Stueve A, Phelan J, Moore RE, Struening E: Lifetime and five-year prevalence of homelessness in the United States, *Am J Public Health* 84(12):1907-1912, 1994.

Malloy C: Children and poverty: America's future at risk, *Pediatr Nurs* 18(6):553-557, 1992.

Masson V: *Just who,* Washington, DC, 1993, Crossroad Health Ministry.

Masson V: When sugarplums go sour: will health care reform help the poor? *J Christ Nurs* 11(3):17-18, 46, 1994.

Merton V, Merton RK, Barber E: Client ambivalence in professional relationships: the problem of seeking help from strangers. In DePaulo B, Nadler A, Fisher J, editors: *New direction in helping,* vol 2, New York, 1983, Academic Press.

Mihaly LK: *Homeless families: failed policies and young families,* Washington, DC, 1991, Children's Defense Fund.

Miller D, Lin E: Children in sheltered homeless families: reported health status and use of health services, *Pediatrics* 81(5):668-673, 1989.

Miller HP: *Poverty American style,* Belmont, Calif, 1966, Wadsworth.

Moccia P, Mason DJ: Poverty trends: implications for nursing, *Nurs Outlook* 34(1):20-24, 1986.

Nightingale F: *Health teaching in towns and villages, rural hygiene,* London, 1894, Spottiswoode.

Pappas G: Elucidating the relationships between race, socioeconomic status, and health, *Am J Public Health* 84(6):892-893, 1994.

Plotnick R, Skidmore F: *Progress against poverty: a review of the 1964-1974 decade,* New York, 1975, Academic Press.

Price J: More mouths, more money, *Washington Times,* April 19, 1994, p A6.

Raspberry W: Several kinds of poverty, *Washington Post,* May 27, 1994, p A25.

Roy C, Andrews H: *The Roy adaptation model: the definitive statement,* East Norwalk, Conn, 1991, Appleton & Lange.

Schorr L, Schorr D: *Within our reach: breaking the cycle of disadvantage,* New York, 1989, Doubleday.

Sebastian J: Vulnerable populations in the community. In Stanhope M, Lancaster J, editors: *Community health nursing: process and practice for promoting health,* ed 3, St Louis, 1992, Mosby.

Sherman A: Wasting America's future: the children's defense fund report on the costs of child poverty, Boston, 1994, Bacon Press.

Sidel R: *Women and children last: the plight of poor women in affluent America,* New York, 1987, Viking-Penguin.

US Bureau of the Census: *Income, poverty and valuation of noncash benefits,* Current population report P-60, 188, Washington, DC, 1993, US Department of Commerce.

Velsor-Friedrich B: Poverty; its effects on children and their families, *J Pediatr Nurs* 7(6):412-413, 1992.

Velsor-Friedrich B: Homeless children and their families: Part I, The changing picture, *J Pediatr Nurs* 8(2):122-123, 1993a.

Velsor-Friedrich B: Homeless children and their families: Part II, Federal programs and health care delivery systems, *J Pediatr Nurs* 8(3):190-192, 1993b.

Vladeck BC: Health care and the homeless: a political parable for our time, *J Health Polit Policy Law* 15(2):305-317, 1990.

Vredevoe DL, Shuler P, Woo M: The homeless population, *West J Nurs Res* 14(6):731-740, 1992.

Wagner J, Menke E: The depression of homeless children: a focus for nursing intervention, *Issues Compr Pediatr Nurs* 14(1):17-29, 1991.

Wagner J, Menke E: Case management of homeless families, *Clin Nurse Specialist* 6(2):65-71, 1992.

Wallsten SM: Geriatric mental health: a portrait of homelessness, *J Psychosoc Nurs* 30(9):20-24, 1992.

Wiecha JL, Dwyer JT, Dunn-Strohecker M: Nutrition and health services needs among the homeless, *Public Health Rep* 106(4):364-374, 1991.

Wiley DC, Ballard DJ: How can schools help children from homeless families? *J Sch Health* 63(7):291-293, 1993.

Wilson WJ: *The truly disadvantaged: the inner city, the underclass, and public policy,* Chicago, 1987, University of Chicago Press, p 165–167.

Wolch JR, Dear M, Akita A: Explaining homelessness, *Am Plan Assoc J* 54:443-453, 1988.

Wright J, Weber E: *Homelessness and health,* Washington, DC, 1987, McGraw-Hill.

Youings J: *Sixteenth-century England,* London, 1984, Penguin.

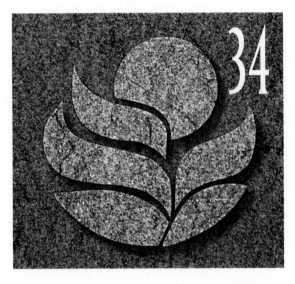

34 Teen Pregnancy

Dyan Aretakis

Objectives ▼

After reading this chapter, the student should be able to do the following:

- ◆ Discuss approaches that could be used in working with the adolescent client.
- ◆ Identify trends in adolescent pregnancy, births, abortions, and adoption in the United States.
- ◆ Discuss reasons that may affect whether a teenager becomes pregnant.
- ◆ Explain some of the deterrents to the establishment of paternity among young fathers.
- ◆ Develop nursing interventions for the prevention of pregnancy problems that adolescents are at risk of experiencing.
- ◆ Identify community health nursing activities that may contribute to the prevention of adolescent pregnancy.

Key Terms ▼

abortion
adoption
birth control
coercive sex
gynecological age
low birth weight
paternity
peer pressure
prematurity
prenatal care
repeat pregnancy
sexual debut
sexual victimization
weight gain

Outline ▼

Teen pregnancy is an area of great public concern. The cause for this concern is not due to dramatic changes in the numbers of pregnant and parenting teenagers but because the impact on communities has become difficult to ignore. Resources to support the special needs of pregnant teenagers are decreasing, and the costs of sustaining young families over time is prohibitive. Many teenagers who become pregnant have been caught in a cycle of poverty, school failure, and limited life options. Other teens will face these issues after a pregnancy occurs. Even under the ideal circumstances of adequate finances, loving and supportive families, and good birth outcomes, a teenager beginning parenthood may need to circumvent necessary developmental tasks in order to raise a child.

There is neither a uniform reason that teens become pregnant nor a universally acceptable solution. The causes of teen pregnancy are diverse and affected by changing moral attitudes, sexual codes, and economic circumstances. The strain that teen pregnancy places on the health care and social service systems is enormous. Social concern also is raised about the lost potential for young parents when pregnancy occurs and the academic and economic disadvantages that their children will experience. Community health nurses are in a key position to understand the impact of teen pregnancy on both the individual and the community and to influence current trends.

This chapter presents a variety of issues associated with teen pregnancy and proposes interventions that community health nurses can use to promote healthy outcomes for individuals and communities.

Did You Know?

The public costs of adolescent pregnancy are staggering. Fifty-nine percent of the families receiving support from Aid for Dependent Children (AFDC), the federal welfare program, began when the mother was a teenager. These families tend to remain on welfare longer than families started when the mother was over age 20. However, states that have the highest AFDC payments per family also have the lowest teen pregnancy rate.

THE ADOLESCENT CLIENT

Adolescents have limited experience independently seeking health care. When they do seek care, it is often to discuss concerns about a possible pregnancy or to find a birth control method. These teens also may need assistance negotiating complex health care systems, and special approaches in both the client interview and subsequent client education are often warranted. The behavior of adolescents toward the community health nurse can range from mature and competent at one visit to hostile, rude, or distant at other times, since the behavior often reflects intense anxiety over what they are experiencing.

Since client interviews usually begin with evaluation of a chief complaint, teens need to know that their concerns are heard. Health care providers may have their own opinions about what teenagers need and may fail to take the chief complaint seriously. For example, when a teen expresses a desire to become pregnant, this should be discussed in depth even though the community health nurse may feel uncomfortable providing information about how to conceive to a young teen. During the interview the nurse can provide preconceptual counseling and emphasize the need to achieve good health and to establish a health-promoting life-style before pregnancy. Not only does information presented this way demonstrate that the nurse has heard what the teen is saying, but it also allows the nurse to provide useful health information that may encourage the teen to examine her plans carefully, seriously, and maturely.

The nurse should pay attention to what the teen fails to verbalize. Knowledge of adolescent health care issues is valuable so that the nurse can anticipate other health concerns and provide an environment in which the adolescent feels safe in raising other concerns. By creating a caring and understanding atmosphere, the nurse can encourage the young person to discuss concerns about family violence, drugs, alcohol, or dating.

Discussing reproductive health care is a sensitive matter for both teens and many adults. Teens may have difficulty expressing themselves because of a limited sexual vocabulary or embarrassment due to their lack of knowledge. The community health nurse must recognize this potential deficit and embarrassment and assist teens by anticipating concerns and by allowing them to express themselves in their own language, which may include crude or offensive words. Nurses must learn about common slang expressions and common misconceptions so they do not miss important concerns that a teenager might have. The nurse can offer more appropriate terms once trust is established.

Teens may have difficulty discussing topics that provoke a judgmental reaction, such as discussing sexually transmitted diseases (STDs; see box on p. 667, top left). It is important for the nurse to choose neutral words to elicit symptoms (e.g., "Has there been a change in your typical vaginal discharge?"). This approach also gives the nurse a chance to educate the young client about normal anatomy and physiology.

Considerable debate exists over whether adolescents should make reproductive health care decisions without their parents' knowledge. As seen in box on p. 667, top right, the adolescent's right to privacy, and thus her right to contraceptive treatment, is federally protected. Obstacles to services do exist, however, and

Sexually Transmitted Diseases and Teen Pregnancy

Sexually transmitted diseases (STDs) affect 25% of sexually experienced teenagers each year. STDs are more easily transmitted to women than men and can be more difficult to detect. STD infections among women can contribute to infertility, cancers, and ectopic pregnancy. When a young women is pregnant, these infections can cause premature rupture of membranes, premature labor, and postpartum infection. Also, the baby can be affected by all STDs in several ways: prematurity and low birth weight, febrile infection after delivery, and long-term infection and even death (e.g., exposure to viral infections such as HPV, HSV, HBV, and HIV).

The pregnant adolescent is at high risk for acquiring an STD because of not using contraceptives such as condoms. During the pregnancy, she will require periodic STD screening. STD education and counseling should accompany this screening. Information given should include ways to reduce one's risk, such as maintaining a mutually monogamous relationship and using latex condoms.

Reproductive Health Care and Adolescents' Rights

No federal regulation requires a young person to have parents involved in decisions on contraception services provided by federal programs. States cannot prohibit an adolescent access to contraception. Several Supreme Court decisions protect this access:

1965: *Griswold v. Connecticut*—the right to prevent pregnancy through the use of contraceptives is protected by the right to privacy.

1972: *Eisenstad v. Baird*—the right to privacy in contraceptive use is extended to unmarried individuals.

1977: *Carey v. Population Services International*—the right to privacy is specifically extended to minors.

Modified from Center for Population Options: *Adolescent abortion and mandated parental involvement: the impact of back alley laws on young women*, Washington, DC, 1993, The Center.

this may result in a teen not receiving contraceptive information and treatment. Obstacles can include lack of transportation to a health care facility, money to pay for services, or permission to leave school early to attend an appointment.

Abortion services for adolescents are not clearly defined. No federal protection is extended to adolescents requesting abortion services, and the adolescent's right to privacy and ability to give consent varies by state, as seen in the box at right.

Confidential care to teenagers may mean the difference between preventing a pregnancy, an unwanted pregnancy, an abortion, or a birth. This care can influence whether prenatal visits begin in the first trimester versus the second or third trimester. Teens have varied reasons for pursuing confidential care, including their attempt at independence as well as serious and well-founded concerns about a parent's potential reaction, such as with an abusive parent. The nurse should identify the reason for confidential care and work with the teen to discuss reproductive health care needs with the family. First, clarify family values about sexuality and family communication styles with the teen. In a dysfunctional family, referral to additional community agencies (e.g., child protective services, Al-Anon) may be necessary. However, the nurse may need to honor the adolescent's need for confidentiality for an unknown period of time and proceed with the usual interventions, such as pregnancy testing, options counseling, and referral for clinical care.

TRENDS IN ADOLESCENT SEXUAL BEHAVIOR AND PREGNANCY

More than 1 million teens become pregnant each year, and more than half go on to have babies. Births

Abortion and Adolescent Rights

Parental consent laws: the parents of a young woman who is under 18 years of age seeking an abortion must give permission to the abortion provider before the abortion is performed. These laws are enforced in 12 states: Alabama, Indiana, Louisiana, Massachusetts, Michigan, Mississippi, Missouri, North Dakota, Rhode Island, South Carolina, Wisconsin, and Wyoming.

Parental notification laws: one or both parents of a young woman seeking an abortion must be notified by the abortion provider before the abortion is performed. These laws are enforced in 10 states: Arkansas, Georgia, Kansas, Maryland, Minnesota, Nebraska, Ohio, Tennessee, Utah, and West Virginia.

Judicial bypass: in a 1979 Supreme Court decision, it was ruled that any mandatory parental consent law must allow the young woman an opportunity to be granted an exception or waiver to the law. A young woman could appeal directly to a judge, who would decide either that she was mature enough to make this decision or that the abortion would be in her best interest. In three states (Maryland, Maine, Connecticut) an adult other than a judge can substitute for parental consent.

Modified from Center for Population Options: *Adolescent abortion and mandated parental involvement: the impact of back alley laws on young women*, Washington, DC, 1993, The Center.

to teenagers compose 24% of all first births in the United States (Moore and Snyder, 1994). The numbers of teens who become pregnant are generally identified in the following way: by age group (less than 15, ages 15 to 17, ages 18 to 19); by pregnancy outcomes (birth, induced abortion or spontaneous abortion); by rates (number of pregnancies, births, and abortions per 1000 young women); and by race/ethnicity (black, white, Hispanic). Birth rates are highest among older teens and decrease with age.

Healthy People 2000 Objectives Related to Adolescent Reproductive Health

1. Reduce pregnancies among girls aged 17 and younger; special population targets are black and Hispanic girls aged 15 to 19.
2. Reduce rape and attempted rape of young women.
3. Increase calcium intake to three or more servings daily of foods rich in calcium for youth aged 12 to 24 and for pregnant and lactating women.
4. Reduce the proportion of adolescents who have engaged in sexual intercourse.
5. Increase abstinence from sexual activity for the previous 3 months among sexually active adolescents aged 17 and younger.
6. Increase contraceptive use, especially those methods that prevent pregnancy and provide barrier protection against disease, among sexually active young people aged 19 and younger.
7. Increase the proportion of sexually active unmarried young women whose partner used a condom at last intercourse.
8. Increase the proportion of sexually active unmarried men aged 15 to 19 who used a condom at last intercourse.
9. Increase the proportion of persons aged 10 to 18 who have discussed human sexuality, including values surrounding sexuality, with their parents and/or have received information through another parentally endorsed source, such as youth, school, or religious programs.
10. Increase the proportion of primary care providers who provide age-appropriate preconception care and counseling.
11. Increase discussions among persons aged 10 and older with family members on topics related to nutrition, physical activity, sexual behavior, tobacco, alcohol, other drugs, or safety.

Modified from *Healthy People 2000: national health promotion and disease prevention objectives*, Washington, DC, 1991, USDHHS, Public Health Service.

Pregnancy rates have increased steadily among teens of all ages from 1986 to 1991, but the total number of pregnancies to teens has declined recently as the population of teenagers has decreased (Spitz et al., 1993).

Birth rates are highest among black teens and are more than double the rate for white teens. Hispanic teens have the next highest rate and have had the greatest increase over the past 5 years (Spitz et al., 1993). Sixty-nine percent of teens are unmarried at the time of their child's birth, a number that has quadrupled since 1960 (Moore and Snyder, 1994).

Healthy People 2000 (1991) established a baseline rate for 1985 of 71.1 pregnancies per 1000 girls aged 15 to 17 and seeks to reduce this to 50 per 1000 adolescents (see box above). By 1990, almost half the states reporting data had reached this goal. The goal for special adolescent populations, such as black and Hispanic girls, is 120 pregnancies per 1000 and 105 pregnancies per 1000, respectively. Less progress has been made toward this goal, with only two of 24 re-

porting states reaching the goal for black adolescent females and nine of 19 reporting states reaching the goal by 1990 for Hispanic adolescent females (*Healthy People 2000,* 1991; Spitz et al., 1993).

Striking geographical differences exist in the distribution of birth rates among teens. The southern states account for a disproportionate number of births to teens. In 1985, almost 50% of babies born to teenagers were from the South, and more than half of either repeat teen births or births to teens under age 15 were among southern teens (*Adolescent pregnancy in the South,* 1989). In 1990 the states with pregnancy rates greater than 50 per 1000 teens ages 15 to 17 were Arizona, Arkansas, Colorado, District of Columbia, Georgia, Hawaii, Kentucky, Louisiana, Maryland, Michigan, Mississippi, Missouri, Nevada, New Mexico, New York, North Carolina, Oregon, Rhode Island, South Carolina, Tennessee, Texas, Virginia, and Washington (Spitz et al., 1993).

Forty-one percent of pregnancies to teenagers are ended by elective abortion (Henshaw, 1993) and 12% by spontaneous abortion (Spitz et al., 1993). Elective abortion rates for teenagers increased from the time of legalization in 1973. From 1986 to 1990, there was a 21% decrease in abortions to teens and a 20% increase in births (Spitz et al., 1993). This decrease may partly result from laws that have required parental notification for minors requesting abortion services in some states. Black and white teens choose abortion at similar rates. Adolescents who terminate their pregnancies by abortion differ from those who give birth in the following ways: more likely to complete high school, more successful in school, higher education aspirations, and more likely to come from a family of a higher socioeconomic status (Alexander and Guyer, 1993).

The United States leads the developed world in rates of teenage pregnancy, teen births, and teen abortions. Teens in Sweden have the highest rate of sexual activity (the United States is second), but they experience fewer pregnancies, births, and abortions. If these same comparisons are made with only white teens, the United States still leads in the number of pregnancies, births, and abortions. Comparisons with statistics in other countries suggests that much of this difference is caused by the limited use of contraceptives among teens as well as a general ambivalence about providing comprehensive sexuality education at home and at school for children and adolescents in the United States (Hatcher et al., 1994).

| What Do You Think? |

Elimination of welfare benefits to school-age parents will reduce adolescent pregnancy.

BACKGROUND FACTORS IN TEEN PREGNANCY

Many adults have difficulty understanding why young people would jeopardize their career and personal potential by becoming pregnant during the teen years. Adolescents, however, view the world differently than do adults. Teens often feel invincible and therefore do not anticipate any risk for the consequences related to their behaviors. That is, they may not believe that sexual activity will lead to pregnancy. When teens become pregnant, they do not think that the negative outcomes they are advised of could come true. Each teen believes he or she is unique and different—the person for whom everything will work out fine. Pregnant teens often express an attitude that they can do it all: school, work, parenting, and socializing.

The characteristics of the teens who are giving birth is changing. A disproportionate number of teens who give birth are poor (more than three quarters), have limited educational achievements, and see few advantages in delaying pregnancy since they do not expect that their circumstances will improve at a later time (Nord et al., 1992). Most teens report that their pregnancy was unplanned, and they typically say they think a pregnancy should be delayed until people are older, have completed their education, and are employed and married (Hatcher et al., 1994). Their behaviors, however, do not support the opinions they express. In fact, some teens actually seem ambitious about becoming pregnant. Several of the factors that often contribute to pregnancy are discussed next.

Sexual Activity and Use of Birth Control

Teens increasingly have their **sexual debut,** or first experience with intercourse, at an earlier age. The proportion of sexually active teens has also increased, although the velocity of this increase is declining. By the 9th grade, 40% of teens are sexually active; by 10th grade, 48%; by 11th grade, 57%; and by 12th grade, 72% (Centers for Disease Control and Prevention [CDC], 1992). Boys reported a dramatic increase in sexual experience between ages 13 and 14; girls reported this dramatic increase between ages 14 and 15 (Leigh et al., 1994). The age of onset varies by residence, race/ethnicity, and family income.

The *Healthy People 2000* goal for adolescents who have engaged in sexual intercourse is a reduction to no more than 15% by age 15 and no more than 40% by age 17 (baseline of 27% girls and 33% boys by age 15; 50% girls and 66% boys by age 17, reported in 1988). Progress has not been made toward these goals because the percentages of sexually active teens continues to rise.

Although more teens have begun using **birth control** in the past 10 years, there still is progress to be made; 65% of adolescent women (Hatcher et al., 1994) report use of birth control at first coitus, and 77% of young men report use of birth control at most recent intercourse (Marsiglio, 1993). Half of all first-time pregnancies occur within 6 months of initiating intercourse (Hatcher et al., 1994). Teens harbor many myths that contribute to poor use of birth control, such as believing you cannot get pregnant the first time, or they may have erroneous knowledge about a woman's fertile time. Failure to use birth control by teens can also reflect their embarrassment in discussing this practice with partners, friends, parents, and health care providers and the obstacles they encounter finding facilities that provide confidential and affordable birth control (Hatcher et al., 1994).

The earlier the sexual debut, the less likely a birth control method will be used, since younger teens have less knowledge and skill related to sexuality and birth control. School-based sex education can come too late or not at all. Birth control is usually discussed in the secondary-school curriculum, but this could be 8th grade in one school district and 10th in another; school curricula are not standardized. Younger teens may falsely believe that they are too young to purchase birth control methods such as condoms. Confidential reproductive health care services may be available for teens, but problems are still associated with transportation, school absences, and costs of care that ultimately restrict access to these services.

Inconsistent use of birth control can reflect teens' willingness to take risks, their dissatisfactions with available birth control methods, and their ambivalence about becoming pregnant. Real and perceived side effects of birth control methods can discourage use. The newer birth control methods such as Depo-Provera (an intramuscular injection every 3 months) and Norplant (a 5-year implant) appeal to some women because the method is less directly tied to coitus. These newer methods may have nuisance-type side effects (e.g., irregular bleeding) that are unappealing to many women.

The use of alcohol and other substances is common among adolescents and can contribute to unplanned pregnancy. Mood-altering effects may reduce inhibitions about engaging in intercourse and interfere with the proper use of a chosen birth control method.

Peer Pressure and Partner Pressure

Peer pressure among teens is not a new phenomenon, but many of the influences have become more serious. Influence has expanded from fashion and language to cigarettes, substance abuse, sexuality, and pregnancy. Teens are more likely to be sexually active if their friends are sexually active (Perkins, 1991). Peers reinforce teen parenting by exaggerating birth control risks, discouraging abortion and adoption, and glamorizing the impending birth of the child.

Both young men and women may think that allowing a pregnancy to happen verifies one's love and commitment for the other. In addition, young men from socioeconomically disadvantaged backgrounds may be more likely to say that fathering a child would make them feel more manly and are less likely to use an effective contraceptive (Marsiglio, 1993).

Other Factors

Other factors influencing teen pregnancy include (1) history of sexual victimization, (2) family structure, and (3) parental influences.

Adolescent women who have a history of sexual abuse are at risk for earlier initiation of voluntary sexual intercourse, are less likely to use birth control, are more likely to use drugs and alcohol at first intercourse, and are more likely to have older sexual partners (Boyer and Fine, 1992). The youngest women are more likely to experience **coercive sex** (74% of women who had intercourse before age 14 reported that it was involuntary) (Alan Guttmacher Institute, 1994). Young women may also become pregnant as a result of forced sexual intercourse. A history of **sexual victimization** will influence a young woman's ability to exert control over future sexual experiences, which will affect the use or nonuse of birth control and rejection of unwanted sexual experiences. Several studies have found that more than half of pregnant teenagers have experienced sexual abuse either before or during the pregnancy (Parker, 1993). In addition, young women who have experienced a lifetime of economic, social, and psychological deprivation may think that a baby will bring joy into an otherwise bleak existence. Some women mistakenly think that a baby can provide the love and attention that her family has not provided.

Family structure can influence adolescent sexual behavior and pregnancy. Adolescents from single-parent families may be more likely to have intercourse than those from two-parent families. Adolescents in families in which there is a divorce and remarriage are also at increased risk (East and Felice, 1992). The age of a young woman when the family structure changes is also important. The most vulnerable age for a family change to occur is 14 (Hollander, 1993).

Parenting styles can influence a young woman's risk for early sexual experiences and pregnancy. Parents who are extremely demanding and controlling or neglectful and having low expectations are least successful in instilling parental values in their children. Parents who have high demands for their children to act maturely and who offer warmth and understanding with parental rules have children more likely to exhibit appropriate social behavior who delay early sexual experiences and pregnancy. Children of parents who are neglectful are the most sexually experienced, followed by parents who are very strict. Further, parents who discuss birth control, sexuality, and pregnancy with their children can positively influence delay of sexual initiation and effective birth control use. Parents who do not communicate about sexuality with their teens may find them more at risk for sexual permissiveness and pregnancy (East and Felice, 1992).

YOUNG MEN AND PATERNITY

One in 15 males becomes a father during the teen years. While one-third of the fathers of babies born to teens are teens themselves, more than half the fathers are between ages 20 and 24. Most fathers of babies born to adolescent mothers are 2 to 3 years older than the mother (Robinson, 1988).

Paternity, or fatherhood, is legally established at the time of the birth when a teen is married. However, it is more difficult to establish paternity among nonmarried couples. Some of the difficulty lies in the complexity of the specific state system for young men to acknowledge paternity. In some states, a young man may have to work with the judicial system outside of the hospital after the birth, and if he is under age 18, he may need to involve his parents.

Some young couples do not attempt to establish paternity and prefer a verbal promise of assistance for the teen mother and child. Although a verbal commitment may be acceptable when the child is born, the mother may become more inclined to pursue the establishment of paternity later when the relationship ends or for reasons related to financial, social, or emotional needs of the child. Young women who receive state or federal assistance (e.g., Aid for Dependent Children, Medicaid) may be asked to name the child's father so the judicial process can be used to establish paternity.

Young men react differently on learning that the partner is pregnant. The reaction often depends on the nature of the relationship before the pregnancy. Many young men will accompany the young woman to a health care center for pregnancy diagnosis and counseling. A large percentage of young men will continue to accompany the young woman to some prenatal visits and may even attend the delivery (Robinson, 1988). These young men may also want to and need to be involved with their children regardless of changes that they may experience in their relationships with the teen mother. It is not unusual for a young man to be excluded or even rejected by the young woman's family (usually her mother), and he may not be motivated or courageous enough to resolve these conflicts.

It is important for the community health nurse to acknowledge and support the young man as he develops in the role of father. His involvement can positively affect his child's development and provide greater personal satisfaction for himself and greater role satisfaction for the young mother (Castiglia, 1990b). The immediate concerns revolve around his financial responsibility, living arrangements, relationship issues, school, and work. Establishing an opportunity to meet with the young man and both families is helpful to clarify these issues and begin to identify roles and responsibilities.

Young men who grow up in poor families are more likely to believe that fathering a child would make them feel manly and are more likely to be pleased with a pregnancy than their affluent counterparts. These young men are also less likely to use or to discuss birth control with a partner. Young men who had previously impregnated a young woman are more likely to feel and act this way (Marsiglio, 1993).

EARLY IDENTIFICATION OF THE PREGNANT TEEN

Some teens delay seeking pregnancy services because they fail to recognize signs such as breast tenderness and a late period because they are experiencing a variety of other pubertal changes. Most young women, however, suspect pregnancy as soon as a period is late. These young women may still delay seeking care, since they falsely hope that the pregnancy will just simply go away. A teen also may delay seeking care to keep the pregnancy a secret from family members, who may pressure her to terminate the pregnancy, or because of fears about gynecological examinations (Cartwright et al., 1993).

Community health nurses must be sensitive to subtle cues that a teenager may offer about sexuality and pregnancy concerns. Such cues include questions about one's fertile period or requests for confirmation that one need not miss a period to be pregnant. Once the nurse identifies the specific concern, information can be provided about how and when to obtain pregnancy testing. The nurse should determine how a teenager would react to the possible pregnancy before completing the test. If the test is negative, the nurse should take the opportunity to assess whether the young woman would consider counseling to prevent pregnancy. A follow-up visit is important after a negative test to determine if retesting is necessary or if another problem exists.

A young woman with a positive pregnancy test requires a physical examination and pregnancy counseling. It is advantageous to offer these at the same time so that the nature of the counseling will be consistent with the findings of the examination. The purpose of the examination is to assess the duration and well-being of the pregnancy as well as to test for sexually transmitted infection. The pregnancy counseling should include the following: information on adoption, abortion, and childrearing; an opportunity for assessment of support systems for the young woman; and identification of the immediate concerns she might have.

The availability of affordable **abortion** services up to 13 weeks' gestation will vary from community to community, whereas second-trimester services may be available locally or involve extensive travel and cost. The community health nurse should be knowledgeable about abortion services and provide information or refer the pregnant teenager to a pregnancy counseling service that can assist.

Guidelines for Adoption Counseling

1. Assess your own thoughts and feelings on adoption. Do not impose your opinion on the decision-making process of teen mothers.
2. Be knowledgeable about state laws, local resources, and various types of adoption services.
3. Choose language sensitively. For example:
   a. Avoid saying "giving away a child" or "putting up for adoption." It is more appropriate and positive to say "releasing a child for adoption," "placing for adoption," or "making an adoption plan."
   b. Avoid saying "unwanted child" or "unwanted pregnancy." A more appropriate term may be "unplanned pregnancy."
   c. Avoid saying "natural parents" or "natural child," since the adopted parents would then seem to be "unnatural." The terms "biological parents" and "adopted parents" are more appropriate.
4. Assess when a discussion of adoption is appropriate. It can be helpful to begin with information on adoption, then explore feelings and concerns over time. Individuals will vary in how much they may have already considered adoption, and this will influence the counseling session.
5. Assess the relationship between the pregnant teen and her partner and what role she expects him to play. Discuss the reality of this.
6. It may be helpful for a pregnant teen to talk with other teens who have been pregnant, are raising a child, have released a child for adoption, or have been adopted themselves.
7. A young woman can be encouraged to begin writing letters to her baby. These can be saved or given to the child when released to the adoptive family.

Modified from Brandsen CK: A *case for adoption*, Grand Rapids, Michigan, 1991, Bethany.

The pregnant teenager needs information about **adoption,** such as current policies among agencies that allow for continued contact with the adopting family. Also, church organizations, private attorneys, and social service agencies provide a variety of adoption services with which the community health nurse should be familiar. The box above lists guidelines for adoption counseling. *Healthy People 2000* objectives include efforts to increase to 90% the proportion of pregnancy counselors who offer positive, accurate information about adoption to their unmarried clients with unintended pregnancies (baseline: 60% of pregnancy counselors in 1984). At this time, 5% of unmarried adolescent women relinquish custody of their children (Nichols, 1991).

Pregnancy counseling requires that the nurse and young woman explore strengths and weaknesses for personal care and responsibility during a pregnancy and parenting. Young women vary in their interest to include the partner or their parents in this discussion. Issues to raise include educational and career plans, family finances and qualifications for outside assistance, and personal values about pregnancy and parenting at this time in their life. Often it is difficult to focus on counseling in any depth at the time of the initial pregnancy testing results. A follow-up visit is usually more productive and should be arranged as soon as possible.

As decisions are made about the course of the pregnancy, the community health nurse is instrumental in referral to appropriate programs such as WIC (Supplemental Food Program for Women, Infants, and Children), Medicaid, and prenatal services. The young woman and her family will also need to know about expected costs of care, and if there is a family insurance policy, whether it will cover the pregnancy-related expenses of a dependent child. For those without insurance, the family can apply for Medicaid or determine if local facilities offer indigent care programs (e.g., Hill-Burton programs for assistance with hospital expenses). The community health nurse can also begin prenatal education and counseling on nutrition, substance abuse/use, exercise, and special medical concerns.

SPECIAL ISSUES IN CARING FOR THE PREGNANT TEEN

Pregnant teenagers are considered high-risk obstetrical clients. Many of the complications of their pregnancy result from poverty, late entry into prenatal care, and limited knowledge about self-care during pregnancy. Community health nursing interventions through education and early identification of problems may dramatically alter the course of the pregnancy and birth outcome.

Initiation of Prenatal Care

Pregnant adolescents differ remarkably from pregnant adults in initiation and compliance with **prenatal care.** Inadequate prenatal care has been negatively associated with health risks to both the mother and the fetus. Half of all pregnant teens delay entering prenatal care until after the first trimester, whereas one-quarter of women of all ages delay until after the first trimester (Children's Defense Fund, 1994; VanWinter and Simmons, 1990). Teens report that the greatest barrier to care is cost, whether it is perceived or real (Cartwright et al., 1993). Other barriers include denial of the pregnancy, fear of telling parents, transportation, dislike of providers' care, and attitudes among clinic staff toward pregnant teens (Cartoof et al., 1991; VanWinter and Simmons, 1990).

Once a teen is enrolled in prenatal care, the community health nurse becomes an important liaison between personnel at the clinical site and the young woman. Confusion and misunderstandings easily occur when teens do not understand what a health care provider says to them. Often these misunderstandings are based on lack of knowledge about basic anatomy and physiology. For example, a teen may be told as she gets close to term that the head of the baby is down and it can be felt. This is an alarming piece of information for a young woman who imagines the entire baby could just pop out any time!

Cooperation between the community health nurse and the clinical staff can also maximize the client's compliance with special health or nutritional needs. For example, a teen who has premature contractions may be placed on bed rest and instructed to increase fluids. The community health nurse who makes home visits can provide additional assessment of the teen's condition and can problem solve about self-care, hygiene, meals, and school.

Low-Birth-Weight Infants and Preterm Delivery

Teens are more likely than adult women to deliver babies weighing less than $5\frac{1}{2}$ pounds or to deliver before 37 weeks' gestation. The risk of **low birth weight** or **prematurity** is greater for younger teens and for a second birth to a teen, especially if it is within 1 year of the first. These low-birth-weight and premature babies are at greater risk for death in the first year of life and are more at risk for long-term physical, emotional, and cognitive problems (Nord et al., 1992). For example, low-birth-weight and premature babies can be more difficult to feed and soothe. This challenges the limited skills of the young mother and can further strain relations with other members of the household, who may not know how to offer support or assistance.

The risk of low-birth-weight and premature births can be averted by the teen's early initiation into prenatal care. Although such births still occur, it is important to work closely with the teen mother as soon as she is identified as pregnant to try to promote compliance with prenatal care visits and self-care during the pregnancy. After the pregnancy, these babies and their mothers will benefit from frequent nursing supervision to ensure that their care is appropriate and that everyone in the home is coping adequately with the strain of a small baby.

Nutrition

The nutritional needs of a pregnant teenager are especially important. First, the teen life-style does not lend itself to overall good nutrition. Fast foods, frequent snacking, and hectic social schedules limit nutritious food choices. Snacks, which account for approximately a third of a teen's daily caloric intake, tend to be high in fat, sugar, and sodium and limited in essential vitamins and minerals. Second, the nutritive needs of both pregnancy and the concurrent adolescent growth spurt require the adolescent to change her diet substantially. The growing teen must increase caloric nutrients to meet individual growth needs as well as allow for adequate fetal growth. Third, poor eating patterns of the teen and her current growth requirement may leave her with limited reserves of essential vitamins and minerals when the pregnancy begins. The community health nurse can assess the pregnant teenager's current eating pattern and provide creative guidance. For example, protein can be increased at fast-food establishments by ordering milkshakes instead of soft drinks and cheeseburgers or broiled chicken sandwiches instead of hamburgers. Snack foods can be purchased for eating on the way to school in the morning and for midmorning snacks (Story, 1990).

The recommended nutritional needs of the adolescent depend on the **gynecological age** of the teen, that is, the number of years between her chronological age and her age at menarche. Young women with a gynecological age of 2 or less years have increased nutrient requirements because of their own growth. Further, the younger and still growing teen may compete nutritionally with the fetus. Fetuses may show evidence of slower growth in young women ages 10 to 16 years (Story, 1990). The community health nurse in collaboration with the WIC nutritionist can determine the nutritional needs of the pregnant teenager to tailor education appropriately.

Weight gain during pregnancy is one of the strongest predictors of infant birth weight. Although precise weight gain goals in adolescence are controversial, pregnant adolescents who gain 26 to 35 pounds have the lowest incidence of low-birth-weight babies (Story, 1990). Younger teen mothers (ages 13 to 16), because of their own growth demands, may need to gain more weight then older teen mothers (ages 17 and over) to have the same-birth-weight baby. Adolescents who begin the pregnancy underweight and have a low pregnancy weight gain are at the greatest risk of a low-birth-weight baby (Story, 1990). Teenagers who begin the pregnancy at a normal weight should be counseled to begin weight gain in the first trimester and average gains of 1 pound per week for the second and third trimesters (Gutierrez and King, 1993). Table 34-1 shows the recommendations established by the Institute for Medicine for adolescent gestational weight gain by prepregnant weight categories.

Table 34-1   Gestational Weight Gain Recommendations for Adolescents*

Prepregnant weight categories[†]	Recommended total gain	
	kg	lb
Underweight (BMI 19.8)	12.5-18	28-40
Normal weight (BMI 19.9-26)	11.5-16	25-35
Overweight (BMI 26-29)	7.0-11.5	15-25
Very overweight (BMI 29)	7.0-9.1	15-20

From Gutierrez Y, King JC: *Pediatr Ann* 22(2):99-108, 1993.
*Very young adolescents (less than or equal to 14 years of age or less than 2 years postmenarche) should strive for gains at the upper end of the range.
[†]BMI (body mass index) is calculated as weight (kg)/height squared (m).

It is important for the community health nurse to assess the attitudes of the pregnant teen about weight gain and to follow her progress. Studies indicate that most teenagers view prenatal weight gain positively (Matsuhashi and Felice, 1991). However, teens who are overweight before pregnancy may have negative attitudes about weight gain. Family support of the pregnant teen can be a strong influence in adequate weight gain and good nutrition during the pregnancy (Stevens-Simon et al., 1993). Nutrition education should emphasize what accounts for weight gain and how fetal growth will benefit.

Iron deficiency is the most common nutritional problem among both pregnant and nonpregnant adolescent females (Story, 1990). The adolescent may begin a pregnancy with low or absent iron stores because of heavy periods, a previous pregnancy, growth demands, poor iron intake, or substance abuse. The increased maternal plasma volume and increased fetal demands for iron (especially in the third trimester) can further compromise the adolescent. Iron deficiency in pregnancy may contribute to increased prematurity, low birth weight, postpartum hemorrhage, maternal headaches, dizziness, shortness of breath, and so on (Story, 1990). The community health nurse can reinforce the need for the teen to take prenatal vitamins during the pregnancy and after the baby's birth; these should contain 30 to 60 mg elemental iron daily. The nurse should educate about iron-rich foods and foods that promote iron absorption, such as those containing vitamin C.

Infant Care

Many adolescents have cared for babies and small children and feel confident and competent. Few teens are ever prepared, however, for the reality of 24-hour care of an infant. The community health nurse can help prepare the teen for the transition to motherhood while she is still pregnant. The nurse can enlist the support of the teen's parents in education about infant care and stimulation. A young father-to-be would benefit from this education as well. The nurse may become aware of child-rearing beliefs and practices that are deeply embedded in the family's values and may need to gently work to change these beliefs. For example, a family may believe that corporal punishment is a necessary component of child rearing.

Adolescents may also have unrealistic expectations about their children's development; for example, they may expect their children to feed themselves at an early age (Castiglia, 1990a). The teen parents often lack knowledge about infant growth and development, as seen in their limited verbal communication with their children, limited eye contact, and the tendency to display frustration and ambivalence as mothers (Koniak-Griffin and Verzemnieks, 1991). Over time, adolescents can improve their ability to foster their children's emotional and social growth. Children of adolescent mothers have also been found to be at risk for academic and behavior problems in late childhood and adolescence (Klerman, 1993). These risks can be reduced when the teen mother receives professional intervention and supervision in the area of infant cognitive development (Ruff, 1990).

Abusive parenting is more likely to occur when the parents have limited knowledge about normal child development. It may also be more likely to occur among parents who cannot adequately empathize with a child's needs. Younger teens are particularly at risk for being unable to understand what their infant or child needs, and this frustration often is exhibited by abusive behavior toward the child (Marshall et al., 1994).

After the birth of the baby, the community health nurse should observe how the mother responds to infant cues for basic needs and distress. The box at right lists specific techniques the new mother can be instructed to use in early child care. It is important to begin parenting education as early as possible. Adolescents who feel competent as parents have enhanced self-esteem; which in turn positively influences their relationship with their child (Censullo, 1994). Recognizing these good parenting skills and providing positive feedback help a young mother gain confidence in her role.

 Research Brief

Arenson JD: Strengths and self-perceptions of parenting in adolescent mothers, J *Pediatr Nurs* 9(4):251-258, 1994.

This study sought to move beyond the negative association with adolescent parenting by having young women discuss how they see themselves as parents and identify their strengths in coping with adolescent parenting.

Study participants were teenage mothers attending a health department pediatric clinic with their children. The format used was open-ended interviews that were later analyzed to identify themes and categories. These young women found that having a child brought positive changes to their lives, such as helping them feel better about themselves. They were also found to have a high degree of hope for both their own and their child's future. Another finding in this study was that most of these young women had an unhappy and destructive past with poor family relationships. The birth of their children brought a notable change in these behaviors, and relationships within the family were dramatically improved.

The implications of this study encourage nurses to recognize the positive outcomes from adolescent birth experiences. For example, the nurse can be more sensitive to the adolescent's perspective of her life and general contentment. This can include anticipatory guidance that meets the needs of the child-rearing young mother.

 Guidelines for Teen Mother/Newborn Interactions

1. Make eye contact with your baby. Position your face 8 to 10 inches from your baby's face and smile.
2. Talk to your baby often. Use simple sentences, but try to avoid baby talk. Allow time for your baby to "answer." This will help your baby acquire language and communication skills.
3. Babies often enjoy when you sing to them, and this may help soothe them during a difficult time or help them fall asleep. Experiment with different songs and melodies to see which your baby seems to like.
4. Babies at this age cannot be spoiled. Instead, when babies are held and cuddled, they feel secure and loved.
5. Babies cry for many reasons and for no reason at all. If your baby has a clean diaper, has recently been fed and is safe and secure, he or she may just need to cry for a few minutes. What works to calm your baby may be different from other babies you have known. You can try rocking, gentle reassuring words, soft music, or quiet.
6. Make feeding times pleasant for both of you. Do not prop the bottle in your baby's mouth. Instead, you should sit comfortably, hold your baby in your arms, and offer the bottle or breast.
7. When babies are awake, they love to play. They enjoy taking walks and looking at brightly colored objects or pictures and toys that make noises, such as rattles and musical toys.

Repeat Pregnancy

Teen mothers who experience a closely spaced second pregnancy, or **repeat pregnancy,** have poorer educational and economic outcomes. Twenty-four percent of teens will have a second birth within 24 months, and the younger the teen, the greater the risk of an early second pregnancy (Kalmuss and Namerov, 1994). Community health nurses should recognize the risk factors for a second teen pregnancy: teens from disadvantaged backgrounds, teens from large families, those who are married, and those who had discontinued their education after the delivery of the first child. Also, teens who reported a planned first pregnancy are more likely to have a second pregnancy within 24 months to complete their family. Parenting adolescents who return to school after the birth of their first child, regardless of prior school performance, are least likely to repeat a pregnancy and more likely to use birth control (Kalmuss and Namerov, 1994).

Discussions about family planning should be initiated during the third trimester of the current pregnancy. Contraceptive options should be reviewed, and the young woman should begin identifying the methods she is most likely to use. It is helpful to determine at this time the methods she has used in the past, her satisfaction or dissatisfaction, and reasons for use or nonuse. Many teens express unrealistic goals, such as "I am never going to have sex again" or "I need a break from guys," and they may erroneously believe that they are unable to conceive for some time after the delivery. After delivery, the community health nurse should follow up on the young woman's plan. Obstacles to obtaining contraceptives may exist, and the nurse can identify these and help problem solve with the new mother.

Schooling and Educational Needs

Adolescents who become parents may have had limited school success before the pregnancy. As noted previously, the potential for a closely spaced second birth may be delayed by return to school. Federal legislation passed in 1972 prohibits schools from excluding students because they are pregnant. Greater emphasis is placed on keeping the pregnant adolescent in school during the pregnancy and returning as soon as possible after the birth. Several factors may positively influence a young woman's return to school. These include her parents' level of education and their marital stability, small family size, whether there have been reading materials at home, whether her mother is employed, and if the young woman is African-American (Ahn, 1994; Klerman, 1993). A practical challenge for young parents is locating and affording quality child care; difficulties with this may prevent the highly motivated teenager from returning to school. In the past 30 years, the percentage of parenting teens who return to school and graduate has improved significantly (Nord et al., 1992).

Young women who have pregnancy complications may seek home instruction. This decision is made according to regulations issued by the state boards of education. Some young women have difficulty attending school because of the normal discomforts of pregnancy or because of social and emotional conflicts associated with the pregnancy. Teens who leave school without parental or medical excuses may face legal problems because of truancy. This increases the potential for them to become school dropouts. The community health nurse can determine if this has happened and try to coordinate with the school personnel (and school nurse if one exists) to tailor efforts for a particular pregnant teen to keep her in school. Specific needs to address may be using the bathroom frequently, carrying and drinking more fluids or snacks to relieve nausea, climbing stairs, carrying heavy bookbags, and fitting comfortably behind stationary desks. Schools that are committed to keeping students enrolled are generally helpful and will assist in accommodating special needs.

TEEN PREGNANCY AND THE COMMUNITY HEALTH NURSE

The community health nurse can influence teen pregnancy through appropriate interventions at home and in the community.

Home-based Interventions

Young women at risk for pregnancy can be identified in families currently receiving services by the community health nurse. Younger sisters of pregnant teens are at a twofold increased risk for becoming pregnant themselves (East and Felice, 1992). Anticipatory guidance that addresses sexuality issues can be offered to the parents of all preteens and teens during home visits to increase their knowledge and awareness.

Visiting the pregnant teen in her home allows the community health nurse to obtain an assessment of the facilities available at home for management of her pregnancy needs and suitability of the environment for her child. Some specific areas to assess are adequacy of heating and cooling, a source of water, cleanliness of the home, cooking facilities, and food storage. The nurse may find it more convenient for parents and other family members to participate in education and counseling sessions in their own home. Also, the need for financial assistance and other social service support may be more easily identified. It has been demonstrated that home visiting by community health nurses during a young woman's pregnancy is positively associated with increases in birth weight and increased utilization of prenatal care and support services (Deal, 1994).

When a teen pregnancy occurs, the family dynamics can shift. Families may go through stages of reactions. First, a crisis stage may occur, characterized by many emotions and conflict. By the third trimester, a honeymoon stage may occur, with greater acceptance and understanding of the teen and the impending birth. Finally, after the infant's birth, reorganization may occur, during which conflict may emerge again over issues of child care and the young woman's role. The community health nurse can facilitate family coping and resolution of these stages by treating the family as client and assessing each person's role and strengths. Ultimately, family support for a teen parent can positively influence both mother and infant (Wilkerson, 1991).

Community-based Interventions

Broad-based coalitions and planning councils are forming in many areas to facilitate a comprehensive approach to teen pregnancy. These groups usually include health care professionals, social workers, clergy, school personnel, businessmen, legislators, and members of other youth-serving agencies. The community health nurse can have a significant role on this team by participating in or organizing community assessments, public awareness campaigns, group education (for professionals, parents, and youth), and interdisciplinary programs for high-risk youths. Community acceptance is more likely when there is a broad base of support for activities directed at the reduction of teen pregnancy or reduction of consequences.

Healthy Communities 2000: Model Standards use the objectives of *Healthy People 2000* and allow for modification of programs to tailor them to each community. These model standards can be used by a broad-based coalition or by a lead agency, such as the public health department. Initially an assessment of need is done, followed by a determination of local priorities. Goals for the individual community can then be established and a plan of action developed. Efforts should be evaluated on a regular basis.

The community health nurse can also be a valuable asset to schools. Family life education programs are strongly recommended or mandated in 46 states, and all 50 states recommend or mandate AIDS education (Kirby et al., 1994). Health teachers may call on community health nurses for educational materials or assistance with classroom instruction, especially in the areas of family planning, STDs, and pregnancy. Schools that do not have nurses may arrange to have the community health nurse available for health consultations with students during school hours. Schools may also request that community health nurses par-

ticipate on their health advisory boards.

School-based clinics are operating in more than 400 middle and high schools in the United States. The services offered may include counseling, referrals, general health evaluations, and family planning. Some of these programs have been found to delay the onset of intercourse and increase the use of contraception (Kirby et al., 1994). The community health nurse can assist school systems to design these programs and can also refer young women in need of reproductive health care services.

Community health nurses bring their knowledge about youth and reproductive behavior to any organization or group that has teens, their parents, or other professionals working with teens. Churches are becoming increasingly interested in addressing the needs of their youth, especially since teen sexual activity, pregnancy, and parenting are affecting more of its members.

Community coalitions can look to the *Healthy People 2000* for planning and the *Healthy Communities 2000* standards for modifying these goals to meet the needs of individual communities.

 ## Clinical Application

The community health nurse is often the first health care professional to recognize a teenager's pregnancy. This may follow a pregnancy test done through the local family planning clinic or may occur accidentally, as with 15-year-old Linda, who was home from school with nausea on the day of the community health nurse's visit to her older sister.

In talking with Linda, the community health nurse discovered that she had been feeling tired and nauseated. Linda has not told her mother that she suspected pregnancy because she had been told repeatedly that she was not to follow in her sister's footsteps and become pregnant while she was a teenager. Her mother had previously taken Linda to the family planning clinic for a gynecological examination and birth control pills. Linda became pregnant before she could begin taking the pills.

The following day at the clinic, the urine pregnancy test was positive. In follow-up counseling, the nurse reviewed the options for abortion, adoption, and child-rearing that Linda could consider. They discussed talking with Linda's mother, but Linda was insistent that the nurse not tell her mother until the pregnancy was obvious. Linda decided not to tell her boyfriend yet either. Linda did agree to attend prenatal care and classes at the community health center, did agree to stop drinking her weekend wine coolers, and said she would try to cut down on her smoking. She also agreed to attend a WIC appointment for nutritional counseling. The nurse gave Linda condoms to prevent contracting an STD during the pregnancy and demonstrated correct use. The nurse

and Linda also discussed how she would get transportation to the appointment.

Throughout the pregnancy, the nurse contacted Linda after each prenatal visit to clarify information Linda received from her health care provider and to chart her weight gains on standardized growth charts for pregnancy. Her weight gain curve was good, but from a nutritional assessment, the nurse recognized that Linda was deficient in certain minerals. To increase Linda's calcium, the nurse recommended increasing milk and cheeses, and to increase her iron, she suggested a bowl of enriched farina, Cream of Wheat daily. At each visit the nurse reviewed the problem signs during pregnancy and instructed Linda to call her health care provider if she noticed any sign. The nurse also began to prepare Linda for labor and delivery and develop a birthing plan.

At 22 weeks the nurse discussed adoption again with Linda. At this time, Linda was beginning to doubt her desires to be a parent. After telling her boyfriend she was pregnant, he said he needed time to think about their relationship. Her mother was now aware of the pregnancy and agreed to assist and support Linda in whatever course she chose. Placing her baby with a stable and loving couple seemed like a positive choice, and Linda was scheduled to talk with an adoption counselor.

At 34 weeks' gestation, Linda began to experience great pelvic pressure and called her community health nurse and health care provider. An appointment was immediately arranged, and tests revealed a urinary tract infection and some cervical change,

Clinical Application—cont'd

which put her at risk for premature labor. Linda was placed on pelvic rest for 3 weeks. The nurse arranged for homebound instruction to begin and educated Linda on the importance of fluids, bed rest, and no intercourse. At this time, Linda changed her mind about adoption; her mother and sisters held a baby shower for her the next week. At 37 weeks', Linda delivered a healthy 7-pound boy by normal spontaneous vaginal delivery.

The nurse visited Linda 2 days after discharge from the hospital. She evaluated Linda's amount of bleeding and pain and reassured her it was within normal limits. She also checked the baby's weight and evaluated his feeding and elimination patterns. During this visit the nurse observed Linda interact with the baby and told Linda that the way she held the baby and spoke to him were excellent. She also addressed infant safety issues, such as not leaving him on the bed unattended or alone with the other two young children in the house. The nurse also evaluated the site of the contraceptive implant that had been placed in Linda's arm before hospital discharge and reviewed the need to avoid coitus for 6 weeks.

Over the next year the nurse continued to visit Linda and her son every 2 weeks. She anticipated his developmental milestones and educated Linda about ways to stimulate him. Linda was referred by the nurse to a parenting group for teenagers held at the high school, and this reinforced her school attendance. Linda graduated high school 2 years later.

Key Concepts

◆ The provision of reproductive health care services to adolescents requires sensitivity to the special needs of this age group. This includes being knowledgeable about state laws regarding confidentiality and services for birth control, pregnancy, abortion, and adoption.

◆ Pregnant teenagers have a substantial percentage of the first births in the United States and are more likely to deliver prematurely and have a baby of low birth weight. This risk can be reduced by early initiation of prenatal care and good nutrition.

◆ Factors that can influence whether a young woman becomes pregnant include a history of sexual victimization, family dysfunction, substance use, and failure to use birth control. Several factors may overlap.

◆ Nutritional needs during pregnancy can be challenged if the teenager has unhealthy eating habits and begins the pregnancy with limited reserves of vitamins and minerals. With education, the adolescent can make good food choices while still snacking or eating fast foods. Weight gain during pregnancy is a significant marker for a normal-weight baby.

◆ Young men need special attention and preparation as they become fathers. The interventions include information about pregnancy and delivery, declaration of paternity, care of infants and children, and psychosocial support in this role.

◆ The pregnant teen will need support during her pregnancy and in child-rearing. Families may provide most of this support. However, many communities have a variety of services available for adolescents. These services include financial assistance for medical care, nutritional programs, and school-based support groups.

◆ Adolescent parents have unrealistic expectations about their children and consequently do not know how to stimulate emotional, social, and cognitive development. The children born to adolescents are at risk of academic and behavioral problems as they become older. Teens who receive education on normal development and child care will be more likely to avert these problems with their children.

◆ During a pregnancy, teenagers are expected to attend school. Homebound instruction is reserved for those with medical complications. Teen mothers who return to school and complete their education after the birth of their child are less likely to have a repeat pregnancy. Problems finding child care and the need to have an income can create an obstacle to school return.

◆ Community coalitions, which include community health nurses, can have a significant impact on teen pregnancy. These coalitions generally have diverse representation from the community, and therefore their activities meet with more community support.

Critical Thinking Activities

1. Become familiar with statistics on teen pregnancy, births, miscarriages, and abortions in your area. Collect information also on utilization of prenatal care, low-birth-weight and premature deliveries, high school completion, and repeat pregnancies.

2. Call or visit local schools and interview the school nurse or guidance counselors about teen pregnancy. Determine what resources are available through the schools for pregnancy prevention. Assess the family life education curriculum, and identify a teaching project for nursing students.

3. Design and offer a childbirth preparation class for pregnant teens and their support persons. Include a plan for identifying potential participants, select a site that is accessible, and develop an evaluation method.

4. Assess reproductive health care services to young men in your community. Design an awareness campaign targeting young men on paternity issues and the prevention of pregnancy.

Bibliography

Adolescent pregnancy in the South: breaking the cycle. A report of the Southern Regional Project on Infant Mortality in cooperation with Southern Governor's Association and Southern Legislative Conference, Washington, DC, 1989.

Ahn N: Teenage childbearing and high school completion, *Fam Plann Perspect* 26(1):17-21, 1994.

Alan Guttmacher Institute: *Sex and America's teenagers,* New York, 1994, The Institute.

Alderman EM, Fleischman AR: Should adolescents make their own health care choices? *Contemp Pediatr,* January 1993, pp 65-82.

Alexander CS, Guyer B: Adolescent pregnancy: occurrence and consequences, *Pediatr Ann* 22(2):85-88, 1993.

American Public Health Association: *Healthy Communities 2000: model standards,* ed 3, Washington, DC, 1991, The Association.

Arenson JD: Strengths and self-perceptions of parenting in adolescent mothers, *J Pediatr Nurs* 9(4):251-258, 1994.

Boyer D, Fine D: Sexual abuse as a factor in adolescent pregnancy and child maltreatment, *Fam Plann Perspect* 24(1):4-11, 1992.

Brandsen CK: *A case for adoption,* Michigan, 1991, Bethany.

Burke PJ: Methodological issues for adolescent pregnancy research, *J Pediatr Nurs* 6(1):30-37, 1991.

Cartoof VG, Klerman LV, Zazveta VD: The effect of source of prenatal care on care-seeking behavior and pregnancy outcomes among adolescents, *J Adolesc Health* 12:124-129, 1991.

Cartwright PS, McLaughlin FJ, Martinez AM, Caul DC, Hogan IG, Reed GW, Swafford MS: Teenagers' perceptions of barriers to prenatal care, *South Med J* 86(7):737-741, 1993.

Castiglia PT: Adolescent mothers, *J Pediatr Health Care* 4(5):262-264, 1990a.

Castiglia PT: Adolescent fathers, *J Pediatr Health Care* 4(6):311-313, 1990b.

CDC: Sexual behavior among high school students—US, 1990, *MMWR* 40(51 and 52):885-888, 1992.

Censullo M: Strategy for promoting greater responsiveness in adolescent parent/infant relationships: report of a pilot study, *J Pediatr Nurs* 9(5):326-331, 1994.

Center for Population Options: *Adolescent abortion and mandated parental involvement: the impact of back alley laws on young women,* Washington, DC, 1993, The Center.

Children's Defense Fund: *The state of America's children yearbook,* Washington, DC, 1994, CDF.

Custer M: Adoption as an option for unmarried pregnant teens, *Adolescence* 28(112):891-902, 1993.

Deal LW: The effectiveness of community health nursing interventions: a literature review, *Public Health Nurs* 11(5):315-323, 1994.

East PL, Felice ME: Pregnancy risk among the younger sisters of pregnant and childbearing adolescents, *J Dev Behav Pediatr* 13(2):128-136, 1992.

Fleming BW, Munton MT, Clarke BA, Strauss SS: Assessing and promoting positive parenting in adolescent mothers, *Matern Child Nurs J* 18:32-37, 1993.

Geronimus AT, Korenman S: Maternal youth or family background? On the health disadvantages of infants with teenage mothers, *Am J Epidemiol* 137(2):213-225, 1993.

Gutierrez Y, King JC: Nutrition during teenage pregnancy, *Pediatr Ann* 22(2):99-108, 1993.

Hatcher RA, Trussell J, Stewart F, Stewart GK, Kowal D, Guest F, Cates W Jr, Policar MS: *Contraceptive technology,* New York, 1994, Irvington.

Healthy People 2000: national health promotion and disease prevention objectives Washington, DC, 1991, USDHHS, Public Health Service.

Henshaw SK: Teenage abortion, birth and pregnancy statistics by state, 1988, *Fam Plann Perspect* 25(3):122-126, 1993.

Hollander D: Family instability, stress heighten adolescents' risk of premarital birth, *Fam Plann Perspect* 25(6):284-285, 1993.

Kalmuss DS, Namerow PB: Subsequent childbearing among teenage mothers: the determinant of a closely spaced second birth, *Fam Plann Perspect* 26(4):149-153, 159, 1994.

Kirby D, Short L, Collins J, Rugg D, Kolbe L, Howard M, Miller B, Sonenstein F, Zabin LS: School-based programs to reduce sexual risk behaviors: a review of effectiveness, *Public Health Rep* 109(3):339-359, 1994.

Klerman LV: Adolescent pregnancy and parenting: controversies of the past and lessons for the future, *J Adolesc Health* 14:553-561, 1993.

Koniak-Griffin D, Verzemnieks I: Effects of nursing intervention on adolescents' maternal role attainment, *Issues Compr Pediatr Nurs* 14(2):121-138, 1991.

Leigh BC, Morrison DM, Trocki K, Temple MT: Sexual behavior of American adolescents: results from a US national survey, *J Adolesc Health* 15:117-125, 1994.

Marshall E, Alexander J, Cull V, Buckner E, Jackson K, Powell K: Parenting and childrearing attitudes among high school students, *J Community Health Nurs* 11(4):239-248, 1994.

Marsiglio W: Adolescent males' orientation toward paternity and contraception, *Fam Plann Perspect* 25(1):22-31, 1993.

Matsuhashi Y, Felice ME: Adolescent body image during pregnancy, *J Adolesc Health* 12(4):313-315, 1991.

Moore KA, Snyder NO: *Facts at a glance.* Sponsored by The Charles Stewart Mott Foundation, Flint , Mich, 1994, Child Trends, Washington, DC.

Nichols FH: Secondary prevention with the pregnant adolescent, *Birth Defects* 27(1):33-43, 1991.

Nord CW, Moore KA, Morrison DR, Brown B, Myers DE: Consequences of teenage parenting, *J Sch Health* 62(7):310-318, 1992.

Parker B: Abuse of adolescents: what can we learn from pregnant teenagers? *AWHONNS Clin Issues Perinat Womens Health Nurs* 4(3):363-370, 1993.

Perkins JL: Primary prevention of adolescent pregnancy, *Birth Defects* 27(1):33-43, 1991.

Robinson B: *Teenage fathers,* Lexington, Mass, 1988, Heath.

Ruff CC: Adolescent mothering: assessing their parenting capabilities and their health education needs, *J Natl Black Nurses Assoc* 4(1):55-62, 1990.

Spitz AM, Ventura SJ, Koonin LM, Strauss LT, Frye A, Heuser RL, Smith JC, Morris L, Smith S, Wingo P: Surveillance for pregnancy and birth rates among teenagers, by state—United States, 1980 and 1990, *MMWR* 42(SS-6):1-27, 1993.

Stevens-Simon C, Nakashima I, Andrews D: Weight gain attitudes among pregnant adolescents, *J Adolesc Health* 14(5):369-372, 1993.

Story M, editor: *Nutrition management of the pregnant adolescent,* Washington, DC, 1990, National Clearinghouse.

VanWinter JT, Simmons PS: A proposal for obstetric and pediatric management of adolescent pregnancy, *Mayo Clin Proc* 65:1061-1066, 1990.

Wilkerson NN: Family focused secondary prevention, *Birth Defects* 27(1):33-43, 1991.

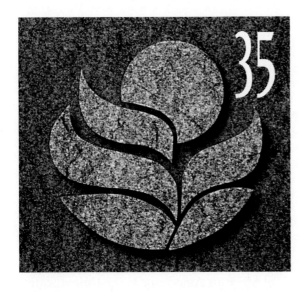

35 Migrant Health Issues

Kim Dupree Jones ◆ Cheryl Pandolf Schenk*

Objectives ▼

After reading this chapter, the student should be able to do the following:

◆ Define the term *migrant farm worker* and discuss the difficulty in determining the definition.
◆ List common health problems of the migrant farm worker and farm worker families.
◆ Recognize the barriers to migrant farm workers and their families in securing health care.
◆ Discuss successful programs that encourage health promotion among migrant farm workers and their families.
◆ Determine the role of the community health nurse in planning and providing care to migrant farm workers and their families.
◆ List legislation that has assisted in the provision of health care services for these groups.
◆ Discuss proposed health reform legislation and the effects of the provision of health care services on migrant farm workers and their families.
◆ Recognize the cultural needs of migrant farm workers and their families, and list methods of providing culturally based nursing care through assessment, planning, intervention, and evaluation.

Key Terms ▼

bicultural/bilingual
collectivism
curandera
East Coast migrant stream
familialism
machismo
Midwest migrant stream
migrant farm worker
Migrant Health Act
National Advisory Council on Migrant Health
personalismo
seasonal farm worker
simpatia
West Coast migrant stream

Outline ▼

*We are grateful to Lynda Crawford, RN, PhD and Jo M. Jones, RN, PhD for their valuable contributions to this chapter.

Imagine yourself working in the tobacco fields 14 hours a day in temperatures over 100° F with no drinkable water or bathrooms. After work, you come home to a two-bedroom trailer shared with 15 other workers. Your home has no indoor plumbing or air conditioning. You expect to have a stiff back and aching knees from your day's labor but are fearful that the constant skin rashes and eye irritation are from pesticides sprayed in the fields. Although a neighboring county has a health care facility for migrant farm workers, no one there speaks Spanish, you have no transportation, and the luxury of a paid sick day does not apply to you. What would you do?

Migrant farm workers and their families are one example of a vulnerable population. Vulnerable populations are characterized by unique social, economic, and health risks that lead to disenfranchisement, victimization, and helplessness. *Healthy People 2000* (1991), a document containing national strategies to promote health and prevent disease over the coming decade, does not specifically address migrant farm workers. However, the objective for clinical preventive services (number 21.5) is to "assure that at least 90 percent of people for whom primary care services are provided directly by publicly funded programs are offered, at a minimum, the screening, counseling, and immunization services recommended by the U.S. Preventive Task Force" (Healthy People 2000, 1991, p. 539). Community and migrant health centers are an example of publicly funded primary care centers that provide some services to migrant farm workers and their families and fall under the objective to incorporate at least 90%. Other *Healthy People 2000* objectives that could be extrapolated to include migrant farm workers involve the health of Hispanic individuals, lower-income individuals, and farm and agricultural workers as an extension of occupational safety and health.

DEFINITION OF MIGRANT

A **migrant farm worker** is defined as a laborer whose principle employment involves moving from farm to farm and planting or harvesting agriculture and attaining temporary housing. A **seasonal farm worker** works during certain seasons in agriculture but does not relocate from area to area to obtain work. For the purposes of this chapter, only the migrant farm worker is discussed. Also, this text refers to migrant workers of Mexican heritage unless otherwise noted.

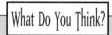

What Do You Think?

Substandard wages paid to migrant farm workers allow Americans to pay less for their fruits and vegetables.

Although migrant farm workers have been a vital link in putting food on the American dinner table for decades, little is known about them. For example, much debate surrounds the actual number of migrant workers. The Office of Migrant Health indicates there are an estimated 4.2 million persons in migrant and seasonal farm work, of which only approximately 12% to 15% are served by federally supported migrant health centers (U.S. Department of Health and Human Services [DHHS], 1993). Other sources, however, report the number of migrant and seasonal farm workers to be between 3 and 5 million (Duggar, 1990). Crawford (1994) demonstrates major flaws in the manner in which migrant workers have traditionally been counted and tracked, particularly in the Hispanic Health and Nutrition Examination Survey (HHANES), the only existing comprehensive study of the health of Mexican-Americans in the United States.

Migrant farm workers have traditionally followed one of three migratory (migrant) streams, each of which has unique characteristics (Table 35-1).

MIGRANT HEALTH PROBLEMS

At a 1993 farm worker hearing before the National Advisory Council on Migrant Health, past and present migrant farm workers indicated that the problems that most concern them involve health and health care, work conditions, pesticide exposure, housing, women, and children and youth. Some of their actual testimonies, first names, and states of residence are given in the box on p. 683.

Health and Health Care

Although migrant farm workers are concerned about specific illnesses, the themes of fundamental economic, societal, and political conditions that lead to poor health are more often discussed. Quality, cost, and accessibility of health care are often discussed in the farms and fields. Some criticize migrant health centers for their inadequate number of bilingual (much less bicultural) staff, limited hours, and inadequate transportation and outreach services. Furthermore, dental, mental health, and pharmacy services are grossly lacking.

The National Migrant Resource Program, Inc. (1990), reports that in the United States, "Migrant farm workers' infant mortality rate is 25% greater than the national average; their life expectancy is 49 rather than 75 years; the rate of parasitic infection among some sets of farm workers approaches 50 times that of the total population." Also, many migrant farm workers are 300 times more likely to contract hepatitis. Studies reporting the frequency and severity of health problems for which migrant workers and their families seek care include the following, in descending order: dental problems, eye problems, back pain, and stress (Littlefield and Stout, 1989). Other leading causes of morbidity and mortality among migrants in-

Table 35-1 Characteristics of Migratory Streams

Migrant stream	Primary residence	Member's origin	Characteristics
East Coast	Southern Florida	Mexican-American, Mexican, Central American, Puerto Rican, and less often, American black, Haitian, and Appalachian white	Headed by a "crew leader," who is paid directly by the grower and redistributes the money to the pickers minus cost of meals and transportation
Midwest	Southern Texas (largest population in the nation)	Mexican-American, Mexican, and more recently Southeast Asian	Families, friends, and single males live together in "colonies," which are not required to have water, sewer, or electricity services. The "truckero" usually transports personal possessions of the workers, who follow in car caravans.
West Coast	Southern California	Mexican-American, Mexican, and a small percentage of American black, nonHispanic white, Southeast Asian, and Central American (many Southeast Asian workers quickly settle in the area and leave the migrant stream)	Individual families and single males often travel independently in cars, trucks, and vans. West Coast housing is known as "the best of the best and the worst of the worst," meaning the work and general living conditions vary widely.

What Migrants Say About . . .

HEALTH AND HEALTH CARE

"What we have to do is reeducate our people and let them know that we have many rights to live and work and to educate and to have health care. And without health care, we cannot have the other three."

Unidentified Male Farm Worker, California

WORK CONDITIONS

"We're used to working. We don't want to be given things. We just want to be respected and to be paid the salaries."

Teresa, California

"Right now, because I'm here today (testifying at hearing on work conditions), I may not have my job. Possibly I may not have my job tomorrow."

Jose, California

PESTICIDE EXPOSURE

"You go to the fields and you think that it's a foggy day because it's so pretty and it's white, but it's actually the chemicals that have been sprayed."

Adelaide, California

"Pesticides presently occupy us tremendously during our work. We wear rubber gloves and that in itself creates a problem because it takes flesh, pieces of flesh from our hands."

Guadalupe, California

HOUSING

"My slogan is, there must be a way to build houses. I believe we have the right to live in a decent way. We are the labor force. It's like

we are foreigners—I am a U.S. citizen. Farmworkers come here with hope, but go home worse off than before."

Unidentified Male Farmworker, Colorado

"We have no coolers in the summer and no heaters in the winter. Temperatures range up to 100 degrees in the summer and 30 degrees in the winter. We work out in the open for 12 or more hours and after working there for more than 12 hours, we have no place to rest. This creates a tremendous amount of frustration, not being able to provide the children with the minimum for comfort."

Margarita, California

"The foremen even charged (the farmworkers) for sleeping under the trees."

Teresa, California

WOMEN

". . . Another thing I would like to mention is the way we are treated as women. As women we are discriminated with our co-workers because they see us as insignificant beings. The men think that they are superior."

Maria, California

CHILDREN AND YOUTH

". . . (the children) go out to the fields. They lay under the trees and there is a residue falling on the children. They are picking grapes, what happens? The sprayers are there with the residue falling on the children."

Irma, Oregon

"We have worked in the fields!!! Well, I'm not very young but I've left some of my youth in the work."

Juliana, Washington

From Galarneau C, editor: *Under the weather: farm worker health*, Austin, Texas, 1993, National Advisory Council on Migrant Health, Bureau of Primary Health Care, U.S. Department of Health and Human Services.

clude infectious diseases such as tuberculosis (TB) and human immunodeficiency virus (HIV) disease. Although traditional health care services perceive problems concerning TB tracking and medication compliance to be important, migrant families are often unable to complete treatment because of extreme poverty, frequent moves, and cultural norms that encourage use of medication only for pain.

Work Conditions

The literature is replete with references to unsafe working conditions in agriculture, especially involving migrant farm workers. Migrant farm workers are faced with questionable farmer payment practices, inadequate record keeping, below minimum wage salary, and lack of enforcement regarding legislation for field sanitation and safety regulations. The U.S. Office of Safety and Health Administration (OSHA) inspectors and Wage and Hour personnel are sometimes related to the farmers because persons growing up in these rural areas usually hold those jobs. Also, the vast number of farms covered by a single government inspector make upholding the standards for workers' safety and for fairness virtually impossible.

The physical demands of harvesting crops 12 to 14 hours a day take their toll on the musculoskeletal system. For example, a worker using improper body mechanics to stoop over with straight legs and pull up weeds or produce will inevitably suffer back pain, whereas the worker who lifts 50-pound crates of produce onto a truck bed all day will complain of shoulder and wrist pain. Naturally occurring chemicals or applied poisons will cause irritation to the skin (contact dermatitis) or to the eyes (allergic or chemical conjunctivitis). This is especially prevalent when working with tobacco, one of the most lucrative crops to harvest.

| Did You Know? |

In many states, workers' compensation benefits are not available to migrant farm workers for on-the-job injuries (Helsinki Commission, 1993).

Because such luxuries as paid vacation, sick days with pay, or workers' compensation do not exist for most migrants, they often work in pain. Simply stated, if they don't work, they don't make money. It is understandable, therefore, why they may not choose to leave the fields to seek health care during working hours. Furthermore, people who live with chronic pain do not sleep well and are more likely to make mental mistakes in the fields that further endanger

their health. Working with automated machinery is especially risky under these circumstances.

Pesticide Exposure

The vast majority of the North American food supply is treated with pesticides. Farm workers are exposed not only to the immediate effects of working in fields foggy or wet with pesticides but also to the unknown long-term effects of chronic exposure to pesticides. Some of the more immediate effects include skin rashes and eye irritation. More chronic exposure may lead to cancer, blindness, Parkinson's disease, infertility or sterility, and liver damage. Although legislation is in effect to minimize pesticide risk, some of the problems that workers typically encounter include:

◆ Nighttime spraying to avoid detection
◆ Failure to post precautions or inadequate posting only in English
◆ Premature field entry after spraying

Housing

Housing for migrant farm workers and their families is a problem of both quality and quantity. When asked where they had lived since working in the United States, migrant farm workers relayed the following list to members of the National Advisory Council on Migrant Health: trailers, dirt floor houses, cabins, labor camps, garages, cars, caves, boxes, ditch banks, tents, chicken coops, under trees, bridges, tarps, orchards, parks, fields, yards, streets, and next to highways and railroad tracks.

Cost and cramped living conditions are also problematic. The weekly rent for a trailer may be $150. The farm worker may only make $25 a day. Therefore, it is not unusual to find 10 to 15 people living in a single dwelling designed to accommodate three or four.

A final and perhaps most crucial point related to housing is that the worker's home is usually tied to his or her job. Therefore, when a job is completed, the worker becomes simultaneously homeless and unemployed. This forced migration leaves little time or energy to seek out and improve living standards.

Women

Hispanic women, as with most women throughout the world, are subject to oppression through both political action and expectations of their own families and communities. Migrant women who work in the fields report sexual harassment and rape. They are concerned about working with pesticides that may cause birth defects and miscarriage. Furthermore, whether women work in the fields or at the camps at home, child care is their responsibility.

Some women describe the necessity to bring infants and small children into the fields and tell horror stories about children being maimed or killed by farm equipment. Day care is not an option for most women working in agriculture because the cost of a single day's care often exceeds a day's wages. State and nationally sponsored summer school programs for farm workers' children over 3 years of age are helping in some areas.

Some women stay at the camp and care for several children whose parents are in the fields. These women suffer from isolation, depression, and anxiety. Many report being forbidden to leave the children except for a single hour 1 day a week, which is to be spent buying food and clothing for the family. A small number of programs have been funded to educate the women to be lay health care workers. These women serve as a link between existing health care agencies and the farm worker families.

Children and Youth

Migrant farm worker parents are deeply invested in the hope of a better future for their children. In fact, this strong hope was the catalyst for many farm workers leaving their country of origin. These children often appear to the outsider as happy, outgoing, and inquisitive. On the surface, they may look like children in any other aggregate. However, these children have many special commonalities, such as the following health care deficits: malnutrition (vitamin A, iron), infectious diseases (upper respiratory infection, gastroenteritis), dental carries (prolonged use of the bottle, bottle propping), inadequate immunization status, pesticide exposure, accidents, and limited access to drug and alcohol prevention and rehabilitation programs.

Did You Know?

Farm worker children are excluded from the protection of the 1938 Child Labor act. Children as young as 10 can work in the fields. Annually, 300 children die in work-related injuries, and 25,000 are injured (Helsinki Commission, 1993).

Children of migrant farm workers may need to work for the family's economic survival. Many work in the fields; others care for the children left at home. They face special challenges in education, including the necessity of being fluent in two languages and competent in two cultures. This is especially difficult for children who may attend many different schools in a single year and miss several days because of travel. Some federally funded summer programs exist to offer supplemental schooling for children of migrant farm workers.

BARRIERS TO MIGRANT HEALTH CARE

"[F]arm workers unmet needs for basic health care is not only a national disgrace, but also a national challenge" (USDHHS p. 20 [1993 Recommendations]).

The Migrant Health Act funds more than 100 migrant health projects in the United States that have 364 actual clinic sites serving more than 500,000 farm workers and their families located in 40 states and in Puerto Rico. Recent surveys indicate that only 12% to 15% of eligible migrants utilize clinic services (Decker and Knight, 1990; DHHS, 1993; Galarneau, 1993; Helsinki Commission, 1993). Factors that inhibit adequate provision of health care services include:

1. *Lack of knowledge.* Many migrant farm workers and their families live in a clustered environment close to work. Minimal outreach by bicultural/bilingual workers to this community is a frequently cited reason for the limited knowledge that services exist.

2. *Lack of income.* The average reported farm worker income in the United States is about $7500 per year based on hourly wages *or* by amount of produce harvested each day. Earning potential may be compromised by broken machinery, drought or rain, and lack of transportation to the next work site. Also, crew leaders are often paid by the farmer and expected to distribute wages to the workers. It is reported that some crew leaders keep a portion of workers' salaries for themselves. Some farm owners deduct Social Security monies, which may or may not be submitted to the government. They may also withdraw wages for substandard housing and charge high interest rates to workers who borrow money from them, then expect the workers to reimburse them by working in the field. All these inequities create a viscous cycle of poverty for the farm worker. Studies contend that two-thirds of farm workers can subsist on money earned, but there is no money for health care and emergencies (Caudle, 1993; Helsinki Commission, 1993).

3. *Lack of state and federal support.* Eligibility criteria for Medicaid and Aid to Families with Dependent Children (AFDC) vary from state to state and are linked to family income and state residency. Many workers earn just enough income to prevent eligibility. Furthermore, workers may not remain in a geographical area long enough to be considered for benefits or may lose benefits when they relocate to a state with different eligibility standards. Federal funding for Migrant Health Services has not kept pace with escalating costs and is equivalent to $100 per user per year, which is inadequate to meet minimal health needs (Duggar, 1990; Helsinki Commission, 1993; *Medicaid,* 1991).

4. *Location of services.* The site of health care services may be located far from work or home. Trans-

portation to and from sites may be nonexistent. Privacy is compromised when migrant workers depend on employers to provide transportation to clinics (Casseta, 1994; Caudle, 1993; DHHS, 1993).

5. *Hours.* Services are generally during work hours and inconvenient to workers, who are only paid when picking; therefore, securing care reduces earnings (Bishop and Harrison, 1987). In the authors' experience, evening appointments are full, whereas daytime appointments often remain unused.

6. *Child care.* Lack of affordable and accessible child care compromises safety. For example, some infants and small children are locked in the cab of a pickup truck near the fields while parents work. This has resulted in overheating or even death. Also, health care services are less readily obtained without available child care.

7. *Mobility and tracking.* Although families move from job to job, their health care records do not. This results in fragmented services in such areas as TB treatment and immunizations.

8. *Discrimination.* Although migrant farm workers and their families bring in much needed revenue to the community, they are perceived as poor, uneducated, transient, ethically distinct, and shiftless. In the authors' experience, even children experience discrimination when they are segregated by being told to sit in the back of the school bus away from other children. Interviews with migrant families reveal a hesitancy in securing care when they interpret treatment by health care staff as not accepting of them (Decker and Knight, 1990; DHHS, 1993; Helsinki Commission, 1993).

9. *Documentation.* Many farm workers and their families are legal residents of the United States. However, some workers are "illegal" and not in compliance with Immigration and Naturalization Service regulations. Some illegal workers fear that securing services in a federally funded or state-funded clinic may lead to discovery and deportation.

10. *Lack of bicultural/bilingual health care staff.* The recruitment and retention of **bicultural/bilingual** health care provider staff is a priority of the National Advisory Council on Migrant Health (1993). Many sources and interviews with migrant workers and their families agree that lack of culturally competent staffing is a factor in utilizing services.

SOCIAL AND CULTURAL CONSIDERATIONS IN MIGRANT HEALTH CARE

Recognition of societal norms and respecting of culture are central to succeeding and thriving in one's environment. This may be evidenced by gaining employment, accessing education, and receiving health

Research Brief

Padgett R, Barrus AG: Registered nurses' perceptions of their communication with Spanish-speaking migrant farmworkers in North Carolina: an exploratory study, *Public Health Nurs* 9(3):193-199, 1992.

A survey was conducted with 55 nurses from 12 state health care agencies that serve migrant farm workers in North Carolina. The purpose of the exploratory study was to determine how nurses communicate with Spanish-speaking migrant farm worker clients. Data were collected with a mailed 30-item questionnaire. Results revealed that most agencies in this study have no bilingual nursing staff and limited bicultural knowledge. The following implications and recommendations for nursing practice were yielded from the study:

1. Teach nurses Spanish. (Speaking even a limited amount of Spanish can convey sincerity and interest.)
2. Appropriately train and use medical interpreters. (Caution is warranted, however, when relying too heavily on nonmedical personnel to translate health care problems and their treatments.)
3. Increase the supply of Hispanic and bilingual nurses. (Implications for recruiting more Hispanics into nursing are discussed.)
4. Improve the overall cultural and language sensitivity of community health agencies. (This ensures cultural competence by networking with existing community agencies.)

care. Acknowledging and providing for the unique culture and values of migrant farm workers and their families are essential in planning and providing care for this aggregate.

Work Ethic and Gender Roles

The male worker in the family is responsible for providing food, clothing, and housing and protecting the family from harm. **Machismo,** the male quality of dominance and chauvinism, is a recurring theme in the migrant family. Machismo is defined as courage, strength, honor, virility, pride, and dignity (de la Rosa, 1989; Decker and Knight, 1990). Because these workers identify with machismo, situations that may compromise the worker's ability to "fit" the machismo definition may undermine self-concept. Being unable to work because of health problems or not being consulted regarding important decisions may be examples of this.

The wife/mother often makes the determination that health care services are needed. She still maintains the traditional role of child caregiver with meal, shopping, and household responsibilities. The male head of the family is in charge of finances and transportation and makes the final decision of whether or not to secure health care services.

Family

All decisions must have the approval and sanction of the male head of the family. Family needs are a priority over individual needs. This is defined as **familialism.** Illness or disability of a family member is a family issue; the decision to seek care is made by the family. At times, an illness or other problems may be kept solely within the family. For example, substance abuse is often considered a moral illness and a family responsibility. Furthermore, some farmers pay their workers with beer.

Love of their children, rather than concern for their own health, may encourage migrant parents to adopt healthier life-styles. One example is when the parents of a child with asthma choose not to continue smoking (Marin, 1990). Health care may not be sought if there is a question of pride or a concern that seeking care is seen as a weakness or irresponsibility on the part of the family and the patriarch. Approval of the intervention by the family and especially the male head of the family will more likely lead to compliance (Caudle, 1993; Smith, 1988).

Health Values

Health is seen as a harmonious relationship between the social and spiritual sides of being. Illness occurs when this relationship is disrupted or a break occurs with cultural norms. Although some traditional health care practices are acknowledged and accepted, farm worker families also believe in seeking treatment from family members and from folk healers or, if from Mexico, **curanderas** (Caudle, 1993; Smith, 1988). Folk remedies are tried first and may remain a mainstay of therapy even if traditional care is sought later. Prayer is extremely important, since most families are Roman Catholic and healing is considered a gift from God.

Interactive Styles

In seeking a health care provider, clients prefer **personalismo,** a provider with a similar background, culture, and language as themselves. Emotionality of the language and the nuances of slang are difficult to translate and may be limited if the services of an interpreter are used. Culturally, there is a goal of a polite, respectful, nonconfrontational relationship with others. This may be defined as **simpatia.** At times, because of simpatia, families may appear to understand what is being said to them when they do not. During the visit to the clinic, family and friends **(collectivism)** may want to witness the examination and discuss the treatment plan (Caudle, 1993; Marin, 1990).

HEALTH PROMOTION AND ILLNESS PREVENTION

Most farm workers do not view illness as a problem unless the condition prevents working. If health care is sought, the expectation (and need) is that a quick and complete recovery with no delay in resuming work will result. Health promotion and disease prevention are difficult concepts to embrace with limited education, lack of future orientation, and compromised access to health care. The authors saw this issue repeatedly in several situations:

◆ A farm worker with peptic ulcer disease and blood in his stools wanted relief from pain but would not acknowledge that cigarette smoking and alcohol consumption aggravated his condition.

◆ A young worker who was nauseated and vomiting while working with tobacco wanted relief from vomiting. He was not receptive to the news that nicotine poisoning may be causing his illness.

◆ Another worker had heat exhaustion because of refusing to drink water during the course of a 12-hour day in 90° temperatures. If she were hydrated, she would earn less money because of time away from the fields to void. She is also at risk for cystitis and pyelonephritis.

Health promotion begins by informing the farm worker family about the resources available. Several migrant health programs have used outreach workers and lay camp aides who have volunteered or been recruited to assist in outreach and health education of the workers. Outreach, as defined by the Migrant Health Program, should ". . . improve utilization of health services, improve effectiveness of health services, provide comprehensive health services, be accessible, be acceptable, and be appropriate to the population served" (DHHS, 1993, p. 54). Outreach programs succeed because they recognize the diversity of this group and the need for flexibility in the provision of services. Because these outreach workers are members of the migrant community, they are trusted and know the culture and the language (Larson and Watkins, 1990; Watkins and Larson, 1991).

The Department of Maternal and Child Health of the School of Public Health at the University of North Carolina at Chapel Hill initiated an outreach program with the Tri-County Community Health Center, a federally funded migrant health clinic. Lay health advisors from the farm workers camps educated workers and their families in the camps and helped to determine those in need of health services. Women were recruited who had leadership ability, respect, caring, and interest in learning about health issues and the importance of sharing that knowledge (Larson and Watkins, 1990). With some training on child health needs, environmental concerns, and resources available, they became ready resources within the camp. Lay workers reported several contacts each week with farm workers who sought out information on health care and resources. While actual statistical data showed no change in specific disease rates in camps, some anecdotal evidence suggests that their presence had a positive impact on health. Information would be further disseminated as women moved from camp to camp. Women involved reported an increased sense of self-esteem and empowerment (Watkins and Larson, 1991). A similar program is sponsored by the Midwest Migrant Health Information Office in conjunction with the Catholic Consortium for Migrant Health Funding.

Education sessions taught by camp aides at the Salud Clinic Outreach program in Oregon focused on concepts of hygiene to prevent the spread of gastrointestinal problems. Farm worker women involved in these sessions were willing to learn these concepts because they were unaware that hygiene and the spread of disease were related (Bishop and Harrison, 1987). La Clinica del Carino in Hood River, Oregon, recruited farm worker women and developed a culturally competent mental health and substance abuse education program for women and adolescents. The Family Health/La Clinica in Washington State developed "Las Comadres," a support network for farm worker women who had been removed from the feminine support network they had at home. Camp health aides and lay health advisors remain identified with their culture, promote preventive health care, and encourage their neighbors to learn about and take responsibility for their health care (Larson and Watkins, 1990).

ROLE OF THE COMMUNITY HEALTH NURSE

The community health nurse understands that a clients' total health status is a function of their ecology: all that "touches" them. The nurse keeps a finger on the pulse of the community by remaining active in those political, social, religious, and employment realms that involve the client. Acting as a community educator, knowledgeable about how to obtain the latest information and resources, the community health nurse can work to assess the infrastructure of the community. These actions sound straightforward, but several barriers must be overcome. For example, in rural communities where most persons are well known to each other, where farmers hold the community "purse strings," and where migrant workers

are exploited, discriminated against, and ostracized, how can nurses make a difference in the health of migrant farm workers and their families?

The community health nurse can be a catalyst for change and may employ the nursing process to assess farm worker needs continually, direct members in search of health care services, and evaluate the success of their efforts. For example, the community health nurse may undertake a community analysis and determine that health care should be offered to farm worker families from 6 PM to 9 PM weekdays (see box below, left). The nurse would then work with other health care agencies to write grants and hire culturally competent personnel to provide these services. Services could include minor acute care and stable chronic care. The needs assessment might also indicate inadequate child and adult immunizations, which may be best provided in the fields, camps, and schools. The nurse may create an immunization tracking system to share information with other counties and states as the farm workers migrate. Culturally specific health promotion and disease prevention materials would be provided, as well as information about referral sources. The box below, right lists selected resources for the community health nurse working with migrant farm workers.

 Resources for the Community Nurse Working with Migrant Farm Workers

FILMS AND VIDEOS

"Health of America's Harvesters: The Migrant Health Program." Produced by Alan McGill, 1990. (Contact the National Migrant Resource Program.)

"Frontline: New Harvest, Old Shame." Produced by Hector Galan, PBS, 1990. (Contact your public or university library.)

WRITTEN MATERIALS

Johnston HL: *Health for the nation's harvesters: a history of the migrant health program in its economic and social setting,* Farmington Hills, Mich, 1985, National Migrant Worker Council.

National Advisory Council on Migrant Health: 1993 *recommendations of the National Advisory Council on Migrant Health,* Rockville, Md, 1993, The Council.

Rust GS: Health status of migrant farmworkers: a literature review and commentary, Am J *Public Health* 80(10):1213-1217, 1990.

Wilk VA: *The occupational health of migrant and seasonal farmworkers in the United States,* ed 2, Washington, DC, 1986, Farmworker Justice Fund.

ORGANIZATIONS

Bureau of Primary Health Care
Migrant Health Program
4350 East West Highway, 7th Floor
Bethesda, MD 20814
(301) 594-4303
National Migrant Resource Program, Inc.
and/or Migrant Clinicians Network, Inc.
1515 Capital of Texas Hwy. South, Suite 220
Austin, TX 78746
(512) 328-7682

 Example of Assessment with Migrant Workers

The authors and community health nursing and family nurse practitioner students relocated to a rural southeastern U.S. county to provide health care to migrant farm workers. During the 2-week experience, the authors noted that migrant workers were most receptive to obtaining health services after 4 PM. The authors also realized that a mobile health van located in the camps where the workers lived was utilized more often than a better equipped migrant health care facility located farther away.

LEGISLATIVE ISSUES

In the late 1930s and 1940s, the Farm Security Act (later part of the U.S. Department of Agriculture) constructed migrant farm worker housing and provided basic health services. In 1946, this program provided health care services to more than 100,000 workers and worker families. This program dissolved in 1947 with all other war relief programs. Farm worker services were without any federal regulations until September 1962, when President John F. Kennedy signed the **Migrant Health Act,** funded under Section 329 of the Public Health Service Act, which provided primary and supplemental health services to migrant workers and their families. This act provides for professional and lay health workers, outreach, transportation, and environmental services, although not all services are provided at all clinic sites.

During 1992, more than 535,000 migrant farm workers and their families received services. The act was funded at $57.3 million in 1993. Average funding is equivalent to $100 per user per year. As mentioned earlier, this act funds more than 100 migrant health projects that support 364 sites located in 40 states and Puerto Rico. The act encourages cooperative agreements with state agencies and state and regional primary care associations to augment health care services and delivery. Partnerships are promoted between migrant health centers and state and local health departments, area health education centers, hospitals, specialty and social service providers, and residency programs. The migrant health centers are part of the Bureau of Primary Health Care, Health Resources and Services Administration, Public Health Service in the Department of Health and Human Services.

The **National Advisory Council on Migrant Health** meets three times a year to advise, consult with, and make recommendations concerning the organization, operation, selection, and funding of migrant centers. Recommendations for 1993 were as follows (DHHS, 1993):

1. *Housing.* The council advocated appropriate and safe housing for migrant farm workers and their families, with no less than 10,000 units per year over the next 10 years. As a result of this recommendation, a work group called the National Hispanic Housing Council was formed and developed criteria and recommendations addressing the needs of worker housing. This recommendation urged that Section 8 HUD funds for housing be available to migrant farm workers.

2. *Appropriations and reauthorization.* The council recommended an annual appropriation of $100 million for the Migrant Health program and perinatal services. Current funding is approximately $57.7 million per year, with a penetration rate of about 12% to 15% (i.e., only 12% to 15% of those who are eligible use the migrant program services).

3. *Mental Health.* The council urged full integration of mental health services into migrant health programs. NOTE: 1994 recommendations urged that $5 million in funding for mental health services be allocated.

4. *Family issues.* The council recommended that all special projects take into consideration the farm worker family. Specific issues revolve around adequate schooling for children, lack of prenatal care for women, domestic violence, child abuse, and day-care needs. NOTE: As a result of this recommendation, there has been an interagency Memorandum of Agreement between the Migrant Health Program and the Migrant Head Start Program to allow interaction when planning direct service delivery.

5. *Health reform.* The council urged that all migrant farm workers and their families, regardless of immigration status, should be serviced by any reform. Benefits would be portable, and there would be state-by-state reciprocity for Medicaid. NOTE: Additional information published in a 1994 update to the recommendations stated a reinforced need for portable benefits, no limitations on out-of-area coverage in that this may directly limit benefit to the highly migratory migrant farm worker, a definition of employer that could be used by the migrant farm worker, and mandatory coverage for the undocumented worker (DHHS, 1994).

6. *Outreach.* The council recommended increased resources for outreach programs and urged that all new federal initiatives include a migrant component and a special allocation for this population.

7. *Occupational and environmental health.* The council recommended the establishment of an interagency group with the Department of Labor, OSHA, and the Social Security Administration to address the enforcement of regulations and laws protecting the farm workers' health and safety. NOTE: Full implementation of the Environmental Protection Agency's Worker Protection Standards were instituted on Jan. 1, 1995. These standards include (DHHS, 1994):

   A "right to know" section so that information on pesticides will be available to the farm worker
   Strict rules on field reentry after pesticide use
   Readily available decontamination facilities for the farm worker

8. *Health professions.* The council recommended incentives to increase the recruitment and supply of health care workers, with emphasis on bicultural/bilingual providers.

9. *Research.* The council recommended the accumulation of hard data on the population and basic health status indicators of migrant farm workers, with cooperative efforts from other state and federal agencies.

10. *Oral health.* The council recommended the inclusion of oral health care into Section 329 of the Public Health Service Act, as well as oral health being listed as a Medicaid benefit (DHHS, 1994).

Clinical Application

Luis, age 53, is a migrant farm worker harvesting vegetables during late July on a large farm in the southeastern United States. One evening, Luis asks if he can talk with Terry, a community health nurse, who is in the medical van parked outside the trailer camp where Luis lives. Luis states he has had continuous upper abdominal pain for the last 3 weeks and is losing weight. He tells Terry that he had this problem in Mexico and that the doctor has given him pills so he can work. He must work as he supports his wife, who recently fell from some farm machinery and has not been able to work because of the resulting pain in her hip. Luis claims he is also responsible for 10-year-old twins, his grandchildren, since their parents were killed in a car accident 6 months ago. His grandchildren attend school when there is no work in the fields. He does not know the last time the children were examined or if they have had their immunizations. Luis believes his grandchildren are healthy but does notice that they cough frequently, especially when he smokes or it is dusty outside. Luis' main concern is his abdominal pain. Terry asks Luis to go inside the van to be evaluated by the nurse practitioner. Concerned about his wife and grandchildren, Terry asks Luis if she can visit their home. Luis reluctantly gives his permission for the visit and wants to be present. They agree that midday the next day would be an agreeable time.

After being evaluated by the nurse practitioner, Luis leaves. The nurse practitioner and Terry discuss Luis and his family. The nurse practitioner is concerned about Luis in that he had significant abdominal tenderness and a positive test for occult blood in his stool. He needs further evaluation and diagnostic tests. She discussed the need for further evaluation, but Luis is very resistant. Terry is concerned about Luis' wife and the health of the grandchildren. She is also concerned that the environment at the camp might be affecting the children's health. The nurses know Luis and his family are not eligible for support programs such as Medicaid or workers' compensation. Both are familiar with the Migrant Health Program in their community and will use this as a resource for Luis and his family. Together, they agree that during the home visit, Terry can discuss their concerns and see to what Luis and his family might agree.

The next day, Terry visits the trailer where Luis and his family live. With Luis there, his wife Eugelia greets the nurse warmly. Eugelia states she fell about 10 days ago and had some pain in her right hip and difficulty moving her leg. She has gradually resumed moving about in the trailer and is feeling better. The nurse notes there is no bruising or compromise to neurological functioning and there is full range of motion of lower extremities without pain. With Luis' permission, they discuss the results of the examination yesterday. Luis comments he has no transportation and no money, and he does not want the farmers to know he is sick. He fears that the farmers will not allow him to work if they know he is ill. Terry asks if he would consider it if she could arrange a doctor to evaluate him after work hours. She also assures him of confidentiality. Terry asks Luis and Eugelia if she can visit again to bring more information. Luis tells Terry she can visit Eugelia only if he knows when she is coming.

When Terry is leaving the trailer, Eugelia tells her that she is very concerned about her husband. She is also concerned about her grandchildren; they often cough and have used "nose and breathing medicine" in the past. The children have been working through most of the year and have fallen behind in school. She states she wants a better life for her grandchildren. In looking at the trailer and trailer park, Terry has environmental concerns for this family as well. It is dusty, and trash surrounds the camp. Terry notes that there is a broken window in the trailer and that the window air-conditioning unit is not functioning.

Returning to the health department, Terry arranges an appointment with the physician who has evening hours at the health clinic that serves farm workers and their families. A van can pick up Luis at his camp and transport him back to his home. Felipe, the outreach worker from the Migrant Health Program, agrees to accompany Terry to visit Luis' family. Felipe also tells Terry that he and members of a local Hispanic church go to local trailer camps to clean the grounds and do some repair. Terry also talks with teachers involved in the summer education program for migrant children. She finds that the 10-year-old twins can participate, and a bus serves the camp. The twins can be evaluated by the nurse practitioner who goes to the school once a week for a clinic.

The next day, Terry sees Luis next to the trailer park convenience store eating his lunch. She asks if she can visit him and Eugelia the next day with Felipe. They agree on a time later in the week.

During the visit, Felipe and Luis talk about the services of the Migrant Health Program. Eugelia is delighted to learn of the opportunity for the children to attend school and be evaluated. She has seen the school bus stop by the camp gate in the past. Eugelia states she is hoping to return to work the next week. Luis agrees to keep his appointment at the health clinic for later in the week after Felipe states that he has seen this doctor himself and that the doctor is a good listener and respectful. Concerned that the children may have reactive airway disease based on what Eugelia has told her and because smoking may further exacerbate Luis' health problems, Terry discusses the need to stop smoking with Luis. He states he will try to stop so his grandchildren will not cough. Felipe also mentions that the church group he works with is coming to the camp next week and asks if Luis would consider having the group fix the window and the air conditioner. Terry shares with Eugelia and Luis that dust and hot air may also contribute to the cough of their grandchildren. With this information, Luis agrees to allow the repairs.

Key Concepts

- A migrant farm worker is a laborer whose principal employment involves moving from farm to farm planting or harvesting agriculture and attaining temporary housing.
- An estimated 3 to 5 million migrant farm workers are in the United States. These numbers are controversial because of the inconsistency in defining farm workers and limitations in obtaining data.
- The life expectancy of the migrant farm worker is 49 years compared with 75 years for U.S. residents.
- Health problems of migrant farm workers are linked to limited access to health services and education and lack of economic opportunities.
- Migrant farm workers are faced with questionable farmer payment practices, inadequate record keeping, below minimum wage standards, and lack of enforcement regarding legislation for field sanitation and safety regulations.
- Farm workers are exposed not only to immediate effects in the fields (foggy or wet with pesticides), but also to unknown long-term effects of chronic exposure.
- When harvesting is completed, the farm worker becomes simultaneously homeless and unemployed. Forced migration to find employment leaves little time or energy to seek out and improve living standards.
- Hispanic women are subject to oppression through both political action and expectations of their own families and communities.
- Children of migrant farm workers may need to work for the family's economic survival.

Critical Thinking Activities

1. Interview health care workers and determine their definition of migrant farm worker. Health care workers could include social workers, nurses, physicians, and registered dietitians. Compare and contrast their definitions.
2. Interview community leaders to determine the presence of migrant farm workers in your area. Compare and contrast information about migrant farm workers by interviewing teachers, clergy, and politicians versus migrant outreach workers, Wage and Hour personnel, Department of Labor personnel, and Migrant Head Start program employees.
3. Consult your library to review vital statistics and census track data to confirm the presence of migrant workers documented in your area. Are there any contradictions between documented statistics and your interview in activity 2? Why is it difficult to account for (much less track) migrant farm workers?
4. Determine eligibility for Medicaid and Aid to Families with Dependent Children services. You may consult the county health department and the state office. Do migrant workers in your state qualify?
5. Design a clinic to provide health care to migrant workers in your area. What services would you provide? What hours would you operate?

Bibliography

Bishop M, Harrison M: *Farm labor camp outreach project: a step toward meeting the healthcare needs of the Hispanic farm worker in Oregon.* Unpublished report, 1987.

Cassetta R: Needs of migrant health workers challenge RNs, *Am Nurse* 6(6):34, 1994.

Caudle P: Providing culturally sensitive health care to Hispanic clients, *Nurse Pract* 18(12):40-51, 1993.

Crawford LH: *Linkages between the health care system and Mexican-American migrant farm workers.* Unpublished doctoral dissertation, Atlanta, 1994, Georgia State University.

de la Rosa M: Health care needs of Hispanic Americans and the responsiveness of the health care system, *Health Soc Work* 14:105-113, 1989.

Decker S, Knight L: Functional health assessment: a seasonal migrant farm worker community, *J Community Health Nurs* 7(3):141-151, 1990.

Duggar B: *Access of migrant and seasonal farm workers to Medicaid covered health care services.* Unpublished paper, 1990.

Galarneau C, editor: *Under the weather: farm worker health,* Austin, Texas, 1993, National Advisory Council on Migrant Health, Bureau of Primary Health Care, US Department of Health and Human Services.

Healthy People 2000: national health promotion and disease prevention objectives, Washington, DC, 1991, USDHHS, Public Health Service.

Helsinki Commission: *Migrant farm workers in the United States: briefings of the Commission on Security and Cooperation in Europe,* Washington, DC, 1993, US Government Printing Office.

Larson K, Watkins E: *Migrant and lay health programs: their role and impact,* Chapel Hill, NC, 1990, University of North Carolina at Chapel Hill Press.

Littlefield C, Stout C: A survey of Colorado's migrant farm workers: access to healthcare, *Int Migration Rev* 21(3):688-707, 1989.

Marin B: AIDS prevention for non Puerto Rican Hispanics. In Leukefeld C, Batjes R, Amsel Z, editors: *AIDS and intravenous drug use: community interventions and prevention*, New York, 1990, Hemisphere.

Medicaid and migrant farm worker families: analysis of barriers and recommendations for change, Washington, DC, 1991, National Association of Community Health Centers.

National Migrant Resource Program, Inc: *Migrant and seasonal farm worker health objectives for the year 2000*, Austin, Texas, 1990.

Smith K: The hazards of migrant farm work: an overview for the rural public health nurse, *Public Health Nurs* 3:48-56, 1986.

Smith LS: Ethnic differences in knowledge of sexually transmitted diseases in North American blacks and Mexican American migrant farm workers, *Res Nurs Health* 11:51-58, 1988.

Staff, Division of Community and Migrant Health, Bureau of Primary Care, US Department of Health and Human Services.

US Department of Health and Human Services: *1993 recommendations of the National Advisory Council on Migrant Health*, Austin, Texas, 1993, National Advisory Council on Migrant Health, National Migrant Resource Program.

US Department of Health and Human Services: *1994 update to the recommendations of the National Advisory Council on Migrant Health*, Austin, Texas, 1994, National Advisory Council on Migrant Health, National Migrant Resource Program.

Watkins E, Larson K: *Migrant lay health advisors: a strategy for health promotion, a final report*, Chapel Hill, NC, 1991, University of North Carolina at Chapel Hill.

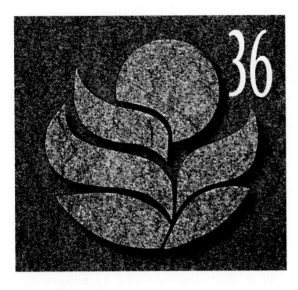

36 Mental Health Issues

Patricia B. Howard

Objectives ▼

After reading this chapter, the student should be able to do the following:

◆ Summarize the evolution of community mental health from historical perspectives and predictions about the future.
◆ Discuss essential mental health services and corresponding national objectives for healthier people by the year 2000.
◆ Evaluate standards, models, concepts, and research findings useful for guiding community mental health nursing practice.
◆ Describe the role of the community mental health nurse with individuals and groups at risk for psychiatric–mental health problems.
◆ Apply the nursing process in community work with clients diagnosed with psychiatric disorders, families at risk for mental health problems, and vulnerable populations.
◆ Explore ways to improve the mental health of people increasingly at risk in a vulnerable society.

Outline ▼

Key Terms ▼

Americans with Disabilities Act (ADA)
community mental health
Community mental health centers (CMHCs)
consumer advocacy
deinstitutionalization
institutionalization
mental health problems
National Alliance for Mental Patients (NAMP)
National Alliance for the Mentally Ill (NAMI)
National Institute for Mental Health (NIMH)
national mental health objectives
psychiatric–mental health disorders
relapse management
severe mental disorders
vulnerability-stress-coping-competence model

Challenges in the mental health field pertain to issues of care for people with problems that range from severe, disabling mental disorders to mental health problems that are less incapacitating but also long term in nature. Other factors that contribute to nursing challenges include the scope and chronicity of mental illness and the uncertainty about specific cause, cure, and treatment for most severe mental disorders. Limited resources compound the problems and present challenges in community mental health work.

Types of services and treatment in various countries are influenced by cultural beliefs and generally parallel economic development; yet two universal truths exist: services for people with mental disorders are inadequate in all countries, and the impact of mental illness on families, communities, and nations is profound. Therefore specialized knowledge and skills about severe mental illness and mental health problems are necessary for effective community nursing practice. Helpful information includes knowledge about the organization of mental health services from historical perspectives as well as trends in current health care demands and delivery. Knowledge about populations at risk for psychiatric–mental health problems and insight about illness outcomes in terms of biopsychosocial consequences are even more important. Finally, it is necessary to refine and broaden nursing process skills in treatment planning to include the impact of mental illness on families and the community.

This chapter focuses on the development of community mental health services, current health objectives for mental health and mental disorders, and the role of the nurse in community settings. Frameworks and concepts useful in community mental health nursing practice are also presented. Because other chapters in this book are devoted to risk groups such as the homeless population and those with substance abuse problems, this chapter focuses on populations who have long-term, severe mental disorders and groups who are vulnerable to mental health problems. **Severe mental disorders** are determined by diagnosis and criteria that include degree of functional disability (American Psychiatric Association, 1994) whereas **mental health problems** are difficulties related to an individual's inability to negotiate the daily challenges of life without experiencing undue social isolation, emotional distress, or behavioral incapacity (Healthy People 2000, 1991).

EVOLUTION OF COMMUNITY MENTAL HEALTH CARE

In the United States today, **community mental health** is the primary model of care for people with mental illness. Components of the model include team care, case management, outreach, and prevention. In most states the model is implemented through comprehensive **community mental health centers (CMHCs),** yet neither the model and its components nor the CMHCs are refined processes and systems of care. Rather, the model continues to evolve in this era of health care reform as the CMHCs react to societal, political, and fiscal pressures. Historically, reform movements influenced the development of mental health services and models of care whether they were located in hospital or community settings.

Historical Perspectives

Early treatment of people with mental disorders was cruel and inhumane (Isaac and Armat, 1990; LaFond and Durham, 1992). Before the eighteenth century, practices were based on superstitions or beliefs that mentally ill people were possessed by demons and both cause and cure were attributed to witches and magicians. Near the end of the eighteenth century, in a movement influenced by Philippe Pinel (1759 to 1820) in France and Benjamin Rush (1745 to 1813) in America, the first revolution in mental health care, known as humanitarian reform, took place (Donahue, 1985; Taylor, 1994).

Humanitarian Reform

Before the humanitarian reform movement, people with mental illness were often housed in jails because health and social services had not been developed. Also, although a result of the reform movement was development of hospitals as a site of treatment, during much of the period, people with mental disorders were neglected and mistreated. For example, the first hospital in the United States was built in Williamsburg, Virginia, in 1773, but approximately 50 years passed before widespread construction of facilities in other states took place (Taylor, 1994). During that 50-year time span, people with mental disorders were removed from the community, placed in poorhouses or almshouses, subjected to cruel treatment, and sometimes sold at public auction (Donahue, 1985). One person in particular, Dorothea Dix, led reform efforts to correct these types of practices (Kalisch and Kalisch, 1986; Bendiner, 1991).

Dorothea Lynde Dix (1802 to 1887) focused attention on three populations: criminals, those with mental disorders, and victims of the Civil War (Donahue, 1985; Kalisch and Kalisch, 1986; Bendiner, 1991). She fostered the idea that people with mental disorders needed health and social services, and her efforts resulted in improved organization of mental health services. Moreover, her work during the Civil War led to the development of hospitals as the primary site of care where she influenced standards for hospital administration and nursing care. Because of her lifetime efforts, often through political action, treatment for mentally infirm persons was altered on both the North American and European continents (Donahue, 1985).

Table 36-1 Legislation that Influenced Community Mental Health Services

Year	Legislation	Focus
1955	Mental Health Study Act	Resulted in Joint Commission on Mental Illness and Health that recommended transformation of state hospital systems and establishment of community mental health clinics
1963	Community Mental Health Centers Act	Marked beginning of community mental health centers concept and led to deinstitutionalization of large psychiatric hospitals
1975	Developmental Disabilities Act	Addressed the rights and treatment of people with developmental disabilities and provided foundation for similar action for individuals with mental disorders
1977	President's Commission on Mental Health	Reinforced importance of community-based services, protection of human rights, and national health insurance for mentally ill persons
1978	Omnibus Reconciliation Act	Rescinded much of the 1977 commission's provisions and shifted funds for all health programs from federal to state governments
1986	Protection and Advocacy for Mentally Ill Individuals Act	Legislated advocacy programs for mentally ill persons
1990	Americans with Disabilities Act	Prohibited discrimination and promoted employment opportunities for people with disabilities, including mental disorders

Hospital Expansion, Institutionalization, and the Mental Hygiene Movement

Psychiatric hospitals constructed during the expansion era were located in rural areas. In general, individuals admitted to the hospitals had severe mental disorders such as schizophrenia or were elderly people with dementia (Grob, 1991). When admitted, they were essentially separated from the community and isolated from their families; many were institutionalized for the rest of their lives, largely in response to a continued fear of people with mental disorders. Even though the hospital movement was intended to bring about a more humane form of treatment, **institutionalization** of large numbers of people combined with minimal information about cause, cure, and care resulted in overcrowded conditions and exploitation of patients (LaFond and Durham, 1992).

At the turn of this century, institutional conditions were reported by Clifford Beers, a patient who knew about psychiatric hospital treatment from personal experiences (Isaac and Armat, 1990). His writings urged reform and influenced the founding of the National Committee for Mental Hygiene. During the mental hygiene movement, attention shifted to ideas about prevention, early intervention, and the influence of social and environmental factors on mental illness. Hospital construction declined, and community services, including child guidance clinics, emerged (Isaac and Armat, 1990). Nonetheless, the community model developed slowly and seldom addressed the problems of severe mental illness. Rather, people with severe mental disorders continued to be hospitalized in existing institutions. In spite of the slow growth of community-based mental health services, an important concept began to take shape during the mental hygiene movement, namely, the idea of a multidisci-

plinary team approach to treatment in community settings (Grob, 1991). Another important outcome of the mental hygiene movement was increased understanding about mental illness. Understanding about the scope of mental illness became even more evident during World War II when men were screened for military service in the United States.

Many men screened for military service during World War II were found to have neurological and psychiatric–mental health disorders. Even more military personnel required treatment for mental health problems associated with social and environmental stress during and after the war. At the same time the community mental health model continued to expand slowly while populations consisting of individuals with severe mental disorders and elderly persons with dementia grew larger in the state hospitals (Grob, 1991). Demands for mental health services in communities, concerns about conditions of state psychiatric hospitals, and disparity in funding for needed services at state levels prompted federal legislation that influenced development of the community mental health concept.

Federal Legislation for Mental Health Services

The first major piece of legislation that influenced mental health services was the Social Security Act passed in 1935, before World War II. The Social Security Act shifted the responsibility of care for ill people from the state to the federal government (LaFond and Durham, 1992). When the demand for mental health services increased during World War II, the federal government's role expanded. Key points of legislation that influenced the development of community mental health services are summarized in Table 36-1.

Post–World War II Legislation

Shortly after World War II the National Mental Health Act was passed and the **National Institute for Mental Health (NIMH)** was designated to administer its programs (Isaac and Armat, 1990; Taylor, 1994). Objectives included development of education and research programs for community mental health treatment approaches. The education provisions of the Act included financial incentives for training grants to increase the number of professional workers, including nurses, in mental health services. Education and research programs materialized readily, but the community mental health approach to services expanded slowly. In effect, psychotherapy, the medical model, psychiatric units in general hospitals, and outpatient clinics expanded while most treatment services for severe mental disorders remained in state hospitals. Concerns about conditions and costs of institutional treatment, advances in science and technology, and the development of psychotropic medications led to legislation that would ultimately force the expansion of the community mental health model (LaFond and Durham, 1992; Keltner and Folks, 1993).

In 1955 the Mental Health Study Act was passed and the Joint Commission on Mental Illness and Health was established by the NIMH (Isaac and Armat, 1990; Taylor, 1994). The commission consisted of representatives of numerous mental health service organizations who studied national mental health needs and submitted a report entitled *Action for Mental Health* to Congress. Recommendations of the report included continued development of research and education programs along with early and intensive treatment for acute mental illness. The report emphasized the importance of reducing the size and populations of large psychiatric hospitals and shifting care of severely mentally ill persons to psychiatric wards in general hospitals and to community mental health clinics. Components of community services that were recommended included a range of aftercare services following hospitalization for individuals with major mental illness (Isaac and Armat, 1990; Grob, 1991). Additional legislation reinforced the shift in the locus of care from state hospitals to community systems.

Legislation for Community Mental Health Centers

In 1963 President John F. Kennedy focused the attention of the nation on mental illness and mental retardation. As a result the Community Mental Health Centers Act (CMHC) was passed and the CMHC concept was formalized. Federal funds were designated to match state funds in constructing CMHCs and in starting up programs. To qualify for funding, CMHCs had to offer specific services, including short-term and partial hospitalization, aftercare, emergency services, outpatient treatment, rehabilitation, and vocational counseling. Some states had less funds than others, and many CMHCs, especially those in poor and rural areas, were unable to generate adequate money for continuing their start-up programs. The deinstitution-

alization of people with severe mental disorders was well underway before some of these shortcomings were recognized.

Deinstitutionalization. Deinstitutionalization involved moving large numbers of patients out of the state psychiatric hospitals. The cost of institutional care was perhaps the main reason for the movement; other influences included discovery of psychotropic medications and civil rights activism (Bachrach, 1990; Isaac and Armat, 1990; Grob, 1991; LaFond and Durham, 1992; Keltner and Folks, 1993). Its purpose was to improve the quality of life for people with mental disorders by providing services in the communities where they lived rather than in large institutions. To change the locus of care, large hospital wards were closed and people with severe mental disorders returned to the community to live. Many patients were discharged to the care of family members; others went to nursing homes. Still others were placed in apartments or other types of adult housing; some of these were supervised settings, and others were not (Bachrach, 1990).

Not surprisingly, as with any abrupt, dramatic change, problems related to unexpected service gaps between the hospitals and CMHCs led to continuity-of-care problems. For example, families were not prepared for treatment responsibilities they had to assume, but few mental health systems offered them education and support programs. Also, although many elderly patients were admitted to nursing homes and personal care settings, education programs were seldom available for staff, who often lacked the skills necessary for treatment of people with mental disorders. And finally, some clients found themselves in independent settings such as rooming houses and single-room occupancy hotels, with little or no supervision. For these persons, quality of life did not improve because of their inability to obtain health services or even suitable living conditions (Bachrach, 1990; Isaac and Armat, 1990).

As a result of these and similar problems, deinstitutionalization fell short of its projected goals. Clients, families, communities, and the nation suffered as poor living and social conditions were associated with mental disorders (LaFond and Durham, 1992). These types of issues prompted additional legislation and advocacy efforts.

Civil Rights Legislation for People with Mental Disorders

Naturally, the development of CMHCs was based on the principle that people with mental disorders had a right to treatment in the least restrictive environment (Bachrach, 1990; Perlin, 1994). Although CMHCs did prove less restrictive than the institutional model, they lacked some much-needed services. For example, people with severe mental disorders require daily monitoring or hospitalization during acute episodes of illness. Even though hospital services were available, many individuals expressed their rights to refuse treatment and resisted admission; moreover, transitional care following discharge for those persons who were admitted to hospitals was not available in most communities (LaFond and Durham, 1992). In addition to the right to refuse treatment, advocates for mentally ill individuals focused on such civil rights issues as segregated services, inhumane practices in psychiatric hospitals, and failure to include clients in treatment planning. Activism for minorities and handicapped persons also influenced civil rights legislation for people with mental disorders. In particular, during the 1970s institutional conditions of people with developmental handicaps prompted the Developmental Disabilities Assistance Act and Bill of Rights Act. Other legislation shifted funding from the federal to the state level.

State systems of mental health services developed in diverse ways. Frequently they were inadequate. In general, individuals with severe mental disorders were vulnerable and neglected and either lacked or were unable to access health and social services. In an effort to offset these problems, in 1986 the federal Protection and Advocacy for Mentally Ill Individuals Act was legislated. Advocacy programs for mentally ill persons became part of the same state advocacy systems developed earlier under the Developmental Disability Act (Wilk, 1993). In spite of advocacy efforts and legislation, the CMHCs were unable to meet the increased and diverse demands for mental health services in their communities. The lack of services combined with concerns about discrimination against all people with disabilities led to additional legislation.

The Americans with Disabilities Act of 1990

In 1990 the **Americans with Disabilities Act (ADA)** was passed. The ADA mandated that individuals with mental and physical disabilities be brought into the mainstream of American life (Perlin, 1994). To promote the mainstreaming process, the ADA addressed three major issues: (1) employment; (2) public services, programs, and activities; and (3) public accommodations (Brazelon Center for Mental Health Law, 1994; Perlin, 1994). For example, the ADA seeks to end discrimination against people with mental impairment or other disabilities in areas of employment, including job application, hiring, advancement, and discharge practices. Also, the ADA mandates that state and local governments administer services in ways that are integrated and applicable for specific populations, including people with **psychiatric–mental health disorders.** Violations of the ADA are considered similar to violations of the Equal Protection Clause of the Constitution (Perlin, 1994).

Even so, implementing the law may not be a smooth process (Shore, 1993; Wilk, 1993). History reveals that past legislation promoted the rights of people with mental disorders, but litigation was also responsible for the lack of growth, if not decline, in community mental health services (Isaac and Armat, 1990; LaFond and Durham, 1992; Wilk, 1993; Perlin,

1994). The community mental health nurse is in a position to advocate for clients to ensure equality in access to health services, housing, and employment. In recent years consumers of mental health services and family members have led advocacy efforts and influenced legislative action.

Did You Know?

The Americans with Disabilities Act (ADA) of 1990 prohibits employment discrimination against people with mental disabilities. Since the ADA went into effect, many people with mental disorders have filed discrimination charges. Employers need assistance in understanding functional limitations commonly associated with mental disorders. Limitations include difficulty concentrating and dealing with stress.

Consumer Advocacy. In this discussion the *consumer* refers to persons who are current or former recipients of mental health services. As in all areas of health care, the rights and wishes of consumers are important in planning and delivering services. However, consumers of mental health services have traditionally had difficulty advocating for themselves. For example, in the past, treatment programs fostered passivity in clients and excluded them from the treatment planning process. In addition, family members were responsible for care in the home, but they lacked resources and even information about treatment (Isaac and Armat, 1990). Like consumers, family members suffered from the stigma of mental illness and public attitudes that contributed to self-advocacy problems. In contrast, self-advocacy and involvement in treatment planning foster self-confidence, promote participation in service, and may influence policy decisions. Consumer and family groups foster these objectives (Isaac and Armat, 1990; LaFond and Durham, 1992).

Family members led self-advocacy efforts in the 1970s when small groups organized efforts to challenge and change mental health services. These early efforts resulted in the formation of the **National Alliance for the Mentally Ill (NAMI),** which today has both state and local affiliates. During the 1980s consumer groups formed. The **National Alliance for Mental Patients (NAMP)** is an example of a consumer organization. Today there is evidence of consumer and family advocacy in service development and in the political arena.

For example, beginning in 1991, along with other mental health organizations, family and consumer groups asserted leadership for mental health services during the national health care reform debate. Early in reform discussions, the unified efforts of consumer, family, and provider groups resulted in a wide range of mental health benefits in the Clinton administration's health care reform proposal. Although comprehensive coverage for mental health services was not included in the Clinton administration's proposal late in 1994, the unified coalition did establish credibility in the political arena (Scallet and Havel, 1994). Clearly, consumer and family groups are valuable resources for nurses and the community.

CURRENT AND FUTURE PERSPECTIVES IN MENTAL HEALTH CARE

Today agreement is widespread that health care services are lacking both nationally and internationally. In the United States, large segments of the population do not have basic health care services or insurance to cover both expected and unexpected illnesses (American Nurses Association, 1991; Griffith, 1993; Feingold, 1994; Manderscheid and Henderson, 1994; Navarro, 1994). Moreover, grave concerns exist among consumers, family members, and health care providers alike about issues pertaining to basic treatment, continuity of care, housing, and costs for acute and long-term mental health services (Bachrach, 1993; Hatfield, 1993; Krauss, 1993; Lazarus, 1994). Therefore health care reform is a major political, social, and economic issue of the current decade.

If changes or reform mandates occur, they will almost certainly be a long-term process because they will involve alterations in the current health care delivery system. In the meantime, nurses working in communities must understand the scope of mental illness and be familiar with national health objectives designed to promote the health and welfare of people with mental health problems.

National Objectives for Mental Health Services

Goals of the community mental health movement are consistent with health promotion and disease prevention objectives outlined in *Healthy People 2000* (Healthy People 2000, 1991). Overall, the **national mental health objectives** emphasize the importance of personal responsibility in developing patterns of healthy living. They also address healthy issues of vulnerable populations, including people with mental disorders. Table 36-2 gives target populations and problems. As indicated in Table 36-2, objectives focus on all age groups, identify specific target populations, and highlight the grave nature of problems associated with mental illness.

Other national objectives were proposed by an advisory committee to the NIMH in 1991 (National Institute of Mental Health, 1991). An aim of the NIMH objectives was to improve services for people with severe mental disorders. Components of services that were emphasized included comprehensive assessment for accurate diagnosis and coordinated treatment and rehabilitation. The NIMH and national health objectives dovetail. For example, target populations of the NIMH objectives are people with schizophrenia, the

Table 36-2 Problems and Populations Targeted in National Health Objectives for Mental Health

Problem	Target population
Persistent mental disorders	Children Adolescents Adults
Adverse health effects from stress	Adults
Injurious suicide attempts	Adolescents
Suicide	Adolescents Adult and elderly men Native Americans and Alaska natives in reservation states
Maltreatment	Children and youth aged 18 yr and younger
Assault injuries	Children aged 12 yr and older Adults
Physical abuse	Women
Rape and attempted rape	Women and adolescents aged 12 yr and older
Homicide	Children aged 3 yr and younger Spouses African-American men and women Hispanic-American men Native Americans and Alaska natives in reservation states

Modified from *Healthy People 2000: national health promotion and disease prevention objectives*, Washington, DC, 1991, USDHHS, Public Health Service.

major mood disorders, and various forms of these two conditions. Suicide, a problem identified in national health objectives, is not uncommon among these groups. Moreover, they and their caregivers are subject to stress, another problem that is targeted. Clearly, these objectives and services are compatible with nursing process activities, are important guides for practice, and fit the role of the nurse in community mental health services. Standards for implementing national objectives are also available for use in community work.

Model Standards for Implementing National Objectives

Useful guidelines for implementing *Healthy People 2000* objectives are available in *Healthy Communities 2000: Model Standards* (American Public Health Association, 1991). The standards cover the priority areas and populations identified in the *Healthy People 2000* objectives, and they are recommended for use in determining needs at state and community levels. Overall, the goal for mental health and mental disorders emphasizes prevention, maintenance, or restoration of mental health and independent functioning. Another goal is to decrease disparities in health among population segments, including those listed in Table 36-2. However, as previously mentioned, individuals with mental health problems have historically lacked adequate services and frequently lack accessible services today. Also, preventive mental health programs are essentially nonexistent today (Krauss, 1993), although they were recommended as early as the mental hygiene movement. The model standards can be used to slow or reverse these trends. For example, psychiatric mental health nurses can (1) promote use of the standards in the agencies where they are employed; (2) use the standards in community assessment activities; and (3) introduce information about the standards to other groups and agencies, including local consumer and family organizations. Other ways to use the standards with specific populations are included in the discussion about the scope of mental illness.

Scope of Mental Illness

Mental illness is prevalent in all segments of societies both nationally and internationally. In the United States an estimated 23 million noninstitutionalized adults in the United States have cognitive, emotional, or behavioral disorders, not including alcohol and other drug abuse problems (Healthy People 2000, 1991). For discussion, the scope of mental illness may be broken into two useful classifications: severe mental disorders and mental health problems.

Severe Mental Disorders

Severe mental disorders strike at the human qualities of thought and behavior. They are persistent and disabling and affect people of all ages, races, and socioeconomic levels. Examples of severe mental disorders that nurses will encounter in the community are major depression and schizophrenia. Detailed information about these conditions is readily available in psychiatric–mental health nursing textbooks and in the *Diagnostic and Statistical Manual of Mental Disorders* (American Psychiatric Association, 1994).

In the United States alone, 4 million people have severe mental disorders; of those, 900,000 are in institutions and the rest live in communities (National Institute of Mental Health, 1991). Factors that contribute to the large numbers of persons living in the community include ongoing deinstitutionalization activities, changes in approaches to acute mental illness that have resulted in reduced hospital admissions along with fewer days spent in hospitals, slow development of services for transition from the hospital to the community, and lack of community services and resources.

In the community today, as in past decades, many people with severe mental disorders live in poverty because they lack the ability to earn or maintain a suitable standard of living. For example, as many as one-third to one-half of the homeless population, which averages 600,000 persons daily, are affected with a severe mental disorder (National Institute of Mental Health, 1991); Krauss, 1993). These estimates suggest that important sites of nursing services are in shelters, soup kitchens, and other places where people seek food and protection. Even those persons who live with family caregivers or who are in supervised housing are at risk for inadequate services since the long-term care they require frequently depletes human and fiscal resources. Indeed, even caregivers may be at risk for mental health problems (Biegel et al., 1991; Norbeck, et al., 1991; Howard, 1994). Types of community resources important for the community mental health nurse include crisis intervention services, intensive care services for those who are a danger to themselves or others, rehabilitation services, and follow-up or continuing care in clinics and home settings (American Public Health Association, 1991).

Mental Health Problems of High-Risk Populations

As indicated in the definitions at the beginning of this chapter, mental health is a dynamic process that enables and promotes the individual's physical, cognitive, affective, and social functioning. Some authors refer to mental health as the empowerment force that motivates the individual in the pursuit and fulfillment of life's goals (Haber et al., 1992). In contrast, threats to mental health create stress that undermines functional, interpersonal, and intrapersonal interactions and diminishes the individual's ability to pursue and achieve life's goals. Both internal and external factors influence an individual's mental health status. Internal factors include the biopsychosocial makeup or personality characteristics of the individual. External factors involve socioenvironmental forces, including the values, beliefs, and material assets of communities. Values and beliefs influence the allocation of resources for neighborhoods and schools and can contribute to or undermine the mental health of people in communities.

Mental health problems are manifested in many ways. Untoward incidents or even anticipated life events can diminish physical, cognitive, affective, and social functioning. For example, in most situations, either anticipated or unexpected death of a family member results in grief that may temporarily interrupt functional activities of surviving family members. Loss of appetite, sadness, difficulty making decisions, and disturbed sleep patterns are common during bereavement. Given adequate support and adaptation, mentally healthy people resume functional life-styles following the death of a loved one. When people do not have adequate resources, or when bereavement is complicated because of the conditions of the situation, there is an increased risk for threats to the mental health of surviving family members.

In this same example, cause of death and age of survivors are two conditions that place people at risk during this particular life event. If the cause of death was suicide, family members may have bereavement complications from reactions such as guilt. If the death was acquired immunodeficiency syndrome (AIDS) related, bereavement complications may be associated with a stigma that increases stress and slows adaptation of surviving family members. On the age continuum, death of a family member can affect survivors in various ways. Infants and youth may be deprived of significant nurturing and care that will result in long-term emotional deficits, adults are at increased risk for stress related to role changes, and elderly persons are vulnerable to social isolation as relatives and friends die.

However, bereavement is not the only cause of diminished mental health. Other causes include but are not limited to physical health problems, disabilities resulting from trauma, exposure to violence in the neighborhood, job loss and unstable employment, and unanticipated environmental disasters that result in loss. Since multiple threats to mental health exist, it is useful to organize the study of problems according to risk. Populations are at risk at all ages along life's continuum.

Children and Adolescents. Approximately 12% of the 63 million children under 18 years of age in the United States have a mental disorder (Krauss, 1993). Some are at risk for acute or chronic mental health problems from neglect, and still others develop problems even in the presence of positive parenting. For example, risks during the prenatal period may be a result of exposure to maternal health deficits such as inadequate nutrition or poor physical health; and children may develop depression associated with loss following divorce even though both parents may provide nurturing and attention.

Types of mental health problems typically diagnosed during childhood are depression, anxiety, and attention deficit disorder. Examples of chronic disorders commonly seen are mental retardation, Down syndrome, and autism. Children are also at increased risk for acute and chronic mental health problems resulting from situations in their environment. Examples of environmental factors include crowded living conditions, violence, separation from parents, and lack of consistent caregivers. These problems have an impact on growth and development and influence mental health during adolescence.

The incidence of suicide suggests that many problems during adolescence are profound. Moreover, studies reveal a steady increase in the number of suicides during adolescence (Healthy People 2000, 1991). Among males between the ages of 15 and 19 years, it is the second leading cause of death (Krauss, 1993). Among adolescent girls, anxiety and phobia are not uncommon, and suicidal behavior, if not actual suicide, is associated with depression. Serious public health problems associated with violence in society and in families also take their toll on adolescents. Teenagers are among those who are most likely to be victims of homicide or experience mental health problems related to intrafamilial violence (Healthy People

2000, 1991). For example, target populations for health and service objectives related to reducing rape and attempted rape include female children 12 years and older, those pertaining to assault injuries including both males and females over 12 years of age, and those designed to interrupt the intergenerational cycle of abuse are directed at children of both genders regardless of age (Healthy People 2000, 1991). Other common problems during adolescence include conduct disorders, eating disorders, and substance abuse.

Children and adolescents require a variety of mental health services including crisis intervention and both short- and long-term counseling. Prevention, education, and including parents in program planning are keys to offsetting problems. When conditions are identified, early intervention and continuity of care can promote optimal functioning and may offset chronic conditions. Since it is apparent that many children and adolescents lack services or access to them, community mental health assessment activities are essential. Assessment activities should include identifying types of programs available or lacking in places where children and adolescents spend time. In addition to homes of clients served in programs, assessment sites to include are schools, day-care centers, churches, and organizations that plan and guide age-specific play and entertainment programs. The model standards also emphasize access to preschool programs, school health education, and health promotion in postsecondary institutions to reduce the risk of mental health problems (American Public Health Association, 1991). Assessment data are essential for planning and developing these types of programs that address mental health problems prevalent from the prenatal period through adolescence because preventing problems during these developmental periods also addresses mental health issues of adulthood.

Adults. The scope of mental illness among adults is revealed in information about the number of people who have a disorder. In 1990 approximately one in five adults, or 41.2 million Americans, had a mental disorder (Krauss, 1993). In addition to severe disorders such as major depression and schizophrenia, adults suffer from multiple sources of stress that contribute to their mental health status. Sources of stress include multiple role responsibilities, job insecurity, and unstable relationships. These and other conditions can undermine mental health and contribute to domestic violence and substance abuse in all populations regardless of income or culture. Other mental health problems during adulthood are caused by factors similar to those of childhood.

For example, environmental and intrafamilial violence threatens the lives of adults. Homicide rates in the United States exceed those of any other developed country and, along with suicide, account for more than one-third of the 145,000 deaths related to injuries that occur in the United States annually (Healthy People 2000, 1991). Women in particular are at risk in situations involving domestic violence. Each year, between 2 and 4 million women are physically abused by spouses, ex-husbands, and boyfriends, and more than 1 million women seek medical assistance for battery-related injuries (Healthy People 2000, 1991). Other mental health problems of adults include eating disorders, psychosocial problems related to AIDS and other medical conditions, and posttraumatic stress disorders. These and other disabling conditions all have an impact on family members.

Most family caregivers are women who care for a spouse, aging parent, or child with a long-term disabling illness (Biegel et al., 1991). Research reveals important information about the impact of disabling disorders on family caregivers. Research findings about women caring for adult children with schizophrenia suggest they were at risk for increased threats to mental health across the continuum of their adult years and into old age (Howard, 1994). Other findings about caregivers of persons with severely disabling mental disorders suggest sources of threats to mental health are guilt (Natale and Barron, 1994), lack of social support (Norbeck et al., 1991), and chronic strain (Reinhardt, 1994). Other chronic conditions that threaten the mental health status of caregivers are Alzheimer's disease and human immunodeficiency virus (HIV)/AIDS. Research findings reveal that care givers of older relatives with Alzheimer's are at increased risk for strain and burden (Kuhlman et al., 1991; Pallett, 1990) and that those who care for loved ones with HIV/AIDS have high levels of distress (McShane et al., 1994) and heightened anxiety and depression (Wiener et al., 1994). During stressful life events such as these, it is important for caregivers to know how to manage their lives.

Activities to improve the mental health status of adults include public education programs, prevention approaches, and providing mental health services in primary care. Specific approaches include use of community support groups, education about life-style management to reduce stress, and work site programs aimed at reducing employee stress (American Public Health Association, 1991). Nevertheless, most programs currently available for adults with mental health problems are directed at monitoring or restoring health rather than preventing problems. Barriers to preventive services include inadequate financing for mental health services and fragmented care (Krauss, 1993).

Older Adults. In the United States the population over 65 years of age has steadily increased since the turn of this century. Today persons who reach 65 years can expect to live into their 80s. Moreover, the segment of the older adult population that is growing most rapidly in the United States today are persons aged 85 years and older (Healthy People 2000, 1991; Krauss, 1993). Although many older people maintain highly functional lives, others have mental health deficits because of normal sensory losses re-

Research Brief

Howard PB: Lifelong maternal caregiving for children with schizophrenia, *Arch Psych Nurs* 8(2):107-114, 1994.

A lifespan perspective of maternal care giving for adult children with schizophrenia was conducted with middle-aged and older women to identify illness-related life events and adaptations to the events. Interviews and diaries were primary sources of data. Data analysis involved coding and classifying study themes, constant comparison, and saturating theme categories. Findings suggested stages and concepts of care giving. Concepts of the theme about stages of learning to live with a child who had schizophrenia were (1) perceiving a problem, (2) searching for solutions, (3) enduring the situation, and (4) surviving the experience. Implications for nursing practice from study recommendations were as follows:

1. Home care services and transition programs from the hospital to community services are important for families with relatives who have severe mental disorders.
2. Interventions with families should include education, respite services, and stress management.

lated to aging, failing physical health, difficulty performing activities of daily living, and social deprivation or isolation. For example, life changes related to work roles and retirement often result in reduced social contacts and support. Other previously described losses are associated with the deaths of a spouse, other family members, and friends. Reduced social networks and contacts brought about by these life events can influence mood and contribute to serious states of depression.

Depression has an impact on functional independence and contributes to suicide. In the United States, men between age 65 and 74 years are in the highest risk category for suicide (Healthy People 2000, 1991). Another factor linked to suicide in this age group is chronic illness. Common physical problems of older adults include terminal illnesses associated with cancer and chronic conditions such as arthritis, osteoporosis, and cardiovascular and respiratory disease. Brain disorders such as Alzheimer disease, dementia, and stroke are also common among older adults. All these conditions have an impact on the mental health status of individuals and their family caregivers.

Healthy aging activities improve the mental health of older adults. Healthy aging activities include developing habits that promote balanced nutrition and physical activity along with establishing social networks. Last, like those in age groups across the lifespan, older adults are victims of violence in the environment and in their homes. Therefore national health objectives related to these issues include reducing the incidence of abuse (Healthy People 2000,

1991). Strategies that address these problems include early screening for risk factors in all primary care settings and organizing health promotion programs through senior centers or other community-based settings that serve older adults (American Public Health Association, 1991).

Low-Income, Ethnic, and Minority Groups. Although all socioeconomic and cultural groups have mental health problems, any discussion about vulnerable populations must include mention of those with low income because they often lack minimal resources for basic needs that are necessary for physical and mental health. Ethnic and minority groups also deserve mentioning because mental well-being is influenced by the conditions of reference groups, and historically these groups have lacked access to adequate, culturally sensitive services (Campinha-Bacote, 1991; Baker et al., 1993).

People who live in poverty or have low incomes live in substandard, overcrowded conditions that contribute to stress in activities of daily living. In single-parent families, a subgroup of the low-income population, depression is not uncommon. In one study, findings suggested that more than half (59.6%) of a sample of low-income single mothers ($N = 255$) had high depressive symptoms. In addition, depression was associated with fewer social resources and greater everyday stressors and was a predictor of parenting attitudes (Hall et al., 1991).

Substandard living conditions also compromise children. For example, elevated blood lead levels that can result in serious mental and physical impairments are not uncommon among children in low-income families. Even more serious, children in low-income families are more vulnerable to death from fire and drowning and all age groups in low-income families are at risk because of violence in their neighborhoods (Healthy People 2000, 1991).

Physical illness, infectious disease, and hazards in the environment also contribute to the mental health status of any individual or group. Nonetheless, individuals in low-income groups are at increased risk for serious illness and infectious disease including tuberculosis and HIV infections (Healthy People 2000, 1991). Homeless mentally ill people who live in poverty are at increased risk for both of these infectious diseases because of their self-care and cognitive deficits combined with overcrowded, unsanitary living conditions (Colson et al., 1994).

Even though data about ethnic and minority groups are limited, epidemiology reveals that many members of minority groups are also members of low-income groups, many with earnings at or below the poverty line (Healthy People 2000, 1991; Krauss 1994). In addition, these groups are at increased risk for mental health problems because they lack access to mental health services (Campinha-Bacote, 1991; Padgett et al., 1994).

The predominant minority populations in the United States are African-Americans, Hispanics, Asian- and Pacific Islander–Americans, native Americans, and Alaska natives (Healthy People 2000, 1991). Within each of these groups are subgroups with unique cultural differences that have been shaped by social, political, and historical factors. Therefore it is important to avoid simplification and overgeneralization in discussions about the characteristics and problems of minorities. Rather, it is critical to conduct community assessments to determine unique characteristics and factors that contribute to mental health deficits within specific aggregates of the population (American Public Health Association, 1991). The information presented here is intended to stimulate thinking and awareness for developing nursing process activities in individual communities.

Today, African-Americans make up the largest minority group in the United States. African-Americans live in all regions of the United States and are represented in all socioeconomic groups, yet one-third live in poverty and one-half are exposed to the high stress of inner-city conditions (Healthy People 2000, 1991; Padgett et al., 1994). Among the many subgroups of the African-American population, African-American elders (aged 65 years and older) represent a unique reference group when it comes to health care. This group had few health care facilities available to them before and during desegregation. This experience and other complex socioenvironmental issues shaped their health beliefs and influenced their awareness about services that may be available for their quality of life and mental well-being (Baker, et al., 1993).

Factors affecting the mental health status of a significant number of African-Americans are similar to those described for low-income families. Still others are exposed to urban problems such as violence. As illustrated in Table 36-2, ethnic groups are target populations for both homicide and suicide. These conditions suggest that violence, stress, despondency, and other severe emotional conditions are influenced by environmental conditions. Similar problems threaten the mental health status of the second largest minority group in the United States.

Hispanic-Americans are the second largest and fastest growing minority group in America with 87% living in urban areas (the largest concentrations are in western states, Florida, and New York [Healthy People 2000, 1991]). Migrant farm workers are also an important subpopulation among Hispanics. As discussed in Chapter 35, migratory living patterns marked by low income, poor education, and lack of health services contribute to stressful living conditions. Hispanic-Americans living in low-income urban areas are subject to many of the conditions described for low-income and disadvantaged African-American families. Outcomes of these living conditions are also similar. For example, the high rates of unintentional injuries and homicide among young Hispanic men (Healthy

People 2000, 1991) not only reveal serious stressful living conditions but also suggest strain, loss, and potential bereavement complications for family members.

Eleven million Asian- and Pacific Islander–Americans who speak over 30 different languages and have diverse cultures make up the third largest minority group in the United States (Healthy People 2000, 1991). Approximately three quarters are from Southeast Asia, and many are refugees. The largest number of this population lives in California. Whereas Asian- and Pacific Islander–Americans, like other minority groups, are represented in all socioeconomic strata, many are in the lower-income groups. The lower-income groups include refugees and recent immigrants who are dealing with displacement issues. Displacement issues involve loss, adjustment, and adaptation. Losses often involve forfeiture of family, traditions, and life-styles for cultures that may seem alien. Adjustments and adaptations include those basic to daily living: learning new languages, laws, and monetary systems and locating support systems. Finding support systems includes acquainting oneself with the health care delivery system. Assessment, planning, and interventions with members of this population and those with diverse languages, customs, and beliefs must include information about their health beliefs and an understanding of the health care system in the United States and of the services that are available to them.

Diversity also characterizes the numerous tribes that make up the native American and Alaska native population. These descendants of the original North American residents number approximately 1.6 million and are the fourth largest minority group in the United States today. About one-third of native Americans live on reservations or historic trust lands, whereas approximately 50% live in urban areas (Healthy People 2000, 1991). Approximately 25% of this minority group live below the poverty line and have threats to mental health that are similar to those described for all low-income groups. Other problems are similar to those described for other minority groups. For example, suicide, homicide, and unintentional injuries are common (see Table 36-2). These problems suggest serious mental health deficits that are important to address when working in communities. More detailed information is available from the Indian Health Service. Community assessments that include data about specific populations from organized agencies such as the Indian Health Service are important since assessment data guide role activities during all steps of the nursing process.

ROLE OF THE NURSE IN COMMUNITY MENTAL HEALTH

The role of the nurse in community mental health was shaped by the evolution of services and the work of nursing pioneers. Development of a knowledge base for the nursing discipline and changes in practice settings prompted recent redefinitions of the scope of psychiatric–mental health clinical practice (American Nurses Association, 1994). The practice standards reflect the values of the profession, describe the responsibilities of nurses, and provide direction for the delivery and evaluation of nursing care with specific populations. Target populations are consistent with those identified in national health objectives. The statement also describes the roles of nurses in both advanced and basic level practice.

Advanced practice psychiatric nurses have graduate level education. They provide primary, secondary, and tertiary care to individuals, groups, families, adults, children, and adolescents. Depending on state laws, some prescribe medications and have hospital admission privileges (Talley and Caverly, 1994). Nurses prepared at the undergraduate level provide basic-level primary, secondary, and tertiary services that are equally valuable. Specific roles and functions of nurses at the basic level are listed in the box below. The functions suggest the overlapping roles of practitioner, educator, and coordinator.

Practitioner

Objectives of the practitioner role are to help the client maintain or regain coping abilities that promote functioning. This involves using the nursing process to guide the diagnosis and treatment of human responses to actual or potential mental health problems (American Nurses Association, 1994). Role functions at the basic practitioner level include case management, counseling, milieu therapy, and psychobiologic interventions with individuals and with groups. Prac-

 Roles and Functions in Psychiatric–Mental Health Nursing Practice

ROLES	FUNCTIONS
Practitioner	Advocacy
Educator	Case finding and referral
Coordinator	Case management
	Community action
	Counseling
	Crisis intervention
	Health maintenance
	Health promotion
	Health teaching
	Home visits
	Intake screening and evaluation
	Milieu therapy
	Psychobiological interventions
	Self-care activities

Modified from American Nurses Association: *A statement on psychiatric-mental health clinical nursing practice and standards of psychiatric-mental health clinical nursing practice,* Washington, DC, 1994, American Nurses Publishing.

titioner skills are used in a variety of settings including the home and often with large groups of people in specific neighborhoods, schools, and public health districts.

For example, many clients who have schizophrenia live in personal care homes. The majority of these clients require psychobiological interventions related to medication management, milieu management for improved social interaction, and assistance with self-care activities for community living such as use of public transportation (Liberman et al., 1993; Murphy and Moller, 1993). Also, the practitioner increasingly coordinates these activities with staff members in community settings. Therefore coordination of care is often the means for promoting treatment plan outcomes and enhancing quality of life for clients. These activities can also result in positive outcomes for others in the community at large.

For example, family members are a primary support system for individuals with schizophrenia. Whether the client lives in a personal care home, family residence, or another setting, counseling family members and the client about the illness may offset the stressors of caregiving. Moreover, educating the public may reduce the stigma and offset social isolation for both clients and families. For the community, implications of these basic-level functions may include public support for needed services and decreased costs of health care resulting from reduced hospitalization. As suggested in these examples, practitioner and educator roles overlap.

Educator

The educator role involves using principles of the teaching-learning process to enhance understanding about the various dimensions of mental illness and mental health. The educator role is foundational to functions such as health maintenance, health promotion, and community action. For example, teaching clients about illness symptoms and the benefits of medications promotes health maintenance and may reduce the risk for illness relapse (Murphy and Moller, 1993). Similar education programs for family members increase their ability to monitor illness symptoms and identify events that lead to relapse (Murphy and Moller, 1993).

At the community level, both formal and informal teaching is important. One important objective for health promotion is to teach positive coping skills. An example of an ineffective coping skill among individuals is overmedicating. Teaching groups about the consequences of this type of medication misuse addresses, in part, the serious public health problem of chemical dependency. Coordinating teaching plans and programs with representatives of consumer groups will facilitate efforts and enhance movement toward community and national health objectives.

Coordinator

Coordination of care is a basic principle of the multidisciplinary team approach in community mental health services. Yet the phenomenon of homelessness suggests there is lack of coordination as well as limited services in most communities. Therefore, at minimum, the role of coordinator must include case finding, referral, and follow-up to evaluate system breakdown and deficits. Because of current system deficits, nurses in community mental health must include in their practice important coordinator role functions such as intake screening, crisis intervention, and home visits. Other objectives of the coordinator role are to enhance the client's health and well-being by promoting independence and self-care in the least restrictive environment. These functions are consistent with descriptions of case management that emphasize continuity of care for individuals who need complex services (Brower, 1992; Bachrach, 1994).

To approximate all these objectives and improve services, the nurse must work with a variety of professionals including advanced practice nurses, social workers, physicians, psychologists, occupational and vocational therapists, and rehabilitation counselors. Since nonlicensed paraprofessionals are frequently involved in direct care activities, their services must be directed, coordinated, and evaluated within the context of treatment planning. Finally, coordination also involves work with individuals who may not have formal preparation but who are essential for positive treatment outcomes. These individuals include family members, volunteers in shelters, a variety of consumer support groups, and community leaders who can influence development of services. The coordinator role clearly offers the nurse an opportunity to identify health system effectiveness and ineffectiveness.

In combination with theoretical and conceptual frameworks, coordinator, educator, and practitioner role activities can enhance the quality of life for the groups who are the direct recipients of community mental health nursing service.

Frameworks

A basic principle of the community mental health movement was that people had a right to mental health services; another principle asserted that those with disorders had a right to services in the least restrictive environment. Moreover, prevention has been emphasized since the inception of the movement. Theories and concepts that help to explain relationships or the dynamics of mental illness provide useful frameworks for fostering these objectives.

Systems Theory

Systems theory is a useful framework for community mental health practice because it emphasizes the relationship of the elements of a unit to the whole. To understand either the element or the whole, one must examine the interactions and relationships that exist between them. A holistic view of system and subsystems can be applied in a variety of ways in community mental health practice. One example of subsystems in a community are its cultural groups. Subsystems of the cultural groups are families; subsystems of the families are individuals. Using systems theory to explore the background, conditions, and context of situations will reveal information about the positive and negative forces that either promote or undermine the well-being of any unit in the system.

Other useful theories to enhance understanding of the multidimensional aspects of community mental health nursing are those that explain biological systems, personality, lifespan development, and family dynamics.

Prevention

Health promotion and illness prevention are fundamental to community mental health practice as well as national objectives previously described (Healthy People 2000, 1991; American Public Health Association, 1991). Therefore the concepts of primary, secondary, and tertiary levels of prevention are useful in practice.

Primary prevention refers to the reduction of health risks. It involves the identification of conditions that have the potential of causing stress and illness. Most functions of the educator role are aimed at primary prevention. Examples include giving education and life-style management classes for caregivers of individuals with severe mental disorders.

Secondary prevention refers to activities aimed at reducing the prevalence or pathological nature of a condition. Many functions of the practitioner role are aimed at secondary prevention. Providing individual and group psychotherapy, case referral, and follow-up to determine the need for additional services and coordinating services following crisis intervention are all examples of secondary prevention.

Tertiary prevention refers to restoration and enhancement of functioning. Many practitioner and coordinator role activities are aimed at tertiary prevention. They include monitoring illness symptoms and treatment responses, coordinating transition from the hospital to the community, and identifying respite care options for caregivers.

Vulnerability-Stress Model

The **vulnerability-stress-coping-competence model** of major mental disorders was designed for use in the rehabilitation of individuals with severe mental illness (Liberman et al., 1993). Within the context of biological, environmental, and behavioral factors, the model explains the onset, course, and outcome of severe mental illness, emphasizing the importance of social skills development necessary for community living.

Liberman et al. (1993) explained that individuals with severe mental disorders have psychobiological

vulnerabilities because of the interplay between genetic brain impairments, not yet fully understood, and stressful life events. According to the theory, biological vulnerability inhibits social skills development during the early years of life. Also, social skills deficits combined with stressful life events can overwhelm the individual's coping ability and result in illness symptoms. Protective factors, another concept of the theory, are important moderators of vulnerability and stress (Liberman et al., 1993). Coping and competence are viewed as essential protective factors. Moreover, coping and competence are "exercised" by "families," "natural support systems," and "professional treatment" as well as the individual who is ill (Liberman et al., 1993). Other protective factors are rehabilitation programs, housing programs, and case management. Relapse management is central to many of the programs and activities that enhance coping skills and competence.

Relapse Management

As a case manager it is important for the community mental health nurse to foster coping and competency aimed at managing illness symptoms with consumers, family members, and other caregivers. The aim of managing illness symptoms is to offset relapse. Since **relapse management** is a major goal of interventions in community mental health nursing, the Moller-Murphy Symptom Management Assessment Tool (MM-SMAT) (Murphy and Moller, 1993) may be especially useful during nursing process activities.

The MM-SMAT was developed to provide consumers, family members, and professionals with a common framework for managing neurobiological disorders such as schizophrenia, bipolar disorder, and major depression (Murphy and Moller, 1993), and it is compatible with vulnerability-stress models of mental illness. Categories of the MM-SMAT focus on the frequency, intensity, and duration of symptoms for the purpose of identifying health, environmental, and behavioral triggers that may lead to illness relapse. Examples of triggers are poor nutrition, poor social skills, hopelessness, and poor symptom management. Once triggers are identified, interventions aimed at fostering effective coping skills can be introduced to offset relapse of symptoms. For example, an intervention that may promote effective coping to offset social isolation is guiding the client to organized consumer group activities available in the community. Another is to promote consumer and family efforts at job training through community vocational agencies. Still another is to promote competency in family members by coordinating services that enhance their understanding of the illness, provide social support, and include respite when needed. Finally, medication management is an important intervention for offsetting relapse.

Scientific advances that led to the use of lithium in the treatment of mania, chlorpromazine (Thorazine) in the treatment of schizophrenia, and imipramine (Tofranil) in antidepressant therapy revolutionized mental health care and services (Keltner and Folks, 1993). More recently in the United States, risperidone (Land and Salzman, 1994) and clozapine (Keltner and Folks, 1993; Clarke and Yaeger, 1994) were introduced for treatment of clients who experienced severe side effects or who did not respond to more traditional antipsychotic drugs (Breier et al., 1993). New antidepressant agents referred to as selective serotonin reuptake inhibitors (SSRIs) have also been introduced. Although these new drugs have dramatically improved the lives of many people with mental disorders, they are not without controversy. Perhaps the greatest controversy is to prescribe medications without incorporating other relapse management approaches. In the nursing process, psychopharmacology should be used with social, behavioral, and psychotherapeutic interventions that take into consideration the cultural dimensions of the client (Keltner and Folks, 1993; Kotcher and Smith, 1993; Clarke and Yaeger, 1994).

What Do You Think?

Although psychopharmacology has dramatically improved the lives of people with severe mental illness since its inception in the 1950s, controversies exist related to medication side effects and the cost of monitoring some of the more serious side effects. For example, side effects of antipsychotic drugs can result in central and peripheral nervous system manifestations. Peripheral nervous system effects include hypotension, urinary retention, sedation, and weight gain. Central nervous system side effects include parkinsonian symptoms such as tremors and rigidity and even more serious manifestations: tardive dyskinesia and neuroleptic malignant syndrome. Do the benefits offered by these medications justify their side effects?

 ## Clinical Application

CASE

Mary, a 62-year-old grandmother, and John, her 66-year-old husband, live in a four-room house in a rural area not far from a large city. Their 28-year-old daughter Ann and her 6-year-old son Jason live with Mary and John. Ann was diagnosed with schizophrenia when she was 20 years old, divorced a short time later when Jason was an infant, and moved home to live with her parents. Ann has been hospitalized frequently for treatment of her psychiatric disorder. Most of the time, she was hospitalized because symptoms of her illness recurred after she quit keeping appointments at the CMHC and refused to take her antipsychotic medications. Other patterns of behavior included leaving home unannounced, seeking rides with strangers, and going into the city, where she lived on the streets for days at a time. Because of these problems, Ann was incarcerated in the legal system and declared mentally incompetent when Jason was 2 years old. At that time, Mary and John legally adopted Jason.

Although there have been few changes in Ann's course of illness during the time since the court ruling, some recent self-care activities suggested that she was more accepting of her illness and treatment plan, including medications. A community mental health nurse from a home health agency was assigned case management activities during Ann's last hospitalization. During the hospitalization, infectious diseases, including HIV, were ruled out, but Ann was identified to be at risk because of her life-style. The nurse established rapport with Ann during hospitalization and began home visits during the week of discharge. Case management activities were to include education and family support. Following in-depth assessment activi-

ties in the home, including use of the MM-SMAT with Ann and her parents, the nurse developed a comprehensive treatment plan incorporating levels of prevention for members of the family.

With Ann, tertiary prevention activities included a plan to help her to identify situations and behaviors that put her at risk for illness relapse, monitoring of medications, teaching about risks for infectious disease including HIV, and exploring options for psychosocial rehabilitation. Tertiary prevention activities for Mary and John included referral to the local NAMI affiliate for supportive services and encouragement of continued work with teachers at Jason's school. The comprehensive plan also revealed the importance of secondary and primary prevention measures.

Because of her multiple roles and limited support outside the family, Mary was at increased risk for continued stress. She also had early signs of depression that included tearfulness, sleep disturbance, loss of appetite, and inability to concentrate. Therefore the nurse arranged for immediate intake and assessment for services at the CMHC. With encouragement, John took over more of the child care activities with Jason. In time, these tertiary and secondary activities resulted in a more stable environment for the family, and since all family members were in agreement, the nurse began to explore supervised housing options for Ann.

In the meantime, John and Mary became more active in the local NAMI affiliate and asked the nurse to recommend someone who could help with education sessions at the agency. The nurse addressed these primary prevention activities with the NAMI group by giving a talk about life-style management and by recom -

Clinical Application—cont'd

mending an advanced psychiatric nurse consultant for more comprehensive program development. During evaluation activities, the nurse identified that the family and consumer groups were important resources for promoting many of the objectives outlined in the model standards for developing healthier communi-

ties. In particular, one community deficit was lack of suitable housing for Ann. Others included lack of consumer education programs about risks for infectious disease and lack of respite services for family caregivers. These shortcomings became targets of program planning and service development.

Key Concepts

- ◆ Reform movements and subsequent federal legislation influenced the development of the current community mental health model that includes team care, case management, prevention, and rehabilitation components of service.
- ◆ During the current decade, federal legislation in the United States focused on mainstreaming people with mental disabilities into American life by legislating access to employment, services, and housing.
- ◆ People are at risk for threats to mental health at all ages across the lifespan. Low income and minority groups are often at increased risk because they lack access to services and because programs may lack cultural sensitivity.
- ◆ Homelessness and substandard living conditions contribute to psychosocial problems related to social isolation and also increases the risk for infectious diseases, including tubercu-

losis (TB) and HIV, among people with severe mental disorders.
- ◆ National health objectives to promote health and services for people who have mental health problems and severe mental disorders illustrate the scope of mental illness and provide direction for community mental health practice.
- ◆ Guidelines for attaining national health objectives were designed to help individuals at regional and local levels establish health priorities that include those for mental illness.
- ◆ Recent redefinitions of ANA standards provide a framework for the roles and functions of community mental health nurses.
- ◆ Frameworks that are useful in community mental health nursing include primary, secondary, and tertiary levels of prevention, vulnerability-stress models, and relapse management.

Critical Thinking Activities

1. For 1 week, keep a list of incidents related to mental health problems that you read about in local newspapers or hear about on the radio and television. Categorize the incidents according to age, gender, socioeconomic, and ethnic or minority status.
2. Visit a local shelter or organization that offers temporary protection for people with mental disorders. Determine services that are available or lacking for children, women, and men.
3. Visit with representatives of your local self-help organizations for consumers to determine types of problems they have and adequacy of resources for people with severe mental disorders and their caregivers.
4. Interview a school nurse, an occupational health nurse, an emergency room nurse, or a hospice nurse in your community to discuss types of mental health problems they deal with in their practice settings.

Determine resources that are available or lacking for primary, secondary, and tertiary prevention.
5. Interview a nurse working in a local community mental health agency to discuss roles, functions, programs, and resources available or lacking for primary, secondary, and tertiary prevention. Compare findings about prevention programs with information obtained from the preceding interview.
6. As a class activity, arrange for a panel of speakers representing the minority populations described in this chapter. Discuss their views about the way culture shapes thinking about mental illness and determine types of culturally sensitive services that are available or lacking in your community.
7. Review articles in at least four research journals to determine current research findings about severe mental disorders and mental health problems.

Bibliography

American Nurses Association: *Nursing's agenda for health care reform*, Pub No PR 3 220M, Washington, DC, 1991, American Nurses Publishing.

American Nurses' Association: *A statement on psychiatric-mental health clinical nursing practice and standards of psychiatric-mental health clinical nursing practice*, Washington, DC, 1994, American Nurses Publishing.

American Psychiatric Association: *Diagnostic and statistical manual of mental disorders*, ed 4, Washington, DC, 1994, The Association.

American Public Health Association: *Healthy communities 2000: model standards, guidelines for community attainment of the year 2000 national health objectives*, ed 3, Washington, DC, 1991, The Association.

Bachrach LL: Deinstitutionalization and the future: the past as prologue. In Cohen N, editor: *Psychiatry takes to the streets: outreach and crisis intervention for the mentally ill*, New York, 1990, The Guilford Press.

Bachrach LL: Continuity of care and approaches to case management for long-term mentally ill patients, *Hosp Community Psych* 44(5):465-468, 1993.

Bachrach LL: The Carter commission's contributions to mental health service planning, *Hosp Community Psych* 45(6):527-528, 543, 1994.

Baker FM, Lavizzo-Mourey R, Jones BE: Acute care of the African-American elder, *J Geriatr Psych Neurol* 6:66-70, 1993.

Bazelon Center for Mental Health Law: Mental disability law in 1993, *Clearinghouse Review*, pp 1322-1330, March 1994.

Bendiner E: Champion of the helpless in our midst, *Hosp Pract* 26(1):139-148, 153-154, 1991.

Biegel DE, Sales E, Schulz R: *Family caregiving in chronic illness*, Newbury Park, Calif, 1991, Sage.

Bower KA: *Case management by nurses*, Pub No NS-32 14M, Washington, DC, 1992, American Nurses Publishing.

Breier A, Buchanan RW, Irish D, Carpenter WT: Clozapine treatment of outpatients with schizophrenia: outcome and long-term response patterns, *Hosp Community Psych* 44(12):1145-1149, 1993.

Campinha-Bacote J: Community mental health services for the underserved: a culturally specific model, *Arch Psych Nurs* 5(4):229-235, 1991.

Clarke DE, Yaeger SF: Addressing emerging social needs of patients treated with new neuroleptics, *J Psychosoc Nurs* 32(11):19-22, 1994.

Colson P, Susser E, Valencia E: HIV and TB among people who are homeless and mentally ill, *Psychosoc Rehab J* 17(4):157-160, 1994.

Donahue MP: *Nursing: the finest art*, St Louis, 1985, Mosby–Year Book.

Feingold E: Health care reform: more than cost containment and universal access, *Am J Pub Health* 84(5):727-728, 1994.

Goren S, Orion R: Space and sanity, *Arch Psych Nurs* 8(4):237-244, 1994.

Griffith HM: Needed: a strong nursing position on preventive service, *Image J Nurs Scholarship* 25(4):272, 1993.

Grob GN: *From asylum to community*, Princeton, NJ, 1991, Princeton University Press.

Haber J, McMahon AL, Price-Hoskins P, Sideleau BF: *Comprehensive psychiatric nursing*, ed 4, St Louis, 1992, Mosby–Year Book.

Hall LA, Gurley DN, Sachs B, Kryscio RJ: Psychosocial predictors of maternal depressive symptoms, parenting attitudes, and child behavior in single-parent families, *Nurs Res* 40(4):214-220, 1991.

Hatfield AB: A family perspective on supported living, *Hosp Commun Psych* 44(5):496-497, 1993.

Healthy People 2000: national health promotion and disease prevention objectives, Washington, DC, 1991, USDHHS, Public Health Service.

Howard PB: Lifelong maternal caregiving for children with schizophrenia, *Arch Psych Nurs* 8(2):107-114, 1994.

Isaac RJ, Armat VC: *Madness in the streets*, New York, 1990, The Free Press.

Kalisch PA, Kalisch BJ: *The advance of american nursing*, ed 2, Boston, 1986, Little, Brown.

Keltner NL, Folks GD: *Psychotropic drugs*, St Louis, 1993, Mosby–Year Book.

Kotcher M, Smith TE: Three phases of clozapine treatment and phase-specific issues for patients and families, *Hosp Community Psych* 44(8):744-747, 1993.

Krauss J: The mental status of health care reform, *Arch Psych Nurs* 8(1):1-2, 1994.

Krauss J: *Health care reform: essential mental health services*, Washington, DC, 1993, American Nurses Publishing.

Kuhlman GJ, Skodol-Wilson H, Hutchinson S, Wallhagen M: Alzheimer's disease and family caregiving: critical synthesis of the literature and research agenda, *Nurs Res* 40(6):331-337, 1991.

LaFond JQ, Durham ML: *Back to the asylum*, New York, 1992, Oxford University Press.

Land W, Salzman C: Resperidone: a novel antipsychotic medication, *J Hosp Community Psychiatry* 45(5):434-435, 1994.

Lazarus A: Managed care: lessons from community mental health, *Hosp Commun Psych* 45(4):301, 1994.

Liberman RP, Wallace C, Blackwell G, et al: Innovations in skills training for the seriously mentally ill: the UCLA social and independent living skills modules, *Innovations Res* 2(2):43-60, 1993.

Manderscheid RW, Henderson MJ: The new informatics of health care reform, *Behav Healthcare Tomorrow*, pp 11-15, Jan/Feb 1994.

McShane RE, Bumbalo JA, Patsdaughter CA: Psychological distress in family members living with Human Immunodeficiency Virus/Acquired Immune Deficiency Syndrome, *Arch Psych Nurs* 8(1):53-61, 1994.

Murphy MF, Moller MD: Relapse management in neurobiological disorders: the Moller-Murphy Symptom Management Assessment Tool, *Arch Psych Nurs* 7(4):226-235, 1993.

Natale A, Barron C: Mothers' causal explanations for their sons' schizophrenia: relationship to depression and guilt, *Arch Psych Nurs* 8(4):228-236, 1994.

National Institute of Mental Health: *Caring for people with severe mental disorders: a national plan of research to improve services* (DHHS publication no. ADM91-1762), Washington, DC, 1991, US Government Printing Office.

Navarro V: The future of public health in health care reform. *Am J Pub Health* 84(5):729-730, 1994.

Norbeck JS, Chafetz L, Skodol-Wilson H, Weiss SJ: Social support needs of family caregivers of psychiatric patients from three age groups, *Nurs Res* 40(4):208-213, 1991.

Padgett DK, Patrick C, Burns BJ, Schlesinger HJ: Ethnicity and the use of outpatient mental health services in a national insured population, *Am J Pub Health* 84(2):222-226, 1994.

Pallett PJ: A conceptual framework for studying family caregiver burden in Alzheimer's-type dementia, *Image J Nurs Scholarship* 22(1):52-58, 1990.

Perlin ML: Law and the delivery of mental health services in the community, *Am J Orthopsych* 64(2):194-208, 1994.

Plaut TF, Arons BS: President Clinton's proposal for health care reform: key provisions and issues, *Hosp Commun Psych* 45(9):871-874, 1994.

Reinhard SC: Perspectives on the family's caregiving experience in mental illness, *Image J Nurs Scholarship* 26(1):70-74, 1994.

Scallet LJ, Havel JT: Reflections on the mental health community's experience in the health care reform debate, *Hosp Commun Psych* 45(9):888-892, 1994.

Shore MF: Social policy: the wheels of change, *Am J Orthopsych* 63(4):498, 1993.

Talley S, Caverly S: Advanced practice psychiatric nursing and health care reform, *Hosp Commun Psych* 45(6):545-547, 1994.

Taylor CM: *Essentials of psychiatric nursing*, ed 14, St Louis, 1994, Mosby–Year Book.

Wiener L, Theut S, Steinberg SM, et al: The HIV-infected child: parental responses and psychosocial implications, *Am J Orthopsych* 64(3):485-492, 1994.

Wilk RJ: Federal legislation for rights of persons with mental illness: obstacles to implementation, *Am J Orthopsych* 63(4):518-525, 1993.

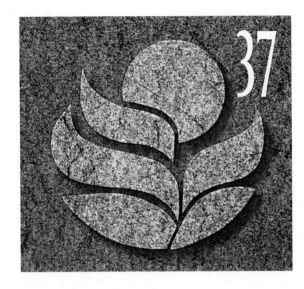

37 Substance Abuse in the Community

Mary Lynn Mathre

Objectives ▼

After reading this chapter, the student should be able to do the following:

◆ Examine personal attitudes toward alcohol, tobacco, and other drug problems to enhance therapeutic effectiveness.
◆ Differentiate among the terms *substance use, abuse, dependence,* and *addiction.*
◆ Discuss the differences among the major psychoactive drug categories.
◆ Discuss the role of the nurse in primary, secondary, and tertiary prevention of alcohol, tobacco, and other drug problems as it relates to individual clients and their families.
◆ Discuss the role of the nurse in primary, secondary, and tertiary prevention of alcohol, tobacco, and other drug problems as it relates to the community.

Key Terms ▼

abstinence
addiction treatment
alcoholism
anhedonia
antiprohibition
blackout
codependency
cross-tolerance
denial
detoxification
drug addiction
drug dependence
enabling
mainstream smoke
polysubstance use or abuse
prohibition
psychoactive drugs
sidestream smoke
substance abuse
tolerance
withdrawal

Outline ▼

Understanding the Problem
 Historical Perspective
 Attitudes and Myths
 Social Conditions
 Definitions
Psychoactive Drugs
 Depressants
 Stimulants
 Marijuana
 Hallucinogens
 Inhalants
Primary Prevention
 Promotion of Healthy Life-styles and Resiliency Factors
 Drug Education
Secondary Prevention
 Assessing for Substance Abuse Problems
 High-Risk Groups
 Codependency and Family Involvement
Tertiary Prevention
 Detoxification
 Addiction Treatment
 Support Groups

Substance abuse is a national health problem that is linked to numerous forms of morbidity and mortality. Between 25% and 40% of all general hospital admissions are related to the effects of alcohol abuse (Institute for Health Policy, Brandeis University, 1993), and a recent study found that one in five dollars of Medicaid is spent on substance abuse (Merrill et al., 1993). More deaths and disabilities annually are attributed to substance abuse than to any other preventable cause. Of the 2 million U.S. deaths each year, one-quarter are attributed to alcohol, illicit drug, and tobacco use (Institute for Health Policy, Brandeis University, 1993). The substance abuser is not only at risk for personal health problems, but also may pose a threat to the health and safety of family members, coworkers, and other members of the community.

Substance abuse and addiction affect all ages, races, sexes, and segments of society. As seen in Appendix A.1, *Healthy People 2000* (1991) lists "tobacco" and "alcohol and other drugs" as separate priority areas, with 35 related objectives. This chapter defines substance abuse as the abuse of alcohol, tobacco, and other drugs. Community health nurses can play a significant role in the reduction of alcohol, tobacco, and other drug (ATOD) problems for individuals, families, and communities.

This chapter gives a historical perspective on ATOD problems. In addition, various attitudes, myths, and current social conditions are examined to differentiate drug problems from those created by lack of information and unfounded fears. Relevant terms are defined to decrease the confusion caused by frequent misuse of terms. The major drug categories are also described, including information on onset and duration of action, main effects and side effects, adverse reactions, overdose effects, and nursing actions and considerations. The remainder of the chapter looks at the role of the community health nurse in primary, secondary, and tertiary prevention of ATOD problems.

UNDERSTANDING THE PROBLEM

ATOD abuse and addiction can cause multiple health problems for individuals. Heavy ATOD use has been associated with many problems, including neonates with low birth weight and congenital abnormalities; accidents, homicides, and suicides; chronic diseases, such as cardiovascular diseases, cancer, and lung disease; violence; and family disruption. Factors that contribute to the substance abuse problem include lack of knowledge about the use of drugs; the labeling of certain drugs (alcohol, nicotine, and caffeine) as nondrugs; lack of quality control of illegal drugs; and drug laws that label certain drug users as criminals.

Community health nurses have a responsibility to seek the underlying roots of various health problems and plan action that is realistic, nonjudgmental, holistic, and positive.

Historical Perspective

Psychoactive drug use has been endemic to virtually all cultures since the beginning of humanity. Often a culture encourages use of some drugs while discouraging the use of others. Coffee, alcohol, and tobacco are socially acceptable drugs in the United States and Canada, whereas other cultures prohibit their use. Conversely, marijuana, cocaine, and heroin use is not accepted in mainstream U.S. society, although these substances are considered sacred and their use is encouraged in various other cultures.

The United States' primary solution to various "drug problems" has been **prohibition.** During alcohol prohibition from 1920 to 1933, the United States experienced a sharp increase in violent crime and corruption among law officials secondary to the illicit marketing of alcohol. Distilled beverages were pushed because of the higher profit margin per bottle of liquor than for beer or wine. Severe health problems were caused by the high alcohol content in illicit moonshine.

Similar problems are occurring with the current prohibition on marijuana, cocaine, and other drugs. An increase in violent crime and corruption among law officials as a result of the illicit market is becoming a major national problem. Stronger drugs are pushed because of their greater profits. Marijuana (bulky and distinctly odorous) is more difficult to obtain than cocaine (compact and odorless). Crack (smokeable cocaine) is replacing cocaine powder because it is more addictive and yields a higher profit margin. Many deaths are occurring as a result of the lack of any quality control to identify the content and strength of these drugs.

In the past decade, the U.S. war on drugs has escalated. Persons who use illegal drugs are arrested and given a choice of jail or treatment. This punitive approach to illicit drug use hinders open communication between the health care professional and the drug user. Those who are abusing drugs, experiencing secondary health problems, or possibly becoming addicted may not seek help for fear of being arrested or confined.

Debates continue as to whether ATOD abuse and addiction are health care or criminal justice problems. Current support for legalization (more appropriately termed **antiprohibition**) suggests that problems with ATOD abuse are health care problems and that the prohibition of drugs causes greater societal problems than the use of those drugs. Newer laws are creating mandatory sentences, destroying civil liberties, and putting most resources into law enforcement rather than drug education and treatment (Heather et al., 1993; Hoffman and Goldfrank, 1990; Vallance, 1993) (Figure 37-1); yet a study of California drug treatment centers found that for every dollar spent on treatment, the public saves 7 dollars in health care and crime costs (National Opinion Resource Center, 1994).

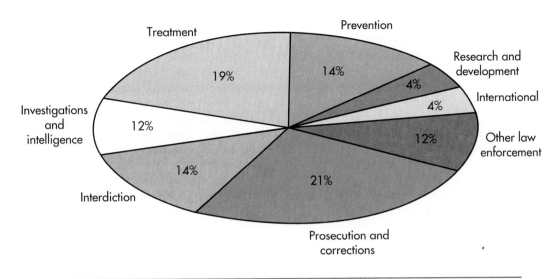

FIGURE 37-1

Federal drug control budget for 1994.

The American Public Health Association is currently reviewing the "harm reduction" model, an approach used in Great Britain, the Netherlands, and Australia. This approach accepts the reality that psychoactive drug use is endemic, and subsequently the focus is on pragmatic interventions, especially education, to reduce the adverse consequences of drug use. The U.S. has already taken this approach with tobacco and alcohol. Educational campaigns are used to inform the public about the health risks of tobacco use. Warnings have appeared on tobacco product labels since 1967 as a result of the surgeon general's 1966 report on the dangers of smoking. In 1971 a ban on television and radio cigarette advertising was imposed. Cigarette smoking has decreased from 42% of the population in 1965 to 26% in 1991 (Institute for Health Policy, Brandeis University, 1993).

Education is beginning to address the dangers of alcohol abuse and establish guidelines for safe alcohol use. Alcohol consumers are choosing lower alcohol-content products such as beer and wine coolers rather than distilled products (Kinney and Leaton, 1995). Research shows that responsible, moderate use of alcohol may have some long-term health benefits (Coate, 1993). The box at right provides an historical overview of the prevention approaches.

Attitudes and Myths

Attitudes are developed through cultural learning and personal experiences. Attitudes toward ATOD problems are influenced by the way society categorizes drugs as either "good" or "bad." In the United States, good drugs are over-the-counter (OTC) drugs or those prescribed by a health care provider, yet this makes them no less problematic or addictive. Bad drugs are the illegal drugs, and persons who use these drugs are considered criminals regardless of whether or not the drug has caused any problems.

The Evolution of Prevention

Prevention approaches have evolved since the 1960s, when a high level of illegal drug use was well noted in the media. The first response was to use *scare tactics*. Drugs were only depicted as harmful, and the information was often exaggerated or inaccurate. Information from peers often invalidated these scare tactics and caused distrust of the "experts." During the early 1970s, some professionals began using the strategy of giving *accurate information* to young people. This strategy may have increased usage rates, creating educated drug users. By the late 1970s, the focus was on teaching young people *life skills*, which included personal self-awareness, independent living, job skills, and communication skills. In the early 1980s, *healthy alternatives* to ATOD use looked at natural highs through recreational experiences. Also in the 1980s, emphasis was placed on changing *policies* to decrease drug use. These policy changes centered around legislative and law enforcement efforts. And by the late 1980s the new approach was *community involvement*, which attempts to bring societal pressure to bear on the problem. The strategy for the 1990s is a *comprehensive* approach that combines all of the previous approaches with the exception of scare tactics.

From Nurse Training Course, "Prevention of Alcohol, Tobacco, and Other Drugs," developed by the National Nurses Society on Addictions, Macro International Inc, and J & E Associates, under contract by the Center for Substance Abuse Prevention, 1994.

Americans have come to rely heavily on prescription and OTC drugs to relieve (or mask) fear, tension, fatigue, and physical or emotional pain. Rather than learning nonmedicinal methods of coping, many people choose the "quick fix" and take pills to deal with their problems or negative feelings.

Americans also rely on drug use to enhance their social activities. Alcohol is clearly the nation's drug of choice for most social occasions, and the marketing of alcohol focuses on the enjoyment and relaxation associated with alcohol consumption. Among some wealthy groups, cocaine (intranasal) was considered the drug of choice at parties during the 1970s and 1980s. For many college students and middle-class adults, marijuana has been a drug to be shared among friends since the 1960s.

Addicts are often viewed as immoral, weak-willed, or irresponsible people who should try harder to help themselves. Although alcoholism was recognized as a disease by the American Medical Association in 1954 and drug addiction was recognized as a disease some years later, the public and many health care professionals have failed to change their attitudes and accept alcoholics and addicts as ill persons in need of health care.

Community health nurses must examine their attitudes toward ATOD use, abuse, and addiction before working with this health problem. To be therapeutic, the nurse must develop a trusting, nonjudgmental relationship with the client. Systematic assessment for ATOD problems is based on an awareness that there may be problems with legal drugs as well as illegal drugs. If the nurse's attitude toward a client with a drug abuse problem is negative or punitive, the issue may never be directly addressed or the client may be avoided. If the client senses the negative attitude of the health care provider, either by words or tone of voice, communication may cease and information thus withheld (Tweed, 1989). To develop a therapeutic attitude, the nurse must realize that any drug can be abused, that anyone may develop a drug dependence, and that drug addiction can be successfully treated.

Myths develop over years, and if myths are not questioned, many attitudes may be formed based solely on fiction rather than fact. Some common myths are as follows: "An alcoholic is a skid row bum"—yet less than 5% of persons with alcoholism fit this description. "If you teach people about drugs, they will abuse them"—although it is true that people may choose to use drugs if they have knowledge about them, it is more likely that people who use drugs without knowledge about them will abuse them. "Addiction is a sin or moral failing"—addiction is recognized as a health problem involving biopsychosocial factors, and persons who use drugs do not do so with the intent to become addicted.

Social Conditions

Social conditions influence the use of drugs. The fast pace of life, competition at school or in the workplace, and the pressure to accumulate material possessions are daily stressors. Pharmaceutical, alcohol, and tobacco companies are continuously bombarding the public with enticing advertisements pushing their products as a means of feeling better, sleeping better, having more energy, or just as a "treat." People grow up believing that most of life's problems can be solved quickly and easily through the use of a drug.

For persons of a lower socioeconomic background and with minimal education or employment possibilities, many of life's opportunities may seem out of reach. For these people, psychoactive drug use may offer a way to numb the pain or escape from their hopeless reality. These people rarely seek relief through a physician's prescription or other therapeutic measures. Instead, they rely on alcohol or illicit drugs, which are more readily available. For some, illicit-drug dealing may appear to be the only way out of the poverty and unemployment rut.

The solution of "just say no" is both simplistic and misleading. Indiscriminant use of "good" drugs has caused more health problems as a result of side effects, adverse reactions, drug interactions, dependence, addiction, and overdoses than use of "bad" drugs. The black market associated with illicit drug use puts otherwise law-abiding citizens in close contact with criminals, prevents any quality control of the drugs, increases the risk of acquired immunodeficiency syndrome (AIDS) and hepatitis secondary to needle sharing, and hinders health care professionals' accessibility to the abuser or addict.

The community health nurse is in a key position to reduce the problem of substance abuse. By approaching substance abuse as a health problem, community health nurses can use their knowledge and skills to assist individuals, families, and the community in alleviating this problem.

Definitions

The terms *drug use* and *drug abuse* have virtually lost their utility because the public and government have narrowed the term *drug* to include only illegal drugs, rather than including prescription, OTC, and legal recreational drugs. The current phrase *alcohol, tobacco, and other drugs (ATOD)* reminds us that our leading drug problems are with alcohol and tobacco. The term *substance* broadens the scope to include alcohol, tobacco, legal drugs, and even foods. **Substance abuse** is the use of any substance that threatens a person's health or impairs his or her social or economic functioning. This definition is more objective and universal than the government's definition of drug abuse, which is the use of a drug without a prescription or any use of an illegal drug. Although any drug or food can be abused, this chapter focuses on **psychoactive drugs:** drugs that affect mood, perception, and thought.

Drug dependence and drug addiction are frequently used interchangeably, but they are not synonymous. **Drug dependence** is a state of neuroadaptation (a physiological change in the central nervous system [CNS]) caused by the chronic, regular administration of a drug in which continued use of the drug becomes necessary to prevent withdrawal symptoms (Jaffe, 1990). This happens when persons are given an opiate such as morphine on a regular basis for pain management. To prevent withdrawal symptoms, the morphine should be gradually tapered rather than abruptly stopped.

Drug addiction is a pattern of abuse characterized by an overwhelming preoccupation with the use (compulsive use) of a drug, securing its supply, and a high tendency to relapse if the drug is removed. Frequently, addicts are physically dependent on a drug, but there also appears to be an added psychological component that causes the intense cravings and subsequent relapse. In general, anyone can develop a drug dependence caused by regular administration of drugs that alter the CNS; however, only 7% to 15% of the drug-using population will develop a drug addiction. The reason some people develop a drug addiction and others do not is not completely understood and continues to be an area of much research.

Alcoholism is addiction to the drug called alcohol. Alcoholism and drug addiction are recognized as illnesses under a biopsychosocial model. Simply stated, the disease concept of addiction and alcoholism identifies them as chronic and progressive diseases in which a person's use of a drug or drugs continues despite problems it causes in any area of life—physical, emotional, social, economical, or spiritual.

Many theories exist on the etiological factors of addiction, and no consensus exists on specific causes. The underlying etiological factors include the belief that addiction is a disease, a moral failing, a psychological disturbance, a personality disorder, a social problem, a dysbehaviorism, or a maladaptive coping mechanism. The reality may be that different persons develop addiction in different ways. For example, some alcoholics have made statements such as, "I knew I was an alcoholic from my first drink; I drank differently than others." These people may be genetically predisposed to alcoholism, and their chemical makeup is such that the disease will begin simply by consuming the drug. Others have no family history of addiction but suffer from great stress (chronic pain,

significant losses, or abusive relationships resulting in low self-esteem) and find that drugs offer an escape from stress. Over time, heavy use of one or more drugs to cope with the stress may develop into addiction. The biopsychosocial model provides a framework to understand addiction as the result of the interaction of multiple causes.

PSYCHOACTIVE DRUGS

Although any drug can be abused, ATOD abuse and addiction problems generally involve the psychoactive drugs. Because they can alter emotions, these drugs are used in social and recreational settings and for personal use to self-medicate uncomfortable feelings. Psychoactive drugs are divided into categories according to their effect on the CNS and the general feelings or experiences the drugs may induce. A pharmacology text will provide detailed information on these drug categories (e.g., depressants, stimulants, hallucinogens). Often if persons cannot obtain their drug of choice, another drug from the same category will be substituted. For example, a person who cannot drink alcohol may begin using a benzodiazepine as an alternative because both are CNS depressants. Table 37-1 ranks commonly used drugs regarding the severity of withdrawal, the reinforcement potential, degree of tolerance, dependence (addiction) potential, and level of intoxication.

In addition to the specific drug being used, two other major variables influence the particular drug experience: set and setting (Weil and Rosen, 1993). *Set* refers to the expectations, including unconscious expectations, a person has about the drug being used. *Setting* is the influence of the physical, social, and cultural environment within which the use occurs. To understand various patterns of drug use and abuse by

Table 37-1   Ranking* of Risks of Six Commonly Used Drugs†‡

	Withdrawal		Reinforcement		Tolerance		Dependence		Intoxication	
	NIDA	UCSF	NIDA	UCSF	NIDA	UCSF	NIDA	UCSF	NIDA	UCSF
Nicotine	3	3	4	4	2	4	1	1	5	6
Heroin	2	2	2	2	1	2	2	2	2	2
Cocaine	4	3	1	1	4	1	3	3	3	3
Alcohol	1	1	3	3	3	4	4	4	1	1
Caffeine	5	4	6	5	5	3	5	5	6	6
Marijuana	6	5	5	6	6	5	6	6	4	4

*Ranking Scale: 1 = most serious; 6 = least serious.

†Ranking by: Dr. Jack E. Henningfield of the National Institute on Drug Abuse (NIDA) and Dr. Neal L. Benowitz of the University of California at San Francisco (UCSF).

‡Explanation of terms: withdrawal—presence and severity of characteristic withdrawal symptoms; reinforcement—substance's ability, in human and animal tests, to get users to take it repeatedly and instead of other substances; tolerance—amount of substance needed to satisfy increasing cravings and level of plateau that is eventually reached; dependence (addiction)—difficulty in ending use of substance, relapse rate, percentage of people who become addicted, addict's self-reporting of degree of need for substance and continued use in face of evidence that it causes harm; intoxication—level of intoxication associated with addiction, personal and social damage that substance causes.

individuals, all three factors (drug, set, and setting) should be considered.

Depressants

Depressants lower the body's overall energy level, reduce sensitivity to outside stimulation, and, in high doses, induce sleep. Low doses of depressants may produce a feeling of stimulation caused by initial sedation of the inhibitory centers in the brain. In general, depressants decrease heart rate, respirations, muscular coordination, and energy and dull the senses. Higher doses lead to coma and, if the vital functions shut down, death. Major categories include alcohol, barbiturates, tranquilizers, and the opiates.

Alcohol

Alcohol (ethyl alcohol or ethanol) is the oldest and most widely used psychoactive drug in the world. Approximately 80% of Americans consume alcohol, and of those approximately 10 million are considered problem drinkers and another 10 million are considered alcoholics (Long, 1993). Alcohol abuse ranks third following coronary diseases and cancer as the major cause of death in the United States. The life expectancy of a person with alcoholism is reduced by 15 years, and mortality is 2 1/2 times greater than that of persons without alcoholism (Kinney and Leaton, 1995). Alcohol abuse costs billions of dollars in lost productivity, property damage, medical expenses from alcohol-related illnesses and accidents, family disruptions, alcohol-related violence, and neglect and abuse of children.

The concentration of alcohol in the blood is determined by the concentration of alcohol in the drink, the rate of drinking, the rate of absorption (slower in the presence of food), the rate of metabolism, and a person's weight and gender. The amount of alcohol the liver can metabolize per hour is equal to about 3/4 ounce of whiskey, 4 ounces of wine, or 12 ounces of beer. Figure 37-2 shows the effects on the CNS as the blood alcohol concentration (BAC) increases. However, with chronic consumption, tolerance will develop and a person can reach a high BAC with minimal CNS effects.

Gender affects the BAC in that females have less alcohol dehydrogenase activity than men (except for males with chronic alcoholism). Because this enzyme detoxifies alcohol, a deficiency results in a higher bioavailability of alcohol. Consequently, females suffer the long-term effects of alcohol intake at much lower doses in a shorter time span (Frezza et al., 1990; Talashek et al., 1994).

Chronic alcohol abuse exerts profound metabolic and physiological effects on all organ systems. Gastrointestinal (GI) disturbances include inflammation of the GI tract, malabsorption, ulcers, liver problems, and cancers. Cardiovascular disturbances include cardiac dysrhythmias, cardiomyopathy, hypertension, atherosclerosis, and blood dyscrasias. CNS problems include depression, sleep disturbances, memory loss, organic brain syndrome, Wernicke-Korsakoff syndrome, and alcohol withdrawal syndrome. Neuromuscular problems include myopathy and peripheral neuropathy. Males may experience testicular atrophy, sterility, impotence, or gynecomastia, and females may reproduce neonates with fetal alcohol syndrome (FAS) or fetal alcohol effects (FAE). Some of the metabolic disturbances include hypokalemia, hypomagnesemia, and ketoacidosis. Also, endocrine disturbances may result in pancreatitis or diabetes.

Barbiturates

Since barbituric acid was discovered in 1864, hundreds of derivatives have been developed. These drugs are generally known as sleeping pills or "downers." High doses help people sleep, and low doses have a calming effect.

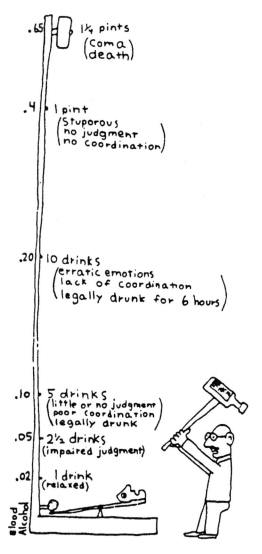

FIGURE 37-2

Blood alcohol level and related CNS effects of a normal drinker (160-lb male) according to the number of drinks consumed in 1 hour. (From Kinney J, Leaton G: *Loosening the grip*, ed 5, St Louis, 1995, Mosby–Year Book.)

The short-acting barbiturates, similar to alcohol in their effects, are frequently abused. These drugs are not as toxic to the body's organ systems as alcohol; however, the tolerance that develops is more dangerous. Tolerance to the effects on mood develop faster than the physical tolerance to the lethal dose, resulting in a greater risk of accidental overdose. When barbiturates are used in combination with alcohol, a synergistic reaction occurs and the risk of overdose is greatly increased.

Benzodiazepines

Benzodiazepines were introduced in the 1960s and marketed to housewives as the cure for everyday stress. More than 88 million benzodiazepine prescriptions, or 1 in 20 prescriptions, were written in a recent year. Of controlled substance prescriptions, 37% were for benzodiazepines. At one time, diazepam (Valium) and chlordiazepoxide (Librium) were marketed for the treatment of alcoholism, but it soon became apparent that these drugs produced an alcohol-like effect and that persons with alcoholism became addicted to these drugs.

These drugs continue to be misprescribed for long-term therapy rather than treating the underlying stress. The benzodiazepines have a relatively safe therapeutic index (difficult to overdose), but withdrawal can be life threatening.

Opioids

Opiates include the natural drugs found in the opium poppy, namely, opium, morphine, and codeine. Opioids are synthetic drugs, such as heroin (semisynthetic), meperidine, methadone, oxycodone, and propoxyphene, that mimic the effects of the natural opiates. Opiates are by far the most effective drugs for pain relief.

The United States has approximately 1 million regular users of heroin, 500,000 heroin addicts, and more than 2 million people who have tried it. The typical heroin addict is male, is from a poor socioeconomic background, and began use between 16 and 19 years of age (Foley, 1993). Heroin is usually consumed intranasally, subcutaneously, or intravenously and costs $10 to $100 per bag. Other opioid abusers (including health care professionals) take prescription opioid analgesics obtained legally (present with false or exaggerated complaints of pain) or illegally (forged prescriptions or diversion).

Tolerance develops quite readily with opioids and can reach striking levels. Tolerance to one opioid extends to other opioids, and thus **cross-tolerance** can occur. Physical dependence also develops quite quickly; less than 2 weeks of continuous use can cause withdrawal symptoms if not tapered. Chronic abuse of the opioids causes few physiological problems except for constipation. The negative consequences primarily result from their illegal status. Lack of quality control (varied strength and purity) often results in unexpected overdoses or secondary effects of the impuri-

ties. A synthetic analog of fentanyl (3-methylfentanyl) marketed as "heroin" is 6000 times as potent as morphine. Unsafe methods of administration (contaminated needles) lead to local and systemic infections. The high cost on the black market leads to crime to support the addiction.

Stimulants

The primary reason most individuals use a CNS stimulant is that it makes them feel more alert or energetic by activating or exciting the nervous system. An increase in alertness and energy results as the stimulant causes the nerve fibers to release noradrenaline and other stimulating neurotransmitters. However, these drugs do not simply give the person more energy; they only make the body expend its own energy sooner and in greater quantities than it normally would.

If used carefully, stimulants are useful and have few negative health effects. The body must be allowed time to replenish itself after use of a stimulant. The "cost" for the "high" is the "down" state following the use of a stimulant: a feeling of sleepiness, laziness, mental fatigue, and possibly depression. Many persons abusing stimulants soon find themselves in a vicious cycle of avoiding the down feeling by taking another dose and can become physically dependent on the stimulant to function. Common stimulants include caffeine, cocaine, amphetamines, and nicotine.

Caffeine

Caffeine is the most widely used psychoactive drug in the world with a U.S. daily per capita consumption of 211 mg. Caffeine is found in coffee, tea, chocolate, soft drinks, and various medications (Table 37-2).

Moderate doses of caffeine from 100 to 300 mg per day probably have little negative effect on health and serve to increase mental alertness. Higher doses can lead to insomnia, irritability, tremulousness, anxiety, cardiac dysrhythmias, and headaches. Regular use of high doses can lead to physical dependence, and the withdrawal symptoms may include headaches, slowness, and occasional depression (Strain et al., 1994). Treating afternoon headaches with analgesics containing caffeine may in reality be preventing a withdrawal symptom from heavy morning coffee consumption.

Cocaine

Cocaine comes from the coca shrub found on the eastern slopes of the Andes and has been cultivated by the South American Indians for thousands of years. The Indians chew a mixture of the coca leaf and lime to get a mild stimulant effect similar to coffee. By 1860 cocaine was isolated from the plant as a hydrochloride salt. It could be dissolved in water and used intravenously or orally when mixed in soft drinks. By the early 1900s the common route of administration of the white powder was intranasal "snorting" (Weil and Rosen, 1993).

In the 1970s, "freebasing" was introduced. This in-

Table 37-2   Caffeine Content in Commonly Consumed Substances

Substance	Caffeine content (mg)
COFFEE (5 OZ)	
Brewed	60-180
Instant	30-120
Decaffeinated	1-5
CHOCOLATE	
Cocoa (5 oz)	2-20
Semisweet (1 oz)	5-35
TEA (5 OZ)	
Brewed	20-90
Iced	67-76
SOFT DRINKS (12 OZ)	
Colas	40-45
Mountain Dew	53
Orange, ginger ale, root beer	0
PRESCRIPTION DRUGS	
Propoxyphene (Darvon)	32.4
Fiorinal	40
Ergotamine (Cafergot)	100
OVER-THE-COUNTER DRUGS	
Aqua-ban	100
Anacin	32
Excedrin	65
No Doz	100
Vivarin	200

volved making the hydrochloride salt a more volatile substance using highly flammable substances such as ether to convert the powder to a crystal that could then be smoked in a pipe. By the early 1980s, another form of smokeable cocaine was introduced. Cocaine was dissolved in water, mixed with baking soda, and then heated to form rocks, or "crack."

Approximately 90% of cocaine users have snorted cocaine, 33% have smoked it, and 10% have injected it (Warner, 1993). Intranasal cocaine has been a popular recreational drug among the "rich and famous," but the cheaper crack form, sold in small quantities at $2 to $20, has become popular, particularly among inner-city black populations. The number of current cocaine users in the United States has increased from 1.6 million in 1991 to 1.9 million in 1992, and much of this increase is believed to be the result of the use of crack (Weiss et al., 1994).

Cocaine produces a feeling of intense euphoria, increased confidence, and a willingness to work for long periods. Smoking cocaine gives intense effects because the drug quickly reaches the brain through the blood vessels in the lungs.

Cocaine's interaction with dopamine seems to be the basis for the addictive patterns. The extreme euphoria is believed to be caused by cocaine's effect of dopaminergic stimulation. Chronic administration can lead to neurotransmitter depletion (especially of dopamine), which results in an extreme dysphoria characterized by apathy, sadness, and **anhedonia** (lack of joy). Thus a cocaine user can get caught up in a dangerous cycle of gaining an extreme high followed by an extreme low and avoiding that low by consuming more cocaine. Crack addiction develops rapidly and is expensive, with addicts needing between $100 and $1000 per day. Users soon learn that their ill health and drug use are related, but overwhelmed by cravings, they may resort to criminal activities (theft or prostitution) to get the money to buy the drug.

Street cocaine ranges in purity from 5% to 60% and may be cut with other drugs, such as procaine or amphetamine, or any white powder, such as sugar or baby powder. The incidence of cocaine-related emergency room visits increased twelvefold from 1985 to 1992. Some of this increase is the result of the lack of quality control; however, most is the result of the use of crack (Weiss et al., 1994). High doses can cause extreme agitation, hyperthermia, hallucinations, cardiac dysrhythmias, pulmonary complications, convulsions, and possibly death (Das and Laddu, 1993; Warner, 1993).

Amphetamines

Amphetamines are a class of stimulants similar to cocaine, but the effects last longer and the drugs are cheaper. Amphetamines have a chemical structure similar to adrenaline and noradrenaline and are generally used to decrease fatigue, increase mental alertness, suppress appetite, and create a sense of well-being. Amphetamines were issued to American soldiers during World War II to decrease fatigue and increase mental alertness. They are currently popular among truck drivers and college students.

These drugs are taken orally, intranasally, or by injection, or they are smoked. When taken intravenously, they quickly induce an intense euphoric feeling (a "rush"). The user may speed for several days (go on a "speed run") and then fall into a deep sleep for 18 or more hours ("crash"). "Ice," a smokeable form of crystallized methamphetamine, was introduced in the late 1980s as an alternative to crack because it can be easily manufactured and the effects last up to 24 hours.

Other drugs containing caffeine, ephedrine, or phenylpropanolamine (singly or in combination), referred to as "look alikes," gained attention on the market after access to amphetamines was controlled by prescription. These chemicals are often found in OTC cold remedies as a nasal decongestant and in diet pills (e.g., Dexatrim).

Nicotine

One in five deaths in the United States is attributed to cigarettes (Institute for Health Policy, Brandeis University, 1993). In 1991 the Centers for Disease Control estimated that 434,000 deaths per year are caused by complications of cigarette smoking, including 30% of all heart disease deaths, 90% of all lung cancer victims, and about 90% of all chronic obstructive pulmonary disease deaths (Fiore, 1993). Figure 37-3 compares mortality for tobacco with other drugs. The *Morbidity and Mortality Weekly Report* (*MMWR*, July 8, 1994) estimated 1993 smoking-related medical costs at $50 billion. In an analysis of 1987 data, the *Report* found that more than 40% of total annual medical care expenditures were attributable to smoking. Cancer mortality could be reduced by approximately 25% if smoking were eliminated.

Currently, the prevalence of cigarette smoking has dropped to 31.7% for men and 26.8% for women. Most of the decline has occurred among better educated and white populations. However, more women are becoming new users than men, and by the year 2000 it is estimated that more women will smoke than men (Fiore, 1993; U.S. Department of Health and Human Services, 1989).

Nicotine, the active ingredient in the tobacco plant, is one of the most toxic drugs known. To protect itself, the body quickly develops tolerance to the nicotine. If a person smokes regularly, tolerance to nicotine develops within hours, compared with days with heroin or months with alcohol. Pipes and cigars are less hazardous than cigarettes because the harsher smoke discourages deep inhalation. However, pipes and cigars increase the risk of cancer of the lips, mouth, and throat.

Smoke can be inhaled directly by the smoker **(mainstream smoke),** or it can enter the atmosphere from the lighted end of the cigarette and be inhaled by others in the vicinity **(sidestream smoke).** Sidestream smoke contains greater concentrations of toxic and carcinogenic compounds than mainstream smoke. Diseases and conditions associated with smoking include cancer, cardiovascular and pulmonary problems, and perinatal effects. Smoking bans are being adopted with the intent to reduce the discomfort and health hazards among nonsmokers. A *Healthy People 2000* public health objective is to enact comprehensive clean indoor air laws in all 50 states.

Nicotine can also be taken in the form of chewing tobacco, or snuff. Marketed as "smokeless tobacco," a wad is put in the mouth and the nicotine is absorbed sublingually. Higher doses of nicotine are delivered in the smokeless forms because the nicotine is not destroyed by heat. Nevertheless, this form is less addictive because nicotine enters the bloodstream less directly.

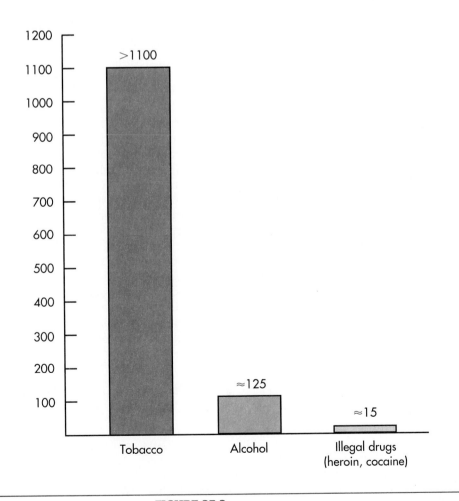

FIGURE 37-3
Drug-related deaths per day.

Marijuana

Marijuana (cannabis sativa or cannabis indica) is the most widely used illicit drug in the United States. Estimates of regular users range from 20 to 30 million Americans, and as many as 60% of those between the ages of 18 and 25 years have tried marijuana at some time (Doweiko, 1990).

In the United States, marijuana was a popular plant grown for its fiber (hemp), seed (popular birdseed), oil, and medicinal as well as psychoactive properties. During World War II the hemp fiber was so valuable that farmers were required to grow marijuana to ensure a supply. Tincture of cannabis was listed in the *U.S. Pharmacopoeia* through 1941 for such ailments as migraines, spasticity, and dysmenorrhea and in the treatment of heroin or cocaine addiction.

Compared with the other psychoactive drugs, marijuana has little toxicity and is one of the safest therapeutic agents known (Randall, 1988). However, because of its illegal status, there is no quality control and a user may consume contaminated marijuana. Users enjoy a mild euphoria, a relaxed feeling, and an intensity of sensory perceptions. Side effects include dry and reddened eyes, increased appetite, dry mouth, drowsiness, and mild tachycardia. Adverse reactions include anxiety, disorientation, and paranoia.

The greatest physical concern for chronic users is possible damage to the respiratory tract. Tolerance can develop as well as physical dependence; however, the withdrawal symptoms are quite benign. Addiction can occur for some chronic users and is difficult to treat because the progression tends to be quite subtle.

In 1970 marijuana was placed in the Schedule I category of drugs by the passage of the Controlled Substances Act and has not been available for medicinal use. The only legal access to this medicine has been through the U.S. Food and Drug Administration's (FDA's) Investigational New Drug Program. In 1992 this program was closed and there are only eight remaining legal patients. In response to this complete prohibition, some health care organizations are supporting access to this medication, including the Virginia Nurses Association (resolution passed in 1994, "Legalizing Marijuana for Medical Purposes") and the National Nurses Society on Addictions (*Access to Therapeutic Cannabis,* 1995).

Hallucinogens

Also called *psychedelics* (mind vision), hallucinogens are capable of producing hallucinations. Many of these drugs have been used for centuries in religious ceremonies and healing rituals and used by many cultures to produce euphoria and as aphrodisiacs (Doweiko, 1990). For these drugs, the user's mood, basic emotional makeup, and expectations (set) along with the immediate surroundings (setting) will have a great influence on the mental effects experienced by the user.

The physical effects are more constant and produce CNS stimulation.

The two broad chemical families of hallucinogens are the indole hallucinogens and the phenylethylamines. The indoles are related to hormones (serotonin) made in the brain by the pineal gland and include such drugs as lysergic acid diethylamide (LSD), psilocybin mushrooms, and morning glory seeds. The phenylethylamines, which closely resemble adrenalin and amphetamines, include peyote and mescaline and MDMA (Ecstasy). Phencyclidine (PCP) is in a class by itself. LSD and PCP will be discussed.

Lysergic Acid Diethylamide

LSD is the most well-known drug in the hallucinogen category. It is one of the most potent drugs known: as little as 25 μg in a single dose will last 10 to 12 hours. It is administered orally in small tablets, in gelatin chips ("window panes"), or on pieces of paper soaked with the drug or stamped with ink containing LSD.

The desired effects include euphoria, a heightened sense of awareness, distorted perceptions, and synesthesia (a mixing of senses, i.e., sounds appearing as visual images). Adverse reactions to LSD include depersonalization, hypertension, panic, and psychosis. Another adverse reaction may be a flashback, or a recurrence of the "trip" weeks or months after the LSD has been ingested. Flashbacks can be frightening, especially because of their unpredictability, but will decrease in frequency over time.

Phencyclidine

PCP is a potent anesthetic and analgesic with CNS depressant, stimulant, and hallucinogenic properties. A high incidence of PCP use was seen in the early 1980s and was focused primarily in the metropolitan areas of Los Angeles, Washington, D.C., and New York City (Brust, 1993). PCP comes in pill or powder form and has often been sold as mescaline, psilocybin, THC, or other drugs. "Angel dust" is PCP sprinkled on a marijuana joint.

The mental effects vary but often include a feeling of disconnection from the body and reality, apathy, disorganized thinking, a drunklike state, and distortions of time and space perception. Adverse reactions include combative behavior, inability to talk, a rigid robotic attitude, confusion, paranoid thinking, catatonia, coma, and convulsions. Unlike the other hallucinogens, phencyclidine can be addicting.

Inhalants

The inhalants do not fit neatly into other categories but include gases and solvents. The three main types of inhalants are organic solvents, volatile nitrites, and nitrous oxide. These substances are inhaled ("huffed") from bottles, aerosol cans, or soaked cloth or put into bags or balloons to increase the concentration of the inhaled fumes and decrease the inhalation of other substances in the vapor (i.e., paint particles).

Organic solvents include rubber cement, model airplane glue, paint thinner, and aerosol products such as spray paint, deodorant, and hair spray. The majority of users are between the ages of 10 and 20 years. These drugs are inexpensive and easy to obtain for that age group.

The effects are similar to alcohol but have a rapid onset and last a short time. The user initially feels stimulated as the inhibitions are depressed; then a drunklike state is experienced and possibly hallucinations. Users may also experience headache, tinnitus, diplopia, abdominal pain, nausea, or vomiting. "Sudden sniffing death" may occur, which appears to be related to acute cardiac dysrhythmia (Dinwiddie, 1994).

Amyl nitrite is the most common of the *volatile nitrites* and is most often used by urban male homosexuals. It is frequently used during sexual activity to intensify the experience and prolong orgasm. This yellow liquid is packaged in cloth-covered glass capsules that have to be popped (hence the common name of "poppers") to release the drug for inhalation.

Often referred to as laughing gas, *nitrous oxide* is widely used in dentistry and minor surgery as a tranquilizer to sedate and create an analgesic effect by changing the patient's mood and interpretation of pain. Nitrous oxide is also found in whipping cream aerosol cans ("whippets") and is released by spraying the can upside down. Dangers with administration increase when inhaling directly from pressurized tanks because the gas is very cold and can cause frostbite to the nose, lips, and vocal cords. Also, if nitrous oxide is not mixed with oxygen, the user may die from asphyxiation (Espeland, 1993).

PRIMARY PREVENTION

Substance abuse is clearly linked to health promotion and disease prevention. Primary prevention for ATOD problems includes (1) the promotion of healthy lifestyles and resiliency factors and (2) education about drugs and guidelines for use. Community health nurses are ideally prepared to use health promotion strategies such as public education about drugs and discussion of healthy alternatives to indiscriminate, careless, and often dangerous drug use practices.

Promotion of Healthy Life-styles and Resiliency Factors

Assisting clients to achieve optimal health includes identifying interventions other than or in addition to the use of drugs whenever possible. Teaching assertiveness skills and decision-making skills helps clients to increase their responsibility for their health and increase their awareness of various options available.

Nagging health problems such as difficulty sleeping, muscle tension, lack of energy, and mood swings are common reasons people turn to medications, especially the psychoactive drugs. The nurse can help clients understand that the medications are only serving to mask these problems rather than solving them. Stress reduction and relaxation techniques along with a balanced life-style can address these problems more directly (Dodge, 1991; Rassool and Winnington, 1993).

Often stress is created by lack of balance in a person's life-style. Lack of sleep, improper diet, and lack of exercise contribute to many health complaints. Assisting clients to balance their rest, nutrition, and exercise on a daily basis can greatly reduce these complaints. The nurse can be resourceful in providing this information to various groups, assisting the development of community recreational resources, or facilitating groups on stress reduction, relaxation, or exercise. Frequently recreational activities are centered around the use of drugs. Nurses can help persons increase their awareness of drug-free community activities and recreational or hobby classes that address this area.

Lack of educational opportunities, job training, or both can contribute to socioeconomical stress and poor self-esteem, which can lead to drug use to escape the situation. Again the community health nurse can assist clients with identifying community resources and problem solving to address these basic needs rather than avoid them.

In addition to decreasing risk factors associated with ATOD problems, emphasis is placed on increasing protective or resiliency factors. It has been found that children from high-risk environments who survive successfully have more resiliency factors than those who do not survive (Kumpfer and Hopkins, 1993). Prevention guidelines to teach parents and teachers how to increase resiliency in youth include the following strategies: helping them to develop an increased sense of responsibility for their own success; helping them to identify their talents; motivating them to dedicate their lives to helping society rather than feeling their only purpose in life is to be consumers; providing realistic appraisals and feedback; stressing multicultural competence; encouraging and valuing education and skills training; and increasing cooperative solutions to problems rather than competitive or aggressive solutions.

The National Nurses Society on Addictions (NNSA), through a grant by the U.S. Center for Substance Abuse Prevention (CSAP), offers primary prevention workshops for nurses and has an independent-study program available for purchase (Jack and Snow, 1994). The workshops and independent study highlight community involvement and cultural diversity issues. See the box on p. 720 for a list of community-based activities in which the community health nurse may get involved.

Drug Education

ATOD problems are much broader than just abuse of psychoactive drugs. Today more than 450,000 different drugs and drug combinations are available. It has been estimated that prescription drugs are involved in almost 60% of all drug-related emergency room visits

Community-based Activities Aimed at ATOD Problem Prevention

Increased involvement and pride in school activities
Student assistant programs
Students Against Drunk Driving (SADD)
Parent awareness and action groups (e.g., MADD)
Increased availability of recreation facilities
Parental commitment to nondrinking parties
Active involvement of religious institutions in conveying nonuse messages and providing activities associated with nonuse
Curtailment of media messages that glamorize drug and alcohol use
Support and reinforcement for antidrug peer pressure
General health screenings, including ATOD use
Collaboration among community leaders to solve problems related to crime, housing, jobs, and access to health care

and 70% of all drug-related deaths. Approximately 25% of elderly hospital admissions result from problems related to noncompliance and drug reactions (Larrat et al., 1990).

Nurses are experts in medication administration and understand the potential dangers of indiscriminant drug use and the inherent inability of drugs to "cure" all problems. The community health nurse can have a powerful impact on the health of clients by destroying the myth of a good drug versus a bad drug. This means (1) teaching clients that no drug is completely safe and that any drug can be abused and (2) helping persons learn how to make informed decisions about their drug use to minimize the potential harm.

We live in a world of ever-growing drug technology, and yet the public receives little information about how to safely use this technology. Harm reduction as a goal recognizes the reality that people consume drugs, and information about the use of drugs and risks involved is necessary for persons to make responsible decisions about their drug use. An effective way to begin drug education on an individual basis is by reviewing the client's prescription medications. Because a physician has prescribed the medication, clients often presume there is little risk involved. Does the client know the name of the medication and how and where it works in the body? Does the client know the importance of taking the correct dose to get the greatest benefit yet limit possible side effects?

Is the client aware of any untoward interactions this drug may have with other drugs being used or food? A common occurrence with drug users is the use of drugs from different categories used together or at different times to regulate how they feel, known as **polysubstance use or abuse.** For example, a person may drink alcohol when snorting cocaine to "take the edge off"; or a person may use barbiturates to assist with sleep after using a stimulant. Polysubstance use can cause various drug interactions that can have additive, synergistic, or antagonistic effects. Indiscriminant polysubstance abuse may lead to serious physiological consequences and can be complicated for the health care professional to assess and treat.

People need to know why they are using a medication. If it is a long-term therapy, will a tolerance develop and the safe dose no longer be effective? Could physical dependence develop, making it difficult or unsafe to abruptly discontinue the use? Some medications are necessary for people to achieve optimal health, such as insulin for a person with diabetes. Some medications are used only to mask the symptoms of an underlying problem that is not being addressed, such as pain medications for headaches induced by stress.

People need to know what questions to ask regarding their personal drug use and should be encouraged to seek the answers to these questions before using any drug. Encouraging clients to ask questions regarding their drug use can increase their responsibility for personal health as well as increase their awareness that drugs will alter their body chemistry. The box below lists seven questions that can assist clients in obtaining the essential information necessary to decrease the possible harm from unsafe medication consumption.

The community health nurse can assist in identifying the various references and community resources available to provide the necessary information. The nurse can also assist in clarifying the information. Griffiths' *Complete Guide to Prescription and Nonprescription Drugs* (1995) offers information regarding drug interactions among medications and other drugs (including alcohol, tobacco, marijuana, and cocaine) and other substances (food and beverages) and serves as an excellent guide for the nurse as well as for the client's personal use.

As clients learn to ask questions about their prescription medications, the nurse can encourage them to ask the same questions regarding self-administration of OTC and recreational drugs. This does not

Drug Consumer Safety Guidelines

1. Determine the chemical being taken.
2. Determine how and where the drug works in the body.
3. Determine the correct dosage.
4. Determine whether there will be drug interactions.
5. Determine if there are allergic reactions.
6. Determine if there will be drug tolerance.
7. Determine if the drug will produce physical dependence.*

From Miller M: *Drug consumer safety rules*, Mosier, Ore, 1994, Mothers Against Misuse and Abuse.
*CAUTION: Approximately 10% of the population may suffer from the disease of addiction. For those persons, responsible use of psychoactive drugs is limited secondary to their disease. Always notify your physician of your addiction if use of psychoactive medicines is being considered in your treatment.

mean that nurses should encourage other drug use but rather that the potential harm from self-medication can be reduced if clients have the necessary information to make more informed decisions.

As parents learn to seek information regarding their use of medications, they begin to act as role models for their children. It can be quite confusing for children and adolescents to be told to "just say no" to drugs, yet at the same time watch their parents or drug advertisements try to "quick fix" every health complaint with a medication.

The simple "just say no" approach does not help young people for several reasons. First, children are naturally curious and drug experimentation is often a part of normal development (Shedler and Block, 1990). Second, children from dysfunctional homes often use drugs to obtain attention or to escape an intolerable environment. And finally, the "just say no" approach does not address the powerful influence of peer pressure (Donaldson et al., 1994).

Drug education is moving into the school curriculum, with Project DARE (Drug Abuse Resistance Education) the most widely used school-based drug-use prevention program in the United States. This program uses law enforcement officers to teach the material, but recent studies find it less effective than other interactive prevention programs (Ennett et al., 1994).

Basic ATOD prevention programs for young people should combine efforts to increase resiliency factors with drug education. Community health nurses can serve as educators or as advisors to the school systems or community groups to ensure all of these areas are addressed. Role-playing can be an effective method of teaching many of these skills.

SECONDARY PREVENTION

To identify substance abuse and plan appropriate interventions, community health nurses must assess each client individually. When drug abuse, dependence, or addiction is identified, nurses must assist clients to understand the connection between their drug use patterns and the negative consequences on their health, their families, and the community.

Illicit drug users are reluctant to seek health care for fear of the consequences. By working within the community, community health nurses can reach those who need health care rather than wait for individuals to seek care. Developing a therapeutic relationship can increase the effectiveness of resources and interventions. Substance abusers will be more honest about their drug use patterns if the nurse can offer assistance rather than judgment.

Assessing for Substance Abuse Problems

Assessing for substance abuse problems should be included in health assessments. An assessment of self-medication practices as well as recreational drug use should be done at the time of the medication history.

This puts all relevant drug use history together and aids in the assessment of drug use patterns. When working with a client over time, periodic assessment of drug use patterns will alert the nurse to any changes requiring intervention.

After obtaining a medication history, follow-up questions will help to determine if any problems exist. For prescription drug use, is the client following the directions correctly? Be especially inquisitive about any prescribed psychoactive drug use: How long has the client been taking the drug? Has the client increased the dosage or frequency above the prescription?

When assessing self-medication and recreational or social drug use patterns, the reason for use should be elicited. Some underlying health problems (i.e., pain, stress, weight, or insomnia) may be alleviated by non-pharmaceutical interventions. Amount, frequency, duration of use, and route of administration of each drug (the 4 H's: how much, how often, how long, and how taken) must be explored.

Assess for the occurrence of blackouts. A **blackout** is an interval of temporary memory loss during which an alcohol-intoxicated person remains conscious and active and may even appear sober but later has no recollection of where he or she was and what has been done or said. Blackouts are considered a "red flag" for alcoholism.

To establish the presence of a substance abuse problem, the nurse must determine if the drug use is causing any negative health consequences or problems with relationships, employment, finances, or the legal system. The box below provides examples of questions

Assessment Questions to Determine Socioeconomical Problems Secondary to Substance Abuse

1. Do your spouse, parents, or friends worry or complain about your drinking or using drugs?
2. Has a family member gone for help about your drinking or using drugs?
3. Have you neglected family obligations secondary to drinking or using drugs?
4. Have you missed work because of your drinking or using drugs?
5. Does your boss complain about your drinking or using drugs?
6. Do you drink or use drugs before or during work?
7. Have you ever been fired or quit secondary to drinking or using drugs?
8. Have you ever been charged with driving under the influence (DUI) or drunk in public (DIP)?
9. Have you ever had any other legal problems related to drinking and using drugs, such as assault and battery, breaking and entering, or theft?
10. Have you had any accidents while intoxicated, such as falls, burns, or motor vehicle accidents?
11. Have you spent your money on alcohol or other drugs instead of paying your bills (telephone, electricity, rent, etc.)?

to ask clients to determine the presence of socio-economical problems that are often secondary to substance abuse.

If a pattern of chronic, regular, and frequent use of a drug is revealed, the nurse must assess for a history of withdrawal symptoms to determine if there is physical dependence on the drug. A progression in drug use patterns and related problems will alert the nurse to the possibility of addiction.

Denial is a primary symptom of addiction. Methods of denial include lying about use, minimizing use patterns, blaming or rationalizing, intellectualizing, changing the subject, using anger or humor, and "going with the flow" (agreeing there is a problem, stating behavior will change, but not demonstrating any behavior changes). Suspect a problem if the client becomes defensive or exhibits other behavior indicating denial when asked about alcohol or other drug use.

Drug Testing

During the 1980s preemployment or random drug testing gained popularity. Drug testing can be done by examining a person's urine, blood, saliva, breath (alcohol), or hair. The limitations of drug testing must be understood to yield any benefits.

When is drug testing appropriate? Drug testing secondary to documented impairment may be helpful in substantiating the cause of the impairment, thus being used as a backup rather than the primary screening method. Another time it is useful is for recovering addicts. Part of their treatment is to abstain from psychoactive drug use; therefore a urine test yielding positive results for a drug indicates a relapse.

The most common method of drug screening is urine testing. Urine testing only indicates past use of certain drugs, not intoxication. Thus persons can be identified as having used a certain drug in the recent past, but the degree of intoxication and extent of performance impairment cannot be determined with urine testing. Also, most drug-related problems in the workplace are due to alcohol, and alcohol is not always included in a urine drug screen.

Blood, breath, and saliva drug tests have the benefit of indicating current use and amount. Any of these tests can be helpful to determine alcohol intoxication, and they often are used to substantiate suspected impairment. A serum drug screen can be very useful when overdose is suspected to determine the specific drug ingested. The testing of hair is gaining attention because the results can provide a long history of drug use patterns.

Employee assistance programs (EAPs) are gaining popularity among many work settings, with at least 30% of U.S. workers having access to an EAP. Roughly 86% of work sites with 5000 or more employees have EAPs (Callery, 1994). These programs are set up to identify health problems among employees and offer counseling or referral to other health care providers as necessary. Early identification of and intervention for substance abuse problems are often addressed through EAPs. These programs also offer services to their employees to reduce stress and provide health care or counseling so that they may prevent substance abuse problems from developing. Nurses frequently develop and run these programs.

High-Risk Groups

Identifying high-risk groups helps the community health nurse to design programs to meet their specific needs and to help mobilize community resources to meet these needs most effectively.

Pregnant Women

During pregnancy the fetus is at risk for negative effects from most drugs. Thus the use of any drug during pregnancy should be discouraged unless medically necessary. Fetal alcohol syndrome (FAS) has been identified as the third leading cause of birth defects and the leading cause of mental retardation in the United States with a 1992 estimate of 5.2 cases per 10,000 live births (Cordero et al., 1994; Peterson and Lowe, 1992). Although it appears an epidemic of drug use (other than alcohol) occurred among pregnant women during the 1980s, with a leveling off in 1988 through 1990, both the size and severity of the epidemic have been overstated. A review of the data from the National Hospital Discharge Survey found that about half (53%) of the discharged infants of drug-using parturient women were drug-affected newborns (Dicker and Leighton, 1994).

Despite the increased focus in the health care system on interventions for drug abuse, many pregnant women with drug problems do not receive the help they need. Reasons for not receiving treatment may include ignorance, poverty, lack of concern for the fetus, lack of available services, and fear of the consequences. The fear of criminal prosecution may push addicted women further away from the health care system, cause them to conceal their drug use from medical providers, and cause them to deliver their babies in out-of-hospital settings, thus further jeopardizing the pregnancy outcome (Chavkin and Kandall, 1990; Fiesta, 1991; Hutchings, 1993; Kain et al., 1993).

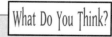

What Do You Think?

Pregnant women who are using illicit drugs should be reported to child welfare services because of the potential harm to the fetus.

Adolescents

Studies have shown that the younger a person is when beginning intensive experimentation with drugs, the more likely dependence will develop.

Heavy drug use during adolescence can interfere with normal development.

Recent reports from annual high school drug surveys monitor the national trends among youth. By the eighth grade, 67% have tried alcohol, 45% smoked cigarettes, more than 12% tried marijuana, and less than 3% tried cocaine. By twelfth grade, about 87% have used alcohol, 62% smoked cigarettes, 57% used marijuana, and 6% tried cocaine (National Institute on Drug Abuse, 1994). These figures are probably low in that they do not include high school dropouts.

The greatest single variable influencing substance use among adolescents is peer pressure. Decreased emphasis on religion, low value on achievement, poor school performance, delinquency, and a high value on risk taking are other factors that are linked with adolescent substance abuse. Research suggests that successful social influence–based prevention programs may be driven by their ability to foster social norms that reduce an adolescent's social motivation to begin using ATOD (Donaldson et al., 1994).

Elderly Persons

Elderly persons (65 years of age and older) represent 12% of the U.S. population and are the fastest growing segment of U.S. society. They consume approximately 25% to 30% of all prescribed drugs, and between 35% and 40% of OTC drugs are purchased by them (McMahon, 1993). Twenty-five percent of the elderly population consume psychoactive drugs. Factors such as slowed metabolical turnover of drugs, age-related organ changes, enhanced drug sensitivities, a tendency to use drugs over long periods of time, and a more frequent use of multiple drugs all contribute to greater negative consequences from drug use among the elderly population.

The increased use of prescription drugs and alcohol by elderly persons may be related to coping problems. Problems of relocation, possible loss of independence, retirement, illness, death of friends, and lower levels of achievement contribute to feelings of sadness, boredom, anxiety, and loneliness.

Two types of elderly persons with alcoholism have been identified: (1) those who have a chronic history of alcohol abuse and (2) those whose excessive drinking is a reaction to the stresses of aging. Often alcohol abuse is not identified because its effects on cognitive abilities may mimic changes associated with normal aging or degenerative brain disease. Also, depression may simply be attributed to the more frequent losses rather than the depressant effects of alcohol, and the elderly person may subsequently receive medical treatment for depression rather than alcoholism.

IV Drug Users

In addition to the problem of addiction, intravenous (IV) drug users are at risk for other health complications. IV administration of drugs always carries a greater risk of overdose because the drug goes directly into the bloodstream. With illicit drugs the danger is increased because the exact dosage is unknown. In addition, the drug may be contaminated with other chemicals that can cause negative consequences. Often IV drug users make their own solution for IV administration and any particles present can result in complications from emboli.

The sharing of needles has been a common practice among addicts. The spread of human immunodeficiency virus (HIV) through needle sharing has become a great public health risk. Hepatitis and other blood-borne diseases can also be transmitted through contaminated needles. Infections and abscesses may develop secondary to dirty needles or poor administration techniques.

IV drug users represent the most rapidly growing source of new AIDS cases and are the greatest risk for

 Research Brief

Watters JK, Estilo MJ, Clarke GL, Lorvick J: Syringe and needle exchange as HIV/AIDS prevention for injection drug users, JAMA 271(2):115-120, 1994.

A study was conducted to evaluate an all-volunteer syringe exchange program in San Francisco. The data were collected from syringe exchange program records, semiannual surveys administered over a 5.5-year period (December 1986 to June 1992), and interviews with injection drug users recruited in two 21-day drug detoxification clinics and three street settings.

The main outcome measures were use of the syringe exchange program and self-reported data regarding sources of syringes, frequency of injection, initiation into drug injection, and frequency of syringe sharing.

Results: In spring 1992, 45% reported "usually" obtaining injection equipment from the syringe exchange and 61% reported using the program within the past year. During the 5.5 years the median reported frequency of injection declined from 1.9 injections per day to 0.7 injection per day, the mean age increased from 36 to 42 years, and the percentage of new initiates into injection drug use decreased from 3% to 1%. Protective factors from syringe sharing were use of the syringe exchange, having received HIV testing and counseling, condom use, older age, and African-American race. Injection of cocaine was a predictor of syringe sharing. The strength of association between use of the syringe exchange program and not sharing syringes was greatest in injection drug users younger than the median age of 40 years.

Conclusions: The syringe exchange program was rapidly adopted by injection drug users. Health interventions associated with not sharing needles included use of the syringe exchange program and voluntary, confidential HIV testing and counseling. The data did not support the hypothesis that a syringe exchange program would stimulate increased drug abuse in terms of frequency of injection or recruitment of new or younger users.

spread of the virus in the heterosexual community. Primarily because of this trend, emphasis is being placed on reducing the transmission of this disease through contaminated needles. Abstinence is ideal but unrealistic for many addicts. Using the harm reduction model, the nurse should provide education on use of bleach to clean needles between use and needle exchange programs to decrease the spread of the virus. Studies indicate that needle exchange programs have not resulted in an increase in IV drug abuse but have, in fact, increased the number of people entering treatment programs (Schwartz, 1993).

Codependency and Family Involvement

Drug addiction is often referred to as a family disease, with one in four Americans experiencing family problems related to alcohol abuse. People in a close relationship with the addict often develop unhealthy coping mechanisms to continue the relationship. This behavior is known as **codependency,** a stress-induced preoccupation with the addicted person's life, leading to extreme dependence and excessive concern with the addict (Talashek et al., 1994).

Strict rules typically develop in a codependent family to maintain the relationships: don't talk, don't feel, don't trust, don't lose control, and don't seek help from outside the family. Codependents try to meet the addict's needs at the expense of their own. Codependency may underlie many of the medical complaints and emotional stress seen by health care providers such as ulcers, skin disorders, migraine headaches, chronic colds, and backaches.

When the addicted person refuses to admit the problem, the family continues to adapt to emotionally survive the stress of the addict's irrational, inconsistent, and unpredictable behavior. Members of the family will consequently develop various roles that tend to be gross exaggerations of normal family roles. Members cling irrationally to these roles, even when they are no longer functional.

One of the most significant roles a family member may assume is that of an enabler. **Enabling** is the act of shielding or preventing the addict from experiencing the consequences of the addiction. As a result the addict does not always understand the cost of the addiction and thus is "enabled" to continue to use.

Although codependency and enabling are closely related, a person does not have to be codependent to enable. Anyone can be an enabler: a police officer, a boss or coworker, and even a drug treatment counselor. Nurses who do not address the negative health consequences of the drug use with the addicted person are enablers.

The community health nurse can assist families to recognize the problem of addiction and help them confront the addicted member in a caring manner. Whether or not the addicted family member is agreeable to treatment, the family members should be given some guidance about the literature and services that are available to help them cope more effectively. The community health nurse can help identify treatment options, counseling assistance, financial assistance, support services, and (if necessary) legal services for the family members. Children of ATOD abusers or addicts are themselves at a greater risk for developing addiction and must be targeted for primary prevention.

TERTIARY PREVENTION

The community health nurse is in a pivotal position to help the addict and the addict's family. The nurse's knowledge of community resources and how to mobilize them can significantly influence the quality of care clients will receive.

Many persons with alcoholism and drug addiction become lost in the health care system. If satisfactory care is not provided in one agency or the waiting list is months long, the person may give up rather than seek alternative sources of care. The community health nurse who knows the client's history, environment, and support systems and who knows the local treatment programs can offer guidance to the most effective treatment modality. Brief interventions by health care professionals who are not treatment experts have been found to be quite effective in helping ATOD abusers and addicts reduce their consumption or follow through with treatment referrals (Bien et al., 1993; Minicucci, 1994). The following box describes six elements commonly included in brief interventions using the acronym FRAMES.

After the client has received treatment, the community health nurse can coordinate aftercare referrals and followup on the client's progress. The nurse can provide additional support in the home as the client and family adjust to changing roles and the stress involved with such changes. The community health nurse can support addicted persons who have experienced relapse by reminding them that relapses may well occur, yet encouraging them and their families to continue to work toward recovery and an improved quality of life.

 Brief Interventions Using the FRAMES Acronym

Feedback: Provide the client direct feedback about the potential or actual personal risk or impairment related to drug use.
Responsibility: Emphasize personal responsibility for change.
Advice: Provide clear advice to change risky behavior.
Menu: Provide a menu of options or choices for changing behavior.
Empathy: Provide a warm, reflective, empathetic, and understanding approach.
Self-efficacy: Provide encouragement and belief in the client's ability to change.

From Bien TH, Miller WR, Tonigan JS: *Addictions* 88:315-336, 1993.

Detoxification

Detoxification refers to the process of clearing one or more drugs from the person's body and managing the withdrawal symptoms. Depending on the particular drug and the degree of dependence, the time period may range from a few days to several weeks. Because withdrawal symptoms vary (depending on the drug used) and range from uncomfortable to life threatening, the setting for and management of **withdrawal** depend on the drug used.

Drugs such as marijuana, stimulants, and opiates may produce withdrawal symptoms that are uncomfortable but not life threatening. Detoxification from these drugs does not require direct medical supervision, but medical management of the withdrawal symptoms increases the comfort level. For detoxification from cigarettes, nicotine supplements are available in patches, gum, and nasal sprays.

On the other hand, drugs such as alcohol, benzodiazepines, and barbiturates may produce life-threatening withdrawal symptoms. These clients should be under close medical supervision during detoxification and should receive medical management of the withdrawal symptoms to ensure a safe withdrawal. For those persons who develop delirium tremens, 15% may not survive despite medical management; therefore close medical management should be initiated as the blood alcohol level begins to fall.

A general rule in detoxification management is to wean the person off the drug by gradually reducing the dosage and frequency of administration. Thus a person with chronic alcoholism could be safely detoxified by a gradual reduction in alcohol consumption. In practice, however, the switch to another drug, usually a benzodiazepine, often offers a safer withdrawal from alcohol as well as an abrupt end to the intoxication from the drug of choice. For example, chlordiazepam (Librium) is commonly used for alcohol detoxification. Home detoxification is being initiated throughout the United States, and the monitoring of the client's status can be effectively managed by the community health nurse.

Did You Know?

Because of cost-containment efforts, more primary care providers and drug treatment programs are initiating outpatient or home detoxification for persons requiring medical detoxification for alcohol withdrawal. Community health nurses can provide the necessary monitoring and evaluation of the client's health status in the home environment to reduce the risk of medical complications related to alcohol withdrawal as well as provide encouragement and support for the client to complete the detoxification.

Addiction Treatment

Addiction "treatment" differs from the management of negative health consequences of chronic drug abuse, overdose, and withdrawal. **Addiction treatment** focuses on the addiction process: helping clients recognize the addiction as a chronic disease and assisting them to make life-style changes to halt the progression of that disease process. According to the disease theory, addicts are not responsible for the symptoms of their disease; they are, however, responsible for treating their disease. On any given day, more than 800,000 persons receive addiction treatment in specialized programs. In 1991 most clients (82%) were outpatients (Institute for Health Policy, Brandeis University, 1993).

Most treatment facilities are multidisciplinary because the intervention strategies require a wide range of approaches and most programs involve interactions among the addict, family, culture, and community. Included in the strategies are medical management, education, counseling, vocational rehabilitation, stress management, and support services. In general, there are two basic approaches to addiction treatment: (1) medical management or controlled use and (2) total abstinence. The key to effective treatment is to match individual clients with the interventions most appropriate for them. Understanding the stages of change (see box on p. 726) and recognizing which stage a client is in are important factors in determining which interventions and programs may be most helpful to the client (Prochaska et al., 1992).

Controlled Use and Medical Management

For those addicted individuals unwilling or unable to completely abstain from psychoactive drugs, other drugs have been used to assist them in abstaining from their drug of choice. Up to the early 1900s U.S. physicians sometimes prescribed morphine for alcoholic persons because of the extensive physical damage or aggressive behavior caused by the alcohol. The person with alcoholism would instead become addicted to morphine but would not suffer the negative physical or behavioral consequences (Brecher, 1972).

A similar philosophy is applied today with the methadone maintenance program for treatment of heroin addiction. Methadone, when administered in moderate or high daily doses, produces a cross-tolerance to other narcotics, thereby blocking their effects and decreasing the craving for heroin. The advantages of methadone are that it is long acting, effective orally, and inexpensive and has few known side effects.

The oral use of methadone offers a solution to the danger of the spread of AIDS and other blood-borne infections that commonly occur among needle-sharing addicts. More recently, trends indicate that many persons with IV heroin addiction are also "shooting" (taking intravenously) cocaine, and since methadone does not affect the cocaine cravings, a heroin-addicted individual on a methadone maintenance program

Stages of Change

PRECONTEMPLATION

At this stage the individual has no intention to change in the foreseeable future. The person is often unaware of any problem. Resistance to recognizing or modifying a problem is the hallmark of precontemplation.

CONTEMPLATION

At this stage the individual is aware that a problem exists and is seriously thinking about overcoming it but has not yet made a commitment to take action. In this stage the nurse can encourage the individual to weigh the pros and cons of the problem and the solution to the problem.

PREPARATION

Preparation was originally referred to as decision making. At this stage the individual is prepared for action and may make some reduction in the problem behavior but has not yet taken effective action (i.e., cuts down amount of smoking but does not abstain).

ACTION

At this stage the individual modifies his or her behavior, experiences, or environment to overcome the problem. The action requires considerable time and energy. Modification of the target behavior to an acceptable criterion and significant overt efforts to change are the hallmarks of action.

MAINTENANCE

In this stage the individual works to prevent relapse and consolidate the gains attained during action. Stabilizing behavior change and avoiding relapse are the hallmarks of maintenance.

From Prochaska JO, DiClemente CC, Norcross JC: Am Psychologist 47(9):1102-1114, 1992.

---

may still continue with IV drug use. Although not recognized as a cure for heroin (or other opiate) addiction, methadone maintenance reduces deviant behavior and introduces addicted persons to the health care system. This may ultimately lead to total abstinence.

For some persons, medical treatment is used to negate the high from their drug of choice or deter use by negative interactions. Naltrexone (Trexan) can be used with opiate addiction. It is a pure opiate antagonist that blocks the effects of all opium-derived compounds. The usual dose is 50 mg orally each morning. This can help the client by preventing the psychological and physical reinforcements of opiates if a person should slip and use an opiate. More recently, Naltrexone also has been found to be effective in blocking the pleasure produced by alcohol (Volpicelli et al., 1995).

Disulfiram (Antabuse) may be prescribed for the recovering alcoholic as a deterrent to drinking. Ingesting alcohol while disulfiram is in the body produces negative health effects including blurred vision, nausea, vertigo, anxiety, and cardiovascular effects, such as hypotension, palpitations, tachycardia, and flushing of the face and neck. The reaction is believed to be caused by disulfiram's inhibition of acetaldehyde dehydrogenase—the enzyme necessary for the breakdown of ac-

etaldehyde, a product of the metabolism of alcohol.

Clients taking disulfiram need to be educated about the risks involved and the hidden sources of alcohol such as in other medicines, recipes using sherry or other alcohol, flavorings, and mouthwashes. Disulfiram treatment should be considered as an adjunct to a recovery program on a limited basis for persons who believe it will prevent them from a relapse during their initial recovery period.

Total Abstinence

Total **abstinence** is the most recommended treatment for drug addiction. Those clients who are addicted to a particular drug (e.g., cocaine) are advised to abstain from the use of all psychoactive substances. The use of another drug may simply reinforce the craving for the original drug and result in relapse. More commonly, the addiction merely transfers to the replacement substance.

Treatment may be on an inpatient or outpatient basis. In general, the more advanced the disease is, the greater the need for inpatient treatment. Inpatient treatment programs usually last 28 days, although they may range from less than 1 week to 90 days. Once a person has completed detoxification, the programs use counseling and group interaction to help him or her stay clean long enough for the body chemistry to rebalance. This is often a difficult time for persons recovering from addictions because they may experience mood swings and difficulty sleeping and dealing with emotions.

The educational segment of the program focuses on providing information about the disease concept and how drugs affect a person physically and psychologically. Clients are informed of the various life-style changes that they must make and learn about tools to assist them in making these changes. Discharge planning continues throughout treatment as clients build the support systems that they will need when they leave the controlled environment of a treatment center and face pressures and temptations (triggers) that may lead to relapse.

Halfway houses have been developed to ease the person recovering from an addiction back into society. These facilities provide continued support and counseling in a structured environment for persons needing long-term assistance in adjusting to a drug-free life-style. The residents are expected to secure employment and take responsibility in managing their financial obligations.

Outpatient programs are similar in the education and counseling offered, but they allow the clients to live at home and continue to work while undergoing treatment. This method is very effective for persons in the earlier stages of addiction who feel confident that they can abstain from drug use and have established a strong support network.

Most programs have incorporated family counseling and education. In addition, specific programs are being developed to address the needs of various populations such as adolescents, women during pregnancy, specific ethnic groups, and health care professionals.

Recovery from addiction involves a lifetime commitment and may include periods of relapse. The addicted person must realize that modern medicine has not found a cure for addiction; therefore returning to drug use may ultimately reactivate the disease process.

Smoking Cessation Programs

The two basic types of smoking cessation methods are self-help strategies and assisted strategies. Most successful quitters (90%) have used the self-help techniques, which include a gradual tapering or stopping abruptly (cold turkey), how-to literature, or OTC drugs. Assisted strategies include smoking cessation clinics, hypnosis, acupuncture, nicotine patches, and other programs involving health care professionals (Rienzo, 1993; Sees, 1990). The most effective way to get people to stop smoking and prevent relapse involves multiple interventions and continuous reinforcement.

Many resources are available on smoking cessation programs and support groups (see box below). Helping the client develop a plan to stop smoking can increase the likelihood of success. *Nursing Care of the Patient Who Smokes* (Rienzo, 1993) provides further information on how to quit smoking.

Support Groups

The development of Alcoholics Anonymous (AA) in 1935 began a strong movement that recognized the important role of peer support in the treatment of a chronic illness. AA groups have developed throughout the world, and their success has led to the development of other support groups such as Narcotics Anonymous (NA) for persons with narcotic addictions and Pills Anonymous for persons with polydrug addictions. Similar programs have been developed for process addictions, such as Overeaters Anonymous and Gamblers Anonymous.

AA and NA assist persons with addictions in developing a daily program of recovery and reinforce the recovery process. The fellowship, support, and encouragement among AA members, all of whom are abstaining alcoholics, provide a vital social network for the person recovering from an addiction.

Al-Anon and Alateen are similar self-help programs for spouses, parents, children, or others involved in a painful relationship with an alcoholic (Nar-Anon for those in relationships with persons with narcotic addictions). Al-Anon family groups are available to anyone who has been affected by their involvement

---

 Smoking Cessation Resources

American Cancer Society

777 3rd Ave
New York, NY 10017
(see local telephone directory)
◆ "Smart Move" (video and literature)
◆ "Fresh Start" smoking cessation program

American Heart Association

7272 Greenville Ave.
Dallas, TX 75231
(214) 373-6300
(see local telephone directly)
◆ "In Control: Freedom from Smoking" program

American Lung Association

1740 Broadway
New York, NY 10019
(see telephone directly)
◆ "Freedom From Smoking for You and Your Family"

Americans for Nonsmokers Rights

2054 University Ave. #500
Berkley, CA 94704

Anti-Tobacco Initiative

American Public Health Association
1015 Fifteenth St., N.W.
Washington, DC 20005

ASH (Action on Smoking and Health)

2013 H St. N.W.
Washington, DC 20006

Five Day Plan to Stop Smoking (general headquarters)

Seventh Day Adventist Church
Narcotics Education Division
6840 Eastern Ave. N.W.
Washington, DC 20012

National Interagency Council on Smoking and Health

Room 1005, 291 Broadway
2BB:New York, NY 10007

Office of Cancer Communications

National Cancer Institute
National Institutes of Health
Bethesda, MD 20205
(800) 638-6694
(800) 492-6600 in Maryland

Office on Smoking and Health

U.S. Department of Health and Human Services
Room 1-58
5600 Fishers Lane
Rockville, MD 20857
(800) 232-1311
◆ "Action Guide to Second-hand Smoke"
◆ "African American Quitting Guide"

SmokEnders

Memorial Parkway
Phillipsburg, NJ 08864
(908) 454-4357

STAT (Stop Teenage Addiction to Tobacco)

511 East Columbus Ave.
Springfield, MA 01105
(413) 732-7828

with an alcoholic person. The purposes of Alateen include providing a forum for adolescents to discuss family stressors, learn coping skills from one another, and gain support and encouragement from knowledgeable peers. Adult Children of Alcoholics (ACOA) groups are also available in most areas to address the recovery of adults who grew up in alcoholic homes and are still carrying the scars and retaining dysfunctional behaviors.

For some persons the AA program places too much emphasis on a higher power or focuses too much on the negative consequences of past drinking. Women for Sobriety focuses on rebuilding self-esteem, a core issue for many women with alcoholic problems (Kaskutas, 1994). Rational Recovery has a cognitive orientation and is premised on the assumption that ATOD addiction is caused by irrational beliefs that can be understood and overcome (Galanter et al., 1993).

 ## Clinical Application

A 6-week prenatal class was developed by a community health nurse for pregnant women from an inner-city, low-rent housing area. The program was designed because so many women in the area did not have the resources to get routine prenatal care and were identified as a high-risk group.

One of the classes focused on drug use during pregnancy. After the class, Jenny, a 23-year-old single black woman in her first trimester, approached the nurse. She did not know where to begin, except she wanted the nurse to know that she really wanted her baby but was afraid she may have already harmed the fetus. She admitted that she had used crack on a regular basis and had been trying to quit but that she had used it again over the weekend when a friend brought some by. She also smokes cigarettes but had cut back from one pack per day to one-half pack. Teary-eyed, Jenny stated she did not know where to go or who to see but that she wanted to get help.

The nurse sat down with Jenny and continued to assess Jenny's crack use and other drug use patterns and obtained a thorough biopsychosocial history. Her mother had died, and her father had a history of alcoholism. There was no supportive family member nearby, and her older sister's husband would not let her stay with them because she had stolen money and property from them on more than one occasion to buy crack. Jenny was not sure who the father of her baby was because she had multiple partners in exchange for cocaine. She was currently living with friends who also used crack. She was afraid that if she returned to her environment she would not be able to stay clean.

The nurse was aware of a treatment program that was affiliated with a hospital that was able to take pregnant women but realized there may be a waiting list. The nurse worked with the community services board to find housing in a homeless shelter until Jenny could get into treatment. The nurse counseled Jenny about getting tested for the HIV virus and other sexually transmitted diseases (STD's), and on Jenny's request blood tests were arranged through the public health department. The nurse contacted the treatment program, and Jenny was admitted a few days later into their inpatient program where she would also get prenatal care as necessary. The facility was smoke free, and Jenny could smoke only during designated smoke breaks outside. She used this structured program to gradually taper her use, and after the first week she stopped completely.

While in treatment, Jenny was encouraged to develop an aftercare program, and finding a place to live was of great concern. The treatment team encouraged Jenny to consider a halfway house in a nearby city that was designed for pregnant women. She would have to agree to abide by their rules, attend specific classes on child care and parenting, and attend AA and NA meetings on a daily basis. If the baby had any complications secondary to Jenny's crack use, the staff at the halfway house were prepared to assist Jenny in meeting the baby's health care needs. Jenny decided to go to the halfway house and subsequently delivered a 6-pound baby girl 1 week before her due date. The baby was healthy, and Jenny remained at the halfway house with her daughter for another 4 months.

This case study shows how a community health nurse can make a difference by determining high-risk groups within the community and developing a plan of care to bring knowledge and care into the client's environment. Jenny may not have been aware of the full impact her crack addiction could have on the fetus and may not have sought help so early in her pregnancy. After identifying Jenny's addiction problem, the nurse was able to mobilize community resources to find her a safe place to live, get her screened for possible STDs that could require treatment, and make an appropriate referral to a treatment program that would also offer prenatal care. Although relapse is still possible, Jenny was able to abstain from further crack or other drug use during her pregnancy and therefore decreased the possibility of permanently damaging her baby in utero.

The nurse provided Jenny with much encouragement to stop smoking, obtained smoking cessation literature from the American Lung Association for Jenny, and talked with Jenny about the dangers of sidestream smoke if Jenny resumed smoking after her pregnancy. Relapse with smokers who try to quit happens frequently, but it is hoped that Jenny will try to quit again if she does relapse, and at least she has new information that makes her determined to never smoke in a confined area with her baby.

Key Concepts

- Substance abuse is a national health problem that is linked to numerous forms of morbidity and mortality.
- Harm reduction is a new approach to the substance abuse problem that deals with substance abuse primarily as a health problem rather than a criminal problem.
- All people have attitudes about the use of drugs that influence their actions.
- Social conditions such as a fast-paced life, excessive stress, and the availability of drugs influence the incidence of substance abuse.
- Important terms to understand when working with individuals, groups, or communities for whom substance abuse is prevalent are drug dependence, drug addiction, alcoholism, psychoactive drugs, depressants, stimulants, marijuana, hallucinogens, and inhalants.
- Primary prevention for substance abuse includes education about drugs and guidelines for use, as well as the promotion of healthy alternatives to drug use for either recreation or to relieve stress. Community health nurses can play a key role in developing community prevention programs.
- Secondary prevention depends heavily on careful assessment of the client's use of drugs. Such assessment should be part of all basic health assessments.
- High-risk groups include pregnant women, young people, elderly persons, and intravenous drug users.
- Drug addiction is often a family, not merely an individual, problem. Codependency describes a companion illness to the addiction of one person in which the codependent member is addicted to the addicted person.
- Brief interventions by the community health nurse can be as effective as treatment. Community health nurses are in ideal roles to assist with tertiary prevention for both the addicted person and the family.

Critical Thinking Activities

1. Read your local newspaper for 4 days, and select stories that illustrate the effect of substance abuse on individuals, families, and the community.
2. For each of the stories in the newspaper related to substance abuse, describe preventive strategies that a community health nurse might have tried before the problem reached such a dire state.
3. Looking at your local community resources directory (or the telephone book), identify agencies that might serve as referral sources for individuals or families for whom substance abuse is a problem.
4. In groups of three to five students discuss your personal attitudes toward drinking, smoking, and drug abuse. Discuss each category of substance abuse separately. Consider the following areas: sex, age, amount, time, occasion, place where substance abuse occurs, companions, motivation, and incentives.
5. Review popular magazine and television advertisements for alcohol, tobacco, and other medicines (e.g., sleepers, analgesics, laxatives, stimulants). In small groups discuss the messages conveyed in the advertisements and what the implications would be for patient education to reduce possible harm from misuse and abuse of these substances.
6. Attend an open AA or NA meeting and an Al-Anon meeting. Go alone if possible or with an alcoholic or a drug-addicted friend. As the members introduce themselves, give your first name and state, "I am a visitor." Plan to listen and do not attempt to take notes. Respect the anonymity of the persons present. Discuss your experiences later in a group.
7. In groups of four or five, review the national health objectives in *Healthy People* 2000 (Appendix A) under "Tobacco" and "Alcohol and Other Drugs." Pick an objective from each section, and brainstorm about possible community efforts a nurse could initiate to reach that objective.

Bibliography

Bien TH, Miller WR, Tonigan JS: Brief interventions for alcohol problems: a review, *Addiction* 88:315-336, 1993.

Brecher EM: *Licit and illicit drugs*, Boston, 1972, Little, Brown.

Brust JCM: Other agents: phencyclidine, marijuana, hallucinogens, inhalants, and anticholinergics, *Neurol Clinics* 11(3):555-561, 1993.

Callery YC: Chemical abuse rehabilitation for hospital employees, *AAOHN J* 42(4):67-75, 1994.

Chavkin W, Kandall SR: Between a "rock" and a hard place: perinatal drug abuse, *Pediatrics* 85(2):223-225, 1990.

Coate D: Moderate drinking and coronary heart disease mortality: evidence from NHANES I and the NHANES I follow-up, *Am J Pub Health* 83(6):888-890, 1993.

Cordero JF, Floyd RL, Martin ML, et al: Tracking the prevalence of FAS, *Alcohol Health Res World* 18(1):82-85, 1994.

Das G, Laddu A: Cocaine: friend or foe? I, *Intern J Clin Pharmacol Ther Toxicol* 31(9):449-455, 1993.

Dicker M, Leighton EA: Trends in the US prevalence of drug-using parturient women and drug-affected newborns, 1979 through 1990, *Am J Pub Health* 84(9):1433-1438, 1994.

Dinwiddie SH: Abuse of inhalants: a review, *Addiction* 89(8):925-939, 1994.

Dodge VH: Relaxation training: a nursing intervention for substance abusers, *Arch Psychiatr Nurs* 5(2):99-104, 1991.

Donaldson SI, Graham JW, Hansen WB: Testing the generalizability of intervening mechanism theories: understanding the effects of adolescent drug use prevention interventions, *J Behav Med* 17(2):195-216, 1994.

Doweiko HE: *Concepts of chemical dependency*, Pacific Grove, Calif, 1990, Brooks/Cole.

Ennett ST, Tobler NS, Ringwalt CL, Flewing RL: How effective is drug abuse resistance education? a meta-analysis of Project DARE outcome evaluation, *Am J Pub Health* 84(9):1394-1401, 1994.

Espeland K: Inhalant abuse: assessment guidelines, *J Psychosoc Nurs Ment Health Serv* 31(3):11-14, 1993.

Fiesta J: Mother vs child: a legal controversy, *Nurs Management* 22(10):14-17, 1991.

Fiore MC: Treatment options for smoking in the '90s, *J Clin Pharmacol* 34(3):195-199, 1993.

Foley KM: Opioids, *Neurol Clinics* 11(3):503-521, 1993.

Frezza M, di Padova C, Pozzato G, et al: High blood alcohol levels in women: the role of decreased gastric alcohol dehydrogenase activity and first-pass metabolism, *N Engl J Med* 322(2):95-99, 1990.

Galanter M, Egelko S, Edwards H: Rational recovery: alternative to AA for addiction? *Am J Drug Alcohol Abuse* 19(4):499-510, 1993.

Griffiths WH: *Complete guide to prescription and nonprescription drugs*, New York, 1995, Putnam-Berkley.

Healthy People 2000: national health promotion and disease prevention objectives, Washington, DC, 1991, USDHHS, Public Health Service.

Heather N, Wodak A, Nadelmann E, O'Hare P, editors: *Psychoactive drugs and harm reduction: from faith to science*, London, 1993, Whurr.

Hoffman RS, Goldfrank LR: The impact of drug abuse and addiction on society, *Emerg Med Clin North Am* 8(3):467-480, 1990.

Hutchings DE: The puzzle of cocaine's effects following maternal use during pregnancy: are there reconcilable differences, *Neurotoxicol Teratol* 15:281-286, 1993.

Institute for Health Policy, Brandeis University: *Substance abuse: the nation's number one health problem, key indicators for policy*, Princeton, NJ, 1993, The Robert Wood Johnson Foundation.

Jack L, Snow D: *Prevention of alcohol, tobacco, and other drug problems: an independent study for nurses*, Raleigh, NC, 1994, US Center for Substance Abuse Prevention and the National Nurses Society on Addictions.

Jaffe JH: Drug addiction and drug abuse. In Gilman AG, Rall TW, Nies AS, Taylor P, editors: *Goodman and Gilman's the pharmacological basis of therapeutics*, ed 8, New York, 1990, Pergamon Press.

Kain ZN, Rimar S, Barash PG: Cocaine abuse and the parturient and effects on the fetus and neonate, *Anesth Analg* 77(4):835-845, 1993.

Kaskutas LA: What do women get out of self-help? Their reasons for attending Women for Sobriety and Alcoholics Anonymous. *J Subst Abuse Treat* 11(3):185-195, 1994.

Kinney J, Leaton G: *Loosening the grip*, ed 5, St Louis, 1995, Mosby.

Kumpfer KL, Hopkins R: Prevention: current research and trends, *Psychiatr Clin North Am* 16(1):11-20, 1993.

Larrat EP, Taubman AH, Willey C: Compliance-related problems in the ambulatory populations, *Am Pharmacy* NS30(2):18-23, 1990.

Long MC: Overview of substance abuse: implications for the primary care nurse practitioner, *Nurs Pract Forum* 4(4):191-198, 1993.

McMahon AL: Substance abuse among the elderly, *Nurs Pract Forum* 4(4):231-238, 1993.

Medical-care expenditures attributable to cigarette smoking—US, 1993, *MMWR* 43(26):469-472, 1994.

Merrill J, Fox K, Chang H: *The cost of substance abuse to America's health care system. Report 1: Medicaid hospital costs*, New York, 1993, Center on Addictions and Substance Abuse at Columbia University.

Miller M: *Drug consumer safety rules*, Mosier, Ore, 1994, Mothers Against Misuse and Abuse (MAMA).

Minicucci DS: The challenge of change: rethinking alcohol abuse, *Arch Psychiatr Nurs* 8(6):373-380, 1994.

National Institute on Drug Abuse: Trends in adolescent drug use, *NIDA Notes* 9(1):19, 1994.

National Opinion Research Center: *Evaluating recovery services: the California drug and alcohol treatment assessment*, Chicago, National Opinion Research Center, 1994.

Peterson PL, Lowe JB: Preventing fetal alcohol exposure: a cognitive behavioral approach. *Int J Addict* 27(5):613-626, 1992.

Prochaska JO, DiClemente CC, Norcross JC: In search of how people change, *Am J Psychol* 47(9):1102-1114, 1992.

Randall R: Marijuana, medicine, and the law, *Nurs Times*, Washington, DC, 1988, Galen Press.

Rassool GH, Winnington J: Using psychoactive drugs, *Nurs Times* 89(47):38-40, 1993.

Rienzo PG: *Nursing care of the patient who smokes*, New York, 1993, Springer.

Schwartz RH: Syringe and needle exchange programs worldwide, *South Med J* 86(3):323-327, 1993.

Sees KL: Cigarette smoking, nicotine dependence, and treatment, *West J Med* 152(5):578-584, 1990.

Shedler J, Block J: Adolescent drug use and psychological health: a longitudinal inquiry, *Am Psychol* 45(5):612-630, 1990.

Strain EC, Mumford GK, Silverman K, Griffiths RR: Caffeine dependence syndrome: evidence from case histories and experimental evaluation, *JAMA* 272(13):1043-1048, Oct 5, 1994.

Talashek ML, Gerace LM, Starr KL: The substance abuse pandemic: determinants to guide interventions, *Pub Health Nurs* 11(2):131-139, 1994.

Tweed SH: Identifying the alcoholic client, *Nurs Clin North Am* 24(1):13-31, 1989.

US Department of Health and Human Services: *Reducing the health consequences of smoking: 25 years of progress. A report of the Surgeon General*, Washington, DC, 1989, US Government Printing Office.

Vallance TR: *Prohibition's second failure: the quest for a rational and humane drug policy*, Wesport, Conn, 1993, Greenwood Publishing Group.

Volpicelli JR, Watson NT, King AC et al: Effect of Naltrexone on alcohol "high" in alcoholics, *Am J Psychiatry* 152(4):613-615, 1995.

Warner EA: Cocaine abuse, *Ann Intern Med* 119(3):226-235, 1993.

Weil A, Rosen W: *Chocolate to morphine: understanding mind-active drugs*, Boston, 1993, Houghton Mifflin.

Weiss RD, Mirin SM, Bartel RL: *Cocaine*, ed 2, Washington, DC, 1994, American Psychiatric Press.

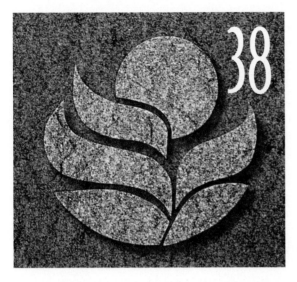

38 Violence and Human Abuse

Jacquelyn Campbell ◆ Kären Landenburger

Objectives ▼

After reading this chapter, the student should be able to do the following:

◆ Discuss the scope of the problem of violence in American communities.
◆ Describe at least three factors existing in most communities that influence violence and human abuse.
◆ Identify at least three types of common community facilities that can help mitigate violence.
◆ Identify typically noticed indicators of child abuse.
◆ Define the four general types of child abuse: neglect, physical abuse, emotional abuse, and sexual abuse.
◆ Discuss abuse of elderly persons as a growing community health problem.
◆ Evaluate the role that community health nurses can assume with rape victims.
◆ Identify primary preventive nursing interventions for community violence.
◆ Describe the different responses that a nurse would expect to see in a battered woman from the beginning of the abuse until after the relationship has ended.
◆ Discuss the principles of nursing intervention with violent families.
◆ Identify specific nursing interventions with battered women.

Key Terms ▼

assault
battered child syndrome
child neglect
elder abuse
emotional abuse
emotional neglect
empowerment
helplessness
homicide
incest
physical abuse
physical neglect
powerlessness
rape
sexual abuse
spouse abuse
suicide
survivors
violence
wife abuse

Outline ▼

The word "violence" comes from the Latin violare, meaning to violate, injure, or rape. Indeed, violence is a violation, with both emotional and physical effects. American society is unfortunately quite violent by most measures. Statistics indicate that the United States has the fifth highest homicide rate in the world. Newspaper headlines and television reports are rife with news of violence. Although considerable progress has been made in decreasing rates of death from all other causes since 1940, the risk of homicide in the United States is actually increasing (Healthy People 2000, 1991). The violence in our streets and in our homes threatens the health and well-being of our entire population.

It is not clear from research if violence stems from an innate aggressive drive or is primarily learned behavior. However, it *is* clear that all human beings have the capability for violence. It is also clear that some entire societies are basically nonviolent (Counts, et al., 1991). Therefore it is important to understand under what conditions aggression and violence are exacerbated and, conversely, what keeps them in check and promotes nonviolent conflict resolution. From a community health standpoint, nurses should be interested in these forces at a family, an aggregate, and a community level.

Violence is a community health nursing concern. Significant mortality and morbidity result from violence, and extensive violence within a community is distressing to all inhabitants. Communities across the United States are voicing anger and fear about rising crime and violence rates. Medical, nursing, psychology, and social service professionals have been slow in developing a response to violence that is integral to their daily professional lives. As a result, the estimated 4 million victims of violence annually may not receive the best care possible. In addition, the extent of their pain that could have been avoided by community health prevention efforts is unknown.

Violence is generally defined as those nonaccidental acts, interpersonal or intrapersonal, that result in physical or psychological injury to one or more persons. A consensus is emerging among epidemiologists that violent behavior is predictable and thus is preventable (Rosenberg and Fenley, 1991). Within the past 5 years, public opinion polls indicate the average person's perception of violence has converged with that of the public health community: violence can be prevented, particularly by community action. This perception has been shaped by a large body of research showing that violence is a major cause of premature mortality and lifelong disability and that violence-related morbidity is a significant factor in the rising costs of health care. Violence is the twelfth leading cause of death in the United States and the sixth leading cause of premature mortality (Healthy People 2000, 1991). A section of the *National Objectives for the Year 2000* is now devoted to violence, providing official recognition of the need for health professionals to address this issue (see Appendix A).

This chapter examines violence as a public health problem and discusses how the community health nurse can help families, groups, and the community cope with and reduce violence and human abuse. Community health nurses have access to clients in a wide variety of settings, including the home. They are in key positions to detect and intervene in community and family violence. It is important that nurses understand community-level influences on all types of violence as a beginning point for addressing this important problem.

SOCIAL AND COMMUNITY FACTORS INFLUENCING VIOLENCE

Numerous variables within a community can support or minimize violence. Changing social conditions, multiple demands on people, economic conditions, and institutions that make up a given society or community influence the level of violence and human abuse. The following discussion of selected contemporary social conditions provides a basis for understanding factors that influence violent behavior.

Work

Productive and paid work is an expectation in mainstream American society, especially for men. Work can be fulfilling and thus can contribute to a sense of well-being, but it can also be frustrating and unfulfilling, contributing to stress that may lead to aggression and violence. Unemployment is also associated with violence both within and outside the home.

When jobs are repetitive, boring, and lacking in stimulation, frustration mounts. Some work environments discourage creativity and reward conformity and "following the rules." In many work settings people try to get ahead regardless of the cost to others. Workers often go home feeling physically and psychologically drained. They may have worked at a backbreaking pace all day only to be yelled at by the boss for what seemed like a trivial oversight. It is hard to separate feelings generated at work from those in the home environment.

For example, a father arrives home feeling tired, angry, and generally inadequate because of a series of reprimands from his boss. Soon after he sits down, his 4-year-old son runs through the house pretending to fly a wooden airplane. After about three loud trips past his father, who keeps shouting for the child to be quiet and go outside, the airplane hits the father in the head. The father may strike out in frustration and anger.

During economic downturns, people are often afraid to give up jobs that are frustrating, are boring, or create stress. Family needs may necessitate that they keep the hated job. They feel trapped and may resent those who depend on them. This frustration and resentment may lead to violence.

Unemployment also often precipitates aggressive outbursts. The inability to secure or maintain a job may lead to feelings of inadequacy, guilt, boredom, dissatisfaction, and frustration. Unemployment does not fit the image of the ideal man in American society, and these men are more likely to commit violence both within and outside the family (Tolman and Bennett, 1990).

Young, minority males have the highest rates of unemployment in the United States, ranging close to 50%. This group also has the highest rate of violence. They are described as young men living in a world of oppression, with lack of opportunity and enormous anger as a "subculture of exasperation." The norms developed by this group are a response to being pushed out of mainstream society and of being on the receiving end of the fallout of policies that ignore their dilemmas and give them no stake in mainstream America. Most analyses conclude that the differential rates of violence between blacks and whites in the United States have more to do with economic realities, such as poverty, unemployment, and overcrowding, than with race (Hawkins, 1993; Straus and Gelles, 1990).

Education

In recent years schools have assumed many responsibilities traditionally assigned to the family. Schools teach sexual development, discipline children, and often serve as a place to "dump" children who have no other place to go. Large classes often mean that teachers spend more time and energy monitoring and disciplining children than challenging and stimulating them to learn. In large classes, isolation is often the primary method of dealing with children who do not conform to norms of expected behavior. The nonconforming child is simply removed from the classroom because time does not permit concerted efforts toward helping the child learn alternative ways of behavior.

It is ironic that parents often punish children for hitting or biting other children by spanking them. Corporal punishment is also still used in many U.S. schools. Such punishment only reinforces the child's tendency to strike out at others.

Prince (1980) contends that five basic human needs—stimulation, power, intimacy, interdependence, and "anger outlets"—could be provided by major social institutions but in most cases are not. She believes that the education system, especially in urban areas, fails to meet these needs largely because of a lack of financial resources. Thus schools are often places where the stressors and frustrations that can contribute to violence are rampant, and violence is learned rather than discouraged; yet school has the potential to be a powerful contributor to nonviolence. Classes have been designed to help adolescents learn peaceful conflict resolution, to help students understand the issues of date rape, and to help young children deal with the threat of sexual abuse (Gelles and Conte, 1990; Webster, 1993). Parents can be advised of the availability of these kinds of programs, and school boards should be urged to adopt them into the curriculum.

Media

The media can be instrumental in campaigns against violence. Recent television programs, both documentaries and dramatizations, and print articles have heightened public awareness about family violence. Abused women and rape victims have especially benefited from media attention, which tends to lessen the stigma of such victimization. The media are also useful in publicizing services. However, the media have often served as a source of frustration to poor persons in U.S. society, as a cause of public apathy, and as a model of violence to be emulated.

Television, movies, newspapers, and magazines portray happy, fun-loving people. Television parades all the wonders money can provide; yet for many Americans, the hope of buying many of these nonessentials seems unrealisitic. Such polarization between what is available and what is possible provides fertile ground for the development of abusive patterns. Frustration, unfilled dreams, and unmet wishes are often handled through hurting someone who is limited in the ability to fight back.

The media cater to children by advertising products intended to stimulate their curiosity and desire to purchase. Parents subsequently may get angry when their children request the foods, toys, and clothes they see on television, in magazines, or in newspapers or hear advertised on the radio. In addition, many toys and video games encourage violence through play.

Not only does the media tantalize children and adults with a vast array of possible items to buy and things to do, but also both television and newspapers often portray the world as a violent place. When the public is convinced that violence is rampant, there are two possible results. People may become blasé about violence and no longer feel outraged and galvanized to action when terrible things happen in their community. On the other hand, some become frightened of their neighbors, isolate themselves, and refuse to become involved when someone needs help. Neither response is useful in any community-action program.

Hitting, kicking, stabbing, and shooting are seen daily as ways to handle anger and frustration. By the age of 18 years, the average child has seen 1800 murders and countless acts of nonfatal violence on television. Often in these acts of violence, the good guys conquer the bad ones. Thus violence is often seen as justified when the perpetrator views the cause to be worthy. Frequent violent television viewing by children has been associated with aggressive behavior in longitudinal research (Campbell and Humphreys, 1993).

Organized Religion

Three of the human needs cited by Prince (1980) are often provided by the church—stimulation, a sense of worth or power, and some degree of closeness and intimacy. Religion also usually encourages nonviolent conflict resolution between adults; and the church, clergy, and church groups often provide positive role models and reinforcement for peaceful behavior.

However, a seemingly contradictory relation exists between abuse and religion in a historical perspective. For example, many religious groups uphold the philosophy of "spare the rod, spoil the child." Also, some faiths uphold the victimization of people with their disapproval of divorce. Family members may stay together, although they are at emotional or physical war with one another, because of religious commitments (Prince, 1980).

Although controversial, the role of guilt as a form of victimization needs to be considered. Some religious bodies seem more concerned about using religious beliefs to keep members "in line" than offering suggestions and encouragement for behavior. Rigid guidelines complete with predictions of dire spiritual consequences can produce guilt and lowered self-esteem.

Population

A community's population can influence the potential for violence. Two significant factors are density and diversity.

High–population-density communities can have a positive or negative influence on violence. Those with *a sense of cohesiveness* may have a lower crime rate than areas of similar size that lack social and cultural groups to support unity among members. Bonds formed among church groups, clubs, and professional organizations may promote harmony among members. Such groups provide members an opportunity to talk about stressors rather than to respond through violence. For example, residents of public housing often form neighborhood associations to deal with situations common to many or all residents. Tension can often be released in a productive way through projects carried out by the association.

Some high-population areas experience a community feeling of **powerlessness** and **helplessness** rather than one of cohesiveness. Fear and apathy may cause community residents to withdraw from social contact. Withdrawal can foster crime because many residents assume someone else will report suspicious behavior, and residents fear reprisals for such reports.

Youths often attempt to deal with feelings of powerlessness by forming gangs. A number of these young adults have attempted to deal with their feelings by turning to crime against people and property to release frustration. In many cities these gangs have been highly destructive.

Other high-population areas may be characterized by a *sense of confusion,* resulting in disintegration and disorganization. These areas often have transient populations who have limited physical or emotional investment in the community. Lack of community concern allows crime and violence to go unchecked and may become a norm for the area. Also, as crime increases, residents who are able to move leave the area. This increases community disintegration because the residents who leave are often the most capable members of the population.

The potential for violence also tends to increase among highly diverse populations. Differences in age, socioeconomic status, ethnicity, religion, or other cultural characteristics may disrupt community stability. Highly divergent groups may neither accept nor understand one another. They may not communicate effectively. Many such groups become hostile and antagonistic toward one another. Each group may see the other as different and not belonging. The alienated group may become the focal point for the others' frustrations, anger, and fears. Isolation or hostile attacks increase tension and decrease the potential for community cohesiveness and integration.

Community Facilities

Communities differ in the resources and facilities they provide to residents. Some are more desirable places to live, work, and raise families and have facilities that can reduce the potential for crime and violence. Recreational facilities such as playgrounds, parks, swimming pools, movie theaters, and tennis courts, provide socially acceptable outlets for a variety of feelings, including aggression.

Spectator sports, such as football or hockey, also allow members of the community to express feelings of anger and frustration. However, viewing sports can encourage a sense of violence as participants hit or shove one another.

Although the absence of such facilities can increase the likelihood of violence, their presence alone does not prevent violence or crime. These facilities are adjuncts and resources to be used by residents for pleasure, personal enrichment, and group development.

Familiarity with factors contributing to a community's violence or potential for violence enables community health nurses to recognize them and intervene accordingly. It is the nurse's responsibility to work with the citizens and agencies of the community to correct or improve deficits.

VIOLENCE AGAINST INDIVIDUALS OR ONESELF

The potential for violence against individuals (e.g., murder, robbery, rape, and assault) or oneself (e.g., suicide) is directly related to the level of violence in the community. Persons living in areas with high rates of crime and violence are more likely to become victims than those in more peaceful areas. The major categories of violence addressed in this chapter can be described in terms of the scope of the problem in the United States and underlying dynamics.

Homicide

Homicide is the eleventh leading cause of death for all Americans, and the number one cause of death for young (age 15 to 34 years) black men *and* women (U.S. Public Health Service, 1990). However, the black homicide rate has decreased significantly since 1970, whereas the white homicide rate has increased (U.S. Public Health Service, 1990). Although the data are not adequate, it also appears that Hispanic-American males have a much higher rate of homicide than non–Hispanic-American whites. Homicide is increasing the most among adolescents, but even among very young children in the United States, homicide occurs at an alarming rate. In 1986, 4.2 per 100,000 children age 3 years and younger were killed by another person, usually a family member (U.S. Public Health Service, 1990). Only 12.4% of all homicides in the United States occur as a result of a stranger killing someone in the context of a crime (e.g., burglary, rape) (O'Carroll and Mercy, 1986). Many of these homicides are related to the illegal substance-abuse network. Efforts directed toward eliminating that problem by the criminal justice system will also help in decreasing violence against strangers.

The majority of homicides, however, are perpetrated by a friend, acquaintance, or family member during an argument. Therefore prevention of homicide is at least as much an issue for the public health system as for the criminal justice system (Mercy and O'Carroll, 1988).

Homicide Within Families

At least 13% of the homicides in the United States occur within families (Bachman, 1994) and half of these occur between spouses. These numbers, however, do not include unmarried couples who are living together or those who are either divorced or estranged, a group at higher risk. Husbands comprised about 60% of perpetrators in spousal homicides, and self-defense is involved approximately seven times as often when wives kill their husbands than vice versa (Campbell, 1991; Bachman, 1994).

An alarming aspect of family homicide is that small children often witness the murder or find the body of a family member. No automatic follow-up or counseling of these children occurs through the criminal justice or mental health system in most communities. These children are at great risk for emotional turmoil and for becoming involved in violence themselves.

The underlying dynamics of homicide within families vary greatly from those of other murders. Homicide within families is most often preceded by abuse of a family member (Campbell, 1991). Thus prevention of family homicide involves working with abusive families. The chance of eventual homicide must always be kept in mind when working with these families. Nurses have a "duty to warn" family members of the possibility of homicide when severe abuse is present, just as they warn of the hazards of smoking (Campbell, 1995). Other nursing care issues are discussed further in the section on family violence.

Assault

The death toll from violence is indeed staggering; yet the physical injuries and emotional costs of **assault** are equally important issues in terms of the acute health care system and both public health nursing and home health care. At least 100 nonfatal assaults occurs for each homicide that occurs in the United States (U.S. Public Health Service, 1990). Of all simple and aggravated assaults, 33% resulted in injury (Reiss and Roth, 1993). The greatest risk factor for an individual's victimization through violence is age, with youth at significantly higher risk. Whereas more males than females are victims of homicide and assault, women are more likely to be victimized by a relative, especially a male partner (Bachman, 1994). Sometimes the difference between a homicide and an assault is only the response time and quality of emergency transport and treatment facilities. Whatever community measures are used to address homicide are also useful to combat assault. In addition, nurses find that assaulted persons are often seen in home health care with long-term health problems such as head injuries, spinal cord injuries, and stomas from abdominal gunshot wounds. In addition to physical care, nurses must also address the emotional trauma resulting from a violent attack by helping victims talk through their traumatic experience and try to make some sense of the violence and by referring them for further counseling if anxiety, sleeping problems, or depression persists after the assault.

Rape

Currently **rape** is one of the most underreported yet fastest growing forms of human abuse in the United States. Rape is the one category of violent crime that continued to increase between 1975 and 1990. The rates of completed and attempted rape are equivalent (Reiss and Roth, 1993). In 1986 there were 120 rapes per 100,000 people (Healthy People 2000, 1991). One factor influencing an increase in the incidence of rape is higher victim reporting. Hospital, emergency personnel, and police have improved the protocols for use with victims of rape. Although an emphasis has been placed on the collection of information leading to prosecution, a major focus of the protocols has been ensuring respectful and supportive treatment for all victims. Another important factor is the recognition of date and marital rape. Official recognition of rape regardless of a victim's relationship to the perpetrator has led to an increased number of women reporting rape. There is also a growing recognition that rape often happens to men, especially boys and young men, but the statistics on the incidence of male rape vary. A major problem in obtaining statistics is that the definition of rape adopted by the Federal Bureau of Investigation for compiling the Uniformed Crime Reports is limited to penile-vaginal penetration only (Koss and Harvey, 1991). Although much more research on male rape is needed, beginning studies suggest that the emotional trauma to a male rape victim is at least as serious as that for a woman.

For reported rapes, cities constitute higher risk areas than do rural areas; and the hours between 8 PM and 2 AM, weekends, and the summer are the most critical times. In about one-half of rapes the victim and the offender meet on the street, whereas in other cases the rapist either gains entry to the victim's home or somehow entices or forces the victim to accompany him.

Prevention of rape, as in other forms of human abuse, requires a broad-based community focus for educating both the community as a whole and key groups such as police, health providers, educators, and social workers. Research has shown connections between rape rates and community-level variables such as community approval and legitimization of violence (e.g., violent network television viewing and permitting corporal punishment in schools), which underscores the need for community-level intervention (Baron et al., 1988).

Attitudes

The first priority is to change attitudes about rape and about victims. Rape is a crime of violence, not a crime of passion. The underlying issues are hostility, power, and control rather than sexual desire. The defining issue is lack of consent of the victim. When a woman or man refuses any sexual activity, that refusal means "no." People have the right to change their mind, even when they seemed initially acquiescent. Pressure in the form of physical contact, threats, or deliberate inducement of drug or alcohol intoxication is a violation of the law. There must also be an end to the myths that women say "no" to sex when they really mean "yes" and that the victims of rape are culpable because of the way they dress or act.

Pornography

There is persuasive evidence that viewing pornographic material depicting violence against women within the context of sex is correlated with aggressive and sexual behavior (Sommers and Check, 1987). More research is needed in this area before definitive public policy recommendations can be made concerning laws governing pornography. However, there is enough evidence to recommend keeping violent pornography illegal, especially for minors. Prevention also involves providing information to women about self-protection, including self-defense procedures, avoiding high-risk locations, and safeguarding one's home against unwanted entry.

The Victim

During the act of rape, victims are often hit, kicked, stabbed, and severely beaten. It is this violence that most traumatizes the victim—because of the fear for her life and her helplessness, lack of control, and vulnerability.

People react to rape differently, depending on their personality, past experiences, background, and support received after the trauma. Some victims cry, shout, or discuss the experience. Others withdraw and fear discussing the attack. During the immediate as well as the follow-up stages, victims tend to blame themselves for what has happened. It is important while working with rape victims that community health nurses assist them in identifying the issues behind self-blame. Although fault should not be placed on the victim, it is essential to teach mechanisms that enable a victim to take control, learn assertiveness, and therefore believe that she has steps she can take to prevent future rapes. Victims need to talk about what happened and to express their feelings and fears in a nonjudgmental atmosphere. Therefore nonjudgmental listening is an essential nursing measure.

In any psychological trauma, the right to privacy and confidentiality is of the utmost importance. Victims should be given privacy, respect, and assurance of confidentiality. Victims also should be apprised of health care procedures conducted immediately after the rape and should be linked with proper resources for ease of reporting. Nurses are responsible for providing continuous care once the victim enters the health care system. Because many victims deny the event once the initial crisis is past, a single-session debriefing should be completed during the initial examination. The physical assessment, examination, and debriefing should be carried out by specially trained providers (Koss and Harvey, 1991).

In several states nurses perform the physical examination in the emergency department to gather evidence (e.g., hair samples and skin fragments beneath the victim's fingernails) for criminal prosecution (Lenehan et al., 1983). This is an important intervention mode because physicians are often impatient with the time required for this procedure and nurses can take advantage of this opportunity to provide therapeutic communication. Nurses can be trained to conduct the examination easily, and their evidence is credible and effective in resultant court proceedings (Dinitto et al., 1987). Community health nurses can lobby for changes in hospital policies and state laws to make this strategy a reality in all states.

Rape is a situational crisis for which advance preparation is rarely possible. Therefore nursing efforts are directed toward helping victims maximize their ability to cope with the stress and disruption of their lives caused by the attack. Counseling focuses on the crisis and the concomitant fears, feelings, and issues involved. The goal is to help the victim use problem-solving skills to develop ways to regroup personal forces. If posttraumatic stress disorder has developed, professional psychological or psychiatric treatment is indicated.

Many rape victims need follow-up mental health services to help them cope with the short- and long-term effects of the crisis. The time after a rape is one of disequilibrium. Common, everyday tasks often overtax an individual's resources. Many individuals forget or fail to keep appointments. Therefore community health nurses must not only make appropriate referrals but also obtain permission from the victim to remain in contact through telephone conversations. In this manner the ongoing needs of the victim can be assessed and support, encouragement, and resources can be offered as needed (Koss and Harvey, 1991).

Did You Know?

Forty to forty-five percent of physically abused women are also being forced into sex. This has implications for the prevention of unintended and adolescent pregnancies, human immune virus (HIV), acquired immunodeficiency syndrome (AIDS), and repeat sexually transmitted diseases (STDs), as well as for women's healthy sexuality and self-esteem.

Suicide

Thirteen percent of deaths for persons ages 15 to 19 years were due to **suicide** (MMWR, 1992). Suicide is more likely to lead to death for young people than any other cause except motor vehicle accidents (Public Health Improvement Plan, 1994). The risk for death by suicide is greater than for death by homicide (Reiss and Roth, 1993). Approximately 11.6 suicides per 100,000 people occur in the United States (US Public Health Service, 1990). The incidence of suicide increases with age, reaching a high of 40 per 100,000 among persons over 75 years of age.

Among adolescents the incidence of actual suicide is equally alarming. According to the National Institute of Mental Health, more than 6000 adolescents kill themselves each year. This figure means that every 90 minutes an adolescent commits suicide; in addition, it is estimated that every day 1000 more will attempt it (Oliphant, 1986). Leading risk factors for adolescent suicide are low self-esteem, chronic depression, incest, and extrafamilial sexual and physical abuse (Eggert, 1994; Hernandez et al., 1993).

Males commit suicide three times more frequently than females, although females attempt suicide more often. The number one risk factor for actual and attempted suicide in adult women is spouse abuse (Stark and Flitcraft, 1991). Suicide is four times more frequent among whites than among blacks. Affluent and educated people have higher rates of suicide than do the economically and educationally disadvantaged.

Nursing care must focus on family members and friends of suicide victims. **Survivors** often feel angry toward the dead person yet frequently turn the anger inward. Likewise, survivors frequently question their own liability for the death. The impact of suicide can affect family, friends, co-workers, and the community. Survivors may have difficulty dealing with their feelings toward the dead person. They may have difficulty concentrating and may limit their social activities because it is often difficult for both survivors and their friends to talk about the suicide. Community health nursing intervention can help survivors cope with the trauma of the loss and may include referral to a counselor or support groups.

FAMILY VIOLENCE AND ABUSE

Family violence is also reponsible for significant injury and death. Reported child abuse increased during the 1980s, a decade that also witnessed more attention to wife abuse and the beginning of documentation of elder abuse (U.S. Public Health Service, 1990). The most recent random-sample family-violence survey indicates that at least 10.5 million Americans are severely assaulted by a family member each year; however, this survey excluded elder abuse (Straus and Gelles, 1990). Although no national survey of elder abuse has been conducted, estimates of the number of elders abused by a relative per year range from 1 million to 2.5 million (Pillemer and Finkelhor, 1986). These rates of family violence suggest that at least 10% of all American families are violent and that community health nurses should be actively intervening in abuse or potential abuse situations in more than 10% of their cases.

Family violence can include **sexual** and **emotional abuse,** as well as **physical abuse.** These three forms tend to occur together as part of a system of coercive control. Generally, violence within families is perpetrated by the most powerful against the least powerful. Thus approximately 90% of all "spouse abuse" is directed primarily toward wives (although they may physically fight back), whereas approximately 7% to 8% is mutual violence, and 2% to 3% is husband abuse (Campbell and Humphreys, 1993).

Recognizing the battered child or spouse in the emergency room is relatively simple after the fact. It is unfortunate that, by the time medical care is sought, serious physical and emotional damage may have been done. Community health nurses are in a key position to predict and deal with abusive tendencies. By understanding factors contributing to the development of abusive behaviors, nurses can identify abuse-prone families.

Development of Abusive Patterns

Factors that characterize people who become involved in family violence include upbringing, living conditions, and increased stress. Understanding how these factors influence the development of abusive behavior can help the nurse deal with abusive families.

Upbringing

Of all the factors that characterize the background of abusers, the most predictably present is previous exposure to some form of violence (Straus and Gelles, 1990). As children, abusers were often beaten themselves or witnessed the beating of siblings or a parent. Children raised in this way may abhor the use of violence, but they have had no experience with other models of family relationships.

Repeated research has demonstrated that even what is considered "normal" physical punishment of children is associated with future abuse of both children and spouses (Straus and Gelles, 1990). Childhood physical punishment teaches children to use violent conflict resolution as an adult. A child may learn to associate love with violence because parents are usually the first persons to hit a child. Children can come to believe that those who love them also are those who hit them. The moral rightness of hitting other family members thus may be established when physical punishment is used to train children, especially when it is used frequently and severely. This type of experience predisposes children ultimately to use violence with their own children.

People who become abusers may also learn parenting skills from dysfunctional role models. Their parents may have set unrealistic goals, and when the children failed to perform accordingly, they were criticized, demeaned, punished, and denied affection. These children may have been told how to act, what to do, and how to feel, thereby discouraging the development of autonomy, problem-solving skills, and creativity (Scharer, 1979). Children raised in this way grow up feeling unloved and worthless. They may want a child of their own so that they will feel assured of someone's love.

To protect themselves from feelings of worthlessness and fear of rejection, abused children form a protective shell and grow increasingly hostile and distrustful of others. The behavior of potential abusers reflects a low tolerance for frustration, emotional instability, and the onset of aggressive feelings with minimal provocation. Because of their emotional insecurity, they often depend on a child or spouse to meet their needs so that they may be valued and feel secure. When their needs are not met by others, they become overly critical. Critical, resentful behavior and unrealistic expectations of others lead to a vicious cycle. The more critical these people become, the more they are rejected and alienated from others. Abusive individuals tend to perceive that the target of their hostility is "out to get them." These distorted percep-

tions can be detected when parents talk about an infant crying or keeping them up at night "on purpose."

Increased Stress

A perceived or actual crisis may precede an abusive incident. Because crisis reinforces feelings of inadequacy and low self-esteem, it is often a number of events occurring in a short time that precipitates abusive patterns. Factors such as unemployment, strains in the marriage, or an unplanned pregnancy may set off violence.

The daily hassles associated with raising young children, especially in an economically strained household, intensify an already stressed atmosphere for which an unexpected and difficult event provides a catalyst for violence. Research by Straus and Gelles (1990) showed associations among stressful life events, poverty, the number of small children, and family violence.

Crowded living conditions may also precipitate abuse. The presence of numerous people in a small space tends to heighten tensions and to reduce privacy. Tempers flare because of the constant stimulation from others.

Social isolation is associated with abuse in families (Straus and Gelles, 1990). Such isolation reduces social support, decreasing a family's ability to deal with stressors. The problem may be intensified if a violent family member tries to keep the family isolated to escape detection. Therefore when a family misses clinic or home visit appointments, community health nurses need to keep in mind that abuse may be present. Community health nurses can encourage involvement in community activities and can help neighbors reach out to neighbors to help prevent abuse.

Frequent moves disrupt social support systems, are associated with an overall increased stress level, and tend to isolate people, at least briefly. Mobility can have a serious negative impact for the abuse-prone family. These families do not readily seek out new relationships, leaving only the family to turn to for support. Resources may be unfamiliar or inaccessible to them. Because frequent moving may be both a risk factor for abuse and a sign of an abusive family trying to avoid detection, community health nurses should assess such families carefully for abuse.

Types of Family Violence

It is important to realize that the various forms of family violence and violence outside the home frequently occur together. When nurses detect child abuse, they should also suspect other forms of family violence. When elderly parents report that their (now adult) child was abused or has a history of violence toward others, the nurse should recognize the potential for elder abuse. Physical abuse of women is frequently accompanied by sexual abuse both inside and outside marital relationships. Severe wife abusers are likely to have a history of other acts of violence. Families who are extremely verbally aggressive in conflict resolution (e.g., using name calling, belittling, screaming, and yelling) are more likely to be physically abusive. Although the various forms of family violence are discussed separately, they should not be thought of as totally separate phenomema.

No member of the family is guaranteed immunity from abuse and neglect. Spouse abuse, child abuse, abuse of elderly persons, serious violence among siblings, and mutual abuse by members all occur. Although these examples are not inclusive, they demonstrate the scope of family violence.

Child Abuse

A recent national survey projected that nearly 1.5 million children and adolescents are subjected to abusive physical violence each year (Straus and Gelles, 1990). This is probably a conservative figure, since only the most severe cases are reported. Child maltreatment was rarely discussed in medical literature until Henry Kempe et al. published their classic article in 1962, which coined the term **battered child syndrome.**

Kempe and his associates (1962) were highly successful in generating public and professional concern over child maltreatment. Their work led to the passage in 1974 of the Child Abuse Prevention and Treatment Act, which mandated reporting by professionals of child maltreatment.

The presence of child abuse signifies ineffective family functioning. Abusive parents who recognize their problem are often reluctant to seek assistance because of the stigma attached to being considered a child abuser.

Children are frequent victims of abuse because they are small and relatively powerless in the family hierarchy. In many families only one child is abused. Parents may identify with this particular child and be particularly critical of that child's behavior. In some cases the child may have certain qualities such as looking like a relative, being handicapped, or being particularly bright and capable, that provoke the parent.

Abusive parents tend to be very controlling of their children's behavior and insensitive to their needs (Houck and King, 1989). They often have unrealistic expectations of the child's developmental abilities. The nurse must not only teach them what is normal but also tend to their underlying emotional needs. The box above lists some of the behavioral indicators of potentially abusive parents. These parents often experience pain and poor emotional stability. They are in need of intervention as much as their children.

Foster Care. When child abuse is discovered, the child is often placed in a foster home. It is unfortunate that there is not enough good foster care for all abused children, and many foster care situations are also abusive. Abused children generally want to return to their parents, and the goal of most agencies is to keep natural families together as long as it is safe for the child.

 Behavioral Indicators of Potentially Abusive Parents

The following characteristics in couples expecting a child constitute warning signs of actual or potential abuse.

1. Denial of the reality of the pregnancy, as evidenced by a refusal to talk about the impending birth or to think of a name for the child
2. An obvious concern or fear that the baby will not meet some predetermined standard: sex, hair color, temperament, or resemblance to family members
3. Failure to follow through on the desire for or seeking of an abortion
4. An initial decision to place the child for adoption and a change of mind
5. Rejection of the mother by the father of the baby
6. Family experiencing stress and numerous crises so that the birth of a child may be the "straw that broke the camel's back"
7. Initial and unresolved negative feelings about having a child
8. Lack of support for the new parents
9. Isolation from friends, neighbors, or family
10. Parental evidence of poor impulse control or fear of losing control
11. Contradictory history
12. Appearance of detachment
13. Appearance of misusing drugs or alcohol
14. Shopping for hospitals or health care providers
15. Unrealistic expectations of the child
16. Abuse of mother by father, especially during pregnancy
17. Child is not biological offspring of male stepfather or mother's current boyfriend

Many times the community health nurse's role involves helping to monitor a family in which a formerly abused child has been returned after a time in foster care. Keen judgment and close collaboration with social services are necessary in these situations. The nurse must ensure the safety of the child, while working *with* the parents in an empathetic way. The nurse's goal is to enhance their parenting skills, not to be viewed as yet another watchdog.

Another point to keep in mind about abusive parents is that the wish to replace a child who has been removed by the courts because of abuse is a normal response to the grief of losing a child. Rather than regarding another pregnancy as a sign of continued poor judgment or pathological behavior, the pregnancy can be perceived by the community health nurse as an opportunity for intensive intervention to prevent the abuse of the expected child. Generally, the parents are equally eager to avoid further problems if enlisted as partners in the project.

Indicators of Child Abuse. It is essential that community health nurses recognize the physical and behavioral indicators of abuse and neglect. The box on p. 740 summarizes indicators of physical abuse, physical neglect, sexual abuse, and emotional maltreatment. Child abuse ranges from violent physical attacks to passive

Indicators of Actual or Potential Abuse

1. An unexplained injury
   a. Skin: burns, old or recent scars, ecchymosis, soft tissue swelling, human bites
   b. Fractures: recent or ones that have healed
   c. Subdural hematomas
   d. Trauma to genitalia
   e. Whiplash (caused by shaking small children)
2. Dehydration or malnourishment without obvious cause
3. Provision of inappropriate food or drugs (alcohol, tobacco, medication prescribed for someone else, foods not appropriate for the child's age)
4. Evidence of general poor care: poor hygiene, dirty clothes, unkempt hair, dirty nails
5. Unusually fearful of nurse and others
6. Considered to be a "bad" child
7. Inappropriately dressed for the season or weather conditions
8. Reports or shows evidence of sexual abuse
9. Injuries not mentioned in history
10. Seems to need to take care of the parent and speak for the parent
11. Maternal depression
12. Maladjustment of older siblings

neglect. Violence such as beating, burning, kicking, or shaking may often result in severe physical injury. Passive neglect may result in insidious malnutrition or other problems. Abuse is not limited to physical maltreatment but includes emotional abuse such as yelling at or continually demeaning and criticizing the child.

Emotional Abuse. Extreme debasement of feelings may result in the child feeling inadequate, inept, uncared for, and worthless. Victims of emotional abuse learn to hide their feelings to avoid incurring additional scorn. They may act out by performing poorly in school, becoming truant, and being hostile and aggressive.

Physical symptoms of physical, sexual, or emotional stress may include hyperactivity, withdrawal, overeating, dermatological problems, vague physical complaints, stuttering, enuresis (bladder incontinence), and encoporesis (bowel incontinence). It is ironic that bed-wetting is often a trigger for further abuse, which makes for a particularly vicious cycle. When a child displays physical symptoms without clear physiological origin, ruling out the possibilty of abuse should be part of the community health nurse's assessment process.

Child Neglect. The two categories of child neglect are: physical and emotional. **Physical neglect** is defined as failure to provide adequate food, proper clothing, shelter, hygiene, or necessary medical care (Campbell and Humphreys, 1993). Physical neglect is most often associated with extreme poverty.

In contrast, **emotional neglect** is the omission of basic nurturing, acceptance, and caring essential for healthy personal development. These children are largely ignored or in many cases are treated as nonpersons. Such neglect usually affects the development of self-esteem. It is difficult for a neglected child to feel a great deal of self-worth because the parents have not demonstrated that they value the child.

Neglect is much more difficult to assess and evaluate than abuse because it is more subtle and may go unnoticed. Astute observations of children, their homes, and the way in which they relate to their caregivers can provide clues of neglect.

Sexual Abuse. Child abuse also includes sexual abuse. Approximately one of four female children and one of ten males in the United States will be subject to some form of sexual abuse by the time they reach 18 years of age. The exact prevalence is difficult to obtain because developmentally children do not have the cognitive ability to articulate these experiences (Wyatt and Powell, 1988). This abuse ranges from unwanted sexual touching to intercourse. The majority of childhood sexual abuse is perpetrated by someone known to the child. Between one-half and one-third of all sexual abuse involves a family member (Convington, 1989). The long-term effects of sexual abuse are depression, sexual disturbances, and substance abuse (Stein et al., 1988).

Research has shown that many of the characteristics of physically abusive and sexually abusive parents, such as unhappiness, loneliness, and rigidity, are shared by both groups (Milner and Robertson, 1990). However, sexually abusive parents report fewer family problems and a more positive view of the child than do physically abusive parents.

It is estimated that at least 1 girl in 100 is abused sexually by her father or stepfather (Brunngraber, 1986). Many cases of parental **incest** go unreported because victims fear punishment, abandonment, rejection, or family disruption if they acknowledge the problem.

Incest is not limited to "backwoods" people but occurs in all races, religious groups, and socioeconomic classes. Incest is receiving greater attention because of mandatory reporting laws, yet all too often, its incidence remains a family secret.

Because nurses, particularly community health nurses, are often involved in helping women deal with the aftermath of incest, it is crucial to understand the typical patterns and the long-term implications. The most typically encountered case scenario presents as follows. The daughter involved in paternal incest is usually about 11 years of age at the onset and is often the oldest or only daughter. The father seldom uses physical force. He most likely relies on threats, bribes, intimidation, or misrepresentation of moral standards or exploits the daughter's need for human affection (Brunngraber, 1986).

Nurses must be aware of the incidence, signs and symptoms, and psychological and physical trauma of incest. An extensive review of research (Rew, 1989) identified clusters of affective symptoms, including low self-esteem, depression, and intrusive imagery. Somatic symptoms include headaches, eating and sleeping disorders, menstrual problems, and gastrointestinal distress. Other symptoms include difficulties in social situations, especially in forming and maintaining close relationships with men, and behavioral symptoms such as substance abuse and sexual dysfunction.

Adolescents may display inappropriate sexual activity or truancy or may run away from home. Running away is usually considered a sign of delinquency, but community health nurses should be alert to the possibility that an adolescent who runs away is displaying a healthy response to a violent family situation. Therefore assessment should include an inquiry about sexual and physical abuse at home and appropriate intervention.

In their impressive review of the literature on child maltreatment effects, Houck and King (1989) stress that the effects of any kind of child maltreatment can be lessened if the child has a nonoffending parent, another relative, or an adult outside the family to provide stable, ongoing support and emotional nurturance.

Abuse of Female Partners

Although women do abuse men, by far the greatest proportion of what is often discussed as spouse abuse or domestic violence is actually wife abuse. At least 1.8 million women are battered by their husbands each year in the United States (Straus and Gelles, 1990). Neither the term **wife abuse** nor **spouse abuse** takes into account violence in dating or cohabiting relationships. Spousal or partner violence can be used as a more inclusive term to refer to all kinds of violence between partners, and all adults should be assessed for violence in their primary intimate relationships. However, abuse of female partners has the most serious community health ramifications because of the greater prevalence, the greater potential for homicide (Campbell, 1995), the effects on the children in the household, and the more serious long-term emotional and physical consequences.

Victims of child abuse and individuals who witnessed their mothers being battered are at risk of using violence toward an intimate partner, whether one is male or female (Straus and Gelles, 1990). However, using evidence of a violent childhood to identify women at risk of abuse is less useful. Much evidence now suggests that abuse cannot be predicted based on characteristics of the individual woman. It is the violent background of an abusive male, combined with his tendencies to be possessive, controlling, and extremely jealous, that is most predictive of abuse. Substance abuse is also associated with battering, although it cannot be said to "cause" the violence.

Signs of Abuse. Battered women often have bruises and lacerations of the face, head, and trunk of the body. Attacks are often carefully inflicted on parts of the body that can easily be disguised by clothing. This pattern of proximal location of injuries (breasts, abdomen, upper thighs, and back) rather than distal is extremely characteristic of abuse (Campbell and Sheridan, 1989). When a woman has a black eye or bruises about the mouth, the nurse should ask, "Who hit you?" rather than, "What happened to you?" The latter implies that the nurse is not knowledgeable or not comfortable with violence, and this may prompt the woman to fabricate a more acceptable cause of her injury.

Once abused, women tend to exhibit low self-esteem and depression (Campbell, 1989a). They exhibit significantly more physical symptoms of stress than women in troubled relationships and also frequently complain of chronic pain. Both of these symptoms may be related to repeated injuries, as well as to the intense stress of a violent relationship (Campbell, 1989; Campbell and Humphreys, 1993).

Abuse as a Process. Research by both Landenburger (1989) and Campbell et al., (1994) suggests that there is a process of response to battering over time wherein the woman's emotional and behavioral reactions change. At first there is a great need to minimize the seriousness of the situation. The violence usually starts with a slight shove in the middle of a heated argument. All couples fight, and if there is any physical aggression, both the man and woman tend to blame the incident on something external such as a particularly stressful day at work or drinking too much. The male partner usually apologizes for the incident, and as with any problem in a relationship, the couple tries various strategies to improve the situation. Although marital counseling may be useful at this very early stage, it is generally contraindicated at all other stages because of the risk to the woman's safety. Unfortunately, abuse tends to escalate in frequency and severity over time, and the man's remorse tends to lessen (Walker, 1984).

Because women have often been taught to take responsibility for the success of a relationship, they usually go through a period in which they tend to change their behavior to end the violence. They may even blame themselves for infuriating their spouse. Women who blame themselves for provoking the abuse are more likely to have low self-esteem and be depressed than those who do not blame themselves. The majority of battered women do not blame themselves for provoking the abuse, and any self-blame tends to decrease over time (Campbell, 1989a; Frieze, 1983). Women find that no matter what they do, the violence continues. During this period the woman tends to try to hide the violence because of the stigma attached. She tries to placate her spouse and feels she is losing her sense of self (Landenburger, 1989; Ulrich, 1989). Women are also typically very concerned about their children. An abused woman worries about the well-being of her children if she leaves and about their safety if she stays.

Some abuse escalates to the point that the woman is kept in terror, similar to a prisoner of war (Okun, 1986). She is constantly subjected to emotional degradation, absolute financial dependency, sadistic physical and sexual violence, and control of all her activities. She is in terror that her partner will try to kill her, her children, or both if she attempts to leave. This fear is, in fact, often justified. Clinically, she may be suffering from learned helplessness, traumatic stress syndrome, or both and will need intensive therapy. She may kill herself or her abuser to escape because she sees no other way out (Campbell, 1992). A nurse encountering an abusive situation such as this needs to be fairly directive in arranging for the safety of the woman and her children. The woman will need an order of protection, a legal document specifically designed to keep the woman's abuser away from her. She will also need help in getting to a safe place, such as a wife abuse shelter. At the very least, the woman must design a carefully thought-out plan for escape and arrange for a neighbor or an adolescent child to call the police when there is another violent episode.

The more frequently encountered battered woman is one who has tried several times to leave. She will eventually successfully do so or otherwise manage to end the violence (Campbell et al., 1994; Okun, 1986). Each attempt to leave is a gathering of resources, a trial of her children's ability to survive without a father, and a testing of her partner's promises to reform. When and if it becomes clear that he is not going to change and she has the emotional support and the financial resources to do so, she will end the relationship. Often this will involve using a shelter for abused women or individual advocacy and support groups (Bowker, 1983).

An alternative to ending the relationship is the male partner's attendance at programs for batterers. These programs have been shown to be most effective if they are court mandated and if the man's underlying values about women are addressed, as well as his violence (Dutton, 1988; Gondolf and Hanneken, 1987). Abused women need affirmation, support, reassurances of the normalcy of their responses, accurate information about shelters and legal resources, and brainstorming about possible solutions. These needs can be met by other women in similar situations and professionals such as nurses (Campbell et al., 1993). Women should not be pushed into actions they are not ready to take.

After the abuse has ended, a period of recovery ensues. This includes a normal grief response for the relationship that has ended and a search for meaning in the experience (Landenburger, 1989). Thus a formerly battered woman who is feeling depressed and lonely after the relationship has ended is exhibiting a normal response for which support is needed.

Sexual Abuse. Because 40% to 45% of battered women are also sexually abused (Campbell, 1989b), the nurse must carefully assess for this form of violence in women in ongoing relationships. In fact, between 10% and 14% of all American women have been raped within a marriage. This sexual abuse is not always accompanied by physical abuse (Finkelhor and Yllo, 1985).

The notion that men have a right to force their wives to have sex comes from traditional English law that stated that a woman gave irrevocable and perpetual consent to her husband on marriage to have sex whenever and however he wanted. This legal tradition was reflected in the laws of 47 states in the United States as recently as 1980 as a marital rape exemption. In other words, a man could not be charged with rape if the victim was his wife. By 1994 only 7 states still retained this provision, but the fact that it is still legal for a man to rape his wife in any state is alarming. Serious physical and emotional damage has been documented from marital rape (Campbell, 1986b; Campbell and Alford, 1989). There is also an alarming incidence of date rape, the dynamics of which may parallel marital rape.

To assess for sexual assault, the question of "Have you ever been forced into sex you did not wish to participate in?" should be used in all nursing assessments. This will allow for the ascertainment of marital rape, date rape, or rape of a male.

Abuse During Pregnancy. Battering during pregnancy has serious implications for the health of both women and their children. Approximately one of six pregnant women is physically battered during pregnancy, with a larger proportion (20%) of adolescents abused during pregnancy than adult women. Although abuse during pregnancy occurs across ethnic groups, white women experience a significantly higher severity of abuse than black or Hispanic women (McFarlane et al., 1993). These women are at risk for spontaneous abortion, premature delivery, low-birth-weight infants, substance abuse during pregnancy, and depression (Bullock and McFarlane, 1989; Campbell et al., 1992; McFarlane et al., 1994). Abuse before pregnancy was identified as the most important risk factor for abuse during pregnancy.

Generally, the same dynamics of coercive control are operating when a woman is battered during pregnancy. The largest group of one sample of 76 battered women were subject to the same abuse whether or not they were pregnant. About 20% escaped abuse during pregnancy, although they were abused again after the baby was born. Another 35% indicated that their perception of the reason for abuse during pregnancy was that their partner was jealous of or angry at the baby (Campbell et al., 1993). It could be anticipated that this group of infants would be at particularly high risk of child abuse after they are born. The main difference found between women who were battered during pregnancy and those who were not was that those women battered during pregnancy had been battered more frequently and severely previous to their pregnancy (Campbell et al., 1993). The clear implication is that all pregnant women should be assessed for abuse at each prenatal care visit, and postpartum home visits should include assessment for child abuse and partner abuse.

 Research Brief

Parker B, McFarlane J, Soeken K, et al: Physical and emotional abuse in pregnancy: a comparison of adult and teenage women, Nurs Res 42:173-178, 1993.

Nursing Researchers asked 691 black, Hispanic, and white pregnant women about abuse at their first prenatal care visit. A higher percentage (21.7%) of teens said that they were abused during the pregnancy than did the adult women (15.9%). Another 10% of the adolescents were abused before the pregnancy. However, the adult women were more severely emotionally and physically abused than the adolescent women. Since one out of five pregnant adolescents is abused during pregnancy, nurses need to include domestic violence in school health programs and adolescent pregnancy programs, as well as assess *all* pregnant women for abuse.

Abuse of Elderly Persons

Elder abuse is a form of family violence that is only recently being documented and explored. Statistics show that 4% of senior citizens suffer from some form of abuse, neglect, or exploitation (Weith, 1994). Similar to spouse abuse and child abuse, most cases of elder abuse go unreported. As with other forms of human abuse, elder maltreatment includes emotional, sexual, and physical neglect, financial abuse, and violation of rights (Weiner, 1991). In addition, similar to spouse abuse, alcohol abuse is used as an excuse (Anetzberger et al., 1994).

Types of Elder Abuse. The elderly are neglected when others fail to provide adequate food, clothing, shelter, and physical care and to meet physiological, emotional, and safety needs.

Roughness in handling elderly people can lead to bruises and bleeding into body tissues because of the fragility of their skin and vascular systems. It is often difficult to determine if the injuries of elderly persons result from abuse, falls, or other natural causes. Careful assessment both through observation and discussion assists in determining the cause of injuries. Other ways in which elderly persons are physically abused occur when caregivers impose unrealistic toileting demands and when the special needs and previous living patterns of the elderly person are ignored.

Elderly persons can also be abused with regard to nutrition. They may be given food that they cannot chew or swallow or that is contraindicated because of dietary restrictions. Caregivers may overlook food preferences or social or cultural beliefs and patterns

about food. Elderly people may become undernourished if they can neither prepare their own food nor eat the food that is prepared for them.

Caregivers occasionally give elderly people medication to induce confusion or drowsiness so that they will be less troublesome, will need less care, or will allow others to gain control of their financial and personal resources. Once medicated, elderly persons have few ways to act on their own behalf.

The most common form of psychological abuse is rejection or simply ignoring elderly people. This kind of treatment conveys that they are worthless and useless to others. Elderly persons may subsequently regress and become increasingly dependent on others, who tend to resent the imposition and demands on their time and life-styles. The pattern becomes cyclical: the more regressed the person becomes, the greater the dependence. Further, the elderly people's past accomplishments and present abilities are not consistently acknowledged, causing them to feel even less capable. Indicators of actual or potential elder abuse are listed in the box below.

Precipitating Factors for Elder Abuse. Caregivers abuse elderly people for a variety of reasons. Elderly family members may impose a physical, emotional, or financial burden on the caregiver, leading to frustration and resentment. The abuser may be reversing earlier family patterns, whereby the abuser was previously abused by the elderly person (Anetzberger et al., 1994).

Many persons tend to think of abused elderly individuals as dependent on others for their care. A factor that increases the risk of elder abuse is the dependency of a significant other on the elderly person (Lang, 1993). The single most important risk factor was that the abuser had a history of violence (Pillemer and Finkelhor, 1988). In addition, a significant pro-

 Indicators of Potential or Actual Elder Abuse

Unexplained or repeated injury
Fear of the caregiver
Untreated sores or other skin injuries, such as decubitus ulcers, excoriated perineum, burns
Overall poor care (e.g., unclean, given inappropriate food)
Withdrawal and passivity
Periods of time when elderly person is unsupervised
Failure to seek appropriate medical care
Contractures resulting from immobility or restraint
Unwillingness or inability of caregiver to meet elderly person's needs
Improper home repair
Unsafe home situation (e.g., poor heating, ventilation, dangerous clutter)

Modified from Phillips LR: J Adv Nurs 8:379, 1983; and Ferguson D, Beck C: Geriatr Nurs 4:301, 1983.

portion of female abused elderly persons are battered women who have become old. Thus, although it is important to assess for elder abuse when the elderly person is in need of care from family members, all elderly persons should be assessed for abuse.

A subgroup particularly vulnerable to abuse are confused and frail elderly persons. Large numbers of frail elderly people, many with serious physical or mental impairments, live in the community and are cared for by their families. Recent research indicates that individuals with Alzheimer's disease and other dementias have a greater risk for physical abuse than elderly persons with other illnesses. These illnesses resulted in a high burden on the caregiver and subsequent depression of the caregiver (Coyne et al., 1993). Living with and providing care to a confused elderly person are difficult, round-the-clock tasks that often exhaust family members. Family stress increases as members must work harder to fulfill their other responsibilities in addition to the needs of the elderly person.

Prevention Strategies. Fulmer (1989) suggests the following prevention strategies for communities: (1) develop new ways to provide assistance to caregiving families, including helping them with decisions about discontinuing caregiving at home; (2) publicize existing supports for caregiving families; and (3) involve all community organizations in developing new supports and training, such as Neighborhood Watch programs for families with elderly persons. In addition, community health nurses must help families who are contemplating taking care of an elderly member at home to fully evaluate that decision and prepare for the stressors that will be involved. A plan for regular respite care for the elderly person is absolutely necessary. Strategies for the primary and secondary prevention of abuse of elderly persons include victim support groups, senior advocacy volunteer programs, and training for providers working with elderly persons (Wolf et al., 1994).

Elderly people need to retain as much autonomy and decision-making ability as possible. Community health nurses have multiple avenues for detecting abuse among elderly persons and have skills and responsibility for discovering abuse, giving treatment, and making referrals. Many families who care for elderly members exhaust their resources and coping ability. Community health nurses can assist in finding new sources of support and aid.

COMMUNITY HEALTH NURSING INTERVENTION
Primary Prevention

To prevent violence and human abuse, a community approach is essential. First, the community can take a stand against violence and make sure their elected officials and the local media are clear that nonviolence is a priority in their area. In their roles as community advocates, nurses can help with this process. In the legislative arena, laws are needed to outlaw physical punishment in schools and marital rape. State laws are needed to enforce mandatory arrest for abusers, which has been shown to decrease repeat offenses, at least for men who are employed (Edleson and Tolman, 1992).

Cultural analysis of family violence suggests that strong community sanctions against violence in the home are effective in keeping abuse levels low (Counts et al., 1991; Levinson, 1989). Neighbors keeping an eye out and working together to address problems in other families is not an invasion of privacy but a sign of community cohesiveness. Nurses need to work with advocate groups to make sure police deal with assault within marriage as swiftly, surely, and severely as assault between strangers (Carmody and Williams, 1987). Nurses can encourage others to interfere when they see children beaten in a grocery store, notice that an elderly person is not being properly cared for, see a neighborhood bully beat up his classmates, or hear a neighbor hitting his wife.

Second, persons can take measures to reduce their vulnerability to violence by improving the physical security of their homes and learning personal defense measures. Community health nurses can encourage people to keep windows and doors locked, trim shrubs around their homes, and keep lights on during high-crime periods. Many neighborhoods organize crime watch programs, posting signs to that effect, in addition to signs indicating that certain homes will assist children who need help; these homes are identified by the sign of a hand, usually posted in a window. Other neighbors informally agree to monitor one another's property and safety. Also, many law enforcement agencies evaluate homes for security and teach individual or neighborhood safety programs. Individuals install home security systems, participate in personal defense programs such as judo or karate, and purchase firearms for their protection.

Unfortunately, handguns are far more likely to kill family members than intruders (Kellerman and Reay, 1986). Accidental firearm death is a leading cause of death for young children, and handguns kept in the home are unfortunately easy to use in moments of extreme anger with other family members or extreme depression. The majority of homicides between family members and most suicides involve a handgun. All community health nursing assessments should include a question about guns kept in the home, and the family should be made aware of the risk that a handgun holds for family members. If the family feels that keeping a gun is necessary, safety measures should be taught, such as keeping the gun unloaded and in a locked compartment, keeping the ammunition separate from the gun and also locked away, and instructing children about the dangers of firearms. Lobbying for handgun-control laws is a primary prevention effort that would significantly decrease the rate of death and serious injury caused by handguns in the United States.

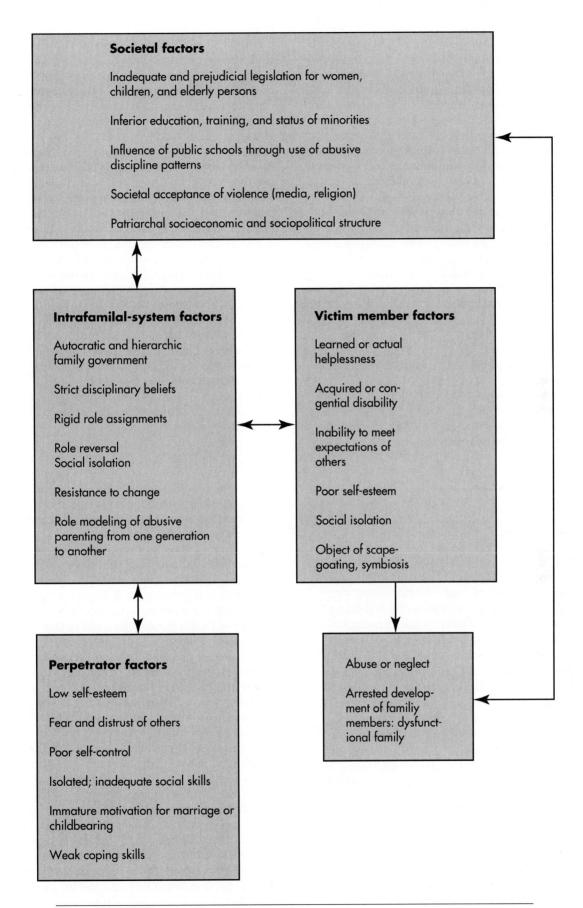

FIGURE 38-1

Factors to include when assessing an individual's or family's potential for violence.

Assessment for Risk Factors

Identification of risk factors is an important part of primary prevention. Although abuse cannot be predicted with certainty, a variety of factors tend to influence the onset and support the continuation of abusive patterns. Community health nurses are in an excellent position to identify potential victims of abuse because these nurses see clients in a wide variety of settings.

Factors to include in an assessment of an individual or family's potential for violence are categorized by Logan and Dawkins (1986) as illustrated in Figure 38-1.

The nurse must also be able to identify "red-flag" antisocial behaviors that might lead to abusive patterns. According to Klingbeil (1986), high-risk categories of behavior include the following:

1. Psychiatric diagnosis such as depression
2. Pattern of substance abuse
3. Loss and grief after death of a loved one
4. Isolation
5. Lack of support system
6. Homelessness
7. Previous history of assaultive or suicidal behavior
8. Chronic unemployment
9. Presence or use of weapons; previous arrests
10. History of runaways
11. Single-care auto accidents
12. Psychosomatic complaints

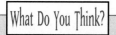

What Do You Think?

Most experts on violence agree that all women entering the health care system should be asked about domestic violence and sexual assault experience; yet men are also victimized by violence, even though little is known about their responses to such experiences. Some experts feel that health care professionals should be asking men if they are perpetrators of violence as a secondary prevention activity, reasoning that if identified early, such behavior may be more amenable to interventions. Others are concerned that since we are not sure what health care system interventions are most effective for male perpetrators or victims of violence, it is premature to do routine screening. There is also some concern that perpetrators of domestic violence or child abuse may become angry if asked about their violent behavior and retaliate against the family member.

Individual and Family Strategies for Primary Prevention

Primary prevention of abuse includes strengthening individuals and families so they can cope more effectively with multiple life stressors and demands and reducing the destructive elements in the community that support and encourage the use of human violence. In their work in schools, community groups, employee groups, day-care centers, and other community institutions, nurses can foster healthy developmental patterns and identify signs of potential abuse.

Many clinicians believe that providing support and psychological enrichment to at-risk individuals and families prevents the onset of health disruption. For example, community health nurses have varied opportunities to strengthen and even teach parenting abilities. Basic skills such as diapering, feeding, quieting, and even holding and rocking a baby can be the focus of a class or home or clinic visit. Parents also need to learn acceptable and workable ways to discipline children so that limits are maintained without causing the child emotional or physical harm.

Mutual support groups are valuable for new parents, families with special children, or abused people themselves. Such groups have variable formats and can provide information, support, and encouragement. Nurses can help begin such groups or can actually serve as group leaders. Chapter 23 describes the role of the community health nurse in working with community groups.

Secondary Prevention

When abuse occurs, community health nurses can initiate measures to reduce or terminate further abuse. Both developmental and situational *crises* present opportunities for abusive situations to develop. The occurrence of violence represents a family crisis and should be handled using the crisis intervention strategies.

Nursing intervention is directed toward helping participants discuss the problem and seek alternatives for dealing with the tension that led to the abusive situation. Injured persons must be temporarily or permanently placed in a safe location. Secondary preventive measures are most useful when potential abusers recognize their tendency to be abusive and seek help. For children, there is often a need for 24-hour child protection services or caregivers who can take care of the child until the acute family or individual crisis has been resolved. Respite care is extremely important in families with frail elderly members. Telephone crisis lines can be used to provide immediate emergency assistance to families.

Effective *communication* with abusive families is important. Typically, these families are not eager to discuss their problems. Many members of such families are embarrassed to be involved in an abusive situation. Often considerable guilt is involved. Effective communication must be preceded by an attitude of acceptance. It is often difficult for nurses to value the worth of an individual who willfully abuses another. The behavior, not the person, must be condemned. The nurse must radiate caring, acceptance, understanding, compassion, and a nonjudgmental attitude.

Additionally, families do not always know how to have fun. Nurses can assess how much recreation is integrated into the family's life-style. Through community assessment, the nurse will know what resources and facilities are available and how much they cost. Families may need counseling about the value of recreation and play in reducing tension and appropriately channelling aggressive impulses.

Tertiary Prevention: Therapeutic Intervention with Abusive Families

It is extremely difficult to form a trusting relationship with abusive families, but the community health nurse is often in a key position to act as case manager, coordinating the other agencies and activities involved. Principles of giving care to families who are experiencing violence include the following: (1) intolerance for violence, (2) respect and caring for all family members, (3) safety as the first priority, (4) absolute honesty, and (5) **empowerment.** Nurses must clearly indicate that any further violence, degradation, and exploitation of family members will not be tolerated, but that all family members are respected, valued human beings. However, everyone must understand that the safety of every family member is the first priority.

Abusers often fear they will be condemned for their actions, so it is often difficult to make and maintain contact with abusive families. Although community health nurses convey an attitude of caring and concern for them, families may doubt the sincerity of this concern. They may avoid being home at the scheduled visit time out of fear of the consequences of the visit or an inability to believe that anyone really wants to help them. If the victim is a child, parents may fear that the nurse will try to remove the child.

Nurses are mandatory reporters of child abuse, even when only suspected, in all states. They are also mandatory reporters of elder abuse and abuse of other physically and cognitively dependent adults in most states. The mandatory reporting laws also protect reporters from legal action on cases that are never substantiated. Even so, physicians and nurses are sometimes reluctant to report abuse. They may be more willing to report abuse in a poor family than in a middle-class one, or they may think that an elderly person or child is better off at home than in a nursing home or foster home. Referral to protective service agencies should be viewed as enlisting another source of help, rather than an automatic step toward removal of the victim or criminal justice action. This same attitude can be communicated to families so that reporting is done *with* families rather than without their knowledge and prior input. Absolute honesty about what will be reported to officials, what the family can expect, what the nurse is entering into records, and what the nurse is feeling is essential.

To further empower the family, the nurse needs to recognize and capitalize on the violent family's strengths, as well as to assess and deal with its problems. The nurse must use a nurse-family partnership rather than a paternalistic or authoritarian approach. The family is generally capable of generating many of its own solutions, which will be much more culturally appropriate and individualized than those the nurse may generate. Victims of direct attack need information about their options and resources and reassurance that abuse is unfortunately rather common and that they are not alone in their dilemma. They also need reassurance that their responses are normal and that they do not deserve to be abused. Continued support for their decisions must be coupled with nursing actions to ensure their safety.

Nursing Actions

The community health nurse can meet the family's therapeutic needs in a variety of ways. Beside referral to appropriate community agencies, nurses can act as role models for the family. During clinic and home visits, nurses can demonstrate constructive adult-child interactions. Nurses often teach mothers child-care skills such as proper feeding, calming a fretful child, effective discipline, and constructive communication.

Nurses can demonstrate good communication skills and discipline by teaching both parents and children in a calm, respectful, and informative manner. Caregivers, especially those caring for children, handicapped people, or elderly persons, may need to learn age-appropriate expectations. It is unreasonable to expect a 14-month-old infant to be able to differentiate between what is right and wrong. Children at this age do not deliberately annoy caregivers by breaking delicate pieces of china. Likewise, a person with poor sphincter control does not willingly soil clothes or bedding.

Role modeling can be used with abuse victims of all ages. When providing nursing care to abused spouses or to elderly persons, nurses can demonstrate communication skills, conflict resolution, and skill training. For example, adult children often become abusive toward their parents when they become frustrated and taxed in their abilities to care for the elderly person. During home visits, nurses can demonstrate ways to physically and psychologically care for family members. The nurse can work with caregivers to help them develop approaches that are acceptable to the individual elderly person. Assessment, creativity, and critical thinking help the nurse, family, and client devise ways together of meeting client and family needs, without causing undue stress and frustration.

The emotional investment and sheer drain of energy required to effectively work with abusers and victims of abuse cannot be disregarded. Abusers present difficult clinical challenges because of their reluctance to seek help or to remain actively involved in the helping process.

Referral is an important component of tertiary prevention. Community health nurses should know about available community resources for abuse victims and perpetrators (see box on p. 748 for a list of common

Common Community Services

Child protective services
Child abuse prevention programs
Adult protective services
Parents Anonymous
Wife abuse shelter
   Program for children of battered women
   Community support group
   24-Hour hotline
   Legal advocacy or information
Stat coalition against domestic violence
Batterer treatment
Victim assistance programs
Sexual assault programs

community services). If attitudes and resources are inadequate, it is often helpful to work with local radio and television stations and newspapers to provide information about the nature and extent of human abuse as a community health problem. This also helps to acquaint people with available services and resources. Frequently, people fail to seek services early in an abusive situation because they simply do not know what is available to them. Ideally, a program or planned emphasis for abused people begins with a needs assessment to identify potential clients and to determine how to effectively serve this group. Community health nurses serve as catalysts for getting programs started and as a major source of public education.

Nursing Interventions Specific to Female Partner Abuse

Although women in abusive relationships seek care through a variety of means and their entry into health care can be from any point in a system, it is more likely that if a woman seeks care for injuries, it will be in an emergency setting, a private physician's office, or a prenatal clinic (Tilden, 1989). Generally, these women are seeking assistance for injuries sustained during physically abusive episodes (Tilden and Shepard, 1987). Although abused women are most likely to enter the health care system via the emergency department, there is a widespread lack of recognition of battering by health personnel. Despite the overall incidence of battering and its resultant physical and emotional health problems for women, health professionals fail to identify abused women, use derogatory labeling, and are generally seen as judgmental, insensitive, and less effective and helpful than agencies who have personnel trained to deal with the needs of battered women.

Because of the stigma involved, women and health care providers are often reluctant to initiate discussion about abuse. However, the majority of battered women say they would have liked to talk about the issue with a health care professional if they were asked (Campbell and Humphreys, 1993). Because abuse is often insidious, starting with minor psychological abuse and building to more severe physical incidents,

it often remains unrecognized by victims and health care providers alike until a severe episode forces attention on the situation. Stigma and inadequate assessment lead to women continually seeking care with the problem being virtually unmentioned.

It has been suggested that the quality of health care that a battered woman receives often determines whether she follows through with referrals to legal, social service, and health care agencies. Within emergency departments alone, at least 18% of women presenting with trauma have been abused (Tilden, 1989). Care in the emergency department is often fragmented and necessarily oriented toward life and death situations. Therefore women are not adequately assessed, and thus they receive little or no emotional support or intervention specific to their needs. It can be surmised that the cost to the health care system is phenomenal with little or no positive outcome. A cycle persists in which women seek care and receive either no interventions or interventions that are grossly ineffective. This cycle perpetuates feelings of anger and inadequacy within health care providers, resulting in blame placed on women for their lack of compliance to remedies offered.

Many battered women are reluctant to identify themselves as victims of domestic violence for a number of complex reasons, such as fear that revelation will further jeopardize their safety, increase their sense of shame and humiliation, and minimize the repetitive or serious nature of the violence. This hesitation to speak out often makes it very difficult for the emergency department staff to identify the battered woman. In addition, the very nature of the systems in which victims of violence introduce themselves during crisis can be barriers. Emergency departments, shelters, and health departments are busy places. Staff members are working hard to maintain the functioning of these facilities, and the reality is they may not want to be "kept from their work" by completing data collection tools. Sometimes it is difficult in this often chaotic setting for staff members to realize that they may be the first or only health provider to recognize violence in their clients' lives (Senter, 1993).

Studies have found that only a small percentage of battered women in emergency department settings were identified and treated, despite the reality that the prevalence of domestic violence in emergency department populations has been demonstrated to be between 22% and 35% of all women presenting with physical trauma (Campbell and Sheridan, 1989).

Battered women present for treatment in a number of ways. If they present with injuries, they may not ascribe these injuries to a battery. If they do say, for example, that they were beaten, kicked, or stabbed, they may be reluctant to reveal their relationship to the assailant. Battered women may present with psychosomatic complaints related to the chronic stress of living in an abusive situation. They may be unaware of the relationship of their symptoms to the violence in their lives. For the battered woman and the emergency department staff to begin to make the connection between like situations and her presenting complaints, the staff needs to ask direct questions in a supportive, open, and concerned manner (King and Ryan, 1989).

Assessment. Assessment for all forms of violence against women should take place for all women entering the health care system. The assessment should be ongoing and stress confidentiality. A thorough assessment gathers information on physical, emotional, and sexual trauma from violence, risk for future abuse, cultural background and beliefs, perceptions of the woman's relationships with others, and stated needs. The assessment should be conducted in private. Other adults who are present should be directed to the waiting area and told that it is policy that initially women are seen alone. Women should be asked directly if they were in an abusive relationship as a child or are currently in an abusive relationship as an adult. They should also be asked if they have ever been forced into sex that they did not wish to participate in. Shame and fear often make disclosure difficult. Verbal acknowledgment of the situation and emotional and physical support assist women in talking about past or current circumstances.

Women can be categorized into three groups: no, low, or moderate to high risk. Women with no signs of current or past abuse are considered at no risk. At the initial assessment a woman may hesitate to speak of concerns she has. Future visits should include questioning a woman about whether there have been any changes in her life or whether she has additional information or questions about topics discussed at previous visits.

Women at low risk show no evidence of recent or current abuse. Education that helps a woman gain perspective on her situation and her needs should be discussed. Resource materials including group and individual formats can be suggested. The risk level should be recorded, and preventive measures and teaching should be documented.

Assessment of moderate to high risk includes evaluation of a woman's fear for both psychological and physical abuse. Lethality potential should be assessed (Campbell, 1995). Risk factors for lethality include behaviors such as stalking or frequent harassment, threats or an escalation of threats, use of weapons or threats with weapons, excessive control and jealousy, and public use of violence. Statements from an abuser such as "If I can't have you, no one can" should be taken seriously. In all cases a history of abuse and alcohol and drug use should be collected and carefully documented. The determined risk level should also be documented along with any past or present physical evidence of abuse from prior or current assault; this evidence should be photographed, shown on a body map, or described narratively. It is important that the assailant be identified in the record; this can take the form of either quotes from the woman or subjective information. These records can be very important for women in future assault or child custody cases, even if the woman is not ready to make a police report at the present time.

Immediate care for a woman in a potentially harmful or present abusive situation involves the development of a safety plan. A woman can be assisted to look at the options available to her. Shelter information, access to counseling, and legal resources should be discussed. If a woman wants to return to her partner, she can be helped in the development of plans that can be carried out if the abuse continues or becomes more serious.

Whenever there is evidence of sexual assault within the prior 24 to 48 hours, a rape kit examination should be performed. Lists of resources such as rape crises clinics and support groups for survivors of physical and emotional abuse should be made available.

Prevention. Prevention, public policy, and social attitudes are intertwined. Our society has taken a major step toward the secondary prevention of abuse through the establishment of programs that encourage women and children to speak about their experiences. Nurses need to support these programs further by believing the experiences they are told. In the development of laws that punish child and woman abuse, society has given some support to the victims of abuse, but often the very victims are again victimized by disbelief of their experiences, the devaluing of the effects of these assaults on their persons, and a focus on assisting the perpetrators of the crimes. Primary prevention should encompass a total attitudinal change within the values of society. Both girls and boys need to be taught human values of interdependence, respect for human life, and a commitment to empathy and strength in the development of the human species regardless of gender, race, or socioeconomic status. We must urge continued progress toward eliminating the feminization of poverty and ensuring gender parity in economic resources. In addition, local communities must make it clear that violence against women is not tolerated by eliminating pornography, mandating arrests of abusers, and creating a general climate of nonviolence.

Abused women need assistance in making decisions and taking control of their lives. Community health, prenatal, planned parenthood, primary care, and emergency department nurses are involved with women at key times when they can be screened for the presence or absence of abuse. Mechanisms for screening women who are either abused or at risk for abuse are available (Campbell and Sheridan, 1989; McFarlane, 1993; McFarlane et al., 1991). To intervene effectively, nurses must understand abuse as a cumulative process that must be examined as a continuum within the context of a relationship (Landenburger, 1989). During this process the abuse, the relationship, and a woman's view of self change, requiring time-specific interventions. Research indicates that women are often given blame and responsibility for the abuse inflicted on them by their male partners (Landenburger, 1993). Subsequently women are either assisted in a way that discounts their feelings and further devalues them, or the abuse is ignored.

Significance. Nurses in all health settings must become actively involved in identifying women at risk for abuse. Abuse often begins or escalates at the time of family transitions or crises (Campbell and Humphreys, 1993). In planned parenthood clinics, prenatal care settings, primary care, and hospital emergency departments, it should be a routine practice to assess all women for signs and symptoms (Campbell and Sheridan, 1989). If necessary, women should be offered information from which they can learn more about abusive relationships and available resources. Efforts must center not only in helping a woman to make decisions about her relationship but also in developing safety plans for when the abuse takes place and in conveying to the woman the effects of an abusive environment on her children. Women need to understand the criminal justice options open to them, such as orders of protection and court-mandated batterer treatment. Understanding the experiences of women over time can assist in the assessment and identification of the needs of women, leading to more effective health care interventions to meet these needs. It may be that women's responses to abuse are sufficiently different because of socioeconomic status, patterns of living and environment, or cultural background and beliefs. For that reason, the models currently being used for intervention may not be helpful to all battered women.

Strategies Addressing Education for Health Professionals. A variety of strategies have been reported that address the knowledge deficit of health practitioners on abuse issues. The National March of Dimes Birth Defects Foundation has sponsored a variety of train-ing sessions for health professionals and produced several audiovisual tape and slide productions that address violence against women and battering during pregnancy (McFarlane, 1989; Helton et al., 1987).

Helton et al. (1987) report that 6 months after receiving 20 hours (2 1/2 days) of training, 75% of the 841 health professionals who participated in the course were routinely assessing for battering during pregnancy or were in the process of developing an assessment protocol within their practices. Tilden and Shepard (1987) instituted a battered women identification training program for emergency department personnel in a large urbal medical center and reported that the incidence of recorded positive histories of adult family violence rose from 9.72% before training to 22.97% after the education program and implementation of an interview protocol.

After inception of a hospital-based family violence program housed in an urban emergency department, Sheridan et al. (1985) demonstrated that the number of positive and probable battered women rose from 242 in 1986 to 337 in 1987, approximately a 40% increase in identification. The program included ongoing in-service training of all emergency department personnel including nonmedical support staff (i.e., unit secretaries, housekeepers, and security guards), as well as daily chart audits and telephone follow-up calls.

Clinical Application

Mrs. Smith, a 75-year-old bedridden woman, consistently became rude and combative when her daughter, Mary, attempted to bathe her and change her clothes each morning. During a home visit, Mary told the nurse, Mrs. Jones, that she had gotten so frustrated with her mother on the previous morning that she had hit her. Mary felt terrible about her behavior. She stressed that her mother's incontinence made it essential that she be kept clean; her clothes had to be changed every day for her own safety and physical well-being.

Mrs. Jones, in taking Mrs. Smith's vital signs and examining her skin turgor, engaged her in a conversation. She learned that Mrs. Smith felt stiff and seemed to have more joint pain from her arthritis in the mornings. By late afternoon, her joints were more flexible and less painful. Nurse, daughter, and client discussed their options and decided that Mary would wash only her mother's anal area in the morning and put clean pads under her if indicated. Total hygienic care would be done in the late afternoon.

Mrs. Jones demonstrated to Mary alternative ways to move, turn, and wash her mother to minimize the strain on her arthritic joints and to incorporate some effective exercise into the bath. They also decided that, on two mornings each week, a home health care aide would be employed to stay with Mrs. Smith. Mary could then do family shopping and errands and participate in activities in which she had previously been involved.

Nursing intervention was based on the principles introduced earlier. The nurse listened carefully to the pain and anguish the daughter felt about hitting her mother. She conveyed a nonjudgmental attitude and helped the daughter and mother explore ways in which both of their needs could be more effectively met. She provided information and resources to allow the daughter some respite from constant caretaking and a way to continue her own activities. The nurse also taught her ways to improve her mother's physical care. Mrs. Jones will need to monitor the situation carefully for any further signs of abuse. Any further instance of violence must be discussed with the daugher and immediately reported. In a subsequent visit, the nurse evaluated the effectiveness of her teaching and learned that Mary and her mother were working much more cooperatively on Mrs. Smith's care.

Key Concepts

- Violence and human abuse are not new phenomena, but they have increasingly become community health concerns.
- Communities throughout the United States are voicing anger and frustration about increasing levels of violence.
- The community health nurse is in a position to evaluate and intervene in incidents of community and family violence; to intervene effectively, the community health nurse must understand the dynamics of violence and human abuse.
- Factors influencing social and community violence include changing social conditions, economic conditions, population density, community facilities, and institutions within a community, such as organized religion, education, the mass communication media, and work.
- The potential for violence against individuals or against oneself is directly related to the level of violence in the community. Identification and correction of factors affecting the level of violence in the community constitute one way of reducing violence against family members and other individuals.

- Violence and abuse of family members can happen to any family member: spouse, elderly person, child, or developmentally disabled person.
- People who abuse family members are often persons who were themselves abused and who react poorly to real or perceived crises. Other factors that characterize the abuser are the way the person was raised and the unique character of that person.
- Child abuse can be physical, emotional, or sexual. Incest is a common and particularly destructive form of child abuse.
- Spouse abuse is usually wife abuse. It involves physical, emotional, and, frequently, sexual abuse within a context of coercive control. It usually increases in severity and frequency and can escalate to homicide of either partner.
- Community health nurses are in an excellent position to identify potential victims of family abuse because they see clients in a variety of settings, such as schools, businesses, homes, and clinics. Treatment of family abuse includes primary, secondary, and tertiary prevention and therapeutic intervention.

Critical Thinking Activities

1. For 1 week keep a log or diary related to violence.
   a. Make a note of each time you feel as though you are losing your temper. Consider what it might take to cause you to react in a violent way.
   b. Think back; when was the last time you had a violent outburst? What precipitated it? What were your thoughts? What were your feelings? How might you have handled the situation or those feelings without reacting in a violent way?
   c. During this same week make note of the episodes of violent behaviors you observe. For example, do parents hit children in the supermarket? What seems to precipitate such outbursts? What alternatives might exist for reacting in a less violent way?
2. If you learned, after a careful assessment of your community, that family violence is a significant community health problem, what plan of action might you take to intervene? Remember that the goal is to promote health; outline a plan of action with objec-

   tives, timetables, implementation strategies, and evaluation plans for intervening in family violence in your community.
3. Complete a partial community assessment to determine the actual incidence and types of violence in your community.
4. What resources are available in your community for victims of violence? Interview a person who works in an agency that seeks to aid victims of violence. What is the role of the agency? Do its services seem adequate? Who is eligible? Is there a waiting list? What is the fee scale?
5. Cut out all stories about violence in your local newspaper every day for 2 weeks. Note the patterns. Is the majority of the violence perpetrated by strangers or family members? How are the victims portrayed? What kinds of families are involved? What kinds of stories and families get front page treatment rather than a few lines in the back of the paper?

Bibliography

Anetzberger GJ, Korbin JE, Austin: Alcoholism and elder abuse, *Journal of Interpersonal Violence* 9(2):184, 1994.

Bachman R: *Violence against women: a national crime victimization survey report*, Washington, DC, 1994, US Department of Justice, Office of Justice Programs, Bureau of Justice Statistics.

Baron LS, Straus MA, Jaffee D: Legitimate violence, violent attitudes, and rape: a test of the cultural spillover theory, *Ann NY Acad Sci* 528:80, 1988.

Bowker LH: *Beating wife-beating*, Lexington, Mass, 1983, Lexington Books.

Brunngraber BS: Father-daughter incest: immediate and long-term effects of sexual abuse, *ANS* 8(4):15, 1986.

Bullock L, McFarlane J: Higher prevalence of low birthweight infants born to battered women, *Am J Nurs* 89(9):1153, 1989.

Burgess A, Holmstrum L: *Rape: crisis and recovery*, Bowie, Md, 1979, Brady.

Campbell, JC: *Assessing dangerousness: potential for further violence of sexual offenders*, Newbury Park, Calif, 1995, Sage.

Campbell JC: A test of two explanatory models of women's responses to battering, *Nurs Res* 38(1):18, 1989a.

Campbell, JC: Battered woman syndrome: a critical review, *Violence update* 1(4):1, 1990.

Campbell JC: Women's responses to sexual abuse in intimate relationships, *Health Care Women Int* 10:335, 1989b.

Campbell JC: "If I can't have you, no one can": homicide in intimate relationships. In Radford J, Russell DEH, editors: *Femicide: the politics of woman killing*, Boston, 1992, Twayne Publishers.

Campbell JC: In Sampselle CM, editor: *Violence against women: nursing research, education, and practice issues*, Washington, DC, 1991b, Hemisphere Publishing.

Campbell JC, Alford P: The dark consequences of marital rape, *Am J Nurs* 89:946, 1989.

Campbell JC, Humphreys J: *Nursing care of survivors of family violence*, St Louis, 1993, Mosby.

Campbell JC, Miller P, Cardwell MM, Belknap RP: Relationship status of battered women over time, *J Fam Viol* 9:99, 1994.

Campbell JC, Oliver C, Bullock L: Why battering during pregnancy? *AWHONN's Clinical Issues in Perinatal and Women's Health Nursing*, 4(3):343-349, 1993.

Campbell JC, Poland M, Waller J, Ayer T: Correlates of battering during pregnancy, *Res Nurs and Health* 15:219, 1992.

Campbell JC, Sheridan DJ: Clinical articles: emergency nursing interventions with battered women, *J Emerg Nurs* 15(1):12, 1989.

Campbell J, Smith McKenna L, Torres S, Sheridan D, Landenburger K: Nursing care of abused women. In Campbell J: Humphreys J editors: *Nursing care of survivors of family violence*, St. Louis, 1993, Mosby, pp 248-289.

Carmody DC, Williams KR: Wife assault and the perceptions of sanctions, *Violence Victims* 2(1):25, 1987.

Counts D, Brown J, Campbell J: *Sanctions and sanctuary*, Boulder, Col, 1991, Westview Press.

Covington CH: Incest: the psychological problem and the biological contradiction, *Issues Ment Health Nurs* 10:69, 1989.

Coyne AC, Reichman WR, Berbig LJ: The relationship between dementia and elder abuse, *Am J Psychiatry* 150(4):643, 1993.

Dietz P: Social factors in rapist behavior. In Roda R, editor: *Clinical aspects of the rapist*, New York, 1978, Grune & Stratton.

Dinitto DM, et al: Nurses conduct the rape kit examination, *Response* 10(2):10, 1987.

Dutton DG: *The domestic assault of women*, Newton, Mass, 1988, Allyn & Bacon.

Edleson JL, Tolman RM: *Intervention for men who batter*, Newbury Park, Calif, 1992, Sage.

Eggert LL, Thompson EA, Herting JR, Nicholas LJ: Prevention research program: reconnecting at-risk youth, *Issues Meut Health Nurs* 15(2):107-135, 1994.

Elder abuse, Washington DC, 1980, National Clearing House on Aging.

Finkelhor D, Yllo K: *License to rape: sexual abuse of wives*, New York, 1985, The Free Press.

Frieze IR: Investigating the causes and consequences of marital rape, *J Women Culture Soc* 8(3):532, 1983.

Fulmer T: Mistreatment of elders, assessment, diagnosis, and intervention, *Nurs Clin North Am* 24(3):707, 1989.

Gelles R, Conte J: Domestic violence and sexual abuse of children: a review of research in the eighties, *J Marriage Fam* 52(4):1045, 1990.

Gondolf EW, Hanneken J: The gender warrior: reformed batterers on abuse, treatment, and change, *J Fam Violence* 2(2):177, 1987.

Hawkins DF: Inequality, culture, and interpersonal violence, *Health Affairs* 12(4):80-95, 1993.

Healthy People 2000: national health promotion and disease prevention objectives, Washington, DC, 1991, USDHHS, Public Health Service.

Helton AS, McFarlane J, Anderson ET: Battered and pregnant: a prevalence study, *Am J Pub Health* 77(10):1337, 1987.

Helton A, McFarlane J, Anderson E: Prevention of battering during pregnancy: focus on behavioral change, *Public Health Nurs* 4(3):166-174, 1987.

Hernandez JT, Lodico M, DiClemente RJ: The effects of child abuse and race on risk taking in male adolescents, *J Natl Med Assoc* 85(8):593-7, 1993.

Hotaling GT, Sugarman DD: An analysis of risk markers in husband to wife violence: the current state of knowledge, *Violence Vict* 1(20):101, 1986.

Houck GM, King MC: Child maltreatment: family characteristics and developmental consequences, *Issues Ment Health Nurs* 10:193, 1989.

Kempe CH et al: The battered child syndrome, *JAMA* 181:17, 1962.

Kellermann AL, Reay DT: Protection or peril? an analysis of firearm-related deaths in the home, *N Engl J Med* 314(24):1557, 1986.

King M, Ryan J: Abused women: Dispelling myths and encouraging intervention, *Nurse Pract*, 14:47-58, 1989.

Klingbeil K: Interpersonal violence: a comprehensive model in a hospital setting—from policy to program. In *The Surgeon General's workshop on violence and public health report*. DHHS Pub No HRS-D-MC 86-1, Washington DC, 1986, Health Resources and Services Administration, US Public Health Service, US Department of Health and Human Services.

Koss MP, Harvey MR: *The rape victim: clinical and community intervention*, 2nd ed. Newbury Park, Calif, 1991, Sage.

Landenburger K: A process of entrapment in and recovery from an abusive relationship, *Issues Ment Health Nurs* 10:209, 1989.

Lang SS: Finding refute traditional views on elder abuse, *Human Ecology Forum* 21(3):30, 1993.

Lenehan G, Bowie S, Ruksnaitis N: Rape victim protocol and chart for use in emergency department, *J Emerg Nurs* 9:83, 1983.

Levinson D: *Family violence in cross-cultural perspective*, Newbury Park, Calif, 1989, Sage.

Logan BB, Dawkins CE: *Family-centered nursing in the community*, Menlo Park, Calif, 1986, Addison-Wesley.

McFarlane J: Battering during pregnancy: tip of an iceberg revealed, *Women Health* 15:69-83, 1989.

McFarlane J: Abuse during pregnancy: the horror and hope, *AWHONN's Clinical Issues in Perinatal and Women's Health Nursing*, 4(3):350-362, 1993.

McFarlane J: Abuse during pregnancy: the horror and the hope. *AWHON's Clinical Issues in Perinatal and Women's Health Nurs* 4(3):350, 1993.

McFarlane J, Christoffel K, Bateman L, Miller V, Bullock L: Assessing for abuse: self-report versus nurse interview, *Public Health Nurs*, 8: 245-250, 1991.

McFarlane, J, Parker B, Soeken K: Abuse during pregnancy: effects on maternal complications and birthweight in adult and teenage women, *Obstet Gynecol* 84(3):323, 1994.

Mercy JA, O'Carroll PW: New directions in violence prediction: the public health arena, *Violence Vict* 3(4):285, 1988.

Milner JS, Robertson KR: Comparison of physical child abusers, intrafamilial sexual child abusers, and child neglecters, *J Interpersonal Violence* 5(1):37, 1990.

MMWR, 41(41):760-2, 771-2,1992.

O'Carroll PW, Mercy JA: Regional variation in homicide rates: why is the West so violent? *Violence Vict* 4(1):17, 1986.

Okun LE: *Woman abuse: facts replacing myths*. Albany, NY, 1986, State University of New York Press.

Oliphant C, editor: *Health scene*. Pendleton, OR, 1986, Pendleton Community Hospital.

Phillips LR: Abuse/neglect of the frail elderly at home: an exploration of theoretical relationships, *J Adv Nurs* 8:379, 1983.

Pillemer K, Finkelhor D: The prevalence of elder abuse: a random sample survey, *Gerontologist* 28:51, 1988.

Prince J: A systems approach to spouse abuse. In Lancaster J: *Community mental health nursing: an ecological perspective*. St Louis, 1980, Mosby–Year Book.

Public Health Improvement Plan. Olympia, WA, 1994, Washington State Department of Health.

Reiss AJ, Roth JA, editors: *Understanding and preventing violence*, Washington, DC, 1993, National Academy Press.

Rew L: Childhood sexual exploitation: long-term effects among a group of nursing students, *Issues Ment Health Nurs* 10:181, 1989.

Rosenberg ML, Fenley MA, editors: *Violence in America: a public health approach*, New York, 1991, Oxford.

Rosenberg ML, Mercy JA: Homicide and assaultive violence. In *Violence as a public health problem*, Atlanta, 1985, US Public Health Service.

Scharer K: Nursing therapy with abusive and neglectful families, *J Psychiatr Nurs* 17(9):12, 1979.

Sengstock MC, Barrett S: Elder abuse. In Campbell J, Humphreys J, editors: *Nursing care of survivors of family violence*, St Louis, 1993, Mosby–Year Book.

Senter S: *Program planning manual for implementing a response to domestic violence in hospital emergency departments*, Seattle, Wash, 1993, Seattle-King County Department of Public Health.

Sheridan D, Belknap L, Katz S, Kelleher P: *Guidelines for the treatment of battered women victims in emergency room settings*, Chicago, 1985, Chicago Hospital Council.

Sommers EK, Check J: An empirical investigation of the role of pornography in the verbal and physical abuse of women, *Violence Vict* 2:189, 1987.

Stark E, Fitzcraft A: Spouse abuse. In Rosenberg ML, Finley MA: *Violence in America*, New York, 1991, Oxford.

Stein JA, Golding JM, Siegel JM, Burnam MA, Sorenson SB: Long term psychological sequelae of child sexual abuse. In GE Wyatt, GJ Powell, editors: *Lasting effects of child sexual abuse*, Newbury Park, CA, 1988, Sage, pp 135-154.

Straus MA, Gelles RJ: *Physical violence in American families: risk factors and adaptations to violence in 8,145 families*. New Brunswick, NJ, 1990, Transaction.

Tilden VP: Response of the health care delivery system to battered women, *Issues Ment Health Nurs*, 10:309-320, 1989.

Tilden VP, Shepard P: Increasing the rate of identification of battered women in an emergency department: use of a nursing protocol, *Res Nurs Health* 10:209-215, 1987.

Tolman RM, Bennett LW: A review of research on men who batter, *Journal of Interpersonal Violence* 5(1):87, 1990.

Ulrich YC: Cross-cultural perspective on violence against women, *Response Victimiz Women Child* 12(1):21, 1989.

US Department of Justice: *Murder in families: violence against women*, Washington, 1994, Bureau of Justice Statistics.

US Surgeon General: *Workshop on violence and public health report*, DDHS Pub No HRS-D-MC 86-1, Washington, DC, 1986, Health Resources and Services Administration, US Public Health Service, US Department of Health and Human Services.

Walker LE: *The battered woman syndrome*, New York, 1984, Springer.

Webster DW: The unconvincing case for school-based conflict resolution, *Health Affairs* 12(4):126-141, 1993.

Weiner A: A community based education model for identification and prevention of elder abuse, *J Gerontol Soc Work* 16(3-4):107-119, 1991.

Weith ME: Elder abuse: a national tradegy, *FBI Law Enforcement Bulletin* 63(2):24-26, 1994.

Wolf RS, Pillemer K, Wilson NL: What's new in elder abuse programming, *Gerontologist* 34(1):126-129, 1994.

Wyatt GE, Powell GJ, editors: Identifying the lasting effects of child sexual abuse. In *Lasting effects of child abuse*. Newbury Park, Calif, 1988, Sage, pp 11-18.

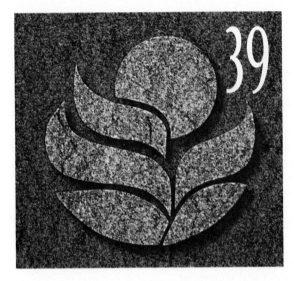

39

Communicable Disease Risk and Prevention

Francisco S. Sy ◆ Susan C. Long-Marin

Objectives ▼

After reading this chapter, the student should be able to do the following:

◆ Discuss the current impact and threats of infectious diseases on our society.
◆ Explain the agent-host-environment triad and how its components interact to cause infectious diseases.
◆ Discuss the factors leading to the emergence or reemergence of infectious diseases.
◆ Define and discuss the implications of immunity in terms of active immunity, passive immunity, and herd immunity.
◆ Define surveillance and discuss the functions and elements of a surveillance system.
◆ Explain why tuberculosis is once more on the rise in this country, and discuss diagnostic tools, treatment, prevention, and control measures.
◆ Discuss the risk of foodborne illness and appropriate prevention measures giving special attention to *Salmonella* and *E. coli 0157:*H7.
◆ Explain the rise in parasitic infections, the population particularly at risk, and possible preventive measures.
◆ Discuss the three levels of prevention and give appropriate examples of preventive interventions.
◆ Discuss the multisystem approach to control of communicable diseases.

Key Terms ▼

- acquired immunity
- active immunization
- agent
- common vehicle
- communicable period
- control
- disease
- elimination
- emerging infectious diseases
- endemic
- environment
- epidemic
- epidemiologic triad
- eradication
- herd immunity
- horizontal transmission
- host
- incubation period
- infection
- infectiousness
- natural immunity
- nosocomial infections
- pandemic
- passive immunization
- resistance
- surveillance
- vertical transmission
- zoonosis

Outline ▼

Continued.

Outline—cont'd

The topic of communicable diseases includes the discussion of a wide and complex variety of organisms; the pathology they may cause; and their diagnosis, treatment, prevention, and control. This chapter presents an overview of the communicable diseases with which community health nurses deal most often. Diseases are grouped according to descriptive category (by modes of transmission or means of prevention) rather than by individual organism (*E. coli*) or taxonomic group (viral, parasitic). Detailed discussion of sexually transmitted diseases, HIV/AIDS, and viral hepatitis are discussed in Chapter 40. Although not all infectious diseases are directly communicable from person to person, the terms infectious diseases and communicable diseases are used interchangeably throughout this chapter. Because this discussion is intended as an overview and only selected diseases are included, it is suggested that those seeking more information on communicable diseases consult standard textbooks, such as *Principles and Practice of Infectious Diseases* (Mandell et al., 1995) and the American Public Health Association's *Control of Communicable Diseases in Man* (Benenson, 1990).

HISTORICAL AND CURRENT PERSPECTIVES

In 1900 communicable diseases were the leading cause of death in the United States. Now nearing the end of the century, improved nutrition and sanitation, vaccines, and antibiotics have put an end to the epidemics that once ravaged entire populations. In 1900 tuberculosis was the second leading cause of death; in 1990 it caused 1810 total deaths. In general, individuals live longer, and heart disease, cancer, and stroke have replaced infectious diseases as the leading killers. Infectious diseases, however, have not vanished from our lives. They are still the leading cause of death worldwide. Infectious diseases account for 25% of all physician visits each year and antibiotics are the second most prescribed type of drugs in the United States (CDC, 1994a).

Did You Know?

During the past decade, as rates of infectious disease have increased, the use of antibiotic drugs has grown significantly. Antibiotics are now the second most prescribed group of drugs in the United States. With the introduction of new antibiotic drugs comes new forms of antibiotic drug resistance, a problem that is further exacerbated by inappropriate use of antibiotics.

New killers are emerging, and old familiar disease forms are taking on new, more virulent characteristics. Consider the following recent developments. The advent of the AIDS epidemic in the 1980s reminds us of plagues from the past and challenges our ability to contain and control infection like no other disease in this century. In 1995, AIDS replaced accidents as the leading killer of young men 20 to 44 years of age. Tuberculosis, though nowhere near the threat it posed in the past, is reappearing with more frequency and with a new twist—resistance to once effective drug therapy. Legionnaire's Disease and Toxic Shock Syndrome have become new additions to our vocabulary. In the summer of 1993 in the southwestern United States, healthy young adults were stricken with a mysterious, unknown and often fatal respiratory disease that came to be known as Hantavirus Pulmonary Syndrome. Methicillin-resistant *Staphylococcus aureus* is now resistant to all but one antibiotic, vancomycin. A severe, invasive strain of *Streptococcus pyogenes Group A,* referred to by the press as the flesh-eating bacteria, drew public attention in 1994. Children dying from eating poorly cooked hamburgers containing *Escherichia coli 0157:H7* at fast food restaurants (CDC, 1994a) is yet another example of the threat posed by infectious diseases.

It is estimated that 90,000 people per year die from microbial causes separate from AIDS-associated illnesses (McGinnis and Foege, 1993). The economic burden of infectious diseases is staggering. The annual combined direct cost and lost productivity attributable to intestinal infections is estimated at $30 billion while the annual treatment cost for sexually transmitted diseases, excluding AIDS, is $5 billion. Annual direct medical cost attributable to nosocomial infections is $4.5 billion, and the combined medical cost and lost productivity for influenza is $17 billion per year. The yearly estimated expenditure from antimicrobial resistance is $4 billion (CDC, 1994a).

Because of the morbidity, mortality, and associated cost from infectious diseases, *Healthy People 2000,* the compilation of health promotion and disease prevention goals for the nation, includes in its section on infectious disease objectives for reducing the incidence of (1) indigenous cases of vaccine-preventable disease, (2) epidemic-related pneumonia deaths among people 65 years of age or older, (3) viral hepatitis, (4) tuberculosis, (5) nosocomial infections, (6) selected diseases of international travelers, (7) bacterial meningitis, (8) diarrheal diseases of children in day care, (9) acute middle ear infections in young children, and (10) pneumonia-related days of restricted activity. An objective for reducing salmonellosis and other foodborne infections is found in the section for food and drug safety. Although infectious diseases may not be the leading cause of death, they continue to present varied, multiple, and complex challenges to all health care providers. The community health nurse must be knowledgeable about these diseases in order to play an effective role in their diagnosis, treatment, prevention, and control.

TRANSMISSION OF COMMUNICABLE DISEASES

Agent, Host, and Environment

The transmission of communicable diseases depends on the successful interaction of the infectious agent, host and environment. These three factors are referred to as the **epidemiologic triad.** Changes in the characteristics of any of these three factors may result in disease transmission (Benenson, 1990; Evans, 1989). Consider the following examples. Antibiotic

therapy not only may eliminate a specific pathologic agent but also may alter the balance of normally occurring organisms in the body so that one of these agents overruns another, and disease, such as a yeast infection, occurs. HIV performs its deadly work not by directly poisoning the host but by destroying the host's immune reaction to other disease-producing agents. Individuals living in the temperate climate of the United States do not contract malaria at home, but they may become infected if they change their environment by traveling to a climate where malaria-carrying mosquitos thrive. As these examples illustrate, the balance between agent, host, and environment is often precarious and may be unintentionally disrupted. As we approach the twenty-first century, the potential results of such disruption should command considerable contemplation as advances in science and technology, destruction of natural habitat, explosive population growth, political instability, and a worldwide transportation network combine to alter the balance between our environment, ourselves, and the agents that produce disease.

Agent Factor

There are four main categories of infectious agents that may cause infection or disease: bacteria, fungi, parasites, and viruses. The individual **agent** may be described by its ability to cause disease, and the nature and the severity of the disease. Terms commonly used to characterize infectious agents are defined in the box below.

Host Factor

A human or animal **host** may harbor an infectious agent. The characteristics of the host that may influence the spread of disease are host resistance, immunity, herd immunity, and infectiousness of the host. **Resistance** is the ability of the host to withstand infection. This resistance may be due to natural or acquired immunity. **Natural immunity** refers to species-determined innate resistance to an infectious agent. **Acquired immunity** is the resistance acquired by a host as a result of previous natural exposure to an

 Six Characteristics of an Infectious Agent

1. Infectivity	The ability to enter and multiply in the host.	
2. Pathogenicity	The ability to produce a specific clinical reaction after infection occurs.	
3. Virulence	The ability to produce a severe pathological reaction.	
4. Toxicity	The ability to produce a poisonous reaction.	
5. Invasiveness	The ability to penetrate and spread throughout a tissue.	
6. Antigenicity	The ability to stimulate an immunologic response.	

infectious agent, for example, immunity to measles resulting from prior infection with measles virus.

Acquired immunity may be induced by active or passive immunization. **Active immunization** refers to the immunization of an individual by administration of an antigen (infectious agent or vaccine) and usually is characterized by the presence of antibody produced by the individual host. Vaccinating children against diseases of childhood is an example of inducing active immunity.

Passive immunization refers to immunization through the transfer of specific antibody from an immunized individual to a nonimmunized individual, such as the transference of antibody from mother to infant or by administration of an antibody-containing preparation (immune globulin or antiserum). Passive immunity from immune globulin is almost immediate, but it is short-lived. It is often induced as a stop-gap measure until active immunity has time to develop after vaccination. Examples of commonly used immunoglobulins include those for hepatitis A, rabies, and tetanus.

Herd immunity refers to the immunity of a group or community. It is the resistance of a group of people to the invasion and spread of an infectious agent. Herd immunity is based on the resistance to infection of a high proportion of individual members of a group. It is the basis for increasing immunization coverage for vaccine-preventable diseases. Higher immunization coverage will lead to greater herd immunity, which in turn will block the further spread of the disease.

Infectiousness is a measure of the potential ability of an infected host to transmit the infection to other hosts. It is concerned with the relative ease with which the infectious agent is transmitted to others. For example, a droplet-spread infection like tuberculosis is more infectious than a tickborne infection like Lyme disease.

Environment Factor

The **environment** refers to all that is external to the human host, including physical, biological, social, and cultural factors. These environmental factors facilitate the transmission of an infectious agent from an infected host to other susceptible hosts. Reduction in communicable disease risk can be achieved by altering these environmental factors. Using mosquito nets and repellants to avoid arthropod bites, installing sewage systems to prevent fecal contamination of water supplies, and washing utensils after contact with raw meat to reduce bacterial contamination are all examples of altering the environment to prevent disease.

Modes of Transmission

Infectious diseases can be transmitted horizontally or vertically. **Vertical transmission** refers to passing the infection from parent to offspring via sperm, placenta, milk, or contact in the vaginal canal at birth. Examples of vertical transmission are transplacental transmission of HIV and syphilis. **Horizontal transmission** refers to person-to-person spread of infection through one or more of the following four routes: direct/indirect contact, common vehicle, airborne, or vectorborne. Sexually transmitted diseases are spread by direct sexual contact. Enterobiasis or pinworm infection can be acquired through direct contact or indirect contact with contaminated objects, such as toys, clothing, and bedding. **Common vehicle** refers to trans-portation of the infectious agent from an infected host to a susceptible host via water, food, milk, blood, serum, or plasma. Hepatitis A can be transmitted through contaminated food and water, hepatitis B through contaminated blood products. Legionellosis and tuberculosis are both spread via contaminated droplets in the air. Vectors can be arthropods, such as ticks and mosquitos, or other invertebrates, such as snails, that can transmit the infectious agent by biting or depositing the infective material near the host.

Disease Development

Exposure to an infectious agent does not always lead to an infection. It is also true that infection does not always lead to disease. It depends on the infective dose, infectivity of the infectious agent, immunity, and immunocompetence of the host. It is important to differentiate infection and disease as clearly illustrated by the HIV/AIDS epidemic. **Infection** refers to the entry, development, and multiplication of the infectious agent in the susceptible host. **Disease** is one of the possible outcomes of infection, and it may indicate a physiological dysfunction or pathological reaction. In an example from the sports world, compare the case of Magic Johnson with that of Greg Louganis. Both publicly announced that they had tested positive for HIV, but whereas Johnson was asymptomatic, Louganis had developed the clinical signs of AIDS. Or in other words, Johnson was infected but not diseased; Louganis was both infected and diseased.

Incubation period and communicable period are not synonymous. **Incubation period** refers to the time interval between invasion by an infectious agent and the first appearance of signs and symptoms of the disease. The incubation period of infectious diseases vary from 2 to 4 hours for staphylococcal food poisoning to 10 to 15 years for AIDS. **Communicable period** refers to the time interval during which an infectious agent may be transferred directly or indirectly from an infected person to another person. The period of communicability for influenza is 3 to 5 days after the clinical onset of symptoms. Hepatitis B infected persons are infectious many weeks before the onset of first symptoms and remain infective during the acute phase and chronic carrier state, which may persist for life.

Disease Spectrum

Persons with infectious diseases may exhibit a broad spectrum of disease that ranges from subclinical infection to severe and fatal disease. Those with subclinical or inapparent infections are important from the public health point of view because they serve as a source of infection and may not be cared for like those with clinical disease. They should be targeted for early diagnosis and treatment. Those with clinical disease may exhibit localized or systemic symptoms and mild to severe illness. The final outcome of a disease may be recovery, death, or something in between including a carrier state, complications requiring extended hospital stay, or disability requiring rehabilitation. At the community level, the disease may occur in endemic, epidemic, or pandemic proportion. **Endemic** refers to the constant presence of a disease within a geographic area or a population. Measles is endemic in the United States. **Epidemic** refers to the occurrence of a disease in a community or region in excess of normal expectancy. Although people tend to associate large numbers with epidemics, even one case can be termed epidemic if the disease is considered previously eliminated from that area. **Pandemic** refers to an epidemic occurring worldwide and affecting large populations. HIV/AIDS can be classified as both epidemic and pandemic since the number of cases is growing rapidly across various regions of the world, as well as in the United States.

SURVEILLANCE OF COMMUNICABLE DISEASES

Surveillance is a system of close observation of all aspects of the occurrence and distribution of a communicable disease through systematic collection, orderly consolidation and analysis, and prompt dissemination of all relevant data. The surveillance system must be current, accurate, complete, purposeful, and dynamic to be useful for effective planning, implementation, and evaluation of disease prevention and control programs (Benenson, 1990; Evans, 1989).

Elements of Surveillance

The basic 10 elements of surveillance are the routine sources of data on disease occurrence, which include mortality registration, morbidity reporting, epidemic reporting, epidemic field investigation, laboratory reporting, individual case investigation, surveys, utilization of biologics and drugs, distribution of animal reservoirs and vectors, and demographic and environmental data.

Community health nurses may be involved at different levels of the surveillance system. They play important roles in collecting data, making diagnoses, reporting cases, and providing feedback information to the general public. Examples of possible activities include investigating sources and contacts in outbreaks of diseases, such as measles, in school settings or shigellosis in day care; TB testing and contact tracing; collecting and reporting information pertaining to notifiable communicable diseases; and providing morbidity and mortality statistics to those who request them, including the media, the public, those planning services, and those writing grants.

List of Reportable Diseases

Requirements for disease reporting in the United States are mandated by state laws and regulations. The

---

 Infectious Diseases Designated as Notifiable at the National Level

AIDS	Hepatitis, non-A, non-B	Rheumatic fever*
Amebiasis*	Hepatitis, unspecified	Rocky Mountain spotted fever (Typhus fever, tickborne)
Anthrax	Legionellosis	
Aseptic meningitis	Leprosy (Hansen disease)	Rubella
Botulism	Leptospirosis	Salmonellosis*
Brucellosis	Lyme disease	Shigellosis*
Chancroid*	Lymphogranuloma venereum*	Syphilis
Cholera	Malaria	Syphilis, congenital
Congenital rubella syndrome	Measles	Tetanus
Diphtheria	Meningococcal infection	Toxic shock syndrome
Encephalitis	Mumps	Trichinosis
Escherichia coli 0157:H7	Pertussis	Tuberculosis
Gonorrhea	Plague	Tularemia
Granuloma inguinale*	Poliomyelitis	Typhoid fever
Haemophilus influenzae	Psittacosis	Varicella (chickenpox)*†
Hepatitis A	Rabies, animal	Yellow fever*
Hepatitis B	Rabies, human	

From Centers for Disease Control and Prevention: *MMWR* 43(43):800, 1994b.
*Reports of these diseases are not printed weekly in Table I or Table II of the *MMWR*.
†Although varicella is not officially a nationally notifiable disease, the Council of State and Territorial Epidemiologists encourages transmission of information about cases of varicella to CDC.

list of reportable diseases in each state varies. The state health departments report the cases of selected diseases to the Centers for Disease Control and Prevention (CDC) in Atlanta, Georgia. The diseases included in the National Notifiable Diseases Surveillance System (NNDSS) at CDC are listed in the box on p. 759. The NNDSS data are collated and published weekly in the *Morbidity and Mortality Weekly Report (MMWR)*. Final reports are published annually in the *Summary of Notifiable Diseases* (CDC, 1994b).

EMERGING INFECTIOUS DISEASES
Emergence Factors

Emerging infectious diseases are those diseases in which the incidence has actually increased in the past two decades or has the potential to increase in the near future. These emerging diseases may include new or known infectious diseases. Consider the following examples. Identified only in the past two decades when sporadic outbreaks occurred in Sudan and Zaire, Ebola virus is a mysterious new killer with a frightening mortality rate that sometimes reaches 90%, no known treatment, and no known reservoir in nature. It appears to be transmitted through direct contact with bodily secretions, and as such potentially can be contained once cases are identified. Why outbreaks occur is not understood. Ebola is an example of new viruses that may appear as civilization intrudes farther and farther into previously uninhabited natural environments, changing the landscape and disturbing ecological balances that may have existed unaltered for hundreds of years.

Closer to home, Hantavirus was first detected in the southwestern United States in 1993 when a mysterious and deadly respiratory disease appeared to be targeting young, healthy Native Americans. The disease was soon discovered to be a variant of, but to exhibit very different pathology from, a rodentborne virus previously known only in Europe and Asia. It also was recognized that the virus has no particular predilection for Native Americans. One explanation for the outbreak in the Southwest is that an unseasonably mild winter had resulted in an unusual increase in the rodent population, exposing more people than usual to a virus that had until that point gone unrecognized in this country. Hantavirus now has been diagnosed in sites across the United States. The best protection against it seems to be avoiding rodent-infested environments.

Not only is HIV/AIDS a new disease, but the resultant immunocompromise is largely responsible for the rising numbers of previously rare opportunistic infections, such as cryptosporidiosis, toxoplasmosis, and pneumocystis pneumonia. It is theorized that HIV may have existed in isolated parts of sub-Saharan Africa for years and emerged only recently into the rest of the world as the result of a combination of factors, including new roads, increased commerce, truck drivers, and prostitutes. Tuberculosis is a familiar face turned newly aggressive. After years of decline, it is on the increase once more because of drug resistance and infection secondary to HIV/AIDS.

Several factors, operating singly or in combination, can influence the emergence of these diseases as shown in Table 39-1. Except for microbial adaptation and changes made by the infectious agent, such as those likely in the emergence of *Escherichia coli 0157:H7*, most of the emergence factors are consequences of activities and behavior of the human hosts and environmental changes, such as deforestation, urbanization, and industrialization. The rise in households with two working parents has increased the number of children in day care, and with this shift has come an increase in diarrheal diseases, such as shigellosis. Changing sexual behavior and illegal drug use

Table 39-1 Factors that May Influence the Emergence of New Infectious Diseases

Categories	Specific examples
Societal events	Economic impoverishment; war or civil conflict; population growth and migration; urban decay
Health care	New medical devices; organ or tissue transplantation; drugs causing immunosuppression; widespread use of antibiotics
Food production	Globalization of food supplies; changes in food processing and packaging
Human behavior	Sexual behavior; drug use; travel; diet; outdoor recreation; use of child care facilities
Environmental changes	Deforestation/reforestation; changes in water ecosystems; flood/drought; famine; global warming
Public health infrastructure	Curtailment or reduction in prevention programs; inadequate communicable disease surveillance; lack of trained personnel (epidemiologists, laboratory scientists, vector and rodent control specialists)
Microbial adaptation and change	Changes in virulence and toxin production; development of drug resistance; microbes as cofactors in chronic diseases

From Centers for Disease Control and Prevention: *Addressing emerging infectious disease threats: a prevention strategy for the* US, Atlanta, 1994a, CDC.

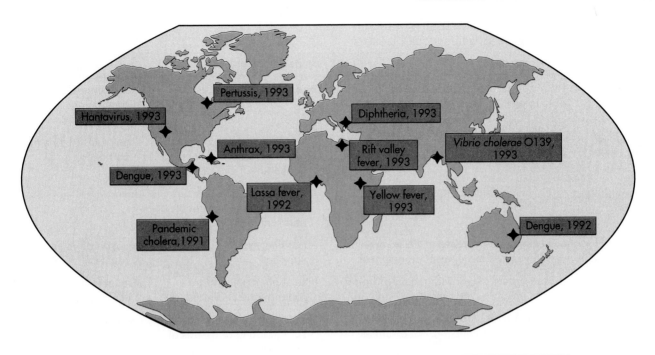

FIGURE 39-1

Examples of emerging and resurgent infectious diseases in the 1990s. (From Centers for Disease Control and Prevention: *Addressing emerging infectious disease threats: a prevention strategy for the* US, Atlanta, 1994a, CDC.)

play a role in the spread of HIV/AIDS and other sexually transmitted diseases. Before the era of large airconditioning systems with cooling towers, legionellosis was virtually unknown. Immigrants, legal and illegal, as well as travelers, bring with them a variety of known and potentially unknown diseases. In the efforts to prevent and control these emerging diseases, it will be important to focus on developing more effective ways to educate people and change their behavior and on the development of drugs and vaccines. In addition, it is vital that current surveillance systems should be strengthened and expanded to improve the detection and tracking of these diseases.

Examples of Emerging Infectious Diseases

Examples of emerging and resurgent infectious diseases in the 1990s in the world are depicted in Figure 39-1 (CDC, 1994a). Selected emerging infectious diseases, including a brief description of the diseases and symptoms they cause, their modes of transmission, and causes of emergence are listed in Table 39-2.

PREVENTION AND CONTROL OF COMMUNICABLE DISEASES

Communicable diseases can be prevented and controlled. Communicable disease **control** programs aim to reduce the prevalence of a disease to a level at which it no longer poses a major public health problem. In some cases, diseases may even be eliminated

or eradicated. **Elimination** focuses on removing a disease from a large geographic area, such as a country or region of the world. **Eradication** refers to the irreversible termination of all transmission of infection by extermination of the infectious agents worldwide (Last, 1983; CDC, 1993b). The World Health Organization (WHO) officially declared the global eradication of smallpox on May 8, 1980 (Evans, 1985). After the successful eradication of smallpox, the eradication of other communicable diseases became a realistic challenge. Polio appears to have been eliminated from the Americas (CDC, 1994d). No cases of indigenous polio caused by wild-type virus have been reported in the United States since 1979. The WHO has adopted a resolution for eradication of paralytic poliomyelitis and dracunculiasis (guinea worm infection) from the world by the year 2000.

Primary, Secondary, and Tertiary Prevention

Prevention of communicable diseases can be attained at three levels: primary, secondary, and tertiary (Last, 1983). Primary prevention is aimed at reducing the incidence of disease through health promotion and education or, in other words, preventing disease before it happens. Examples of primary prevention include immunization against communicable diseases, malaria chemoprophylaxis, the adoption of universal precautions by health care workers, the promotion of safer sex, and making water and the environment safe.

Table 39-2 Examples of Emerging Infectious Diseases

Infectious agent	Diseases/Symptoms	Mode of transmission	Causes of emergence
Borrelia burgdorferi	Lyme Disease: rash, fever, arthritis, neurologic and cardiac abnormalities	Bite of infective Ixodes tick	Increase in deer and human populations in wooded areas
Escherichia coli 0157:H7	Hemorrhagic colitis; thrombocytopenia; hemolytic uremic syndrome	Ingestion of contaminated food, especially undercooked beef and raw milk	Likely caused by a new pathogen
Ebola-Marburg Viruses	Fulminant, high mortality, hemorrhagic fever	Direct contact with infected blood, organs, secretions, and semen	Unknown
Legionella pneumophila	Legionnaires' disease: malaise, myalgia, fever, headache, respiratory illness	Air cooling systems, water supplies	Recognition in an epidemic situation
Hantaviruses	Hemorrhagic fever with renal syndrome; pulmonary syndrome	Inhalation of aerosolized rodent urine and feces	Human invasion of virus ecologic niche
Human immuno-deficiency virus HIV-1	HIV infection; AIDS/HIV disease; severe immune dysfunction, opportunistic infections	Sexual contact with or exposure to blood or tissues of infected persons; perinatal	Urbanization; life-style changes; drug use; international travel; transfusions; transplants
Human papillomavirus	Skin and mucous membrane lesions (warts); strongly linked to cancer of the cervix and penis	Direct sexual contact, contact with contaminated surfaces	Newly recognized; changes in sexual life-style
Cryptosporidium	Cryptosporidiosis; infection of epithelial cells in gastrointestinal and respiratory tracts	Fecal-oral, person-to-person, waterborne	Development near watershed areas; immunosuppression
Pneumocystis carinii	Acute pneumonia	Unknown; possibly airborne or reactivation of latent infection	Immunosuppression

Modified from Ledeberg J, Shope RE, Oaks SC: *Emerging infections: microbial threats to health in the* US, Washington DC, 1992, National Academy Press and Centers for Disease Control and Prevention: *MMWR* 43(RR-7):1, 1994c.

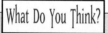

What Do You Think?

Refusal of preventive health care to illegal immigrants may prove a threat to the public's health.

Secondary prevention is aimed at reducing prevalence of disease or diminishing the morbidity of the disease through early diagnosis and treatment. Examples of secondary prevention are skin testing for tuberculosis, serological screening for HIV, screening for sexually transmitted diseases (STDs), contact investigation in tuberculosis control programs, and partner notification in AIDS and STD programs.

Tertiary prevention is aimed at reducing complications and disabilities related to the disease through treatment and mental and physical rehabilitation. Two examples of tertiary prevention are *Pneumocystis carinii* pneumonia (PCP) chemoprophylaxis for people with

AIDS and providing footwear and gloves to leprosy patients to prevent trauma to their insensitive and deformed hands and feet.

Multisystem Approach to Control

Communicable diseases represent an imbalance in the harmonious relationship between the human host and the environment, providing the infectious agent an opportunity to cause greater morbidity and mortality in the human population. Realizing the multifactorial causes of communicable diseases, a multisystem approach to control of these diseases, as illustrated in Table 39-3, must be developed.

VACCINE—PREVENTABLE DISEASES

Vaccines are one of the most effective methods of preventing and controlling communicable diseases. The vaccine against smallpox, which left distinctive scars on so many of our shoulders, is no longer in use

Table 39-3   A Multisystem Approach to Communicable Disease Control

Goal	Example
Improve host resistance to infectious agents and other environmental hazards	Improved hygiene, nutrition, and physical fitness; increased immunization coverage; provision of chemoprophylaxis and chemotherapy; stress control and improved mental health
Improve safety of the environment	Improved sanitation, provision of safe water and clean air; proper cooking and storage of food; appropriate control of vectors and animal reservoir hosts
Improve public health systems	Increased access to health care; adequate health education; improved surveillance systems
Facilitate social and political changes to ensure better health for all people	Individual, organizational, and community action; legislation

From Wenzel RP: In Last JM, and Wallace RB, editors: *Public health and preventive medicine*, ed 13, Norwalk, 1992, Appleton and Lange.

because the smallpox virus has been declared totally eradicated from the world's population. Diseases, such as polio, diphtheria, pertussis, and measles, which earlier in the century occurred in epidemic proportions, today are controlled through routine childhood immunization. They have not, however, been eradicated. Therefore, it is important that vigilance be maintained in insuring that children continue to be immunized against these diseases. In the United States, "No shots, no school" legislation has resulted in the immunization of most children by the time they enter school. However, many infants and toddlers, the group must vulnerable to these potentially severe diseases, are not receiving scheduled immunizations despite the availability of free vaccines. Inner-city children from minority and ethnic groups appear to be at particular risk for incomplete immunization.

In 1993, President Clinton initiated the Childhood Immunization Initiative (CII), a comprehensive national response to underimmunization that set national goals for immunization coverage for 1996 as an interim step in achieving immunization goals set by *Healthy People 2000* and provided federal money for vaccines, immunization delivery programs, and immunization research. State governments and health departments across the country have responded to this initiative by making immunization a top health priority. Since a large number of children receive their immunizations at public health departments, community health nurses play a major role in the effort to increase immunization coverage of infants and toddlers. These nurses can track children known to be at risk for underimmunization and call or send reminders to their parents. They can help avoid missed immunization opportunities by checking the immunization status of every young child they encounter whether the clinic or home visit is immunization-related or not. In addition, they can organize community immunization outreach activities that deliver immunization services; provide answers to parents' questions and concerns about immunization; and educate parents about why immuniza-

tions are needed, inappropriate contraindications to immunization, and the importance of completing the immunization schedule on time.

 Research Brief

Bates AS, Fitzgerald JF, Dittus RS, Wolinsky FD: Risk factors for underimmunization in poor urban infants, JAMA 272(14):1105-1110, 1994.

Researchers evaluated the relationship between financial access, personal characteristics, mother's health beliefs, and underimmunization by following the immunization status of infants born at a large municipal teaching hospital in the Midwest.

The study consisted of 464 healthy, full-term newborn infants who were to be discharged to the care of their mothers. The mothers were interviewed 24 to 72 hours postpartum regarding personal and financial characteristics and 9 to 12 months later to determine where immunizations were received. The immunization status of the infants was checked at 3 and 7 months of age.

Despite availability of free vaccine to most infants, only 67% had received their first set of immunizations by 3 months of age, and only 29% were up-to-date by 7 months of age. Marital status, coresidence with the infant's grandmother, adequacy of prenatal care, and poverty were some of the factors predictive of immunization status.

The implications for community health nurses from the study recommendations are
1. The provision of free vaccine alone will not guarantee adequate immunization of children, and
2. Poor urban infants of single mothers and of mothers who received inadequate prenatal care, and those not living with their grandmothers should be targeted for tracking and follow-up to ensure adequate immunization.

Table 39-4 Recommended Childhood Immunization Schedule

Vaccine	Birth	2 Months	4 Months	6 Months	12^b Months	15 Months	18 Months	4-6 Years	11-12 Years	14-16 Years
Hepatitis B^c		HB-1								
		HB-2		HB-3						
Diphtheria, Tetanus, Pertussis^d		DTP	DTP	DTP	DTP or DTaP at ≥ 15 months			DTP or DTaP	Td	
H. influenzae type b^e		Hib	Hib	Hib	Hib					
Poliovirus		OPV	OPV	OPV				OPV		
Measles, Mumps, Rubella^f					MMR			MMR or MMR		

From Centers for Disease Control and Prevention, *MMWR* 43(51, 52):959, 1995.

^{a}Recommended vaccines are listed under the routinely recommended ages. Shaded bars indicate range of acceptable ages for vaccination.

^{b}Vaccines recommended in the second year of life (i.e., 12-15 months of age) may be given at either one or two visits.

^{c}Infants born to hepatitis B surface antigen (HBsAg)-negative mothers should receive the second dose of hepatitis B vaccine between 1 and 4 months of age, provided at least 1 month has elapsed since receipt of the first dose. The third dose is recommended between 6 and 18 months of age. Infants born to HBsAg-positive mothers should receive immunoprophylaxis for hepatitis B with 0.5 ml Hepatitis B Immune Globulin (HBIG) within 12 hours of birth, and 0.5 ml of either Merck Sharpe & Dohme (West Point, Pennsylvania) vaccine (Recombivax HB) or of Smith Kline Beecham (Philadelphia) vaccine (Engerix-B) at a separate site. In these infants, the second dose of vaccine is recommended at 1 month of age and the third dose at 6 months of age. All pregnant women should be screened for HBsAg during an early prenatal visit.

^{d}The fourth dose of diphtheria and tetanus toxoids and pertussis vaccine (DTP) may be administered as early as 12 months of age, provided at least 6 months have elapsed since the third dose of DTP. Combined DTP-Hib products may be used when these two vaccines are administered simultaneously. Diphtheria and tetanus toxoids and acellular pertussis vaccine (DTaP) is licensed for use for the fourth and/or fifth dose of DTP in children aged ≥ 15 months and may be preferred for these doses in children in this age group.

^{e}Three *H. influenzae* type b conjugate vaccines are available for use in infants: 1) oligosaccharide conjugate Hib vaccine (HbOC) (HibTITER, manufactured by Praxis Biologics, Inc. [West Henrietta, New York], and distributed by Lederle-Praxis Biologicals, [Wayne, New Jersey]); 2) polyribosylribitol phosphate-tetanus toxoid conjugate (PRP-T) (ActHIB, manufactured by Pasteur Mérieux Sérums & Vaccins, S.A. (Lyon, France), and distributed by Connaught Laboratories, Inc. [Swiftwater, Pennsylvania], and OmniHIB, manufactured by Pasteur Mérieux Sérums & Vaccins, S.A., and distributed by SmithKline Beecham); and 3) *Haemophilus* b conjugate vaccine (Meningococcal Protein Conjugate) (PRP-OMP) (PedvaxHIB, manufactured by Merck Sharp & Dohme). Children who have received PRP-OMP at 2 and 4 months of age do not require a dose at 6 months of age. After the primary infant Hib conjugate vaccine series is completed, any licensed Hib conjugate vaccine may be used as a booster dose at age 12-15 months.

^{f}The second dose of measles-mumps-rubella vaccine should be administered EITHER at 4-6 years of age OR at 11-12 years of age.

Recommended Childhood Immunization Schedule

Children in the United States are routinely immunized against the following nine diseases: hepatitis B, diphtheria, pertussis, tetanus, paralytic poliomyelitis (polio), *Hemophilus influenzae* type B (Hib), measles, mumps, and rubella. Diphtheria, pertussis, and tetanus (DTP) are usually given in combination, as are measles, mumps, and rubella (MMR). To achieve recommended immunization levels by 2 years of age, most of these immunizations should begin when an infant reaches 2 to 3 months of age. Live vaccines—measles, mumps, rubella, and polio—should be completed by 18 months of age. Table 39-4 provides the immunization schedule recommended by the Advisory Committee on Immunization Practices, American Academy of Pediatrics, and the American Academy of Family Physicians (CDC, 1995).

To the undoubted relief of parents who fear many days of work lost to caring for children miserable with chicken pox, a vaccine against the chickenpox-causing varicella virus was licensed for general use in April, 1995. Other vaccines are available for use in special circumstances against the following diseases: cholera influenza, hepatitis A, meningococcal meningitis, plague, pneumococcal pneumonia, rabies, and yellow fever.

Measles

Measles is an acute, highly contagious disease that is considered a childhood illness but is seen more and more frequently in the United States in adolescents and young adults. Symptoms include fever, sneezing and coughing, conjunctivitis, small white spots on the inside of the cheek (Koplik spots), and a red, blotchy rash beginning several days after the respiratory signs. Measles is caused by the rubeola virus and is transmitted by inhalation of infected aerosol droplets as from sneezing, direct contact with infected nasal or throat secretions, or with articles freshly contaminated with the same nasal or throat secretions. Its very contagious nature combined with the fact that patients are most contagious before they are aware they are infected makes measles a disease that can spread rapidly through the population. Infection with measles confers lifelong immunity.

Measles and malnutrition form a deadly combination for many children in the developing world, but cases in the United States have been dramatically reduced since the introduction of the live attenuated measles vaccine in 1963. Before the advent of the vaccine, 200,000 to 500,000 cases of measles were reported yearly. In 1983 reported cases dropped to an all-time low of 1497. Then in the late 1980s, the incidence of measles began to climb again. In 1990 more than 25,000 cases of measles and 89 measles-associated deaths were reported. This increase was largely attributed to low immunization coverage rates among preschool-aged children, and was countered with efforts to increase immunization rates and the routine use of two doses of measles vaccine for all children (Mandell et al., 1995).

In 1993, reported measles cases again dropped to an all time low, but 1994 saw incidence once more beginning to increase. However, in contrast to the 1989 to 1991 measles resurgence, the 1994 measles outbreaks occurred predominantly among high school- and college-aged persons, many of whom had received only one previous dose of measles vaccine. From 1991 to the beginning of 1994, reported measles cases among children less than 5 years of age dropped by 50%; this decrease was attributed to systematic efforts to increase measles immunization coverage among children 24 months of age. Other patterns that have emerged in measles cases since 1991 include the importance of cases brought into this country from abroad and the spread of measles in groups that do not routinely accept immunization—45% of reported cases during the first half of 1994 occurred among members of groups with philosophic or religious objections to immunization (CDC, 1994f).

Healthy People 2000 calls for the sustained elimination of indigenous measles in the United States. Efforts to meet this goal include (1) rapid detection of cases and implementation of appropriate outbreak control measures, (2) achievement and maintenance of high levels of vaccination coverage among preschool-aged children in all geographic regions, (3) greater implementation and enforcement of the two-dose schedule among young adults, and (4) the determination of the source of all outbreaks and sporadic infections (CDC, 1994e). The roles of community health nurses involved in these efforts are to receive reports of cases, investigate and initiate control measures for outbreaks, and to use every opportunity to immunize adolescents and young adults who lack documentation of two doses of measles vaccine. Those who work in regions where illegal immigration is common and/or where groups obtain exemption from immunization on religious grounds need to be especially

alert for cases and the need for prompt outbreak control among these particularly susceptible populations.

Rubella (German Measles)

The rubella virus causes a mild febrile disease with enlarged lymph nodes and a fine, pink rash that is often difficult to distinguish from measles or scarlet fever. In contrast to measles, Rubella is only a moderately contagious illness. Transmission is through inhalation of or direct contact with infected droplets from the respiratory secretions of infected persons. Children may show few or no constitutional symptoms, whereas adults usually experience several days of low-grade fever, headache, malaise, runny nose, and conjunctivitis before the rash appears. Many infections occur without a rash.

Although still primarily a childhood disease, rubella occurs more often in adolescents than do measles or chickenpox. When children are well immunized, infections in these older populations become more important with outbreaks in institutions, universities, and the military. Infection confers lifelong immunity. Rubella is most common in winter and spring.

Prior to the availability of a vaccine, rubella occurred in epidemic proportions at fairly regular intervals. In 1964 in the United States, an epidemic of rubella infected an estimated 12,500,000 persons. Following licensure of the live attenuated rubella vaccine in 1969, cases declined steadily to an all-time reported low of 225 cases in 1988 (Mandell et al., 1995). During 1989 to 1991, rubella, like measles, experienced a resurgence (though small compared to that of measles). During 1992 and 1993, cases fell once more to an all-time low of 160 and 190 respectively (CDC, 1994f). Since then outbreaks have continued to occur.

For many years, because it caused only a mild illness, rubella was considered to be of minor importance. Then in 1941, the link between maternal rubella and certain congenital defects was recognized, and this disease suddenly assumed major public health significance. Congenital rubella syndrome (CRS) occurs in more than 25% of infants born to women who are infected with rubella during the first trimester of pregnancy (Mandell et al., 1995). Rubella infection, in addition to intrauterine death and spontaneous abortion, may result in anomalies that can affect single or multiple organ systems. Defects include cataracts, congenital glaucoma, deafness, microcephaly, mental retardation, cardiac abnormalities and diabetes mellitus.

The CDC maintains a national CRS registry. Recent cases of CRS have followed the rise and decline of rubella from 1989 to 1993. In 1991, 31 cases of confirmed indigenous CRS were reported in the United States, 20 of which occurred in Pennsylvania. A 1991 survey to determine the risk for CRS among babies born to unimmunized Amish mothers in one Pennsylvania county indicated the rate of CRS was 14 per 1000 live births compared with 0.006 for the total U.S.

population. No cases of CRS were reported in 1993. Eight imported cases of CRS were reported among babies born during 1991 to 1993 (CDC, 1994f).

Healthy People 2000 calls for the sustained elimination of both indigenous rubella and CRS. Preventing rubella and CRS will require many of the same efforts discussed with measles, including achievement and maintenance of high rates of immunization among preschoolers, early detection and outbreak control, taking advantage of opportunities like high school and college entrance to immunize susceptible adolescents, extending immunization opportunities to religious groups that traditionally do not seek health care, and targeting adolescent and young adults who are particularly susceptible because they come from or are exposed to persons from countries that do not routinely vaccinate against rubella.

Influenza

Influenza is a viral respiratory infection often indistinguishable from the common cold or other respiratory diseases. Transmission is airborne and through direct contact with infected droplets. Unlike many viruses that do not survive long in the environment, the "flu" virus is thought to survive for many hours in dried mucus. Outbreaks are common in the winter and early spring in areas where people gather indoors, such as in schools and nursing homes. Gastrointestinal signs are common as are respiratory symptoms. Because symptoms do not always follow a characteristic pattern, many viral diseases that are not influenza are often called flu. The most important factors to note about influenza are its epidemic nature and the mortality that results from its pulmonary complications, especially in the elderly.

There are three types of influenza viruses, A, B, and C. Type A is usually responsible for large epidemics, whereas outbreaks from type B are more regionalized, and those from type C are less common and usually only result in mild illness. These influenza viruses have the ability to frequently change the nature of their surface appearance or alter their antigenic makeup. Types B and C are fairly stable viruses, but type A is constantly changing. Minor antigenic changes are referred to as antigenic *drift* and are responsible for yearly epidemics and regional outbreaks. Major changes, such as the emergence of new subtypes, are called antigenic *shift;* these only occur with type A viruses. This antigenic shift and drift results in epidemic outbreaks every few years and pandemic outbreaks every 10 to 40 years. Mortality rates associated with epidemics may be higher than those in nonepidemic situations. During the 1918 to 1919 pandemic, the largest on record, 21 million deaths were reported worldwide, among them 549,000 in the United States (Mandell et al., 1995).

Influenza vaccines are prepared each year based on the best possible prediction of what type and variant of virus will be most prevalent that year. Because of the changing nature of the virus, immunization is necessary yearly and is given in the early fall before the flu season begins. Immunization is highly recommended for the elderly, individuals with chronic respiratory disease, and individuals with other chronic disease conditions that impair the immune system, as well as health-care workers and anyone involved in essential community services. Although immunization is recommended for the previously mentioned groups, any individual may benefit from this protection. Flu shots do not always prevent infection, but they do result in milder disease symptoms. Immunization of adults involves one injection. Children less than 12 years of age may initially receive two doses 1 to 2 weeks apart and subsequently one dose on a yearly basis. Sensitivity to eggs is a contraindication to immunization, and pregnant women should avoid immunization in the first trimester of pregnancy (Benenson, 1990).

Unlike the immunizations for childhood diseases, flu shots are largely targeted at an adult population. Because over 80% to 90% of all influenza-associated deaths in the United States occur in people 65 years of age and older, *Healthy People 2000* has targeted this age group to reduce epidemic-related pneumonia and influenza deaths. Obstacles to meeting this objective include an estimated 20% immunization coverage rate in the over-65 age group, partial antigenic mismatches of vaccine and circulating virus because of the continual emergence of new virus strains, and decreased immune response to vaccine with increasing age.

Since adults outside of health care facilities do not utilize health care services on the regular basis that children do, different approaches may be required to reach higher immunization coverage rates among adults. Public health nurses often spearhead community influenza immunization campaigns. Examples of innovative approaches for immunizing adults of all ages include nurses stationed at polling places during elections and nurses working in the parking lots of health departments, churches, and schools to conduct "drive-up" clinics. And as with children, nurses should check immunization history and encourage immunization for every adult encountered whether the clinic or home visit is immunization related or not.

FOODBORNE AND WATERBORNE DISEASES

Foodborne illness or "food poisoning" often is categorized as food infection or food intoxication. Food infection results from bacterial, viral, or parasitic infection of food. Examples of food infections are salmonellosis, hepatitis A, and trichinosis. Food intoxication results from toxins produced by bacterial growth, chemical contaminants (heavy metals), and a variety of disease-producing substances found naturally in

Table 39-5   Commonly Encountered Food Intoxications

Causal agent	Incubation period	Duration	Clinical presentation	Associated food
Staphylococcus aureus	30 min-7 hr	1-2 days	Sudden onset of nausea, cramps, vomiting, and prostration often accompanied by diarrhea; rarely fatal	All foods, especially those most likely to come into contact with foodhandlers hands that may be contaminated by purulent discharges from infections of the eyes and skin
Clostridium perfringens (strain A)	6-24 hr	1 day or less	Sudden onset of colic and diarrhea, maybe nausea; vomiting and fever unusual; rarely fatal	Inadequately heated meats or stews; food contaminated by soil or feces becomes infective when improper storage or reheating allows multiplication of organism
Vibrio parahemolyticus	4-96 hr	1-7 days	Watery diarrhea and abdominal cramps; sometimes nausea, vomiting, fever and headache; rarely fatal	Raw or inadequately cooked seafood; period of time at room temperature usually required for multiplication of organism
Clostridium botulinum	12-36 hr, sometimes days	slow recovery, maybe months	CNS signs; blurred vision, difficulty in swallowing and dry mouth followed by descending symmetrical flaccid paralysis of an alert person; "floppy baby" w/infant botulism; fatality <15% w/antitoxin and respiratory support	Home-canned fruits and vegetables that have not been preserved with adequate heating; infants have become infected from ingesting honey

From Benenson AS, editor: *Control of communicable diseases in man*, ed 15, Washington, DC, 1990, American Public Health Association.

certain foods, such as mushrooms and some seafood. Examples of food intoxications are botulism, mercury poisoning, and paralytic shellfish poisoning. Table 39-5 presents some of the most common agents of food intoxication, their incubation period, source, symptoms, and pathology. Although not a hard and fast rule, food infections are associated with incubation periods of 12 hours to several days after ingestion of the infected food, whereas intoxications often make themselves known within minutes to hours after ingestion. Botulism is a clear exception to this rule with an incubation period of a week or more in adults. The expression "ptomaine poisoning" enjoys popular usage when discussing foodborne illness but does not refer to a specific causal organism.

It is estimated that somewhere between 6.5 and 81 million cases of foodborne illness occur every year (Mandell et al., 1995). This range is so wide because most cases go unreported. National estimates of deaths from foodborne illness range from the hundreds to the thousands. Recent publicity has surrounded the deaths of individuals from a virulent strain of *E. coli, 0157:H2,* which has been found in hamburger. Whereas the very young, the very old, and the very debilitated are must susceptible, all individuals can acquire foodborne illness regardless of socioeconomic status, race, sex, age, occupation, educa-

tion, or area of residence. However, a new, particularly susceptible population is emerging as a result of the increasing older population, the increasing numbers of immunocompromised individuals (resulting from chemotherapy, immunosuppressive drugs, and AIDS), and the larger numbers of children surviving debilitating illness. At the same time our centralized food production and processing system with its widespread distribution network increases the potential for any contamination to result in a large-scale foodborne disease outbreak.

Ten Golden Rules for Safe Food Preparation

Protecting the nation's food supply from contamination by all virulent microbes is a very complex issue that will be incredibly costly and time consuming to address. However, much foodborne illness, regardless of causal organism, can be prevented easily through simple changes in food preparation, handling, and storage that will destroy or denature contaminants and prevent their further spread. Because these measures are so important in preventing foodborne disease, *Healthy People 2000* has included an objective directed toward them, and the World Health Organization has developed the "Ten Golden Rules for Safe Food Preparation" presented in the box on p. 768.

Ten Golden Rules for Safe Food Preparation

1. Choose food processed for safety.
2. Cook food thoroughly.
3. Eat cooked food immediately.
4. Store cooked food carefully.
5. Reheat cooked foods thoroughly.
6. Avoid contact between raw foods and cooked foods.
7. Wash hands repeatedly.
8. Keep all kitchen surfaces meticulously clean.
9. Protect foods from insects, rodents, and other animals.
10. Use pure water.

From Benenson AS, editor: *Control of communicable diseases in man*, ed 15, Washington, DC, 1990, American Public Health Association.

Salmonellosis

Salmonellosis is a bacterial disease characterized by a sudden onset of headache, abdominal pain, diarrhea, nausea, sometimes vomiting, and almost always fever. Onset is typically within 48 hours of ingestion, but the clinical signs are impossible to distinguish from other causes of gastrointestinal distress. Diarrhea and lack of appetite may persist for several days, and dehydration may be severe. Although morbidity can be significant, death is uncommon except among infants, the elderly, and the debilitated. The rate of infection is highest among infants and small children. It is estimated that only a small proportion of cases are recognized clinically and that only 1% of clinical cases are reported. The number of salmonella infections yearly may actually number in the millions (Benenson, 1990).

Outbreaks occur commonly in restaurants, hospitals, nursing homes, and institutions for children. The transmission route is ingestion of food derived from an infected animal or contaminated by feces of an infected animal or person. Meat, poultry, and eggs are the foods most often associated with salmonellosis outbreaks. Animals are the common reservoir for the various *Salmonella* serotypes although infected humans also may fill this role. Animals are more likely to be chronic carriers. Reptiles, such as iguanas, have been implicated as salmonella carriers along with small pet turtles, poultry, cattle, swine, rodents, dogs, and cats. Person-to-person transmission is an important consideration in day-care and institutional settings.

Escherichia coli 0157:H7

Escherichia coli 0157:H7 belongs to the enterohemorrhagic category of *E. coli* serotypes which produce a strong cytotoxin that can cause a potentially fatal hemorrhagic colitis. This pathogen was first described in humans in 1992 following the investigation of two outbreaks of illness that were associated with con-

sumption of hamburger from a fast-food restaurant chain. Since then, more than 12 outbreaks have been reported in the United States. Undercooked hamburger has been implicated in several outbreaks, as less commonly have roast beef, unpasteurized milk and apple cider, and municipal water. Person-to-person transmission in day-care centers also has been documented (CDC, 1994g). Infection with *0157:H7* causes bloody diarrhea, abdominal cramps, and infrequently fever. Children and the elderly are at highest risk for clinical disease and complications. Hemolytic uremic syndrome is seen in 5% to 10% of cases and may result in acute renal failure. The case-fatality rate is 3% to 5%.

Hamburger appears to be involved in outbreaks so often because the grinding process exposes pathogens on the surface of the whole meat to the interior of the ground meat, effectively mixing the once exterior bacteria thoroughly throughout the hamburger so that that searing the surface is no longer sufficient to kill all the bacteria. Tracking the contamination is complicated by the fact that hamburger is often made of meat ground from several sources. The best protection against this pathogen, as with most foodborne pathogens, is to thoroughly cook food before eating it.

Waterborne Disease Outbreaks and Pathogens

Waterborne pathogens usually enter water supplies through animal or human fecal contamination and frequently cause enteric disease. They include viruses, bacteria, and protozoans. Hepatitis A virus is probably the most publicized waterborne viral agent although other viruses also may be transmitted by this route (enteroviruses, rotaviruses, and paramyxoviruses). The most important waterborne bacterial diseases are cholera, typhoid fever, and bacillary dysentery. However, other *Salmonella* types, *Shigella*, *Vibrio* and various coliform bacteria including *E. Coli 0157:H7* may be transmitted in the same manner. In the past, the most important waterborne protozoans have been *Entmoeba histolytica* (amebic dysentery) and *Giardia lamblia*, but recent outbreaks of cryptosporidiosis like that in the Milwaukee water supply have pushed *Cryptosporidium* into the debate over how to best safeguard municipal water supplies. Protozoans prove especially problematic to municipal water managers because they do not respond to traditional chlorine treatment as do enteric and coliform bacteria.

The CDC defines an outbreak of waterborne disease as an incident in which two or more persons experience similar illness after consuming water that epidemiologic evidence implicates as the source of that illness. Only a single incident is required in cases of chemical contamination. The CDC and the Environmental Protection Agency (EPA) maintain a collaborative surveillance program for collection and periodic reporting of data on the occurrence and causes of waterborne disease outbreaks. During 1991 and 1992,

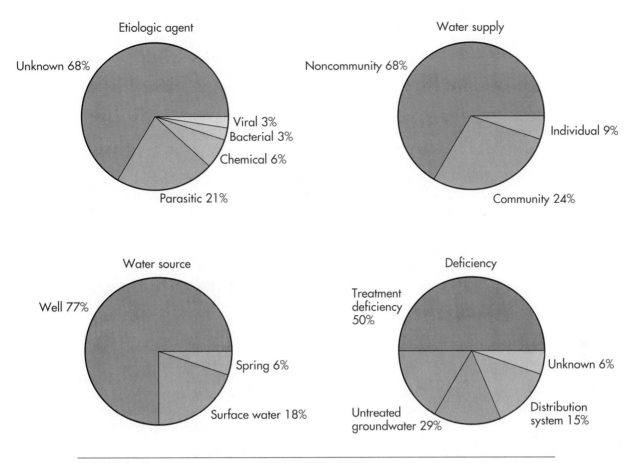

FIGURE 39-2

Outbreaks associated with drinking water in the United States from 1991 to 1992. (From Moore AC, et al: *MMWR* 42(SS-5):1, 1993.)

the CDC reported that 17 states and territories reported 34 outbreaks associated with water intended for drinking that resulted in illness in an estimated 17,464 persons. As shown in Figure 39-2, the majority of the outbreaks were associated with unknown infectious agents (68%), noncommunity water supply (68%), well water sources (77%), and water treatment deficiency (50%) (Moore et al., 1993). Of the 11 outbreaks for which an etiologic agent was established, seven were determined to have been caused by *Giardia* or *Cryptosporidium*. Twenty-one states reported 39 outbreaks associated with recreational water in which an estimated 1825 persons became ill. Of 11 outbreaks of swimming-associated gastroenteritis, six were caused by *Giardia* or *Cryptosporidium,* including three outbreaks associated with chlorinated, filtered pool water. The first reported outbreak of *E. coli 0157:H7* infection associated with recreational exposure occurred during this period (Moore et al., 1993).

VECTORBORNE DISEASES

Vectorborne diseases are diseases transmitted by vectors, usually insects, either biologically or mechani-

cally. With biologic transmission, the vector is necessary for the developmental stage of the infectious agent. An example would be mosquitos that carry malaria. Mechanical transmission occurs when an insect simply contacts the infectious agent with its legs or mouth parts and carries it to the host. An example would be flies and cockroaches that may contaminate food or cooking utensils.

Vectorborne diseases commonly encountered in the United States are those associated with ticks, such as Lyme disease and Rocky Mountain spotted fever. Community health nurses who work with large immigrant populations or with international travelers may encounter malaria and dengue fever, both carried by mosquitoes. Plague *(Yersinia pestis)* is carried by fleas of wild rodents. More rarely seen are babesiosis *(Babesia microti),* ehrlichiosis *(Ehrlichia chafeensis),* tularemia *(Francisella tularensis),* and Q fever *(Coxiella burnetii),* all associated with ticks.

Lyme Disease

Parents in Lyme, Connecticut, concerned about the unusual incidence of juvenile rheumatoid arthritis in their children, first brought attention to the tickborne infection that is now referred to as Lyme disease. Although first described in 1975, Lyme disease is now the most common vectorborne disease in the United States. The causative agent, the spirochete *Borrelia burgdoferi,* was not identified until 1982. Lyme disease is transmitted by Ixodid ticks that are associated with white-tailed deer *(Odocoileus virginianus)* and the white-footed mouse *(Peromyscus leucopus).* Lyme disease has been reported throughout the United States, but cases are concentrated in northeastern, north-central and Pacific coast states. It usually occurs in summer.

The clinical spectrum of Lyme disease can be divided into three stages. Stage I is characterized by erythema chronicum migrans, a distinctive skin lesion often called a bull's eye lesion because it begins as a red macule or papule at the site of the tick attachment and spreads outward in an annular fashion as the center clears. About 50% to 70% of infected persons will develop this lesion 3 to 30 days after a tick bite. The skin lesion may be accompanied or preceded by fever, fatigue, malaise, headache, muscle pains, and a stiff neck, as well as tender and enlarged lymph nodes and migratory joint pain. Most patients diagnosed in this early stage respond well to 10 to 14 days of oral tetracycline or penicillin.

If not treated during this first stage, Lyme disease can progress to stage II, which may include additional skin lesions, headache, and neurological and cardiac abnormalities. Patients may progress to stage III, which consists of recurrent attacks of arthritis and arthralgia, especially in the knees, that may begin months to years after the initial lesion. The clinical diagnosis of classical Lyme disease with the distinctive skin lesion is straightforward. Illness without the lesion is more difficult to diagnose since serological tests are more accurate in stages II and III than in stage I (Mandell et al., 1995).

Rocky Mountain Spotted Fever

Contrary to its name, Rocky Mountain spotted fever (RMSF) is seldom seen in the Rocky Mountains, and most commonly occurs in the Southeast, Oklahoma, Kansas, and Missouri. The infectious agent is *Rickettsia rickettsii.* The tick vector varies according to geographic region. The dog tick, *Dermacentor variabilis,* is the vector in the eastern and southern United States. RMSF is not transmitted from person to person. It is thought that one attack confers lifelong immunity.

Clinical signs include sudden onset of moderate to high fever, severe headache, chills, deep muscle pain, and malaise. About 50% of cases, beginning on the third day, experience a rash on the extremities, which then spreads to most of the body. Some cases of what has been referred to as "spotless" RMSF are now believed to be caused by a newly identified tickborne organism, *Ehrlichia chafeensis.* RMSF responds readily to treatment with tetracycline. Definitive diagnosis can be made with paired serum titers. Since early treatment is important in decreasing morbidity and mortality, treatment should be started in response to clinical and epidemiological considerations rather than waiting for laboratory confirmation (Benenson, 1990).

Prevention and Control of Tickborne Diseases

Vaccines are not available for any tickborne diseases except tularemia. The best preventive measures are wearing protective clothing when engaging in outdoor activities and conducting tick searches afterwards. Protective clothing calls for long sleeve shirts and long pants tucked into socks. Ticks require a prolonged period of attachment (6 to 48 hours) before they start blood feeding on the host. Therefore, prompt tick discovery and removal can help prevent transmission of disease. Ticks should be removed with steady, gentle traction on tweezers applied to the head parts of the tick (Mandell et al., 1995). The tick's body should not be squeezed during the removal process to avoid infection that could be transmitted from resultant tick feces and tissue juices. When outdoors, tick repellents containing diethytoluamide (DEET) can offer effective protection, but significant toxicity, including skin irritation, anaphylaxis, and seizures, has been reported in children.

DISEASES OF TRAVELERS

Individuals traveling outside of the United States need to be aware of and take precautions against potential diseases to which they may be exposed. Which diseases and what precautions will depend on the individual's health status, the particular travel destination, the reason for travel, and the length of travel. Persons who plan to travel in remote regions for an extended period of time may need to consider rare diseases and take special precautions that would not apply to the average traveler. Consultation with public health officials can provide specific health information and recommendations for a given situation.

Upon return from visiting exotic places, travelers may bring back with them an unplanned souvenir in the form of disease. Therefore, in a presenting patient, a history of travel should always be closely considered. Even the apparently healthy returned traveler, especially if residing in a tropical country for sometime, should undergo routine screening to rule out acquired infections. Likewise, refugees and immigrants may arrive with infectious health problems ranging from helminth infections to diseases of major public health significance, such as tuberculosis, malaria, cholera, and hepatitis. Community health nurses may find themselves dealing with these diseases since refugees are often processed and treated through the public health system.

Malaria

Caused by the bloodborne parasite *Plasmodium,* malaria is a potentially fatal disease characterized by regular cycles of fever and chills. Transmission is through the bite of an infected *Anopheles* mosquito. The word *malaria* is based on an association between the illness and the bad air of the marshes where the mosquitos breed. Malaria is a very old disease that first appears in recorded history in 1700 BC China. Literary references to malaria occur in the works of Homer, Chaucer, and Shakespeare. Through the sixteenth to the nineteenth centuries, European travelers to India, Africa, and the western hemisphere were ravaged by malaria. The disease was endemic in Canada and the United States during the eighteenth and nineteenth centuries, and at the beginning of the twentieth century there were more than 500,000 cases of malaria per year in the United States. Malaria has been a major factor in every American-involved war since the American Revolution. It is estimated that in Vietnam, U.S. military personnel lost more combat days from malaria than from battle wounds (Mandell et al., 1995).

Today, malaria poses a major health risk to inhabitants, as well as travelers, in many areas of the world. At present, there is no vaccine available to protect against this disease that causes as many as 200 to 300 million cases and 1 to 2 million deaths per year. Interestingly, in sub-Saharan Africa where *Plasmodium falciparum* malaria kills a million children a year, it is hypothesized that more children do not die than do because those who carry a positive sickle cell trait are somehow protected from the full onslaught of the disease (Mandell et al., 1995). This hypothesis has developed from the observation that in many areas of sub-Saharan Africa, 25% more children than expected are heterozygous for the sickle cell gene. The postulated explanation is that the selection for and maintenance of such a potentially harmful gene must have occurred because this same trait offered protection against some other powerful force, such as *Plasmodium falciparum* malaria.

Prevention of malaria is dependent on protection against mosquitoes and appropriate chemoprophylaxis. Of the four types of human malaria, two, *Plasmodium ovale* and *Plasmodium vivax* can result in relapsing malaria; more seriously, a third, *Plasmodium falciparum,* is drug-resistant. Thus, decisions about antimalarial drugs must be tailored individually, based on the types of malaria in the specific area of the country to be visited, the purpose of the trip, and the length of the visit. The CDC and the World Health Organization publish guides to the status of malaria and recommendations for prophylaxis on a country-by-country basis. At this time, there is no one drug or drug combination known to be safe and efficacious in preventing all types of malaria. Antimalarials are generally started a week to several weeks before leaving the country and are continued for 4 to 6 weeks after

returning. Despite appropriate prophylaxis, malaria may still be contracted. Travelers should be advised of this fact and urged to seek immediate medical care if they exhibit symptoms of cyclic fever and chills upon return home. Immigrants and visitors from areas where malaria is endemic also may become clinically ill after entering this country. Since the malaria parasite is bloodborne, blood donors should be questioned about a history of exposure to malaria.

Foodborne and Waterborne Diseases

As in the United States, since much foodborne disease can be avoided if the traveler eats thoroughly cooked foods prepared with reasonable hygiene; eating foods from street vendors may not be a good idea. Trichinosis, tapeworms, and fluke infections result from eating raw or undercooked meats. Raw vegetables may act as a source of bacterial, helminth, or protozoal infection if they have been grown with or washed in contaminated water. Fruits that can be peeled immediately before eating, such as bananas, are less likely to be a source of infection. Dairy products should be pasteurized and appropriately refrigerated.

Water in many areas of the world is not potable (safe to drink), and drinking this water can lead to infection with a variety of protozoal, viral, and bacterial agents, including amoeba, *Giardia, Cryptosporidium,* hepatitis, cholera, and various coliform bacteria. Unless traveling in an area where the piped water is known to be safe, only boiled or bottled water should be consumed. Ice also must be avoided since freezing does not inactivate these agents. Water must be boiled to render it safe for drinking. Some controversy exists over the amount of time to boil. The CDC recommends bringing water to a roiling boil for at least 1 minute to inactivate all major waterborne bacterial pathogens, protozoans, and hepatitis A (CDC, 1994h). An alternative to boiling is disinfection or water purification with iodine or chlorine compounds, allowing sufficient contact time for these chemical agents to work effectively. Filtration alone does not remove all bacteria, and chemically treated community water may be free of coliform bacteria but still contain protozoa. In some circumstances, such as when water is not factory bottled, bottled water also may be contaminated. Therefore, when potability is in question and circumstances allow, boiling is probably the best way to insure safe drinking water. If the water is questionable, choose coffee or tea made with boiled water, carbonated beverages without ice, beer, wine, or canned fruit juices.

Diarrheal Diseases

Travelers frequently suffer from diarrhea, so much so that colorful names, such as Montezuma's Revenge, Turista, and Colorado Quickstep, to name a few, exist in our vocabulary to describe these bouts of intestinal upset. Some of these diarrheas do not have infectious causes and may result from various factors, including stress, fatigue, schedule changes, and eating foods to which one is not accustomed. Acute infectious diarrheas are usually of viral or bacterial origin. *E. coli* probably causes more cases of traveler's diarrhea than all other infective agents combined (Mandell et al., 1995). Protozoal induced diarrheas, such as those resulting from *Entamoeba* and *Giardia,* are less likely to be acute and more commonly to present once the traveler returns home. Whether contaminated by bacteria, virus, or parasite, food and water are most likely to be the source of much infectious travelers' diarrhea. Thus carefully watching what one eats and drinks remains the best way to decrease the likelihood of contracting this unpleasant traveling companion.

Treatment for travelers' diarrhea, like that for other diarrheas, involves supportive care with fluid replacement and a diet that contains potassium and avoids fats and alcohol. Bananas are a good source of potassium. Oral rehydration solutions can be used if electrolyte replacement is a concern. Prepackaged oral rehydration salts are commonly available in pharmacies, but if they cannot be located a reasonable substitute can be created by mixing one-half teaspoon of table salt (sodium chloride), one-half teaspoon of sodium bicarbonate (baking soda), and four tablespoons of sucrose (table sugar) in one quart of carbonated water. If carbonated water is not available, boiled tap water is an appropriate substitute (Larson, 1990). This drink should be consumed over the course of a day as a supplement to a clear liquid diet. Drugs commonly used to combat diarrhea include diphenoxylate (Lomotil) and loperamide (Immodium). They are not recommended for young children. Medication should be discontinued and a doctor consulted if diarrhea does not respond in 2 days, if diarrhea is accompanied by fever, chills and severe cramps, or if blood and mucus appear in the stool.

ZOONOSES

A **zoonosis** is an infection transmitted from a vertebrate animal to a human under natural conditions. The agents that cause zoonoses do not need humans to maintain their lifecycles; infected humans have simply somehow managed to get in their way. Means of transmission include animal bites, inhalation, ingestion, direct contact, and arthropod intermediates. This last transmission route means that some vectorborne diseases also may be zoonoses. Other than vectorborne diseases, some of the more common zoonoses in the United States include toxoplasmosis *(Toxoplasma gondii),* cat scratch disease *(Rochalimaea henselae),* brucellosis *(Brucella* species), listeriosis *(Listeria monocytogenes),* salmonellosis *(Salmonella* serotypes), and rabies (Family *Rhabdoviridae,* genus *Lyssavirus).*

Rabies (Hydrophobia)

Rabies is probably the zoonosis that has received the most publicity. Movies and books like *Old Yeller* and *To Kill a Mockingbird,* are filled with images of mad dogs, and many families have at least one member who can relate a story about seeing a rabid dog shot. One of the oldest known human diseases, rabies was recognized and documented by Middle Eastern Civilizations as early as 2300 BC. Rabies was not reported in the western hemisphere before the arrival of the Europeans and may have been introduced by dogs that accompanied the conquistadors. In first century Rome, Celsus, the celebrated medical encyclopediast, recommended cautery of animal bites with a hot iron to protect against hydrophobia. Cautery remained the treatment of choice until Pasteur developed a rabies vaccine in 1885 (Mandell et al., 1995). The name hydrophobia comes from the common choking, gagging, and resultant anxiety that may follow a symptomatic patient's attempt to drink.

One of the most feared of human diseases, rabies has the highest case fatality rate of any known human infection, essentially 100%. In the 1970s three cases of presumed rabies recovery were reported. All had received pre-or postexposure prophylaxis. Since that time, despite the intensive medical care available in the United States, no survivors have been reported. A significant public health problem worldwide with an estimated 30,000 deaths a year, rabies in humans in the United States is a rare event because of the widespread vaccination of dogs begun in the 1950s. Today the major carriers of rabies in the United States are not dogs but wild animals—raccoons, skunks, foxes, and bats. Rodents, rabbits and hares, and opossums rarely carry rabies. Epidemiological information should be consulted for information on the potential carriers for a given geographic region. The east coast of the United States is presently experiencing an epizootic (epidemic) of raccoon rabies.

Rabies is transmitted to humans by introducing virus-carrying saliva into the body usually via an animal bite or scratch. Transmission also may occur if infected saliva comes into contact with a fresh cut or intact mucous membranes. Rabies is found in neural tissue and is not transmitted via blood, urine, or feces. Airborne transmission has been documented in caves with infected bat colonies. Transmission from human to human is theoretically possible but has not been documented except for six cases of rabies acquired by receiving corneal transplants harvested from individuals who died of undiagnosed rabies (Mandell et al., 1995). Guidelines for organ donation now exist to prevent this possibility.

The best protection against rabies remains vaccinating domestic animals—dogs, cats, cattle, and horses. If an individual is bitten, the bite wound should be thoroughly cleaned with soap and water and a physician consulted immediately. Suspicion of rabies should exist if the bite is from a wild animal or an unprovoked attack from a domestic animal. Even when there is no suspicion of rabies, a physician should be contacted since tetanus or antibiotic prophylaxis may be indicated.

No successful treatment exists for rabies once symptoms appear, but if given promptly and as directed, postexposure prophylaxis with human rabies immune globulin and rabies vaccine is effective in preventing the development of the disease. The human diploid cell vaccine currently in use in the United States is administered in a series of five, 1-ml doses injected into the deltoid muscle. Reactions to the vaccine are fewer and less serious than with previously used vaccines. Individuals who deal frequently with animals, such as zookeepers, lab workers, and veterinarians, may choose to receive the vaccine as preexposure prophylaxis. The decision to administer the vaccine to a bite victim depends on the circumstances of the bite and is made on an individual basis.

Recommendations for providing postexposure prophylaxis treatment are provided by the Advisory Committee for Recommendations on Immunization Practices available through local public health officials or the CDC. In general, cats and dogs that have bitten someone and have verified rabies vaccinations are confined for 10 days for observation. Treatment is initiated only if signs of rabies are observed during this period. If the animal is known to be or suspected to be rabid, treatment is begun immediately. If the animal is unknown to the victim and escapes, then public health officials should be consulted for help in deciding whether treatment is indicated. With wild animal bites, treatment is begun immediately. With bites from livestock, rodents, and rabbits, treatment is considered on an individual basis. Decisions to treat become more complicated for possible nonbite exposure to saliva from known infected animals, and again public health officials are helpful in making these treatment decisions (CDC, 1991a).

PARASITIC DISEASES

Parasitic diseases are more prevalent in developing countries than the United States because of tropical climate and inadequate prevention and control measures. A lack of cheap and effective drugs, poor sanitation, and a scarcity of funding lead to high reinfection rates even when control programs are attempted. Parasites are classified into four groups: nematodes (roundworms), cestodes (tapeworms), trematodes (flukes), and protozoa (single-celled animals). Nematodes, cestodes, and trematodes are all referred to as helminths. Table 39-6 presents examples of diseases caused by parasites from these groups.

Community health nurses and other health professionals should be aware of the increasing detection of parasitic infections in the United States. Several factors that have affected these recent developments include increases in each of the following areas:

1. international travel;
2. immigration of persons from developing countries;
3. incidence of AIDS with secondary parasitic opportunistic infections, such as pneumocystis carinii pneumonia, cryptosporidiosis, and toxoplasmosis;
4. recognition of giardiasis and cryptosporidiosis as common infectious agents in day care centers and water-borne disease outbreaks;
5. incidence and recognition of sexually transmitted parasitic enteric infections acquired through oral-anal sex; and
6. recognition of cryptosporidium species as pathogens in immunocompetent individuals as a result of improvement in stool examination techniques (Kappus et al., 1994).

Intestinal Parasitic Infections

Enterobiasis (pinworm) is the most common helminth infection in the United States with an estimated 42 million cases a year. Pinworm infection is most common among children and most prevalent in crowded and institutional settings. Pinworms resemble small pieces of white thread and can be seen with the naked eye. Diagnosis is usually accomplished through pressing cellophane tape to the perianal region early in the morning. Treatment with oral vermicides results in a cure rate of 90% to 100% (Mandell et al., 1995).

A recent study found intestinal parasites in 20% of 216,275 stool specimens examined by state diagnostic

Table 39-6 Selected Parasite Categories

Category	Parasite and disease
Intestinal nematodes	*Ascaris lumbricoides* (roundworm)
	Trichuris trichiura (whipworm)
	Ancylostoma, Necator (hookworm)
	Enterobius vermicularis (pinworm)
Blood and tissue nematodes	*Wuchereria bancrofti* (filariasis)
	Onchocerca volvulus (river blindness)
Cestodes	*Taenia solium* (pork tapeworm)
	Taenia saginata (beef tapeworm)
Trematodes	*Schistosoma* species (schistosomiasis)
Protozoans	*Giardia lamblia* (giardiasis)
	Entamoeba histolytica (amebiasis)
	Plasmodium species (malaria)
	Leishmania species (leishmaniasis)
	Trypanosoma species (African sleeping sickness, Chagas' disease)
	Toxoplasma gondii (toxoplasmosis)

From Brown H, Neva FA: *Basic clinical parasitology*, ed 5, Norwalk, Conn, 1983, Appleton-Century-Crofts.

laboratories with the commonly identified parasites being: *Giardia lamblia, Entamoeba histolytica,* hookworm, *Trichuris trichiura,* and *Ascaris lumbricoides* (Kappus et al., 1994). The opportunities for widespread indigenous transmission of these intestinal parasites are limited because of the improved sanitary conditions in this country. Effective drug treatment is available for these intestinal parasitic infections.

Parasitic Opportunistic Infections

Some of the common parasitic opportunistic infections in AIDS and other immunocompromised patients include *Pneumocystis carinii* pneumonia, cryptosporidiosis, microsporidiosis, and isosporiasis. Pneumocystis carinii pneumonia (PCP) occurs in 80% of AIDS patients. It is probably spread by an airborne route. It is found in the lungs and causes severe pneumonia in immunocompromised patients. It does not cause infection in immunocompetent persons. Effective drugs for treatment and prophylaxis of PCP are available, including trimethoprim-sulfamethoxazole and pentamidine isethionate (Martinez et al., 1992).

Cryptosporidiosis, microsporidiosis, and isosporiasis are intestinal protozoans transmitted by the fecal-oral route. Microsporidiosis has been reported in 7.5% of AIDS patients in New York City. The prevalence of cryptosporidiosis among people with AIDS is 4% in the United States and 50% in Haiti and Africa. The prevalence of isosporiasis among AIDS patients is 1% in the United States and 15% in Haiti. There is no effective drug treatment for cryptosporidiosis and microsporidiosis. Trimethoprim-sulfamethoxazole is effective for isosporiasis (Naficy and Soave, 1992).

Control and Prevention of Parasitic Infections

Community health nurses and other health care workers can make a correct diagnosis and provide appropriate treatment and patient education in an effort to prevent and control parasitic infections. Diagnosis of parasitic diseases is based on history of travel, characteristic clinical signs and symptoms, and the use of appropriate laboratory tests to confirm the clinical diagnosis. Knowing what specimens to collect, how and when to collect these specimens, and what laboratory techniques to use are important in interpreting the laboratory results. Effective drug treatment is available for most parasitic diseases. High drug cost, drug resistance, and toxicity are some of the common therapeutic problems. Measures for prevention and control of parasitic diseases include early diagnosis and treatment, improved personal hygiene, safer sex practices, community health education, vector control, and improvement in sanitary control of water, food, waste disposal, and living and working conditions (Brown and Neva, 1983).

NOSOCOMIAL INFECTIONS

Nosocomial infections are infections that are acquired during hospitalization or are developed within a hospital setting. They may involve patients, health care workers, visitors, or anyone who has contact with a hospital. Hospitalized patients are more susceptible than healthy persons because of their underlying illnesses, their exposure to virulent infectious agents from other patients, and their exposure to indigenous hospital flora of the hospital staff. They are also subjected to numerous invasive diagnostic and surgical procedures, and frequently given multiple broad-spectrum antibiotics and immunosuppressive drugs for treatment of neoplastic or chronic diseases. Studies suggest that at least 5% of patients admitted to hospitals in the United States will develop nosocomial infections. These infections result in an average hospital stay extension of 4 days, directly account for 60,000 deaths per year, and add $10 billion to the national health care expenditure (Mandell et al., 1995). The CDC maintains the National Nosocomial Infection Surveillance (NNIS) system, which is the only source of national data on the epidemiology of nosocomial infections in the United States. In the 1970s, CDC initiated the Study on the Efficacy of Nosocomial Infection Control (SENIC) Project to examine the effectiveness of the nosocomial surveillance and control programs in U.S. hospitals (CDC, 1992c).

The infection control practitioner plays a key role in a hospital infection surveillance and control program. Without a qualified and well-trained person in this position, the infection control program will not be effective. Over 95% of infection control practitioners are nurses. Their common job titles are infection control nurse, infection control coordinator and nurse epidemiologist. Nosocomial infections are relevant to the community health nurse in that they are an indicator of the health of one part of the community and as such fall under surveillance and reportable disease categories.

Universal Precautions

In 1985, in response to concerns regarding the transmission of HIV infection in health care settings, CDC developed a strategy of universal blood and body fluid precautions. It emphasizes strict adherence to universal precautions in handling blood and body fluids of *all* patients as if they contain HIV and other blood-borne pathogens. Health care workers must always wash their hands; wear gloves, masks, protective clothing, and other personal protective barriers as indicated; and properly use and dispose of all needles and sharp instruments to prevent exposure to potentially hazardous body fluids (CDC, 1989). CDC also made recommendations for preventing HIV and hepatitis B virus during exposure-prone invasive procedures including medical, surgical and dental procedures (CDC, 1991b).

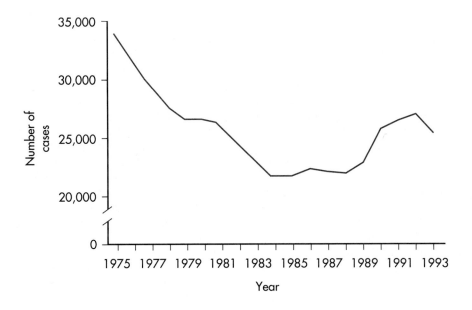

FIGURE 39-3

Number of reported tuberculosis cases in the United States from 1975 to 1993. (From Centers for Disease Control and Prevention: *MMWR* 43(20):361, 1994i.)

TUBERCULOSIS

Tuberculosis is a mycobacterial disease caused by *Mycobacterium tuberculosis*. It is mainly transmitted by exposure to tubercle bacilli in airborne droplets from persons with pulmonary tuberculosis during talking, coughing, or sneezing. The common symptoms of tuberculosis are cough, fever, hemoptysis, chest pains, fatigue, and weight loss. The incubation period is 4 to 12 weeks. The most critical period for development of clinical disease is the first 6 to 12 months after infection. About 5% of those initially infected may develop pulmonary tuberculosis or extrapulmonary involvement. The infection in about 95% of those initially infected becomes latent and may be reactivated later in life. Reactivation of latent infections is common in the elderly, immunocompromised patients, substance abusers, underweight and undernourished persons, and those with diabetes, silicosis, or gastrectomies (Benenson, 1990).

Resurgence of Tuberculosis

Among adults worldwide, tuberculosis is the leading cause of death from a single infectious agent. It is estimated that if global control of tuberculosis remains at the 1990 level during the next 10 years that 30 million people will die from this disease by the year 2000 (Raviglione, et al., 1994). The incidence of tuberculosis in the United States showed a steady decline in the 1970s and early 1980s but began to increase in 1989 as shown in Figure 39-3 (CDC, 1994i). This increase is believed to be due to the increasing incidence of tuberculosis among people with AIDS, the homeless,

substance abusers, the elderly, immigrants, and people in nursing homes and correctional facilities. Several outbreaks attributable to multidrug-resistant *Mycobacterium tuberculosis* (MDRTB) have occurred. These patients with MDRTB exhibited mortality rates from 43% to as high as 89% (CDC, 1994j).

Diagnosis and Treatment

The screening tests used are the tuberculin skin test and chest radiographs for positive skin reactors with pulmonary symptoms. False negative skin test reactions attributable to anergy may occur in persons who are immunosuppressed by drugs or who have diseases, such as advanced tuberculosis, AIDS, and measles. Confirmatory tests include stained sputum smears and other body fluids with demonstration of the acid-fast bacilli (for presumptive diagnosis) and culture of the tubercle bacilli for definitive diagnosis.

The absence of a reaction to the tuberculin skin test does not rule out the diagnosis of tuberculosis disease or infection. In immunosuppressed persons, delayed-type hypersensitivity responses, such as tuberculin reactions, may decrease or disappear. This condition, known as anergy, may be caused by many factors, such as HIV infection, overwhelming miliary or pulmonary TB, severe or febrile illness, measles or other viral infection, Hodgkin's disease, sarcoidosis, live-virus vaccination, and the administration of corticosteroids or immunosuppressive drugs.

On average, 10% to 25% of patients with tuberculosis disease test negative on TB skin tests. Approxi-

Tuberculin Skin Test Classification Guidelines

Use intradermal Mantoux test with 0.1ml of 5 TU PPD tuberculin.
Read reaction 48 to 72 hours after injection.
Measure only induration.
Record results in millimeters.
Test is positive if greater than or equal to 5 mm in
- Persons known or suspected to have HIV infection.
- Persons who have a chest radiograph suggestive of previous TB.
- Close contacts of a person with infectious TB.

Test is positive if greater than or equal to 10 mm in
- Persons with certain medical conditions, excluding HIV.
- Persons who inject drugs (if HIV negative).
- Foreign-born persons from areas where TB is common.
- Medically underserved, low-income populations.
- Residents of long-term care facilities.
- Children younger than 4 years of age.

Test is positive if greater than or equal to 15 mm in
- All persons with no risk factors for TB.

From Centers for Disease Control and Prevention: *Screening for TB disease and infection, core curriculum on tuberculosis,* ed 3, 1994k.

mately one-third of patients with HIV infection and more than 60% of patients with AIDS may have skin test reactions less than 5-mm even if they are infected with *M. tuberculosis.*

Since community health nurses usually perform the tuberculin skin test, they need to know the correct procedure in administering and interpreting the test results. (See box at left for TB skin test guidelines.) They need to educate patients to adhere to the long duration of therapy. Community health nurses may be involved in directly observed therapy (DOT), urine testing to check compliance, or contact investigation of cases in the community.

Patients with tuberculosis should be treated promptly with the appropriate multiple combination of antimicrobial drugs. Effective drug regimens currently used in the United States include isoniazid (INH) combined with rifampin (RIF), with or without pyrazinamide (PZA) for at least 6 months. Treatment failure is largely due to poor compliance to taking medications over the entire treatment period and development of drug resistance (Benenson, 1990).

Clinical Application

One of the biggest problems with tuberculosis prevention and control programs is the required lengthy therapy using multiple drug combinations. Failure to comply with therapy over the entire treatment period may result in treatment failure and the development of drug resistance. The South Carolina Department of Health and Environmental Control, Tuberculosis Control Division developed an innovative program in collaboration with the American Lung Association, South Carolina Chapter to provide incentives to clients to adhere to their treatment regimens (Pozsik, 1995). Incentives are monetary or nonmonetary, but are tailored to the wishes of the individual client. Examples of incentives include food, clothing, fish bait, and books. Tuberculosis control nurses personally administer each dose of treatment drugs to the client, and upon completion of an agreed upon number of treatments, present the client with an incentive item. Each nurse has a regular caseload of clients with whom she meets as the treatment schedule demands. Meetings may be at home or at designated meeting places, such as parking lots, fishing holes, or fast-food restaurants. The incentive program has been so successful in increasing treatment compliance that several other states have replicated this innovative approach. In addition to direct observation of drug therapy, these nurses also aggressively conduct contact investigation of their clients. This investigation may actually involve observing the client's daily activities to identify possible contacts. The vigorous efforts of these community health nurses assigned to the tuberculosis control unit have paid off in the steady decline of tuberculosis cases in South Carolina over the past 10 years.

Key Concepts

- The burden of infectious diseases is high in both human and economic terms. Preventing these diseases must be given high priority in our present health care system.

- The successful interaction of the infectious agent, host, and environment is essential for disease transmission. Knowledge of the characteristics of each of these three factors is impor-

Key Concepts—cont'd

tant in understanding the transmission, prevention and control of these diseases. Effective intervention measures at the individual and community levels must be aimed at breaking the chain linking the agent, host, and environment. An integrated approach attacking all three factors simultaneously is an ideal goal to strive for but may not be feasible for all diseases.

◆ We must constantly be aware of our vulnerability to threats posed by emerging infectious diseases. Most of the factors causing the emergence of these diseases are influenced by human activities and behavior.

◆ Communicable diseases are preventable. Preventing infection through primary prevention activities is the most cost-effective public health strategy.

◆ We must always apply infection control principles and procedures in our work environment. We must strictly practice the universal blood and body fluid precautions strategy to prevent transmission of HIV and other blood-borne pathogens.

◆ Effective control of communicable diseases must use a multisystem approach focusing on improving host resistance, improving safety of the environment, improving public health systems, and facilitating social and political changes to ensure health for all people.

◆ Communicable disease prevention and control programs must move beyond providing drug treatment and vaccines. Health promotion and education aimed at changing human behavior must be emphasized.

◆ Community health nurses play a key role in all aspects of prevention and control of communicable diseases. Close cooperation with other members of the interdisciplinary health care team must be maintained. Mobilizing community participation is essential to successful implementation of programs.

◆ The successful global eradication of smallpox proved the feasibility of eradication of communicable diseases. We must support the current global eradication campaigns against poliomyelitis and dracunculiasis as health professionals and concerned citizens of the global village.

Critical Thinking Activities

1. Ride with a nurse who makes home visits. Discuss living situations and other risk factors that may contribute to the development of infectious diseases, as well as possible points where the nurse may intervene to help prevent these diseases, such as checking the immunization status of all individuals in the household.

2. Spend time with the persons who are responsible for reporting communicable disease for your county or city. To become familiar with the reportable diseases that are a problem in the area, look at how many cases have been reported during the past month, 6 months, and year. Contrast these numbers with national statistics. Discuss outbreak procedures that may accompany the reporting of some of these diseases. If possible go on an outbreak investigation.

3. Accompany a TB outreach nurse to observe case investigation, contact tracing, and directly observed therapy.

4. Visit a clinic that serves a refugee, immigrant, or migrant labor population to observe the infectious diseases commonly seen in these groups. Compare and contrast this visit with a visit to a clinic that serves an inner-city population and a visit to a clinic that serves a rural population.

5. Sit in a clinic waiting room for immunization services and talk with parents about the concerns they may have and the barriers they may perceive in obtaining immunizations for their children.

6. Spend time with a school nurse to see what infectious diseases are routinely encountered in the educational setting. Discuss risk factors for disease in school-aged youth and the strategies employed to prevent infectious diseases in this age group.

7. Visit a day-care center. Observe potential situations for the communication of infectious diseases and discuss with the director the steps taken to prevent and control infection, including immunization requirements and procedures for hand washing and food preparation.

Bibliography

Bates AS, Fitzgerald JF, Dittus RS, Wolinsky FD: Risk factors for underimmunization in poor urban infants, *JAMA* 272(4):1105-1110, 1994.

Benenson AS, editor: *Control of communicable diseases in man,* ed 15, Washington, DC, 1990, American Public Health Association.

Brown H, Neva FA: *Basic clinical parasitology,* ed 5, Norwalk, Conn, 1983, Appleton-Century-Crofts.

Centers for Disease Control and Prevention (CDC): Guidelines for prevention of transmission of HIV and Hepatitis B virus to health care and public safety workers, *MMWR* 38(S-6):1, 1989.

Centers for Disease Control and Prevention (CDC): International Task Force for Disease Eradication, *MMWR* 39(13):209, 1990.

Centers for Disease Control and Prevention (CDC): Rabies Prevention—US, 1991, *MMWR* 40 (RR-3):1, 1991a.

Centers for Disease Control and Prevention (CDC): Recommendations for preventing transmission of HIV and Hepatitis B virus to patients during exposure-prone invasive procedures, *MMWR* 40(RR-8):1, 1991b.

Centers for Disease Control and Prevention (CDC): Update: International Task Force for Disease Eradication 1990 and 1991, *MMWR* 41(3):40, 1992a.

Centers for Disease Control and Prevention (CDC): Eradication of Paralytic Poliomyelitis in the Americas, *MMWR* 41(36):681, 1992b.

Centers for Disease Control and Prevention (CDC): Public health focus: surveillance, prevention and control of nosocomial infections, *MMWR* 41(42):783, 1992c.

Centers for Disease Control and Prevention (CDC): Tuberculosis Control Laws, 1993: Recommendations of the Advisory Council for the Elimination of Tuberculosis (ACET), *MMWR* 42(RR-15):1, 1993a.

Centers for Disease Control and Prevention (CDC): Recommendations of the International Task Force for Disease Eradication, *MMWR* 42(RR-16):1, 1993b.

Centers for Disease Control and Prevention (CDC): *Addressing emerging infectious disease threats: a prevention strategy for the US,* Atlanta, 1994a, CDC.

Centers for Disease Control and Prevention (CDC): National Notifiable Disease Reporting, 1994, *MMWR* 43(43):800, 1994b.

Centers for Disease Control and Prevention (CDC): Laboratory management of agent associated with Hantavirus pulmonary syndrome: interim biosafety guidelines, *MMWR* 43(RR-7):1, 1994c.

Centers for Disease Control and Prevention (CDC): Certification of poliomyelitis eradication—the Americas, 1994, *MMWR* 43(39):720, 1994d.

Centers for Disease Control and Prevention (CDC): Measles—United States, first 26 weeks, 1994, *MMWR* 43(37):673-676, 1994e.

Centers for Disease Control and Prevention: Rubella and congenital rubella syndrome—United States, January 1, 1991-May 7, 1994, *MMWR* 43(21):391-401, 1994f.

Centers for Disease Control and Prevention: *Escherichia coli* 0157:H7 outbreak linked to home-cooked hamburger—California, July 1993, *MMWR* 43(12):214-215, 1994g.

Centers for Disease Control and Prevention: Assessment of inadequately filtered public drinking water—Washington, DC, December 1993, *MMWR* 43(36):663, 1994h.

Centers for Disease Control and Prevention: Expanded tuberculosis surveillance and tuberculosis morbidity—US, 1993, *MMWR* 43(20):361, 1994i.

Centers for Disease Control and Prevention: Guidelines for preventing the transmission of *mycobacterium tuberculosis* in health care facilities, 1994, *MMWR* 43(RR-13):1, 1994j.

Centers for Disease Control and Prevention: *Screening for TB disease and infection, core curriculum on tuberculosis,* ed 3, 1994k.

Centers for Disease Control and Prevention: Recommended childhood immunization schedule—US, January, 1995, *MMWR* 43(51, 52):959, 1995.

Evans AS: The eradication of communicable diseases: myth or reality? *Am J Epidemiology* 122(2):199, 1985.

Evans AS, editor: *Viral infections of humans,* ed 3, New York, 1989, Plenum Medical Book.

Gibson JJ, editor: *Reportable diseases in South Carolina,* Columbia, 1995, South Carolina Department of Health and Environmental Control.

Haley RW: Incidence and Nature of Endemic and Epidemic Nosocomial Infections. In Bennett JV, Brachman PS, editors: *Hospital infections,* ed 2, Boston, 1986a, Little, Brown, & Co.

Haley RW, Garner JS: Infection surveillance and control programs. In Bennett JV, Brachman PS, editors: *Hospital infections,* ed 2, 1986b, Little, Brown, & Co.

Hopkins DR, Ruiz-Tiben E, Ruebush T, Agle AN, Withers PG: Dracunculiasis eradication: March, 1994 Update, *Am J Trop Med Hyg* 52(1):14, 1995.

Kappus KD, Lundgren RG, Juranek DD, Roberts JM, Spencer HC: Intestinal parasitism in the US: update on a continuing problem, *Am J Trop Med Hyg* 50(6):705, 1994.

Larson DE, editor: *Mayo Clinic family health book,* New York, 1990, William Morrow and Company.

Last JM, editor: *A dictionary of Epidemiology,* New York, 1983, Oxford University Press.

Ledeberg J, Shope RE, Oaks SC, editors: *Emerging infections: microbial threats to health in the US,* Washington DC, 1992, National Academy Press.

Mandell GL, Bennett JE, Dolin R, editors: *Principles and practice of infectious diseases,* ed 4, New York, 1995, Churchill-Livingstone.

Martinez A, Suffredini AF, Masur H: Pneumocystis carinii disease in HIV-infected persons. In Wormser GP, editor: *AIDS and other manifestations of HIV infection,* ed 2, New York, 1992, Raven Press.

McGinnis JM, Foege WH: Actual causes of death in the US, *JAMA* 270(18):2207, 1993.

Moore AC, Herwaldt BC, Craun GF, Calderon RL, Highsmith AK, Juranek DD: Surveillance for waterborne disease outbreak—US, 1991-1992, *MMWR* 42(SS-5):1, 1993.

Naficy AB, Soave R: Cryptosporidiosis, isosporiasis and microsporidiosis in AIDS. In Wormser GP, editor: *AIDS and other manifestations of HIV infection,* ed 2, New York, 1992, Raven Press.

Pozsik C: Personal communication, 1995.

Raviglione MC, Snider DE Jr, Kochi A: Global epidemiology of tuberculosis: morbidity and mortality of a worldwide epidemic, *JAMA* 273(3):220, 1994.

Wenzel RP: Control of communicable diseases: overview. In Last JM, Wallace RB, editors: *Public Health and Preventive Medicine,* ed 13, Norwalk, 1992, Appleton and Lange.

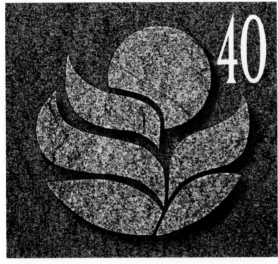

40

HIV, Hepatitis, and Sexually Transmitted Diseases

Patty J. Hale

Objectives

After reading this chapter, the student should be able to do the following:

◆ Describe the natural history of human immunodeficiency virus (HIV) infection and appropriate client education at each stage.
◆ Describe the clinical signs of the major sexually transmitted diseases.
◆ Identify the trends in incidence of the major sexually transmitted diseases and groups that are at greatest risk.
◆ Identify behaviors that place people at risk of contracting sexually transmitted diseases (STDs).
◆ Describe community health nursing activities to prevent and control STDs.
◆ Explain the various roles of community health nurses in providing care for those with chronic STDs.

Key Terms

acquired immunodeficiency syndrome (AIDS)
chancroid
chlamydia
genital herpes
genital warts
gonorrhea
hepatitis B virus (HBV)
HIV seronegative
HIV seropositive
HIV seroprevalence
human immunodeficiency virus (HIV)
human papillomavirus (HPV)
incubation period
partner notification
pelvic inflammatory disease (PID)
seroconversion
sexually transmitted diseases (STDs)
syphilis

Outline

The study of **sexually transmitted diseases (STDs)** has changed dramatically in recent years. For several decades following the development of antibiotics in the 1940s, STDs were considered to be a problem of the past. Recently, the increase in viral STDs and emerging antibiotic-resistant strains have posed new challenges. There is also greater understanding of how coinfection with one STD can increase susceptibility to other STDs, such as **human immunodeficiency virus (HIV).**

This renewed concern about STDs has prompted the development of standards for STDs and HIV in *Healthy People 2000* (1991). The box at right gives some of the goals used to evaluate progress toward diminishing STDs as a health threat and providing related services by the year 2000.

Nearly all STDs are acquired through behaviors that can be avoided or changed, and thus intervention efforts by community health nurses have focused on primary prevention. This is challenging because the population at risk for acquiring STDs has grown, as has the number of people who are sexually active and use injection drugs (Centers for Disease Control, 1993b). Thus there is greater urgency than ever to develop effective methods to prevent and control STDs. Among other activities, community health nurses counsel clients on how to make their behavior more healthful.

This chapter describes several STDs and their nursing management. It concludes with implications for community health nursing care for primary, secondary, and tertiary prevention.

HUMAN IMMUNODEFICIENCY VIRUS INFECTION

HIV infection and **acquired immunodeficiency syndrome (AIDS)** have had an enormous political and social impact on society. Numerous controversies have arisen over many aspects of HIV. The public's fears about HIV have affected many issues and are magnified by the fact that this disease has commonly afflicted two groups that have been largely scorned by society: homosexuals and injection drug users. Debates have arisen over how to control disease transmission and how to pay for related health services. One ongoing debate involves whether clean needles should be distributed to prevent the spread of HIV.

Economic costs are growing as HIV causes premature disability and death. Eighty-eight percent of afflicted persons are between the ages of 20 and 49 years, resulting in disrupted families and lost creative and economic productivity at a period of life when growth is the norm. The health care delivery costs of this group are supported largely by Medicaid, rather than private insurance or Medicare (Schur and Berk, 1994). This is because many people with HIV are either indigent or fall into poverty when paying for

Selected *Healthy People 2000* Objectives Pertaining to Sexually Transmitted Diseases

INFECTION RATES

1. Reduce gonorrhea to an incidence of no more than 225 cases per 100,000 people. (201.6 per 100,000 population in 1992)
2. Reduce *Chlamydia trachomatis* infections as measured by a decrease in the incidence of nongonococcal urethritis to no more than 170 cases per 100,000 people. (182.6 per 100,000 population in 1992)
3. Reduce primary and secondary syphilis to an incidence of no more than 10 cases per 100,000 people. (13.7 per 100,000 population in 1992)
4. Reduce congenital syphilis to an incidence of no more than 50 cases per 100,000 live births. (94.7 per 100,000 population in 1992)
5. Reduce sexually transmitted hepatitis B infection to no more than 30,500 cases. (rate unavailable)

RISK REDUCTION OBJECTIVES

1. Reduce the proportion of adolescents who have engaged in sexual intercourse to no more than 15% by 15 years of age and no more than 40% by 17 years of age.
2. Increase to at least 50% the proportion of sexually active, unmarried people who used a condom at last sexual intercourse.

SERVICE OBJECTIVES

1. Include instruction in STD transmission prevention in the curricula of all middle and secondary schools, preferably as part of quality school health education.
2. Increase to at least 90% the proportion of primary care providers treating patients with STDs who correctly manage cases, as measured by their use of appropriate types and amounts of therapy.

health care over the course of the illness. It is estimated that the total lifetime health care costs for an individual with HIV infection are $119,274 (Hellinger, 1993).

In 1990 the Ryan White Comprehensive AIDS Resource Emergency (CARE) Act was passed to provide services for persons with HIV infection. This program provides funds for health care in geographical areas with the largest number of AIDs cases. Health services that are covered include emergency services, services for early intervention and care (sometimes including coverage of health insurance), and drug reimbursement programs for HIV-infected individuals.

Pathogenesis

HIV infection is caused by a retrovirus, the human immunodeficiency virus, which was discovered in 1983. Retroviruses produce an enzyme called reverse transcriptase that transcribes the viral genome onto the DNA of the host cell. This results in viral replication by the infected cell. HIV causes immunological deficiencies that leave the host susceptible to opportunistic infections and cancers.

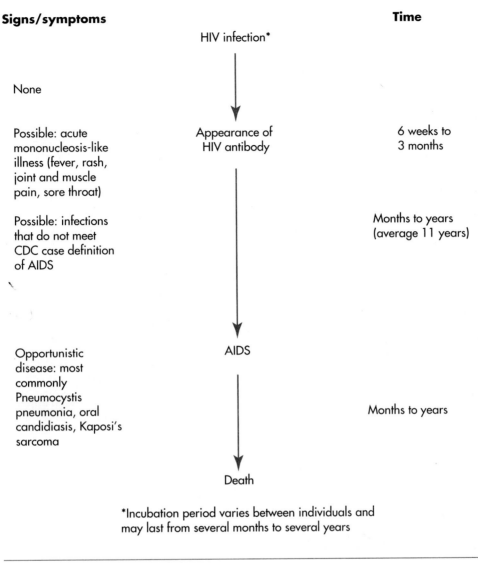

Signs/symptoms   **Time**

HIV infection*

None

Possible: acute
mononucleosis-like   Appearance of   6 weeks to
illness (fever, rash,   HIV antibody   3 months
joint and muscle
pain, sore throat)

Possible: infections   Months to years
that do not meet   (average 11 years)
CDC case definition
of AIDS

Opportunistic   AIDS
disease: most
commonly
Pneumocystis
pneumonia, oral   Months to years
candidiasis, Kaposi's
sarcoma

                                  Death

*Incubation period varies between individuals and
may last from several months to several years

FIGURE 40-1

Natural history of human immunodeficiency virus.

HIV infects many cells, including the dendritic cells, endothelial cells, Langerhans' cells, lymphocytes, monocytes, and macrophages. The greatest damage is from the infection of the CD4, or helper T-, lymphocyte, the cell that induces nearly every immune response. The progressive decline in numbers of CD4 lymphocytes causes disruptions in immune functioning. For example, HIV adversely affects antibody production and decreases intracellular killing of pathogens following phagocytosis.

Natural History of HIV

The natural history of HIV is described in Figure 40-1. On entering the body, HIV infects mostly lymphoid cells and becomes latent for several months or years, so the person is seemingly well and symptom free. It takes an average of 11 years to develop symptomatic disease, and during this prolonged **incubation period,** clients have a gradual deterioration of the immune system. They also carry and are able to transmit the virus.

About 4 weeks after infection and during the time of antibody production, some individuals experience a short-term mononucleosis-like illness. This is a self-limiting illness with the symptoms of lymphadenopathy, myalgias, pharyngitis, lethargy, rash, and fever (Pantaleo et al., 1993).

After a variable period of time—commonly from 6 weeks to 3 months—HIV antibodies appear in the blood. Although most antibodies serve a protective role, HIV antibodies do not. However, their presence helps in the detection of HIV infection because tests show their presence in the bloodstream.

AIDS is the last stage on the long continuum of HIV infection and may result from damage caused by HIV, secondary cancers, or opportunistic organisms. AIDS is defined as a disabling or life-threatening illness caused by HIV, or a CD4 T-lymphocyte count of less than $200/\mu L$ with documented HIV infection. The

Table 40-1   Clinical Manifestations of AIDS

Disease	Clinical signs
INFECTIONS	
Isosporiasis, chronic interstitial (>1 mo)	Diarrhea
Coccidioidomycosis	Fever, fatigue, shortness of breath
Histoplasmosis	Fever, chest pain, dyspnea
Recurrent salmonella septicemia	Fever, vasogenic shock
Candidiasis (respiratory or esophageal)	White patches on tongue, difficulty eating
Cryptococcal meningitis	Fever, headache, stiff neck
Pneumocystis carinii pneumonia or recurrent bacterial pneumonia	Shortness of breath, dry cough, fever, fatigue
Toxoplasmosis of brain	Hemiparesis, seizures, aphasia
Cryptosporidium enteritis infection (>1 mo)	Diarrhea, weakness
Mycobacterium tuberculosis infection (pulmonary or extrapulmonary)	Productive, purulent cough; fatigue; weight loss
Mycobacterium avium complex or other mycobacterium	Septicemia, diarrhea
Cytomegalovirus retinitis or CMV disease	Visual blurring
Herpes simplex virus infection	Chronic vesicles (>1 mo), bronchitis
Pulmonary tuberculosis	Hemoptysis, night sweats
CANCERS	
Invasive cervical cancer	Cervical dysplasia
Kaposi's sarcoma	Purple skin lesions, localized edema
Lymphoma (Burkitt's or primary of brain)	Weight loss, fever, night sweats
SYNDROMES	
Wasting syndrome caused by HIV	Diarrhea, decreased appetite
HIV-related encephalopathy	Decline in cognition, behavior, or coordination
Progressive multifocal leukoencephalopathy	

CD4 T-lymphocyte is the most common mode of tracking progression of the infection, and antiretroviral therapy is begun when the CD4 count falls to 500/μL.

Many of the AIDs-related opportunistic infections are caused by microorganisms that are commonly present in healthy individuals but that do not cause disease in persons with an intact immune system. These microorganisms proliferate in persons with HIV infection because of a weakened immune system.

Opportunistic infections may be caused by bacteria, fungi, viruses, or protozoa. The most common opportunistic diseases are *Pneumocystis carinii* pneumonia and oral candidiasis. On January 1, 1993, an expanded case definition for AIDS was implemented to include pulmonary tuberculosis, invasive cervical cancer, or recurrent pneumonia (Centers for Disease Control, 1992c). Table 40-1 describes diseases commonly associated with AIDS and their clinical manifestations.

Tuberculosis, an infection that is becoming more prevalent because of HIV infection, can spread rapidly among immunosuppressed individuals. Thus HIV-infected individuals who reside in close proximity to one another—such as in long-term care facilities, prisons, drug treatment facilities, or other settings—must be carefully screened and deemed noninfectious before admission to such settings. For more indepth coverage of tuberculosis, see Chapter 39.

Transmission

HIV transmission occurs through exposure to blood, semen, vaginal secretions, and breast milk. HIV is not transmitted through casual contact; thus it is safe to touch or hug someone or shake hands with someone who has HIV infection. HIV is also not transmitted by insects, coughing, sneezing, sharing office equipment, or sitting next to or eating with someone who has HIV infection. Except for those persons who had blood or other body fluid exposure or sexual or needle-sharing contact with an infected person, no one has developed infection (Centers for Disease Control, 1994c). The modes of transmission are listed in the box below. The exposure categories of AIDS are shown in Table 40-2.

Potential donors of blood and tissues are screened through the *HIV antibody test* and interviews to assess for a history of high-risk activities. Blood or tissue is not used from individuals who have a history of high-risk behavior or who are **HIV seropositive** (antibodies of HIV present in the serum). In addition to screening, coagulation factors used to treat hemophilia and other blood disorders are made safe through heat treatments to inactivate the virus. Such screening has significantly reduced the risk of transmission of HIV by blood products and organ donations. It is estimated that the odds of contracting HIV infection through receiving a blood transfusion are 1 in 100,000 units of blood transfused (Perkins, 1993).

Table 40-2 AIDS Cases by Exposure Category Reported Through December 1993, United States

Adult and adolescent exposure category	%*	Pediatric (13 yr of age and younger) exposure category	%
Male homosexual and bisexual contact	54	Hemophilia and coagulation disorder	4
Injectable drug use (heterosexual)	25	Mother with or at risk of HIV infection	89
Injectable drug use and male homosexual and bisexual contact	7	Receipt of blood transfusion, blood components, or tissues	6
Hemophilia and coagulation disorder	1	Undetermined	1
Heterosexual contact	7		
Blood transfusion, blood components, or tissue	2		
Other and undetermined†	5		

Modified from Centers for Disease Control: *HIV/AIDS Surveillance Report* 5(4):3-33, 1994.
*The total of 101% is due to rounding errors.
†Refers to 12 health care workers who developed AIDS after occupational exposure to HIV-infected blood, as documented by evidence of seroconversion; to four patients who developed AIDS after exposure to HIV within the health care setting; to three persons who acquired HIV infection perinatally and were diagnosed with AIDS after 13 yr of age; and to one person with intentional self-inoculation of blood from an HIV-infected person.

When a client is infected with other STDs, it increases the risk of HIV infection, and HIV may also affect other STDs. This is referred to as epidemiological synergy and may result from any of the following: open lesions providing entry of pathogens, STDs decreasing host immune status and changing the progression of HIV infection, and HIV changing the natural history of STDs or the effectiveness of medications used in treating STDs (Clottey and Dallabetta, 1993).

The community health nurse serves as an educator about the modes of transmission, as well as a role model for how to behave toward and provide supportive care for those with HIV infection. An understanding of how transmission does and does not occur will help family and community members feel more comfortable in relating to and caring for persons with HIV (see box at right).

Distribution and Trends

Community health nurses must identify the trends of infection in the populations they serve, so they can recognize clients who may be at risk and so they can adequately plan prevention programs and illness care resources. For example, knowing that AIDS disproportionately affects minorities assists the nurse in setting priorities and planning services to these groups. Factors such as geographical location, age, and racial distribution are tracked to more effectively target programs and are discussed below.

In 1981, five homosexual men in Los Angeles were recognized as having AIDS. By 1994 the epidemic had grown to 393,975 persons. Initially the groups with the highest incidence of HIV infection were homosexual and bisexual males, injection drug users and their sexual partners, and hemophiliacs (Centers for Dis-

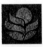 Modes of HIV Transmission

HIV can be transmitted in the following ways:
1. Sexual contact, involving the exchange of body fluids, with an infected person
2. Transfusions or other exposure to HIV-contaminated blood or blood products, organs, or semen
3. Perinatal transmission from an infected mother to her fetus during pregnancy or delivery or to an infant when breast-feeding
4. Sharing or reusing needles, syringes, or other equipment used to prepare injectable drugs

ease Control, 1989). Although homosexual men still make up the largest group infected with HIV, the number of heterosexual women with AIDS is increasing at a faster rate.

It is estimated that 1 million people are infected with HIV in the United States and 13 million people are infected worldwide (Centers for Disease Control, 1990a; World Health Organization, 1993). HIV infection is a leading cause of death among persons 25 to 44 years old in the United States (Centers for Disease Control, 1993e). As of October 1994, 47% of all persons reported to have AIDS in the United States had died (American Health Consultants, 1994).

Gender

From 1991 to 1992, the reported cases of AIDS in women increased by 9.8%, whereas for men the increase was only 2.5%. The rate is much higher in Hispanic and black women than in white women. In 1992, for the first time, heterosexual transmission was greater than injection drug use transmission in women (Centers for Disease Control, 1993d). As the infection rate climbs in women, there is a parallel increase in pediatric AIDS cases, making the disease a family disease. Although the number of pediatric cases (5234) is a fraction of the adult cases, it is of growing concern. AIDS ranks among the top 10 causes of death for those from 1 to 4 years old; and the number of deaths from AIDS in this age group is likely to increase (Kilbourne et al., 1990).

Age

The largest number of reported AIDS cases (46%) is in the age group from 30 to 39 years, and nearly 90% are between the ages of 20 and 49 years of age (Centers for Disease Control, 1994b). Because the incubation period is so long, the infection is likely to have occurred during adolescence and young adulthood. This period of life is characterized by experimentation with various roles and behaviors that may include injectable drug use, sexual experimentation, and other activities that place adolescents and young adults at risk.

Race and Ethnicity

AIDS has disproportionately affected minority groups. African-Americans made up 12.1% of the total U.S. population according to the 1990 census, but they represent 31.8% of those reported to have AIDS (Centers for Disease Control, 1994b). This overrepresentation is associated with urban residence, poverty, transmission through the use of injection drugs, and prostitution (Aral and Homes, 1990).

Geographical Distribution

The geographical distribution of AIDS is clustered in urban areas, but increasingly it is moving into rural areas. Locations with the highest prevalence of AIDS are Florida, New York, New Jersey, California, the District of Columbia, and Texas. Regionally, the Northeast section of the United States and some U.S. territories (e.g., Puerto Rico) reflect the highest rates (Centers for Disease Control, 1994b).

Seroprevalence Studies

AIDS is a reportable condition within the United States. However, the reporting of HIV infection varies among states (Table 40-3). Study of already diagnosed cases of AIDS does not necessarily reveal current HIV infection patterns because of the long interval between infection with HIV and the onset of disease. Moreover, identification of new cases of AIDS does not distinguish between those recently infected and those infected several years ago.

HIV seroprevalence studies involve the anonymous screening of populations for the HIV antibody. This type of study can provide information about the number of HIV carriers and how the virus is spreading within populations. This screening has

Table 40-3   Reporting Requirements for Human Immunodeficiency Virus (HIV) Infection*

By name of infected person	Anonymous	Not required
Alabama	Georgia	Alaska
Arizona	Iowa	California
Arkansas	Kansas	Delaware
Colorado	Kentucky	Florida
Idaho	Maine	Hawaii
Illinois	Montana	Louisiana
Indiana	New Hampshire	Maryland‡
Michigan	Oregon	Massachusetts
Minnesota	Rhode Island	Nebraska
Mississippi	Texas	New Mexico
Missouri		New York
Nevada		Pennsylvania
New Jersey†		Vermont
North Carolina		Washington‡
North Dakota		District of Columbia
Ohio		
Oklahoma		
South Carolina		
South Dakota		
Tennessee†		
Utah		
Virginia		
West Virginia		
Wisconsin		
Wyoming		

Modified from US Department of Health and Human Services, Agency for Health Care Policy and Research: *Early HIV infection, clinical practice guidelines.* AHCPR Pub No 94-0572, Rockville, MD, AHCPR, 1994.
Current as of March 1, 1993. All states require reporting of acquired immunodeficiency syndrome (AIDS) cases by name at the state and local level.
†Implementation date: January 1992.
‡Requires reports of symptomatic HIV infection by name.

been conducted in emergency rooms, family planning clinics, and in military clinics or settings. Based on seroprevalence studies, estimates of HIV infection have been calculated in several groups. For example, the HIV seroprevalence rate for prisoners was found to range from 2.1% to 14.7% (Centers for Disease Control, 1992b). Early detection of infected persons enables medical personnel to develop treatment services and decide where to focus prevention efforts.

HIV Testing

The HIV antibody test is the most commonly used test for determining infection. This test does just as its name implies: it does not reveal whether an individual has AIDS, nor does it isolate the virus. It does indicate the presence of the antibody to HIV. The most commonly used form of this test is the enzyme-linked immunosorbent assay (ELISA). The ELISA effectively screens blood and other donor products. In cases of false-positive results, a confirmatory test, the Western blot, is used to verify the results. False-negative results may also occur after infection before antibodies are produced. This is sometimes referred to as the window period and can last from 6 weeks to 3 months.

What Do You Think?

HIV home test kits, where results will be available by telephone, should be made available to the general public.

Testing for HIV infection is offered at many sites, including health departments, STD clinics, family planning clinics, and freestanding HIV-counseling and HIV-testing sites. Voluntary screening programs for HIV may be either confidential or anonymous: the process for each is unique. With confidential testing the person's name and address are obtained, but the information is considered privileged. With anonymous testing the client is given an identification number that is attached to all records of the test results. Demographical data such as the person's sex, age, and race may be collected, but there is no record of the client's name and address. Anonymous testing may increase the number of people who are willing to be tested, because many of those at risk are engaged in illegal activities. The anonymity eliminates their concern about the possibility of arrest or discrimination.

Perinatal HIV Infection

Women who are HIV infected must consider the risk of perinatal infection and should be counseled to prevent pregnancy. It is estimated that 13% to 40% of those women infected with HIV who become pregnant will pass the virus on to their infants (St Louis, et al., 1993). A study investigating the use of zidovudine

in a test group initiated therapy from 14 to 34 weeks' gestation in pregnant women and in their infants after birth. Results demonstrated that these subjects experienced a significant decrease in transmission compared to a group that was not administered the drug (Centers for Disease Control, 1994g). Recommendations based on this research include the need to identify HIV status early in pregnancy and to weigh the risks versus the benefits of administering the drug. Because of the positive effect of zidovudine, some states are considering mandatory HIV testing and counseling about the benefit of early HIV detection for pregnant women. Health officials at the Centers for Disease Control and Prevention (CDC) recommend mandatory counseling and voluntary testing for pregnant women.

Obviously, some questions remain. Studies are inconclusive about whether pregnancy increases the likelihood of progression to AIDS. Alterations in cell-mediated immunity during pregnancy make the progression to AIDS possible; pregnant women must consider who will care for their children if they become ill. If pregnancy occurs, the decision of whether to terminate it through therapeutic abortion will be influenced by the woman's personal beliefs and values, legal parameters, and the availability of health care and financial resources.

Pediatric HIV Infection

The clinical picture of pediatric HIV infection differs greatly from that of adults. The incubation period in infants is shorter—they usually become symptomatic within the first year of life. Children develop different physical signs and symptoms from adults. These include failure to thrive, diarrhea, developmental delays, and bacterial infections such as otitis media and pneumonia. Children also have a shorter survival period. Because 89% of children with AIDS contract the disease through maternal transmission, many die within the first 3 years of life (Centers for Disease Control, 1994b).

Detection of HIV infection in infants of seropositive mothers is made by using different tests from those used in children over 18 months of age. The ELISA test is not valid because it tests for antibodies that reflect maternal antibodies, and thus even a seronegative infant may show a positive test result. Thus testing is done by either HIV culture, HIV antigen, or polymerase chain reaction (PCR).

Despite having an infected mother, many children will not acquire AIDS perinatally. However, there remains the potential for loss of one or both parents from HIV infection. Many children with AIDS come from impoverished families with limited financial, emotional, and health care resources. The added strain of this illness makes many families unable to provide for the emotional, physical, and developmental needs of affected children.

Did You Know?

Because of impaired immunity, children with HIV infection are more likely to get childhood diseases and suffer serious sequelae. Therefore DPT (diptheria-pertussis-tetanus), IPV (inactivated polio virus), and MMR (measles-mumps-rubella) vaccines should be given at regularly scheduled times for children infected with HIV. HIb (Haemophilus influenza type B), hepatitis B, pneumonoccal, and influenza vaccines may be recommended after medical evaluation.

AIDS Resources

National AIDS Hotline	1-800-342-2437
National AIDS Clearinghouse	1-800-458-5231
CDC Business Responds to AIDS Resource	1-800-458-5231
AIDS Clinical Trials Information Service	1-800-874-2572
Hemophilia and AIDS/HIV Network for Dissemination of Information (HANDI)	1-800-424-2634
Teens Teaching AIDS Prevention Program	1-800-234-8336
AIDS Treatment News	1-800-873-2812

AIDS in the Community

Because AIDS is a chronic disease, afflicted individuals live and function in the community. Much of their care is provided in the home. The community health nurse teaches families and significant others about personal care and hygiene, correct medication administration, universal precautions to ensure infection control, and healthy life-style behaviors such as adequate rest, balanced nutrition, and exercise.

Persons with AIDS have bouts of illness interspersed with periods of wellness when they are able to return to school or work. Policies regarding school and work site attendance have been developed by most communities and some businesses. These policies provide direction for the community's response when an individual develops HIV infection. Among the roles of the nurse is identifying resources such as social and financial support services and interpreting school and work policies.

Businesses are often unprepared and uninformed about how to deal with situations involving HIV infection (Hale, 1990). The 1974 Vocational Rehabilitation Act protects employees from termination of employment or other discriminatory action based solely on the presence of the disease. Community health nurses can assist employers by identifying the importance of sponsoring educational programs on HIV. Educating managers on how to deal with sick or infected workers is vital to reduce the risk of breach of confidentiality or wrongful actions such as termination. Revealing a worker's infection to other workers, terminating employment, and isolating an infected worker are examples of situations that have resulted in litigation between employees and employers.

Children who are HIV infected should be allowed to attend school because the benefit of attendance far outweighs the risk of transmitting or acquiring infections. None of the cases of HIV infection in the United States are known to have been transmitted in a school setting. Decisions regarding educational and care needs should be based on an interdisciplinary team that includes the child's physician, public health personnel, and the child's parent or guardian (Centers for Disease Control, 1988).

Individual decisions about risk to the infected child or others should be based on the behavior, neurological development, and physical condition of the child. Attendance may be inadvisable in the presence of cases of childhood infections, such as chickenpox or measles, within the school, because the immunosuppressed child is at greater risk of suffering complications. Alternative arrangements, such as homebound instruction, might be instituted if a child is unable to control body secretions or displays biting behavior.

Resources

As the number of individuals with AIDS has increased, many needs have evolved. Voluntary service organizations, often referred to as community-based organizations or AIDS support organizations, have developed to address these needs. Services commonly provided by these groups include client and family counseling, support groups, legal aid, personal care services, housing programs, and community education programs. Community health nurses collaborate with workers from community-based organizations in the client's home and may serve to advise these groups in their supportive work.

Each state has established an AIDS hotline. In addition, the federal government and organizations have established toll-free numbers to meet a variety of needs. These are listed in the box above.

ADDITIONAL SEXUALLY TRANSMITTED DISEASES

In recent years the incidence of many other STDs has increased. The common STDs in Table 40-4 are categorized by their biological origin: those caused by bacteria and those caused by viruses. The bacterial infections include gonorrhea, syphilis, chlamydia, and chancroid. Most of these are curable with antibiotics with the exception of the newly emerging antibiotic-resistant strains of gonorrhea.

STDs caused by viruses cannot be cured. These are frequently chronic diseases that result in years of symptom management and infection control. The viral infections include herpes simplex virus, hepatitis B virus, and human papillomavirus (HPV), also referred to as genital warts.

Table 40-4 Summary of Sexually Transmitted Diseases

Disease/ pathogen	Incubation	Signs and symptoms	Diagnosis	Treatment	Nursing implication
BACTERIAL					
Chlamydia: *Chlamydia*	3-21 days	Male: nongonococcal urethritis (NGU): painful urination and urethral discharge; epididymitis Female: none or mucopurulent cervicitis, vaginal discharge. If untreated, progresses to symptoms of pelvic inflammatory disease (PID): diffuse abdominal pain, fever, chills	Tissue culture; Gram stain of endocervical or urethral discharge	Tetracycline, doxycycline, or azithromycin	Refer partner(s) of past 60 days; counsel client to use condoms and to avoid sex until therapy is complete and symptoms are gone in both client and partners; medication teaching
Gonorrhea: *Neisseria gonorrhoeae*	3-21 days	Male: urethritis, purulent discharge, painful urination, urinary frequency; epididymitis Female: none or symptoms of PID	Culture of discharge; Gram stain of urethral discharge, endocervical or rectal smear	Ceftriaxone or doxycycline Penicillinase-producing *N. gonorrhoeae* (PPNG): spectinomycin or ceftriaxone	Refer partner(s) of past 60 days for evaluation; return for reevaluation if symptoms persist; medication teaching; avoid sex until therapy is complete and symptoms gone in both client and partner(s)
Syphilis: *Treponema pallidum*	10-90 days	Primary: usually single, painless chancre; if untreated, heals in few weeks	Visualization of pathogen on dark-field microscopic examination; single painless ulcer (chancre) FTA-ABS* or MHA-TP† VDRL‡ (reactive 14 days after appearance of chancre)	Benzathine penicillin G	Counsel to be tested for HIV; screen all partners of past 3 months; reexamine client at 3 and 6 mo
	6 wk-6 mo	Secondary: low grade fever, malaise, sore throat, headache, adenopathy, and rash	Clinical signs of secondary syphilis	For those allergic to penicillin, tetracycline hydrochloride (do not administer to pregnant women, those with neurosyphilis or congenital syphilis)	
	Within 1 yr of infection	Early latency: asymptomatic; infectious lesions may recur	VDRL;FTA-ABS or MHA-TP	Benzathine penicillin G	
	After 1 yr from date of infection	Late latency: asymptomatic; noninfectious except to fetus of pregnant women	Lumbar puncture, cerebrospinal fluid (CSF) cell count, protein level determination and VDRL		

*Fluorescent treponemal antibody absorption test.
†Microhemagglutination–*Treponema pallidum.*
‡Venereal Disease Research Laboratory test for syphilis.

Continued.

Table 40-4　Summary of Sexually Transmitted Diseases—cont'd

Disease/ pathogen	Incubation	Signs and symptoms	Diagnosis	Treatment	Nursing implication
Syphilis: *Treponema pallidum* (cont'd)	Late active 2-40 yr 20-30 yr 10-30 yr	Gummas of skin, bone, and mucous membranes, heart, liver CNS involvement: paresis, optic atrophy Cardiovascular involvement: aortic aneurysm, aortic valve insufficiency			
Chancroid: *Haemophilus ducreyi*	3-7 days	Small, irregular papule progressing to deep, painful ulcer that drains pus or blood on penis, labia, or vaginal opening; inguinal tenderness, dysuria	Visual inspection of lesion	Azithromycin, erythromycin, or ceftriaxone	Return for examination 3-7 days after treatment begins; partners who had sex within 10 days before client's onset of symptoms should be evaluated; condom use
VIRAL					
Hepatitis B virus (HBV)	4 wk	Varies greatly from subclinical infection to cirrhosis, fulminant hepatitis, hepatocellular carcinoma	Serum IgM alpha-HBc	Hepatitis B immune globulin within 14 days of last exposure; followed by regular three-dose immunization series	Partner(s) should receive HBIG prophylaxis within 14 days after exposure followed by 3-dose immunization series
Genital warts: human papillomavirus (HPV)	4-6 wk most common; up to 9 mo	Often subclinical infection; painless lesions near vaginal opening, anus, shaft of penis, vagina, cervix; lesions are textured, cauliflower appearance; may remain unchanged over time	Visual inspection for lesions; Papanicolaou smear; colposcopy	No cure; one-third of lesions will disappear without treatment Topical podofilox podophyllin or trichloroacetic acid; cryotherapy with liquid nitrogen, laser, or surgical removal	Warts and surrounding tissues contain HPV so removal of warts does not completely eradicate virus; examination of partner(s) not necessary since treatment is only symptomatic; condom use may reduce transmission
Genital herpes: herpes simplex virus 2 (HSV-2)	2-20 days; average 6 days	Vesicles; painful ulcerations of penis, vagina, labia, perineum, or anus; lesions last 5-6 wk and recurrence is common; may be asymptomatic	Presence of vesicles; viral culture (obtained only when lesions present and before they have scabbed over)	No cure; acyclovir for partial control of signs and symptoms and to accelerate healing; lidocaine jelly as topical anesthetic	Refer partner(s) for evaluation; teach client about likelihood of recurrent episodes and ability to transmit to others even if asymptomatic; condom use; annual Pap smear

Gonorrhea

Neisseria gonorrhoeae is a gram-negative intracellular diplococcus bacterium that infects the mucous membranes of the genitourinary tract, rectum, and pharynx. It is transmitted through genital-genital contact, oral-genital contact, and anal-genital contact.

Gonorrhea is identified as either uncomplicated or complicated. Uncomplicated gonorrhea refers to limited cervical or urethral infection. Complicated gonorrhea includes salpingitis, epididymitis, systemic gonococcal infection, and gonococcal meningitis. The signs and symptoms of infection in males are purulent and copious urethral discharge and dysuria, although it is estimated that 10% to 20% of males are asymptomatic. In females it is thought that 25% to 80% have no symptoms, but there may be minimal vaginal discharge or dysuria (Hook and Handsfield, 1990). The asymptomatic state is dangerous because individuals who are unaware of their infection may continue to infect others, whereas those who are symptomatic usually cease sexual activity and seek treatment.

Up to 45% of those infected with gonorrhea are coinfected with *Chlamydia trachomatis*. Therefore selection of a treatment that is effective against both organisms, such as doxycycline or azithromycin, is recommended (Centers for Disease Control, 1993f).

Gonorrhea is the most commonly reported STD. Despite a decrease in the annual incidence of reported gonorrhea between 1990 and 1993, it has increased among adolescents (Centers for Disease Control, 1993b, 1994f). Groups with the highest reported incidence of gonorrhea include blacks and persons 15 to 24 years of age (Centers for Disease Control, 1993b). The CDC estimates the actual number of annual cases to be 1.5 million. The discrepancy between actual and reported cases occurs because gonorrhea may be unreported by health care providers. In addition, infected clients who are asymptomatic do not seek treatment and are therefore not identified.

The number of antibiotic-resistant cases of gonorrhea in the United States is rising at an alarming rate. Penicillin-resistant gonorrhea was first identified in 1976 when 15 cases were reported. By 1990, 64,972 cases were reported (Phillips, 1976; Blount, 1991). After that, a strain of tetracycline-resistant *N. gonorrhoeae* developed. Between 1992 and 1994, another strain was isolated in the United States that is resistant to ciprofloxacin, an antibiotic currently effective against both penicillin- and tetracycline-resistant gonorrhea (Centers for Disease Control, 1994a). The increase in antibiotic-resistant infections is partially attributed to the indiscriminate or illicit use of antibiotics as a prophylactic measure by those with multiple sexual partners (Zenilman et al., 1988). To ensure proper treatment and cure, persons diagnosed with gonorrheal infection should return if symptoms persist; a rescreening test 1 to 2 months after completing therapy is also recommended.

The development of **pelvic inflammatory disease (PID)** is a risk for women who remain asymptomatic and do not seek treatment. PID is an infection of the fallopian tubes (salpingitis) and is the most common of all complications of gonorrhea but may also result from chlamydia infection. PID can result in ectopic pregnancy and infertility as a result of fallopian-tube scarring and occlusion. It may also cause stillbirths and premature labor. It has been estimated that the cost of the complications resulting from PID is more than $2.7 billion annually (Centers for Disease Control, 1991b). Symptoms of PID include fever, abnormal menses, and lower abdominal pain.

Syphilis

Syphilis is caused by a member of the *Treponeme* genus of spirochetes called *Treponema pallidum*. It infects moist mucosal or cutaneous lesions and is spread through direct contact, usually by sexual contact or from mother to fetus. In sexual transmission, microscopic breaks in the skin and mucous membranes during sexual contact create a point of entry for the bacteria.

The number of reported cases of syphilis decreased from 50,578 in 1990 to 33,973 in 1992 (Centers for Disease Control, 1993c). The incidence remains drastically higher than in recent decades: in 1988, the total cases reached just over 40,000, the highest rate in the 40 preceding years. The highest incidence is in blacks and adolescents (Centers for Disease Control, 1993b).

Syphilis is divided into early and late stages. As defined by the U.S. Public Health Service, the early stage is defined as the first full year after infection. The late stage is the time after this first year. The early stage includes primary, secondary, and early latent stages; late syphilis includes late latency and tertiary syphilis. Latency may occur during the early and late phases. During latency there are no clinical signs of infection, but the person has historical or serological evidence of infection. The possibility of relapse remains.

Primary Syphilis

When syphilis is acquired sexually, the bacteria produce infection in the form of a chancre at the site of entry (Figure 40-2). The lesion begins as a macula, progresses to a papule, and later ulcerates. If left untreated, this chancre persists for 3 to 6 weeks and then heals spontaneously.

Secondary Syphilis

Secondary syphilis occurs when the organism enters the lymph system and spreads throughout the body. Signs include rash, lymphadenopathy, and mucosal ulceration. Symptoms of secondary syphilis include sore throat, malaise, headaches, weight loss, variable fever, and muscle and joint pain.

Tertiary Syphilis

Tertiary syphilis may involve the complications of blindness, congenital damage, cardiovascular damage, or syphilitic psychoses. Another potential outcome of tertiary syphilis is the development of lesions of the

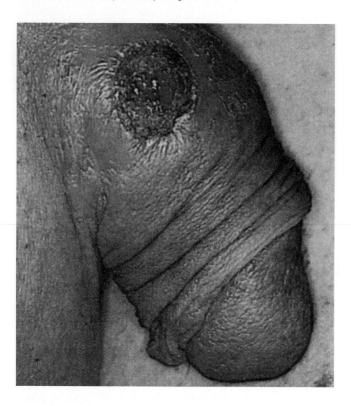

FIGURE 40-2
Primary syphilitic chancre on penile shaft. (Photograph used with permission of Lewis Kaminester, M.D. Reproduced with permission of Burroughs-Wellcome Co.)

bones, skin, and mucous membranes, known as gummas. Tertiary syphilis usually occurs several years after initial infection and is rare in the United States because the disease is usually cured in its early stages with antibiotics. Tertiary syphilis does, however, remain a major problem in developing countries.

Congenital Syphilis

Syphilis is transmitted transplacentally and if untreated can cause premature stillbirth, blindness, deafness, facial abnormalities, crippling, or death. The current treatment is penicillin. However, close follow-up is necessary because some treatment failure has occurred.

Chlamydia

Chlamydia infection results from the bacterium *Chlamydia trachomatis*. It infects the genitourinary tract and rectum of adults and causes conjunctivitis and pneumonia in neonates. Transmission occurs when mucopurulent discharge from infected sites, such as the cervix or urethra, comes into contact with the mucous membranes of a noninfected person. As with gonorrhea, the infection is commonly asymptomatic in women and if left untreated can result in PID. When symptoms of chlamydial infection are present in females, they include dysuria, urinary frequency, and purulent vaginal discharge. In males the urethra is the most common site of infection, resulting in nongonococcal urethritis (NGU). The symptoms of NGU

are dysuria and urethral discharge. Epididymitis is a possible complication.

Chlamydia trachomatis is the most prevalent bacterial STD in the United States, with 4 million infections occurring every year. It is a major area of concentration for prevention in the 1990s because of its association with PID and neonatal complications (Centers for Disease Control, 1993a). Rates of *Chlamydia* have increased in recent years, partly because of improved diagnosis and reporting. Risk factors that positively correlate with chlamydial infection include young age and oral contraception use, multiple sexual partners, and the presence of gonorrhea (Centers for Disease Control, 1993a). The high frequency of chlamydial infections in individuals infected with gonorrhea requires that effective treatment for both be administered when a gonorrhea infection is identified (Centers for Disease Control, 1993f).

Chancroid

Chancroid is caused by *Haemophilus ducreyi* and is spread from person to person through sexual contact. Chancroid is characterized by a type of ulcerative lesion occurring on the penis, labia, or clitoris or at the vaginal orifice. About 1 week after infection, a small papule develops and soon progresses to a painful, deep ulceration (Figure 40-3). The infection spreads to the inguinal lymph nodes and causes tenderness. Usually one or two lesions occur, but there may be as many as 10. In the United States, chancroid is a less-frequent cause of genital ulcers than herpes simplex virus 2 (HSV-2) or syphilis. Although reported cases of chancroid have decreased from 4891 in 1988 to 1886 in 1992, there is documented underreporting of the infection because of lack of mandated reporting in some states, inadequate laboratory testing, and unclear definition of what signs confirm diagnosis (Centers for Disease Control, 1992a). Although chancroid is not as commonly reported as other STDs in the United States, it is much more prevalent worldwide than gonorrhea or syphilis.

Hepatitis B Virus

The Hepatitis B Virus (HBV) is spread in ways other than sexual contact, as well as via sexual transmission. Because the spread of HBV is similar to that of HIV, it is discussed here.

The number of new cases of **hepatitis B virus (HBV)** in the United States increased by 37% between 1979 and 1989, and it is estimated that 200,000 to 300,000 new cases occurred annually between 1980 and 1991 (Centers for Disease Control, 1991a). The groups with the highest prevalence are immigrants and refugees and their descendants who came from areas where there is a high endemic rate of HBV, health care workers, persons with multiple sex partners, and users of injection drugs.

The HBV is spread through blood and body fluids and, like HIV, is referred to as a blood-borne pathogen.

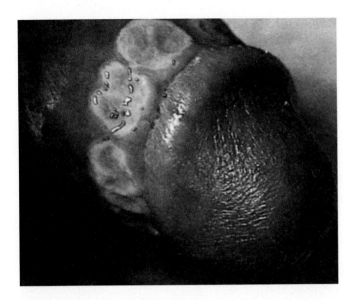

FIGURE 40-3
Chancroid: multiple, punched-out ulcers on penile shaft. (Photograph used with permission of Lewis Kaminester, M.D. Reproduced with permission of Burroughs-Wellcome Co.)

It has the same transmission properties as HIV, and thus individuals should take the same precautions to prevent both HIV and HBV spread. A major difference is that HBV remains alive outside the body for a longer period of time than does HIV and thus has greater infectivity. The virus can survive for at least 1 week dried at room temperature on environmental surfaces (Centers for Disease Control, 1990b).

Infection with HBV results in either acute or chronic HBV infection. The acute infection is self-limiting, and individuals develop an antibody to the virus and successfully eliminate the virus from the body. They subsequently have lifelong immunity against the virus. Symptoms range from mild symptoms that resemble flu to a more severe response that includes jaundice, extreme lethargy, nausea, fever, and joint pain. Any of these more severe symptoms may result in hospitalization. A second possible outcome from infection is chronic HBV infection. These individuals are unable to rid their bodies of the virus and remain lifelong carriers of the hepatitis B surface antigen (HBsAg). As carriers, they are able to transmit the HBV to others. They may develop hepatic carcinoma or chronic active hepatitis. The signs and symptoms of *chronic* hepatitis B include anorexia, fatigue, abdominal discomfort, hepatomegaly, and jaundice.

Strategies for preventing HBV infection include immunization, prevention of occupational exposure, and prevention of sexual and injection drug use exposure. Vaccination is recommended for persons with occupational risk, such as health care workers, and for children. The series of vaccines required for protection from HBV consists of three intramuscular injections, with the second and third doses administered 1 and 6 months after the first (Centers for Disease Control, 1991a). It has been recommended that all pregnant women be tested for hepatitis B surface antigen (HBsAg), which indicates whether they carry and are able to transmit HBV. This test can identify newborns who require hepatitis B immune globulin in addition to hepatitis B vaccine at birth (Centers for Disease Control, 1994e). Hepatitis B immune globulin is an immunizing agent given after exposure to prevent infection.

OSHA *Regulations*

In 1992 the Occupational Safety and Health Administration (OSHA) released the standard "Occupational Exposure to Bloodborne Pathogens," (OSHA 1992) which mandates specific activities to protect workers from HBV and other blood-borne pathogens; these mandates ultimately save lives. Potential exposures for health care workers are needle-stick injuries and mucous membrane splashes. The OSHA standard requires employers to identify the risk of blood exposure to various employees. If employees are deemed to be potentially exposed to others' body fluids, employers are mandated to offer annual educational programs on preventing HBV and HIV exposure in the workplace. Employers are further required to offer the HBV vaccine to the employee at the employer's expense. The employee has the right to refuse the vaccine.

Herpes Simplex Virus 2

Herpes virus infects genital and nongenital sites. Herpes simplex virus 1 (HSV-1) primarily causes nongenital lesions such as cold sores that may appear on the lip or mouth. Herpes simplex virus 2 (HSV-2) is the primary cause of **genital herpes.**

Because there is no cure for HSV-2 infection, it is considered a chronic disease. The virus is transmitted through direct exposure and infects the genitalia and surrounding skin. After the initial infection, the virus remains latent in the sacral nerve of the central nervous system and may reactivate periodically with or without visible vesicles.

Signs and symptoms of HSV-2 infection include the presence of lesions that begin as vesicles and ulcerate and crust within 1 to 4 days (Figure 40-4). Lesions may occur on the vulva, vagina, upper thighs, buttocks, and penis and have an average duration of 11 days. The vesicles can cause itching and pain and may be accompanied by dysuria or rectal pain. Although infectivity is higher with active lesions, some individuals can spread the virus even when they are asymptomatic. Approximately 50% of people experience a prodromal phase. This may include a mild, tingling sensation up to 48 hours before eruption or shooting pains in the buttocks, legs, or hips up to 5 days before eruption (Corey, 1990).

The prevalence of HSV-2 is difficult to determine because of the large proportion of subclinical cases and the difficulty in making a diagnosis. Based on serological studies, 30 million persons in the United States are infected with HSV-2 (Centers for Disease Control, 1993b).

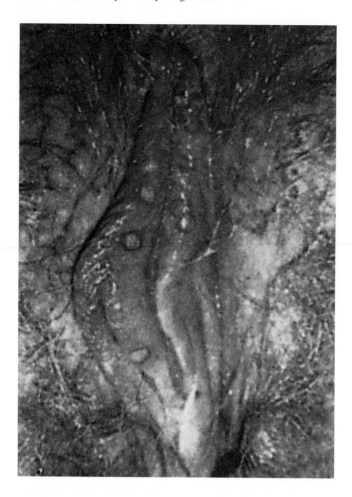

FIGURE 40-4
Pustular herpes simplex virus vulvar lesions. (Photograph used with permission of Lewis Kaminester, M.D. Reproduced with permission of Burroughs-Wellcome Co.)

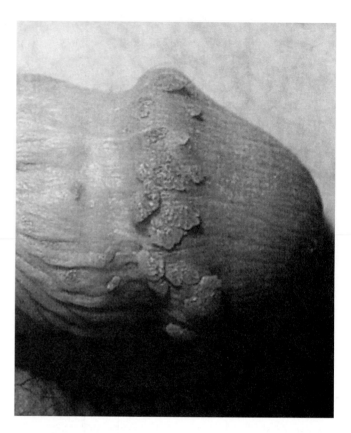

FIGURE 40-5
Genital warts. (Photograph used with permission of Lewis Kaminester, M.D. Reproduced with permission of Burroughs-Wellcome Co.)

The consequences of HSV-2 are of particular concern for women and their children. HSV-2 infection is linked with the development of cervical cancer. There is also an increased risk of spontaneous abortion and risk of transmission to the newborn during vaginal delivery (Puligheddu et al., 1988). A pregnant woman who has active lesions at the time of birth should have a cesarean delivery before the rupture of amniotic membranes to avoid fetal contact with the herpetic lesions. Viral cultures may also be done before delivery, but the results may take 2 to 3 days to return. Mortality for infected neonates is estimated to be as high as 80%, and neurological damage is a major complication (Martens, 1994). The possibility of intrauterine transmission has not been eliminated because some infected neonates are born to women who are asymptomatic at delivery or have had no history of genital HSV (Stone et al., 1989).

Human Papillomavirus Infection

Human papillomavirus (HPV), also called **genital warts,** can infect the genitalia, anus, and mouth.

Transmission of HPV occurs through direct contact with warts that result from HPV. However, HPV has been detected in semen, and exposure to the virus through body fluids is also possible. Genital warts are most commonly found on the penis and scrotum in men and the vulva, labia, vagina, and cervix in women. Figure 40-5 shows the textured surface of the lesions, sometimes described as a cauliflower appearance. The warts are usually multiple and vary between 1 and 5 mm in diameter. They may be difficult to visualize, so careful examination is required.

The prevalence of genital HPV infection is estimated to be between 10% and 20% of American women of childbearing age and between 5% and 19% of women visiting family planning and university student health clinics (Aral and Holmes, 1990). As with genital herpes, the actual prevalence is difficult to ascertain because it is not a reported disease, and many infections are subclinical.

Complications of HPV infection are especially serious for women. The link between HPV infection and cervical cancer has been established and is associated with specific types of the virus. It is estimated that 15% of untreated high-grade lesions resulting from HPV develop into cervical cancer (Crum and Nuovo, 1991). HPV infection is exacerbated in both pregnancy and old age as a result of a decrease in cell-mediated immune functioning. HPV may infect the fetus during pregnancy and can result in laryngeal papilloma that can obstruct the infant's airway. Genital warts may enlarge and become friable during pregnancy, and therefore surgical removal may be recommended.

Because there is no cure for HPV, the goal of therapy is to eliminate the lesions. Genital warts spontaneously disappear over time, as do skin warts. However, because the condition is worrisome for the client and HPV may lead to the development of cervical neoplasia, treatment of the lesions through surgical removal, cytotoxic agents, or immunotherapies is often used.

COMMUNITY HEALTH NURSE'S ROLE IN PREVENTING STDS AND PROVIDING RELATED SERVICES

From prevention to treatments the community health nurse functions as a counselor, educator, advocate, case manager, and primary care provider. Appropriate interventions for primary, secondary, and tertiary prevention are reviewed. The following discussion of primary prevention applies the nursing process to the care of clients with STDs.

Primary Prevention

Primary prevention consists mainly of activities to keep people healthy before the onset of disease. This begins with assessing for risk behavior and providing relevant intervention through education on how to change risky behaviors.

Assessment

Assessing a client's risk of acquiring an STD should be done with all sexually active individuals. Such risk assessment should be included as baseline assessment data of those attending all clinics and those who receive school health, occupational health, public health, and home nursing services. To assess the risk of acquiring STDs, the nurse obtains a sexual and injection drug use history for clients and their partners. The sexual history provides information about the need for specific diagnostic tests, treatment modalities, and partner notification. It also facilitates evaluation of risk factors and is necessary for the nurse to be able to provide relevant education for the client's life-style.

A thorough sexual history should include information about the types of relationships, the number of sexual partners and encounters, and types of sexual behaviors practiced. The confidential nature of the information and how it will be used should be shared with the client to establish open communication and a purposeful interaction.

Most clients feel uneasy disclosing such personal information. The community health nurse can ease this discomfort by remaining supportive and open during the interview to facilitate honesty about intimate activities. The nurse serves as a model for discussing sensitive information in a candid manner. When discussing precautions, direct and simple language should be used to describe specific behaviors. This encourages the client to openly discuss sexuality during this interaction and with future partners.

Community health nurses who are uncomfortable discussing topics such as sexual behavior or sexual orientation are likely to avoid assessing risk behaviors with the client. They will, consequently, be ineffective in identifying risks and in assisting the client in modifying them. It is important that nurses become adept at these skills to prevent and control STDs. Understanding one's own values and feelings regarding sexuality and realizing that the purpose of the interaction is to improve the client's health can help community health nurses gain confidence in conducting sexual risk assessments. The nurse's comfort in discussing sexual behavior can be enhanced through role-playing assessments of sexual and injection drug–using behavior and contracting for behavioral change.

Identifying the total number of sexual and injection drug–using partners and the number of contacts with these partners provides information about the client's risk. The chance of exposure decreases as the number of partners decreases, so people in mutually monogamous relationships are at low risk for acquiring STDs. This information can be obtained by asking, "How many sex (or drug) partners have you had over the past 6 months?" It is important to avoid assumptions about the sexual partner or partners based on the client's gender, age, race, or any other factor. Stereotypes and assumptions about who people are and what they do are common problems that keep interviewers from asking the right questions that lead to obtaining useful information. For exam-ple, it should not be taken for granted that if a male is homosexual he always has more than one partner. Be aware also that the long incubation of HIV and the subclinical phase of many STDs lead some monogamous individuals to assume erroneously that they are not at risk.

It is important to identify whether the person has sexual contact with men, women, or both. This information can be obtained by simply asking, "Do you have sex with men, women, or both?" This lets the client know that the nurse is open to hearing about these behaviors, and thus the nurse is more likely to obtain information that is relevant to sexual practices and risk. Women who are exclusively lesbian are at low risk for acquiring STDs, but bisexual women may transmit STDs between male and female partners. In addition, it is possible for men to have sexual contact with other men and not label themselves as homosexual. Therefore risk reduction education campaigns that are aimed at homosexual males will not be heeded by this group. In such situations the nurse can ask, "When was the last time you had sex with another male?"

Certain sexual practices are more likely to result in exposure to and transmission of STDs. Dangerous sexual activities include unprotected anal or vaginal intercourse, oral-anal contact, and insertion of finger or fist into the rectum. These practices introduce a high risk of transmission of enteric organisms or result in physical trauma during sexual encounters. The nurse can obtain information about sexual encounters by asking, "Can you tell me the kinds of sexual practices in which you engage? This will help determine what risks you may have and the type of tests we should run." Clients who engage in genital-anal, oral-anal, or oral-genital contact will need throat and rectal cultures for some STDs as well as cervical and urethral cultures.

Drug use is linked to STD transmission in several ways. Sexual enhancers, such as alcohol or other drugs, put people at risk because they can impair judgment about engaging in risky behaviors. Drugs such as crack cocaine or amyl nitrate (also referred to as poppers) can cause an ability to have multiple orgasms. This increases both the frequency of sexual contacts and the chances of contracting STDs. Addiction to a drug may lead to intense craving of the drug and to trading sex for the drug. Thus the community health nurse should obtain information on the type and frequency of drug use and the presence of risk behavior.

The use of oral contraception or Norplant is also important to ascertain, because many clients will believe they are safe and do not have to use barrier precautions such as condoms. Use of contraceptives has been found to decrease condom use (Frank et al., 1993).

Condom Use Instructions

Correct use of a latex condom requires the following:
1. Using a new condom with each act of intercourse
2. Carefully handling the condom to avoid damaging it with fingernails, teeth, or other sharp objects
3. Putting on the condom after the penis is erect and before any genital contact with the partner
4. Ensuring no air is trapped in the tip of the condom
5. Ensuring adequate lubrication during intercourse, possibly requiring use of exogenous lubricants
6. Using only water-based lubricants (e.g., K-Y Jelly or glycerin) with latex condoms; oil-based lubricants (e.g., petroleum jelly, shortening, mineral oil, massage oils, body lotions, or cooking oil) that can weaken latex should never be used
7. Holding the condom firmly against the base of the penis during withdrawal and withdrawing while the penis is still erect to prevent slippage

Condoms should be stored in a cool, dry place out of direct sunlight and should not be used after the expiration date. Condoms in damaged packages or condoms that show obvious signs of deterioration (e.g., brittleness, stickiness, or discoloration) should not be used regardless of their expiration date.

Modified from Centers for Disease Control: *MMWR* 42(30):520, 1993.

Intervention

Based on the information obtained in the sexual history and risk assessment, the community health nurse is able to identify specific education and counseling needs of the client. Nursing intervention focuses on contracting with clients to change behavior.

Safer Sex. Sexual abstinence is the best way to prevent STDs. However, for many people, sexual abstinence is undesirable; thus information about making sexual behavior safer must be taught. Safer sexual activities include masturbation on intact skin, dry kissing, touching, fantasy, and vaginal and oral sex with a condom.

The use of condoms can prevent the exchange of body fluids during sexual activity. If used correctly and consistently, condoms can prevent both pregnancy and STDs. Although the failure rate of condoms has been estimated to be 3.1%, this is related to incorrect use rather than condom failure (Novello et al., 1993). Thus information about their proper use and how to communicate about them with a partner is also necessary. The nurse has many opportunities to counsel individuals about this information. Instruction about how to use condoms is shown in the box below, left. The box below, right, discusses the pros and cons of using condoms that have chemical lubricants.

Condom use may be viewed as inconvenient, messy, or decreasing sensation. Moreover, alcohol use may accompany sexual activity, which also may decrease condom use (Kasen et al., 1992; Hale, 1994). The community health nurse can encourage clients to become more skilled in discussing safer sex through role modeling and can suggest that condom application be incorporated as part of foreplay. Table 40-5 describes common reasons for refusing to use condoms and ways clients can encourage partners to use them.

Female condoms can also serve as a barrier to body fluid contact and therefore protect against pregnancy and STDs. The advantage of the female condom is that its use is controlled by the woman. It consists of a sheath over two rings, with one closed end that fits over the cervix (Figure 40-6). See Figure 40-7 for detailed instructions on inserting a female condom.

Condoms and Chemical Barriers

Most agency protocols recommend the use of condoms that are lubricated with nonoxynol-9, a spermicide that is believed to have virucidal properties. The effectiveness of chemical barriers such as nonoxynol-9 has not yet been determined. There is greater emphasis being placed on researching potential chemical barriers as a method of preventing STDs because women control their use. However, for some women, chemical barriers may result in extravasation of the vaginal lining and cervix and therefore may provide breaks in tissue to facilitate transmission of some STDs (Berer, 1992).

Table 40-5 Discussing Condoms with Resistant, Defensive, or Manipulative Partners

Partner response	Rejoinder
YOU DON'T NEED IT	
"I'm on the pill, you don't need a condom."	"I'd like to use it anyway. It protects us both from infections we may not realize we have."
"I *know* I'm clean (disease free); I haven't had sex with anyone in X months."	"Thanks for telling me. As far as I know, I'm disease free too. But I'd still like to use a condom since either of us could have an infection and not know it."
"I'm a virgin."	"I'm not. This protects us both *and* the relationship."
IT'S A TURNOFF	
"I can't feel a thing when I wear a condom; it's like wearing a raincoat in the shower."	"I know there is some loss of it, but there's still plenty of sensation left."
"I'll lose my erection by the time I stop and put it on."	"Maybe I can help you put it on—that might give you extra sensations, too."
"By the time you put it on, I'm out of the mood."	"I know it's distracting but what we feel for each other is strong enough to help us stay in the mood."
"It destroys the romantic atmosphere."	"It doesn't have to be that way. It may be a little awkward the first time or two, but that will pass."
"It's so messy and smells funny."	"Well, sex is that way. But this way, we'll be safe."
"Condoms are unnatural, fake, a total turnoff."	"There's nothing great about genital infections either. Please let's try to work this out—either give the condom a try or let's look for alternatives."
ALTERNATIVES	
"What alternative do you have in mind?"	"Just petting and maybe some manual stimulation. Or we could postpone orgasm, even though I know we both want it."
MANIPULATIVE PLOYS	
"This is an insult! You seem to think I'm some sort of disease-ridden slut or gigolo."	"I didn't say or imply that. I care about us both and about our relationship. In my opinion, it's best to use a condom."
"None of my other boyfriends use a condom. A *real* man is not afraid."	"Please don't compare me to them. A real man cares about the women he dates, himself, and their relationship."
"You didn't make Jerry use a condom when you went out with him."	"It bothers me that you and Jerry talk about me that way. If you believe everything Jerry says, I won't argue with you."
"I love you! Would I give you an infection?"	"Not intentionally, of course not. But many people don't know they're infected. I feel this is best for both of us at this time."
"Just this once."	"Once is all it takes."
"I don't have a condom with me."	"I do" or "This time, we can satisfy each other without intercourse."
"You carry a condom around with you?! You were planning to seduce me!"	"I always carry one with me because I care about myself. I made sure I had one with me tonight because I care about us both."
"I won't have sex with you if you're going to use a condom."	"Let's put it off then, until we have a chance to work out our differences" or "OK. But can we try some other things besides intercourse?"

From Greico A: *Medical Aspects Hum Sex* 21:78, 1987.

Clients should understand that it is important to know the risk behavior of their sexual partners, including a history of injectable drug use and STDs, bisexuality, and any current symptoms. This is because each sexual partner is potentially exposed to all the STDs of the persons that the other partner has been sexually active with.

Drug Use. Injection drug use is risky because the potential for injecting pathogens exists when needles and syringes are shared. During injection drug use, small quantities of drugs are repeatedly injected. Blood is withdrawn into the syringe and is then injected back into the user's vein. Individuals should be advised against using injectable drugs and sharing needles, syringes, or other drug paraphernalia. If equipment is shared, it should be in contact with full-strength bleach for 30 seconds and then rinsed twice with water to prevent injecting bleach (Centers for Disease Control, 1994d).

Injection drug users are difficult to reach. Effective ways to use outreach programs include using community peers, increasing accessibility of drug treatment programs combined with HIV testing and counseling, and long-term repeat contacts after completion of the program (Centers for Disease Control, 1990c).

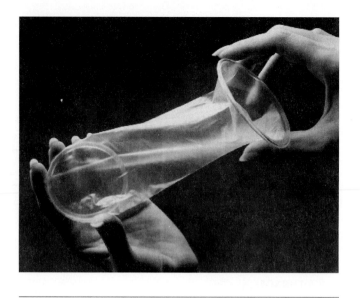

FIGURE 40-6

Female condom. (Photograph courtesy Wisconsin Pharmacal Co. Reprinted with permission of Burroughs Wellcome Co.)

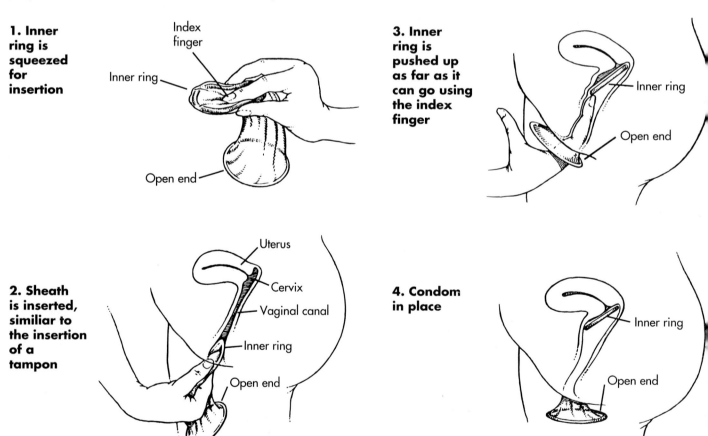

1. Inner ring is squeezed for insertion

Index finger

Inner ring

Open end

2. Sheath is inserted, similiar to the insertion of a tampon

Uterus

Cervix

Vaginal canal

Inner ring

Open end

3. Inner ring is pushed up as far as it can go using the index finger

Inner ring

Open end

4. Condom in place

Inner ring

Open end

FIGURE 40-7

Insertion and positioning of the female condom. (Reproduced with permission of Burroughs Wellcome Co.)

Community Outreach. Because of the illegal nature of injectable drugs and the poverty associated with HIV, many people at risk do not have the inclination or resources to seek health care. Community health nurses may work to establish programs within communities, because the opportunities for counseling on the prevention of HIV and other STDs are increased by bringing services into the neighborhoods of those at risk. Workers go into communities to disseminate information on safer sex, drug treatment programs, and discontinuation of drug use or safer drug use practices (e.g., cleaning equipment with bleach and water or using new needles and syringes with each injection). Some programs provide sterile needles and syringes, bleach for cleaning needs, condoms, and literature on anonymous test sites.

Community Education. The dissemination of accurate health information to large numbers of people is vital for preventing the spread of STDs. Community health nurses often provide educational sessions to community groups about HIV and other STDs. Such educational sessions are most effective in settings where groups normally meet and may include schools, businesses, or churches. When addressing groups about HIV infection, it is important to cover the number of people who are diagnosed with AIDS, the number infected, modes of transmission of the virus, how to prevent infection, common symptoms of illness, the need for a compassionate response to those afflicted, and available community resources. Teaching about other STDs can be incorporated into these presentations because the mode of transmission (sexual contact) is the same. Other information on these diseases can include the distribution, incidence, and consequences of the infection for individuals and society.

Evaluation

Evaluation is based on whether risky behavior is changed to safe behavior and, ultimately, whether illness is prevented. Condom use is evaluated for consistency of use if the client is sexually active. Other behaviors can be evaluated for their implementation, such as abstinence or monogamy. At the community level, behavioral surveys can be done to measure reported condom use and condom sales, and measures of STD incidence and prevalence can be calculated to evaluate the effectiveness of intervention (American Public Health Association, 1991).

Secondary Prevention

Secondary prevention includes the early identification and treatment of STDs, as well as follow-up with sex and drug-using partners to prevent further spread. In general, client teaching and counseling should include preventing reinfection with a curable STD, managing symptoms, and preventing the infection of others with chronic STDs. Testing and counseling for HIV are discussed below.

Testing for HIV

The community health nurse should recommend that persons who have engaged in high-risk behavior be tested. The following people are considered at risk and should be offered the HIV antibody test: those with a history of STDs (which are transmitted through the same behavior and may decrease immune functioning), multiple sex partners, or injection drug use; those who have intercourse without using a condom; those who have intercourse with someone who has another partner and those who have had sex with a prostitute; males with a history of homosexual or bisexual activity; those who have been a sexual partner to anyone in one of these groups; and those who underwent blood transfusion between January 1978 and March 1985.

If HIV infection is discovered before the onset of symptoms, the disease process can be monitored for changes, such as a decrease in the CD4 lymphocyte count, which signals the need for early treatment. Antiretroviral therapy, such as zidovudine, may be given early in the infection to delay the onset of symptomatic illness. Testing enables patients to benefit from early detection and treatment, as well as risk reduction education.

HIV Test Counseling

An important facet of client care is counseling regarding the HIV antibody test. It is essential that the client understand that the test is not diagnostic for AIDS but is indicative only of HIV infection. The key activities performed by the community health nurse during counseling include the following: assessing risk, discussing risk behaviors and how to overcome barriers to change, contracting between the client and the nurse to implement a risk reduction plan, and establishing the follow-up appointment to receive test results and posttest counseling.

Pretest Counseling. It is during pretest counseling that the nurse conducts the actual risk assessment, along with relevant teaching as described in the primary prevention section earlier in this chapter. Other activities include exploring how clients will cope with a positive test and assessing support systems. Asking clients to review how they have handled difficult situations in the past can determine how they might cope with learning they are HIV seropositive.

Also, during this time, the patient is told who will have access to the test results. Although AIDS is reported nationally, the reporting of HIV infection varies among states. States that mandate the reporting of HIV infection differ as to whether the client's name must accompany the report.

Because there is no cure or vaccine available, preventing the transmission of HIV requires a risk assess-

Responsibilities of Persons Who Are HIV Seropositive

Have regular medical evaluations and follow-ups.
Do not donate blood, plasma, body organs, other tissues, or sperm.
Take precautions against exchanging body fluids during sexual activity.
Inform sexual or injection drug–using partners of their potential exposure to HIV or arrange for notification through the health department.
Inform health care providers.
Consider the risk of perinatal transmission and follow up with contraceptive use.

ment of the client's behavior and counseling on how to reduce identified risks. Sexually active individuals who have multiple partners must be encouraged to abstain, to enter a mutually monogamous relationship, or to use condoms. Injection drug users should be advised to enter a treatment program or discontinue drug use. If they continue to use drugs, they should be warned to not share needles, syringes, or any other drug paraphernalia.

Posttest Counseling. Persons who have a negative test result are said to be **HIV seronegative,** and they should be counseled about risk reduction activities to prevent any future transmission. It is important that the client understand that the test may not be truly negative, because it does not identify infections that may have been acquired several weeks before the test. As noted earlier, **seroconversion** takes from 6 to 12 weeks. The client must be aware of the means of viral transmission and how to avoid infection.

If pretest counseling was adequate, clients are likely to have contemplated the meaning of a positive test result. All clients who are antibody positive should be counseled about the need for reducing their risks and notifying partners. If the client is unwilling or hesitant to notify past partners, partner notification or contact tracing, as described below, is often done by the community health nurse. The client should visit a primary health care provider so physical evaluation can be performed and, if indicated, antiviral or other therapies begun. The box above describes responsibilities of an individual who is HIV seropositive.

Psychosocial counseling is indicated when positive HIV test results precipitate acute anxiety, depression, or suicidal ideation. Follow-up counseling sessions and telephone calls are important to monitor the client's status. The client should be informed about available counseling services. The person should be cautioned to consider carefully who should be informed of the test results. Many individuals have told others about their HIV-seropositive status, only to experience isolation and discrimination. Plans for the future should be explored, and clients should be advised to avoid stressors, drugs, and infections to maintain optimal health.

Research Brief

Strader MK, Beaman ML: Theoretical components of STD counselor's messages to promote clients' use of condoms, *Pub Health Nurs* 9(2):109-117, 1992.

The purpose of this study was to identify the types of messages about condom use that STD counselors give to clients. The investigators had STD counselors read vignettes describing clients, and counselors were asked to describe how they would persuade each client to use condoms. The vignettes described clients who were resistant to using condoms for many reasons including the following: they decrease sensation, they interrupt lovemaking, and they are clumsy. Counselors' messages were found to provide information, stress a moralistic tone, or focus on fear. Some of the counselors provided information that was irrelevant to the needs of the clients described in the vignette. Moralistic messages included statements such as "you should do . . ." or "don't you feel bad about what you are doing to your family?" These are not effective ways to promote behavior change; clients who feel reprimanded by the counselor are unlikely to listen to the rest of what the counselor has to say. More effective ways to facilitate behavior change include focusing on behaviors the client can adopt instead of simply advising the cessation of risky behavior. This may work to develop a more positive attitude toward condom use. Counselors would benefit by identifying their own values to understand if client behaviors affect their ability to be non-judgmental.

Partner Notification

Partner notification, also known as contact tracing, is a public health intervention aimed at controlling STDs. It is done by confidentially identifying and notifying exposed sexual and injection drug–using partners of those found to have reportable STDs. Partner notification programs usually occur in conjunction with reportable disease requirements and are carried out by most health departments.

Individuals diagnosed with a reportable STD are asked to provide the names and locations of their partners so that they can be informed of their exposure and obtain the necessary treatment. Clients may be encouraged to notify their partners and to encourage them to seek treatment. If the client agrees to do so, suggestions on how to tell partners and how to deal with possible reactions may be explored. In some instances, clients may feel more comfortable if the nurse notifies those who are exposed. If clients contact their partners about possible infection, the community health nurse contacts health care providers or clinics to verify examination of exposed partners.

If the client prefers not to participate in notifying partners, the nurse contacts them—often by a home visit—and counsels them to seek evaluation and treatment. The client is offered literature regarding treatment, risk reduction, and the test site's location and hours of operation. The identity of the infected client who names sexual and injection drug–using partners cannot be revealed. Maintaining confidentiality is critical with all STDs but particularly with HIV, because antidiscrimination laws may not be in place or may be inadequate.

Tertiary Prevention

Tertiary prevention can apply to many of the chronic STDs, such as HSV, HIV, and untreated syphilis. For viral STDs, much of this effort focuses on managing symptoms and psychosocial support regarding future interpersonal relations. Many clients report feeling contaminated, and support groups may be available to help clients cope with chronic STDs.

Much of the effort in tertiary prevention focuses on clients with AIDS who return home and are unable to provide care for themselves because of progressing illness. The community health nurse conducts physical assessments and makes recommendations to the family about obtaining additional care services or maintaining the client in the home. Case management is important in all phases of HIV infection but is a particularly important activity in this stage to ensure that clients have adequate ser-vices to meet their needs. This may include ensuring that medication can be obtained through identifying funding resources, identifying sources of respite care for caretakers, or referring clients for home or hospice care.

Nursing interventions include teaching families about managing symptomatic illness by preventing deteriorating conditions such as diarrhea, skin breakdown, and inadequate nutrition.

Universal Precautions

The importance of teaching caregivers about infection control in home care is vital. Concerns about the transmission of HIV may be expressed by clients, families, friends, and other groups. Whereas fear may be expressed by some, others who are caring for loved ones with HIV may not take adequate precautions such as glove wearing because of concern about appearing as though they do not want to touch a loved one. Others may believe myths that suggest they cannot be infected by someone they love. Inadequate protection of home-based caregivers has become a concern as a result of eight cases of documented transmission of HIV by individuals living with and caring for an HIV-infected person (Centers for Disease Control, 1994c).

Universal precautions must be taught to caregivers in the home setting. All blood and articles soiled with body fluids must be handled as if they were infectious or contaminated by blood-borne pathogens. Gloves should be worn whenever hands will be expected to touch nonintact skin, mucous membranes, blood, or other fluids. A mask, goggles, and gown should also be worn if there is potential for splashing or spraying of infectious material during any care.

All protective equipment should be worn only once and then disposed. If the skin or mucous membranes of the caregiver come in contact with body fluids, the skin should be washed with soap and water, and the mucous membrances should be flushed with water as soon as possible after the exposure. Thorough hand washing with soap and water—a major infection control measure—should be conducted whenever hands become contaminated and whenever gloves or other protective equipment (mask, gown) is removed. Soiled clothing or linen should be washed in a washing machine filled with hot water using bleach as an additive and dried on a hot air cycle of a dryer.

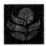 ## Clinical Application

Consider the case of Yvonne Jackson, a 20-year-old woman who visits the Hopetown City Health Department's maternity clinic. Examination reveals she is at 14 weeks' gestation. She is single but has been in a steady relationship for the past 6 months with Phil. She states that she has no other children. The HIV test done as part of the routine prenatal workup is positive.

1. *What questions need to be asked regarding Yvonne's ability to cope with the test result?*
2. *What questions does the nurse need to ask regarding controlling the spread of HIV to others?*
3. *What information should the nurse give to Yvonne?*

Yvonne reacts with an expression of disbelief about the test results. Understanding that this is a common reaction and that Yvonne will not be able to concentrate on all of the questions and information that need to be covered, the nurse prioritizes essential information to obtain and provide during this visit.

Information is gathered from Yvonne about past injection drug–using and sexual partners. The nurse evaluates Yvonne's comfort in sharing the information with Phil as she explores what she believes Phil's response might be. The nurse offers to role-play the situation of Yvonne telling Phil about the possibility of his infection, risks, and the importance of testing for the HIV antibody. Rather than contacting other previous sexual and drug-using partners herself, Yvonne requests that health department staff contact them about possible infection. She gives the community health nurse the names and addresses of two additional drug-using partners.

The most immediate concerns for Yvonne are the need to seek ongoing care to monitor the HIV infection and to decide whether to continue the preg-

Continued.

Clinical Application—cont'd

nancy. The nurse evaluates whether Yvonne has a primary health care provider, provides a list of providers, and stresses the importance of establishing an ongoing relationship with a primary health care provider for follow-up of the HIV infection. She tells her that important information about Yvonne's health may be identified that will help to determine her ability to carry and deliver the baby if she chooses to continue the pregnancy. The community health nurse discusses the meaning of the test results with her and how they may affect the infant's and mother's health.

The nurse explains that transmission to the fetus is possible during the pregnancy and that the mother may have a greater chance of progressing from asymptomatic infection to symptomatic HIV disease but that promising findings have been found with the use of new medications. The nurse explores possibilities with Yvonne about the decision regarding her ability to physically, emotionally, and financially cope with rearing a child that possibly may be ill. Family members and other potential resources are assessed. The need for Yvonne to tell health care

providers or blood handlers about the HIV infection is reviewed. The nurse schedules a second appointment for follow-up counseling 1 week after the initial test results are given. She also gives Yvonne the telephone number of the local AIDS support group and arranges to make a home visit to her in 2 days.

At the follow-up home and clinic visits, specific information is given regarding infection control in the home and safer sexual relations. The community health nurse ensures that Yvonne is taking steps toward receiving prenatal care and medical care for the HIV infection. The nurse reviews information about how to maintain health and avoid stressors and contracts with Yvonne to initiate home visits to provide reinforcement of adequate prenatal nutrition and teaching and to assess Yvonne's physical health as the pregnancy progresses.

1. *What questions need to be asked regarding Yvonne's use of drugs?*
2. *What options are available to the pregnant woman who is HIV infected? What strategies would you use to assist Yvonne in making her decision about the pregnancy?*

Key Concepts

- Nearly all STDs are preventable because they are transmitted through specific, known behaviors.
- STDs are one of the most serious public health problems in the United States. HIV infection has been identified as the most urgent public health problem of this century, and there is an increased incidence of drug-resistant gonococcal infection, chancroid, and chlamydial infections.
- STDs affect certain groups in greater numbers. Factors associated with risk include being under 25 years of age, being a member of a minority group, residing in an urban setting, being impoverished, and using crack cocaine.
- The increasing incidence, morbidity, and mortality of STDs document the need for community health nurses to educate clients about STD prevention.
- Many STDs do not produce symptoms in clients. Other STDs, such as genital warts, HIV, and genital herpes, are associated with cancer.
- Aside from death, the most serious complications caused by STDs are pelvic inflammatory disease, infertility, ectopic pregnancy, neonatal morbidity and mortality, and neoplasia.

- AIDS is the most extreme stage of HIV infection. As more is learned about methods to prevent disease progression, such as antiretroviral therapy, stress reduction, and proper nutrition, more emphasis is being placed on early detection and management of HIV infection.
- HIV testing plays an important role in early detection and treatment and provides opportunities for risk assessment and preventive counseling.
- Partner notification, also known as contact tracing, may be done by the infected client or by the health professional. It is done by identifying, contacting, and encouraging evaluation and treatment of sexual and injectable drug–using partners.
- AIDS has created an entirely new group of people needing health care. This rapidly growing population is straining a health care system that is already unable to meet the needs of many.
- Most of the care that is provided, both home and outpatient care, is done within the community setting, which reduces direct health care costs but increases the need for financial support of home and community health services.

Critical Thinking Activities

1. Identify the number of reported cases of AIDS and the number of reported cases of HIV infection within your state and locale (if reportable in your state). How are the cases distributed by age, sex, geographical location, and race?
2. Identify the location or locations of HIV testing services in your community. Are the test results anonymous or confidential? Describe how and to whom the results are reported.
3. Identify counseling and home care services that are available for the person with HIV infection within your community. Are they adequate to meet the needs of those infected? How much do these services cost?
4. Form small groups and role-play a nurse-client interaction involving a risk assessment and counseling regarding safer sex and injection drug–using practices.

Bibliography

American Health Consultants: *AIDS Alert* 9(10):148, 1994.

American Public Health Association: *Healthy communities 2000 model standards*, ed 3, Washington, DC, 1991, The Association.

Aral SO, Holmes KK: Epidemiology of sexual behavior and sexually transmitted diseases. In Holmes KK, et al, editors: *Sexually transmitted diseases*, New York, 1990, McGraw-Hill.

Berer M: Adverse effects of nonoxynol-9, *Lancet* 340:615-616, 1992.

Blount J: Personal communication, 1/18/1991.

Centers for Disease Control: Chancroid—United States, 1981-1990: evidence for underreporting of cases, *MMWR* 41(SS-3):57-61, 1992a.

Centers for Disease Control: Decreased susceptibility of Neisseria gonorrhoeae to fluoroquinolones—Ohio and Hawaii, 1992-1994, *MMWR* 43(18):325-327, 1994a.

Centers for Disease Control: First 100,000 cases of acquired immunodeficiency syndrome: United States, *MMWR* 38:561, 1989.

Centers for Disease Control: Guidelines for effective school health education to prevent the spread of AIDS, *MMWR* 37(S-2):1-14, 1988.

Centers for Disease Control: Hepatitis B virus: a comprehensive strategy for eliminating transmission in the United States through universal childhood vaccination—ACIP, *MMWR* 40(RR-13):1-25, 1991a.

Centers for Disease Control: HIV prevalence estimates and AIDS case projections for the United States: report based upon a workshop, *MMWR* 39(RR-16), 1990a.

Centers for Disease Control: HIV prevention in the correctional system, 1991, *MMWR* 41(22):389-391, 397, 1992b.

Centers for Disease Control: HIV/AIDS surveillance report, *MMWR* 5(4):3-33, 1994b.

Centers for Disease Control: Human immunodeficiency virus transmission in household settings—United States, *MMWR* 43(347):353-356, 1994c.

Centers for Disease Control: Knowledge and practices among injecting-drug users of bleach use for equipment disinfection—New York City, 1993, *MMWR* 43(24):439, 445-446, 1994d.

Centers for Disease Control: Maternal hepatitis B screening practices—California, Connecticut, Kansas, and US, 1992-1993, *MMWR* 43(17):311, 317-320, 1994e.

Centers for Disease Control: 1993 revised classification system for HIV infection and expanded surveillance case definition for AIDS among adolescents and adults, *MMWR* 41(RR-17), 1992c.

Centers for Disease Control: 1993 sexually transmitted diseases treatment guidelines, *MMWR* 42(RR-14), 1993f.

Centers for Disease Control: Nosocomial transmission of hepatitis B virus associated with a spring-loaded fingerstick device—California, *MMWR* 39(35):610-613, 1990b.

Centers for Disease Control: Pelvic inflammatory disease: guidelines for prevention and management, *MMWR* 40(RR-5):1-25, 1991b.

Centers for Disease Control: Recommendations for the prevention and management of chlamydia trachomatis infections, 1993, *MMWR* 42(RR-12), 1993a.

Centers for Disease Control: Special focus: surveillance for sexually transmitted diseases, *MMWR* 42(SS-3), 1993b.

Centers for Disease Control: Summary of notifiable diseases, *MMWR* 41(55):3-73, 1993c.

Centers for Disease Control: Summary of notifiable diseases, US 1993, *MMWR* 42:53, 1994f.

Centers for Disease Control: The second 100,000 cases of acquired immunodeficiency syndrome—United States, June, 1981-December 1991, *MMWR* 41(2):28-29, 1992d.

Centers for Disease Control: Update: acquired immunodeficiency syndrome—United States, 1992, *MMWR* 42(28):547-551, 557, 1993d.

Centers for Disease Control: Update: reducing HIV transmission in intravenous-drug users not in drug treatment—United States, *MMWR* 39(31):529, 536-538, 1990c.

Centers for Disease Control: Update: mortality attributable to HIV infection/AIDS among persons aged 25-44 years—United States, 1990 and 1991, *MMWR* 42(25):481-486, 1993e.

Centers for Disease Control: Zidovudine for the prevention of HIV transmission from mother to infant, *MMWR* 43(16):285-287, 1994g.

Clottey C, Dallabetta G: Sexually transmitted diseases and human immunodeficiency virus, *Infect Dis Clin North Am* 7(4):753-770, 1993.

Corey L: Genital herpes. In Holmes KK, Mardh PF, Sparling PF, Wiesner PJ, editors: *Sexually transmitted diseases*, New York, 1990, McGraw-Hill.

Crum CP, Nuovo GJ: *Genital papillomaviruses and related neoplasms*, New York, 1991, Raven Press.

Frank ML, Bateman L, Poindexter AN: Planned condom use by women with norplant implants, *Adv Contraception* 9:227-232, 1993.

Hale PJ: Employer response to AIDS in a low prevalence area, *Fam Community Health* 13(2):38, 1990.

Hale PJ: Women's self-efficacy for the prevention of sexual risk behavior, 1994 (unpublished doctoral dissertation, University of Maryland).

Healthy People 2000: national health promotion and disease prevention objectives, Washington, DC, 1991, Public Health Service.

Hellinger F: The lifetime costs of treating a person with HIV, *JAMA* 270:474-478, 1993.

Hook E, Handsfield H: Gonococcal infections in the adult. In Holmes KK, Mardh P, Sparling PF, Wiesner PJ, editors: *Sexually transmitted diseases*, New York, 1990, McGraw-Hill.

Kasen S, Vaughan RD, Walter HJ: Self-efficacy for AIDS preventive behaviors among tenth grade students, *Health Educ Q* 19(2):187-202, 1992.

Kilbourne BW, Buehler JW, Rogers MF: AIDS as a cause of death in children, adolescents, and young adults, *Am J Pub Health* 80(4):499-500, 1990.

Martens KA: Sexually transmitted genital tract infection during pregnancy, *Emerg Med Clin North Am* 12(1):91-113, 1994.

Novello AC, Peterson HB, Arrowsmith-Lowe JT, et al: Condom use for the prevention of sexual transmission of HIV infection, *JAMA* 269(22):2840, 1993.

Occupational Health and Safety Administration: *Occupational exposure to bloodborne pathogens*, Richmond, Virginia, Department of Labor and Industry, 1992. Standard 1910.1030.

Pantaleo G, Grazioso C, Fauci AS: The immunopathogenesis of human immunodeficiency virus infection, *N Engl J Med* 328(5):327-335, 1993.

Perkins HA: Safety of the blood supply, *J Clin Apheresis* 8:110-116, 1993.

Phillips I: Beta-lactamase producing, penicillin-resistant gonococcus, *Lancet* 2:656-657, 1976.

Puligheddu P, Nieddu R, Medda F, et al: HSV-2 and cervical intraepithelial neoplasia: cytological, histological and serological features, *Clin Obstet Gynecol* 15(3):88-93, 1988.

St Louis ME, Kamengo M, Brown C, et al: Risk for perinatal HIV-1 transmission according to maternal immunologic virologic, and placental factors, *JAMA* 269(22):2853-2859, 1993.

Schur CL, Berk ML: Health insurance coverage of persons with HIV-related illness: data from the ACSUS screener. In *AIDS cost and services utilization survey (ACSUS) Report* No 2, Rockville, Md, 1994, Agency for Health Care Policy Research.

Stone K, Brooks C, Guianan ME, Alexander E: National surveillance for neonatal herpes simplex virus infections, *Sex Trans Dis* 16(3):152-156, 1989.

Strader MK, Beaman ML: Theoretical components of STD counselor's messages to promote clients' use of condoms, *Pub Health Nurs* 9(2):109-117, 1992.

World Health Organization: *The HIV/AIDS pandemic: 1993 overview.* WHO Global Programme on AIDS, Pub No WHO/GPA/CNP/EVA/93-1, Geneva, 1993, The Organization.

Zenilman J, Bonner M, Sharp K, et al: Penicillinase-producing Neisseria gonorrhoea in Dade County, Florida: evidence of core-group transmitters and the impact of illicit antibiotics, *Sex Trans Dis* 15(1):45-50, 1988.

Part Seven Community Health Nurses: Roles and Functions

At one time the role of the community health nurse primarily included visiting clients at home and identifying cases of communicable disease; over the decades the role has become multi-faceted. As the health care system has changed, the need for a comprehensive, population-focused public health system has become more evident. Nurses are able to provide care to individuals, families, and communities in a wide variety of settings and roles.

With increasing emphasis being placed on the community as the client, community health nurses recognize that, in order to address community health issues, the nurse must be able to meet the needs of the individuals, families, and groups who are the nucleus of the community. Unlike in the past, when the primary practice setting for the nurse was the hospital or public health agency, nurses find their clients in many settings. Regardless of the type of client, practice setting, specialty area of practice, or the functional role of the nurse, the community health nurse acts as advocate for clients in meeting their needs through the health care system.

This section discusses the roles of manager, consultant, case manager, and nurse practitioner with specific emphasis on the development of the advocacy role in community health practice. Throughout the text, content is applicable to a variety of practice settings, including the more traditional public health practice arena such as the health department. Aside from the official agencies, a few multiple practice settings with close association to community health nursing have been chosen for presentation (e.g., school health, occupational health, home health, and primary health care settings). ▼

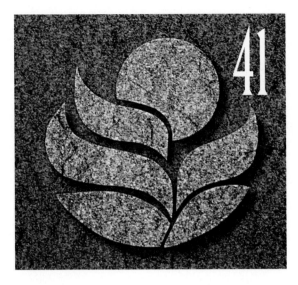

41

Community Health Nurse In Home Health and Hospice Care

Marcia Stanhope*

Objectives

After reading this chapter, the student should be able to do the following:

◆ Define home health care.
◆ List the types of home health agencies.
◆ Analyze the similarities and differences in the types of home health agencies.
◆ Discuss the educational requirements for a home health care nurse.
◆ Relate the nursing process and the standards of community health nursing practice to the home health setting.
◆ Identify the roles and functions of the interdisciplinary health care team.
◆ Describe the regulatory impact on home health care and nursing practice.
◆ Analyze the reimbursement mechanisms and issues relative to home health care.
◆ Describe a hospice care program.
◆ Identify the impact of deregulation on future home health care programs.

Key Terms

accreditation
combination agencies
contracting
direct care
distributive care
documentation
episodic care
facilitator
home health aide
home health care
hospice
hospital-based agencies
indirect care
interdisciplinary collaboration
intermittent care
Medicare
occupational therapists
official agencies
physical therapists
professional competency
proprietary agencies
recertification
regulation
reimbursement
reimbursement system
research
self-care
speech pathologist
voluntary and private nonprofit agencies

Outline

Continued.

*Recognition is given to Eileen Garvey and Jacquelyne Logue for prior contributions to this chapter.

Outline—cont'd

This chapter presents another aspect of community health nursing: home health care. Home health care differs from other areas of health care in that the health care providers practice in the client's environment. Home is a place where nurses have provided care for more than a century in the United States.

When working in a client's home, the nurse is a guest and, in order to be effective, must earn the trust of the family. In this setting nurses have the opportunity to observe family life, a privilege usually reserved for family and friends. Family dynamics, lifestyle choices, communication patterns, coping strategies, responses to health and illness, social, cultural, spiritual, and economic issues are but a few of the factors nurses can assess when visiting in a family's home (Doherty and Hurley, 1994).

Portnoy and Dumas (1994) have suggested that when working with an individual client or family in the home the real work is not just within the boundaries of that household. To provide effective, comprehensive care, nurses will want to analyze the strength that clients gain from their neighborhoods, the social network which can be used to support clients in times of vulnerability and crisis. Therefore, nurses working in the home will also want to gain the trust of the communities by providing for the needs of the clients they serve in that community with caring, honesty, competence, and ethical and cultural sensitivity (Doherty and Hurley, 1994).

The parameters of home health care use in the managed care environment are expected to expand in response to increased demands for cost-effectiveness, consumer preferences, technological advancements, and proven quality of service.

DEFINITION OF HOME HEALTH CARE

Home health care in today's society cannot simply be defined as "care at home." It includes an arrangement of disease prevention, health promotion and episodic illness-related services provided to people in their places of residence. A more comprehensive definition of home health care has been prepared by a Department of Health and Human Services interdepartmental work group (Warhola, 1980):

Home health care is that component of a continuum of comprehensive health care whereby health services are provided to individuals and families in their places of residence for the purpose of promoting, maintaining or restoring health, or of maximizing the level of independence while minimizing the effects of disability and illness, including terminal illness. Services appropriate to the needs of the individual patient and family are planned, coordinated, and made available by providers organized for the delivery of home care through the use of employed staff, contractual arrengements, or a combination of the two patterns.

Home health nursing, according to the American Nurses Association (1992), is a synthesis of community health nursing and selected technical skills from other nursing specialties (see Figure 41-1). It involves the same primary preventive focus of care of aggregates of the community health nurses and the secondary and tertiary prevention foci of the care of individuals in collaboration with the family and other caregivers.

Finally, a third definition, by the NAHC, defines home health care as a broad spectrum of health and social services offered in the home environment to recovering, disabled or chronically ill persons (1994).

These definitions integrate the components of home health care: the client, family, health care professionals (multidisciplinary) and goals to assist the client to return to an optimum level of health and independence. Their differences rest on the fact that interpretation and actual delivery of home health care vary according not only to the client, but also to the provider and reimburser of these services.

Family, which includes any caregiver or significant person who takes the responsibility to assist the client

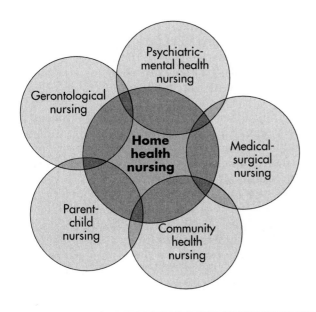

FIGURE 14-1

A conceptual model of home health nursing. (From American Nurses Association: A *statement on the scope of home health nursing practice*, Washington, DC, 1992, The Association.)

in need of care at home, is an integral part of home health care. Roles of the caregiver include supervising clients by ensuring that their basic needs are being met and providing direct care such as personal hygiene, meal preparation, administering medications, and providing treatment that, in the past, would have been done only in the hospital by a health care provider. This person is valuable in providing the needed maintenance care between the skilled visits of the professional provider.

A person's **place of residence** has its own uniqueness in terms of the location for providing care, depending on what the person calls home. It may be a house, an apartment, a shelter, or a car.

The client **goals** are always related to the principles of health promotion, maintenance, and restoration, regardless of the primary health care provider. By maximizing the level of independence, home health care nurses can help the clients function at the best possible level for preventing dependence. This assistance can take the form of teaching or linking the client with community services that provide limited assistance for enabling the client to stay at home. In addition, prevention of complications of chronically ill persons can help to minimize the effects of disability and illness. Countless complications of long-term illness seen in the form of disability are preventable with adequate home health care intervention. Terminal illness, as seen by the development of hospice home care programs, can be handled at home instead of in the hospital if the client and family accept this concept. Alleviation of pain and suffering is possible in the home care setting. Pain control through the use of medications is closely supervised by nurses in the home. They assess the client's response to the medica-

tion and report these findings to the client's physician, who then modifies the medication as needed.

Services can be tailored to any client need or problem. When the client's level of independence increases, the need for service decreases. The services are coordinated through an agency obligated to maintain quality care and provide for continuity. Thus the range of services provided in home health care is extensive. The challenge of home health care to community health nurses can be more fully appreciated by briefly tracing the history of this nursing role.

HISTORY OF HOME HEALTH CARE

Throughout its history, home health care nurses have epitomized Florence Nightingale's philosophy that nurses are "messengers of health as well as ministers of disease" (Woodham-Smith, 1951). The community health nurses working in the homes were social reformers, living in immigrant communities, providing nursing clinics, health education, and care for the sick. They provided for the nutritional needs of their communities as well as clothing, hygiene, and adequate shelter. They provided prenatal care, post-partum visits to new mothers and healthy babies, established hot lunch school programs, preschool clinics, coordinated transportation services, worked with summer camp programs, did tuberculosis screening, blood typing, immunization for polio, and established "sick room" equipment programs. This combination of preventive services and sick care continued until the introduction of Medicare in 1966. This program emphasized a sick-care payment program that influenced the services offered through home health and deleted all emphasis on illness prevention and health promotion, although some home health agencies continued to develop programs to benefit their communities, paying for them through their profits or contributions. Today, with health care reform and the emphasis on managed care, a number of agencies are beginning once again to offer a combination of preventive and sick care services.

Home health care began in the United States around the 1800s. As in England in the early days, so in America were the sick cared for by nuns and sisters. The Sisters of Charity of St. Joseph was established in Maryland in 1809. Aside from the work of the sisters and nuns, the first organized visiting nurse work was done by the Ladies Benevolent Society of Charleston, South Carolina, founded in 1813. This society had a visiting committee of 16 ladies who were allotted a certain portion of the city in which to visit the sick at home. When it became essential, nurses were hired by the visitors to provide nursing care to the sick at home. This society lasted well over 50 years, until the beginning of the Civil War. The society was revived in 1902 when a trained nurse was employed to carry on the work of the society.

In 1832 the Lying in Charity for attending women in their homes was established in Philadelphia. In

1842 this organization was combined with a subsidiary organization called the Nurse Society. These nurses were given training to assist them in their work in the home and were supervised by an active committee of *Philadelphia Ladies.*

Organized visiting nursing, the precursor of modern home care, was first established in the United States in March 1877 when the women's branch of the New York City Mission first sent trained nurses into the homes of the poor and the sick. The first home care nurse, Frances Root, was a member of the first class to graduate from the new training school at Bellevue Hospital. The establishment of the first visiting nurses association in the United States occurred in 1885 when the Buffalo District Nursing Association was begun by Mrs. Elizabeth Marshall. In 1886 Boston formed the Instructive Visiting Nursing Association to promote health education. During this same period, Philadelphia developed a visiting nurses association that led the way for establishing a pay service. This association appointed a nurse superintendent and adopted a uniform for nurses to wear while working with patients.

By 1890, some 13 years after the first nurse was sent out by the New York City Mission, 21 visiting nurses associations existed in the United States, most employing only one nurse each. These associations preceded the development, in 1893, of the Henry Street Settlement, founded in New York by Lillian Wald. After 1894, the use of visiting nurses grew more rapidly with the advent of growing social consciousness.

The Waltham (Massachusetts) Training School was established in 1885 by Dr. Alfred Worcester after he conferred with Florence Nightingale and designed a course to train nurses for private duty. The course included experience in the home. Later, public health nursing with field experience was added to the program. The school was criticized for sending students into homes to earn money for the hospital and for overworking and not supervising the students (Dolan, 1958).

As the demands on public health nurses visiting in the home increased, the question of the nurses' education became more important; hospital training was not sufficient for public health nurses. The demand for nurses experienced in providing care in the home greatly exceeded the supply of trained nurses, and community after community had to begin nursing associations with untrained nurses. Undergraduate education sometimes involved an affiliation with a visiting nurses association that allowed students to leave the hospital for short periods of training in the districts. The first postgraduate course in public health nursing was offered in 1906 by the Instructive District Nursing Association of Boston. Following these very simple training programs, Columbia University, in 1910, offered the first university course in public health nursing. This set a precedent for higher education to become involved in public health nursing education.

In 1909 the Metropolitan Life Insurance Company began offering home nursing services to its millions of industrial policy holders in the United States and Canada. Initially, arrangements were made with Lillian Wald and the Henry Street Settlement to provide these nursing services. By 1912 Metropolitan was offering home nursing services from 589 nursing centers. These centers provided an opportunity not only to develop payment mechanisms based on the exact cost of visits to patients, but also to engage in a number of valuable health studies and to collect data based on statistics kept by the nurses for future projections about the health care needs of the policy holders. Sixteen years later, John Hancock Mutual Life Insurance Company established a similar service for its policy holders.

Following the example of the Visiting Nurse Society of Philadelphia (the first to establish a pay service) and of the insurance companies, other nursing organizations began to develop pay services. In some instances payment was made on an hourly basis, by appointment, or by capitation to meet the needs of those who could pay for nursing services. The introduction of payment for services marked a change in the philosophy of home nursing services—from providing services only to the "worthy" poor to providing services to people with moderate incomes who required continuous nursing care and household assistance.

Industrial nursing also grew out of the early visiting nurses associations. In 1895 Fletcher Proctor, onetime governor of Vermont, and Adamelle Stewart, an 1894 graduate of the Waltham Training School, introduced district nursing into several villages whose residents were employees of the Vermont Marble Company. This service was essentially a home service, with patient referrals coming from physicians.

The number of public health visiting nurses in the United States increased from 136 in 1902 to 3000 in 1912. With funding from both private and public sources, visiting nurses were employed by some 810 agencies, including visiting nurse associations, city and state boards of health and education, private clubs and societies, the tuberculosis leagues, hospitals and dispensaries, business concerns, settlements and day nurseries, churches, charitable organizations, and other organizations.

The 1920s, an economically vital period, saw continued expansion of public health nursing. Then came the dramatic crash of the stock market in October 1929 and the beginning of the financial depression in America. Public health nursing was greatly affected as the budgets of private agencies dwindled and reserve funds disappeared. At the same time, visiting nursing work became more complicated because of the social problems experienced by the patients under care and their families.

This crash ushered in an era of changing philosophy concerning the provision of home care services. Less stress was placed on quantitative growth and more on qualitative measures of care provided. However, because of staff reductions, elimination of staff educational programs, and limited supervision, quality could not be assured—at a time when the country most needed comprehensive and effective services.

At this point, the federal government provided aid to the country and began to develop a new relationship among local communities and the state and federal governments. The Federal Emergency Relief Administration provided for allocation of federal funds to states so that nursing care could be given to the employed sick receiving federal relief. The Civil Works Administration provided funds for the use of nurses who were unemployed. These nurses worked primarily for official agencies and institutions. A large number of nurses found themselves in the field of public health without preparation or experience.

In the 1940s, hospitals began to take a more serious interest in home care as a result of the increased number of chronically ill clients being hospitalized. The Montefiore Hospital Home Care Program in New York began in 1947 and offered comprehensive home care services such as medical nursing and social services. Before enactment of Medicare in 1966, most agencies relied on charity and public contributions for survival.

Home care reached a turning point with the arrival of Medicare, which introduced regulations for home care practice as well as for reimbursement mechanisms. In 1967, one year after Medicare was enacted, there were 1753 Medicare-participating home health agencies in the United States with the majority being either visiting nursing associations or programs in public health departments. By 1980 there were 2924 home health agencies, an increase of about 48%. The Health Care Financing Agency (HCFA) reported 7521 Medicare-certified home health agencies as of 1994, as well as 6047 non-Medicare-certified home health agencies for a total of 13568. The growth in certified agencies alone represents a 429% growth in 28 years (NAHC Report, 1994).

Home health care agencies must provide nursing care as their primary service under Medicare.

TYPES OF HOME HEALTH CARE AGENCIES

Since the beginning of organized home care, many types of organizations have established programs to meet the home care needs of people. Home health agencies are divided into the following five general types based on the administrative and organizational structure: (1) official, (2) private and voluntary, (3) combination, (4) hospital-based, and (5) proprietary. These types differ in organization and administration but are similar in terms of the standards they

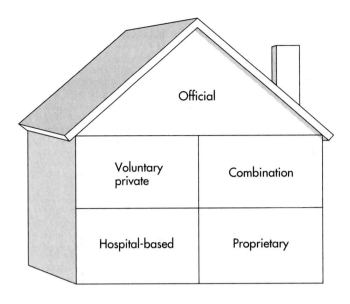

FIGURE 41-2
Types of home health care agencies.

  Home Health Agency Facts

6047 noncertified HHAs
1987—$11.6 billion spent on home care
1994—$23.7 billion spent on home care
 (National Medical Expenditures Survey)
Average per home visit—1987, $49; 1994, $70
Medicare—$13.7 billion in 1994 for 218,595,000 visits to
 3,345,100 clients
Medicaid—$101,707 million in 1994

must meet for licensure, certification, and accreditation. Figure 41-2 shows the types of home health agencies, and Table 41-1 lists the numbers and kinds of home health agencies; also see the box above for facts concerning home health agencies.

Official Agencies

Official agencies (public agencies) include those agencies operated by the state or by local governments (county, city) such as health departments. They are financed primarily by tax funds and are nonprofit entities. Most official agencies, in addition to having a home care component, also provide health education and disease prevention programs to people in the community.

Community health nurses employed in this setting may provide not only general home health care, but also well-child clinics, well-child home visits, immunization, health education programs, and home visits for preventive health care. Official agencies, in addition to being funded for services with local money, are

Table 41-1   Number and Kinds of Home Health Agencies

	Hospital	Rehabilitation Hospital	SNF	Visiting Nurses Association (VNA)	Combination Agency	Private (for Profit)	Proprietary	Private (Non-profit)	Other	Total
1967	133	0	0	549	93	939	0	0	30	1753
1980	359	8	9	515	63	1260	186	484	40	2924
1990	1486	8	101	474	47	985	1884	710	0	5695
1994	2081	3	123	586	45	1146	2892	597	48	7521

HCFA Office of Survey and Certification, 1994, USDHHS.

reimbursed for home care services as are the other types of home health care agencies. Medicare, Medicaid, and private insurance companies reimburse for home health care but not equally or totally in all cases. The **reimbursement system** is complicated and standardized. **Medicare** has the most standardized payment system of all third-party payers. Official agencies have been able to offer more comprehensive types of community health services than other kinds of agencies because of their objectives of health promotion and disease prevention and also because of the additional public funding often available.

Voluntary and Private Nonprofit Agencies

Voluntary and private agencies are grouped together as the nonprofit home health agencies. Voluntary agencies are supported by charities such as United Way, as well as by Medicare, Medicaid, and other third-party payers and client payments. The amount of financial assistance the voluntary agency receives depends on the community it serves. Traditionally, visiting nurses associations were the principal voluntary type of home health agency. With the advent of Medicare in 1966, the private nonprofit agency emerged as a viable establishment. Also emerging were rehabilitation agencies, which were based in rehabilitation facilities and in skilled facilities.

Voluntary and private nonprofit agencies are governed by boards of directors which represent the communities they serve. These agencies are nongovernmental organizations and are exempt from federal income tax. Historically, voluntary agencies were responsible for the initial development of nursing in the home, based on the client's need for service rather than the ability to pay.

Combination Agencies

In some communities, to decrease cost and prevent duplication of services, official and voluntary home health agencies have merged into **combination agencies** to provide home health care. The services remain the same, and the board members come from either one of the two existing agencies or a new board is formed. The

nurse may serve in several community health nursing roles as does the nurse in the official type of agency.

Hospital-Based Agencies

Hospitals have long been a pivotal point for health care services. In the 1970s, **hospital-based agencies** developed in response to the need for continuity of care from the acute care setting and also in response to the high cost of institutionalization.

In 1983 implementation of the prospective payment system and diagnosis related groups (DRGs) by the federal government precipitated a fundamental change in the attitudes of hospital personnel toward home care. Cost containment dictated earlier discharge of sicker patients to control profit margins. Increased liability risks, the desire for better patient management, and the potential for a diversified base of products and services increased the number of hospital-based home care agencies (Cassak, 1984). As of 1994, hospital-based agencies outnumbered all other types of Medicare-certified agencies except for proprietary agencies (HCFA, 1994).

Hospital-based agencies differ from other home health care agencies in that the already-established hospital board of directors is responsible for governing the agency. Moreover, clients of hospital-based home health care have access to existing inpatient services. Whether the agencies are official, voluntary, private nonprofit, or proprietary depends on the hospital structure. Regardless of the form they take, in most cases these agencies are a source of revenue for the hospital and may compete with community-based agencies.

Proprietary Agencies

Agencies ineligible for income tax exemption are called **proprietary** (profit-making) **agencies**. Proprietary agencies can be licensed and certified for Medicare by the state licensing agency. The owner of the agency is responsible for governing. Reimbursement is primarily from third-party payers and individual clients if agencies do not accept Medicare.

Opponents of this type of agency claim that proprietary agencies offer substandard quality of care and are involved only for monetary gains. There is little evidence to support this claim because all agencies that are Medicare-certified must comply with the same conditions. In recent years the number of Medicare-certified proprietary agencies increased significantly as hospitals began implementing "quicker" discharge of "sicker" patients (HCFA, 1994).

Managed care and the development of alliances and networks are changing the structure of the health care delivery system. As discussed in Chapter 5, these changes have introduced managed competition into the health care environment. Agencies are reacting to managed competition with a couple of strategies. The first is the creation of networks of providers who become contracting partners to negotiate as low-cost providers. A second response to managed competition is to acquire or merge with other agencies to gain strength, to lower costs, or to increase power to compete (McClure, 1994).

While home health care represents only 2% of all health care expenses, it is the fastest growing market. With changes in the health care system, it is projected that there will be more home care and community-based services with decreases in institutional services, such as hospitals. Thus home care agencies are expected to move in one of two directions. An agency may very likely either become a contracted partner in a network to provide home care services for a hospital, an HMO, a group of physicians and others; or it might be purchased by other agencies and become the sole provider of home care for that agency. Both of these arrangements are good opportunities for nurses to reintroduce primary prevention and health promotion into their practices. This can reduce the likelihood of their clients needing more costly services such as hospital care offered through their network. As a result, home health agencies and nurses need to participate in case management while understanding the cost of care of each client (Dee-Kelly et al., 1994).

Regardless of the type of home health agency existing in a community, the primary goal should be to provide quality home health care to the community based on the health needs of its people. The development of additional agencies in a community can be an emotional issue to people working in already established home health agencies. Competition in home health care is on the rise. Traditionally, most agencies have remained noncompetitive because of the humanitarian aspect of the service. The competitive issue is the result of the federal government's move to deregulate and deinstitutionalize areas of health care. Competition can be a positive force in developing and maintaining quality home health care programs. Nevertheless, there is profit to be made in home health care, which necessitates utilization review and quality assurance mechanisms (see Chapter 22).

Current changes in home health care have several implications for the community health nurse. Clients are being discharged at earlier stages of treatment, thereby needing a highly skilled level of care. Also, to survive in the competitive arena, agencies must continue to provide quality care and also be cost effective without compromising accountability. These home care criteria require that community health nurses in management have highly developed administrative skills.

EDUCATIONAL REQUIREMENTS FOR PRACTICE

Demonstration of **professional competency** is the foremost requirement for home health care nurses. Home health care nurses come from a variety of educational and practice settings. Differences in both experience and educational preparation influence the contributions that nurses make to home health care.

Home health care nurses should be trained and educated to function at a high level of competency so that they can be relied on not only by their professional colleagues but also by the community. A baccalaureate degree in nursing should be the minimum requirement for entry into professional practice in the community health care setting. Nursing education has the responsibility of producing competent, skillful practitioners. A baccalaureate degree does not ensure a qualified, mature professional nurse, but a quality education does lay the foundation for the development of such important characteristics. Life experience, compassion, and awareness of self are factors that are inherent in the delivery of quality client care and professionalism.

In home health care, the nurse with a baccalaureate degree usually functions in the role of a staff nurse or home health care nurse. The nurse with a master's degree is better prepared for the practitioner, administrator, or teacher role. As home care continues to develop its larger role in community health nursing, the need for specialized nurse clinicians will also increase to meet the ever-increasing, highly technological care that is transposed from the hospital into the home setting. In managed care more clinical specialists will be needed to provide case management and to develop programs to meet the needs of the population served by the network.

SCOPE OF PRACTICE
Objective in Home Health Care

A common misconception of home health care is that it is a "custodial" type of nursing. It is important to remember that home health care nursing is a *division* of community health nursing. Thus health *promotion activities are a fundamental component of practice*. Since the health promotion component of home health care is delivered in the patient's home environment and is *intermittent* care, a primary objective for the home health nurse is to facilitate self-care.

According to Orem (1995, p 104), "Self-care is the practice of activities that individuals initiate and perform on their own behalf in maintaining life, health, and well-being." This definition includes community health nursing activities and, notably, home health care nursing. Home health care nurses use this concept for all clients, regardless of the clients' abilities. For example, a client may be recuperating at home after suffering a stroke and be unable to perform activities of daily living (ADL) without assistance. Although such clients are unable to perform self-care activities, they can be instructed in the performance of these activities in a modified form. In this way they have some control over their life and self-care activities, and they can be taught to prevent possible losses in other self-care areas. This example also supports another definition, which is even more specific to the home health care population. **Self-care** is an action taken by the consumer or client, on their own behalf to maintain life, health and well-being (Goeppenger and Labuhn, 1992).

A primary goal is to help prevent the occurrence of illness and to promote the client's well-being. In the home care setting, the clients possess more control and ability for determining their own health care needs. The client role is active because continuance of service depends a great deal on the client's understanding of plans established jointly by the client and community health nurse. The nurse serves as a **facilitator** for development of positive health behaviors for the individual who has had an episode of illness.

Contracting

Contracting is a vital component of all nurse/client relationships. Constantly evolving legislative guidelines, third-party payer requirements, the high risk of liability, and the intense level of nurse autonomy, require that contracting be reviewed in the home care context (see Chapter 25).

The process of contracting in-home care involves not only the client and the nurse but also the family. **Contracting** refers to any working agreement, continuously renegotiable, between the nurse, client, and family. The process of contracting can be reflected in the client's care plan and clinical notes. Contracting allows the client and family to set their own goals and alleviates the problem of nurses who set expectations without comprehending the needs and wishes of the client and family.

Contracting is directly related to use of the nursing process (Figure 41-3) and can be done at each phase of the nursing process. As an example, during an initial home visit, the nurse gathers data and determines the components of the agreement and plan for subsequent actions by establishing the contract with the client and family. During that visit, if appropriate, portions of the contract may be implemented. If not, subsequent visits will provide such opportunities.

Contracts can be formal (written) or informal (verbal), depending on the client's needs. In either case, the process is recorded in the client's chart. The most important aspect is not the type of contract, but the

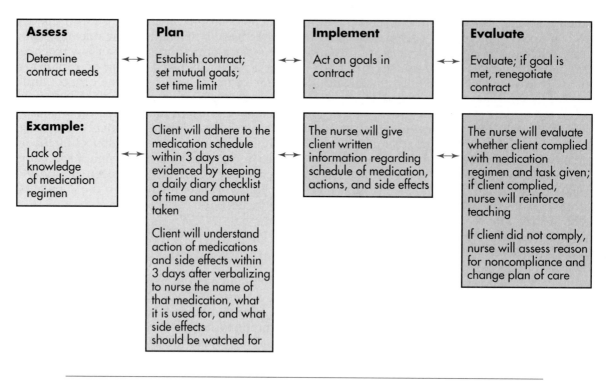

FIGURE 41-3

Contracting in relation to nursing process.

client's actual participation in establishing, implementing, and evaluating the process.

To avoid what is often referred to as the *home visit—ritual or therapy dilemma,* the home care nurse must establish both short-term and long-term goals with the clients and families. The purpose of this is not only for continuity of care but also for evaluating the client's condition and progress toward an optimum level of self-care. A study of community health nurses who made home visits found that half of the purposes of the visit were unknown to the clients since the nurses in the study did not share the purposes for the visits with them. Much of the dialogue failed to show any development of the interrelationship between the client and nurse.

Practice Functions of the Home Health Care Nurse

Home health care nursing involves both direct and indirect functions. In performing these functions, the home health care nurse assumes a variety of roles.

Direct Care

Direct care refers to the actual physical aspects of nursing care, anything requiring physical contact and face-to-face interactions. In home health care, direct care activities include performing a physical assessment on the patient, dressing changes of wounds, injections, insertion of an indwelling catheter, or IV therapy. Direct care also involves teaching clients and family caregivers how to perform a certain procedure or duty. By serving as a role model, the nurse can assist the client and family to develop positive health care behaviors. Technical skill competency must be demonstrated by the nurse to receive reimbursement by Medicare and Medicaid. Nursing care is covered by Medicare and other third-party payers as long as the care being delivered is "skilled." To determine whether a service performed by the nurse is skilled, several factors are evaluated and must be adequately documented:

1. Is the service complex, thereby requiring the knowledge and skill of a registered nurse?
2. Does the client's condition warrant skilled intervention?
3. Can this service be performed by a nonmedical person?
4. Does the instruction of a service to a client involve knowledge, instructions, and demonstrations by a registered nurse?

To adequately answer these questions, the home health care nurse must have a sufficient knowledge base of regulatory mechanisms and also must be competent and experienced to know how to interpret "skilled." These interpretations can be subjective; therefore, objective data are necessary to account for the service.

Some examples of skilled nursing services include the following:

1. Observing and evaluating client's condition, both physical and emotional.
2. Providing direct care in administering treatments, rehabilitative exercises and medications, catheter insertion, colostomy irrigation, and wound care.
3. Assisting client and family toward developing positive coping behavior.
4. Teaching client and family to give these treatments and medications when indicated.
5. Teaching client and family to carry out physician's orders such as use of a special diet, remembering to consider cultural background, financial status, and personal preferences.
6. Reporting to physician any new signs and symptoms relative to client's status and arranging for medical follow-up as indicated.
7. Assisting client and family to identify resources that will help client attain state of optimal functioning.

Indirect Care

Indirect care occurs when a client does not have personal contact with the nurse. This type of care is seen when home health care nurses serve as consultants to other health personnel who provide home care or even to those who provide in-hospital care. Clients often have their own patterns for care (such as ostomy care) and, when hospitalized, need assistance from hospital nurses to continue this program. Hospital nurses frequently contact the home health care nurse for advice on how to accomplish the client's usual method of care. This type of consultation will likely occur more often in managed care arenas.

Team conferences are a means of providing indirect care in home health care. It is an ideal time for increasing coordination and continuity of services for optimal client care and use of resources and services. Advice on how to manage clients with particular problems can be shared with various members of the team. Supervision of home health aides is a direct and indirect function because the home health care nurse may not always see the home health aide performing but can evaluate the care given to the client. Regular supervision of the aide by the nurse for at least 2-week intervals is mandated. There is much indirect care in the home health care setting. It may not be directly visible to the client, but it does exist and it does assist with ensuring quality home health care.

Although Medicare places an emphasis on episodic, or acute, care because of its limitations on benefits and requirements for skilled care, the home health care nurse cannot entirely separate primary, secondary, and tertiary prevention because of the interrelationship. These levels of prevention have been categorized into two levels of care: episodic and distributive.

Episodic Versus Distributive Care

Episodic care refers to the curative and restorative aspect of practice, or secondary and tertiary prevention, and **distributive care** refers to health maintenance and disease prevention, or primary prevention. A clinical example can best illustrate the application of these two aspects in home health care.

Mr. Jones, a 70-year-old white man discharged from the hospital the previous day, is admitted to home health care services for skilled nursing to assess his cardiovascular status after heart surgery for coronary artery disease. The episodic care involves teaching Mr. and Mrs. Jones about medications, exercise, and the signs and symptoms of possible heart problems postoperatively. In addition, the home health care nurse will provide direct care in assessing his cardiovascular status and helping Mr. Jones return to his optimum state of functioning.

Mr. Jones' psychosocial adaptation and needs will also be addressed in addition to assessing his level of self-care and adjustment relative to postcardiac surgery status. In regard to the distributive aspect, the home health care nurse will do additional teaching about ways Mr. Jones can prevent exacerbation of his condition by maintaining medical follow-up and adhering to the programs set up for him.

Nursing Roles

The roles of clinician, educator, researcher, administrator, and consultant are seen in home health care. They can be demonstrated by the experienced home health care nurse, the nursing supervisor, the director of nursing, or the administrator.

Home health care nurses in a staff position are clinicians because they provide direct nursing care to clients and families. Home health care nurses are also educators because they teach clients and families the "how to's" and "why's" of self-care. Formally, they may teach classes to community groups regarding health education topics. The researcher role in home health care has been relatively dormant even though home health care nurses often provide the data required for clinical or administrative change within their agency of employment. The home health care setting abounds with potential research areas. This role needs to take priority in the future if quality and cost effectiveness are to be maintained. A home health care administrator can be a nurse who has had advanced education with community health experience; requirements are stipulated by both federal and state rules and regulations. Finally, consultants may provide advice and counsel to staff and clients. (Refer to Chapter 43 for discussions of specific roles in community health nursing.)

Confusion exists in some health care circles regarding role differentiation between the private duty nurse and the home health care nurse. Even registered nurses who have not been directly exposed to home health care in either their educational or clinical experiences are not aware of the differences.

The only similarity is that both nurses are provided to clients in their homes. Table 41-2 clarifies the different components of private duty nursing and home health care nursing.

STANDARDS OF HOME HEALTH NURSING PRACTICE

The home health care nurse practices in accordance with the Standards of Home Health Nursing Practice developed by the American Nurses Association, Council of Community Health Nurses (ANA, 1986). Table 41-3 represents the relationship between the nursing process and the Standards of Practice. The use of the nursing process in the home care setting is evident by the legal requirement of documentation of all nursing action.

ANA Standard I: Organization

All home health services are planned, organized, and directed by a master's-prepared professional nurse

Table 41-2   Components of private duty and home health care nursing

	Private duty	Home health care
Role and function	One-to-one client care assignment Maintenance Custodial Episodic	Distributive Skilled care Rehabilitative Episodic
Reimbursement	Payment to nurse Third-party insurance (some)	Payment to agency Medicare and Medicaid Third-party insurance
Cost	Daily or hourly rate charge	Per visit or capitated charge
Frequency	Full-time and shift duty	Intermittent visits based on frequency and need of client

From Garvey E, Logue J: In Stanhope M, Lancaster J: *Community health nursing: process and practice for promoting health*, ed 2, St Louis, 1988, Mosby.

with experience in community health and administration.

The nurse executive and nurse manager work together to plan and direct programs that meet the needs of the communities served. The nurse administrators use their community health and administration knowledge and experience to write the mission, philosophy, and goals of the agency and to decide which services are needed by the individuals and families in their community. They establish a budget, personnel policies, and evaluation methods for programs and personnel. They establish, monitor, and use a quality assurance program to revise and improve services, and they assist the organization to maintain compliance with licensing and regulatory agencies.

ANA Standards II-IV: Theory, Data Collection, Diagnosis

The framework for assessment, intervention, and evaluation is based on theoretical concepts derived from nursing, public health, and physical, social, and behavioral sciences (see Table 41-2).

The home care nurse is responsible for assessing the client and family during the initial home visit as well as during all subsequent visits. This process establishes *database* information from the client and family, consisting of both subjective and objective data. Examples of *subjective* data include *information* that the client, family, and physicians relate to the nurse by means of verbal communication. This information is obtained from direct questioning. Information necessary to ob-

Table 41-3 Relationship between nursing process and ANA standards of practice

Nursing process	Standard		Description
Assess	I.	Organization	All home health services are planned, organized, and directed by a master's-prepared professional nurse with experience in community health and administration.
	II.	Theory	The nurse applies theoretical concepts as a basis for decisions in practice.
	III.	Data Collection	The nurse continuously collects and records data that are comprehensive, accurate, and systematic.
	IV.	Diagnosis	The nurse uses health assessment data to determine nursing diagnoses.
Plan	V.	Planning	The nurse develops care plans that establish goals. The care plan is based on nursing diagnoses and incorporates therapeutic, preventive, and rehabilitative nursing actions.
Implement	VI.	Intervention	The nurse, guided by the care plan, intervenes to provide comfort, to restore, improve, and promote health, to prevent complications and sequelae of illness, and to effect rehabilitation.
Evaluate	VII.	Evaluation	The nurse continually evaluates the client's and family's responses to interventions in order to determine progress toward goal attainment and to revise the data base, nursing diagnoses, and plan of care.
	VIII.	Continuity of Care	The nurse is responsible for the client's appropriate and uninterrupted care along the health care continuum, and therefore uses discharge planning, case management, and coordination of community resources.
	IX.	Interdisciplinary Collaboration	The nurse initiates and maintains a liaison relationship with all appropriate health care providers to assure that all efforts effectively complement one another.
	X.	Professional Development	The nurse assumes responsibility for professional development and contributes to the professional growth of others.
	XI.	Research	The nurse participates in research activities that contribute to the profession's continuing development of knowledge of home health care.
	XII.	Ethics	The nurse uses the code for nurses established by the American Nurses Association as a guide for ethical decision-making in practice.

From American Nurses Association: *Standards of home health nursing practice,* Kansas City, Mo, 1986, The Association.

tain a thorough data base for making accurate nursing diagnoses include the following:

1. Diagnosis
2. Present health status
3. Family history
4. Review of systems (health/illness history of cardiovascular, pulmonary, musculoskeletal, gastrointestinal, genitourinary, endocrine, neurological, integumentary systems)
5. Socioeconomic status (source of income, amount, religion, educational level, number of dependents, occupation, support systems, environmental safety)
6. Daily patterns (diet, meal pattern, elimination, rest and sleep, exercise, activity, recreation, interest, hygiene)

Objective data are obtained using a review-of-systems approach and physical assessment skills.

These data are recorded in the client's clinical home care record in the form of a flow sheet or assessment chart. From these baseline data the home health nurse develops nursing diagnoses for the problems identified. It is during the assessment phase that the home health nurse determines that other resources are needed, such as physical therapy, occupational therapy, speech therapy, home health aide, medical social services, Meals on Wheels, transportation assistance, or nutritional counseling. The family is included throughout the entire nursing process because it is they who will assist the implementation and evaluation of the plan of care.

The Omaha System of Classification of Nursing Diagnosis is one of the best approaches to nursing diagnosis in home health (see Chapter 10).

ANA Standard V: Planning

Nursing diagnoses give the home health nurse the necessary information to develop *short-term* and *long-term* goals for the client and family in addition to formulating an individualized *plan* for direct actions. This plan must indicate expected or anticipated outcomes for each identified problem or nursing diagnosis. Its goals must focus on health promotion, maintenance, restoration, and the prevention of complications. The information is documented on the developed client care plan, which serves as a continuous resource for accountability and as a means to promote continuity of care.

ANA Standard VI: Intervention

Implementation of the plan occurs in three phases: before, during, and after the home visit, depending on plan requirements. It is the home health nurse's responsibility to assist the client to return to an optimal level of functioning and health and to ensure that the client and family are active participants in the home care. Instruction, supervision of medications, diet teaching, and evaluation of diabetic management are examples of such actions.

ANA Standard VII: Evaluation

Together the client, family, and home health nurse *evaluate* the client's status and progress toward goal achievement on a continual basis. During subsequent visits, previous goals may be replaced with new ones, based on the client's changing status. The home health nurse prepares the client and family for the client's discharge as early as the initial visit. He or she explains to the client and family the short-term nature of the services. The frequency of visits and the duration of the service are decreased when the client is able to assume self-care or the family has learned how to care for the client. Discharge must include provisions for aftercare on a periodic basis in those cases where the illness episode is not resolved.

The need for *discharge planning* was formally identified in 1972 by the American Hospital Association and legislated by Social Security (1972), JCAH (1977), and HCFA (1978). An adjunct effect of DRG implementation in hospitals has been a reevaluation and expansion of the discharge planner's role in effecting cost containment and facilitating continuity of care. The nursing student's community health curriculum ideally should include experience with this emerging specialty area. Interaction between the student and discharge planner would enhance the significance of home health care and reinforce the process of collaboration in providing continuity in health care services.

Discharge planning begins with the first contact with the client. At the time of assessment, the nurse determines with the client the goals for home care, including moving the client and family toward self-care and independence. At each visit the nurse reinforces the client's progress toward independence and prepares the client for termination of services. Prior to the last visit, the nurse and the client discuss the client's readiness to provide self-care and the data of the last visit. The nurse provides appropriate referral to other community resources, such as social services, if other assistance is needed upon termination of home care. During the episode of care, if the nurse determines the client or family will not be able to care for the client, the nurse must plan with the client about moving toward long-term care with a facility or arranging for the employment of a caregiver in the home.

ANA Standard VIII: Continuity of Care

Home health care nurses are responsible for providing *a system of care that will provide a smooth transition for the client and family from hospital to home.* The nurse does this by coordinating care and community resources the client may need. As such, the nurse is a case manager, referring the client to needed and available community services, following up on the referrals to see that the client's needs are met, and providing a written plan for discharge from the agency.

ANA Standard IX: Interdisciplinary Collaboration

Collaboration about health care in the home health area is particularly important in that a multitude of health team members are needed to successfully manage the care of clients in their homes. The nurse actively collaborates with other health care providers, professionals, and community representatives to assess, plan, implement, and evaluate care.

ANA Standard X: Professional Development

Community health nurses, as described in Chapter 22, actively participate in quality assurance, including peer review, evaluation of oneself and the entire health team. Both the nurse and the employing agency are encouraged to endorse nursing participation in *professional development,* which includes continuing education. Professional development is an increasingly important area since home health care is changing rapidly in order to meet societal and health care needs.

ANA Standard XI: Research

Community health nurses practicing in the home care setting have a variety of opportunities to participate in **research.** Although the home care nurse may not have formalized research training, she may participate in research if administrative support and adequate resources are available.

ANA Standard XII: Ethics

The code for nurses of ANA provides a guide for nurses making *ethical judgments.* The home health nurse acts as client advocate, maintaining the client's confidentiality, promoting informed consent, and making contacts to see that community resources are available to clients. Ethical conflicts and dilemmas are identified and resolved through a formal agency mechanism designed to address such issues. The nurse is responsible for building a trust relationship with the family, determining whether the home is the appropriate place for providing care, and must keep up to date on ethical issues related to home care.

INTERDISCIPLINARY APPROACH TO HOME HEALTH CARE

Interdisciplinary collaboration is required in the home health care setting. Its use is mandated for Medicare-certified home care agencies, and it is also inherent in the definitions of home health care. Without effective collaboration there would be no continuity of care and the client's and family's understanding of the home care program would be fragmented.

The collaborative process for home care may begin in the hospital with the discharge planner and hospital nurse who identify a client's need for home care and then review their observations and plans with the physician for approval and orders. The discharge planner then calls the referral intake coordinator of the home care agency, specifying the services requested by the physician. If persons from several disciplines will be involved such as registered nurses, home health aides, and physical therapists, the director of clinical services notifies the appropriate persons and monitors the interdisciplinary collaboration.

In home care, as in other health care settings, professionals experience stress associated with changing roles and overlapping responsibilities. In collaborating, each home health care provider should carefully analyze the roles of all to determine if overlapping occurs, and then the team should adjust the plan of care accordingly. It is unrealistic to assume that there is a clear-cut way to avoid role stress, ambiguity, or overlapping. Professionals in home care are in a unique setting in which they can truly work together to accomplish the client's care goals.

In terms of legal accountability and compliance with federal regulatory mechanisms, it is the physician who must certify the plan of treatment for the client. However, in most instances, it is other health care professionals who reevaluate the client's status, report the findings to the physician, and then, with the physician, modify the plan of treatment for the client.

Medicare requires that interdisciplinary services be documented. This requirement allows for accountability for each professional and fosters continuity of care. Documentation in the client's chart reflects interdisciplinary collaboration as evidenced by case conferences and contracts made between the caregivers. Documentation is the evidence or means, not the end product of care. Quality assurance mechanisms (chart audits, peer reviews) verify the appropriateness and effectiveness of the collaboration.

Successful interdisciplinary functioning depends on numerous factors, including knowledge, skills, and attitudes, with the foremost characteristic being that the team members must be competent practitioners in their own field. Factors necessary for successful interdisciplinary team functioning are shown in the box on p. 818. Again, regulations require that appropriate resources are used with documentation of collaboration with other disciplines. Care plans and treatments by each discipline are to be built on by other health care providers involved. For example, nurses must reinforce the teaching by the physical therapist of exercise regimen and gait training.

Responsibilities of the Disciplines

The responsibilities and functions of the disciplines in home health care are dictated by Medicare regulations, professional organizations, and state licensing boards. The home health care providers' role dis-

Factors for Interdisciplinary Functioning

KNOWLEDGE

1. Understand how the group process can be used to achieve group goals.
2. Understand problem-solving.
3. Understand role theory.
4. Understand what other professionals do and how they see their roles.
5. Understand the conceptual differences between home care and the practice versus institutional care and practices.

SKILL

1. Use principles of group process effectively.
2. Communicate clearly and accurately.
3. Communicate without using own profession's jargon.
4. Express self clearly and concisely in writing.

ATTITUDE

1. Feel confident in role as a professional.
2. Trust and respect other professionals.
3. Share tasks with other professionals.
4. Work toward conflict resolution effectively.
5. Be flexible.
6. Be "research-minded."
7. Be timely.

cussed in the following sections are different from providers' roles in other health care settings. Other professional services can be provided in the home such as podiatry, pharmaceutical therapy, follow-up nutrition counseling, intravenous therapy, respiratory therapy, and psychiatric or mental health nursing when indicated. Much of these contributions can be provided on a consultant basis in the form of in-service training by direct care.

Physician

Each client in the home care program must be under the current care of a *doctor of medicine, podiatry, or osteopathy* to certify that the client does have a medical problem. A nurse can make an assessment visit without physician approval but must have the physician's *certification* if a plan of care with follow-up is developed. The physician must certify a plan of treatment for the home health agency before care is provided to the client. This plan must be reviewed at least every 62 days.

A plan of care includes diagnosis, mental status, types of services and equipment required, frequency of visits, prognosis, rehabilitation potential, functional limitations, activities permitted, nutritional requirements, medications and treatments, and any safety measures to protect against impairing instructions for timely discharge or referral (NAHC, 1994).

Additionally, the plan of treatment needs to be reviewed by the physician in collaboration with home care professionals at least every 62 days but more of-

ten if the person's condition warrants more frequent assessment and alteration of care. This process is called **recertification**.

Physicians in the community also serve in an advisory capacity to the home health agency by assisting in the development of home care policies and procedures relative to client care. Physician involvement in and acceptance of home health care is necessary if the benefits of this form of health care are to be recognized. The American Medical Association in the early 1960s urged physicians to "participate in organized home health care programs for any patient who can benefit from the program and to promote such programs in their communities." The Physician Guide to Home Health Care (AMA, 1979) explains the important role of home health care and the benefits that clients can receive from this service. Today, some physicians are doing home visits to provide home health care.

Physical Therapist

Physical therapists provide maintenance, preventative, and restorative treatment for clients in the home. Physical therapists must be licensed by the state in which they practice and are graduates of a baccalaureate or master's level physical therapy program. Like home health care nurses, a physical therapist also provides direct and indirect care. Direct care activities include strengthening muscles, restoring mobility, controlling spasticity, gait training, and teaching active-passive resistive exercises. The treatment modalities used include therapeutic exercise, massage, transcutaneous electrical nerve stimulation, heat, water, ultraviolet light, ultrasound, postural drainage, and pulmonary exercises. The therapist is also responsible for teaching the client and family the treatment regimen to promote self-care and responsibility.

Indirect care activities of the physical therapist include consulting with the staff and contributing to client care conferences by sharing skills and area of expertise. Physical therapy assistants provide some therapy under the direction of a registered physical therapist. Assistants are high school graduates who have completed an approved assistants' program and have been licensed.

Occupational Therapist

Occupational therapists (OT) help clients achieve their optimal level of functioning by teaching them to develop and maintain the abilities to perform activities of daily living in their home. Occupational therapists focus most of their treatment on the client's upper extremities by assisting to restore muscle strength and mobility for functional skills. Occupational therapists earn baccalaureate degrees. When the OT becomes registered by the National Occupational Therapy Association, they are subsequently referred to as OTRs.

Direct functions of the OTR include evaluating the client's level of function and ability by testing muscles and joints. The OTR teaches self-care activities, assesses the client's home for safety with possible modifications for removing barriers, and provides adaptive equipment when needed. Indirect care is similar to the other home care professionals' roles of serving as consultants for special client needs regarding self-care activities and adapting the home for the client. Occupational therapy has not been used to its full potential in the home because of the lack of knowledge of health care providers. This discipline is a valuable resource in assisting the client to become independent in self-care, a mutual goal of all home health care professionals.

Certified occupational therapy assistants (COTAs) are high school graduates with an approved continuing education certificate from an occupational therapy program. The COTA works under the supervision of the OTR.

Speech Pathologist

Speech pathologists or therapists are certified by the American Speech, Language, and Hearing Association and are educated at the master's level. Speech pathologists work with people with communication problems related to speech, language, or hearing. Most clients receive direct care services, such as evaluation of speech and language ability, with specific plans being taught to the client and family for follow-up. The goal of speech therapy is to assist individuals to develop and maintain optimum speech and language ability. Speech pathologists also work with eating and swallowing problems. By serving as a consultant to other home care staff members, the speech pathologist can teach other providers of care and families how to encourage development of the best method of communication for clients.

Social Worker

The *social worker* in home health care holds a master's degree in social work (MSW) and has one year of social work experience. The social worker helps clients and families deal with social, emotional, and environmental factors that affect their well-being. Social workers assist directly in intervening or referring clients to appropriate community resources. Often after an episode in the hospital, the clients return home unable to cope with their present state of functioning and need assistance in getting their lives reorganized. Many indirect care duties are performed by the social worker since consultation and referral constitute the major focus of their practice. Other functions include resource identification and application, crisis intervention, and equipment procurement when payment is a problem.

Social work assistants are prepared at the baccalaureate level and function similar to the social worker, who directly supervises the activities of the assistant.

Homemaker/Home Health Aide

With the advent of Medicare, the **home health aide** and the homemaker, became important members of the home health care team. The home health aide (HHA) is directly supervised by the home health care nurse or physical therapist. The role of the HHA is to help clients reach their level of independence by temporarily assisting with personal hygiene. Additional duties include light housekeeping and other homemaking skills. The HHA must be experienced as an aide, be trained, and complete a certification program or a competency evaluation to provide home care services. The HHA implements the plan of care established by the nurse or other professionals to reinforce teaching. The role of the homemaker, as distinct from the HHA, emphasizes housekeeping chores.

The homemaker service is one provided by some home health agencies. While this service is not reimbursed by Medicare, it is a much needed program and may be provided by some third-party payers or be paid for by clients on a sliding scale.

Aide supervision is required every 2 weeks except in the absence of skilled nursing care, then a visit is required every 60 days. A therapist may make the visit only when therapy and personal care services are being given.

ACCOUNTABILITY AND QUALITY ASSURANCE

Quality Control Mechanisms

Since the advent of Medicare, home health agencies have monitored the quality of care to their clients as a mandatory requirement for certification as a home health agency. All agencies are accountable to the clients and families, to their reimbursement sources, to themselves as a health care provider, and to professional standards. Quality is demonstrated through evaluations reflecting that appropriate and needed care has been given to clients in a professional manner.

Clinical records are of paramount importance as the basis for documentation of all the care and services the client receives and of any communication between the physicians and other home health providers. It is in the clinical record that nurses must *prove* that they are delivering quality care and also identify means to *improve* the quality of care. It is a legal method by which quality care can be assessed. This documentation also demonstrates the client's ongoing need for services and shows how the multiple disciplines arrange for continuity and comprehensive care.

Evaluation of the agency is required to monitor the control of cost and quality of care. Standards serve as requirements for the evaluation in accordance with Medicare certification (HCFA, 1994).

Requirements for Evaluation

1. The agency must have written policies requiring an overall evaluation of the agency's total program at

least once a year by a group of professional personnel, agency staff, and consumers, or by professional people outside the agency working in conjunction with consumers.

2. The evaluation must consist of an overall policy, an administrative review, and a clinical record review done at least quarterly.
3. The evaluation will assess the extent to which the agency's program is appropriate, adequate, effective, and efficient in promoting patient care.
4. Results are reported to and acted upon by those responsible for the agency.
5. A written administrative document is maintained.

These standards are viewed as an external means of evaluating each agency because individuals from *outside* the agency evaluate the records. Representatives from appropriate disciplines such as nursing, physical therapy, occupational therapy, speech therapy, and medicine, as well as consumers, objectively report the findings of the review. It is the responsibility of the agency to plan and implement goals for the revision, modification, and correction of deficiencies noted. The evaluative process is valuable to the home health agency. From these reviews the agency can maintain and promote better client care for the consumers in the community. It is the responsibility of the individual agency to devise the method of implementing the process of clinical review.

Documentation of nursing care is central to home care. It affects the home care nurse more than the nurse in any other setting. As an example, during the initial evaluation visit, the home care nurse or other health care professional assesses the client's and family's status, including a history and physical, psychological, and environmental characteristics. This information becomes a permanent part of the clinical record. Subsequent integration of health services must be noted. Besides clinical notes of all home visits, progress notes must be sent to the client's physician, including the assessment of the client to verify the applicability of the plan of care.

Accreditation

Another means of evaluating quality assurance in home health care is **accreditation**. In 1975 the National League for Nursing and the American Public Health Association developed criteria to evaluate home health agencies and community nursing services. The committee represented all personnel who delivered community and home health services. Since then, the criteria was revised and standards for measurement of quality were added.

The purpose of the accreditation process is to evaluate the administrative practices of the agency and conditions based on the major assumption that there is a relationship between the quality of administration and the quality of services delivered to the commu-

 Research Brief

Ellenbecker C, Shea K: Documentation in home health care practice. *Nurs Clin of North Am*, 29(3) Sept 1994, 495-506.

Documentation is an important and essential part of nursing care. It serves a number of purposes: communication among providers, quality assurance, legal justification of practice, evaluation of care, prediction of client outcomes, examination of care trends, and plans for resource allocation. Since the introduction of problem-oriented recording by Weed in the 1970s, many health care organizations have adopted the method. The method requires nurses to SOAP their client notes, providing subjective and objective data followed by actions and a plan for follow-up.

Although documentation is an important part of practice, nurses have historically reported problems, such as constraints and time costs. In addition nurses are consumed with what agencies require them to document versus actual care given because of issues related to financial reimbursement. This study reported on the findings of a study conducted by a home care agency to assist staff to improve and maintain quality documentation. In this agency providing more than 1 million visits per year, many variations of the problem-oriented record have been tried in an attempt to standardize care and forms.

The problem was identified as a gap between what happened with the client in the home and what appeared in the record. Twenty-five (50%) of the agency nurses completed a self-administered questionnaire. The questionnaire asked questions related to problems nurses felt they were having with documentation and nurses' perceptions of colleagues' difficulties and documentation.

While nurses felt the current forms in the agency and the use of SOAP was helpful in documenting client care, potential inhibitors to quality documentation were noted: lack of time, interruptions, redundancy of forms, demands of Medicare, records access, lack of good records, and client emergencies, to name a few. Staff suggested a change in agency philosophy from one that emphasized Medicare demands to one that emphasized the complexities of the family unit and supported nurses for the work they do.

Nurses can use this study to identify staff development issues, need for individual instruction regarding quality documentation, problem-solving, and need for negotiations with management to be responsive to the nurse's need to document actual care versus documentation for Medicaid and Medicare and other reimbursement sources.

nity. Components of an evaluation include (1) community assessment, (2) organization and administration, (3) program, (4) staff, (5) evaluation, and (6) future plans.

The process of self-study is an educational experience for all involved with the home health agency. The board of directors, executive director, professional advisory committee and the entire staff participate in the ongoing process of evaluation since they make up the home care program.

Self-study is a monitoring tool voluntarily imposed on the agency at the agency's discretion. The accreditation decision is based on the data in the self-study, the report of the site visit team, and any additional information. A noteworthy trend for the future may be the requirement of accreditation for certification for licensure of all home health agencies.

Today, home health agencies may be accredited through the Joint Commission for Accreditation of Health Care Organizations (JCAHO) or the Community Health Accreditation Program (CHAP) at the National League for Nursing. Both organizations look at the organizational structure through which care is delivered, the process of care through home visits, and the outcomes of client care focusing on improved health status.

The process involves self-study and a site visit—which involves home visits, clinical records review, telephone surveys, exit conference, policies, and administrative documents.

Regulatory Mechanisms

Regulation in home health care is an important concern to the home health nurse. The home health nurse is responsible on a daily basis for ensuring that the clinical practice is being performed within the guidelines set up by the regulatory agencies. In view of this, the home health nurse must interpret regulations not only to colleagues but also to clients, families, and the community.

The Health Care Financing Administration (HCFA) is accountable for overseeing the Medicare program, federal participation in the Medicaid program, and other health care quality assurance programs. HCFA is responsible for promulgating the regulations that govern two administrative functions: health financing and quality assurance (see box above).

Home health regulation is carried out mainly at the state level, with state health departments certifying home health agencies according to the HCFA Conditions of Participation for Home Health Agencies (1994). These conditions of participation serve as the basis to evaluate each aspect of home health agencies:

Under Medicare regulations, a Home Health Agency is defined as one which meets the following criteria:

1. Primarily engages in providing skilled nursing services and other therapeutic services.
2. Has policies established by a group of professional personnel, including one or more physicians and one or more nurses to govern the services which it provides.

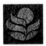 **Medicare Conditions of Participation**

1. Definitions of home health agency terminology
2. Compliance with federal, state, and local laws
3. Organization, services, and administration
4. Group of professional personnel with advisory and evaluation function
5. Acceptance of clients, plan of treatment, and medical supervision
6. Services—skilled nursing, therapies, medical and social work, home health aide
7. Establishment and maintenance of clinical records
8. Evaluation of the agency's total program and behavior
9. Provision of oral and written Clients' Bill of Rights (see box on p. 825)
10. Confidentiality of medical records
11. Disclosure of ownership and management information
12. Compliance with accepted professional standards and principles
13. Qualification to provide outpatient physical or speech pathology services

3. Provides for supervision of services by a physician or registered nurse.
4. Maintains clinical records on all patients.
5. Is licensed by state or local laws.
6. Meets the conditions of participation.

Clients are accepted for treatment on the basis of a reasonable expectation that the client's medical, nursing, and social needs can be met adequately by the agency in the client's place of residence.

Agencies must provide skilled nursing and at least one other service: physical, speech, or occupational therapy, medical, social, or home health aide services. One service must be provided in its entirety by HHA employees. The other services may be contracted.

Client's are confined to home and require skilled nursing care on an intermittent basis or speech therapy, physical therapy, or a continual need for occupational therapy.

Intermittent care is defined as follows:

- Up to and including 28 hours per week of skilled nursing and home health aide services provided on a less than daily basis.
- Up to 35 hours per week of the above services provided on a less than daily basis, subject to review on a case by case basis.
- Up to and including full-time service (8 hours per day) needed 7 days per week for temporary periods of up to 21 days.

The state agencies responsible for licensure and certification of home health agencies use these criteria in evaluating whether the agencies are conforming with federal regulations. Each criterion has minimum standards to which the program should adhere. Failure to meet these conditions can result in loss of licensure and the closing of the agency. Refer to Chapter 22 for further discussion of quality assurance and regulatory control.

FINANCIAL ASPECTS OF HOME HEALTH CARE
Reimbursement Mechanisms

Before federal intervention, home health care was reimbursed by clients who could pay for the service by donations, which subsidized the care provided to those who could pay only a portion or not at all. Now Medicare and Medicaid are the principal funding sources, with third-party health insurance providing another major source.

Medicare

Reimbursement of home health services is handled through insurance companies under contract to the Social Security Administration to pay home care agencies for Medicare-covered services rendered to beneficiaries. To qualify for home health services a beneficiary must be over 65 years of age or disabled and (1) under the care of a physician, (2) confined to the home (homebound), or (3) in need of skilled nursing services, physical therapy, occupational therapy, or speech therapy on an intermittent basis.

The person's attending physician establishes the plan of care and also certifies the necessity of home health services. This plan must be reviewed at least every 62 days; continuance of care requires recertification of the plan by the physician.

Skilled services are those required by an individual that are *reasonable and necessary* for treatment of an illness or injury. The following factors are evaluated in determining the degree of skill: (1) complexity of service and condition of client, (2) performance or supervision of performance by a registered nurse or registered physical therapist, (3) teaching of service by skilled professional, and (4) whether the service can be accomplished by a nonmedical person.

Services directed toward the prevention of illness or injury are not covered by Medicare. This does not mean, however, that these activities cannot be performed. They must be done in conjunction with a "skilled" service. The following are examples of services that are reimbursable and covered under Medicare because they require skill, knowledge, and judgment on the part of the practitioner: (1) observation and evaluation of physical status, (2) teaching and training activities to client or family, caregiver, (3) therapeutic exercises (for restoration or loss of function), (4) insertion and irrigation of a catheter, (5) administration of medications (intravenous and intramuscular injections and teaching of medication regimen), and (6) skin care (extensive decubitus ulcer).

Unlike the general population, Medicare beneficiaries usually suffer from chronic conditions with multiple disease processes. Medicare beneficiaries rely on federal reimbursement criteria that definitely influence the provision of care. Medicare places an emphasis on episodic care because of its limitations in benefits and requirements for skilled care. One of the shortcomings of Medicare is its limited protection. Medicare usually reimburses 80% of "usual, customary and reasonable charges." The remaining 20% must be "coinsured" for protection against excessive expense. The nurse should encourage the elderly client to acquire supplemental health insurance to cover the cost of charges that Medicare may not pay. The use of home health services under Medicare has increased significantly since the passage of the 1972 amendments and since the implementation of the prospective payment system for hospitals in 1983. New rules and regulations are written for Medicare and intermediaries as needed. These changes are published in bulletins sent to agencies.

Medicaid

Authorized by Title XIX of the Social Security Act, Medicaid provides health services to low income persons. It is a medical assistance program for eligible people under Title XVI (Aid to Families with Dependent Children) or title XVI (Supplemental Security Income) of the Social Security Act and also is available for those individuals whose income is insufficient to cover medical services and for disability coverage. Medicaid is administered by the states but is both state and federally subsidized. Providers are directly reimbursed by the state, which is also responsible for monitoring the operations and enforcing the regulations. Medicaid covers home health services, including skilled and unskilled services such as personal care. Needy children are eligible under Medicaid, whereas the elderly usually receive Medicare.

Table 41-4 compares Medicare with Medicaid. If a client has both Medicare and Medicaid or a private insurance plan, Medicare is used as the primary payment source provided the services being delivered to the client are "skilled." When the client is no longer eligible for home care under Medicare, the Medicaid benefits can be used.

Private Insurance

Third-party payers are represented by private insurance companies in which the person subscribes individually or with a group such as an employer. Some states (e.g., Connecticut) have laws that require home health care to be a provision in health insurance coverage. Individuals under 65 years of age who need home care follow-up after surgery or prolonged hospitalization use this benefit the most. This benefit can decrease a client's length of stay in the hospital, thereby assisting clients to return to their former level of functioning.

Table 41-4   Comparison of the Two Major Federally Supported Programs for Home Health Care

Medicare (Title XVIII)	Medicaid (Title XIX)
Federal insurance program administered by Social Security Administration	Federal and state assistance program administered by the state
Age 65 and over or disabled	Income-based eligibility
Conditions of participation	Conditions of participation
Homebound status	Not necessarily homebound status
Intermittent service	Intermittent service
Skilled service	Not necessarily skilled service
Restorative program	Custodial and maintenance program
Physician certification	Physician certification
Therapies, medical, or social service	State option—therapist, medical, or social service
Pays rental and purchase	Pays purchase
Reimbursement—"reasonable cost"	Reimbursement—maximum allowed at state level

Payment by Individual

Some individuals who require home health services but do not have health insurance may pay the home health agency directly. Individuals who do not meet their insurance coverage requirements and still want the services pay the established charge or may be offered the service on a sliding scale or established fee, based on their financial status. For example, clients may no longer require skilled nursing service for assessment of their condition but may still need the help of a home health aide to assist with personal hygiene needs. Some persons may pay for home health services that are needed or desired above and beyond the home health services the Medicare program offers.

Nursing Visit Changes

Home health care is growing because it is assumed to be more cost-effective than hospital care. It is likely that financiers will closely scrutinize the implementation of home health services, and adjustments and restrictions will evolve as needed to maintain cost containment. Several factors influence the cost and charge data: (1) type of service provided, (2) geographical location of the agency, and (3) current community staffing patterns. The term *cost* refers to the dollar amount agencies spend to provide the service. The term *charge* is the dollar amount expected or billed to the client for the service provided.

The Health Care Financing Administration continuously gathers data regarding use of home care services by analyzing factors such as cost, frequency, duration of services, and number of visits. The federal government is interested in cost containment and also in quality of care.

Cost Effectiveness

Refer to Chapter 5 for an in-depth discussion of the economics of health care and its impact on community health nursing. Updated published data are lacking regarding the cost effectiveness of home health care. Public attention is now being focused on home health care as a cost-effective alternative to institutionalization.

Nurses are usually not exposed directly to the financial aspects of health care in their clinical setting. In home health nurses are "cost conscious" because of their responsibility to interpret to clients what Medicare *will* or *will not* pay. It is difficult for the elderly to understand why Medicare will not pay for the nurse to make home visits to take their blood pressures if the client's condition remains stable. Medicare pays for services only if the client's condition remains unstable. The key words to remember for Medicare home health coverage are *skilled, homebound, intermittent* or *part-time* and *unstable.*

Physician's case management frequently conflicts with Medicare guidelines. It should be noted that services or frequencies certified by a physician as being *necessary* for a particular home care Medicare client may not meet Medicare's guidelines of "reasonable and necessary" and, therefore, are not covered by Medicare. For example, a physician might order physical therapy for strengthening exercises for a postsurgical debilitated client. This does not constitute a Medicare-approved physical therapy diagnosis, and therapy would not be provided. However, if skilled nursing is ordered for this same client, and "is reasonable and necessary," during the skilled visit the nurse can instruct the family and client regarding a plan of rehabilitation that is developed in collaboration with the therapist.

IMPACT OF LEGISLATION ON HOME HEALTH CARE SERVICES

The federal government plays a significant role in the delivery of home health care services. The information is organized to present an overview of the historical development of the laws and their effect on home health. The student should remember that congressional activity can change federal legislation regarding home health care. For updated information concerning new amendments or bills presented in Congress, consult the *Federal Register*.

The Social Security Act of 1935 signaled the major entrance of the federal government into the area of social insurance.

The Medicare program was enacted on July 30, 1965, as Title XVIII of the Social Security Act and became effective July 1, 1966. The program offers two coordinated insurance coverages—hospital insurance, referred to as Part A, and supplemental medical insurance, referred to as Part B. Each provides reimbursement for home health agency services. This legislation established requirements for client eligibility, reimbursement costs, physician participation, and agency eligibility.

The Social Security Amendments of 1972 made the following changes in home health coverage to provide incentives for greater use of the benefit:

1. In the supplementary insurance section (Part B) the 20% co-insurance requirement was eliminated for services furnished on or after January 1, 1973.
2. The Secretary of HEW (now DHHS) was authorized to establish by diagnoses the permissible periods of coverage of home health care under Part A for clients with specified conditions.
3. Payments for services that neither the home health agency nor the beneficiary previously knew were covered.
4. Medicare coverage (including home health care) was extended to individuals receiving Social Security benefits based on disability or end-stage renal disease. This coverage began in July 1973.

The early 1980s brought substantial changes in the area of home health care services. In 1980 congress enacted legislation that modified the existing programs of Medicare and Medicaid—the Medicare and Medicaid Amendments of 1980, Title IX of the Omnibus Reconciliation Act of 1980 (PL 96-499). PL 96-499 carries provisions relating not only to home health but also to hospital services, skilled nursing facilities, intermediate care facilities, and physicians who are involved with reimbursement from Medicare and Medicaid.

The Omnibus Reconciliation Act of 1980 broadened Medicare coverage for home health services by instituting changes such as unlimited visits by home health care providers, elimination of a mandatory 3-day hospital stay as a prerequisite to reimbursement, reimbursement for occupational therapy, and involvement of proprietary agencies. Other important features of the Omnibus Reconciliation Act include the establishment of regional intermediaries for home health agencies by the Department of Health and Human Services and the achievement of more effective administration of the home health benefits. (Law, Paragraph 924,097; Committee reports, Paragraph 24,347).

The Medicaid Community Care Act, Section 2176 of the Omnibus Reconciliation Act, recognized and supported the concept of community care as a viable alternative for clients requiring long-term care. The states and providers of home health services were afforded the opportunity to develop their own plan and implement their own ideas without the burden of excessive federal regulations. Some individuals feel, however, that the decrease of federal involvement will foster fraud and abuse in Medicare home care use by some *not-so-honest* entrepreneurs.

The Patient Self-Determination Act (U.S. Code, 1990), part of the Omnibus Reconciliation Act of 1990 (see box on p. 825, top, left), requires all health care agencies including home health to provide written information to their clients about their rights, their options to refuse treatment, and to sign advance directives in compliance with state law. These advance directives must be documented in the client's record or a note must be made of the client's refusal to initiate such directives. These documents signify the client's wishes and take the form of living wills, and durable powers of attorneys. It is the goal of the advance directives to have clients make decisions while they are capable and to initiate the directives when the client is unable to make decisions. The directives can be changed at any time. The durable power of attorney names a person who will make health care decisions when the client is unable, while the living will indicates the client's decision to decline or stop treatment. States differ in the implementation of advance directives. The Kentucky Living Will Directive Act is presented in the box on p. 825, top, right, and an example of a living will directive and a do not resuscitate order from the State of Kentucky are presented in Figures 41-4 and 41-5 respectively. The Omnibus Budget Reconciliation Act of 1993 reduced payments for home health services and hospice services and extended Alzheimer Demonstration projects and the ban on physician referral to self-owned agencies.

TRENDS AND ISSUES IN HOME HEALTH CARE
Legal and Ethical Issues

Any health care subsystem has a potential for illegal and unethical actions. Much publicity has been given to Medicare fraud and abuse with the last decade. This avenue for exploitation has been partially caused by

Client's Bill of Rights

1. Client has the right to be informed of his or her rights. The home health agency must protect and promote the exercise of these rights.
2. The Home Health Agency must provide the client with a written notice of the client's rights in advance of furnishing care to the client or during the initial evaluation visit and before the initiation of treatment.
3. The Home Health Agency must maintain documentation showing that it has complied.
4. The client has the right to exercise his or her rights as a client of the agency.
5. The clients' family or guardian may exercise the client's rights when the client has been judged incompetent.
6. The client has the right to have his or her property treated with respect.
7. The client has the right to voice grievances regarding treatment or care that is (or fails to be) furnished, or regarding the lack of respect for property by anyone who is furnishing services on behalf of the agency and must not be subjected to discrimination or reprisal for doing so.
8. The agency must investigate complaints made by a client or the client's family or guardian regarding treatment or care that is (or fails to be) furnished, or regarding the lack of respect for the client's property by anyone furnishing services on behalf of the agency and must document both the existence of the complaint and the resolution of the complaint.
9. The agency must inform and distribute information to the client, in advance, concerning the policies on advance directives including a description of applicable state law.
10. The client has the right to confidentiality of the clinical records.
11. The agency must advise the client of the agency's policies and procedures regarding disclosure of clinical records.
12. The client has the right to be advised, before care is initiated, of the extent to which payment for services may be expected from Medicare or other sources and the extent to which payment may be required from the client.
13. The client has the right to be advised of the availablity of the toll-free home health agency hotline in the state, the purpose of the hotline, and the hours of operation.

US Congress: *Omnibus reconciliation act of* 1990, Washington, DC, 1990, US Government Printing Office; USDHHS: *Federal Register* Washington, DC, 1990, US Government Printing office.

 Kentucky Living Will Directive Act

Effective as of July 15, 1994
Defines "Advance Directive" as "written." Can be any living will or health care surrogate executed prior to July 15, 1994, any document providing health care directions by the grantor or living will directive in accordance with the 12 sections of the new law.

SECTION ONE
Defines all pertinent terminology.

SECTION TWO
An adult (18 or older) may write a living will directive that does any or all of the following:
   a. Directs the withholding or withdrawal of life-prolonging treatment; or
   b. Directs the withholding or withdrawal of artificially provided nutrition or hydration; or
   c. Designates one (1) or more adults as a surrogate or successor surrogate to make health care decisions on behalf of the grantor. During any period in which two (2) or more surrogates are serving, all decisions shall be by unanimous consent of all the acting surrogates unless the advance directive provides otherwise."
Notification to any "emergency medical responder" of a person's authentic wish not to be resuscitated must be on a standard form (handwritten advanced directives might cause confusion).

SECTION THREE
States the living will directive shall be substantially in the form as quoted in the law. It may, however, include other specific directions (if in accordance with accepted medical practice and not in violation of any other statute). (You will note the last two lines of directions on the Living Will Directive Form refer to restrictions about pregnant women and assisted suicide. Per information Kentucky Legal Research Commission—Health and Welfare Committee.)
An advance directive needs to be (1) in writing; (2) signed by or at the direction of the "grantor"; and (3) witnessed by two or more adults **or** acknowledged before a notary public or other "oath taker."

the increase in available federal money. Examples of such practices include overuse of home health services when the client does not need them, inaccurate billing for services, excessive administrative staff, "kickbacks" for referrals, and billing of noncovered medical supplies. In 1977, the Medicare-Medicaid Anti-Fraud and Abuse Amendments (PL 95-142) were passed to deter such practices.

Home health care nurses can be confronted with multiple issues in everyday practice. The definition of skilled care can be judgmental, and its interpretation can vary. The home health care nurse must abide by the established federal regulations when delivering care to clients. Frequency of visiting poses another issue. Home health care clients require only intermittent visits for evaluation of status. If the frequency increases, then full-time skilled services may be required. Reevaluation of the client and family needs is imperative so that overuse and inappropriate use of services can be avoided. Home health care nurses must be knowledgeable about which medical supplies are covered. This information is readily available to home health care nurses, and as professionals, nurses must work within the regulatory guideline framework and educate the community as to what home health care is and should be.

Stressors in home health care affect practicing nurses. Paperwork, while often overwhelming, is necessary to document accountability. Being accountable can be stressful because the home health care nurse must demonstrate that all actions are valid and justifiable. The expanded role of the home health care nurse

Living Will Directive

My wishes regarding life-prolonging treatment and artificially provided nutrition and hydration to be provided to me if I no longer have decisional capacity, have a terminal condition, or become permanently unconscious have been indicated by checking and initialing the appropriate lines below. By checking and initialing the appropriate lines, I specifically:

Designate _____ as my health care surrogate(s) to make health care decisions for me in accordance with this directive when I no longer have decisional capacity. If _____ refuses or is not able to act for me, I designate _____ as my health care surrogate(s).

Any prior designation is revoked.

If I do not designate a surrogate, the following are my directions to my attending physician. If I have designated a surrogate, my surrogate shall comply with my wishes as indicated below:

_____ Direct that treatment be withheld or withdrawn, and that I be permitted to die naturally with only the administration of medication or the performance of any medical treatment deemed necessary to alleviate pain.

_____ DO NOT authorize that life-prolonging treatment be withheld or withdrawn

_____ Authorize the withholding or withdrawal of artificially provided food, water, or other artificially provided nourishment or fluids.

_____ DO NOT authorize the withholding or withdrawal or artificially provided food, water, or other artificially provided nourishment or fluids.

_____ Authorize my surrogate, designated above, to withhold or withdraw artificially provided nourishment or fluids, or other treatment if the surrogate determines that withholding or withdrawing is in my best interest; but I do not mandate that withholding or withdrawing.

In the absence of my ability to give directions regarding the use of life-prolonging treatment and artificially provided nutrition and hydration, it is my intention that this directive shall be honored by my attending physician, my family, and any surrogate designated pursuant to this directive as the final expression of my legal right to refuse medical or surgical treatment and I accept the consequences of the refusal.

If I have been diagnosed as pregnant and that diagnosis is known to my attending physician, this directive shall have no force or effect during the course of my pregnancy.

I understand the full import of this directive and I am emotionally and mentally competent to make this directive.

Signed this _____ day of _____, 19____.

_____

Signature and address of the grantor.

If our joint presence, the grantor, who is of sound ming and eighteen years of age, or older, voluntarily dated and signed this writing or directed it to be dated and signed for the grantor.

_____

Signature and address of witness.

_____

Signature and address of witness.

OR

STATE OF KENTUCKY

_____ County

Before me, the undersigned authority, came the grantor who is of sound mind and eighteen (18) years of age, or older, and acknowledged that he voluntarily dated and signed this writing or directed it to be signed and dated as above.

Done this _____ day of _____, 19____.

_____

Signature of Notary Public or other officers.

_____

Date commission expires.

Execution of this document restricts withholding and withdrawing of some medical procedures. Consult Kentucky Revised Statutes or your attorney.

FIGURE 41-4

Example of a living will directive.

KENTUCKY EMERGENCY MEDICAL SERVICES PREHOSPITAL DO NOT RESUSCITATE (DNR) ORDER

Patient's Full Legal Name _____

I, the undersigned patient or surrogate who has been designated to make health care decisions in accordance with Kentucky Revised Statutes, hereby direct that in the event of my cardiac or respiratory arrest that this DO NOT RESUSCITATE (DNR) ORDER be honored and that I understand that DNR means that if my heart stops beating or if I stop breathing, no medical procedure to restart breathing or heart function will be instituted by emergency medical services (EMS) personnel.

I understand this decision will NOT prevent emergency medical services personnel from administering other emergency medical care.

I understand that I may revoke this DNR order at any time by physical cancellation, destruction of this form, removal of DNR bracelet, or by expressing a desire to be resuscitated by the EMS personnel. Any attempt to alter or change the content, names, or signatures on the DNR form shall make the DNR form invalid.

I understand that it is my obligation to see that this form, or a standard DNR bracelet, is readily and immediately available to EMS personnel upon their arrival. In the event of my death, the EMS agency which responds shall obtain this form, or the standard DNR bracelet, and it shall become a part of the EMS medical record.

I hereby state that this "Do Not Resuscitate" (DNR) is my authentic wish not to be resuscitated.

_____   _____
Patient/legal surrogate signature   Date

_____
Legal surrogate's relationship to patient

_____   _____
Witness name (print)   Witness signature

This Do Not Resuscitate form has been approved by the Kentucky Board of Medical Licensure. DNR form number (<u>serially numbered</u>).

FIGURE 41-5

Example of a "do not resuscitate" order.

can be complex, since the assumption of nontraditional responsibilities can be viewed as a threat by other health team members. Physician support may be lacking, and home health care may be underused if the hospital orientation views home care as second rate and bothersome because of the excess paperwork it entails. Others view home health care as a service for the poorer classes and therefore find it unappealing.

Cost-effectiveness is another negative phrase to some health care professionals because it is difficult to link cost-effectiveness with quality in all situations. But to exist in the competitive health care arena today, home health care must be competitive. By properly organizing and using decision-making principles, home health care nurses do not have to sacrifice quality for cost-effectiveness.

Issues in the 1990s and Beyond

The 1970s brought an era of regulation, primarily since the government played an important part in financing health care. Regulations have now been accused of jeopardizing the quality of care. In the 1980s, we saw a different trend—that of deregulation. In the

1990s we see a more comprehensive restructuring of the health care system and more emphasis on home health care.

Health care providers and consumers are concerned about high quality and cost-effective alternatives to institutional care. Home health nurses can play a vital role in providing the leadership to see that this realistic dream can come true. Quality care can be provided in the home setting. The benefit of home health care is measurable in terms of evaluating client outcomes, as described in the quality assurance section of this chapter.

The per diem cost of home health care is less than the per diem cost of hospital care. It is assumed that greater self-care is a means to cutting health care costs. Home health care encourages promotion of self-care. If home health care is to exist as a viable alternative to institutionalization, then nurses must not only continue to provide quality care but must participate in research to clarify the contribution of home health care to cost effectiveness in the health care delivery system. Home health care need not be referred to only as an alternative to institutionalization. Rather, it should be the first choice, with institutionalization being an alternative when appropriate.

In 1982, the National Association of Home Health Agencies (NAHHA) and the Council of Home Health Agencies/Community Health Services (CHHA/CHS) merged to form the National Association for Home Care (NAHC). The purpose and definition of the new organization were developed by a National Task Force for Home Health Services. Some of the areas that will influence home health in the year 2000 include increasing political awareness of home health services, participating in legislative and regulatory processes, focusing on the positive aspects of home health care services not only with governmental but also private sector agencies, compiling data, and distributing educational information to the public regarding home health care.

Competition in home health care is on the rise. This factor is based primarily on the slant of federal programs to deinstitutionalize and deregulate areas of health care. Clients are being discharged in a more *acute* condition than previously. The level of care requires a highly skilled practitioner in community health nursing. Administrators of home health agencies are being faced with "selling" home health care to consumers. This task, although seemingly difficult, can be easy if accountability and quality assurance exist in the agencies.

National Health Objectives

In 1991 *Healthy People 2000* documented the nation's health objectives for the year 2000. The document challenged the nation to increase the span of healthy life for Americans, to reduce health disparities among Americans, and to achieve access to preventive services for all. Health promotion, health protection, and preventive services activities are key to meeting these objectives. Because home health nurses are working with clients and families in the home and in the community, they are in a position to promote the achievement of some of the key national health objectives as they relate to the age groups served by the home health nurse. The nurse can assess the client's status as it relates to certain key objectives, assess available resources to meet client needs, and coordinate care with other providers and community agencies. The box on p. 829 highlights the objectives the home health nurse can assist the nation in meeting through their client case management activities.

> ### What Do You Think?
>
> Disease prevention and health promotion are integral to quality home health care.

Obviously, all of these objectives relate to life-style issues. With appropriate health education and referral to community resources for assistance, numerous lives can be saved or prolonged and chronic disabilities reduced. In this way the nurse can contribute to meeting the national health objectives on a one-to-one client-provider level.

On a broader, community-wide level, the accompanying document to *Healthy People 2000, Healthy Communities 2000,* 1991: model standards presents a guide to assist communities in attaining the National Health Objectives. The model standards goal for communities is that they will work to "promote, achieve, and maintain optimum health for all residents through the provision of primary care services, including clinical preventive services and home health care" (p. 329).

Communities are encouraged to set target objectives to ensure available and accessible certified, licensed, or accredited home health agencies; to increase awareness of clients and other providers about home health services; to provide services for those who need them; to ensure quality; to provide staff training; to provide home health assessments and documented care plans which include disease prevention and health promotion services; and to provide services which include in-home convalescence, pre-natal and post-partum home visits, hospice, and mutual health services; and to collaborate with official agencies on communicable diseases, environmental health and other health related problems of the community (pp. 337-341).

The home health nurse can be instrumental in assisting communities to set and meet these objectives through participation in community planning activities and through participation with the home health agency to identify which of the objectives the agency needs to work toward to meet their population needs.

National Health Objectives, Year 2000: Services and Protection Objectives for Home Health Nurse Interventions

2.18	Increase to at least 80% the receipt of home food services by people aged 65 years and older who have difficulty in preparing their own meals or are otherwise in need of home delivered meals.
3.8	Reduce to now more than 20% the portion of children aged 6 years and younger who are regularly exposed to tobacco smoke at home.
3.16	Increase to at least 75% the proportion of primary care providers who routinely advise cessation and provide assistance and follow-up for all of their tobacco-using clients.
4.19	Increase to at least 75% the proportion of primary care providers who screen for alcohol and other drug use problems and provide counseling and referral as needed.
6.3	Increase to at least 75% the portion of primary care providers who include assessment of cognitive, emotional, and behavioral functioning with appropriate counseling, referral, and follow-up.
9.17	Increase the presence of functional smoke detectors to at least one on each habitable floor of all residential dwellings.
9.21	Increase to at least 50% the proportion of primary care providers who routinely provide age-appropriate counseling on safety precautions to prevent unintentional injury.
11.6	Increase to at least 40% the proportion of homes in which home occupants have tested for radon and made modification to reduce health risks.
11.11	Perform lead based paint tests in at least 50% of homes built before 1950.
11.15	Establish programs for recyclable materials and household hazardous waste in 75% of counties.
12.3	Increase to at least 75% the proportion of households that routinely refrain from leaving perishable food out of refrigerator for over 2 hours and wash cabinet counters, cutting boards, and utensils after contact with raw meat and poultry.
12.6	Increase to at least 75% the proportion of primary care providers who routinely review with clients aged 65 years and older all prescribed and over the counter medicines taken by clients each time a new medication is prescribed.
13.14	Increase to 70% the proportion of people over aged 35 years using the oral health care system during each year.
15.13/ 15.14	Increase to 75% and 90% the proportion of adults who have their cholesterol and blood screened within every 2 to 5 years respectively.
16.11/ 16.12	Increase the number of women receiving clinical breast exams, Pap smears, and mammograms.
17.17	Increase to at least 60% the proportion of providers or care for older adults who routinely evaluate for urinary incontinence and impairments of visual, hearing cognition, and functional status.
20.14	Increase to at least 90% the proportion of providers who provide information and counseling about immunization and offer age appropriate immunizations to their clients.

Source: *Healthy People 2000: national health promotion and disease prevention objectives,* Washington, DC, 1991, USDHHS, Public Health Service.

Clinical Preventive Services Task Force

The U.S. Preventive Services Task Force, a multidisciplinary panel of experts appointed by the U.S. Public Health Services, met in the late 1980s to develop scientifically sound recommendations for clinical preventive services for clients. These recommendations are provided by age, gender, and other risk factors. *Healthy People 2000* promotes the use of these protocols for planning care of clients of all ages. Each of these recommendations (protocols) outlines the leading causes of death, health screening, health counseling, immunizations, potential health problems, and high risk categories across the age span. The home health nurse can use these protocols for assessing clients, care planning, and health education (see Appendix A.2).

Indigent Care

There is no legal right to health care in the United States, and no recognized constitutional basis exists to solicit this right. The President's Commission for the Study of Ethical Problems in Medicine showed 34 million people were uninsured during some period of 1983 and determined that clients' inability to pay was a major detriment to obtaining health care services (President's Commission, 1983). This number has risen to 43 million in 1995 (USPHS, 1995). Murphy (1986) observed that health care is provided through a mutual agreement and providers can legally deny services based on an individual's ability or inability to pay for services rendered.

Inadequate health care funding, limited resources of private charitable care, and absence of legal recourse to obtain health care as a basic human right adversely affects the medically indigent and limit their access to home care. Nursing has the opportunity to ameliorate this health deficit through clinical research, public advocacy, and devising cost-reducing strategies.

With health care reform and managed care systems it is hoped that access will be much improved for this population. Many home health agencies use endowment monies, have United Way funds, or have a fund to which the staff contributes to provide indigent home health care. Some states have programs in which home health agencies agree to contribute a certain percentage of their time to provide indigent care (Health Kentucky, 1995).

High Technology Nursing

The DRG incentive for early hospital discharge has created a precipitous transfer of high technology nursing skills from the hospital to the home care setting (Sheldon, 1994). Parenteral nutrition, chemotherapy, IV antibiotic therapy, hydration, pain management, ventilators, apnea monitors, and skeletal traction are examples of current home care technologies. Increased care of the organ transplant client in the home and home surgeries and home births are becoming a reality. The home care nurse must be prepared to execute these high technology skills in the home to maximize professional performance, to deter inherent liability risk, to enhance client rehabilitation, and to use research to secure nursing as a vital element of this rapidly developing component of health care.

In order to provide high technology services in the home, clients must be screened and must meet specific admission criteria. All clients are not suited for home care, and it is up to the nurse to advocate for clients when home care *is* appropriate and when it is *not* appropriate. An example of criteria that clients must meet for home infusion therapy is as follows: (1) appropriate diagnosis and treatment orders; (2) a medically stable client who does not require 24 hour monitoring by the nurse; (3) venous accessibility or a plan for initiation and maintenance; (4) safe and appropriate home environment; (5) client and caregiver capability for learning and willingness to perform necessary care; and (6) financial resources (Sheldon, 1994).

Maternal-Child Home Care

Pediatric home care has changed tremendously over the past few years as children are being treated outside the institutional environment. Policymakers in the United States are beginning to appreciate the relationship between home care and pediatrics. Legislation has been proposed to require that private insurance companies cover home care in employee benefit packages. New programs, resources, and options for funding are beginning to become available for care of children at home.

The family is the key to the successful management of a child at home because children already have a built-in support system to assist with personal care, training, and developmental needs. A supportive and stable home environment for children can contribute to healing and maintenance of health.

Specialized programming for the pediatric population is mandatory. Although infants have been treated in the home for years, the focus on high technology care requires evaluation of key issues such as reimbursement, staffing, and quality assurance programs. Pediatric needs range from an infant who needs observation and treatment with home phototherapy to an infant requiring a sleep monitor, to a child needing ventilator assistance and enteral feeding. Approximately 10 million children are disabled and institutionalized today because of terminal or chronic conditions. Pediatric home care in the future will continue to assist parents in the care of their children at home if resources and interventions continue to be appropriate.

While maternal-child home care is not a new concept, there is a revitalized interest in expanding these home care services to reduce maternal and infant mortality and morbidity. The reemerging home care services target high-risk pregnant mothers and provide health education, short-term skilled nursing care and anticipatory guidance.

Home care of infants focuses on parent education about infant needs, parenting skills, instructions to improve growth and development outcomes, and skilled medical care. These programs are being shown to be cost-effective. Programs to provide skilled home care to addicted mothers and infants include such services as family counseling, medical treatment, emotional support, methods to improve nutritional state and reduce infant irritability, and training in improving maternal-infant interaction (Struk, 1994). Currently hospitals are developing home care programs which provide the nurse the ability to provide continuity of care from hospital to home. The nurse is providing obstetrical inpatient care, which follows the mother and baby to the home to provide post partum care.

Family Responsibility, Roles, and Functions

The family plays an important part in the delivery of home health care. The term *family,* as discussed previously, refers to a caregiver responsible for the client's well-being. An issue being discussed at this time is whether home health care services should be used as a respite, or relief, type of care. Sometimes a family member is debilitated and unable to help the client without assistance. Should supportive services be paid by the federal government? On the other hand, some family members are capable of providing the needed care but are unwilling to do so. Who should pay for the service and who should provide the needed care? Family responsibility is an issue that may not be resolved. The situations vary from one family to another. Assistance from social support systems facilitates coping with the stress of caring for an ill family member. However, the goal is to assist in maintaining the client at home for as long as possible and to provide high-quality care. To do this, resources must be used appropriately and effectively. However, determining this use poses a problem.

Hospice Home Care

Historically, the word **hospice** referred to a place of refuge for travelers. The contemporary meaning refers to palliative care of the very ill and dying, offering both respite and comfort (Gurfolino and Dumas, 1994). Originating in nineteenth century England, the earliest hospices first provided palliative care to terminally ill patients in hospitals and later extended the services into the homes. In 1970 the hospice movement in the United States gained momentum in response to awakened public interest generated by Dr. Elisabeth Kübler-Ross' book, *Death with Dignity.* Public-sponsored hospices, successful in meeting the special needs of the dying patient, attracted congressional attention. After evaluation of a limited trial hospice benefit, Congress enacted legislation in 1985 that provided coverage for hospice services under Medicare. Stringent controls and criteria for quality hospice care are imposed both by the HCFA and the JCAHO.

As a result of the hospice movement, people with terminal diseases now are offered the opportunity to die at home, if it is their choice, with the supportive services that home care can provide. A variety of hospice care models in the United States use institutional services, home care service, or both. Those that use an existing hospital in conjunction with an established home health agency (hospital-based or contracted services) are probably the most cost efficient because each organization can contribute a portion of its resources to this concept of care. In addition to prescribed home care services, core services unique to hospice are a medical director who actively participates as a member of the hospice team, volunteers, chaplain support, respite care, financial assistance with medicines and equipment, and bereavement support of the family after the death of the client.

It should be noted that choosing hospice does not mean a client has chosen to die. It is the goal of hospice to ensure and enhance the quality of remaining life. The hospice team is usually medically directed and nurse coordinated. Pain management and symptom control are primary areas of expertise they offer. One criterion for hospice care is that death is imminent within 6 months. Medicare covers this period and the Hospice usually covers the period after 6 months. A client who improves during care may be discharged and re-admitted when the condition changes. In hospice an on-call nurse is available 24 hours per day to triage changes in client conditions. After the death of the client, hospice provides bereavement benefits and attends to family needs for up to one year. While a home care agency may provide hospice services, today most hospice agencies are free-standing agencies (Gurfolino and Dumas, 1994).

Hospice care requires a team of professionals and paraprofessionals with experience in caring for the terminally ill. Interdisciplinary coordination is imperative for a smooth transfer of clients to the home care setting from the hospital. In keeping clients at home, the primary goal is to help both the client and family in maintaining the client's integrity and comfort. Palliative rather than curative care is the objective. This goal is met by nursing actions such as alleviating symptoms and meeting the special needs of the dying client and client's family.

Health care providers who work with the dying often experience stress which must be identified and appropriately addressed to deliver quality client care and to maintain the care provider's integrity. Employee stress factors related to hospice care differ from general job-related stressors. Understanding these differences will enable the hospice nurse to practice self-care while delivering client care.

The following stress factors may be identified: (1) difficulty accepting the fact that a client's physical and psychosocial problems cannot always be controlled, (2) frustration resulting from investing large amounts of energy for people who then die, (3) anger at being subjected to "higher-than-standard" performance expectations, (4) difficulty deciding when to set limits on involvement with clients and family, and (5) difficulty establishing realistic limitations as to what can be provided by hospice.

The hospice nurse needs a firm foundation in home care skills, knowledge of community resources, the ability to function constructively as a team member, and the mature ability to meet personal emotional needs and the emotional needs of the hospice patient and family.

One of the major issues confronting hospice care is the reimbursement structure in the health care delivery system. Initially, many hospices provided free services as a mission of ministering to the dying. Others accepted available payment from third-party payers for billable services. In November 1983, the federal government legislated a Medicare hospice benefit for reimbursement to Medicare hospice-certified agencies (Federal Register, 1983). Originally, the regulation was to be in effect through September 30, 1986; but additional legislation changed the hospice benefit to a permanent status in April 1986 (PL 99-272, 1986).

The hospice reimbursement benefit is optional for the Medicare-eligible patient. Hospices may bill for *skilled* home care services under regular Medicare Part A benefits if the patient does not want to use the hospice benefit. Responding to the perceived cost-containment potential of hospice care and the public demand for caring services during the terminal illness, third-party payers are following Medicare's lead in providing hospice service options.

Not all terminal clients choose hospice care, and of those who do, not all are eligible for Medicare or covered by private insurance. If reimbursement potential becomes an admission criterion for hospice care, it will no longer be a viable option for all terminal clients. The community health nurse choosing hospice as a specialty area must be prepared to deal with this and other potentially ethical issues. Despite the many unresolved issues (e.g., client choice, hospice availability, reimbursement status, admission criteria), hospice nursing is a rewarding specialty.

Clinical Application

Referrals, or requests for evaluation of need for service, usually come from physicians, social workers, or hospital discharge planners; but clients and family also can make direct inquiries to the agency. The agency's referral intake coordinator receives basic information on the client from the referring source, including name, diagnosis, insurance data, dates of hospital stay, and physician's specific orders for service. Many agencies schedule new admissions within 24 hours of receiving the request for service.

The nurse assigned to make the evaluation visit is given the referral information and the "admission packet," which includes the Clients' Bill of Rights and Advance Directives. He or she then contacts the client by phone to clarify directions to the home and to schedule the time of the visit.

After arriving at the client's home, the nurse explains the philosophy and purpose of the agency and verifies the insurance coverage. If the visits are to be covered by Medicare Part A, the nurse ascertains that Medicare's eligibility requirements for home care are met (homebound with *skilled, intermittent, or part-time care need*). Medicare-approved agencies accept the amount paid by Medicare for services and do not bill patients over and above this amount. If the pay status is private insurance or private pay, the nurse will discuss charges and billing procedures with the client and family. For the noninsured client, services can be provided either free or on a sliding-fee scale, determined by the individual agency's purpose, philosophy, and mission.

Depending on the ease in determining eligibility for home care, the client may sign the insurance release form and release of information form at this point in the interview, or the paperwork may be deferred until after the assessment. The nurse interviews the clients and caregivers and completes both a psychosocial and medical history. A physical examination is done on the first visit, incorporating information gleaned from the interview. Any treatments needed and ordered are performed at this time (e.g., catheter changes or dressing changes). The nurse focuses on teaching from the moment the interview begins until the visit is concluded. This is one major difference between home care and hospital nursing. In the hospital the nurses provide primary hands-on care; in the home the focus is on *teaching* self-care to the client and family.

At this point, the nurse reviews all medications, completes a medication schedule sheet, and teaches the purpose and side effects of the medications. Ideally, a home teaching program is completed on carbonless paper for each problem identified (e.g., catheter care). After reviewing each with the client or caregiver, the nurse has the client sign the form, leaves a copy in the home, and retains a copy for the client's record. The home teaching form, signed by the client or family, is a contract for care and a standard for measuring the client's progress and compliance. If the referral information was complete, the nurse executes the orders as received. If new problems are identified during the visit, the nurse contacts the physician for clarification and new orders. For example, the nurse may have identified a need for home health aide services that the physician had not addressed. The physician's plan of care cannot be altered without his or her approval.

Because third-party payer guidelines for reimbursement change frequently, the home health nurse must maintain current knowledge of the criteria. The nurse coordinates the physician's requests, the client's needs, and the reimbursement available (if applicable) to achieve maximum health services for the homebound client. Client and family needs that exceed standard criteria are referred to the agency social worker. When available, community resources are used as needed to assure a comprehensive plan of care for the client's health care needs.

To conclude the initial visit, the nurse reviews services the physician has ordered, the assessment of the present visit, all home care programs, the plan of treatment, including frequency of visits and duration of each service to be provided, an emergency care plan, including the name and number of the agency. The nurse then establishes the date of the next visit.

An initial home visit takes about 1½ hours; 1 hour is for charting, contacting the physician, and arranging interdisciplinary referrals, and the remainder is for travel time.

The admission visit uses all the home care nurse's professional skills, and, to the extent that a correct assessment is completed and an appropriate plan implemented, the home care program will enhance recovery in the client's own environment.

Key Concepts

♦ Home health care differs from other areas of health care in that the health care providers practice in the client's environment. This unique characteristic affects several components of nursing practice in the home care setting.

♦ Family is an integral part of home health care, which includes any caregiver or significant persons who takes the responsibility to assist the client in need of care at home.

♦ Home care reached a turning point with the arrival of Medicare, which provided regulations for home care practice and reimbursement mechanisms.

♦ Home health agencies are divided into the following five general types based on the administrative and organizational structures: official, private and voluntary, combination, hospital-based, and proprietary.

♦ Regardless of the type of home health agency existing in a community, the primary goal should be to provide quality home health care to the community based on the health needs of people.

♦ Demonstration of professional competency is the foremost requirement for home health care nurses.

♦ Home health care nursing is a *division* of community health nursing. Thus health *promotion activities are a fundamental component of practice.*

♦ There are three accepted components of the concept of self-care: *patient education, patient compliance,* and *self-help.*

♦ Contracting is a vital component of all nurse-client relationships. Contracting refers to any working agreement, continuously renegotiable, between the nurse, client, and family.

♦ The home health care nurse practices in accordance with the Standards of Home Health Nursing Practice developed by the American Nurses Association, Council of Community Health Nurses.

♦ Interdisciplinary collaboration is a required process in the home health care setting. Its use is mandated for Medicare-certified home care agencies, and it is also inherent in the definition of home health care.

♦ In home care, as in other care settings, professionals experience stress associated with changing roles and overlapping responsibilities. In collaborating, home health care providers should carefully analyze each others' roles to determine if overlapping occurs and adjust the plan of care as needed.

♦ Since the advent of Medicare, home health agencies have monitored the quality of care to their clients as a mandatory requirement for certification as a home health agency. All agencies are accountable to clients and families, to their reimbursement sources, to themselves as a health care provider, and to professional standards.

♦ The home care nurse today faces many challenges. Ethical issues (reimbursement criteria and indigent care), role development (high technology and hospice nursing), and opportunities for research (quality of care and cost-effectiveness) affect nursing practice in the home.

♦ The concept of home health care began in the 1800s with an emphasis on health promotion and disease prevention. With the advent of Medicare, the goal became episodic illness care. Today home health is moving back to more of an emphasis on disease prevention and health promotion.

♦ With the development of managed care networks, home health agencies will be contracting with a group of health care organizations to provide care or will be purchased by a larger network and provide care only to the network's clients.

♦ Home care agencies may be accredited through JCAHO or CHAP.

♦ The Omnibus Reconciliation Act of 1990 introduced the home care clients' bill of rights and advance directives to empower clients with control over their own health care.

Critical Thinking Activities

1. Make a joint home visit with an experienced home health care nurse to do the following:
   a. Evaluate the process and content of the nurse/client interaction to determine if the visit was merely ritual or therapeutic, and describe the process of the visit.
   b. Compare actual roles and functions with the Standards of Home Health Nursing Practice.
   c. Assess level of skilled care the clients receive and determine whether the care is needed and appropriate. (Is it within the four criteria described in the section on roles and functions? Answer the four questions in relation to the home visit made.)
2. Make a joint home visit with another home health care professional and assess, as in the preceding activity. Also attend a client care conference meeting and write a summary of the process of the group.
3. Review your state's laws governing advance directives. Consider the legal and ethical advantages and disadvantages of having such directives.
4. Interview a nurse and determine how the client's bill of rights has affected practices.

Bibliography

American Medical Association: *Physician guide to home health care*, Monroe, Wis, 1979, The Association.

American Nurses Association: *A statement on the scope of home health nursing practice*, Washington, DC, 1992, The Association.

American Nurses Association: *Standards of home health nursing practice*, Kansas City, Mo, 1986, The Association.

American Nurses Association: Division of Community Health Nursing: *A conceptual model of community health nursing*, Pub No CH-102M, Kansas City, Mo, 1980, The Association.

American Public Health Association: *Health Communities 2000: model standards*, ed 3, Washington, DC, 1991, APHA.

Cassak D: Hospitals in home health care—an industry in transition, *Health Industry Today* 16:75, July, 1984.

Community Home Health Accreditation Program (CHAP): *Standards of excellence for home care organizations*, NLN, NY, 1993.

Dee-Kelly P, Heller S, Sibley M: Managed care, *Nurs Clin North Am* 29(3):471-481, 1994.

Doherty M, Hurley S: Suburban home care, *Nurs Clin North Am* 29(3):483-493, 1994.

Dolon J: *Goodnow's history of nursing*, Philadelphia, 1958, WB Saunders.

Ellenbacker C, Shea K, Documentation in home health care practice, *Nurs Clin North Am* 29(3): 495-506, 1994.

Ethridge PA: Nursing HMO: Carondelet St Mary's experience, *Nurs Manage* 27(7):22-27, 1991.

Expansion to Wellness Market: the home advantage, 1(4) Andover, Md, 1994, Carney Marketing Resource.

Garvey E, Logue J: Community health nurses: roles and functions. In Stanhope M, Lancaster J, editors: *Community health nursing: process and practice for promoting health*, ed 2, St Louis, 1988, Mosby.

Goeppenger J, Labuhn K: Self health care through risk appraisal and reduction. In Stanhope M, Lancaster J, editors: *Community health nursing: process and practice for promoting health*, 2nd ed, St Louis, 1992, Mosby.

Gurfolino V, Dumas V: Hospice Nursing, *Nurs Clin North Am* 29(3):533-548, 1994.

Harvey C: New systems: the restructuring of cancer care delivery and economics, *Oncol Nurs Foundation* 21(1):72-76, 1994.

Health Care Financing Administration: *Conditions of participation for home health agencies*, Subpart 1, Section 405.1229, Evaluation, Washington, DC, 1994, Department of Health and Human Services.

Healthy People 2000: national health promotion and disease prevention objectives, Washington, DC, 1991, USDHHS, Public Health Service.

Home Health Services: *Commerce Clearing-house Medicare and Medicaid Guide*, Paragraph 1401, Washington, DC, 1982, Department of Health and Human Services.

Joint Commission for Accreditation of Health Organizations (JCAHO): *Accreditation manual for home care, 1995*, Oakbrook Terrace, Ill, 1994.

McClure G: Home care networks, alliances and acquisitions, *Caring* 13:48-53, 1994.

Medicare Program: Hospice care, *Federal Register* 48:560008-36, 1984, US Government Printing Office.

Morrison C: Delivery systems for the care of persons with HIV infection and AIDS, *Nurs Clin North Am* 28(2):317-331, 1993.

Murphy EK: Health Care: right or privilege? *Nurs Econ* 4:66-68, 1986.

NAHC: A providers guide to a medicare home health certification process, ed 3, Washington, DC, 1994, NAHC.

NAHC: *1995 legislative blueprint for action*, Washington, DC, 1995, NAHC.

Orem DE: *Nursing: concepts of practice*, ed 3, St Louis, 1995, Mosby.

Portnoy F, Dumas C: Nursing for the public good, *Nurs Clin North Am* 29(3):371-376, 1994.

President's Commission: *Securing access to health care*, Washington, DC, 1983, US Government President's Office.

Sheldon P: High technology in home care, *Nurs Clin North Am* 29(3):507-519, 1994.

Struk C: Women and children, *Nurs Clin North Am* 29(3):395-408, Sept 1994.

US Congress: *Omibus reconciliation act of 1990*, Washington, DC, 1990, US Government Printing Office.

US Preventive Services Task Force: *Guide to clinical preventive services*. Baltimore, Md, 1989, Williams & Wilkins.

Warhola C: *Planning for home health services: a resource handbook*, Pub No (HRA) 80-14017, Washington, DC, August, 1980, USDHHS, Public Health Service.

Weed L: *Medical records, medical education, and patient care*, Cleveland, 1970, Press of Case Webster Reserve.

Woodham-Smith C: *Lonely crusader*, New York, 1951, McGraw-Hill.

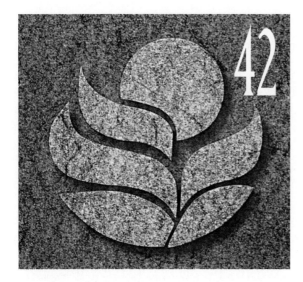

42

Community Health Clinical Nurse Specialist and Family Nurse Practitioner

Molly Rose*

Molly Rose*

Objectives ▼

After reading this chapter, the student should be able to do the following:

◆ Briefly discuss the historical development of the roles of the clinical nurse specialist (CNS) and family nurse practitioner (FNP or NP).
◆ Describe the educational requirements for the community health CNS and NP.
◆ Discuss credentialing mechanisms in nursing as they relate to the role of the CNS and NP.
◆ Compare and contrast the various role functions of the community health CNS and NP.
◆ Identify potential arenas of practice for the CNS and NP.
◆ Explore current issues and concerns relative to the practice of the community health CNS and NP.
◆ Identify five stressors that may affect community health nurses in expanded roles.

Key Terms ▼

administrator
block nursing
certification
clinician
collaborative practice
community health clinical nurse specialist
consultant
educator
family nurse practitioner
health maintenance organizations
institutional privileges
liability
parish nursing
prescriptive authority
professional isolation
protocols
researcher
third-party reimbursement

Outline ▼

Continued.

*The author acknowledges the contributions of Cynthia S. Selleck, Ann T. Sirles, and Rebecca H. Sloan for the chapters in previous editions of this book, from which this chapter is revised.

Outline—cont'd

This chapter explores the roles of the community health clinical nurse specialist (CNS) and family nurse practitioner (FNP or NP). The **community health clinical nurse specialist** is a licensed professional nurse prepared at the master's level to take leadership roles in applying the nursing process and public health sciences to populations or at-risk groups to optimize the health of the community (Association of Community Health Nursing Educators [ACHNE], 1991). The **family nurse practitioner** is generally a master's-prepared nurse who applies advanced-practice nursing knowledge with physical, psychosocial, and environmental assessment skills to respond to common health and illness problems (DiVincenti, 1993). The CNS and NP often work in similar settings. However, their client focus differs. The NP's client is an individual or family usually in a fixed setting. The CNS's client may be individuals, families, at-risk groups, or communities, with the ultimate goal of promoting the health of the community as a whole (American Public Health Association [APHA], 1982). The similarities and differences in the two roles of CNS and NP have been debated over the past decade. The overlapping of functions of CNSs and NPs are becoming more evident, and future programs may prepare a blended "advanced practice nurse" (American Association of Colleges of Nursing [AACN], 1993; Fenton, 1992; Gioiella, 1993; Sparacino, 1993).

What Do You Think?

The overlapping preparation and functions of CNSs and NPs are becoming more evident, and future programs may begin to prepare advanced practice nurses who blend the skills of the CNS and NP.

This chapter provides historical perspectives on the educational preparation of the community health CNS specialist and the NP. Functions in advanced practice and arenas for practice are discussed. Issues and concerns, role negotiation, and areas of role stress relative to the community health CNS and the NP are also discussed.

HISTORICAL PERSPECTIVE

Changes in the health care system and nursing have occurred in the past few decades because of a shift in societal demands and needs. Trends that have influenced the new roles of the CNS and NP include improvements in technology, self-care, cost-containment measures, accountability to the client, third-party reimbursement, and demands for humanizing technological care.

The CNS role began in the early 1960s and grew out of a need to improve patient care. CNSs educate patients and their families, provide social and psychological support to patients, serve as role models to nursing staff, consult with nurses and staff in other disciplines, and conduct clinical nursing research (Elder and Bullough, 1990).

In the United States during the 1960s, a shortage of physicians occurred, and there was an increasing tendency among physicians to specialize. The number of physicians who might have provided medical care to communities and families across the nation was thus reduced. As this trend continued, a serious gap in primary health care services developed (Bullough, 1980).

The NP movement was begun in 1965 at the University of Colorado by Dr. Henry Silver and Dr. Loretta Ford. They determined that the morbidity among medically deprived children could be decreased by educating community health nurses to provide well-child care to children of all ages. Nursing practice for these pediatric nurse practitioners included the identification, assessment, and management of common acute and chronic conditions, with appropriate referral of more complex problems (Silver et al., 1967). As a profession, nursing's priorities have traditionally been to care for and support the well, the worried well, and the ill client, using both physiological support and physical care services previously provided only by physicians. Preparing nurses as primary health care providers was not only consistent with traditional nursing, but also responsive to society's critical need for primary health care services, including health promotion and illness prevention (Kozlowski, 1990).

In 1965, as with the NP role, the physician assistant (PA) role was initiated at Duke University. This program was intended to attract exmilitary corpspersons for training as medical extenders (Fisher and Horowitz, 1977). NPs are often combined into a single category with other nonphysician providers and are erroneously portrayed as physician extenders. This misinterpretation of the intended role is addressed by one of the movement's founders, Dr. Loretta Ford (1986):

> As conceptualized, the nurse practitioner was always a nursing model focused on the promotion of health in daily living, growth and development for children in families as well as the prevention of disease and disability. It evolved from such societal needs and opportunities as nursing's development as a discipline and a profession, not because there was a shortage of physicians. Nor did our early plans include preparing nurses to assume medical functions. Our interests were in health and prevention for aggregate populations in community settings including underserved groups. These were the hallmarks of community health nursing.

A report issued by the U.S. Department of Health, Education, and Welfare (now Department of Health and Human Services, DHHS), *Extending the Scope of Nursing Practice* (1971), helped convince Congress of the value of NPs as primary health care providers. The Nurse Training Act of 1971 (PL 92-150) and the comprehensive Health Manpower Act of 1971 (PL 92-157) provided educational funding for many NP and PA programs through the 1970s and into the 1980s.

EDUCATION

Educational preparation for the community health CNS includes a master's degree and is based on a synthesis of current knowledge and research in nursing, public health, and other scientific disciplines. In addition to performing the functions of the generalists in community health nursing, specialists possess clinical experience in interdisciplinary planning, organizing, delivering, and evaluating services; community empowerment; political and legislative activities; and demonstrated ability to assume a leadership role in interventions that have a positive impact on the community's health. The community health CNS's skills are based on knowledge of epidemiology, demogra-

phy, biometry, community structure and organization, community development, management, program evaluation, and policy development (ACHNE, 1991).

In contrast to the CNS, educational preparation of the NP has not always been at the graduate level. Early NP programs were continuing education certificate programs, and the baccalaureate degree was not always a requirement. The recent trend, however, has been toward graduate education for NPs. The curriculum prepares NPs to perform a wide range of professional nursing functions, including assessment and diagnosing, conducting physical examinations, ordering laboratory and other diagnostic tests, developing and implementing treatment plans for some acute and chronic illness, prescribing medications, monitoring patient status, educating and counseling patients, and consulting and collaborating with and referring to other providers (National Organization of Nurse Practitioner Facilities [NONPF], 1993).

CREDENTIALS

Certification examinations for advanced practice nurses are offered by the American Nurses Association (ANA). The purpose of professional certification is to confirm knowledge and expertise and provide recognition of professional achievement in defined areas of nursing. **Certification** is a means of ensuring the public that nurses who claim competence at an advanced level have had their credentials verified (ANA, 1994). Although certification itself is not mandatory, several state boards of nursing require that nurses in advanced practice, particularly those in an NP role, be nationally certified as a prerequisite to practice.

The ANA began its certification program in 1973 and has offered NP certification examinations since 1974. The NP examination was first offered in 1976. Since 1985, the basic qualifications for certification as an NP have been a baccalaureate degree in nursing and successful completion of a formal NP program. As of 1992, a master's or higher degree in nursing is required for all NP examinations. Examination topics for the family NP certification examination include evaluation and promotion of client wellness, assessment and management of client illness, nurse-client relationships, professionalism, and health policy and organizational issues (ANA, 1994).

The certification examination for CNSs in community health nursing was first offered in October 1990. Qualifications for this examination include a master's or higher degree in nursing with a specialization in community and public health nursing practice. Effective in 1998, eligibility requirements will also include holding a baccalaureate or higher degree in nursing and a master's degree in public health with a specialization in community and public health nursing. Examination topics for the community health CNS include public health sciences, community assessment process, program administration, trends and issues, theory, research, and the health care delivery system. For the community health CNS certification, the applicant must also meet a practice requirement of an average of 12 hours per week and a minimum of 1400 hours in the specialty since receiving the master's degree.

Certification for the community health CNS and NP is for 5 years. To maintain certification, the nurse must submit documentation of current RN licensure and meet a practice and continuing education requirement within the specialty area.

ADVANCED PRACTICE ROLE

Master's degree programs in community health nursing may prepare CNSs or NPs. They may assume some or all of the roles discussed in this section.

Clinician

Most differences between the roles of the community health CNS and NP are seen in clinical practice. Although the CNS's practice includes nursing directed at individuals, families, and groups, the primary responsibility is to take a leadership role in the overall assessment, planning, development, coordination, and evaluation of innovative programs to meet identified community health needs. The CNS provides the direction for community health care, as indicated by identified and documented health needs and resources in a particular community, in collaboration with community health nurse generalists, other health professionals, and consumers (ACHNE, 1991). Practicing within the role of **clinician,** the community health CNS is involved in conducting community assessments; identifying needs of populations at risk; and planning, implementing, and evaluating population-based programs to achieve health goals.

The NP applies advanced practice nursing knowledge and physical, psychosocial, and environmental assessment skills to manage common health and illness problems of clients of all ages and both sexes. The NP's primary "client" is the individual and family. In the direct role of clinician, the NP assesses health risks and health and illness status, as well as the response to illness of individuals and families. The NP also diagnoses actual or potential health problems; decides on treatment plans jointly with clients; intervenes to promote health, protect against disease, treat illness, manage chronic disease, and limit disability; and evaluates with the client and other primary health care team members the effectiveness, comprehensiveness, and continuity of the intervention (NONPF, 1993).

The ability of NPs to diagnose and treat has increased the provision of health care, teaching, and compliance. Although physician input may be necessary at times, the nurse can usually carry out the treatment regimen and establish the relationship of health caregiver (White et al., 1992). Frequently, the NP uses **protocols** or algorithms that have been previously agreed on by the physician and NP. These documents, required by some states, serve as standing orders for the management of certain illnesses. Over the past few years, 45 state legislatures have broadened the authority of NPs to receive direct payment and write prescriptions (Mundinger, 1994).

An important area for both CNSs and NPs to include in their advanced practice is health promotion and disease prevention. Within the past several decades, there has been a growing belief that the most effective way of dealing with major health problems is through prevention. This requires refocusing the health care system, identifying aggregates at risk, introducing risk reduction interventions, teaching people that they control their own health, and encouraging health promotion and disease prevention behaviors. It has been predicted that there will be an even greater emphasis on community-based care and that nursing will increasingly be viewed as the way to address many of the health care problems that plague society in the 1990s (Maraldo, 1990; Mundinger, 1994). The use of *Healthy People 2000: National Health Promotion and Disease Prevention Objectives* (1991) and the *Healthy Communities 2000 Model Standards* (APHA, 1991) is essential for CNSs and NPs in working toward the goal of a healthier nation.

Educator

Nurses in advanced practice function in several indirect nursing care roles. The **educator** role of the community health CNS and NP includes health education within a nursing framework (as opposed to health educators who may not have a nursing background) and professional nursing education.

The CNS identifies groups at risk within a community and implements health education interventions. The CNS and NP enhance wellness and contribute to health maintenance and promotion by teaching the importance of good nutrition, physical exercise, stress management, and a healthy life-style. They provide education about disease processes and the importance of following treatment regimens. In addition, they provide anticipatory guidance and educate clients on the use of medications, diet, birth control methods, and other therapeutic procedures (Burns, 1994). They also counsel clients, families, groups, and the community on the importance of assuming responsibility for their health. This education may occur on an individual, family, or group level in an institutional or ambulatory setting, or it may occur in the community with vulnerable at-risk populations.

As professional nurse educators, the CNS and NP provide formal and informal teaching of staff nurses and undergraduate and graduate students in nursing and other disciplines. They also serve as role models by instructing students in advanced practice in the clinical setting.

Administrator

The community health CNS and NP may function in administrative roles. As a health **administrator,** they may assume the responsibility for all administrative matters within the setting. They may be responsible for and have direct or indirect authority and supervision over the organization's staff and client care. In this capacity, nurses in advanced practice in community health nursing serve as decision makers and problem solvers. They may also be involved in other business and management aspects, such as supporting and managing personnel, budgeting, establishing quality control mechanisms, program planning and influencing policies, public relations, and marketing (ACHNE, 1991; Fenton, 1992; Fenton and Brykczynski, 1993).

Consultant

Consultation is an integral part of practice for the community health CNSs and NPs. The CNS's and NP's work as **consultant** involves problem solving with an individual, family, or community to improve health care delivery. Steps of the consultation process include assessing the problem, determining the availability and feasibility of resources, proposing solutions, and assisting with implementation, if appropriate (Fenton, 1992; NONPF, 1993). The CNS and NP may serve as formal or informal consultants to other nurses, providing them with information on improving client care. They may also consult with physicians and other health care providers or with organizations or schools. For example, nurse consultants are often used at the district or state level of public health departments. They are community health CNSs and NPs who work closely with nurse supervisors, nurse practitioners, and public health nurses to develop programs and improve the services provided to patients at the clinic and in the home. Public health nurse consultants may work with all public health nurses or may be under departments such as maternal child health, chronic diseases, or family planning.

Researcher

Improvement in nursing practice depends on the commitment of nurses to developing and refining knowledge through research. Practicing CNSs and NPs are in ideal positions to identify researchable nursing problems. They can apply their research findings to the community health practice setting.

All CNSs and most NPs are trained as **researchers** and can conduct their own investigations and collaborate with doctorally prepared nurses, answering questions relevant to nursing practice and primary health care (Lyons et al., 1990). The acts of identifying, defining, and investigating clinical nursing problems and reporting findings foster collegial relationships with other professions and contribute to health care policy and decision making (Gilliss, 1991). For example, CNSs in administrative, consultant, or practitioner roles daily encounter situations that warrant further investigation (e.g., noncompliance with certain public health regimens or immunization schedules). They may anecdotally identify a trend, that if examined, could be dealt with through public health strategies. CNSs and NPs collaborate with public health nurses at all levels to develop the research design, collect and analyze the data, and determine the implications for further use of public health nursing interventions identified. It is important for these studies to be shared through nursing literature.

ARENAS FOR PRACTICE

Positions for NPs and CNSs vary greatly in terms of scope of practice, degree of responsibility, power and authority, working conditions, creativity, and reward structure (Lancaster and Lancaster, 1993). These factors and their effect on practice are influenced by nurse practice acts and other legislation (e.g., reimbursement and prescriptive privileges) that govern the legal practice in each state (Pearson, 1993). The following areas include traditional as well as alternative practice settings for community health nursing.

Private and Joint Practices

Research indicates that the opportunities for NPs in private practice settings increased throughout the 1980s. This trend is expected to continue (Safriet, 1992). In medical private practice settings, the NP may be the only professional nurse. Role negotiation is essential before entering into an employment contract in this situation. Clear communication must exist among NPs and physicians so that there is mutual understanding and respect for each practitioner's role and contribution to the care of clients (Kassirer, 1994; Mundinger, 1994). Currently, the CNS role in private or joint practice is not seen as frequently as that of the NP. This may change as health care continues to shift from primarily acute care settings such as hospitals to innovative models of community-based preventive care.

Independent Practice

Nurses form independent practices for several reasons, including personal or professional desire to break new ground for nursing and to meet health care needs within a community. It is important to investigate the state's nurse practice act to determine the limitations and legal ramifications of this arrangement. For example, NPs may provide a more comprehensive array of health services in states where they have legislative authority to prescribe drugs. Currently, no states provide this privilege for CNSs without NP certification. However, nurses in many states have successfully lob-

Research Brief

Pickwell S: The structure, content, and quality of family nurse practice, J *Am Acad Nurse Pract* 5(1):6-10, 1993.

The objective of this study was to review the data from three large surveys of family physician practices and to compare them with three similar smaller studies of NP practice. The research questions were:

What is the frequency of diagnostic categories encountered by NPs?

How do diagnostic categories in an NP practice differ from those encountered by family physicians?

What are the implications of this knowledge for NP education, clinical practice, and research?

The researcher reported a wide spectrum of clinical problems frequently seen by both NPs and physicians. Acute health problems formed the bulk of both practices, with hypertension a prevalent concern. Implications for practice included the importance of NPs monitoring their own clinical practice patterns to observe trends in their development as clinicians and professionals. Education implications revolved around designing curricula based on skills and knowledge needs in actual practice rather than by disease entity only.

---

bied for third-party reimbursement for all RNs who provide currently reimbursable services (Pearson, 1993). The independent practice option is more likely to be chosen by NPs and CNSs in states that have established legislation to facilitate this nursing practice.

Another option for NPs and CNSs interested in independent practice is to contract with physicians or organizations to provide certain services for their clients or staffs. Nurses need to define a service package and market it attractively. An example is providing a home visit to new parents after 2 weeks to assess the newborn, respond to parental concerns, and provide counseling and anticipatory guidance about nutritional, developmental, and immunization needs. This service may be marketed to pediatricians and family practice physicians who would offer or recommend the service to their clients as an option. An NP may negotiate with a local school board to provide preschool children with health examinations or physical assessments before beginning participation in sports. CNSs may develop health and safety programs on accident prevention and health promotion activities for small companies that provide time and resources.

Nursing Centers

Nursing centers or clinics, a type of joint practice developed by advanced practice nurses, provide opportunities for collaborative relationships for CNSs, NPs, baccalaureate-prepared nurses, other health care professionals, and community members (Stein, 1993). Primary health services may be provided by NPs de-

pending on state legislation. Community health CNSs, along with nurses and nursing students, may identify aggregates at risk and work as a partnership with the community to implement risk reduction activities (Christopher et al., 1993). Nursing center models are discussed in more detail in Chapter 18.

Block Nursing

Block nursing is an innovative nursing model designed to allow elderly clients to stay in their homes when they are not totally independent. The beginning of block nursing was seen in the earliest days of professional nursing, when people sought service on a fee basis from nurses who lived in their community. The present model arose from a study by the U.S. General Accounting Office conducted in 1979. The study showed that 20% to 40% of elderly clients in nursing homes could have remained in their own homes if they had received some support services (Martinson et al., 1985). More recent block nursing models involve NPs and CNSs collaborating with baccalaureate-prepared nurses in the case management of individuals and families in a specific geographical area. These individuals and families receive professional nursing assessment and care from the NP, while the CNS mobilizes and coordinates community agencies and volunteers to provide needed supportive services.

An evaluation of a block nursing program in Minnesota revealed that 85% of those served would have been institutionalized without the block nursing services and that the total cost of living for families with block nursing was 24% less than it would have been for custodial care in nursing homes (Jamieson, 1990). Federal agencies and private foundations have granted funds to communities to form block nursing programs. Block nursing may be a future trend that will offer unique opportunities for CNSs and NPs.

Parish Nursing

The concept of **parish nursing** began in the late 1960s in the United States when increasing numbers of churches employed registered nurses (RNs) to provide holistic, preventive health care to the members of their congregations. The parish nurse functions as health educator, counselor, group facilitator, client advocate, and liaison to community resources (Coldewey, 1993). Since these activities are complementary to the population-focused practice of community health CNSs, parish nurses either have a strong public health background or work directly with both baccalaureate-prepared public health nurses and CNSs. In a Midwest community, the *Healthy People 2000* (1991) objectives are being addressed in health ministries through a coalition between public health nurses and parish nurses (King et al., 1993).

Institutional Settings

Ambulatory and Outpatient Clinics

NPs and CNSs may be employed in the primary care unit of an institution (e.g., ambulatory center or outpatient clinic). Ambulatory and outpatient facilities are cost-effective and can improve the hospital's image in community service. Hospital clinics generally provide hospital referral, hospital follow-up care, and health maintenance and management for nonemergent problems. The population served is usually more culturally and economically diverse and represents a larger geographical area than that served by private practices. In these outpatient settings, NPs typically practice jointly with physicians to provide acute and chronic primary health care. Hospital acute care outpatient services may include clinics for general medicine or family practice or specialty-oriented clinics, such as pediatric, obstetrical-gynecological, and ear-nose-throat (ENT) clinics. Outpatient clinics organized for chronic care may be problem oriented (e.g., hypertension, diabetes, or acquired immunodeficiency syndrome [AIDS] clinics).

Emergency Departments

Persons without accessible health care, such as the medically uninsured and the homeless, frequently do not seek health care services until they become ill. Hospital emergency departments are increasingly used for nonemergent primary care. Although this is an inappropriate use of expensive health resources, it is a result of the current system, which limits access to routine and preventive health care.

Emergency services often require long waits for persons with nonemergent problems. Medical treatment is usually provided with little or no counseling or guidance. NPs in these settings see clients with nonemergent problems and provide the necessary treatment and appropriate counseling. CNSs may also help to educate clients on the importance of health care and how to gain access to the health care system. CNSs' knowledge of community health resources helps ensure that, if possible, psychosocial needs are assessed and met. CNSs can act as liaisons for community programs that serve the needs of special populations.

Long-Term Care Facilities

The U.S. Bureau of the Census estimates that 4% to 5% of Americans over age 75 reside in nursing homes. It is estimated that by the year 2025, persons 65 and older will make up approximately 22% of the total U.S. population (Healthy People 2000, 1991).

Gerontology is an increasingly important field of study, and many courses are available on health needs of elderly clients. NPs and CNSs with an interest in geriatrics will need to continue their education in this area to increase their knowledge and skills specific to this at-risk aggregate. Many NPs and CNSs view long-term care facilities as exciting areas for practice and a way of increasing quality of care while containing costs (Brown and Grimes, 1993; Safriet, 1992). Federal legislation provides reimbursement for NPs and CNSs associated with physicians to provide care to clients in Medicare-certified nursing homes and to recertify eligible clients for continued Medicare cover-

age. In long-term care facilities where clients are not ambulatory, NPs and CNSs associated with a medical practice may make regular nursing home rounds, assess clients' health status, and provide care and counseling as appropriate. In long-term care facilities in which the residents are more ambulatory, NPs and CNSs contract with the primary care physicians to provide health maintenance and other primary health care services to their nursing home clients.

Industry

The *Healthy People 2000* (1991) objectives include a section on occupational health and safety with goals to reduce work-related injuries and deaths. Thousands of new cases of disease and death occur each year from occupational exposures.

Community health CNSs and NPs are increasingly useful in occupational health programs as business and industry seek ways to control their health care costs. The CNS in an industrial setting assesses the organization's health needs based on claims data, cost/benefit health research, results of employee health screening, and the perceived needs of employee groups. With their advanced administrative and clinical skills, CNSs plan, implement, and evaluate company-wide health programs (Jackson, 1991).

NPs in occupational settings generally practice independently, with physician consultation as needed. The worker's health and welfare are the major concerns. Responsibilities for maintaining employee health include direct nursing care for on-the-job injuries. Often, clinical responsibility extends to monitoring nonoccupationally related illnesses such as diabetes and hypertension. Employees may elect to see the NP for common problems and see a physician for more complicated problems. The role of the occupational health nurse is discussed in Chapter 45.

Government

U.S. Public Health Service

The U.S. Public Health Services (PHS) operates two services: the National Health Service Corps, which places health practitioners in federally designated areas with shortages of health personnel, and the Indian Health Service, which provides health services to Native Americans.

During the 1970s, both the Corps and the Indian Health Service offered to pay to educate RNs to be nurse practitioners if they would promise to work for a designated time with the PHS. These programs were discontinued during the 1980s, when the emphasis was on physician recruitment. In 1988, Congress reauthorized two loan repayment programs, one with the Corps and one with the Indian Health Service.

The only nurses who are currently eligible for the loan repayment program are experienced bachelor of science in nursing (BSN) graduates and master of science in nursing (MSN) graduates prepared as NPs, midwives, or anesthetists. Nurse practitioners are primarily sought by the Corps, while nurse anesthetists and BSN graduates are the two areas primarily sought by the Indian Health Service at this time.

Depending on the needs of the area, an NP employed by the PHS may be the only health care provider in the setting or may practice with a group of providers to serve a rural or Native-American population.

Armed Services

The increased availability of physicians reduced the active recruitment of nurses in advanced degree programs that the armed forces conducted during the 1980s. Currently, the Army, Navy, and Air Force have programs providing educational leave and tuition to pursue advanced degrees for nurses on active duty. NPs are used in ambulatory clinics serving active duty and retired personnel and their dependents. The Civilian Health and Medical Program of the Uniformed Services (CHAMPUS) provides services to members of the uniformed services and their families when care cannot be obtained from a military hospital. Certified NPs are authorized to provide CHAMPUS services and are directly reimbursed (Mittelstadt, 1993). CNSs use their skills with needs assessment and program planning and evaluation to develop programs aimed at improving the health of the aggregate identified.

Public Health Departments

Public health departments are increasingly employing community health nurses with master's degrees. These CNSs and NPs have administrative and clinical skills to work collaboratively with physicians and to manage and implement clinical services provided by the health departments. Home care and hospice services are nursing sections in many public health departments and require the services of community health nursing specialists.

Health departments also provide primary health care services in well-child clinics, family-planning clinics, and general adult primary health care clinics. A public health department may use NPs and CNSs, depending on the department's size, the department's health priorities in the community, and financial constraints.

Schools

School health nursing, discussed in Chapter 44, involves comprehensive assessment and management of care, with particular emphasis on health education to promote health behaviors in children and their families (Yates, 1994). CNSs and NPs may be employed as school health nurses by school boards or county health departments to provide specific services to schools. These services include confirming that immunization status is current, performing hearing and vision screening, and providing many organizational, assessment, and political functions. More progressive school systems employ an on-site nurse at each school within their jurisdiction. School-based health services may be staffed by CNSs and nurses prepared as school,

pediatric, or family nurse practitioners. Services provided by these advanced practitioners include not only basic health screening, but also monitoring of children with chronic health problems and securing health care for children with limited access to medical care. These nurses work collaboratively with parents, community leaders, educators, and physicians to ensure that each child within the school community receives needed services. Community health CNSs and NPs may be well suited to manage school health services if they meet specific criteria developed by individual states.

Other Practice Arenas

Health Maintenance Organizations

Health maintenance organizations (HMOs) emphasize health promotion and disease prevention services to reduce health risks and avoid expensive medical care. NPs are often employed in HMOs to provide cost-effective basic health care services. Recently, HMOs have been contracting with Medicare to provide services to enrollees. NPs often deliver these services but, in this case, must work in collaboration with a physician (Mittelstadt, 1993).

An example of a nursing HMO, the Carondelet Nursing Network HMO in Southern Arizona, provides community care, including wellness, home health, and hospice services. All high-risk patients are case managed, most dealing with long-term chronic illness or terminal health problems. The Nursing Network also runs 19 community wellness centers. NPs refer patients when needed to a network of physicians who contract with their HMO. These physicians then often refer their patients to the Nursing Network for case management (Miller, 1994).

Home Health Agencies

Major legislative changes in Medicare and third-party reimbursement for hospital services have resulted in unprecedented growth in the home health care industry. Home health care is less expensive than extended hospitalization and thus is an attractive option for third-party payers (Martin and Scheet, 1993). In addition, equipment and drug companies are developing products for home use, physicians and hospitals are exploring the development of home services, and consumers are demanding greater availability of services.

Because of their knowledge and skills in the following areas, NPs and CNSs are well-qualified to provide home health care that yields positive outcomes for clients and their families: (1) public and community health principles, (2) family and individual counseling skills, (3) health education and strategies for adult learning, and (4) increased decision making.

Correctional Institutions

The organizational structure of prisons and jails has long been a barrier to providing or improving health care. Inmates are a population with health needs that can be met by CNSs and NPs.

Community health CNSs are an asset within prison systems, planning and implementing coordinated health programs that include health education as well as health services. Where personnel resources are limited, CNSs provide counseling for inmates and their families to prepare prison clients for transition to the community on their release. NPs often practice in on-site health clinics at prisons, providing both primary health care services and health education programs (Stevens, 1993).

ISSUES AND CONCERNS

Legal Status

The legal authority of nurses in advanced practice is determined by each state's nurse practice act and, in some states, by additional rules and regulations for practice. Community health CNSs have less need than NPs for expanded practice within the traditional nursing domain. The community health CNS role involves acting as a consultant-facilitator, and guidelines for practice are more frequently defined by the nurse practice act (Hanson and Martin, 1990). In the 1970s, regulations for the direct care role performed by NPs, including diagnosis and treatment, were less defined in state nursing laws than they are today, and the legal statutes of NPs were being questioned. Since 1971, when Idaho revised its nurse practice act to include the practice of NPs, states have amended their nurse practice acts or revised their definitions of nursing to reflect the new nursing roles. It was recently reported that NPs in 37 states are regulated by their state boards of nursing through specific regulations. In an additional eight states, NPs function under a broad nurse practice act but with no specific title protection. In six states, however, NPs are still regulated by both the state board of nursing and the board of medicine (Pearson, 1995).

Legislative authority to prescribe has changed dramatically in the last several years. By 1995, NPs in 44 states (including the District of Columbia) had **prescriptive authority,** some with independent prescribing authority and some dependent on physician collaboration (Pearson, 1995). Although legal problems and unresolved disputes still exist in a few states, tremendous gains have been made because of nurses' active involvement in the political and policy-making arenas.

Reimbursement

The **third-party reimbursement** system in the United States, both public and private, is complicated. Since health care costs rise at an average of 10% per year, many people need a third-party payer to receive health care services (Grace, 1990). To practice independently or work collaboratively with physicians, NPs need to be reimbursed adequately. Because states regulate the insurance industry, availability of

third-party private reimbursement depends largely on state statute. Advanced practice nurses require direct access to these third-party payers. The most common mechanism through which NPs and CNSs acquire access to direct payment are mandated-benefits laws and nondiscrimination provisions (Edmunds, 1994; Safriet, 1992).

The Rural Health Clinic Services Act of 1977 (PL 95-210) was the first breakthrough in third-party reimbursement for nurses in primary health care roles. The law authorized Medicare and Medicaid reimbursement to qualified rural clinics for services provided by NPs and PAs, regardless of the presence of a physician (Wasem, 1990). The intent of the act was to improve access to health care in some of the nation's underserved rural areas; however, its use from state to state has varied dramatically. Recent legislative changes, including the coverage of services by certified nurse midwives, clinical psychologists, and social workers, have improved the effectiveness of the Rural Health Clinic Services Act for reimbursement options.

In 1989, Congress mandated reimbursement for services furnished to needy Medicaid recipients by a certified NP or certified pediatric nurse practitioner whether or not under a physician's supervision. Reimbursement under Medicare requires the NP to work in collaboration with a physician and includes four situations: (1) services furnished concomitant with a physician's services, (2) services under an HMO contract, (3) services in a skilled nursing facility, and (4) services in a rural area (Safriet, 1992).

> ### Did You Know?
>
> In . . .
>
> 1989, as part of the Omnibus Budget Reconciliation Act (OBRA), Congress recognized NPs as direct providers of services to residents of nursing homes.
>
> 1990, through OBRA, Congress allowed NP and CNS services to be directly reimbursed when provided in a rural area.
>
> 1990, Congress established a new Medicare benefit through the federally qualified health centers, where services of NPs are directly reimbursed when provided in these centers.

Institutional Privileges

Because of their direct care role, NPs in community health are more concerned than CNSs about **institutional privileges.** It is often difficult for NPs to obtain hospital privileges within institutions where their clients are admitted. The traditional hospital nurse is automatically responsible to and governed by the department of nursing as a condition of employment. However, if an NP is employed in a private joint practice with a physician, there is rarely a mechanism for clinical privileges to be granted by the department of nursing because the nurse is not employed by the hospital. Two reasons exist for providing a mechanism for community-based NPs to gain access to their hospitalized clients. First, if people are allowed to choose or purchase direct nursing care, access by NPs to hospitalized clients is a necessity. Second, nursing must be accountable for and regulate the practice of its practitioners. No other group can knowledgeably review or set forth the standards for nursing practice. Since the nursing department is responsible for establishing and upholding nursing care standards within an institution, nurses should have the authority to grant or deny nursing privileges for all nurses within the setting, regardless of whether they are employed by the institution (Coles and Adamson, 1993).

The importance of state legislation and the role of the professional organization in encouraging institutional privileges cannot be minimized. Legislative action, changes in nurse practice acts, Federal Trade Commission (FTC) intervention, consumer demands, and pressures by nonphysicians will increase NPs' direct client access (Safriet, 1992).

The changing economy and health care trends are altering the role of the traditional hospital. With competition for clients and nonhospital care increasing, hospitals are more willing to consider alternatives to the medical model. Efforts to obtain third-party reimbursement for care provided by NPs must continue.

Employment and Role Negotiation

For NPs and CNSs to provide comprehensive primary health care collaboratively, they must understand and develop negotiation skills. Positive working relationships with health professionals, organizations, and clients require role negotiation, particularly when few guidelines exist or a role is new and undeveloped. NPs and CNSs need to assess the organization's internal politics as part of their role negotiation. Networking is another necessary skill. Forums, joint conferences, collaborative practice, and research provide opportunities to expand their functions (Forbes et al., 1990).

Because NPs and CNSs often seek employment in some locations, as opposed to being sought by employers, assertiveness is needed. Increased economic constraints and new health care legislation have reduced the visibility of job opportunities. NPs and CNSs should feel comfortable about marketing their skills. Marketing strategies should be designed to project an image that reflects achievement. In assessing and analyzing the needs of target markets, they must balance professional, institutional, and target groups' goals.

Methods of obtaining positions and negotiating future roles include providing portfolios of credential documents and samples of professional accomplish-

ments such as audiovisual materials, client education packets, and history and physical tools. NPs and CNSs should keep folders containing examples of their professional activities. Names, addresses, and telephone numbers of professional and personal references should be furnished only after permission has been obtained.

ROLE STRESS

Factors causing stress for advanced practice nurses include legal issues (as discussed previously), professional isolation, liability, collaborative practice, conflicting expectations, and professional responsibilities. NPs and CNSs should identify self-care strategies to cope with predictable stressors, some of which are discussed next.

Professional Isolation

Professional isolation is a source of conflict for NPs and CNSs. Because they practice across all age groups, NPs and CNSs are likely to be sought for practice at remote employment sites. Rural communities unable to support a physician, for instance, may find the NP an affordable and logical alternative for primary health care services. The autonomy of practice in these sites attracts many NPs and CNSs, who may fail to consider the disadvantages of isolated practice. These rural practitioners often experience long drives, long hours, lack of social and cultural activities, and lack of opportunity for professional development. These sources of stress that could lead to job dissatisfaction can be reduced or eliminated by negotiating the employment contract to include educational and personal leaves.

Liability

All nurses are liable for their actions. Because more legal action is appearing in the judicial system, specifically concerning NPs and CNSs, the importance of **liability** or malpractice insurance cannot be overemphasized. Although malpractice insurance is not a prerequisite to functioning as an NP or CNS, most nurses carry their own liability insurance. It is in the best interest of NPs and CNSs to investigate thoroughly the coverage offered by different companies rather than to assume that the coverage is adequate. Practitioners who function without a physician on site are particularly vulnerable. The scope of NP's and CNS's authority determines the liability standards applied. The limits of each practitioner's authority are legislated by individual states (Pearson, 1995).

Collaborative Practice

The future of NPs and CNSs depends on whether they make a recognizable difference in the health of families and communities and on their ability to practice collaboratively with physicians. **Collaborative practice** denotes a collegial relationship with mutual trust and respect. Working out a collaborative practice takes a considerable amount of time and energy. Until such practice relationships evolve within joint practice situations, the quality health care that nursing and medicine can collaboratively provide will not be achieved. The arrangement demands the professional maturity to work together without territorial disputes, and the structure and philosophy of the organization must support joint practice as a mechanism for health care delivery. The growing pains of establishing such a practice produce stress for all involved; however, the results and benefits to clients and professionals are worth the effort.

Collaborative practice for CNSs and NPs involves more disciplines than just medicine. Advanced practice nurses work with baccalaureate-prepared nurses and other nurses, social workers, public health professionals, nutritionists, and community leaders and members to meet their goals for the health of individuals, families, groups, and communities. To work toward the *Healthy People 2000* (1991) objectives, collaboration of multidisciplinary groups is essential. CNSs, NPs, and baccalaureate-prepared nurses can provide leadership in the attainment of this collaborative effort.

Conflicting Expectations

Services provided by NPs and CNSs in health promotion and maintenance are often more time consuming and complex than just the management of clients' health problems. NPs and CNSs frequently experience conflict between their practice goals in health promotion and the need to see the number of clients required to maintain the clinic's economic goals. The problem is compounded when the clinic administrator or physician views NPs or CNSs only as medical extenders and when reimbursement to them is limited. A practice model that can assist nurses in integrating health promotion and maintenance activities as well as medical case management into each client visit uses (1) flexible scheduling, (2) health maintenance flow sheets, and (3) problem-oriented recording with nursing goals and plans prominently displayed in the health record. Being an educator and role model in carrying out *Healthy People 2000* (1991) objectives will also emphasize the importance of health promotion and disease prevention in the health care system.

Professional Responsibilities

Professional responsibilities contribute to role stress. Most states require NPs and CNSs in expanded roles to be nationally certified and to maintain certification. Recertification requires documentation of continuing education hours in primary health care topics. Because the practitioner is in a minority role in nursing, continuing education may not be locally available and may require travel and lodging expenses in addition to time away from practice. Anticipating professional responsibilities and attendant expenses in financial planning decreases these concerns. Negotiating with the employer for education leaves and expenses should be part of any contract.

Quality of client care, however, cannot be measured or ensured by continuing education or credentials. Professional responsibility includes monitoring one's own practice according to standards established by the profession and protocols, if used. A quality assurance process with peer review is another professional responsibility for NPs and CNSs. This process should evaluate need, cost, and effectiveness of care in relation to client outcomes (Cassidy and Friesen, 1990).

TRENDS

In the United States, there are more than 100,000 advanced practice nurses, half of whom are NPs and nurse midwives and half of whom are CNSs (ANA, 1993). Although the trend has been for physicians to be more interested in specialty medicine, nurses have leaned more toward primary health care. Numerous studies have shown that the independent judgments of NPs and physicians were similar. However, nurses were generally more likely to talk with patients about their health and medical regimens in relationship to their family environments and life-styles and were more likely to include health promotion and disease prevention counseling (Mundinger, 1994). The need for NPs and CNSs is increasing, especially in light of health care reform, social changes, and complex specialized health problems (Chinn, 1991; Harrington et al., 1994). More CNSs and NPs may appear in inpatient settings (Aiken, 1994; Keane and Richmond, 1993).

Delivery rates for many preventive services are low in the United States, often falling below 50%, for areas such as immunizations, prophylactic measures, and screening (PHS, 1994). CNSs and NPs in collaboration with nurses, community agencies and members, and other disciplines have the potential to make an impact on health promotion and disease prevention at the individual, family, group, and community levels. Both community health CNSs and NPs are in excellent positions to use the *Healthy People 2000* objectives and the *Healthy Communities 2000 Model Standards* in planning their advanced practice nursing interventions. Other suggestions to increase the use of NPs and CNSs include continued reimbursement of services, direct reimbursement by Medicare in all situations, admitting privileges by hospitals, and more collaborative systems (Aiken and Fagin, 1993; Fagin, 1994).

Clinical Application

Case 1: Family Nurse Practitioner

Julie Andrews is a master's level NP who practices with two board-certified family practice physicians in an urban office. Julie has her own appointment schedule and sees 12 to 20 adults and children on an average day. Although she sees some acutely ill clients, most of her appointments are for routine health maintenance visits. The two physicians also refer clients to Julie for management of stable chronic health problems such as hypertension and diabetes. Referral of these problems by the physicians did not begin until Julie had been with the practice for about a year.

During the first months of practice, Julie assessed the numbers and types of patient problems seen in a typical week. She found that hypertension was the most frequent chronic problem. Julie reviewed a sample of records of hypertensive clients and found that many had recorded blood pressures indicating uncontrolled hypertension. After her assessment, Julie negotiated with the physicians to assign randomly 30 hypertensive clients to her for follow-up care. Nine months later, Julie was able to show that blood pressure measurements were lower in her group of clients than in a randomly selected group of 30 clients managed by the physicians. By doing the study, Julie confirmed her belief that clients with chronic problems have as much or more need for nursing care as medical care. The physicians now also refer clients to Julie for weight, smoking cessation, and diabetes education.

Case 2: Clinical Nurse Specialist

Martha Corley is a community health CNS who coordinates the after-care services for a community hospital's early-discharge patients. Martha has worked with the nursing staff to develop a nursing history form to identify family and social supports available to patients who are likely to need nursing or supportive care for a limited time after discharge. With this and additional information from head nurses, Martha visits selected patients to begin discharge planning. She consults with each patient and family to validate assessed needs. The physician is also consulted about medical therapies to be continued at home. Martha has access to nurses and other resources throughout the community who accept cases on contract. She outlines the initial care plan with nurse case managers assigned to the patient and receives regular progress reports. Martha continually evaluates the after-care service and assesses patient and family satisfaction by questionnaire and telephone. Patient outcome data on medical complications and rehospitalization are also used to evaluate the service.

Evaluation indicates that the after-care program is meeting a need for families in the community. Martha believes that her expertise in community health nursing has been of critical importance to the after-care program.

• • •

As shown by these descriptions, the diverse roles of the CNS and NP are evident in the community and within a structured health care system.

Key Concepts

◆ Changes in the U.S. health care system and nursing have occurred in the past few decades because of a shift in societal demands and needs.

◆ Trends such as an increase in technology, self-care, cost-containment measures, accountability, third-party reimbursement, and demands for humanizing technical care have influenced the new roles of the CNS and NP.

◆ Educational preparation of the CNS has always been at the graduate level, whereas this has not been true of NP preparation; however, the trend is for the NP also to be master's prepared.

◆ Specialty certification through the ANA began in 1976 for NPs and in 1990 for community health CNSs.

◆ The roles of NP and CNS are merging, and many common features exist; however, controversy exists on this blending of roles.

◆ The major role functions of the NP and CNS in community health nursing are clinician, consultant, administrator, researcher, and educator; typically, the NP spends a greater proportion of time in direct care clinical activities and less time in indirect activities than the CNS.

◆ Major arenas for practice for NPs and CNSs in community health include private practice, institutional settings, industry, government, public health agencies, schools, home health, HMOs, correctional health, nursing centers, and health ministry settings.

◆ Legal status, reimbursement, institutional privileges, and role negotiation are important issues

Key Concepts—cont'd

and concerns to nurses who practice in an advanced role in community health nursing.

◆ Major stressors for NPs and CNSs include professional isolation, liability, collaborative practice, conflicting expectations, and professional responsibilities.

◆ The use of *Healthy People 2000* objectives is important in emphasizing health promotion and disease prevention in advanced practice nursing and in improving health in the United States.

Critical Thinking Activities

1. Explore the development of the community health NP and CNS roles locally.

2. Compare and contrast the local, state, and national movement related to advanced practice in community health nursing.

3. Investigate graduate programs in community health nursing within the state or region to determine the requirements for admission, the type of degree awarded, and whether or not NP and CNS preparation is available.

4. Review your state's nurse practice act and any rules and regulations governing advanced practice roles.

5. Negotiate a clinical observation experience with an NP and a CNS in community health nursing, and compare and contrast their roles.

Bibliography

Aiken LH: Charting the future of hospital nursing. In Lee PR, Estes CL, editors: *The nation's health*, ed 4, Boston, 1994, Jones & Bartlett.

Aiken LH, Fagin C: More nurses, better medicine, *New York Times*, March 11, 1993.

American Association of Colleges of Nursing: In search of the advanced practice nurse, *AACN Issue Bulletin*, Washington, DC, 1993, AACN.

American Nurses Association: *Nursing facts: advanced practice nursing: a new age in health care*, Washington DC, 1993, ANA.

American Nurses Association: *Credentializing center certification catalog*, Washington, DC, 1994, ANA.

American Public Health Association: The definition and role of public health nursing practice in the delivery of health care, *Am J Public Health* 72:210, 1982.

American Public Health Association: *Healthy communities 2000 model standards: guidelines for community attainment of the year 2000 national health objectives*, Washington, DC, 1991, APHA.

Association of Community Health Nursing Educators: *Essentials of master's level nursing education for advanced community health nursing practice*, Louisville, Ky, 1991, ACHNE.

Brown SA, Grimes DE: *A metaanalysis of process of care, clinical outcomes, and cost-effectiveness of nurses in primary care roles*, Washington, DC, 1993, American Nurses Association.

Bullough B: *The law and the expanding nursing role*, ed 2, New York, 1980, Appleton-Century-Crofts.

Burns CM: Toward *Healthy People 2000:* the role of the nurse practitioner and health promotion, *J Am Acad Nurse Pract* 6:29-35, 1994.

Cassidy DA, Friesen MA: QA: applying JCAHO's generic model, *Nurs Manage* 21(6):22-27, 1990.

Chinn P: Looking into the crystal ball: positioning ourselves for the year 2000, *Nurs Outlook* 39:251-256, 1991.

Christopher MA, Reinhard S, McConnell K, Mason D: Neighborhood nursing: community as partner, *Caring* 12:44-47, 1993.

Coldewey LJ: Parish nursing: a system approach, *Health Progress* November 1993, pp 54-57.

Coles T, Adamson S: How to obtain hospital privileges, *NP News* 1(4):2, 1993.

DiVincenti M: *Advanced practice nursing roles—to blend or not to blend?* Atlanta, 1993, Southern Council in Collegiate Education for Nursing.

Edmunds M: Inside Washington . . . nurse practitioners . . . ability to care for Medicare patients, *NP News* 2(2):15, 1994.

Edmunds M: State news . . . state legislative activity . . . nurse practitioners, *NP News* 2(2):6, 13, 1994.

Elder RG, Bullough B: Nurse practitioners and clinical nurse specialists: are the roles merging? *Clin Nurse Specialist* 4(2):78-84, 1990.

Fagin CM: Collaboration between nurses and physicians: no longer a choice. In Lee PR, Estes CL, editors: *The nation's health*, ed 4, Boston, 1994, Jones & Bartlett.

Fenton MV: Education for the advanced practice of clinical nurse specialist, *Oncol Nurse Forum* 19(suppl 1):16-20, 1992.

Fenton MV, Brykczynski KA: Qualitative distinctions and similarities in the practice of clinical nurse specialists and nurse practitioners, *J Prof Nurs* 9:313-326, 1993.

Fisher DW, Horowitz SM: The physician's assistant: profile of a new health profession. In Bliss AA, Cohen ED, editors: *The new health professionals*, Germantown, Md, 1977, Aspen.

Forbes KE, et al: Clinical nurse specialist and nurse practitioner core curriculum survey results, *Nurse Pract* 15(4):43, 46-48, 1990.

Ford LC: Nurses, nurse practitioners: the evolution of primary care, *Image* 18:177-178, 1986 (book review).

Gilliss CL: Family nursing research: theory and practice, *Image* 23:19-22, 1991.

Gioiella EC: Meeting the demands for advanced practice nurses, *J Prof Nurs* 9:254, 1993.

Grace H: Can health care costs be contained? *Nurs Health Care* 11:123-130, 1990.

Hanson C, Martin LL: The nurse practitioner and clinical nurse specialist: should the roles be merged? *J Am Acad Nurse Pract* 2(1):2-9, 1990.

Harrington C, Feetham SL, Moccia PA, Smith GR: Health care access: problems and policy recommendations. In Lee PR, Estes CL, editors: *The nation's health*, ed 4, Boston, 1994, Jones & Bartlett.

Healthy People 2000: national health promotion and disease prevention objectives, Washington DC, 1991, Public Health Service.

Jackson LC: Ergonomics and the occupational health nurse: instituting a workplace program, *Occup Health Nurs* 39(3):119-127, 1991.

Jamieson MK: Block nursing: practicing autonomous professional nursing in the community, *Nurs Health Care* 11:250-253, 1990.

Kent HJ, Hanley B: Home health care, *Nurs Health Care* 11:234-240, 1990.

Kassirer JP: What role for nurse practitioners in primary care? *N Engl J Med* 330:204-205, 1994.

Keane A, Richmond T: Tertiary nurse practitioners, *Image* 25:281-284, 1993.

King JM, Lakin JA, Striepe J: Coalition building between public health nurses and parish nurses, *J Nurs Adm* 23(2):27-31, 1993.

Kozlowski D: Nurse practitioners: 25 years of quality health care, *Am Nurses Assoc Council Prim Health Care Nurse Pract Newslett* 13(7):4, 1990.

Lancaster J, Lancaster W: Nurse practitioners: health care providers whose time has come, *Fam Community Health* 16(2):1-8, 1993.

Lyons NB, Stein M, Blackhue S, Tribotti SJ, Withers J: Too busy for research? Collaboration an answer, *Matern Child Nurse* 15(2):67-72, 1990.

Maraldo P: The nineties: a decade in search of meaning, *Nurs Health Care* 11:11-14, 1990.

Martin KS, Scheet NJ: Home health clients: characteristics, outcomes of care and nursing interventions, *Am J Public Health* 83:1730-1734, 1993.

Martinson I, Jamieson M, O'Grady B, Sime M: The block nurse program, *J Community Health Nurs* 2(1):21-29, 1985.

Miller N: An interview with Phyllis Ethridge: challenges for nurse executives, a nursing HMO, chronic patients, and team work, *Nurs Econ* 12(2):65-70, 1994.

Mittelstadt PC: Federal reimbursement of advanced practice nurses' services empowers the profession, *Nurs Pract* 18(1):43-49, 1993.

Mundinger M: Advanced practice nursing—good medicine for physicians? *N Engl J Med* 330:201-212, 1994.

National Organization of Nurse Practitioner Faculties: *Advanced nursing practice: nurse practitioner curriculum guidelines*, New York, 1993, NONPF.

Pearson LJ: 1994-95 update: how each state stands on legislative issues affecting advanced nursing practice, *Nurse Pract* 20:23-38, 1995.

Pickwell S: The structure, content, and quality of family nurse practice, *J Am Acad Nurse Pract* 5(1):6-10, 1993.

Safriet BJ: Health care dollars and regulatory sense: the role of advanced practice nursing, *Yale J Regulation* 9:417-487, 1992.

Silver HK, Ford LC, Stearly SA: A program to increase health care for children: the pediatric nurse practitioner program, *Pediatrics* 39:756-760, 1967.

Sparacino P: The advanced practice nurse: is the time right for a singular title? *Clin Nurse Specialist* 7:3, 1993.

Stein LM: Health care delivery to farmworkers in the Southwest: an innovative nursing clinic, *J Am Acad Nurse Pract* 5(3):119-124, 1993.

Stevens R: When your clients are in jail, *Nurs Forum* 28(4):5-8, 1993.

Streff MB, Netzer R: Third-party reimbursement. In McCloskey JC, Grace, HK, editors: *Current issues in nursing*, St Louis, 1990, Mosby.

Styles NM: Nurse practitioners creating new horizons for the 1990s, *Nurs Pract* 15(2):48-57, 1990.

US Department of Health, Education, and Welfare: *Extending the scope of nursing practice*, Washington, DC, 1971, US Government Printing Office.

US Department of Health and Human Services, Public Health Service: Put prevention into practice: implementing preventive care, *J Am Acad Nurse Pract* 6:257-260, 1994.

Wasem C: The Rural Health Clinic Services Act: a sleeping giant of reimbursement, *J Am Acad Nurse Pract* 2(2):85-87, 1990.

White JE, Nativio DG, Kobert SN, Engberg SL: Content and process in clinical decision making by nurse practitioners, *Nurse Practitioner* 24:153-258, 1992.

Wilbur J, Zoeller LH, Talashek M, Sullivan JA: Career trends of master's prepared family nurse practitioners, *J Am Acad Nurse Pract* 2(2):69-78, 1990.

Yates S: The practice of school nursing: integration with new models of health service delivery, *J Sch Nurs* 10(1):10-14, 16-19, 1994.

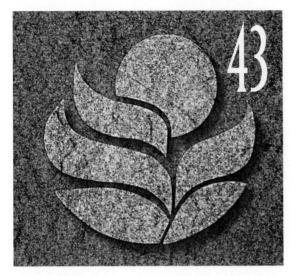

43

Community Health Nurse Manager and Consultant

Juliann G. Sebastian ◆ Marcia Stanhope*

Juliann G. Sebastian ◆ Marcia Stanhope*

Objectives ▼

After reading this chapter, the student should be able to do the following:

◆ Explain why community health nurses need effective leadership, management, and consultation skills in today's health care environment.
◆ Distinguish between community health nursing leadership, management, and consultation.
◆ Explain how major trends in the health care environment influence the roles and functions of community health nurse managers and consultants.
◆ Explain what is meant by empowerment and how it is related to community health nursing management and consultation.
◆ Give examples of ways that micro- and macro-level management theories are used in community health nursing management.
◆ Distinguish between content and process theories of consultation and describe their applicability to community health nursing practice.
◆ Apply the principles of process consultation in community health nursing practice.
◆ Identify consultant and client responsibilities in the various phases of consultation.
◆ Describe the major skills required to be effective in the community health nurse manager and consultant roles.
◆ Examine the impact of funding on community health nurse manager and consultant roles.
◆ Cite educational requirements for community health nurse managers and consultants.

Key Terms ▼

acceptant intervention mode
alliance
catalytic intervention mode
coaching
cognitive theories
community health nursing leadership
community health nursing management
conflict resolution
confrontation intervention mode
consultation
consultative contract
contingency leadership theory
continuous quality improvement
delegation
distributional effects
doctor-patient model
empowerment
ERG theory
Expectancy Theory
Goal-Setting Theory
institutional theory
job enlargement
job enrichment
Job Redesign Theory
leadership
learning organizations
macro-level theories
managed care
micro-level theories
multiskilled
need theory
negotiation

Continued.

Outline ▼

Continued.

Contents of this chapter may reflect contributions of Roberta K. Lee from edition 3 of this text. Excerpts from this chapter were contributed by Rena Alford in edition 3 of this text. The authors gratefully acknowledge the work of both women.

Never have community health nurse managers and consultants been more valuable than in today's hyperturbulent health care environment. Community health nurses are relied on more and more not only to organize clinical services and manage related resources, but also to help *others* perform these two functions. They perform such functions in a variety of settings, including community-based clinics, schools, health maintenance organizations, and public health departments. The roles of manager and consultant are critical to the success of client outcomes—which depend heavily on cost-effective, efficient delivery of care—because so many aspects of health care are moving from institutional settings to the community. For that reason, this chapter examines the roles and functions of community health nurse managers and consultants in the late twentieth and early twenty-first century, emphasizing nursing leadership in clinical practice, personnel management, and consulting with groups and individuals on a variety of issues affecting clinical nursing services in the community.

MAJOR TRENDS AND ISSUES

A number of societal trends and issues are important to community health nurse managers and consultants. One of these is the emphasis on cost containment in health care, which in turn affects a number of related issues. These include the following: job redesign, or changes in the kinds of responsibilities held by individual employees and the ways in which

they are expected to interact with others; the amount and kind of reimbursement available in conjunction with the payors, documentation requirements; and, finally, the way the present health system is organized.

Consider the job redesign dilemma that Elizabeth Schaeffer faces in the following case:

Elizabeth Shaeffer, R.N., is the nurse manager of a mobile health clinic for migrant farmworkers. The clinic is owned by the local health department and is housed in a van that travels to migrant camps in a 10 country area providing outreach, case finding, and primary care services. The clinic employs two nurses, one social worker, one physical therapist, and two lay community health workers. Administration wants to increase efficiency by instituting cross-training. The Commissioner asked Elizabeth whether it would be possible to train the nurses on the van to implement certain physical therapy procedures and train the community health workers to do phlebotomy and run electrocardiograms. Elizabeth is concerned about the effects of redesigning these jobs on quality of care and on employee morale. She begins her analysis by checking on the Standards for Community Health Nursing Practice (ANA) and the standards for physical therapy services. What do you think Elizabeth should do?

Cost concerns have led to an emphasis on managed care. **Managed care** refers to integrating payment for services with delivery of services (Hicks et al., 1993) and emphasizing cost-effective service delivery along a continuum of care. In Figure 43-1, the person at point A may be a low-birth-weight infant requiring multiple, costly service. By the time that individual is an adult (at point B) the extent and expense of his or her service needs may have declined if the care has

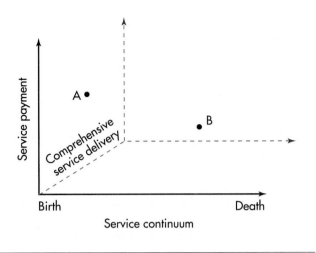

FIGURE 43-1
Managed care.

been managed well. Managed care organizations (MCOs) may both pay for and provide services or they may pay for services and contract with selected health care providers to actually provide services for the enrollees in the MCO. Either way, a close connection exists between service payment and service delivery. In practice, this means that someone functions as a gatekeeper (or case manager) and approves and monitors the delivery of services for individual enrollees. Managed care organizations collect payment from enrollees before services are delivered (usually on a periodic basis, e.g., monthly). Most MCOs are capitated, which means that clinical agencies receive a set payment for each MCO enrollee. Any costs over and above this amount are not reimbursed. Therefore, MCOs have an incentive to keep their enrollees healthy, and when it is necessary to provide illness care, they prefer to provide the least expensive, most effective services. As a result more health services are delivered in community settings, where costs are assumed to be lower. Community health nurse managers and consultants are being challenged to develop new, creative health programs focused on health promotion and disease prevention, and to obtain payment from MCOs for their enrollees. Community health nurse managers and consultants must be able to anticipate the cost of providing nursing services to

---

| What Do You Think? |

Managed care organizations are less likely than other organizations to recruit vulnerable populations, since they are most likely to have complex, expensive health problems (Aiken and Salmon, 1994). Therefore, community health nurse managers and consultants must develop programs to ensure that vulnerable populations receive needed health services.

a certain target population over a specified period of time and to develop a proposal (or bid) for a contract to provide the services. Because managed care organizations have an incentive to enroll the healthiest people, they may be less likely to actively recruit high-risk, disadvantaged groups. This suggests that the public health sector needs to monitor the health needs of vulnerable populations and ensure that these populations receive the health care services they require (Aiken and Salmon, 1994).

In many local areas, the health system is being reorganized to provide a full continuum of services within a seamless system of care. Large, vertically integrated systems are able to do this because they own the full spectrum of services that clients might need. In other cases, free-standing agencies collaborate to achieve seamlessness. Achieving this goal should reduce service fragmentation and be particularly helpful for vulnerable populations, such as people who are homeless or abused, and populations with long-term care needs, such as the frail elderly and their caregivers. Community health nurses traditionally have emphasized coordinating clients' care across agencies, but this trend places added emphasis on more formal interagency liaisons, such as **alliances,** agency partnerships, joint programs, and participation in **service delivery networks** through interagency planning meetings and consortia. Community health nurse managers and consultants actively participate in these groups and need good political and negotiation skills to be effective.

Another important trend is the public's increasing interest in becoming involved in planning for health services and in being active participants in their own care. It is critical for community members to take a partnership role in identifying community health needs and planning how to meet those needs. Community health nurse managers and consultants need to be able to listen well and collaborate with lay community members who often have different priorities than health care professionals.

One way of involving community members more actively is through continuous quality improvement programs. **Continuous quality improvement** has replaced more static methods of quality assurance as the way to make real-time improvements in nursing service delivery processes (Dienemann, 1992). This approach to quality emphasizes combining both formative and summative evaluation methods, actively including consumers in the process, and identifying benchmarks of excellence against which an agency's performance can be judged (Simpson, 1994). Managed care organizations increasingly rely on agency report cards in selecting those agencies with which they will contract. An agency report card is a written listing of how the agency compares with others in the field on certain key indicators of quality, including morbidity and mortality measures, consumer satisfaction, and cost of care.

In order to know whether an agency is performing as expected, community health nurse managers and consultants must be familiar with their professional standards of care, the standards held by accrediting bodies, such as the Joint Commission on Accreditation of Healthcare Organizations, and guidelines for practice, such as those developed by the Patient Outcomes Research Teams sponsored by the federal Agency for Health Care Policy and Research. Nurse managers and consultants also need to know the purposes of clinical and management information systems, and how to use these systems to link patient outcomes with clinical and management processes. They need to be familiar with advances in nursing informatics, and particularly how to use minimum data sets that include nursing diagnoses, the Nursing Interventions Classification (McCloskey and Bulechek, 1992), and related clinical outcomes (McCloskey, 1994).

DEFINITIONS

Community health nursing leadership refers to the influence that community health nurses exert on improving client health, whether clients are individuals, families, groups, or entire communities. **Community health nursing management,** on the other hand, refers to the ways that community health nurses manage resources in the provision of clinical services. These resources might be people, as when a community health nurse coordinates an interdisciplinary team, or financial resources. An example of managing financial resources is when a nurse monitors the budget for an immunization program to ensure that personnel time, supplies, and equipment are being used efficiently. Community health nurses also manage time. For example, home health nurses must manage their time in order to provide clients with direct and indirect nursing services, such as health education and making referrals (respectively).

Consultation has been described as a process in which the helper provides a set of activities that help the client perceive, understand, and act on events occurring in the client's environment (Schein, 1969). Consultation is similar to experiential learning because consultants help "clients find and learn about new or different ways of behaving in order to overcome some problem or difficulty" (Evans et al., 1992, p. 7). Caplan (1970) defined it as a process in which a specialist identifies ways to handle work problems involving the management of clients or the planning and implementation of programs. Management consultation "is any service provided by a qualified person or group of people to increase the effectiveness of a manager or an organization" (Berger et al., 1993, p. 65). Community health nurses have a breadth of knowledge that makes them desirable consultants for colleagues both inside and outside the organizations in which they work. For example, a nurse working in a home health agency might be called upon by a school nurse to give suggestions about the most effective way to intervene with a child using a respirator. Another example that occurs frequently is the informal consultation provided by community health nurses who help nurses working in hospitals learn how to make effective community referrals.

Consultation is closely linked with the idea of **empowerment.** When consultants help clients identify and work through problems and learn new skills that clients see as most important, they are enabling clients to solve more of their own problems. This is very similar to the traditional community health nursing philosophy of empowering individuals, families, groups, and communities to solve their own problems. Empowerment is consistent with Dorothea Orem's nursing theory of self-care (Orem, 1989), in which she states that the nurse's role is to promote clients self-care abilities.

MANAGEMENT

Goals

The goals of community health nursing management are (1) to achieve organizational and professional goals for client services and clinical outcomes, (2) to empower personnel to perform their responsibilities effectively and efficiently, and (3) to develop new services that will enable the organization to respond to emerging community health needs.

Theories of Management and Leadership

Leadership and management theories fall into two general categories: micro-level theories and macro-level theories. Community health nurses use both micro- and macro-level theories work effectively to improve community health. **Micro-level theories** originate in psychology and help explain and predict individual behavior (e.g., motivation theories) and interpersonal dynamics (e.g., leadership theories, communication theories, and theories of group dynamics). **Macro-level theories** use a more sociological approach and explain issues at a broader, organizational level. These theories focus on the best ways to organize work, how to obtain the resources necessary to accomplish organizational goals, organizational change, and power dynamics (e.g., structural contingency, resource dependence, and institutional theories).

Intrapersonal/Interpersonal Theories Applied to Community Health Nursing Management

Many early management theories tried to predict how to encourage workers to be productive and emphasized micro-level approaches. These theories are important to community health nurse managers because the cost-containment and job-redesign trends described earlier in the chapter emphasize productivity. Much uncertainty exists about how to measure productivity in health care and many ethical issues surround decisions about increasing productivity.

Consider this example:

Sharon Myers is the nurse manager of a home health agency that has a contract with a large managed care organization (MCO). The managed care organization wants Sharon's agency to provide services as inexpensively as possible for the enrollees in the MCO. Sharon knows one way to do this is to hire fewer staff and ensure that nurses visit as many people as possible each day. She wonders, however, how many people the nurses can be expected to visit. Is an average of five visits per day adequate? What about seven, or eight? She knows of nurses who are paid per visit who make as many as 10-12 visits per day. Sharon is not sure how many visits a nurse can make and still provide high quality care. She also worries about the effects on staff morale if she asks them to increase their visits beyond a certain point. "What is best?", she wonders. What factors enter into the decision? What are the ethical issues? How would you decide?

Scientific management predicts that the best way to increase worker productivity is to identify the most efficient way to do the task, usually through time and motion studies and then assign a person to do that task repeatedly (Marriner-Tomey, 1992). If an agency is large enough to organize specialized teams of nurses, it might be able to increase productivity by doing this. For example, nurses on an intravenous therapy team in a visiting nurse agency are organized according to this theory because they specialize in tasks related to IV therapy. However, one must be aware that some individuals become bored by repeating the same task, while others enjoy the satisfaction of specializing in an area.

Neoclassical management, also know as the human relations approach (Marriner-Tomey, 1992), argues that managers should pay attention to workers' human needs and group dynamics, and foster cooperation in order to increase productivity. A nurse manager might consider identifying the types of clinical cases nurses are most interested in and assigning only these types of patients. However, this could lead to inefficiency because nurses would not always be able to organize their work geographically and may spend more time than necessary in travel. Furthermore, many clients have multiple problems and community health nurses work with family groups as well as individuals, so it may be difficult to give assignments based solely on clinical interests.

This emphasis on meeting human needs and encouraging cooperation led to the development of theories of motivation and leadership. Motivation theories can be categorized as need theories, cognitive theories, and social/reinforcement theories. The most well-known **need theory** is Maslow's theory of human needs (Maslow, 1970). Clayton Alderfer (1972) modified Maslow's work by proposing that people have only three basic needs: existence, relatedness, and growth needs. His theory became known as **ERG theory.** He argued that people do not constantly strive to meet a higher level need, as Maslow had said. Instead, he said that people often remain at a certain

level. For example, community health nurses who are working in an understaffed, high-stress situation may function at the existence level until their situation changes.

Alderfer's theory was adapted by Hackman and Oldham (1976) to predict how to design jobs to increase worker productivity and job satisfaction. According to Hackman and Oldham's **Job Redesign Theory,** people with high growth need strength are most productive and satisfied when their jobs provide task variety, task identity, task significance, autonomy, and feedback. A clinic nurse whose primary job responsibility is taking patients' vital signs and assigning them to exam rooms does not have a job that is high in either task variety or task identity. A nurse case manager who works with clients over a long period of time and helps them manage comprehensive health care needs has much higher task variety and identity. Most community health nurses see their roles as high in task significance. Community health nurses have a great deal of clinical autonomy, which sometimes poses challenges in terms of delegation of authority and supervision. Finally, certain community health functions involve high levels of feedback; for example, working with children, families, and staff in school settings typically gives the nurse many opportunities for feedback from these groups.

Ensuring that all five job design elements are high is referred to as **job enrichment.** This differs from **job enlargement,** in which only task variety, task identity, and/or task significance are enhanced. Workers often do not find job enlargement to be motivating because they view it as simply adding tasks, whereas job enrichment increases individual responsibility, autonomy, and feedback. This is important for community health nurse managers to consider because many workers who are cross-trained or **multiskilled** may have had their jobs enlarged, rather than enriched. Another implication is that community health nurses who delegate tasks to others and supervise other workers should know whether these workers are more motivated by existence, relatedness, or growth needs and attempt to meet the relevant needs as much as possible. For example, if nursing staff in an adult day care center have high relatedness needs, then these nurses may appreciate opportunities to work together in retreats and committees.

Cognitive theories explain that motivation results from a person's beliefs and expectations about what will occur as a result of their actions. For example, Locke's **Goal-Setting Theory** (Latham and Locke, 1991) says that people are more motivated to achieve goals they participate in setting, that are challenging, and for which they receive regular feedback. Combining this theory with Victor Vroom's (1964) **Expectancy Theory,** the community health nurse manager should identify each worker's goals and their expectations about which actions will lead to goal achievement and whether they believe themselves to be capable of these actions. In this way, the community health nurse manager can identify inaccurate perceptions (e.g., the belief that the nurse manager 'plays favorites' may be erroneous) and ways to help workers achieve their own personal goals while achieving organizational goals.

Social/reinforcement theories say that human motivation results from learning that occurs following a behavior. **Reinforcement theory's** basic premise is that behavior is conditioned by reinforcers applied after the behavior occurs. Reinforcers are often very effective ways of increasing productivity and improving worker morale. For example, the home health nurse manager who thanks staff for a job well done with a note or special acknowledgements is more likely to maintain a positive working environment.

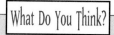

What Do You Think?

Some criticize reinforcement theory for not recognizing that humans behave voluntarily. Others say that reinforcement is simply a way of manipulating behavior and, as such, is unethical.

A related theory is Albert Bandura's **Social Learning Theory** (1977). Bandura says that people learn from role models and that confidence in one's ability to reach a goal is a key component of motivation and the ability to sustain effort to achieve goals. Community health nurses should be aware that they serve as role models for other staff and sometimes for lay workers as well. Community health nurses may wish to consciously model certain behaviors and work with staff to set achievable goals and develop realistic strategies for goal achievement. In this way, they can combine strategies suggested by both cognitive and social/reinforcement motivation theories.

Good **leadership** skills are essential for community health nurse managers and consultants. Although many theories of leadership have been proposed, contingency, path-goal, and transformational leadership theories are especially relevant for community health nurse managers and consultants. **Contingency leadership theory** (Fiedler, 1967) states that the most effective leadership style is contingent (or dependent) on characteristics of the relationships between leaders and followers, the task, and the situation. The most effective leadership style depends on the degree of knowledge and maturity possessed by group members (Hersey and Blanchard, 1988). Contingency theory says that individuals who are less familiar with the task or less self-directed will be more productive when the leader focuses on task accomplishment through coaching, supervision, and follow-up. On the other hand, leaders who are working with individuals who possess technical expertise, are highly motivated, and

are self-directed, primarily need guidance and opportunity from the leader. In this case, the leader functions more as a facilitator and less as a supervisor. Contingency theory is particularly relevant to community health since so many people work independently in clients' homes or in mobile clinics, or other areas where supervision may be difficult. Contingency theory suggests that the community health nurse manager should know the level of skill, motivation, and maturity of the team members and adjust his or her leadership style accordingly.

Path-goal theory (House, 1971) says that good leaders help others identify their goals and then develop ways to help them achieve those goals. In this way, leaders serve as facilitators who identify a path for goal achievement and remove barriers along the path. This theory focuses on individual goals and meeting individual needs and is especially compatible with the role of the community health nurse consultant. A major goal in consultation is helping an individual, program, department, or an entire organization identify its needs and working with it to help it meet those needs.

Finally, **transformational leadership** incorporates both the needs of organizations and individuals. Burns (1978) defined transformational leadership as that form of leadership in which the leader motivates followers to achieve a vision that is compatible with their values. Transformational leaders influence others to work toward achieving something new and as yet unimagined, essentially, a new dream of what is achievable. Whereas contingency and path-goal theories focus on identifying the best way to achieve a given goal, transformational leadership addresses the goal itself and the relationship of the goal to values. The transformational leader is able to transform, or change, the situation to one that differs from the status quo. Transformational leaders sometimes are found in **learning organizations** or organizations that not only learn from past experience but also create new visions for their future (Marriner-Tomey, 1993). The community health nurse manager or consultant who recognizes opportunities for improving the health of the public and who works with others to design creative nursing programs is just one example of a transformational leader.

Organizational-Level Theories Applied to Community Health Nursing Management

The macro-level, or organizational-level theories, that are particularly relevant for community health nurse managers and leaders are structural contingency theory, institutional theory, resource dependence theory, and systems theory. Managers and consultants often ask which form of organizational structure will best foster efficient achievement of organizational goals. **Structural contingency theory** predicts that the most effective structure depends on characteristics in the given situation (Thompson, 1967). Organizational structure refers to the ways people in an agency organize themselves to accomplish the mission and goals of the agency. It is depicted by the organizational chart, which illustrates the formal lines of authority in the agency and is operationalized by written documents, such as the mission, goals, philosophy, policies, procedures, and job descriptions. Together, all of these elements portray what the agency is trying to accomplish and how employees at all levels will work together to do so. Every organization also has an informal structure, which is the way people actually work together; it includes informal communication patterns, informal sources of power, and unwritten rules of conduct. Community health nurse managers and consultants should be familiar with both formal and informal agency structures.

According to structural contingency theory, organizations should have more formal structures, or be more mechanized (Burns and Stalker, 1961), (1) when employees perform routine tasks that are not expected to vary a great deal, (2) when employees do not have high levels of specialized education, and (3) when the industry or environment in which the organization operates is stable and not changing very much. Typically, as an organization grows larger it becomes more highly structured, or formalized. This is often the case in large health departments, home health agencies, school districts, and ambulatory care clinics. On the other hand, organizations that accomplish their goals through the work of highly skilled professionals, that provide individualized services that are expected to vary across clients, and that operate in a turbulent, rapidly changing environment, are more likely to be successful if their structures are more organic (Burns and Stalker, 1961), or loose, allowing employees latitude and autonomy in making decisions. Organically structured organizations are more likely to be decentralized, with much decision-making authority pushed down to the lowest level in the organization where employees have the information needed for making decisions. In the past, organic structures were most often seen in small agencies. Today, health care organizations of all types are moving toward more organic structures, despite sometimes being very large. Individual units, departments, or programs often operate very autonomously within the overall mission and goals of the organization. This places a great deal of authority and responsibility in the hands of nurse managers.

Institutional theory focuses on how formally stated and informally held values and norms affect organizational activity. According to this theory, organizational members are more likely to respond to widely shared values and norms of behavior than they are to formally written policies and procedures (Meyer and Rowan, 1977). For example, norms for treatment of substance abuse differ greatly from norms for treatment of severe mental illness (D'Aunno et al., 1991). Addiction treatment groups tend to value dependence

on a higher authority and admitting powerlessness over the addiction. Mental health professionals, on the other hand, value increasing individual self-reliance and increasing one's control over one's own health. When a community mental health center treats both types of clients, and particularly when treating dually-diagnosed clients who are both drug dependent and severely mentally ill, treatment norms may conflict. In such a situation, the written policies and procedures are not good predictors of the actual treatment practices of individual providers (D'Aunno et al, 1991). Community health nurse managers and consultants must be aware of the powerful influence that values and norms play in organizational work and understand the informal norms that exist.

Resource dependence theory (Pfeffer and Salancik, 1978) says that the primary motivator for organizational behavior is the desire to reduce uncertainty about acquiring the resources necessary to operate. These resources are usually fiscal, but also may include key personnel, seats on influential community boards, or contracts with prestigious organizations. This theory is basically about power and its acquisition and maintenance. In order to be effective, community health nurse managers and consultants must be able to accurately analyze power dynamics both within an organization and within the community. They must be able to predict the resource needs of the organization and how acquiring and maintaining those resources may affect power dynamics within the system.

Systems theory emphasizes the interdependence of organizational players. Nurses often recognize interdependence of units within an organization, but may be less aware of interorganizational interdependence. Economists analyze the **distributional effects** of policies to determine which players in a system will be influenced by policies and how they will be influenced. For example, if the federal government reduces money for health and human services, the recipients of those services may be negatively affected. Employees of service agencies also are affected because agencies are likely to downsize in order to manage the reduced funding. Consequently, employees may either lose their jobs or experience wage cuts. Others likely to be affected include voluntary agencies and religious groups who might be expected to provide more services.

Roy's *Adaptation Model of Nursing* has been extended to include nursing management (Roy and Anway, 1989). Roy argues that organizations are composed of interdependent systems, just as individual clients are. The role of nurse managers is to assist the organization to adapt to changing circumstances in the most effective way possible. Roy's Model is particularly helpful for explaining and predicting how community health nurse managers and consultants can help organizations adapt to change. Community health nurse managers and consultants should analyze how well interdependent subsystems function to achieve organizational goals. Furthermore, nurse managers and consultants function as change agents because they foster organizational adaptation.

The Community Health Nurse Manager Role

First-line community health nurse managers may be team leaders or program directors (e.g., director of a satellite occupational health clinic or director of a small migrant health clinic), while mid-level or executive-level nurse managers may be divisional directors (including multiple programs or departments), local or state commissioners of health, or directors of large home health agencies with multiple offices. They function as coaches, facilitators, role models, evaluators, advocates, visionaries, community health and program planners, teachers, and supervisors. Community health nurse managers have ongoing responsibilities for clients, groups, and community health, and for personnel and fiscal resources under their supervision.

CONSULTATION

Goal

The goal of consultation is to empower clients to take more responsibility, feel more secure, deal constructively with their feelings and with others in interactions, and internalize flexible and creative problem-solving skills. The functions of a consultant differ from those of managers because consultation typically is a temporary and voluntary relationship between a professional helper and a client. This relationship is based on cooperation between consultant and client, who share equally in problem-solving.

The community health nurse's job responsibilities include internal and external consultation. For example, a nurse may be employed to consult with other nurses in the agency about client care problems or as an employee of the health department, may serve as a consultant to a local retirement center about the public health care needs of its residents. If the community health nurse is an internal consultant, the nurse is employed on a full-time salaried basis by a community agency in which the consultation takes place. If the community health nurse is an external consultant, the nurse is employed temporarily on a contractual basis by the client. The client of the external nurse consultant may be a colleague, another health provider, or a community group or organization. The following research belief illustrates the balance of internal and external consulting functions filled by occupational health nurses. The nature of the consultative relationship should not change the goal of consultation.

Theories of Consultation

Several models of consultation have been developed. This chapter focuses on Edgar Schein's models because they are consistent with the nursing process and

Research Brief

Guzik VL, McGovern PM, Kochevar LK: Role function and job satisfaction: a study of nurse graduates of educational resource center programs employed by the health care industry, AAOHN J, 40(11):521-530, 1992.

This study compared role functions and job satisfaction of occupational health nurses (OHNs) who functioned primarily as internal consultants with those who functioned primarily as external consultants. Role theory provided the framework for the study. Data were collected by mailed questionnaires on work situation variables, including tasks, level and type of decision making, role ambiguity, and conflict; intervening variables, such as personal and demographic characteristics; and the outcome variables of job and career satisfaction. The 65 subjects were graduates of masters programs in occupational health nursing and were employed in the health care industry in the United States in 1988 (rather than OHNs employed in other industries, such as manufacturing). Examples of sites in which respondents were employed included ambulatory clinics in health maintenance organizations and specialty physician group practices, medical supply companies, corporate facilities, long-term care, and governmental agencies.

Researchers found that OHNs who functioned primarily as internal consultants provided more direct care services, such as individual physical exams, case management services, counseling, and immunications. Those who functioned more as external consultants engaged in more marketing and management functions, including developing and managing annual operating budgets for the occupational health program, conducting market research to determine the need for occupational health services, pricing services and products, designing marketing tools, developing and managing contracts, and personnel management, including hiring, evaluating, and firing staff. No significant differences in job satisfaction existed between OHNs who functioned primarily as internal consultants and those who functioned more as external consultants. Those who had greater role certainty did report higher levels of job satisfaction. Stress from role ambiguity had a negative impact on job satisfaction, in part because subjects felt overwhelmed and were uncertain about which tasks they did not need to perform. The researchers concluded that OHNs would be able to reduce role ambiguity if they write or revise their own job descriptions, and if they possess good time management, communication, negotiation, and conflict management skills.

with community health nursing values of empowering clients and collaboratively working as partners with clients.

Purchase-of-expertise consultation (Figure 43-2) is defined as the purchase (hiring) of a professional

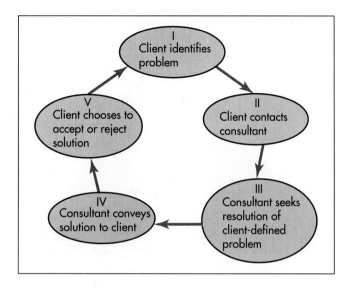

FIGURE 43-2

The purchase-of-expertise consultation model.

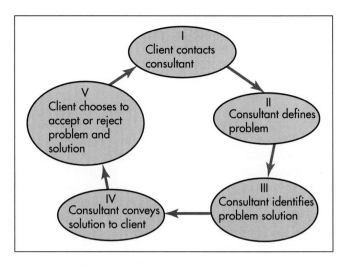

FIGURE 43-3

The doctor-patient consultation model.

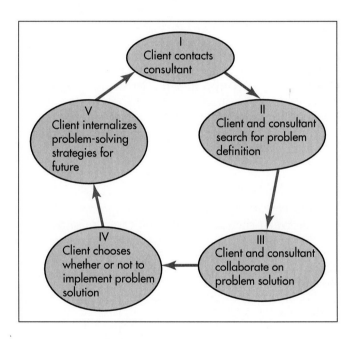

FIGURE 43-4

The process consultation model.

helper by a client to provide expert information or service (Schein, 1969). Buyers may be individuals, groups, or organizations. In this model the client defines the need for the consultant. The need is defined as information the client seeks or an activity the client wants implemented. The advantage of this popular model is that the client does not have to spend time or energy in solving the identified problem, because that is the responsibility of the "expert consultant." The disadvantage is that the client may question the quality of the consultation if the client has identified the wrong problem or does not like the consultant's solution.

Although this model often is used, it may be unsatisfactory in effectively and efficiently identifying and resolving client problems. Once the consultant has implemented steps to solve the problem, the client must live with the consequences of the changes. This model is likely to be effective by itself only when problems are simple and the client needs specific expert information (Rokwood, 1993).

Another popular consultative model is the **doctor-patient model** (Figure 43-3), in which the consultant is employed by the client to diagnose the problem and prescribe solutions without assistance from the client (Schein, 1969). Again, the major advantage of this model from the client's viewpoint is the limited time and energy required of the client. This model is often applied in nursing situations requiring consultative services. For example, the director of nursing at the public health department calls in a nurse consultant from the local university. Nurse performance is poor, according to the director, and the nurse consultant is asked to diagnose what is wrong with the department. If the problem is found to be poor management rather than poor performance by the staff, the administrator may be reluctant to accept the diagnosis. Since the client does not help diagnose the problem, the goals of consultation may not be met.

The purchase-of-expertise and doctor-patient models are *content* models of consultation since they deal with the content (or nature) of the problem. The **process consultation model** focuses on the *process* of problem solving and emphasizes collaboration between consultant and consultee (Rokwood, 1993). The major goal of the process model, as seen in Figure 43-4, is to help the client assess both the problem and the kind of help needed to resolve the problem (Schein, 1969). Process consultation incorporates assessment of the underlying organizational culture that influences the problem and its resolution (Schein, 1990). Both consultant and client participate in the problem-solving steps that lead to changes or to actions for problem solution. The assumptions underlying each of the three models are listed in the box below.

Content and process consultation models do not need to be mutually exclusive (Rokwood, 1993; Schein, 1989). Instead, although consultants should emphasize process consultation, they should be willing to share their expertise when appropriate. Because process consultation is collaborative, Schein (1989) recommends that consultants be willing to offer opinions and advice at various stages of the consultation process. Thus, although the major emphasis should be on process consultation, consultants may find it effective to integrate the three models at selected points.

In the process model, the consultant is a resource person whose primary goal is to provide the client with choices for decision making. As shown in Figure 43-5, the process consultation model includes the same steps as the nursing process, establishing a nurse-client interaction based on trust to assess the problem, plan and implement actions, and evaluate the outcomes of nursing interventions. Nursing interventions may be described as direct client care or as consultation activities, depending on the goal of the intervention. The analysis and synthesis of the process consultation model by Blake and Mouton (1983) serves as the basis for the following discussion and application of this model.

Process Consultation

Process consultation involves a temporary relationship between client and consultant for the purpose of

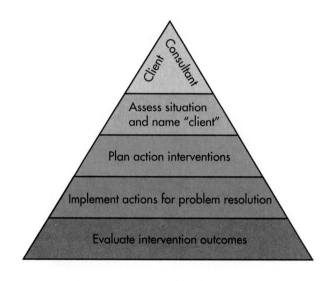

FIGURE 43-5
Integration of the nursing process and the process model of consultation.

bringing about change. Consultation may be proactive or reactive. Proactive consultation is directed toward anticipating a future problem and taking steps to prevent it. Reactive consultation is directed toward curing an existing problem through therapeutic intervention. For example, a parent-teacher council developing a school-based family resource center contacts the community health nurse to assist with options for future nursing and health care for the students and their families. The board wishes to be proactive and plan for the needs of high-risk students and families. Conversely, the administrator of a minimum security prison has found that inmates are missing work for

Assumptions of Schein's Consultation Models

PURCHASE-OF-EXPERTISE MODEL
1. The client correctly diagnoses the problem.
2. The client correctly communicates the needs to the consultant.
3. The client correctly assesses the consultant's expertise to provide the information or perform the service.
4. The client knows the consequences of implementing the services suggested by the consultant.

DOCTOR-PATIENT MODEL
1. The client is willing to reveal information needed by the consultant to make an appropriate diagnosis.
2. The consultant is able to get an accurate picture of the problem through observation.
3. The client accepts the diagnosis and the prescriptions offered by the consultant.

PROCESS MODEL
1. Clients often do not know what the problem is and need assistance in problem diagnosis.
2. Clients are not aware of the services a consultant may offer and need assistance in finding proper help.
3. Clients want to improve situations and need guidance in identifying appropriate methods to reach goals.
4. Clients can be more effective if they learn how to diagnose their own strengths and limitations.
5. Consultants usually cannot spend enough time learning all variables that may help or hinder suggested courses of action, so they need to work with the client, who has intimate knowledge of the effects of proposed courses of action.
6. The client who learns to diagnose situation problems and who engages in decision making about alternative courses of action will be actively involved in implementing actions for problem resolution.
7. The consultant is an expert in problem diagnosis and in establishing an effective helping relationship and passes these skills on to the client.

minor health problems and that health costs are skyrocketing. The community health nurse is asked to help explore solutions to the problem. Prison administration is reacting to an existing problem requiring immediate intervention.

One of the most important decisions a nurse makes before accepting or writing a consultative contract is identifying the client in the situation. The client is identified by determining who in the situation has the problem and needs to change.

The following vignette illustrates this point:

Barry Rubin is a school health nurse who receives an inquiry from the school board about ways to get parents to support a school-based clinic. Barry decides that the consultative contract needs to include representatives of the school board and representatives of the parents' group to find effective answers to the question. He realizes that time would be wasted and resistance to change would still be present if the focus were only on one group at a time. If he was to meet separately with the parent group, they may decide such a clinic should be limited to acute illnesses and injuries, and should include parental permission for all interventions. At the school board meeting he could find that the board is concerned about teenage pregnancy and sexually transmitted diseases and wishes to provide more comprehensive interventions that ensure confidentiality for the students. After expending much energy meeting with both groups separately, he would find that by being a messenger between the two groups rather than a facilitator for problem solving, the consultant role has been diluted. On the other hand, by meeting with both groups together Barry could serve as a resource for helping the parents and school board explore all viewpoints and alternatives for solving the problem. In this case, both the school board and the parents' group are Barry's clients.

Once the client has been identified, the nurse must decide the best method(s) for intervening in the problem situation. Blake and Mouton (1983) describe five basic intervention modes or techniques that can be applied to the process consultation model: acceptant, catalytic, confrontation, prescriptive, and theory-principles. These are summarized in Table 43-1. The **acceptant intervention mode** involves clarifying emotional reactions so that more objective problem solving can begin. This intervention mode benefits the client by improving self-acceptance, emotional health, and the ability to objectively define and deal with problems. Two disadvantages exist with this intervention mode. Expressing emotions may only help the client accept the circumstances leading to the problem rather than taking actions to correct the problem, and this catharsis may be seen by others as hostile and aggressive (Blake and Mouton, 1983).

In the **catalytic intervention mode,** the consultant helps clients broaden their view of the situation by gaining additional information or by integrating existing data (Blake and Mouton, 1983). The consultant helps the client (1) clarify understanding of problems by increasing available information, (2) break down barriers to communication by identifying ineffective communication patterns, and (3) raise the awareness

of all involved regarding the problem. The consultant is a facilitator providing the client with the information needed to solve a problem. Lack of information, however, may be the symptom, not the problem. The disadvantage of having the consultant improve information-flow is that the client may rely on the facilitator for data rather than becoming efficient in finding solutions to future problems (Blake and Mouton, 1983; Caplan, 1970).

The **confrontation intervention mode** presents the client with facts that reveal the client's values and assumptions in ways that are undeniable and indisputable (Blake and Mouton, 1983). This intervention mode provides clients with an objective look at how their values and beliefs control their behavior. By looking at present behavior, the consultant and client can examine alternative values to redirect behavior toward improved methods of problem solving. The disadvantage is that the client may not wish to participate in interactions that could be interpreted as criticism (Blake and Mouton, 1983). For example, a consultant may find that the staff nurses in a local public health department are going to resign their positions because they view the director's decisions as autocratic and uncompromising. On the second visit to the agency, the consultant could confront the director with these observations. The director may deny the behavior and point out evidence of having acted democratically. As a result of the confrontation, the director may regard the consultant's observations as a personal affront or be willing to examine and analyze the discrepancies between the perceived and the actual behavior.

The **prescriptive intervention mode** requires less collaboration between consultant and client because the consultant tells the client how to solve the problem (Blake and Mouton, 1983). This mode is best used along with other intervention modes, such as acceptant or catalytic. If clients do not participate in problem solution, they will not be able to solve future problems and may not follow the prescriptions offered. The advantage of the prescriptive intervention mode is its usefulness in situations where clients have lost confidence in their problem-solving ability or have given up in despair (Blake and Mouton, 1983). In the above example, the nurse consultant could decide that the best method of dealing with the problems between the staff and the director is to present a prescription for behavioral conduct to be implemented by the director and the staff. The consultant tells the group when and how follow-up evaluation will be conducted to look at the progress of both parties in resolving their differences.

Use of the **theory-principles intervention mode** requires that the client learn theories, such as behavioral theory, and their application to problem solving. This intervention mode introduces the theories after clients have shared their usual methods of problem solving. It also allows the client to apply the

Table 43-1   Consultative Intervention Modes

Intervention mode	Definition	Problem example	Consultant actions
Acceptance	Consultant urges client to share feelings to move to more objective problem solving.	1. Low morale 2. Feelings of powerlessness to change a situation	1. Attempt to understand the client's feelings about the situation. 2. Listen actively. 3. Encourage the client to talk. 4. Try to clarify the client's feelings and help the client to accept those feelings. 5. Refrain from agreeing or disagreeing with the client's situation. 6. Encourage the client to explore ways of dealing with the problems. 7. Listen for more data to reveal the total scope of the problem.
Catalytic	Consultant broadens client's knowledge of problem by offering new data or clarifying existing data.	1. Standards are violated or changed 2. Inability to meet goals or objectives	1. Set a nonauthoritarian tone for the interaction by beginning the intervention with social conversation. 2. Ask the client to describe the situation and use the description as a basis for the interaction. 3. Suggest data-gathering techniques that may provide new information of interest to the client. 4. Provide support to the client as the client attempts to accurately perceive the problem. 5. Avoid specific suggestions. 6. Encourage the client to make decisions about problem resolution.
Confrontation	Consultant presents clients with indisputable facts.	1. Additional insight needed 2. Unwillingness to solve problem	1. Continually question clients about their description of the situation. 2. Present data and logic to test clients' chosen courses of action. 3. Challenge clients' chosen courses of action. 4. Probe for motives and causes of present situation. 5. Provide own thoughts about situation without personally attacking client's values.
Prescriptive	Consultant tells client how to solve problem.	1. Inability to cope 2. Needs immediate answer	1. Probe for data about the client's situation. 2. Act authoritatively. 3. Control by telling the client how the problem is to be perceived. 4. Tell the client the best solutions. 5. Remind the client if he/she is procrastinating in implementing actions. 6. Offer praise if the client does what the consultant suggests.
Theory-Principles	Consultant teaches how to solve problem using theories or principles.	1. Additional insight needed 2. Lack of knowledge to solve problem	1. Introduce theories for problem-solving to the client. 2. Use techniques to assist the client to internalize theories. 3. Provide strategies for practical application of the theories, such as problem situations or critiques of application. 4. Offer support when the theory is applied in the actual problem situation.

theories to problem situations while developing skills in problem diagnosis and solution. The major challenge with this mode is determining how to help clients learn practical ways to apply the theory (Blake and Mouton, 1983). This mode can be combined with another mode because consultation involves facilitating client learning (Evans et al., 1992). Evans and colleagues (1992) explain that theory can be used to help clients better understand what the data is saying, better diagnose the problem, and generate more potentially effective decision alternatives. Before using this mode with the health department staff and director, the consultant may present a conference on leadership theories and principles and a discussion of the responsibilities in administrative decision making. The consultant may be able to show both parties how leadership styles should vary with the types of decisions to be made and with the people involved.

The choice of a particular intervention mode depends on the client and the problem. Blake and Mouton (1983) identified four categories of problems: power/authority, morale/cohesion, norms/standards, and goals/objectives. The power/authority problem results from questions about who has the right to supervise and who has the right to make decisions. The morale/cohesion problem occurs when the client has lost confidence in the ability to solve problems and feels powerless. The norms/standards problem occurs when group norms or professional or organization standards are violated or changed. Problems related to goals/objectives involve establishing new goals, changing goals, or being unable to meet goals.

Several intervention modes may be used with each of the problem issues. The most common intervention for morale/cohesion or power/authority problems is the acceptant mode because the issue generally causes feelings that block decision making. The catalytic mode is the best choice with norms/standards and goals/objectives problems because it focuses on strengthening the client's perceptions of the most effective decision-making methods. The theory-principles intervention mode may be helpful regardless of the problem, especially when additional insights are needed. The prescriptive mode may not be helpful unless the client is unable to cope with the situation and needs immediate direction or answers to solve the problem (Blake and Mouton, 1983) or unless the problem is fairly straightforward (Rokwood, 1993).

The Community Health Nurse and Use of Process Consultation

The consultative relationship is based on expectations. The consultant has expectations concerning time, reimbursement, resources, and the participation of the client in the process. Clients have expectations about what they will gain from the consultative relationship. Discussing the terms of the **consultative contract**

makes expectations explicit, reduces the likelihood of violations of contract terms, and reduces the risk of additional demands being made on either party. Areas to include in the written consultative contract are (1) client and consultant goals, (2) the identified problem, (3) the consultant's resources, (4) the time commitment, (5) limitations of the contract, (6) cost, (7) conditions under which the contract may be broken or renegotiated, (8) intervention modes to be used, (9) expected benefits for the client, (10) methods of data collection to be used, (11) client resources, (12) potential interventions, (13) evaluation methods to be used, and (14) confidentiality. An example of a consultation contract appears in Figure 43-6.

Writing a contract for consultative relationships has a number of advantages. The contract terms assist the consultant in determining the number of hours that must be devoted to the interaction and in identifying needed resources and out-of-pocket expenses required to complete the interaction. Negotiation of the contract assists the client in identifying realistic expectations of the consultant and firmly establishes what the consultant will and will not do. The client has the opportunity during the negotiation to place limits on what the consultant can do, and the contract allows for future renegotiation of terms. Pricing methods for consultative services vary with the nature of the services. Consultants may price their services based on the actual number of billable hours required to perform the service, or set a flat fee during the contract negotiation phase. Flat fees are more attractive to clients since they reduce uncertainty over the total cost of the consultation. They create an incentive for consultants to be efficient and to use an accurate method of estimating their services prior to the contract negotiation meeting.

Consultation involves seven basic phases: (1) initial contact with the client, (2) definition of the relationship, (3) selection of a setting and approach, (4) collection of data and problem diagnosis, (5) intervention, (6) reduction of involvement and evaluation, and (7) termination. The initial contact is made when the client or someone in a family, group, or community communicates with the nurse about a potential problem that requires intervention. The communication may be person-to-person during a home visit, may be written, or may occur by telephone. On initial contact, the client and the nurse have an exploratory meeting to define the problem, assess the nurse's ability to help, assess the nurse's interest, and formulate future actions. If the nurse has little experience with the type of problem presented, the client may wish to seek assistance elsewhere. Also, if the nurse is quick to make decisions and has a directive approach, the client with a more laissez faire philosophy may have difficulty accepting the nurse's approach. Conversely, the nurse may conclude that the situation is not within the nurse's expertise and will want to recommend someone else to work with the client.

Client Name: J. Hyde, Nurse Manager Address: Residential Complex Phone: 111-2222	Consultant Name: P. Jones, Nursing Student Address: College of Nursing Phone: 333-4444

Estimated costs (external consultant only): $500
(including phone, secretarial assistance, preparation, supplies, travel expenses, and
  consultant sessions)

Client problem definition: Facility undergoing expansion: residents likely to need more
assistance with health promotion & health monitoring. Average
resident age is 72.3 yrs. Residents have on avg. 2.5 chronic
illnesses each. 10-15 miles from health facilities. Residents
are becoming increasingly homebound.

Suggested intervention mode: Catalytic/Prescriptive

Client goals:
A healthy resident population through
accessible and ongoing health promotion & monitoring.

Scope of consultation (time & no. of sessions):
3 planning & data gathering sessions in 6
weeks; 3 evaluation sessions at
2 to 3 week intervals during data
collection; final evaluation session.

Consultant resources (e.g., computer, secretary, library):
Computer to analyze data; library; assistance
from faculty; staff to collect data (3 students).

Contract renegotiation & termination terms:
Renegotiation at 2 to 3 week evaluation con-
ferences.
Termination at final evaluation conference.

Client resources (e.g., records, secretary, copy):
Project records available to collect data;
secretary type survey questionnaires;
conference room for interviews; final report
typing; supplies.

Anticipated client benefits:
Residential complex will have a plan for
meeting health needs of residents.
Residents will have increased access to health
promotion & health monitoring
services.

Contract limitations (e.g., who, what, when, how data will be shared):
Survey of residents' health needs, and per-
ceptions of staff and administrators by CHN
student. Report to nurse manager,
facility manager, and college faculty.

Potential interventions (e.g., report shared with administration: meetings held with staff):
Meetings with staff and residents to
obtain input on the problem and potential solutions. Review of resources to find the residential complex's ability to manage the problem itself.

Consultant goals:
Collect data as outlined.
Assess and define problem in collaboration
with residents, staff, and administration.
Identify resources for solving the
problem.
Develop a realistic method for solving the
problem in collaboration with residents,
staff, & administration.

Data collection methods:
Interviews: Staff, nurse manager,
                           facility manager, local
                           health care providers
Surveys: Residents
Focus groups: Residents, staff &
                           administrators, faculty
Phone: N/A
Contract evaluation:
                           At the end of 12 weeks
                           will look at potential
                           alternatives; choose one that
                           is satisfactory to residents,
                           staff, & administrators.

FIGURE 43-6
Example of a consultation contract.

Next, the terms of the relationship are discussed. The nurse consultant finds out what the client expects to gain from the relationship and establishes terms for the interaction. Finally, in the initial exploratory meeting the setting for the consultation is decided upon, the time schedule is set, the goals of the interaction are established, and the mode of intervention is chosen.

When the terms of the contract are agreed upon, the data gathering methods will be part of the agreement. Data gathering methods used by consultants include direct observation, individual and group interviews, use of questionnaires or surveys, and tape recordings. One particularly useful data gathering strategy is the focus group (Krueger, 1994). This is a group of eight to 10 people who share a common characteristic, such as staff nurses in the same organization or community members living in the same neighborhood. Focus groups are led by one individual, who has prepared five to six open-ended questions to guide the discussion. A recorder takes thorough notes during the session. Focus group sessions are usually 1 hour in length and include refreshments. After the session, the leader and recorder discuss their observations and impressions in order to capture all important data. The outcomes of focus group discussions can guide the development of written surveys (LoBiondo-Wood and Haber, 1994; McDaniel and Bach, 1994; Morgan, 1993).

While data are being gathered and after the diagnosis has been finalized, the nurse actively engages in the chosen intervention mode. After fulfilling the terms of the contract, the nurse must disengage or reduce the amount of involvement with the client. Decreased contacts allow each side to evaluate the effectiveness of the intervention. During disengagement the nurse reassures the client that future interactions are possible at the client's discretion. When the agreed-upon period of disengagement has passed, the relationship is terminated (Beare, 1988; Blake and Mouton, 1983; Reinert and Buck, 1989; Schein, 1969). The nurse typically provides the consultee with a written summary of the findings and recommendations resulting from the interactions during the disengagement and termination phases (Ingersoll and Jones, 1992).

The consultative relationship entails responsibilities by both the nurse and the client. Although the contract defines the terms of the relationship, the client can assist in making the consultative process a successful interaction. Initially the client must determine whether an internal or external consultant can best assist in solving the problem. An internal nurse consultant knows the organization and the values of the organization and the staff, is a team member, has expertise, and is probably committed to helping solve internal problems. The external nurse consultant brings new ideas and a broader regional or national perspective, has new or proven strategies to offer, can bring objectivity to the problem, and has a short-term, less expensive commitment to the organization (Collins, 1989; Novle and Harvey, 1988).

The client can obtain efficient, effective consultation by recognizing that the problem belongs to the client, and the nurse's role in solving the problem is limited. Once the problem has been accepted, the client can offer an agenda to maximize the nurse's time, identify key people to work with the nurse, and offer a written summary of issues and questions. The client should remain open to all proposed suggestions or solutions, summarize the content of the nurse's visits and need for follow-up, clarify disputed findings and recommendations with the nurse, and try out the proposed solutions after examining the benefits and consequences of implementing them (Berger et al., 1993; Collins, 1989; Greenblatt, 1994; Novle and Harvey, 1988; Schaffner, 1987).

To develop a credible reputation, a nurse must clarify all role expectations with the client and present accurate credentials and skills, maintain a professional image, and complete assignments in an agreed-upon time frame. The nurse also should assess the situation and collect all essential data, be available for follow-up, and use a written evaluation tool to assess the fulfillment of mutual expectations (Beare, 1988; Beecroft, 1988; Reinert and Buck, 1989).

An example of a consultative intervention follows:

Intervention:	Prescriptive
Client:	Director of Nursing
Consultant:	Internal
Problem:	Norms/standards

The client telephoned the state nursing consultant and requested a meeting at the local health unit. The purpose of the meeting was to review serious problems the local nursing staff was having in meeting program standards and requirements, as identified in a recent audit. The nurse consultant, Elizabeth, met with the client, Maggie, and reviewed her findings, sharing her analysis of the problems and contributing factors. The central problem was defined as inconsistent supervision of staff with a need for role clarification of supervisory responsibilities. Maggie was immobilized by the situation. Elizabeth directed Maggie to restructure the supervisory job descriptions to clearly reflect supervisory roles and expectations; she also recommended giving supervisors written performance evaluations and guidelines for improving staff performance. Elizabeth maintained contact with Maggie until termination of the consultation occurred and corrective action was completed.

The Nurse Consultant Role

An agency that delivers care similar to an official generalized community health service will most likely employ a generalist nurse who provides traditional or comprehensive community health nursing consultation for a broad range of community health activities (e.g., a community health nurse clinical specialist). A community health agency that provides a programmatic approach to the delivery of community health services, such as family planning, maternity, child health, handicapped children's services, school health, or home health, will tend to employ specialist consultants; these may have skills and training in specific clinical areas (e.g., a pediatric clinical nurse specialist) in addition to broad community health expertise. Agencies providing primary health care require a consultant with both a knowledge of community health practice and specialized knowledge in a clinical area. This is also a requirement in agencies involved in long-term and home health care.

The community health nurse consultant employed within an official health agency functions as an internal consultant to the employing agency. As a representative of the agency, the nurse provides nursing and community health consultation to colleagues, other disciplines, agency administration, and other health and human service agencies and/or community groups. Two primary roles of the internal consultant are resource person and facilitator (Pati, 1980).

With knowledge of available resources, the nurse consultant can identify deficiencies and gaps in service, identify the critical services provided by the health delivery systems, and promote service integration for meeting health or social needs of the population. The consultant facilitates staff nurse problem-solving about individual client and family needs, health needs of a group of clients, or professional concerns and attitudes. The consultant may assist managers and administrators with solving problems about personnel, program needs, organizational goals, community relationships, and client population needs. The consultant also may facilitate communication across agencies by working with interagency coalitions or alliances.

A generalist nurse in an official community agency is often required to function in a dual supervisor-consultant role. **Supervision** means decision making and implementation of activities in an ongoing relationship, which is the opposite of consultation. Functions of the supervising role could replace the consultative role, and the staff could perceive the supervisor/consultant as being directly aligned with administration. Effective communication is vital.

The internal consultant as a representative of the employing agency has implied authority that may result in conflict between the consultant and the consultee. The amount of conflict depends on the centralization or decentralization of the health agency and the degree of autonomy of the individual units in the organization. One way to decrease potential conflict is to clearly define the role the consultant is to assume. For example, in one state, the state health department has jurisdiction over all the county health departments (centralized). The state has decided to decentralize by making all the county health departments autonomous in their delivery of health services. The state health department will continue to advise the county units about delivery of services but will not supervise the delivery of care. Nursing in the county units will have its own directors, and the nursing consultants at the state level will be used as resource persons and facilitators.

Although the state health department was centralized and provided direct supervision to the counties for delivery of health care, the state family planning consultant was also responsible for supervising the county health department staff members who were responsible for delivery of family planning services. In the decentralized system, the supervisory functions are removed from the consultant's responsibilities and the consultant facilitates the work of other nurses by offering advice and information that will assist them in understanding how to do their work.

The role of external nurse consultant also involves acting as a facilitator or a resource person. The external nurse consultant may represent the employing agency and provide information to the consultee for planning interagency programs to meet population needs. The external nurse consultant may serve as a resource to health educators, school personnel, psychologists, counselors, dentists, social workers, physicians, legislators, and probation officers, providing data about individual client, group, or community needs. The external consultant may be asked to serve as facilitator to an official agency board to solve problems about community health priorities or to serve as a facilitator or resource person to voluntary agencies, such as the American Red Cross or the American Heart Association.

Consultants from federal agencies often are used as external nurse consultants. The nurse consultant from the federal agency may come to the local or state agency to serve on request as facilitator or resource person helping with program planning, development, and implementation. The primary role function of this consultant is to serve as a resource person, although the consultant may facilitate movement toward identifying actual program objectives.

SKILLS REQUIRED BY MANAGEMENT AND CONSULTANT ROLES
Leadership Skills

Community health nurse managers and consultants need effective leadership, interpersonal, organizational, and political skills. Leadership skills that are essential to these roles are the abilities to identify a vision and influence others to achieve the vision, emphasize that client needs are the basis for health services, empower others, balance attention to people and tasks, delegate tasks and manage time appropriately, and make decisions effectively. The Essential Public Health Services Work Group of the United States Public Health Service (1994) articulated the vision and mission of public health in America, the definition of public health, and essential public health services (see box on p. 865). Community health nurse managers should be involved in develop-

Public Health in America

Vision: Healthy People in Healthy Communities
Mission: Promote Health and Prevent Disease

PUBLIC HEALTH

◆ Prevents epidemics and the spread of disease.
◆ Protects against environmental hazards.
◆ Prevents injuries.
◆ Promotes and encourages healthy behaviors.
◆ Responds to disasters and assists communities in recovery.
◆ Assures the quality and accessibility of health services.

ESSENTIAL PUBLIC HEALTH SERVICES

◆ Monitor health status to identify community problems.
◆ Diagnose and investigate health problems and health hazards in the community.
◆ Inform, educate, and empower people about health issues.
◆ Mobilize community partnerships and actions to solve health problems.
◆ Develop policies and plans that support individual and community health efforts.
◆ Enforce laws and regulations that protect health and ensure safety.
◆ Link people to needed personal health services and assure the provision of health care when otherwise unavailable.
◆ Assure an expert public health work force.
◆ Evaluate effectiveness, accessibility, and quality of health services.
◆ Research for new insights and innovative solutions to health problems.

From Essential Public Health Services Work Group, United States Public Health Service: *The Nation's Health* p 3, Dec, 1994.

ing *organizational level vision, mission, and goal statements.* The American Nurses Association Standards for Community Health Nursing Practice (ANA, 1986) and the Standards for Organized Nursing Services (ANA, 1988) both offer guidance in these areas.

Effective community health nursing leaders understand the concept of **service leadership.** Greenleaf (1991) points out that customers come first, and the leader's basic function is to serve customers. Expanded to the health care context, the community health nurse managers and consultants need to remember that clients are the reason for their work, whether clients are individual patients in a primary care clinic; families in a home care caseload; aggregates, such as teachers and staff in a school setting; or entire communities. This means that basic organizational assumptions often must change. For example, the assumption of organizational hierarchy as a pyramid with clients at the bottom and top administration at the apex must be reversed. In a service leadership context, administration is at the bottom of the pyramid, and clients are at the top, with staff who work directly with clients located immediately below clients. This alteration in perspective is more than just semantic; it changes the leader's basic assumptions about

work rules. For example, in a traditional bureaucracy, organizational efficiency is achieved by establishing detailed rules governing how work is done. Often, these rules do not match the needs of individual clients. If a single mother brings her three preschool children to a health department clinic for a check-up for her infant and must return at a different time to obtain immunizations for the 4- and 5-year-old children, her needs and the needs of her children have not been met. On the other hand, if the clinic is organized around family needs, as opposed to specializing in the needs of narrow age groups, then all three of her children can be immunized in one visit and the client's needs have been met.

Leaders *empower* others to make organizations more responsive to client needs. This means giving staff the knowledge, skills, and authority to act on behalf of clients (Manthey, 1991). It means removing organizational barriers to decision making and allowing staff nurses the authority to make client decisions in "real time," as needs demand, rather than requiring nurses to obtain numerous approvals. Empowerment is more than simply increasing workers' authority. It includes ensuring that they have the necessary information, knowledge, and skills to make the decisions for which they are being empowered effectively. For example, community health nurse managers who are responsible for preparing their own department or program budgets and for approving program expenditures must be given the opportunity to learn budgetary concepts. The concept of empowerment underpins the consulting process. Consultants assist others in identifying solutions to problems and, more importantly, in developing the ability to manage problems independently in the future.

A key leadership skill for community health nurse managers and consultants is the ability to balance attention *to people* and *to tasks* (Hersey and Blanchard, 1988). This skill derives from contingency leadership theory and means that effective leaders do not focus all of their attention on simply getting the job done; if they do this, they may appear cold and uncaring and reduce morale. Similarly, effective leaders don't spend all of their time attending to workers' personal needs and problems. If they did this, the goals of the organization would never be met. Effective leaders must balance their focus, depending on the needs and skills of those with whom they work and on the demands of the situation. In situations in which time is a critical factor, such as in disasters, effective leaders emphasize tasks, such as victim triage, meeting basic community needs for safe food and water and shelter. After the emergency has stabilized somewhat, they should attend to long-term mental health needs, such as shock, grief and posttraumatic stress syndrome.

Effective leaders need to be able to delegate appropriately and to manage time well. The purposes of **delegation** include increasing organizational efficiency, developing others' talents, and managing time well

(Poteet, 1984; Sullivan and Decker, 1992). Organization efficiency increases when tasks are assigned to the first level in the hierarchy where employees possess the necessary skills and knowledge to complete the task and where the task is related to the goals of those positions. Delegation develops others' talents and can contribute to job satisfaction. Asking a staff nurse in a community nursing clinic for the homeless to develop a booklet describing community resources for the homeless helps the staff nurse learn more about community resources, the gaps that exist in local resources, and where opportunities exist for interagency collaboration. The staff nurse also is likely to learn about visual presentation, layout and brochure design issues, and how to present material at the appropriate reading level. Finally, delegation is an important tool in *time management*. A school nurse may delegate locating resources for a screening clinic to the parent-teacher association and spend the time he or she saves on developing a teaching plan for volunteers who will help with the actual screening. Strategies for effective delegation and time management tips are listed in the boxes below.

Delegation has become a increasingly important skill for community health nurses whether they have an official role as a manager or not. As more agencies increase their use of unlicensed assistive personnel and lay community workers, community health nurses increasingly are delegating selected aspects of practice to others and supervising the completion of those tasks. Two types of delegation occur in clinical practice. Direct delegation involves speaking to an individual personally and transferring responsibility for a task to that person (ANA, 1994). Indirect delegation results when an agency has policies and procedures in place that stipulate the tasks that may be performed by someone else other than the person ultimately accountable (ANA, 1994). Sometimes nurses mistakenly think that they are not accountable for tasks that are indirectly delegated through agency policies (e.g., policies for cross-training). However, if nursing care has been delegated, then nurses are accountable for the safe and effective completion of that care.

The first source of guidance for delegating tasks to unlicensed individuals is the state nurse practice act. The next source of assistance comes from specialty professional organizations. For example, the National Association of School Nurses in collaboration with three other national groups (The Joint Task Force for the Management of Children With Special Needs, 1990) issued detailed guidelines about the school nurse's responsibility in delegation. In general, any task involving specialized knowledge from advanced education cannot be delegated to an unlicensed person. This includes assessment, data analysis, planning, monitoring, and evaluation (National Council on State Boards of Nursing, 1990). For example, a school nurse would assess a child with physical disabilities and develop a plan of care for that child. Selected aspects of that plan of care, such as assisting with feeding, or emptying a catheter bag and recording output, could be delegated to an assistant; providing that person had received appropriate training and was competent to perform the task. This means that it is not adequate that the nurse knows the individual has been certified as a nursing assistant; he or she also needs to know that the individual is competent to safely perform the delegated task. The nurse retains the legal accountability for safe patient care. This responsibility may be shared with the person to whom one is dele-

Strategies for Effective Delegation

Identify who possesses the knowledge and skills to safely and effectively perform the task.

Identify relevant laws and regulations and what they say about delegation to various levels and categories of personnel.

Explain the purpose and desired outcome of the task and the time frame in which the task is to be completed.

Explain any procedures or important elements for the task.

Ask if there are any questions.

Establish times or checkpoints when you expect feedback on progress toward task completion.

If you do not receive feedback at the agreed-upon times, seek it out yourself. Remember, you are ultimately responsible for the safe and effective accomplishment of the task!

Review the process of task accomplishment with the individual, identifying any barriers or things either of you wish to improve the next time.

Praise the individual for a job well done.

Time Management Tips

List your goals for 5 years, 1 year, and daily.

Prioritize the goals.

Identify the tasks you need to perform in order to accomplish the goals.

Identify the tasks you need to perform in order to accomplish the goals.

Identify tasks that can be delegated.

Group the tasks in some meaningful way, e.g., geographically.

Plan strategies to minimize time wasters, e.g., plan office hours when people may find you in your office available to respond to questions.

Plan to work on tasks at times when you are at your peak level of efficiency, e.g., plan tasks requiring mental alertness in the morning if you are more alert at that time.

Plan plenty of time to accomplish tasks with adequate transitional time between tasks.

Say no to tasks that are not essential to your position or your goals.

Take adequate breaks from your work, including breaks during the day and vacations.

Maintain your personal energy level through good health habits, including proper nutrition and adequate exercise and sleep.

gating, but accountability is never transferred (see the box at right).

Finally, a core leadership skill is the ability to *make decisions* effectively. This is a two-stage process in which community health nurse managers first must decide how much input they will seek from others and, second, generate alternatives for the decision and choose among the alternatives. Including others in the decision-making process is beneficial in part because others may have information and ideas that would lead to a better decision and because others may support the decision more if they are involved in making it. However, participatory decision making is more time consuming than making decisions alone. Vroom and Yetton (1973) found that choosing whether to include others in the decision-making process should be based on the extent to which the manager or consultant needs information and ideas from other people, the extent to which those affected are likely to support a decision they do not participate in making, and the extent to which time pressures are present. This model provides a decision-tree for selecting a leadership style that varies from a unilateral, independent decision process, to progressively more participative styles, with the most participative style involving delegating authority to a group to be responsible for making the decision. Although many assume that autocratic decision making is not effective, in fact, it may be both effective and efficient under certain circumstances, such as emergencies. In other situations, it may be better to seek input from others individually, or as a group, or to seek suggestions for solutions from the group, or simply to turn a problem over to a group to solve on their own.

The next stage of the decision-making process is to generate alternative solutions and to choose among those solutions. Bernhard and Walsh (1995) devel-

Delegating Responsibility

Community health nurse managers share responsibility for any tasks they delegate to others. The nurse manager delegates responsibility for a task, but retains final accountability for the safe, effective outcome of the task (ANA, 1994). It is critical then that the community health nurse manager know that the individual to whom they are delegating responsibility is both prepared and capable of effectively completing the task. The community health nurse manager should plan specific times to obtain progress reports on task completion. This will allow the opportunity to manage problems as they arise and to provide staff with helpful feedback or instruction if needed.

oped a useful decision model for nurses. With this model, the nurse determines what characterizes a good decision in the case at hand and then determines what the goal is for that characteristic. For example, both risk and cost are important dimensions in most situations. The goal is low cost and low risk to clients and staff. Other dimensions might be unique to the situation. Table 43-2 illustrates the process of deciding whether to develop an in-house wellness program for an occupational setting or to contract with a consulting group for that service. After identifying the key dimensions and goals, the community health nurse manager ranks each alternative according to how well it is likely to match the goals. For example, if an alternative poses no risk at all, then it completely matches the goal of low risk and receives a ranking of 1. If it poses moderate risk, the nurse might choose to give it a 0.5 and if it poses a high level of risk, he or she may give it a 0 because it does not match the goal at all. After rating each alternative along every dimension,

Table 43-2 Bernhard and Walsh's Decision-Making Model Example Decision: How to Provide Employee Wellness Services

Dimension	Goal	Solution #1 Provide wellness services using current staff		Solution #2 Contract for wellness services with local consultants		Solution #3 Contract with local consultants only for exercise program	
Feasible	Yes	Probably	0.7	Possibly	0.3	Likely	0.8
Risk	Low	Moderate	0.1	Low	1.0	Moderate	0.2
Cost	Low	Low	1.0	High	0.0	High	0.3
Quality	High	Fair	0.5	Excellent	1.0	Moderate	0.5
Certified instructor	Yes	No	0.0	Yes	1.0	Yes	1.0
Fully utilize staff	Yes	Yes	1.0	No	0.0	Partially	0.5
Consistent with company values	Yes	Yes	1.0	Maybe	0.2	Maybe	0.4
		Total = 4.3		Total = 3.5		Total = 3.7	

Modified from Bernhard LA, Walsh M: *Leadership: the key to the professionalization of nursing*, ed 3, St Louis, 1995, Mosby, p 160.

the scores are added and the alternative with the highest score is the one selected for implementation.

In this example, the occupational health nurse manager would choose to develop the wellness program in house, rather than using a consultant. The advantages of this model are that it allows for staff participation in identifying key dimensions and goals and brainstorming creative solutions; participants' values are built into the dimensions and goals, and it allows for both creative and logical thinking processes. This is a particularly helpful decision model for community health nurse consultants.

Community health nurse managers and consultants must be adept at *critical thinking*. Critical thinking incorporates values, makes assumptions explicit, and encourages creativity and innovation (Tappen, 1995). It includes reflection about the connections between sociocultural and biophysiological aspects of health status and services. Critical thinking may be fostered through the use of guided group discussions, in which group members are assisted to think about the connections just described and about the distributional effects that decisions may have on others. It also is fostered through activities to stimulate creativity, such as brainstorming, brainwriting, and nominal group techniques (Marriner-Tomey, 1992). In the example of the occupational wellness program, the nurse manager would need to critically think about ways to enhance program quality.

Interpersonal Skills

Community health nurse managers and consultants need good interpersonal skills in communication, motivation, appraisal and coaching, contracting, supervision, team building, and managing diversity. Good *communication skills,* including skills in the use of assertiveness techniques are essential to being effective in managerial and consultative roles. Community health nurses have a particular challenge in communicating because many of those with whom they work may be in a different health profession or in a different field altogether. Community health nurses often communicate with lay workers also. It is especially critical to listen carefully, to make underlying assumptions clear, and to speak in the other's language. This may mean avoiding the use of professional jargon and speaking in more commonly shared language, or speaking in the listener's dominant language. For example, a community health nurse manager working in a migrant clinic with a large Hispanic population would find it helpful to be fluent in Spanish. Communication must be culturally sensitive to be effective. Because communication involves words, tone of voice, posture, eye contact, and spatial relationships, cultural norms often influence the meanings given to different aspects of body language. For example, whereas most advise direct eye contact when communicating, in some cultures this may be viewed as aggressive, especially when the eye contact is prolonged. Some cultures prefer closer spatial relationships that may make others feel they are being crowded. Other aspects of the communication context are important as well, such as the appropriate place for reprimands. It is never appropriate to reprimand or criticize in public, although public praise is usually an excellent idea. Community health nurse managers and consultants should be sensitive to the power of written communication and be aware that, although putting a message in writing is a good way to avoid confusion, it also may be seen as aggressive, distrustful, or as a bid for power. On the other hand, managers and consultants must accurately document their assessments and interventions (Ingersoll and Jones, 1992). The key is to ensure that the message that is communicated is the message that was intended. Effective communication skills are listed in the box on p. 869.

One of the more difficult skills to master is *motivating* other people. In fact, one cannot ever really motivate others, since motivation is internal. However, the skillful manager can create a motivating environment, working to ensure that both individual and organizational goals are met to the extent possible. Sometimes individual motivation may be low because employees do not believe they have the skills necessary to achieve their goals or they believe that the system will not allow them to do so. The effective community health nurse manager identifies which perceptions are inaccurate and helps individuals develop plans for improving their personal capacities for achieving goals.

Did You Know?

Community health nurse managers and consultants are more likely to be effective when working with people from cultures different from their own if they take the time to learn as much as possible about the culture. This includes learning the language if possible. For example, nurses who are not Native Americans, but who work with Native Americans, should learn about the culture of the tribal groups with whom they are working. Similarly, nurse managers and consultants who work with Vietnamese immigrants (or any other immigrant group) should try to learn about the culture of that group. This helps clarify underlying beliefs, values, and assumptions that may influence managerial or consultative issues and improves communication effectiveness and the effectiveness of change processes. Nurses who are not Hispanic, but work with many Spanish-speaking Hispanic people, will find it helpful to learn to speak conversational Spanish or at least to hire a translator.

Effective Communication Skills

Active listening
Restating the main points
Speaking in the listener's language
Culturally sensitive eye contact and body language
Appropriate context
Awareness of the power of written communication
Simple, direct words
Use of "I" statements and saying how you feel
Frequent feedback
Reflection on the meaning of the message

Although adequate salaries are clearly important, it is not always possible to increase pay in the short run. Community health nurse managers possess other tools for increasing motivation, even when budgets are tight. One home health aide supervisor is known for the high level of morale among her staff and the unusually low level of turnover, despite low salaries. She makes a point of being available for discussion before the aides leave the agency in the morning and upon their return in the afternoon. Also, she always puts a birthday card and small piece of candy in their mailboxes on their birthdays, and thanks them for a job well done (Raab 1991). Other keys to motivation are listed in the box below.

Employee *appraisal and coaching* are closely related to motivation and individual development. The purpose of performance evaluation is to assist employees to more effectively meet the objectives of their roles and to help them develop their potential in ways that facilitate achievement of organizational goals. Performance evaluation should not take place just before

Keys to Motivation

Identify employee needs and goals.
Identify beliefs about their abilities to meet their goals.
Discuss with employees their strengths and areas for future development.
Discuss how the employee's goals and the organizational goals can be meshed.
Jointly develop job-related goals with employees, including timetable with checkpoints.
Provide frequent, regular feedback to employees.
Identify with the employee his or her key reinforcers.
Provide frequent thanks for a job well done and for progress toward goals.
Facilitate the development of mentor-protege relationships and role modeling.
Provide opportunities for employees to learn new goal-related skills.
Provide tangible signs of recognition, such as merit pay, employee of the month, special bonuses for achievements.

an annual appraisal interview is scheduled. It should be a regular part of the job, with the manager providing regular feedback on employee progress toward goals. Performance appraisal is particularly challenging for community health nurse managers because so many community health workers practice independently in the field. For example, nurse managers in home health must plan either to make visits with the nursing staff on a regular basis, or to obtain other forms of input on employee performance, such as planning telephone or office conferences with staff (Knollmueller, 1988; Lee, 1992).

Coaching involves "directing and closely supervising task accomplishment, and explaining decisions, soliciting suggestions, and supporting progress" (Blanchard et al., 1985, pp. 30,56; cited in Vestal, 1995, p. 73). With coaching, managers retain responsibility for decisions, but request input and explain decisions. They support progress by helping the employee break the task into manageable segments, providing resources for task accomplishment and for acquiring the necessary skills, and praising task accomplishment. Coaching is most useful with people who may not yet be skillful in a particular area and who are not confident about the skills they do have (Blanchard et al., 1985).

Contracting involves identifying expectations and responsibilities by both parties. Some contracts are informal, verbal agreements between individuals, while others (such as the consulting contract at the end of the chapter) are formal, written agreements.

Community health nurse managers who delegate tasks to others must *supervise* the completion of those tasks and build in mechanisms to ensure that the tasks are completed safely and effectively (ANA, 1994). The American Nurses Association defines supervision as "the active process of directing, guiding, and influencing the outcomes of an individual's performance of an activity" (ANA, 1994, p. 9). Supervision may occur either on site when the nurse manager is present while the activity is being performed, or off site when the nurse manager "provides direction through various means of written and verbal communication" (ANA 1994, p. 9). It is important for community health nurse managers to build effective means of providing off-site supervision because so many community health activities do not take place within a single agency (e.g., home health care occurs within individual homes, and school health services are provided within individual schools).

Handling criticism is a difficult skill that involves both the give and take of criticism related to job performance. Community health nurse managers should provide constructive criticism as close as possible to the time they observe a problem with an employee's job performance. Constructive criticism is that which focuses on the behaviors necessary to meet the job expectations and helps identify sources of problems, resources for managing problem behavior, and feedback. For example, if an employee is chronically tardy, the community health nurse manager should speak privately with the employee about the job expectation for promptness, identify why the employee is frequently tardy, establish a behavioral goal with time frames and consequences or achieving or not achieving the goal, and assist the employee to develop a plan for achieving the goal. The employee may simply be unaware of the importance of punctuality and can easily change the behavior. On the other hand, a behavior modification plan may be useful to help share the desired behavior (Marriner-Tomey, 1992). Behavioral consequences may include both positive reinforcers, such as praise, and disciplinary measures, such as oral and written warnings, limited raises, suspension, and termination (Sullivan and Decker, 1992). Suspension and termination normally are used only with problems related to safety, inability to perform job duties, breach of confidentiality, and illegal acts and are detailed in organizational policies and procedures.

Finally, *team building* and *managing diversity* are group-level skills needed by community health nurse managers and consultants. Interdisciplinary teams increasingly are used to assess clients, plan client care or services, and manage quality improvement activities. Teams may include members of multiple health disciplines as, for example, with home infusion teams (Sheldon and Bender, 1994). They also may include people from other backgrounds, including lay community health workers, such as Hispanic nurse extenders (Bray and Edwards, 1994). Community health nurse managers and consultants can facilitate team building by assisting the team to develop goals and ground rules, identifying who will fill various roles and determining how to share leadership, developing strategies for ongoing cooperation and recognition of contributions of each member, and resolving conflict (Larson and LaFasto, 1989).

A key challenge to community health nurse managers is managing diversity in positive, growth-promoting ways that value diversity. Because the demographic profile of the American workforce is changing so rapidly, the nature of the workplace is changing as well. Female and nonwhite groups are increasing the most rapidly in the workforce (AARP, 1993), with projections that 25% of the workforce will be composed of African, Hispanic, and Asian Americans by the year 2005 (Mancini, 1995). Community health nurse managers must understand cultural values and norms in order to communicate effectively and interpret behavior accurately. They must know how to prevent any form of racial, sexual, or ethnic harassment, and ensure a positive and welcoming environment in the workplace.

Organizational Skills

Community health nurse managers and consultants use organizational skills, such as planning, organizing,

implementing and coordinating, monitoring and evaluating, improving quality, and managing fiscal resources. *Planning* includes prioritizing daily activities in order to achieve goals. It also includes long-range planning, such as working with nurses in a department to plan a new program. Because planning is primarily a cognitive activity, community health nurse managers and consultants may deemphasize its importance and allow little time for adequate planning. However, planning is the basis for direct nursing services, so it is important to make adequate time for planning. Several documents are available to help community health nurse managers and consultants plan nursing services. *Healthy People 2000* (Healthy People 2000, 1991) delineates the national health goals for the United States by the year 2000 and should be the basis for program planning. Each community has different needs and strengths that should be incorporated into health planning. *Model Standards for Community Health Programs* (APHA, 1992) provides guidelines for adapting the year 2000 objectives to local conditions and baseline local health indicators. *The Assessment Protocol for Excellence in Public Health (APEX-PH)* (National Association of County Health Officials, 1991) gives detailed suggestions for maximizing a health department's ability to work with the community in meeting the year 2000 objectives. A *Planned Approach to Community Health (PATCH)* (Kreuter, 1992) provides guidelines for ways to work in partnership with the community to develop strategies for improving personal and community health.

Community health nurses and consultants must collaborate with other disciplines to provide *coordinated services* for target populations requiring multiple services from diverse agencies. For example, high-risk students have problems that are not neatly categorized as health or education problems (Igoe, 1994). Therefore, school nurses must work cooperatively with others to plan for comprehensive services. One model for doing this is the Five-Stage Process for Change (Figure 43-7) (Melaville et al., 1993), which is based on a partnership process built on trust. This model includes the following stages: (1) organizing a group of people interested in the problem, (2) building trust and commitment to solving the problem, (3) developing a strategic plan for managing the problem, (4) taking action, and (5) adapting the model to other situations and solidifying the program within the organizational structure.

Organizing involves determining appropriate sequencing and timelines for the activities necessary to achieve goals and arranging for the appropriate people to carry out elements of the plan. Flow sheets and timetables are helpful tools that allow community health nurse managers and consultants to visualize how tasks are organized and to identify gaps in the planning.

Implementing a plan includes not only following the timelines, but also ensuring adherence to relevant

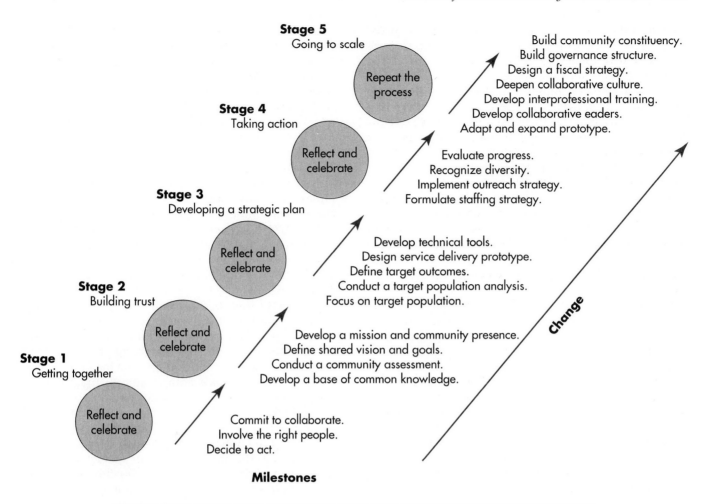

Stage 5
Going to scale

Build community constituency.
Build governance structure.
Design a fiscal strategy.
Deepen collaborative culture.
Develop interprofessional training.
Develop collaborative eaders.
Adapt and expand prototype.

Stage 4
Taking action

Evaluate progress.
Recognize diversity.
Implement outreach strategy.
Formulate staffing strategy.

Stage 3
Developing a strategic plan

Develop technical tools.
Design service delivery prototype.
Define target outcomes.
Conduct a target population analysis.
Focus on target population.

Stage 2
Building trust

Develop a mission and community presence.
Define shared vision and goals.
Conduct a community assessment.
Develop a base of common knowledge.

Stage 1
Getting together

Commit to collaborate.
Involve the right people.
Decide to act.

Change

Milestones

FIGURE 43-7

The five-stage process for change. (From Melaville AI, Blank MJ, Asayesh G: *Together we can: a guide for crafting a pro-family system of education and human services*, Washington, DC, 1993, US Government Printing Office.)

regulations, that appropriate documentation of activities, and coordination of the work of all team members. Community health nurse managers and consultants must ensure that sufficient attention has been given to the change process, by helping those involved identify the need for change, keeping them informed, soliciting their input, and making changes in the plan as necessary.

Monitoring and *evaluating* are critical to community nursing services. Community health nurse managers should monitor nursing services on a regular basis and make improvements as soon as the need for improvements becomes apparent. Professional standards and the standards of various accrediting bodies guide the focus of monitoring and evaluating. The Joint Commission on Accreditation of Healthcare Organizations standards for home health and ambulatory care clinics provides detailed and explicit minimum standards that all such agencies should be expected to meet. Community nursing agencies utilize the National League for Nursing's Community Health Accreditation Program (CHAP) standards for ensuring quality

(Davis, 1992). Specialized regulations are in place for diagnostic laboratory procedures and facilities through the Clinical Laboratory Improvement Amendments (CLIA) (Final CLIA regulations, 1992). Home health agencies must conform to Medicare guidelines (Harris, 1993) and accreditation policies are being developed for occupational health (Yodaiken and Zeitz, 1993).

In addition to professional standards of practice available from the American Nurses Association and specialty nursing organizations, the Agency for Health Care Policy and Research has convened numerous Patient Outcomes Research Teams (PORTs) that have searched the literature to determine which clinical procedures yield the best client outcomes. These best practices have been summarized and published as clinical guidelines for specialized conditions, such as benign prostatic hypertrophy and pain. Although adhering to the clinical guidelines is voluntary, health professionals may need to justify not following them if client outcomes are poor. Managed care organizations are likely to use guidelines in order to standardize the process of care and needs for resources. One of the challenges for the community health nurse manager and consultant is keeping abreast of the numerous standards applicable to his or her practice setting and the changes in those standards.

One example of a guideline that is useful in making programmatic decisions is the concept of screening test sensitivity and specificity. When planning screening clinics, community health nurse managers must choose tests that are both sensitive and specific. A test is sensitive to a health problem when it is likely to detect all cases of the problem, and not give false negatives. On the other hand, to be useful, a test must also be specific to that health problem and not erroneously yield false positives. These concepts provide a useful decision making tool for the community health nurse manager. Formulas for determining sensitivity and specificity, and guidelines for screening programs are in the box below.

Finally, community health nurse managers must be skilled in the area of fiscal management. Community health nurse managers and consultants must be able to forecast the cost of nursing services. This is especially important in a managed care environment because the forecast must include actuarial risk rating of the likely health and illness experiences of a target population. Combining community health assessment skills, epidemiologic projections, and consultation are key steps in this process. After developing a profile of the anticipated health and illness experiences of a target population, the next step is anticipating the amount and kind of nursing resources needed by the population. These skills are basic to the development of proposals for managed care contracts.

Community health nurse managers have taken on more responsibility for developing and monitoring their own department budgets as agencies have decentralized. They must be able to develop a justifiable budget and monitor how actual expenditures compare with planned expenditures. The box on p. 873 lists the usual expenses to be included in an operating budget. It is helpful to obtain staff input when developing a budget in order to make fiscal projections as realistic as possible. It may be necessary to prepare a revenue budget as well if a program anticipates bringing in revenues either from different sources or that vary with the volume of services provided. Combining anticipated volume, revenues, and expenses allows the community health nurse manager to anticipate a break-even point for new services (i.e., determining when a new program can be expected to be financially self-sufficient).

Table 43-3 depicts a portion of a variance report. **Variance analysis** means identifying the variation between actual and planned results, determining the cause of the variation, and correcting problems when they exist. Spending more than anticipated is not always negative; it may simply indicate that client or service volume was higher than anticipated. Higher expenditures than planned are not always under the control of the community health nurse manager. For example, if the prevailing wage rate increases because of changes in the labor market, an agency may spend more than expected on salaries. On the other hand, spending less than predicted does not always indicate that a program is running efficiently. It may be that client volume is down, or that staff are not providing adequate services.

Screening Test Sensitivity and Specificity

$$\text{Sensitivity} = \frac{\text{Number of true-positives}}{\text{Number of true-positives} + \text{Number of false-negatives}} \times 100$$

$$\text{Specificity} = \frac{\text{Number of true-negatives}}{\text{Number of true-negatives} + \text{Number of false-positives}} \times 100$$

Criteria for a Screening Program

- Test has high sensitivity and specificity.
- Test meets acceptable standards of simplicity, cost, safety, and patient acceptability.
- Disease that is focus of screening should be sufficiently serious in terms of incidence, mortality, disability, discomfort, and financial cost.
- Evidence suggests that the test procedure detects the disease at a significantly earlier stage in its natural history than it would present with symptoms.
- A generally accepted treatment that is easier or more effective than treatment administered at the usual time of symptom presentation must be available.

- The available treatment is acceptable to patients as established by studies on compliance with treatment.
- Prevalence of the target disease should be high in the population to be screened.
- Follow-up diagnostic and treatment service must be available and accompanied by an adequate notification and referral service for those positive on screening.

Modified from Valanis B: *Epidemiology in nursing and health care*, ed 2, Norwalk, Conn, 1992, Appleton & Lange, pp 336, 342.

Components of an Operating Budget

Salaries
    Direct salary costs
        Staff
        Fringe benefits
Expenses
    Direct expenses
        Supplies
        Equipment
        Travel
    Other
Overhead
    Administration
    Depreciation
    Ancillary services
    Marketing
    Other

Modified from Finkler SA, Kovner CT: *Financial management for nurse managers and executives,* Philadelphia, 1993, WB Saunders.

Table 43-3   Variance Report

Item	Expected budget	Actual budget	Variance
Salaries	$40,000	$42,000	($2,000)
Supplies	750	1,000	(250)
Travel	1,000	600	400
Total	$41,750	$43,600	($1,850)

In the example in Table 43-3, the community health nurse manager observes that more has been spent on salaries and supplies than originally budgeted and less on travel. Is this desirable or undesirable? In order to analyze the variance the nurse should ask if the prices for labor and supplies were higher than expected (wage rate or price variance) or if the agency has used more nursing time or supplies than planned (quantity variance) (Finkler and Kovner, 1993). The answers to these questions will help determine whether the variance resulted from factors under the manager's control, such as inefficiency, or from factors outside of the manager's control, such as higher wage rates or higher prices than expected. The answers also will help determine if the variance resulted from an increase in patient volume or an alteration in case mix, with the agency serving sicker patients. Whether a volume variance or case mix alteration is seen as desirable will depend partly on whether the agency is paid on a fee-for-service basis or on a capitated basis. In a capitated environment, higher volume will be viewed in a more positive light if the services are primary care, health promotion services and more negatively if the services are inpatient, acute care services. On the other hand, in the traditional fee-for-service environment, there is a stronger incentive to prefer higher volume in the inpatient, acute care areas.

Political Skills and Power Dynamics

Political skills include negotiation skills, conflict resolution skills, and skills in recognizing and managing power dynamics. Principled **negotiation** (Marriner-Tomey, 1992) involves bargaining based on the characteristics of the issues, rather than focusing on participant personalities. This form of negotiation emphasizes collaborative problem solving, rather than rigid adherance to a single position. It does not imply compromising values or goals, but instead emphasizes development of mutually agreeable ways of achieving goals. **Conflict resolution** strategies can result in win-win, win-lose, or lose-lose outcomes. Strategies most likely to create win-win situations include collaboration, confronting problems directly, and ensuring that all parties have adequate opportunity for input (Sullivan and Decker, 1992).

Community health nurse managers and consultants must understand **power dynamics.** Because nurses possess altruistic values, they may believe that being powerful is not necessary. However, it is impossible to create health promoting clinical services without some legitimacy in decision-making arenas. Community health nurse managers need power to ensure that working conditions are conducive to excellent clinical care. Power may originate in information, knowledge, and positioning. Community health nurse managers who are knowledgeable about health care trends and issues, client needs, and clinical services are more likely to possess expert power. Membership on community agency boards and advisory committees positions community health nurse managers to influence service delivery.

Consultants' advice may be followed because of perceived expert power. The client feels that the consultant possesses superior knowledge or skills and is trustworthy and credible. The internal nurse consultant may have legitimate power resulting from his or her role in the organization. The external consultant has only assumed authority, which may result in conflict for the consultant and the client (Polk, 1980). The client may not feel obligated to implement the recommendations. On the other hand, external consultants may possess referent power because of an affiliation with other well-known consultants or a national organization. The consultant's ability to persuade clients by offering reasons, new techniques, or methods of problem solving may establish the consultant's informational power.

EDUCATIONAL REQUIREMENTS

First-line community health nurse managers should have undergraduate preparation in management and leadership theory and in application of these theories in community health agencies. The educational requirements for the community health nurse consultant are determined by the practice setting and the client population. The nurse with undergraduate preparation may serve as a generalist nurse consultant to individuals, families, and groups of clients with identified health problems, such as hypertension or diabetes. The consultant serves either as a facilitator to seek a problem's solution or as a resource to provide community referrals. This nurse also may consult with other health provider agencies involved with client groups, such as hospitals, clinics, and physicians.

 ## Clinical Application

The nurse manager of a nursing clinic in a residential facility for frail elderly approached the local College of Nursing for assistance with health promotion and health monitoring activities for the residents. The facility was undergoing renovation and was expected to more than triple its capacity by the time the renovation was completed. The nurse manager thought the health promotion activities that were already in place would be inadequate to serve the growing needs. Most of the residents were over 70 years of age and had several chronic illnesses each. The residential complex was 10 to 15 miles away from health care facilities. Sheila, the nurse manager, supervised a staff of three nurses and one homemaker aide. She contracted with a local physical therapy firm for services as needed for the residents. Sheila had asked the staff if they thought they could realistically expand their services and they suggested consultation. The staff commented that residents really needed nurses who could provide health monitoring and skilled nursing services in their apartments, because so many were getting increasingly homebound. Staff members were hesitant about expanding into home care themselves because they feared it would mean a cutback in the health promotion activities they were currently engaged in. They thought the needs and the resources that would be required to meet the needs should be evaluated before making any final decisions. The nurse manager thus used a participative approach to making the decision to obtain external consultation. The community health faculty member assigned Patricia, a community nursing student, to *assess* this community's request for consultation.

Patricia met with the nurse manager and the manager of the residential complex to discuss the problem, assess her ability to help, and explore the client's expectations for herself and for the College of Nursing. After careful consideration, Patricia and the nurse manager determined that a survey of residents' needs, community resources, and staff perceptions would assist them in *planning* the alternatives they could explore for providing additional health promotion and health monitoring to the residents.

With the approval of the community health faculty member, Patricia and her fellow students agreed to *implement* a health screening survey project and to collect data about the residential program, such as the physical facilities, the available equipment and supplies, and staff available to provide assistance with health screening and promotion activities. They collected data on existing relationships with community referral sources, including local home care programs, money available to support program expansion at the residential facility, and the attitudes of staff and residents toward expansion. Anticipated outcomes to be *evaluated* for the consultation included recommending to the management of the residential program that home care services be made more accessible for residents using one of several options. The facility might contract for such a program with the College of Nursing, or develop a service contract with the health department for a satellite home care agency on facility grounds, or it might provide space for a proprietary home care agency to operate within the facility.

At the evaluation conference, Patricia and her colleagues shared the results of their data collection. After careful consideration of the data, the nurse manager and the manager of the residential facility agreed that residents needed more access to home care and decided to develop a contract with the College of Nursing for provision of home nursing services on site. This would enable the current staff to devote their energies to aggregate health promotion activities.

Key Concepts

◆ The goals of community health nursing management are (1) to achieve organizational and professional goals for client services and clinical outcomes, (2) to empower personnel to perform their responsibilities effectively and efficiently, (3) to develop new services that will enable the organization to respond to emerging community health needs.

◆ Community health nurses use micro-level management theories to help them function in

Key Concepts—cont'd

leadership roles, facilitate individual and group motivation, and foster effective group dynamics. Macro-level management theories provide direction for planning and organizing work, obtaining resources necessary to achieve organizational goals, and managing power dynamics.

◆ Community health nurse managers may be team leaders or program directors, directors of home health agencies or community-based clinics, or commissioners of health. The function as visionaries, coaches, facilitators, role models, evaluators, advocates, community health and program planners, and teachers. They have ongoing responsibilities for clients, groups, and community health, and for personnel and fiscal resources under their direction.

◆ The goal of consultation is to stimulate clients to take responsibility, feel more secure, deal constructively with their feelings and with others in interaction, and internalize skills of a flexible and creative nature.

◆ Consultation models can be categorized as content or process models. Both purchase-of-expertise and the doctor-patient models are content models. Purchase-of-expertise model consultation involves hiring an expert to provide information or service. In the doctor-patient model of consultation, the client hires the consultant to find the problem and offer solutions without background data or assistance from the client. Process model consultation assists the client with assessing both the problem and the kind of help needed to solve the problem.

◆ Five basic intervention modes or techniques applied to process consultation are acceptant, catalytic, confrontation, prescriptive, and theory principles. The use of a particular intervention mode is based on the client and the problem. Four categories of problems are power/authority, morale/cohesion, norms/standards, and goals/objectives.

◆ Consultation involves seven basic phases: initial contact, definition of the relationship, selection of setting and approach, data collection and problem diagnosis, intervention, reduction of involvement and evaluation, and termination.

◆ Nurse consultants may function as internal consultants within an organization or external consultants outside the client organization.

◆ Community health nurse managers and consultants use a wide variety of skills, including leadership, interpersonal, organizational, and political skills. Leadership skills include abilities to influence others to work toward achieving a vision, empower others, balance attention to people and tasks, delegate tasks, manage time, and make decisions effectively. Interpersonal skills include communication, motivation, appraisal and coaching, contracting, team building, and diversity management skills. Organizational skills include planning, organizing, and implementing community health nursing services, monitoring and evaluating services, quality improvement, and managing fiscal resources. Political skills are those used in negotiation and conflict management and managing power dynamics.

◆ Generally, both community health nurse managers and consultants must hold a baccalaureate degree in nursing or higher. Organizations employing nurses without this credential should help them obtain additional education in the areas of community health nursing, management theories and principles, and theories and principles of consultation.

Critical Thinking Activities

1. Discuss with your class members the implications that managed care has for nurse managers and consultants in community-based organizations and in public health departments. What other implications can you think of in addition to those described in the text?

2. Draft a vision and mission statement for a community health nursing clinic with your classmates. Develop goals and objectives that follow the vision and mission you selected. What type of employees would you need to hire? List some of the policies and procedures you would need to have in such a clinic based on your vision, mission, goals, and objectives.

3. Have several class members obtain the vision, mission, and philosophy statements from several agen-

Continued.

Critical Thinking Activities—cont'd

cies in which students have community health clinical experiences. Compare these statements in terms of the agencies' target populations, basic values, and essential functions.

4. Interview one or more practicing community health staff nurses. Ask them to describe the activities of their jobs that could be categorized as consultation. During the interview, attempt to determine the following:

   a. How they define consultation.

   b. The goals they are attempting to achieve with their consulting activities.

   c. The model they seem to be applying in their consulting activities.

   d. The intervention modes they use.

   e. Whether their activities are of a generalist or a specialist nature and of an internal or external consultative nature.

   f. The strengths and limitations they perceive in themselves regarding their consultative functions (e.g., educational, experiential, organizational, relational, economic).

5. Interview one or more community health nurse consultants. During the interview, attempt to determine the answers to the preceding questions. Compare the responses of the two groups (consultants and staff nurses). Analyze the factors you think account for the similarities and differences.

Bibliography

Aiken LH, Salmon ME: Health care workforce priorities: what nursing should do now, *Inquiry* 31(3):318-329, 1994.

Alderfer CP: *Existence, relatedness, and growth: human needs in organizational settings,* New York, 1972, Free Press.

American Association of Retired Persons (AARP): *America's changing workforce,* Washington, DC, 1993, American Association of Retired Persons.

American Nurses Association (ANA), Council of Community Health Nurses: *Standards of community health nursing practice,* Kansas City, Mo, 1986, American Nurses Association.

American Nurses Association (ANA): *Standards for organized nursing services and responsibilities of nurse administrators across all settings,* Kansas City, Mo, 1988, American Nurses Association.

American Nurses Association (ANA): *Registered professional nurses and unlicensed assistive personnel,* Washington, DC, 1994, American Nurses Publishing.

American Public Health Association (APHA): *Health communities 2000: model standards,* ed 3, Washington, DC, 1992, American Public Health Association.

Bandura A: *Social learning theory,* Englewood Cliffs, NJ, 1977, Prentice-Hall.

Beare P: The ABC's of external consultation, *Clin Nurse Spec* 2(1):35-38, 1988.

Beecroft P: The consultant's image, *J Nurs Adm* 18(2):7-10, 1988.

Berger MC, Ray LN, Del Togno-Armanasco V: The effective use of consultants, *J Nurs Adm* 23(7/8):65-69, 1993.

Bernhard LA, Walsh M: *Leadership: The key to the professionalization of nursing,* ed 3, St Louis, 1995, Mosby.

Blake R, Mouton J: *Consultation,* ed 2, Reading, Mass, 1983, Addison-Wesley.

Blanchard L, Zigmari P, Zigmari D: *Leadership and the one minute manager,* New York, 1985, William Morrow & Co.

Bray ML, Edwards LH: A primary health care approach using Hispanic outreach workers as nurse extenders, *Pub Health Nurs* 11(1):7-11, 1994.

Burns JM: *Leadership,* New York, 1978, Harper and Row.

Burns T, Stalker GM: *The management of innovation,* London, 1961, Tavistock.

Caplan G: *The theory and practice of mental health consultation,* New York, 1970, Basic Books.

Collins B: Do you need an external consultant: a model for decision making, *Clin Nurse Spec* 3(2):91-96, 1989.

Davis CK: Deemed status for CHAP: a new standard for health care, *Nurs Health Care* 13:294-295, 1992.

D'Auno T, Sutton RI, Price RH: Isomorphism and external support in conflicting institutional environments: a study of drug abuse treatment units, *Acad Management Journal* 34:636-661, 1991.

Dienemann J, editor: *Continuous quality improvement in nursing,* Washington, DC, 1992, American Nurses Publishing.

Essential Public Health Services Work Group: Public health in America, *The Nation's Health* pp 1, 3, Dec 1994.

Evans B, Reynolds P, Cockman P: Consulting and the process of learning, *Journal of European Industrial Training* 16(2):7-11, 1992.

Fiedler FE: *A theory of leadership effectiveness,* New York, 1967, Mc-Graw-Hill.

0Final CLIA regulations: Clinical Laboratory Improvement Amendments. *Health Devices* 21:42-425, 1992.

Finkler SA, Kovner CT: *Financial management for nurse managers and executives,* Philadelphia, 1993, WB Saunders.

Greenblatt A: Guiding your consultant, *Association Management* 46(2):63-67, 1994.

Greenleaf RK: *Servant leadership: a journey into the nature of legitimate power and greatness,* New York, 1991, Paulist Press.

Guzik VL, McGovern PM, Kochevar LK: Role function and job satisfaction: a study of nurse graduates of educational resource center programs employed by the health care industry, *AAOHN J,* 40(11):521-530, 1992.

Hackman JR, Oldham GR: Motivation through the design of work, *Organizational Behavior and Human Performance* 16:250-279, 1976.

Harris MD: The peer review organization process revisited, *Home Health Nurse,* 11(5):67-68, 1993.

Healthy People 2000: national health promotion and disease prevention, objectives, Washington, DC, 1991, USDHHS, Public Health Service.

Hersey P, Blanchard K: *Management of organizational behavior,* ed 5, Englewood Cliffs, NJ, 1988, Prentice-Hall.

Hicks LL, Stallmeyer JM, Coleman JR: *Role of the nurse in managed care,* Washington, DC, 1993, American Nurses Publishing.

House RJ: A path-goal theory of leader effectiveness, *Adm Sci Q* 16:321-338, 1971.

Igoe JB: School nursing, *Nurs Clin North Am* 29(3):443-458, 1994.

Ingersoll GL, Jones LS: The art of consultation, *Clin Nurse Spec* 6(4):218-220, 1992.

The Joint Task Force for the Management of Children with Special Health Needs: *Guidelines for the delineation of roles and responsibilities for the safe delivery of specialized health care in the educational setting.*

Unpublished manuscript, Reston, Va, 1990, *The Council for Exceptional Children.*

Knollmueller RN: Reshaping supervisory practice in home care, *Nurs Clin North Am* 23(2):353-362, 1988.

Kohnke M: *The case for consultation in nursing: design for professional practice,* New York, 1978, John Wiley & Sons.

Kreuter MW: PATCH: Its origins, basic concepts, and links to contemporary public health policy, *J Health Educ* 23(3):134-139, 1992.

Krueger RA: *Focus groups: a practical guide for applied research,* ed 2, Thousand Oaks, Calif, 1994, Sage.

Larson CE, LaFasto FMJ: *Teamwork: what must go right/what can go wrong,* Newbury Park, Calif, 1989, Sage.

Latham GP, Locke E: Self-regulation through goal setting. *Organizational Behavior and Human Decision Processes* 50:212-247, 1991.

Lee RK: The community health manager. In Stanhope M, Lancaster J, editors: *Community health nursing: process and practice for promoting health,* ed 3, St Louis, 1992, Mosby.

LoBiondo-Wood G, Haber J: *Nursing research: methods, critical appraisal, & utilization,* ed 3, St Louis, 1994, Mosby.

Mancini M: Managing cultural diversity. In Vestal KW, editor: *Nursing management: concepts and issues,* Philadelphia, 1995, JB Lippincott.

Manthey M: Empowering staff nurses: decision on the action level, *Nurs Manage* 22(2):16-17, 1991.

Marriner-Tomey A: *Guide to nursing management,* ed 4, St Louis, 1992, Mosby.

Marriner-Tomey A: *Transformational leadership in nursing,* St Louis, 1993, Mosby.

Maslow A: *Motivation and personality,* New York, 1970, Harper and Row.

McCloskey JC: The NMDS is a trend, not a fad, *J Prof Nurs* 10(6):332, 1994.

McCloskey JC, Bulechek GM, editors: *Nursing interventions classification,* St Louis, 1992, Mosby.

McDaniel R, Bach C: Focus groups: a data-gathering strategy for nursing research, *Nurs Sci Q* 7(1):4-5, 1994.

Melaville AI, Blank MJ, Asayesh G: *Together we can: a guide for crafting a pro-family system of education and human services,* Washington, DC, 1993, US Government Printing Office.

Meyer JW, Rowan B: Institutionalized organizations: formal structure as myth and ceremony, *Am J Sociology,* 83:340-363, 1977.

Morgan DL: Successful focus groups: advancing the state of the art, Newbury Park, Calif, 1993, Sage.

National Association of County Health Officials: *APEX-PH: assessment protocol for excellence in public health,* Washington, DC, 1991, National Association of County Health Officials.

National Council on State Boards of Nursing: *Concept paper on delegation.* Unpublished manuscript, Chicago, 1990, National Council of State Boards of Nursing.

Novle J, Harvey K: Selecting and using a nursing consultant, *Nurs Econ* 6(2):83-85, 1988.

Orem D: Nursing administration: a theoretical approach. In Henry B, Arndt C, DiVincenti M, Marriner-Tomey A, editors: *Dimensions of nursing administration: theory, research, education, and practice,* Boston, 1989, Blackwell Scientific Publications.

Pati B: Nursing consultation: a collaborative process, *J Nurs Adm* 10(11):33-36, 1980.

Pfeffer J, Salancik GR: *The external control of organizations: a resource dependence perspective,* New York, 1978, Harper & Row.

Polk GC: The socialization and utilization of nurse consultants, *Psychiatr Nurs* 18:33-36, February, 1980.

Poteet G: Delegation strategies: a must for the nurse executive, *J Nurs Adm* 14(9):18-21, 1984.

Raab M: Personal communication, 1991.

Reinert B, Buck E: Issues in liability insurance and the nursing consultant, *Clin Nurse Spec* 3(1):42-45, 1989.

Rokwood GF: Edgar Schein's process versus content consultation models, *J Counseling & Development* 71:636-638, 1993.

Roy SC, Anway J: Roy's adaptation model: theories for nursing administration. In Henry B, Arndt C, DiVincenti M, Marriner-Tomey A, editors: *Dimensions of nursing administration: theory, research, education, and practice,* Boston, 1989, Blackwell Scientific Publications.

Schaffner J: The consultation you don't want: taking charge, *J Nurs Adm* 17(8):6-7, 1987.

Schein EH: *Process consultation: its role in organizational development,* Reading, Mass, 1969, Addison-Wesley.

Schein EH: Process consultation as a general model of helping. *Consulting Psychology Bulletin* 41:3-15, 1989.

Schein EH: Organizational culture, *Am Psychol* 45:109-119, 1990.

Sheldon P, Bender M: High-technology in home care: an overview of intravenous therapy, *Nurs Clin North Am* 6(2):507-519, 1994.

Simpson RL: Benchmarking MIS performance, *Nurs Manage* 25(1): 20-21, 1994.

Sullivan EJ, Decker PJ: *Effective management in nursing,* ed 3, Redwood City, Calif, 1992, Addison-Wesley.

Tappen RM: *Nursing leadership and management: concepts and practice,* ed 3, Philadelphia, 1995, FA Davis.

Thompson JD: *Organizations in action,* New York, 1967, McGraw-Hill.

Valanis B: *Epidemiology in nursing and health care,* ed 2, Norwalk, Conn, 1992, Appleton & Lange, pp 336, 342.

Vestal KW: *Nursing management: concepts and issues,* Philadelphia, 1995, JB Lippincott.

Vroom VH: *Work and motivation,* New York, 1964, John Wiley & Sons.

Vroom VH, Yetton PW: *Leadership and decision-making,* Pittsburgh, 1973, University of Pittsburgh Press.

Yodaiken RE, Zeitz PS: Accreditation policies in occupational health care, *J Occup Med* 35:562-567, 1993.

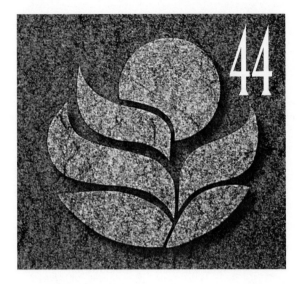

44

Community Health Nurse in the Schools

Judith B. Igoe ◆ Sudie Speer

Objectives ▼

After reading this chapter, the student should be able to do the following:

◆ Describe the functions of school nurses as clinicians and managers.
◆ Examine the three core components of school health.
◆ Identify health-related behaviors and risk factors that contribute to school failure.
◆ Identify and discuss two of the health services provided in schools.
◆ Explain the basic requirements for administration of medications in schools.
◆ Discuss the school health implications of the Individuals with Disabilities Education Act (PL 94:142).
◆ Cite three general goals of health education.
◆ Describe a health education program that empowers the consumer to use the health system effectively.
◆ Explain the four essential steps involved in managing a school health program.
◆ Describe one innovative approach to the planning, organization, and delivery of school health programs.

Key Terms ▼

absenteeism
area education agencies (AEA)
boards of cooperative education services (BOCES)
case-finding
case manager
Certificates of Immunization Status
community health nurse specialist for school-aged children
counseling
Division of Adolescent and School Health (DASH)
Early Periodic Screening Diagnosis and Treatment Program (EPSDT)
environmental health
health education
Individuals with Disabilities Education Act (IDEA)
individualized education plan (IEP)
individualized family service plans (IFSP)
neurodevelopmental evaluations
nontraditional health facilities
primary health care services
school-based health centers (SBHC)
school nurse practitioner (SNP)
screening
vague, nonspecific health complaints

Outline ▼

Health Problems of School-Age Children
History of School Nursing
Components of the School Health Program
    Health Services
    Health Education
    Environmental Health
Roles, Functions, and Credentials for School Nurses
    Specialists
    Credentials
Management of the School Health Program
    The Relationship Between Education Reform and School Health
    Planning
    Organizing
    Directing
    Controlling
Innovations in School Health
    School-Based Health Centers
    Family Resource/Service Centers
    Employee Health

In the United States 46,222,124 children and adolescents attend approximately 110,000 public and private schools (Digest of Educational Statistics, 1989). Although these girls and boys can be described as relatively healthy individuals, the stresses of rapid growth and development and societal pressures create health problems.

"Children as children are constantly growing and developing. This basic dynamic characteristic accounts for both their increased vitality and vulnerability and requires specific health approaches in relation to the child's changing needs" (*Child Health USA 89*, 1989).

HEALTH PROBLEMS OF SCHOOL-AGE CHILDREN

School nurses are in a unique position to help children manage health problems and to provide health education so that children can enjoy good health throughout their school age and adult years. Table 44-1 lists the leading health problems of children, by age groups. It is interesting to note that for school-age children these problems vary substantially between the younger years (5 to 12) and the adolescent years (13 to 19). For children, accidents, cancers (including leukemia), influenza and pneumonia, homicides, upper respiratory infections, malnutrition, and dental disease are the major problems that interfere with their health and school attendance. For adolescents, pregnancy, alcohol and drug abuse, accidents, suicide, homicide, and venereal disease are the most common conditions that lead to school failure.

Since 1977, acute respiratory diseases consistently have been the main reason for absence from school because of illness. Asthma and chronic bronchitis are the leading chronic conditions limiting children's activity (Healthy People 2000, 1991).

The nutritional problems seen in schools may have changed, but they still exist. Today fewer children are undernourished; modern problems are related to overconsumption and imbalances in the types and amounts of food. Many children consume foods high in sugar, fat, and salt and thus increase their risk of becoming obese and acquiring diabetes, heart disease, hypertension, and other chronic degenerative diseases later in life (Guide to Clinical Preventive Services, 1989). Childhood obesity is a serious problem for children aged 2 to 9 years, particularly for females and Hispanic children (*Child Health USA 89*, 1989).

Many children and adolescents have vision and hearing problems. In 1981, state maternal and child health agencies reported that over 250,000 school-age children who received vision screening required treatment. The prevalence rate for myopia ranges from 6% to 20%, with the higher rates occurring in children and youth who are 10 to 14 years of age (Committee on Vision, 1989). The National Society for the Prevention of Blindness (NSPB) estimates that 1 in 500 school children in the United States is partially sighted (Harley, 1983). Hearing loss occurs in 6% of children of all ages, and 0.87% of children are diagnosed as legally deaf (Northern, 1989).

Alcohol is still the most widely abused substance among teenagers, and drug abuse continues. However, recent studies show that alcohol and drug use has declined for this age group. Among high school seniors, 51.0% reported drinking alcohol in the past month and 27.5% reported that they had five or more drinks at one time during the previous 2 weeks in 1993. In 1988, 63.9% of these students reported daily drinking (a decline of 12%), and 34.7% indicated they had five or more drinks in the previous 2 weeks (a decline of 7%) (*Health: United States, 1993*, 1994).

Use of marijuana and cocaine also decreased from 1988 to 1993. The National Center for Health Statistics reported that marijuana use dropped from 18% in 1977 to 15.5% in 1993. Cocaine use by adolescents also was reported to be less, declining from 3.4% in 1988 to 1.3% in 1993 (*Health: United States, 1993*, 1994). Not only is the use of alcohol and drugs among those 12 to 17 years of age reported to be down, the awareness of the risks involved in these behaviors also has generally increased (*Health: United States, 1993*, 1994).

Unfortunately, this profile of declining drug and alcohol use does not hold true for eighth grade and

Table 44-1   Leading Age-Specific Health Problems of Children 1 to 19 Years of Age

Age	Leading causes of death	Common health problems
1-9 years of age	Unintentional injury* Congenital anomalies Malignant neoplasms Homicide Diseases of the heart	Respiratory Injury Infectious and parasitic diseases Digestive system Nervous disorders
10-14 years of age	Unintentional injury* Malignant neoplasms Homicide Suicide Congenital anomalies	Respiratory Injury Digestive system Mental disorders Malnutrition
15-19 years of age	Unintentional injury* Homicide Suicide Malignant neoplasms Diseases of the heart	Pregnancy/childbirth Injury Mental disorders Digestive system Respiratory systems

Modified from US Department of Health and Human Services, Health Resources and Services Administration, Maternal and Child Health Bureau, *Child Health USA '93*, DHHS Pub No HRSA-MCH-94-1. Washington, DC, Mar, 1994 US Government Printing Office.

*Unintentional injury includes motor vehicle accidents, drowning, firearms, fires/burns, falls.

younger students. In 1988 reports of eighth graders' daily drinking habits indicated an increase from 25.1% to 26.2% of eighth grade students in 1993. Marijuana use was reported at 5.1% in 1993. Reports of cocaine use were at 0.7%. (*Health: United States, 1993*, 1994).

In 1985, 1,031,000 teenagers became pregnant; of these, 31,000 were younger than age 15. The outcomes included 477,710 live births; 416,170 induced abortions; and 137,120 spontaneous abortions. For teenagers 15 to 19 years of age, one American in 10 becomes pregnant each year as compared with fewer than one in 20 in Canada, England, and France (*Child Health USA 89*, 1989).

What Do You Think?

Counseling of students with high-risk social behaviors that may result in unintended pregnancy, sexually transmitted diseases, and HIV infection in school districts is considered highly controversial. The health professionals attempting to cope with these issues are viewed negatively and accused of encouraging the very problems they are attempting to resolve.

Each year, 2.5 million teenagers in the United States are infected with a sexually transmitted disease. Seventy-five percent of all sexually transmitted diseases occur among those 15 to 24 years of age. As of 1993, 629 cases of Acquired Immune Deficiency Syndrome (AIDS) were reported in children younger than 13 years of age and there were 456 cases of AIDS reported in adolescents aged 13 through 19 years. Most of the cases in children under 13 years of age involve babies and toddlers. Whereas the majority of cases of AIDS occurring in whites is related to blood product exposure, the majority of cases in blacks and Hispanics is a result of sexual activity and drug use (*Health: United States*, 1993, 1994).

Although adolescents are at risk for HIV infection, they are not well informed about its prevention (Stoto et al., 1990). Consequently, the American School Health Association suggests a broad-based health education approach, addressing the subject of sexually transmitted diseases (STD) in all grades. Financial resources to provide education about AIDS prevention have been substantial, and these funds provide the opportunity for increasing this type of health instruction.

Children do not benefit as much from school when they are not feeling well and are absent. According to Klerman (1988), "Educators believe that students who miss more than 10 days in a 90-day semester (11% of school days) have difficulty in staying at grade level." In 1986, the National Health Survey (NHIS) estimated that students ranging in age from 5 to 17 years lost 226.4 million days of school or 5 days per child. (A missed class day in this instance is classified as an absence only when it occurs as the result of an acute or chronic health condition.) The absentee rate for girls is slightly higher than for boys, and the rate for whites is somewhat higher than for blacks. Children who miss school have a higher rate of visits to the school nurse than other students (Klerman, 1988). Excessive school absence in intermediate and high school often is the result of factors outside the health care sphere. Chaotic family environments, lack of achievement motivation, understaffed and uninviting schools, and other societal problems are the major reasons for repeated absences, school failure, and early school leaving (Klerman, 1988).

Poor children and adolescents are at highest risk for absenteeism and therefore need and deserve special attention from the school nurses. These children often have serious ear infections that will eventually lead to hearing loss if left untreated (Flinn, 1989). Others have repeated upper respiratory infections, bouts with allergies, dental decay, skin disorders, and other clinical disorders that will result in extended periods of absenteeism if diagnostic and treatment services are not readily available. These students are four times as likely to miss school because of their ailments. They are also two to three times more likely to have a health condition that limits their school activity and are twice as likely to have mental health problems (Starfield, 1982). They frequently go without health care because they are uninsured, and they may fail academically, perhaps because adult supervision is lacking. Some are homeless and do not attend school regularly. Others live in homes in which English is a second language and the child does not speak enough English to understand class discussions. Therefore, they soon lose interest in attending school.

Today, 21% of school children in the U.S. are poor; minority youth are most often members of this group (*Health: United States*, 1993, 1994). In 1992, the poverty rate for Hispanics was 2.4 times that for whites but less than the poverty rate for blacks (*Health: United States*, 1993, 1994). Because poor children often are enrolled in the federally sponsored free breakfast and lunch programs offered at schools, school nurses can discreetly use enrollment rosters for these programs to identify those students who are in special need of school health care and access to community health services. Measures should be taken to reduce physical and emotional health problems and poor health habits among these children and youth. Offering diagnostic and treatment services at school may be necessary for these students if no other sources of health care are available in the community. For these girls and boys, these health-related risk factors often set in motion a cycle of absenteeism and school failure.

In addition, children and adolescents want and need to address their own problems. Several surveys of school-age youth reveal that they are interested in learning about health and that health topics are most often at the top of their priority lists. In past surveys of high school students to determine the health needs with which they wanted help, the top five identified were acne, sex education, depression, obesity, and parental disagreements.

The modern health problems of school-age children involve social, emotional, behavioral, and technological issues that require a complex range of services delivered by individuals and systems in a flexible, coordinated, and collaborative manner. Many practitioners, educators, and policymakers have concluded that the school nurse is a key figure in meeting many of the health care needs of students, especially those who are at high risk (Califano, 1986).

The number of students who have disabilities and chronic health conditions and are enrolled in regular school has increased since the enactment of the Education for All Handicapped Children legislation (PL 94-142) in 1975. Over a million more children now have access to a free and appropriate education than previously had access. From 1977 to 1978, about 8.6% of students received special education because of their disabilities; 11.1% received these services in 1987 to 1988. Most of this increase is attributed to the preparation of children identified as learning disabled, which rose from 2% of all children in 1977 to 1978 to 5% of all children in 1987 to 1988 (Digest of Educational Statistics, 1989).

Scientific advances and improved technology make it possible for low-birth-weight babies to survive, for students with chronic and terminal illnesses to enter remission and live with their diseases, and for severely physically disabled youth to communicate with others. Students in the largest category of those eligible for services under PL 94-142 have specific learning disabilities and are usually in good health. However, the health problems experienced by those who do need nursing care at school (related services) have become increasingly complex. The proportion of school-aged children limited in activity by special health needs and reporting to school increased from 4% in 1975 to 6% in 1985 (Kovar, 1988). Among the treatments and procedures some students require at school are medications; bladder catheterization; endotracheal suctioning; colostomy, ileostomy, and ureterostomy care; and nasogastric tube feedings.

At the time of the reauthorization of PL 94-142 in 1991, this legislation was retitled the **Individuals with Disabilities Education Act (IDEA).** This federal law guarantees a free public education and related services for every disabled child from 5 to 21 years of age. The IDEA bill PL 101-476 identifies a number of related services, including health care, physical therapy, occupational therapy, speech therapy, and psychological services. In addition each state has its own plan for implementing this legislation, which can be more specific. In some states, like Colorado, school nursing services are designated as a type of health services that must be available for these students.

HISTORY OF SCHOOL NURSING

Lillian Wald, the nursing director of Henry Street Settlement House in New York City discovered a 12-year-old boy excluded from school because of eczema:

> In the early 1900s, I had been downtown only a short time when I met Louis. An open door in a rear tenement revealed a woman standing over a washtub, a fretting baby on her left arm, while with her right hand she rubbed at the butcher's aprons which she washed for a living.
>
> Louis, she explained was "bad." He did not "cure his head," and what would become of him, for they would not take him into the school because of it? Louis, hanging the offending head, said he had been to the dispensary a good many times. . . . But "every time I go to school Teacher tells me to go home".
>
> It needed only intelligent application for the dispensary ointments to the affected area, and in September I had the joy of securing the boy's admittance to school for the first time in his life (Woodfill and Beyrer, 1991).

Public health efforts in those days concentrated on the control of communicable disease. Thousands of immigrants were crowding into the tenement areas of large cities, such as New York and Boston. With the tenements came the diseases that resulted from poverty and overcrowding. Having identified this child and many more like him, Lillian Wald and her staff carefully compiled a data-based report that soon convinced city officials to introduce physicians into schools to examine students and exclude those with contagious diseases. As an isolated event, these daily inspections created more problems than they solved. Follow-up of treatment and counseling was definitely needed because students and their families were frequently unable to understand the instructions on the exclusion card:

> In many cases the excluded children, not fully understanding the instructions, played on the street with their companions as they came out of school and lost or destroyed the cards. In other instances the cards were taken home, but the parents, often ignorant of the English language, did not understand what the child tried to explain and the Latin names were uncomprehended. . . . In many instances the cards were never looked at but remained in their sealed envelopes while the child played on the street (Rogers, 1908).

After 5 years of medical inspections in schools, thousands of children were excluded because of trachoma, and classrooms were empty. "In a single school three hundred children were out at one time" (Rogers, 1905). Lillian Wald proposed to the boards of health and education that a nurse be sent into the schools. As a demonstration project, Lena Rogers visited four schools daily, spending an hour in each:

Here she dresses or cleanses all such cases as the physician directs, mild cases of conjunctivitis, minor skin infections, such as ring-worm, etc., and the children need not then miss their class-work, as otherwise they would have to do as a matter of protection to the rest. She then visits those who have been sent home, and keeps records of them (Dock, 1902).

Between 1903 and 1904, 39 nurses were recruited by the New York City Health Department, and they were remarkably successful. According to health department records, 98% of students previously excluded from school were retained in classrooms. Improvised dispensaries were set up to treat students on-site. Nurses provided the counseling and instruction necessary to overcome parental fear and indifference. During home visits, nurses found that many students were out of school for social reasons rather than because of disease, and many were "victims of the temptations of the streets" (Struthers, 1917). Others, however, needed clothing and food before they could come to school, and some were caring for younger children while their mothers worked. In a few instances, these children were providing nursing care to family members who were ill. Steps were taken by the nurses to relieve a number of these social problems, and the children returned to school.

By 1909, municipalities throughout the United States were employing school nurses. Initially, the visiting nurse association provided the nursing service on a demonstration basis. If the project was effective, the tax-supported boards of education or health would assume administrative control (Waters, 1909). In 1912 the American Red Cross created a nursing service to meet the school health needs in rural areas (Woodfill, 1991).

The need for school nurses to provide treatment in schools and to focus their efforts almost exclusively on the control of contagious diseases began to diminish around 1916. Different priorities arose with the onset of World War I. In a time when able-bodied men were needed to defend their country, literally thousands of recruits were found to be physically unfit to serve because of poor eyesight, hearing loss, advanced dental disease, or orthopedic defects. Consequently, the importance of early case finding and corrective follow-up during childhood became clear to public health officials. School nurses soon shifted their attention from communicable disease control to primary prevention efforts, such as vision and hearing screening. It was the first organized large scale attempt to proactively improve the long-term health status of American children.

By the 1920s, the role of the school nurse had expanded to include the functions of health educator and counselor. The dual role of school nurse-teacher evolved in 1937. Subsequently, a school nurse-teacher group became a section of the newly formed Department of School Health and Physical Education of the National Education Association (NEA).

Later a separate department of school nurses was formed, which eventually evolved into the National Association of School Nurses (NASN). This organization is now constitutionally separate from the NEA, but a close alliance still exists.

Over the past 40 years, school nurses have been recognized for their humanitarian, preventive, and educational contributions to child and adolescent health. However, the role of school nurse-teacher has been the subject of almost continual debate, and significant clinical roles for school nurses are only now emerging. Fortunately, the duties and functions of school nurses are less ambiguous today, largely because of numerous attempts at standardization of the role and state certification.

During World War II, the nursing shortage became acute, and the school health program became the responsibility of school personnel other than the school nurse and the few physicians who still worked in the field. Consequently, most school nurses gave up their more labor intensive roles as health teachers and counselors to take on the role of health consultant/coordinator/liaison between school, home, and community. Ironically their school assignments doubled and tripled under this arrangement and no extra personnel (e.g., health assistants) were added at the building level to carry out the various screenings, simple health instructions, and follow-up activities. Consequently, the quality of school health programs deteriorated.

By the end of the 1960s, many working mothers and worried school administrators recognized the educational and economic advantages of offering more diagnostic services and treatment services at school. Thus, the clinical role of the school nurse practitioner appeared. Over the last two decades, the importance of the health consultant role and school-teacher roles has diminished, and the school nurse practitioner role has become more prominent. In turn, all school nurses gradually have become more clinically competent and are providing more case management services.

Various studies have shown that success with the school nurse clinician role requires administrative support, clerical and paraprofessional assistance, available medical consultation, and the presence of others to participate in the planning, coordination, operation, and management of the overall school health program (Goodwin, 1981; Meeker et al., 1986). In the past, the only dollars allocated for school health were salaries for school nurses. Consequently, the strategy today for finding the resources necessary to develop a comprehensive school health program, in which the school nurse clinician is a member of an interdisciplinary team, requires reorganization of schools and community health agencies to consolidate child and adolescent health efforts. Therefore, to be truly effective, school health programs need to include, in addition to the nurse, an array of health,

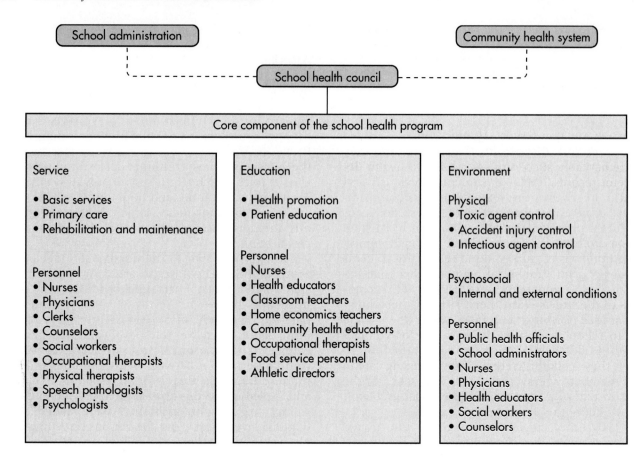

FIGURE 44-1

The organization of the school health program. (From School Health Programs, University of Colorado Health Science Center, 1989).

social service, and education personnel who are prepared to deal with the health-related problems of students. These new developments in school health also present new opportunities for nurses to become school health managers or health coordinators.

With one foot in nursing and the other in education, school nurses often have balanced precariously on the periphery of both fields. Unfortunately, there has been little power or recognition in either field. However, major changes are underway, and these frustrations have become tolerable as the public and policymakers recognize the value of improving health programs in schools. Here it is possible to enhance the health status of all boys and girls and to provide special attention to those who have no other regular source of health care or whose health condition requires special nursing care for them to attend school. The history of school nursing clearly reflects the evolving nature of this role. A chronology of other health, education and social events that have contributed to its development and to the school health movement is in Table 44-2.

COMPONENTS OF THE SCHOOL HEALTH PROGRAM

The three cord components of school health are health services, health education, and a healthy environment. Figure 44-1 illustrates the services and the personnel involved. The rough estimate for 1987 expenditures for basic school health services, not including primary health care and the services of nurse practitioners, was $13/student/year (Walker et al., 1990). This figure is exclusive of the costs involved in providing classroom health education and maintaining a healthy environment. No national estimates for these components of school health are currently available.

The Centers for Disease Control and Prevention, **Division of Adolescent and School Health (DASH)** defines school health according to an eight-component model: (1) health services, (2) health education (3) healthful school environment, (4) physical education, (5) guidance and psychologic services, (6) food services, (7) school community health promotion efforts, and (8) site health promotion for faculty and staff. Difficulties in implementing this definition of school

Text continued on p. 889.

Table 44-2   Chronology: A Listing of Events Significant in the History of School Health Services

Developments in school health services	Developments in education
1800 First school physicians and nurses hired in Europe (1834-1892)	**1800** Child labor reform and emergence of a public education system
1894 First medical inspections began in Boston schools to identify and exclude students with communicable disease; no follow-up	**1890** Responsibility for school health assigned to local school boards because health departments not in existence in every town Minimal school health instruction
COMMUNICABLE DISEASE CONTROL	
1900 Classroom inspections expand to include screening for ringworm, scabies, impetigo, malnutrition Proper hygiene practices demonstrated in school and home Minor cases of contagion treated at school (e.g., dressing changes)	
1902 Home visits for sanitary inspection, follow-up on excluded students, truancy, social problems; as a result, school attendance escalates	
1910 Emergency services now available in schools School inspections expand to individualized medical examinations to identify and correct defects	**1910** School health instruction is combined with medical inspection; teachers rarely participate and health professionals do the health teaching
1920 Red Cross provides school nursing services to rural America	
1924 Employee health services incorporated into school health; Rogers' report recommends teachers have health exams and tuberculin tests	
1930 Mass screenings for early casefinding (i.e., vision, hearing, dental caries, orthopedic defects) increasingly widespread Counseling, health education, and consultation offered in conjunction with health services	**1930** Federal school lunch program starts. (Department of Agriculture)
1934 School nurses/physicians services are overextended and quality of services deteriorates (National Organization of Public Health Nursing [NOPHN] Study)	
HEALTH GUIDANCE AND CONSULTATION	
1940 Nonstatutory ban on school-based diagnosis and treatment widely enforced First/aid emergency services closely identified with school nurses despite their "no more bandaides" campaign to delegate more responsibilities for non-nursing tasks to other school personnel Service more public health oriented (e.g., coordinating community services for students)	**1940** First coordinated integrated health education curriculum developed
1945 School health councils advocated as a means for organizing school health programs	
1950 School health services under review by American Public Health Association (APHA), American Nurses Association (ANA), American School Health Association (ASHA)	

From Office of School Health, University of Colorado Health Sciences Center, 1995.   *Continued.*

Table 44-2   Chronology: A Listing of Events Significant in the History of School Health Services—cont'd

Developments in school health services	Developments in education
PRIMARY CARE	
1960 Comprehensive health histories recommended in lieu of cursory school examinations; record-keeping excessive and not effective for planning purposes	1960 Title I-Elementary and secondary education act authorized provisions for health and nutrition services OED
1969 Introduction of the first pilot for school-based primary health care using school nurse practitioners (Denver Public Schools)	1970 Child Find Screenings begin to identify students eligible for special services under PL 94-142 Handicapped Children's Act
1974 Special services available for students with disabilities, handicaps, chronic illness (i.e., medication administration, catheterization) New school health personnel (clerks, occupational therapist, physical therapist, psychologist, speech pathologist, substance abuse counselors)	White House Conference on Children and Youth recommendations for early childhood education and day care Immigration of Vietnamese/Indo-Chinese refugees with third world health problems; complex cultural and language barriers must be overcome
	1978 School Health Education Study procedures comprehensive curriculum models for health education (Grades K-12)
1979 Private agencies (including hospitals) assume the management of some school health programs on an experimental basis in New York	1979 Growing Healthy curriculum adopted nationwide; well-validated program reported to produce health behavior changes in elementary school students Teenage Health Modules will develop later and also will be disseminated nationally
HEALTH PROMOTION/SPECIAL NEEDS	
1980 National School Health Services Program, Robert Wood Johnson Foundation (1980-1985); demonstrates the effectiveness of school-based diagnosis and treatment by school nurse practitioners. Emphasis on elementary schools	1980 School Reform movement underway; parent participation increases Carnegie Foundation Report *Turning Points* recommends numerous changes in middle school including the establishment of family resource centers and a new role for a health coordinator Student assistance programs to prevent drug and alcohol abuse proliferate under the leadership of guidance counselors
1986 The School Based Adolescent Health Care Program (SBAHC), Robert Wood Johnson Foundation; increased the number of school-based health centers with diagnostic and treatment services (1986-1992); school based clinics now concentrate on adolescent services Main obstacles: conservative public opinion, financing, integration with the rest of school health program Disease prevention, health promotion services flourish: health hazard appraisals; fitness/endurance/cardiovascular risk screening; student health fairs	1987 Youth 2000 campaign launched by the business community to combat the school dropout problem Division of Adolescent and School Health, Center for Chronic Disease Prevention and Health Promotion, Centers for Disease Control established
1990 Clinical services, health education, health promotion, environmental measures increasingly overlap; growing emphasis on environmental health	1990 Numerous initiatives begin to support integrated services between health, education, and social services
1995 Institute of Medicine Study of School Health; proceedings encompass extensive literature review of the field	
1995 School Health Resource Services program opens at the University of Colorado Office of School Health; first National Resource Center, 1-800-669-9954	

Table 44-2 Chronology: A Listing of Events Significant in the History of School Health Services—cont'd

Developments in pediatrics, nursing, public health	Social and legislative developments
1800 Fundamental discoveries in bacteriology	**1897** First appropriation by states for care of handicapped children, Minnesota
1908 First Bureau of Child Hygiene established in N.Y.C.	**1904** Child labor legislation
1909 School nursing services provided from visiting nurse associations First White House Conference recommends Federal Children's Bureau	
1912 Discovery of numerous serious health defects among army recruits	**1912** Act of 1912, Children's Bureau established
1913 School Nursing Committee created within the National Organization for Public Health Nursing (NOPHN) Lina Rogers Struthers, chairman	**1915** Rockefeller Foundation well-child clinics and clean-milk stations
1918 Schools of Public Health open	
1920 All cities with population of 100,000+ have maternal and child health services in most state health departments Second White House Conference advocates standards of MCH; consumer education is stressed School nurse established as faculty member in New York State and referred to as School Nurse-Teacher	**1921** Maternity and Infancy Act (Sheppard-Towner) federal grant-in-aid to the states
1926 National Organization for Public Health Nursing published its first statement on the objectives, scope of work, and methods in school nursing	**1924** An alliance develops between the National Education Association and the American Medical Association "Health education, not health services is the proper role for the schools."
1927 American School Health Association (ASHA) is formed	
1930 American Academy of Pediatrics is formed	**1935** Title V; Social Security Act enacted; Maternal and Child Health Care Services authorized
1937 School nurses became a section of the new Department of School Health and Physical Education of the National Education Association; eventually this section evolved into the National Association of School Nurses	
1939 Crippled Children's Services from State Health Department expand	
1940 Delegation of school nurse tasks to teachers, health clerks, volunteers 50% of all public health nurses are employed in school health	
1941 First edition of *The Nurse in the School* published by the Joint Committee of the National Education Association and the American Medical Association (Second edition released in 1955)	
1944 Selective service reports Army recruits have numerous health defects Committee on School Nursing Policies and Practices of the American School Health Association established (Name changed in 1958 to School Nursing Committee and since the late 1960s referred to as the Study Committee on School Nursing)	
1949 Significant increases in number of school nurses employed by health departments	

Continued.

Table 44-2   Chronology: A Listing of Events Significant in the History of School Health Services—cont'd

Developments in pediatrics, nursing, public health	Social and legislative developments
1950 White House Conference demands a ban on racial public school segregation Concept of school health team develops	1954 *Brown v. Board of Education*; a civil rights case that over-turned the "separate but equal" doctrine in public schools
1960 White House Conference on Children and Youth has youth participation for the first time; profound con-cern about drug abuse, increases in the incidence of venereal diseases, illegitimate births, inadequate opportunities for youth employment, and concern for the environment	1960 "New Frontier," "Great Society," "War on Poverty" Partnership for Health act—comprehensive neigh-borhood health centers
1961 National Institute of Child Health and Human Devel-opment established, a national center for basic re-search in child development	1963 MCH funds authorized for children and youth projects
1962 Two-thirds of school nurses are employed by Boards of Education; number of nurses swell to 30,000	1965 Headstart Title V; Social Security Act; provides preschool health, education Medicaid, medical services for low-income families (Title XIX) National Health Promotion/Disease Prevention Cam-paign underway with release of the Surgeon Gen-eral's report on smoking
1969 School Nurse Practitioner program developed at the University of Colorado in conjunction with Denver Public Schools	
1970 Position Statement "Role of the School Nurse Practi-tioner" developed by various public health, school health and medical associations	1970 Family Planning Services and Population Research Act (PL 94:142); Education of the Handicapped leg-islation Rehabilitation Act of 1973 Early Periodic Screening, Diagnosis and Treatment (EPSDT); (Title XIX, Social Security Act); compre-hensive and preventive health services for diagno-sis and treatment of physical and mental defects
	1973 Child Abuse ACT (PL 934-247)
	1974 The Education of All Handicapped Children Act (PL 94:142) helps states provide a free and appropri-ate public education
1975 National Association of State School Nurse Consultants organized	1975 School-based initiative developed, states improve on child-abuse-reporting laws and include school personnel
1976 23 of 50 states have mandatory school nurse certifica-tion requirements; 10 states have permissive legislation	
1980 AIDS epidemic fully recognized	1980 Refugee Education Assistance Act
1983 *Standards for School Nursing Practice*, a set of guidelines for nursing practice in the schools and developed jointly by five professional health and nursing organizations, published by the American Nurses' Assocation	1981 Select Panel for the Promotion of Child Health
1989 Position statement *Role of the School Nurse in Disease Pre-vention, Health Promotion and Health Protection* receives American School Health Association endorsement	1986 Education of the Handicapped Act Amendments (PL 99-457) (Part H); program for infants and toddlers with handicaps
1990 Bureau of Maternal and Child Health reestablished National Health Agenda and Objectives for the Year 2000 launched	

Table 44-2   Chronology: A Listing of Events Significant in the History of School Health Services—cont'd

Developments in pediatrics, nursing, public health	Social and legislative developments
1991 National School Health/Education Coalition established	
1992 National Health objectives for the year 2000 related to school health established	
1993 Numerous coordinating councils for school health established by Bureau of Maternal and Child Health; Division of Adolescent and School Health (CDC)	
1993 Goals 2000 Educate America Act of 1993: Title 1, Section 102, Public Law 103-227	
1994 National Nurses Coalition for School Health formed; representatives include the National Association of School Nurses, National State School Nurses Consultants Association, American School Health Association, American Public Health Associaton, American Nurses Association	
1995 Child and adolescent health standards established and published *Bright Futures*	

health suggest a simpler explanation of school health is necessary. In addition the eight-component model is heavily weighted toward health education. Currently the rising demand for clinical services at school implies additional resources will be required in this area in the future. Hence the DASH model does not appear to be an accurate representation of how resources should be delegated. The important point here, however, is the principle of "local control" and the fact that local school districts prefer to develop and define their own programs. Consequently models/definitions of school health should be considered as reference materials for local policy makers rather than dictates.

Health Services

School health services generally include health screenings, basic care for minor complaints, administration of medications, surveillance of immunization status, case-finding for the early identification of problems, case management, health counseling, nursing care of students with special health needs, and in some districts, primary health care. All of these activities are family-centered and intended to prevent disease and promote health. School nurses are generally the persons responsible for this component of school health. These nurses may or may not have medical and psychological consultation available to them, depending on the size of their school health program and its level of development.

Recent advances in nursing research have substantially increased the knowledge base for the design and delivery of school health services of high quality. The University of Colorado School Health Programs in Denver, Colorado, manages a resource center, clear-

inghouse, reference collection, and newsletter. School nurses and others interested in school health have access to this information. The system also provides referrals to nurses working in model school health programs throughout the country.

Screening

The school nurse's responsibility in the **screening** process is to work with families and other team members to (1) establish what screening will be done, (2) develop a plan for the screening and a data management system, (3) teach paraprofessionals and others (including students and volunteers) how to conduct the screenings, (4) determine the appropriate resources for additional diagnostic work-up for children with signs and symptoms, (5) refer students in need of further evaluation to other school and community resources, and (6) collaborate with others in implementing and evaluating treatment plans.

Preventive health screenings may include vision, hearing, scoliosis, dental, cardiovascular risk factor analysis, and more comprehensive surveys of personal health habits known as behavioral risk surveys. These screenings usually take place as close to the beginning of the school year as possible to uncover problems that may interfere with learning. The box on p. 890 lists recommended screenings for school-age youth.

Special screening packages for preschool children are also available in school. One such program is the **Early and Periodic Screening Diagnosis and Treatment Program (EPSDT).** This program is a part of the Medicaid program (Title XIX of the Social Security Act), a means-tested entitlement program for medical assistance to needy families with dependent children. All states have an EPSDT program that offers early

Screening and Counseling for School-Age Youth

AGES 7-12

Leading Causes of Death

Motor vehicle crashes
Injuries (nonmotor vehicle)
Congenital anomalies
Leukemia
Homicide
Heart disease

Recommended Screening

Height and weight
Blood pressure
HIGH-RISK GROUPS
Tuberculin skin test (PPD)

Patient and Parent Counseling

Diet and Exercise
Fat (especially saturated fat), cholesterol, sweets and between-meal snacks, sodium
Caloric balance
Selection of exercise program
Injury Prevention
Safety belts
Smoke detector
Storage of firearms, drugs, toxic chemicals, matches
Bicycle safety helmets
Dental Health
Regular tooth brushing and dental visits
Other Primary Preventive Measures
HIGH-RISK GROUPS
Skin protection from ultraviolet light

Remain Alert for:

Vision disorders
Diminished hearing
Dental decay, malalignment, mouth breathing
Signs of child abuse or neglect
Abnormal bereavement

AGES 13-18

Leading Causes of Death

Motor vehicle crashes   Injuries (nonmotor vehicle)
Homicide   Heart disease
Suicide

Recommended Screening

History
Dietary intake   Tobacco/alcohol/drug use
Physical activity   Sexual practices
Physical Exam
Height and weight   Blood pressure
HIGH-RISK GROUPS
Complete skin exam   Clinical testicular exam
Laboratory/Diagnostic Procedures
HIGH-RISK GROUPS
Rubella antibodies   Counseling and testing for HIV
VDRL/RPR   Tuberculin skin test (PPD)
Chlamydial testing   Hearing
Gonorrhea culture   Papanicolaou smear

Patient and Parent Counseling

Diet and Exercise
Fat (especially saturated fat), cholesterol, sodium, iron, calcium
Caloric balance
Selection of exercise program
Substance Use
Tobacco: cessation/primary prevention
Alcohol and other drugs: cessation/primary prevention
Driving/other dangerous activities while under the influence
Treatment for abuse
HIGH-RISK GROUPS
Sharing/using unsterilized needles and syringes
Sexual Practices
Sexual development and behavior
Sexually transmitted diseases: partner selection, condoms
Unintended pregnancy and contraceptive options
Injury Prevention
Safety belts
Smoke detector
Storage of firearms, drugs, toxic chemicals, matches
Bicycle safety helmets
Dental Health
Regular tooth brushing and dental visits
Other Primary Preventive Measures
HIGH-RISK GROUPS
Discussion of hemoglobin testing
Skin protection from ultraviolet light

Remain Alert for:

Depressive symptoms   Tooth decay, malalignment, gingivitis
Suicide risk factors   Signs of child abuse or neglect
Abnormal bereavement

From American School Health Association: *School health in America,*
Kent, Ohio, 1989, The Association.

screening, diagnosis, treatment and periodic follow-up services to children and youth who meet the financial eligibility requirements and who are under 21 years of age.

There are two other preschool programs that include a number of health screenings. Head Start is an early childhood education program for children who are at risk for academic problems because of poverty and lack of sufficient social stimulation. Child Find is the other screening program and is part of the IDEA legislation (PL 104-476). Its purpose is early identification of preschool children who are at risk for school failure because of mental retardation, other disabilities, chronic health conditions, or special health needs. Currently, school administrators including school health personnel face the challenge of combining all of these preschool programs into a more consolidated screening package to control costs and avoid unnecessary duplication. Although the EPSDT, Head Start, and Child Find programs offer services only to selected children, there is a national trend underway to offer early childhood education and health screenings to all students.

Controversy surrounds some screenings. What should be provided, who should do the screening, and who will finance the service are questions that are raised frequently. Persons skilled in epidemiology (most often health department personnel) need to work with schools and school nurses in identifying which screenings are sufficiently valid, reliable, cost effective, simple, and safe. Many states mandate certain screenings through either statutes or regulations. Currently there are serious questions about the high priority assigned to scoliosis screening (Mann, 1990).

In addition to the traditional school health screenings, various circumstances have developed that now necessitate the delivery of more complex clinical services at school. Consequently, selective screening has become available for pregnancy, emotional disorders, and sexually transmitted diseases. In conjunction with this type of screening, students need psychosocial and behavioral counseling and other disease prevention and health promotion services as well as traditional medical treatments.

Case-Finding

Case-finding is a form of selective screening, which involves a search for certain students whose behavior, family circumstances, or health status place them at particular risk for ill health, **absenteeism,** and poor school performance. Instead of mass screening in which all students in various grades are involved, case-finding efforts begin by identifying risk factors and then locating students whose behavior suggests they are at risk for certain problems and in need of further assessment and possible referral. Therefore case-finding techniques are more intensive efforts and usually require the clinical judgment of school nurses to determine whether further assessment and diagnosis is necessary.

Case-finding is carried out by practicing careful, systematic observation of all children with whom nurses come in contact, looking for anomalies or suspect symptoms. **Case-finding** efforts should concentrate on identifying students who have these kinds of risk factors:

1. Students who are absent more than 10% of school days.
2. Students frequently sent to the principal's office for illness.
3. Students frequently sent to the principal's office for "acting out in the classroom."
4. Students who appear chronically ill to the teacher.
5. Students with subtle, as well as obvious, physical defects who are experiencing problems in functioning at school.
6. Students with subtle, as well as obvious, emotional problems.
7. Students who frequently seek out the nurse with vague, nonspecific complaints.
8. Students who have been seriously injured or who have a history of repeated injuries.
9. Students who are genetically predisposed to certain conditions, such as sickle cell disease.

Because the frequency rates for absenteeism, visits to the school nurse's office, injuries, referrals to the principal's office, and the practice of various personal health habits vary a great deal from school to school, the first step in case-finding is to establish these rates for each school building and for the district as a whole. This is done by keeping track of the students seen by the nurse, reviewing screening results and absenteeism records, collecting information from teachers and school administrators, and having students complete personal life-style inventories. Once the overall frequency rates for student behavior in these instances have been established, it becomes possible to determine whether the responses of certain students are the same or different from the rest of their classmates. Within most schools there are school administrators with experience in setting up surveillance systems that can help the school nurse in gathering this type of information and learning how to interpret it if a school health supervisor is not available. In 29 states, there are school nurse consultants located in the state departments of health and education who are also available to help.

The most likely place to begin case-finding efforts is with observation of children who are obviously physically or mentally different; children who are part of a desegregation program or who have moved from rural, mountain, urban, or suburban settings into a totally different social environment; and children from stressful situations where parental expectations may sometimes seem unreasonable for the child's stage of cognitive, physical, and psychosocial development. School nurses are especially concerned with detecting children who are victims of social illness (e.g., neglect or abuse). The nurse's responsibility in working with children suspected of being abused is to provide them with a nonthreatening environment, providing comfort, a safe place, support, encouragement, and compassion. It is also the nurse's responsibility to report the problem to appropriate authorities, such as the Children's Protective Services.

Surveillance of Immunization Status

Legally, entry into school requires that students be currently immunized unless exempted for religious or medical reasons. Consequently, up-to-date **Certificates of Immunization Status** must be presented to school personnel for admission. This usually applies to preschool students as well as to boys and girls who are older. Each of the following vaccines are required: polio, measles, mumps, rubella, and diphtheria/tetanus, and in the instance of preschoolers, pertussis. Because of recent measles outbreaks, an additional booster during adolescence is now recommended and, in many instances, is required by state law.

The school should have a procedure for dealing with immunizations. First, an administrator (or designee, often a secretary or a teacher) who has received the necessary instruction from the school nurse conducts a primary review of the child's health record to determine the immunization status. Next, the information collected from the school is shared with the local county health department. Those children not in compliance with the immunization law are cited with an exclusion order by the health department. This information is then routed back to the school, where administrators exclude the unimmunized students. If students do not return to school in a reasonable length of time (i.e., 3 to 4 days), follow-up measures are taken to investigate the truancy. Often families have no access to immunization services because of poverty. Consequently, some schools have reintroduced school-based immunization clinics to alleviate the problem. Previously, Goodwin found that this alternative was by far the most efficient and economical approach (Goodwin, 1978).

Managing Minor Complaints

Each school building should have first-aid supplies and equipment in accordance with accepted first-aid guidelines. Local district policies, as well as state and federal occupational health regulations, need to be followed. A health room area should be available in which to deliver first aid and emergency care, as well as care for such common complaints as abdominal pain, headaches, earaches, fatigue, nonspecific complaints, and nuisance diseases, such as pediculosis.

Increasingly, nurses have begun to involve teachers and students in the responsibilities associated with first aid. Often first-aid kits are located in the classrooms, and nurses work with school personnel and students to enable them to deal directly with minor injuries. American Red Cross classes are often an excellent means of preparation. This approach is especially important if the nurse is not in the building on a full-time basis.

All school nurses need physical assessment skills and equipment to diagnose, treat, or refer students with common health complaints. This type of information also needs to be recorded on the student's health record at school and, to ensure continuity of care, on written referrals prepared and sent with the student if another health care provider becomes involved. It is also important for the nurse to receive feedback from the community health care provider. Frequently, a regular system of communication has to be worked out to establish this kind of collaboration. Although this is more complicated in larger communities, the place to begin is to identify the students' health care providers. This is handled by having parents complete emergency cards that not only specify where the parent may be located during the day but also the name of their health care provider and the health facility or managed care system they use.

Some creative school nurses have established an ongoing link to community health professionals in various ways, including inviting them to visit and tour the school with the nurse, inviting them to join the school health council, and placing them on the mailing list for the school health newsletter.

Administration of Medications

One type of drug problem that occurs in children is improper use of medication. Based on a recent study by the National Council on Patient Information and Education, "In any two-week period, about 13 million people in the United States under the age of 18 take medicines prescribed or recommended by a physician. Of those, 46% either stop treatment too soon, do not take enough medication, take too much, or refuse to take any at all. When children use medicines improperly, lives are lost, treatable chronic diseases remain uncontrolled, and acute illnesses needlessly continue or recur" (National Council on Patient Information and Education, 1989). Many of these medications are administered in school.

Medication policies are essential in schools today. However, these policies should not serve as a barrier to gaining access to the classroom and learning. Some students with chronic disease (e.g., asthma) are in special self-management programs to help them learn how to function independently. School nurses need to support this approach by individualizing overall medication policies as appropriate. The five basic requirements for administration of medications in schools are the following:

1. Medications are given only with parents' written permission.
2. Medications requiring a prescription are given only on the written authorization of a physician.
3. For medications requiring a prescription there must be an individual, pharmacy-labeled bottle for each student.
4. Medications must be recorded by the school personnel who administer them. This record states the

student's name, medication, dosage, time, and the person administering the medication.

5. Medications must be stored in a secure, locked, clean container or cabinet.

The administration of medications in schools is so prevalent today that in many instances nonnursing personnel have this responsibility. In these cases instruction is needed, and manuals do exist for this purpose (Iowa Department of Education, 1991). States vary in their interpretation of the school nurse role, relationship and responsibility to the persons dispensing the medications. The state board of nursing is the agency responsible for establishing this policy.

Counseling

The ability to counsel students or others skillfully is an art. The counselor's responsibility is to provide information; to listen objectively; and to be supportive, caring, and trustworthy. Counselors do not make decisions; they help clients arrive at the decisions that best suit them. **Counseling** therefore differs from teaching and interviewing. For example, teaching is giving information; interviewing is obtaining information from someone; counseling is helping people arrive at workable solutions to their problems or conflicts. The box on p. 890 lists recommended counseling topics for school-age youth.

Students usually require counseling when they are unable to make decisions about personal concerns that affect their lives, for example, taking medication and changing life-style habits. If the nurse lacks the ability to counsel or to recognize that counseling is needed, the student may be unable to fully comprehend the extent of the problem or to find alternatives to resolve the problem. Students' peers can be used as counselors. However, students who act as counselors must be trained for the role. After providing students who are acting as peer counselors with technical advice, school nurses also should encourage them to use their personal experiences, to role-play, and to be available and accessible to other students.

Students with **vague, nonspecific health complaints** who visit the health room frequently should be of special concern to school nurses. This may be the first warning sign of a student who is not doing well in school and who is at risk for eventually dropping out. Lewis and others have previously identified that children at risk of becoming school dropouts develop this type of maladaptive response to stress (vague health complaints) in early school years. This behavior continues into adulthood, thereby jeopardizing work and school performance (Lewis and Lewis 1990). However, with the right assistance and counseling from the school nurse, which involves making sure the child is not physically ill and developing plans to enhance the student's self-concept, improve their problem-solving skills, and reduce stress levels, these students can be helped to manage their problems more effectively.

Schneider M, Friedman S, Fisher M: Stated and unstated reasons for visiting a high school nurse's office, J *Adolesc Health* 16:35-41, 1995.

Research Brief

A survey of students visiting the school nurse's office was conducted to determine the relationship between presenting complaints and underlying psychosocial problems. For students attending most schools in America the investigators (nonnurses) believe the "nurse's office" will likely remain the primary source of school-based health care for the foreseeable future. It also was assumed the nurse at school could play an important role in providing psychosocial care and follow-up referral to community providers as needed.

The study lasted 5 months, during which time questionnaires were distributed to students in a suburban high school in the East. The questionnaires were anonymous and required 5 to 10 minutes to complete. Students were asked to identify (1) their chief complaints, (2) their perception concerning the likelihood that stress, depression, drugs, etc. were associated with their complaints, (3) the type of help sought from the nurse, (4) demographic information, (5) student's assessment of stress in his or her life and (6) past use of the nurse's office.

One hundred eighty-six students presented to the nurse's office with a variety of complaints including headache, infections, fatigue, abdominal distress. Five students said they had vague complaints. Others associated their complaints with several psychosocial factors, including not sleeping well, family problems, school problems, stress, and depression. Implications for school nursing practice from study recommendations were:

1. School nurses are well positioned to assume an expanded role in meeting the psychosocial needs of students.
2. School nurses should routinely screen for high stress levels that can interfere with academic performance, peer relationships, and motor activities in light of the fact that in this study nearly 30% of students complained of unusual and debilitating amounts of stress in their lives.

Case Management

As a **case manager,** the school nurse performs a number of general activities. Parents need to be contacted to seek permission to discuss their child's health problem with the family physician. The nurse also will need to inform teachers and administrators accurately about the nature and prognosis of the health problem and the specific therapies required during the school day. Situations occurring at school that either interfere with the treatment plan or exacerbate the health condition need to be identified, communicated to the parties involved, and managed. Problems that arise from the student's health condition that deter learning also need to be recognized and handled. This usually involves obtaining and conveying information between health and school personnel. The school nurse is usually the person who bridges this gap through the process of case management.

Primary Health Care

School-wide campaigns to improve diet and physical exercise habits, contraceptive advice, individual and small-group counseling to reduce stress and improve self-image, and social skills training and cognitive therapies to prevent substance abuse and delay the onset of sexual activity are just a few examples of the kind of generalized primary care health services and health promotion activities now available in schools. The American School Health Association also recommends fitness screening, school breakfast and lunch programs, physical education, and mental health programs (Healthy People 2000, 1991). Detailed handbooks are available to assist school nurses and other school health personnel in developing these programs (Allensworth and Wolford, 1988). If school nurse practitioners are available, students also will be able to receive comprehensive health evaluations in schools.

An increasing number of boys and girls today need to obtain additional **primary health care services** in their schools. This type of care includes health history, physical examination, simple laboratory tests, and diagnosis and treatment of minor health problems. A 24-hour a day, 7-day a week, year-round referral system also must be in place in case students' problems require additional medical attention or they become ill when school is closed. The 1984 National Health Interview Survey found that 4.5 million (14%) students 10 to 18 years of age are from poor and minority households. These students are the ones who are least likely to have health insurance and access to primary health care.

Increasingly, school nurse practitioners also are becoming involved in more specialized forms of primary care. For example, some nurses serve as sports trainers, offering evaluations and special interventions to reduce the likelihood of sports injuries. Other nurses who are primary care providers work exclusively with students experiencing emotional disorders or with students who are medically fragile and technology-dependent. Still other school nurse practitioners delivery primary care in special settings, such as the diagnostic center for a school system.

Health Services for Students with Special Needs

According to the IDEA bill (PL 101-476), students eligible for service must have a comprehensive interdisciplinary evaluation followed by the preparation of an **individualized education plan (IEP).** This plan is reviewed and modified at regular intervals during the

school year and throughout the student's school experience. Parent conferences always occur in conjunction with the evaluation and preparation of the IEP. Students frequently join their parents and school staff for these meetings. For students whose health status significantly interferes with their ability to learn, a health care plan is a component of the IEP.

The health component of the IEP includes the following types of information: specific notations of any special preparation and supervision that may be required in caring for the student, health counseling that is necessary for the student to function in the class, and any changes in the school environment that are necessary, such as the removal of architectural barriers. Also included in the health component of the IEP would be safety measures, measures required to relieve pain and discomfort (i.e., suctioning, skin care), special diet, medications, and special assistance with activities of daily living. Finally, any special adaptations of school health activities (i.e., screenings, health education, case-finding) are described so that the student is able to have full access to this program.

School staff members often need preparation and supervision by the school nurse to competently manage health care plans and the special health needs of students. Fortunately, the professional organizations for teachers and school nurses have developed policies to delineate their roles and responsibilities (Guidelines, 1990). Unfortunately, often it is difficult to enforce policies and guidelines that are issued from professional organizations because they have no statutory authority over local school systems.

In 1986, PL 94-142 was amended by PL 99-457, which changed the limit for mandated health and education services to include disabled children 3 to 5 years of age. Moreover, section H of the amendment, called infants and toddlers, the states also were given the option to extend these early intervention services to children from birth to 3 years of age to include those infants and toddlers who are disabled or who have special health needs that could eventually interfere with their ability to learn. In these instances, **individualized family service plans (IFSP)** are developed by a interdisciplinary team in partnership with parents, setting in place an early intervention program to prepare the infant/toddler/preschooler for school. Those states involved in section H also designate one community agency to coordinate these efforts. The school has been the designated agency in some states, however, other agencies also have been selected, including departments of health and social services.

Health Education

During the past decade, **health education** has been closely identified with the health promotion movement. Basically, health promotion is a social concept or campaign, as well as a set of health education activities intended to develop healthy life-styles among Americans (Green, 1984). Although not all health educators agree, many believe that the two areas are practically synonymous or that health promotion is the more encompassing activity and health education is a technique for its achievement. Health education efforts must therefore relate to the values and beliefs of students and their families. Because the potential exists for health education to infringe on the constitutional rights of individuals, health education at school is best developed locally, by committee, and should be open for public inspection and parental approval.

The health education component should include instructional efforts that foster wellness, such as health classes and courses to prevent the spread of infectious diseases like acquired immune deficiency syndrome (AIDS). Health education also includes education for students with chronic health problems who need to learn more about their diseases, self-care, and how to effectively use the health care system. Three general goals for the health education component of school health are: (1) to teach all children about their bodies and how to keep them healthy; (2) to instill in boys and girls lifelong healthy habits and the knowledge to make responsible decisions concerning their own health, the health of their families when they become adults, and the health of their communities (Wold, 1981); and (3) to teach students how to use the health care system wisely and effectively.

There are a number of validated health education curricula available today. Five programs are particularly well known. The Growing Healthy curriculum for elementary grades is a generalized program aimed at improving students' personal life-styles (Kolbe, 1984). At the high school level, the Teenage Health Teaching Modules (THTM) have been widely used (Kolbe and Iverson, 1984). A more targeted type of health instruction is the Know Your Body course, which focuses on making students aware of their own cardiovascular risk factors through screening activities followed by special instruction related to risk reduction (Kolbe and Iverson, 1984). The Quest and Dare programs often are used in schools for drug and alcohol prevention (Kolbe and Iverson, 1984).

The HealthPACT course is a different type of health instruction. Designed as consumer health affairs lessons, it is intended to prepare children to communicate effectively with health professionals during visits for health care. HealthPACT teaches children to communicate effectively by using five basic communication skills: (1) **T**alk with the health care provider; (2) **L**isten and learn; (3) **A**sk questions; (4) **D**ecide what to do, with help from the provider; (5) **D**o follow through. The letters (TLADD) are used as an acronym to help children learn and remember their health consumer responsibilities.

This program may be used as a supplement to an established health education curriculum, or it may be taught to children in a wide range of locations, including school classrooms, clinics, youth organizations, and at home. Since 1971, it has been implemented in varying degrees and at various times by school nurses, general health educators, dentists, teachers, physicians, clinic and hospital staff, parents, nurses, and physicians' assistants. A variety of program evaluations has been done over the years, with successful outcomes (Stember, 1988).

A 3-year national investigation of the HealthPACT program demonstrated that the program was successful in teaching students in elementary grades how to actively participate during visits for health care. Fourth grade is apparently the best age for this type of instruction (Stember, 1988).

The implications from the HealthPACT program and its evaluation are threefold: (1) the role of the patient/consumer is changing; (2) the concept of the patient as partner even during childhood is acceptable; and (3) children can learn consumer behaviors for use in health settings if they have support. The HealthPACT program also demonstrates that a new kind of health education is needed and is acceptable. Starting with instruction about active participation in a health facility, children and youth and their parents also need to learn self-help measures (e.g., how to do their own vision screening, how to use an otoscope), and they also need to know more about the overall health care system and how it operates so that they can successfully negotiate their way around this system and can change its nature and operation if, as citizens, they see the need for change (Igoe, 1990).

Environmental Health

The third component of the school health program is **environmental health,** which involves physical and psychosocial factors, such as infectious agent control and the physical and social environment of children. This component has received little attention until recently. Evaluating the need to improve the social environment in schools today is complex and involves instilling a sense of pride in students and measuring the morale of teachers and parents, as well as evaluating the attitudes of the rest of the school team for signs of apathy, powerlessness, and hostility (Comer, 1988).

The physical environment in schools also needs to be evaluated. School nurses should work closely with local public health officials to ensure that this area of school health is not overlooked. Safety programs are most important. Often nurses enlist the active involvement of students in identifying areas in the school in which injuries are most frequent and in planning intervention strategies to reduce the risk. Incident reports need to be completed by school personnel when injuries occur, and school health personnel should review this information regularly to improve conditions. Asbestos, lead poisoning, and toxic substances in the chemistry and art classrooms are areas of concern to school administrators. Nurses must be well informed and have a close working relationship with the environmental health personnel at the local health department to be a useful resource for school officials. Often the nurse will be involved in surveying areas for risks, collecting information from parents, and providing school administrators, parents, and students with the most current approach to these problems to avoid unnecessary scares and instances of consumer fraud.

ROLES, FUNCTIONS, AND CREDENTIALS FOR SCHOOL NURSES

The majority of the 26,000 registered professional nurses now employed in school health are generalists prepared at the baccalaureate level who function in the consultant/coordinator role. The newer role for school nurses is as school health manager or coordinator. The functions associated with this role include: (1) policy-making activities to ensure a more comprehensive and integrated school health program; (2) case management functions to help families find the help they need; (3) program management duties so that a system of formalized school health activities and protocols develops as an integral part of both the private and public community health system; and (4) health promotion and health protection responsibilities, including health education in the curriculum; health screening, follow-up, and referral for potential child health problems; and participation in activities that will make the school environment safe for children (e.g., adequate lunch programs, asbestos monitoring). Because children's health problems are becoming more complex, knowledge of nursing, pediatrics, adolescent health, and public health is essential. These nurses also must be prepared to identify health-related situations that place the student at risk and that other school personnel might fail to recognize. In

---

Did You Know?

A common misconception about school nurses is that there are fewer of them now than in years past. A 1993 national investigation of school health personnel, however, does not support this idea.

◆ Only 1% of school districts reporting indicated there were fewer nurses now than in the past.

◆ Over 40% of 482 school districts (large and small and throughout the U.S.) reported additional nursing staff were added last year. Despite this finding, insufficient nursing staff remains one of the leading barriers to improved nursing service at school. The complexity of student health problems today requires direct service and difficult case management, all of which is very labor intensive work.

---

addition, school nurses also must be very familiar with community resources and how to gain access to them. 'People' skills also are necessary because this nurse serves as the key link between the school and community health agencies.

A number of school nurses have dual degrees. Although health education has been a popular second degree, the guidance and counseling degree is a new goal for many school nurses. Efforts are underway now to inform school nurses that this content is integrated into graduate nursing programs, which should alleviate the need for school nurses to seek degrees outside of nursing.

Specialists

For nurses wishing to pursue a specialty in school nursing, a graduate degree in nursing is highly recommended. Two types of degree plans are designed specifically for them: the clinician role and the administrative/managerial role. The most common clinical role now seen in schools is as a **school nurse practitioner (SNP)** or as a specialist in such areas as child psychiatry, mental health, rehabilitation, and developmental disabilities. Only 400 certified SNPs are available and employed in schools. Thousands are needed. The number of other nurse specialists working in schools is unknown. The number of nurses in this group is probably much smaller than the number of SNPs but is just as much in demand.

School nurse practitioners are registered professional nurses whose advanced practice area is primary health care. They can serve as primary care providers for students who have no access to health care or whose parents prefer that their child receive this care at school. In addition to working with this group of students, SNPs also evaluate any students coming to their health office with complaints of illness and injuries. Earlier studies have demonstrated that (1) SNPs send home from school 50% fewer students than regular school nurses, (2) parents are more likely to act on the advice of SNPs, (3) SNPs handle 87% of the health complaints referred to them, and (4) SNPs resolve 96% of the health problems they see. In addition the difference in cost in relation to other community health facilities is substantial (Igoe, 1990; Meeker et al., 1986).

In addition to working in a clinical setting, evaluating students in need of primary health care and those who are sick and injured, SNPs are also part of the interdisciplinary team involved in screening students with special health needs who may be eligible for services under the IDEA legislation PL 101-476. One of their unique functions is the performance of **neurodevelopmental evaluations.** These evaluations contribute greatly to the overall assessment of a child by helping primary care providers identify the student's strengths and deficits in processing information. The **community health nurse specialist for school-aged children** is the newest role proposed for school nurses. This role encompasses the functions of the school health manager previously described. These nurses function in **nontraditional health facilities** (alternative health care delivery systems), using various community settings, such as schools, juvenile corrections facilities, group homes for the disabled and chronically ill, day care centers, and shelters for the homeless. Special organizational skills and management expertise are needed to provide more accessible public/community health programs in these settings, especially if the nurse is to have a leadership role. These settings frequently lack the necessary policies and procedures, data management systems, coordinated networks with other community health systems, and effective financing mechanisms to function effectively. Nurses functioning in this role have the organizational and political skills to design and implement health programs in these settings that cut across systems and produce results (Igoe, 1991).

Credentials

In addition to their nurses' license, school nurses often elect to become certified as a school nurse, school nurse practitioner, community health nurse, or other type of clinical nurse specialist through one or more of their national professional nursing associations. In some states the State Department of Education offers an additional state certification program for school nurses. In fact, depending on the state, it may not be possible to be employed in some school systems (or for school administrators to receive any federal reimbursement for school nursing care for students with handicaps) without a state certificate. Currently, many school nurses are striving to establish this type of credentialing to upgrade the quality of school nursing.

MANAGEMENT OF THE SCHOOL HEALTH PROGRAM

A school health program requires good management to operate smoothly and effectively. Four essential steps are involved in reaching this goal: planning, organizing, directing, and controlling the quality of the program through proper evaluation. Planning for school health should be a joint endeavor involving members of a school health council. To ensure broad-based representation, this council should be composed of teachers, school nurses, parents, students, administrators, and community leaders. Members of this team need to set the direction for the program, ensuring that the mission of the school health program is consistent with the goals of the school district and the rest of the community health system. The council plans and sets goals for the school health program and develops and then implements strategies to meet these goals. The council also evaluates the program in view of these goals and makes changes as necessary. A school health council is a valuable support mechanism for the proper development, revision, implementation, and evaluation of the school health program. Although technically school health councils are advisory bodies, the current emphasis in schools on community participation and parental involvement conveys a special sense of authority to the school health council. This influence, if used properly, provides the school health program the support it needs to operate successfully.

The Relationship Between Education Reform and School Health

In 1990 the National Governor's Association established the following goals for education by the year 2000.
1. All children will start school ready to learn.
2. The high school graduation rate will increase to at least 90% for all groups.
3. All students will leave grades 4, 8, and 12 having demonstrated competency over challenging subject matter in English, mathematics, science, history, and geography.
4. U.S. students will be first in the world in mathematics and science achievement.
5. Every adult will be literate and possess the knowledge and skills necessary to compete in a global economy and to exercise the rights and responsibilities of citizenship.
6. Every school in America will be free of drugs and violence and will offer a disciplined environment conducive to learning (U.S. Department of Education, 1990).

The impetus for this action and the need for major reform movements within education in recent years is the result of the growing public awareness that academic achievement scores of American youth are slipping; school dropout rates are rising; violence and drug abuse is threatening the integrity of many school communities; and minority youth and those who are disabled or who have special health needs still do not have equal opportunities for learning. All of these factors threaten the ability of students to become productive adults.

The educational goals for the year 2000 along with *Healthy People 2000: National Health Promotion and Disease Prevention Objectives* (Healthy People 2000, 1991) are the guidelines that set the direction for school health planning. In June 1990 the National Commission on the Role of the School and Community in Improving Adolescent Health issued a designated planning document for school health in secondary schools, *Code Blue: Uniting for Healthier Youth* (Code Blue, 1990). The commission that authored this report was composed of community leaders from health, education, and religious organizations, business, and government. The Commission was cosponsored by the National Association of State Boards of Education

(NASBE) and the American Medical Association (AMA), with funding from the Centers for Disease Control.

Subsequently, Guidelines for Adolescent Preventive Services (GAPS) have been issued and are now being piloted in many settings, including school-based student health centers (Department of Adolescent Health, 1992). In 1991 National Health Objectives Related to School Health were identified (see the box below, left). These objectives provide specific direction, especially in the area of school health education.

Planning

Many school nurses are themselves the managers or coordinators of school health programs. School health requires a unique type of management known as pivot management. Under this plan, nurses organize a school health team using the personnel already in the school system or closely associated with it: teachers, students, parents, administrators, psychologists, health educators, social workers, speech pathologists, counselors, secretarial staff, and maintenance personnel. With the help of a school health council, this team develops a comprehensive school health plan, and a

budget is developed and proposed to school administrators. Program goals, strategies, and activities are designed and organized so that health services, health education, and environmental components of the program are coordinated with one another. If the health program for students with disabilities is separated from the general school health program, special care must be taken to link these two efforts to avoid unnecessary duplication and fragmentation.

A needs assessment is the starting point for program development. It is used to determine the problems requiring attention and the way to best meet these needs. The box below, right, provides an outline of some areas covered in needs assessments for school health.

All three areas of school health must be considered when planning is done, and decisions must reflect innovative and economical ways of combining health services with health education and environmental health measures. Unfortunately, school health programming often is handled haphazardly, with decisions about the health education curriculum made in one department, health services planned and implemented from another office, and the environmental health component attended to in yet another department.

Traditionally, health services have been limited to screening and first aid. However, the advent of school-

---

National Health Objectives Related to School Health

By the year 2000:

1. Increase to at least 50% the proportion of children in grades 1 to 12 who participate in daily physical education activities at school.
2. Increase to at least 90% the proportion of school lunch and breakfast programs with menus consistent with nutritional principles contained in Dietary Guidelines for Americans.
3. Increase to at least 75% the proportion of the nation's schools that provide nutrition education from preschool through twelfth grade.
4. Include tobacco-use prevention in the curricula of all elementary, middle, and secondary schools.
5. Provide children in all primary and secondary schools with educational programs on alcohol and other drugs.
6. Increase to at least 85% the proportion of people 10 to 18 years of age who have discussed human sexuality with their parents or received information from parentally endorsed sources, such as schools.
7. Increase to at least 50% the proportion of elementary and secondary schools that teach nonviolent conflict-resolution skills.
8. Provide academic instruction on injury prevention and control in at least 50% of public school systems.
9. Increase to at least 95% the proportion of schools that have age-appropriate HIV education curricula for children in grades 4 to 12.
10. Include in all middle and secondary schools instruction on preventing sexually transmitted diseases.

From *Healthy people 2000: national health promotion and disease prevention objectives,* Washington, DC, 1991, USDHHS Public Health Service.

School Health Needs Assessment

STUDENT HEALTH

Absenteeism: frequency and nature
Health problems presented at school (for example: illness and the nature, frequency, and location of injuries)
Resolution of health problems: frequency
Chronic health conditions, handicapping conditions
Health status of students
  Immunization level
  Dental
  Vision
  Hearing
  Emotional disorders
  Physical/sexual abuse
  Prevalence of positive health behavior (for example: nutrition, exercise, safety, and avoidance of substance abuse)
Change in health status of students

RESOURCES

Community resources available
Use of community resources (overuse as well as underuse)
Health care/education available in regular curriculum (for example: physical education, home economics, special education, science, and health education)
Health services available through current school health programs

EMPLOYEE HEALTH

Health state of school personnel: absenteeism and nature of disability claims

based health centers, the increased numbers of uninsured students, and the admission of students with complex health care needs—all have affected the development of much more complex school health services. In fact, care now being delivered in schools closely resembles the activities of traditional health facilities, including on-site diagnostic and treatment services and sophisticated nursing care for students with complex health problems. Rehabilitative services also must be available. Consequently, public health codes governing primary health care facilities often apply to school-based health centers. By maintaining a close working relationship with the local public health authorities, the school nurse is aware of local health regulations.

Health education requirements are especially important today because the public health agenda increasingly emphasizes disease prevention and health promotion. By obtaining an aggregated life-style profile for individual schools and for the total school district, school health planners will be more aware of the level of need for health education in their district. This kind of information can be provided through health appraisal questionnaires that ask students about their knowledge, attitudes, and life-style behaviors in relation to diet, nutrition, exercise, dental health, human sexuality, infectious disease, and substance abuse. Also, an audit of student health and school records to determine injury rates and illness-related absences provides administrators and the community with data about the overall health status of the student body. This approach often is effective in gaining school board support for a health education curriculum.

Next, school health planners must decide who will provide the health instruction. Ideally, sufficient numbers of school-employed health educators will teach the classes. More realistically, these same health educators, who are in very short supply, develop the health education curriculum and work with classroom teachers, school nurses, and other community health professionals to implement the program.

A well-organized school health program must have clear and appropriate written policies and procedures. To be effective, these regulations must address the problems of poor students, students with chronic illnesses or disabilities, and sick and disabled infants and toddlers. The "new morbidities" affecting school-aged children cannot necessarily be managed completely by the health care system alone because many problems have psychosocial, political, and physical features. External environmental and sociopolitical forces that lead to these problems must be considered to implement school health programs effectively. Tools for planning, implementing, and evaluating the school health program should describe a general plan and provide regulations for emergencies, such as allergic shock, breathing disorders, drug overdose, and head and spinal injuries. Policies and procedures should address these areas and others, including disaster plans, communicable diseases, reportable diseases required by the state, child abuse, and the warning signs and incidence of suicide. If state school nurse consultants are available, they should be consulted during the planning stage.

Organizing

There are 15,577 public school systems in this country, which are considerably less than the 100,000 districts that existed at the end of World War II around 1945. School nurses are unevenly distributed from one district to the next and from state to state. Although professional organizations recommend a ratio of 1 nurse for every 750 students, a ratio of 1 nurse to 1500 students is more realistic in terms of the supply of prepared nurses that are available and the costs involved. For students with special health needs, the requirements for care are much different; hence, ratios must be adjusted accordingly. However, as yet insufficient data are available about the nursing care required to make any reliable recommendations.

More problematic than the number of students per nurse is the number of school buildings the nurse must visit to come in contact with students. For example, 47% of school districts have a total school enrollment of only 2500 students (Digest of Educational Statistics, 1989). This means that one or two school nurses often make up the total school health team in these districts, with an assignment of 3 to 5 schools each. In large urban "inner city" school districts, the ratio of nurses to students and nurses to buildings is far worse (Igoe, 1991). This organizational dilemma adds to the credibility of a recommendation that came from a President's Commission on School Health in the early 1970s, which advised that health assistants be placed in schools to handle basic care (first aid, minor complaints), with nurses assuming managerial positions.

The intermediate education district is another network for organizing school health. Known as **area education agencies (AEAs)** or **boards of cooperative educational services (BOCES),** these systems frequently provide related services for special education students in school districts of limited size. School nursing, speech, audiology, occupational and physical therapy, and psychological services are some of the services often provided regionally. Nurses working in regional agencies often help local school district personnel develop and implement health care plans for certain students, such as those who are disabled or at high risk for academic difficulty. These specialized school nurses also work with the school nurse in the local district, if there is one, who is responsible for the overall school health program.

School nurses face a tremendous challenge daily in managing their time effectively. Therefore it is important to have a written plan that sets the direction, priorities, and schedule for the school health program. Within this context, the nurse also must organize the day in such a way that low-priority tasks are not crowding out time to work on high-priority activities. For example, many school nurses have discovered that an open-door policy fosters continual interruptions throughout the day. Consequently, school nurses in many school systems now have initiated an appointment system for seeing students and for parent-teacher conferences. Specified sick-call times are often established as another way of cutting down on the number of unnecessary interruptions.

It is also important for school nurses to organize an epidemiological data base that profiles the health status of the student body both individually and collectively. This is accomplished by using a systematic recording system for the problems that nurses see and the care they provide. Well-organized school health programs have policy and procedure manuals that explain the recording system to be used in a particular school system. Software packages for computerized school health records recently have been introduced, and school nurses have begun to include personal computers in their budget requests (Kaplan, 1991). Currently, some effort is underway to coordinate school and community health data systems by having school health personnel use the International Classification of Disease (ICD-9) codes in recording student health problems. Another approach undertaken in the Multnomah County Educational Service District in Portland, Oregon, has been to use the nursing diagnosis classification system developed by the North American Nursing Diagnosis Association (NANDA). This is in keeping with the Oregon nurse practice act, which requires nurses to document their practice in this manner.

Individuals developing new school health programs or revising old ones, also must now consider organizing school health under a single department, office, or division so that needs are met, services do not overlap, and costs are contained. The ideal organizing process would involve and consolidate all health personnel responsible for the care of students in general, for students with special health needs, and for other students at high risk for school failure. Such personnel would include school nurses, speech pathologists, occupational therapists, physical therapists, social workers, clinical psychologists, and counselors, including student assistant personnel. Although most related service personnel are employed by school districts to carry out the provisions of the IDEA bill, this does not mean that school administrators cannot integrate these professionals with other school employees, such as school nurses, to achieve a more comprehensive approach to school health.

There are three barriers to reorganization and consolidation of school health. First, many of the related service personnel do not identify themselves with school health. Second, school nurses may be unaccustomed to a team approach in which the other members of the team are not nurses. Third, bureaucratic turf battles often interfere with interdisciplinary and transdisciplinary efforts in which the students' needs are first identified and then the team decides who is the person best suited to provide the care.

One way of overcoming the natural resistance to change would be to organize related service personnel, including the school nurse, into interdisciplinary teams that service a cluster of schools. This organizational arrangement allows various persons with backgrounds in fields other than education to become members of their own team and to gain a sense of identity. Team development work will be needed to build trust and a sense of how to operate in this kind of an interdisciplinary environment. Nevertheless, this personnel arrangement offers the support system school nurses and other personnel often miss when they function separately.

Once the health service component of school health has been unified, the next step in restructuring school health is to strengthen the link between the health service, health education and environmental health divisions. Regular meetings of the persons responsible for these programs is essential as is the need for them to develop a comprehensive coordinated strategic management plan for school health. The school health council is their advisory body.

Although schools traditionally have employed their own school health personnel or contracted with the public health agency for these services, new partnerships and organizational arrangements are emerging. School nurses in California and New York are forming their own school health companies and contracting directly with schools. Hospitals, both profit and nonprofit, also have begun to contract with schools to administer school health programs.

Directing

Leadership for school health programs needs strengthening at all levels. States currently have school nurse consultants, with approximately 50% of them employed by state health departments and the rest responsible to the state department of education instruction. These individuals frequently provide technical assistance to local school districts, known as local education agencies (LEA), in the form of inservice education and on-site evaluation of the program while performing statewide planning for school health.

At the local level, a school nurse supervisor/coordinator usually oversees the health services program and provides supervision for other school nurses. In a 1986 national survey of school nurse supervisors, 60% were registered professional nurses. Other supervisors for school nurses were school administrators (10%), educators (health and physical educators) (15%), psychologists and counselors (12%), and physicians (3%) (Igoe, 1991). As the health needs of students become increasingly complex and the level of care delivered in school rises, there is an obvious need for the school health program (especially the health service component) to be managed by a health professional who is knowledgeable about the clinical aspects of care.

School health managers/coordinators require certain skills to be effective. Among the most frequently cited skills of effective managers are the following: (1) verbal communication (including listening); (2) managing time and stress; (3) managing individual decisions; (4) recognizing, defining, solving problems; (5) motivating and influencing others; (6) delegating; (7) setting goals and articulating a vision; (8) self-awareness; (9) team building; and (10) managing conflict (Whetten and Cameron, 1991). Individuals seeking to manage school health programs would definitely need these abilities in night of the major changes that most school health programs are undergoing.

The school nurse's role is expanding rapidly in the area of supervision of school health assistants. As the number of children and the complexity of their health needs continues to rise, the need for assessments and care in the school setting increases. This makes it essential that school nurses have available to them a way to train and credential school health assistants working with children with special needs.

Controlling

Efforts to evaluate school health programs are underway, but this area of program management is still in its infancy. Fortunately, practice standards for the school nurse and school nurse practitioner exist, and these serve as useful guides in determining nurses' effectiveness (Guidelines, 1990). Program evaluations also occur (Igoe, 1991). School nurses are beginning to include outcome measures as well as process variables in these evaluations. For example, the number of referred students who now wear glasses should be noted in an evaluation (outcome measures) as should the number of students screened (process variables). Outcome measures of the effectiveness of a particular school health activity also must reflect what impact the activity had on the child's academic performance.

Another way to improve the quality of school health is to mandate or require that certain services, health education, and environmental measures be provided for students. A regulated approach, however, is not always the best way to proceed. This can turn out to be a highly political process and once things are mandated it is often difficult to change them if there is evidence that a practice is no longer necessary. Finally, the area of school health that is probably most in need of quality control is the environment. Generally, environmental health standards are not always relevant, available, or enforced. The box above provides an overview of the environmental health regulations that are currently in effect (Lovato,

Overview of State Regulations That Affect Environmental Health Conditions in Schools

RESPONSIBLE AGENCY

◆ 11 states (21%) responsible party employed by State Education Agency

◆ 15 states (30%) responsible party employed by State Health Department

◆ 18 states (35%) both Department of Education/health agencies

◆ 7 states (14%) Department of Education, State Department of Health, plus other agencies

TRADITIONAL

◆ Ventilation—32 states (63%)
◆ Kitchen—45 states (88%)
◆ Illumination—27 states (53%)
◆ Safety glass—31 states (61%)

INSPECTION REQUIREMENTS

◆ Most frequent—Kitchen (46 states, 61%), restrooms (29 states, 57%)

◆ Less than one-third of states required mandatory inspection of the chemical laboratory, classroom, gymnasium, playground, athletic field

OTHER POLICIES/STANDARDS

◆ New Standards (EPA/Office of Water)—Lead in school drinking water

◆ Asbestos—Containing Materials in Schools Rule EPA (40 CFR Part 763 Subpart E)—25 states (49%) developed plan to meet 1989 federal regulations

From American School Health Association: *School Health in America*, Kent, Ohio, 1989, The Association.

1990). A congressional report issued in 1995 provided additional evidence of the deterioration of school buildings and called for the need for immediate improvements to safeguard student health.

INNOVATIONS IN SCHOOL HEALTH
School-Based Health Centers

School-based health centers (SBHC) were established as a result of several demonstration projects conducted during the past two decades (Meeker et al., 1986). These projects demonstrated that the school can be an effective site for primary health care services because most children and youth attend school and have access to this facility. The projects also demonstrated that nurse practitioners with appropriate physician consultation provide excellent health care, reduce unnecessary referrals, and cut down on the time away from school. This is particularly true if a student's only other access to care is a public clinic where the waiting time is extensive (Kornguth, 1990). Presently, there are an estimated 300 school-based health centers in the U.S. located in secondary schools. No accurate estimates exist of the number that are established in elementary schools, preschools, or in school-based after-school day care centers.

Schools encounter financial problems with even the most basic school health program. Therefore if a community's school-age population is to benefit from the advantages of using the school setting as the student health center, the responsibility for organizing, financing, and delivery of school health services in these sites must be shared with other community health systems, including state and local health departments. School-based health centers are cost effective in comparison to other community health facilities, with estimates ranging from $90/student/year to $150/student/year (Model School Health Programs, 1991). Consequently, financing mechanisms must be found to support SBHCs such as third party reimbursement for services rendered to students who have Medicaid benefits or other health insurance plans as is done in the Hartford, Connecticut, school district (Model School Health Programs, 1991).

School-based health centers change the school nurse responsibilities in several ways. In some instances the school nurse takes on the responsibility for providing the care as a school nurse practitioner. In other settings the school nurse acts as the manager for the center and designs the programs and activities necessary for its operation. In other settings, nurses serve as team members for the center and their responsibility is triage and case management. However, it should be pointed out that the delivery of individualized personal health services is but one aspect of the total school health program. Therefore policy makers would be ill advised to trade away all the rest of their school health program (generalized health services for the entire student body, health education, and a healthy environment) for a school-based health center.

Family Resource/Service Centers

In Florida, Kentucky, New Jersey, and numerous other states the idea of family resource/service centers is attracting attention. Within this organizational structure, a number of school and community resources for families are consolidated into one agency for the sake of efficiency and cost containment. Various public agencies, including the school, pool their child and adolescent health and child care resources and reduce their overhead and management expenses by offering a one-stop shopping arrangement. An extension of the school health program logically belongs within these centers.

Family resource centers may be either geographically located in the school or linked to the school in some other way. In addition to student services, education and employment opportunities for parents also are offered.

Employee Health

Another key aspect of some school health programs is that the program should meet some of the health needs of the teaching staff and other employees of the school system. Currently, a number of school districts have wellness programs for employees, as well as medical services (i.e., physical examinations, counseling for drug and alcohol abuse) and in-house evaluations for workmen's compensation claims. These services are often highly valued by the school board and school administrators because of the potential for health care cost containment and reduction in absences. School nurses also have offered various consumer health education programs, such as an adult version of the HealthPACT course, in an effort to enhance teacher satisfaction with the health care system and to improve their use of their health care benefits.

 ## Clinical Application

A referral was made to the school by Monique's sixth grade teacher. Mr. Mather had noticed that Monique was having increasing problems in the classroom with attention, behavior problems, and poor work, for about the last 2 weeks. Could the nurse see whether any of these problems might be health-related?

Conversation with the teachers revealed that Monique was new to the school, having moved into the district only 2 months ago. Monique was the daughter of an immigrant; the family had been in the U.S. for 10 years. Her mother spoke limited English, but Monique appeared to have a good command of the language. When the teacher spoke with the mother, Monique would assist with interpretation. The teacher stated that Monique did respond to questions appropriately "when she paid attention." He noted that Monique appeared to have few friends

in the class. So far as her behavior was concerned, she would talk or 'day dream' in class instead of listening and was disruptive with her irrelevant remarks.

The nurse agreed that it was appropriate to investigate the possible causes of Monique's classroom difficulties. Parental permission was sought and granted. Plans were made to meet Monique in the school clinic. The findings would be discussed with Monique, her parents, and the teacher.

When seen in the clinic, Monique was a quiet, shy girl, neatly but plainly dressed. At first, she responded only when questioned. Little information was volunteered. However, as the interview progressed she soon relaxed enough to talk more spontaneously with the nurse. Monique was feeling left out of activities with the other students—they had

Clinical Application—cont'd

their own friends to sit with at lunch and she did not really see any of them after school. Sometimes Monique would try to get their attention in class or ask questions about what the teacher said because she could not always understand him. She was "feeling ok" now, but was tired and sometimes her neck and jaw would ache, usually on one side only. Yes, she would get colds every year and her mama would buy "medicine for her ears," but she had not had any for a long time. The nurse noticed that Monique would turn her head to the right side when she was spoken to. Her partial physical examination revealed a low-grade temperature of 99.2° F, caries in a right molar, and a dull right tympanic membrane (tm) with decreased mobility and mild erythema. The left tm showed evidence of scarring from previous infection. The lymph nodes in her neck were enlarged, the right more than the left. She also had nasal congestion with clear nasal drainage. She denied any pain. Her speech was clear.

A quick review of Monique's health records from her previous school indicated that several referrals had been made for earaches and dental care. There were few notations regarding behavior.

Assessment of the information indicated that Monique had acute otitis media (om) and chronic dental caries. The recent onset of classroom difficulties indicated that there was a possible association between these conditions and her behavior in the classroom. A more long-term problem was her sense of isolation from her classmates and acting out behaviors to get their attention.

A call was placed to Monique's mother regarding the nurse's findings. Although Monique's mother spoke limited English, the nurse was bilingual and was able to convey the information that Monique needed treatment for an ear infection and would need to see a dentist because she had cavities. With Monique's additional help with interpretation, the nurse learned that the family was uninsured and had no regular source of medical and dental care. The family would be interested in low cost medical care because they had limited financial resources and no insurance. The transportation to receive medical care would also be a problem because Monique's father would be at work and unable to take her for medical care.

The nurse had the address and phone number of the local community health clinic. She helped call and arrange an appointment time for Monique and her mother to go to the clinic. Monique could be seen the same day that her mother applied for clinic services. No interpreter would be available at the clinic to help with the details of the financial qualifying interview or with the health history. It was apparent that additional assistance was needed since the nurse's schedule prevented her from accompanying the family, and Monique's mother agreed.

The community resource book listed a local agency responsible for assistance to immigrant groups within the community. A call to the agency yielded the name of a representative who could serve as an interpreter. The agent agreed to contact Monique's mother and arrange assistance with transportation for medical care and an interpreter for the visit.

On follow-up with Monique and her mother, the nurse learned that Monique had been seen in the local health clinic and treated for acute otitis media. Future appointments were made for follow-up visits to assess the response to medication, for a complete physical examination, and for dental care. The mother was pleased with the clinic and planned to use the clinic services for regular health care needs for the entire family. Because she had a contact with an agency that would assist with language difficulties, the mother felt more comfortable seeking care for herself and her family.

The nurse also maintained contact with Monique's teacher. He was made aware of the ear infection and in the following weeks reported an improvement in her attention to school work. Behavior problems lessened as Monique's ear infection resolved and she was able to understand what was being said. There were still attempts by Monique to get the attention of other students, so it was agreed that the teacher would use class activities to encourage student interaction and offer opportunities for students to know each other better. The nurse counseled Monique and her mother, encouraging Monique's involvement in activities (both in and out of school) that would foster friendships with her classmates.

As a final step, the nurse and teacher agreed that Monique would be encouraged to develop friendships, and the nurse would be notified if other problems were noted. The previously identified physical problems would be followed through the routine screenings alone in each school, with special attention given to any indications of recurring physical problems.

The preceding case study illustrates the role of the school nurse in providing care to school-age youth. Use of available school and community resources is not only wise but necessary if the nurse is to function effectively. Care of a student requires collaboration between teachers, students and their families, and community resources if needs are to be properly identified and met. The school nurse is a key resource for assessment and preventive health maintenance and coordination of services.

Key Concepts

- The health problems of school-age youth vary substantially between the younger years and the adolescent years.
- Health problems are major risk factors for absenteeism and academic failure.
- Children and adolescents who are poor are at high risk for absenteeism and school failure.
- The three core components of school health are health services, health education, and promotion of a healthy environment.
- School health services generally include health screenings, basic care for minor complaints, administration of medications, surveillance of immunization status, case-finding for the early identification of problems, and nursing care of students with special needs.
- Historically, reducing absenteeism has been the single most important reason for school nursing services. With the current emphasis on education reform and academic performance, reducing absenteeism continues to be a top priority for school nurses.
- The role of the school nurse includes the functions of health education and counseling, as well as the delivery of clinical care to students with disabilities. Coordination of the overall school health program and case management of individual student health problems are other responsibilities of the nurse.
- School health activities are family centered and are intended to promote health and reduce the incidence of disease.

- Although health screenings are an integral component of school health services, nurses must prepare other school personnel, students, and volunteers for this work.
- Administration of medications and clinical care of students with disabilities in school is increasing in frequency. Nevertheless the risks associated with these practices can be managed successfully provided there are well-developed policies and procedures.
- School health education involves health promotion instruction for all students to develop their positive personal health habits; self-help classes for students with special health needs; and consumer education for all so that the next generation will be prepared to use the health care system effectively.
- The school environment requires attention, and certain measures are necessary if the climate at school is to be both physically and psychologically healthy.
- Schools are nontraditional health care settings. Consequently, it is important to establish health policies, procedures, and plans to provide direction for the school health program.
- Planning and operation of the school health program involves parents and community health professionals, as well as school personnel.

Critical Thinking Activities

1. Visit a school. Observe the activities and interactions of students as a group both inside and outside the classroom. What are the advantages and disadvantages of learning collectively as opposed to being tutored? What are the implications for health teaching and counseling?

2. Interview a school nurse, school nurse practitioner, or community health nurse specialist for school-aged youth working in schools. How do they explain their roles in the school? What are the rewards? What are the frustrations?

3. Visit a school with a school nurse. Observe how the nurse works with individual children with disabili-

ties and with boys and girls who are at high risk for academic failure because of chronic illness, poverty, and family problems. Inquire about any special procedures and precautions they observe in caring for these students. Look at the record keeping system. Ask to review an individual education plan (IEP) and an individualized family service plan (IFSP). Find out whether the school nurse is involved with the school district's preschool program. Does the school also have a program for those infants and toddlers 0 to 3 years of age who have disabilities? How is the nurse involved with this effort?

Critical Thinking Activities—cont'd

4. Find a journal or textbook for school teachers. Review the table of contents to determine the areas of interest and importance to them. Select and read one of these articles/chapters. Compare and contrast the school teacher's approach to problem solving with the way nurses solve problems. What benefits and constraints could these differences present when nurses and teachers try to work together?

5. Attend a school board meeting. In preparation for this activity find out whether the board members are appointed or elected. Also find out something about the board members: their names, occupations, special concerns about education. At the time of the meeting, review the agenda, notice the amount of preparatory work the board members must do before meetings, observe the interactions between the board, school administrators, and members of the audience. What are the chief concerns expressed at this meeting? How will this affect the school health program and school nurses?

6. Find a group of children or adolescents. Ask them to draw you a picture of (or explain) the nature of the health program at their school. What services are provided? What health classes are taught? What activities go on at school to keep it a safe and healthy environment for students? Ask the students to identify one change in the school health program that they would like to make.

7. Contact a parent who is a member of the Parent Teachers Organization (PTO). Discover the purpose and functions of this organization. Find out whether the PTO is involved in school health locally or nationally. Also discover whether the PTO represents all parents. Are parents who are poor or from minority groups involved?

8. Is there a state school nurse consultant in your state? Find out by contacting the State Department of Health and the State Department of Education/Instruction. If there is a nurse consultant available, find out the answers to these questions: (1) How many school nurses are there in your state? (2) Is there a current statewide policy/procedure manual for school health that is available to guide the practice of all school health personnel, especially those people working in districts too small to develop their own? How is this manual developed? (3) What is the major school health concern right now in your state and the nurse consultant's strategy for addressing this issue? (4) Where are the school health programs in your state that work well? What are the ingredients in these school systems that make these programs successful?

9. Review the Chronology of School Health Events in Table 44-2 and predict what type of school health program will be needed in the year 2015.

Bibliography

A children's defense budget FY 1989: an analysis of our nation's investment in children, Washington, DC, 1988, Children's Defense Fund.

Allensworth D, Wolford C: *Achieving the 1990 health objectives for the nation,* Kent, Ohio, 1988, American School Health Association.

Benson U, Marano: *Current estimates from the national health interview survey, United States, 1992,* Vital and health statistics, series 10, Washington, DC, 1992, National Center for Health Statistics.

Califano J Jr: *American's health care revolution: Who lives? Who dies? Who pays?* New York, 1986, Random House.

Child Health USA 89, USDHHS Pub No (PHS) Bureau of Maternal and Child Health and Resource Development, Office of Maternal and Child Health HRS-M-CH8915, Washington, DC, 1989, Department of Health and Human Services.

Child Health USA 93, USDHHS Pub No HRSA-MCH-94-1, Washington, DC, March 1994, US Government Printing office.

Children and America's other drug problem: guidelines for improving prescription medicine use among children and teenagers, Washington, DC, 1989, National Council on Patient Information.

Code blue: uniting for healthier youth: a call to action, The National Commission on the Role of the School and Community in Improving Adolescents Health, Alexandria, Va, 1990, NASBE.

Comer J: Educating poor minority children, *Sci Am* 259:42-48, 1988.

Committee on Vision: *Myopia: prevalence and progression,* Commission on Behavioral and Social Sciences and Education, National Research Council, Washington, DC, 1989, National Academy Press.

Current Population Reports, Series P-60, No 161, US Department of Commerce, Washington, DC, 1988, Bureau of the Census.

Department of Adolescent Health, American Medical Association: *Guidelines for adolescent preventive services (GAPS),* Chicago, Ill, 1992, American Medical Association.

Dever A: *Epidemiology of health service management,* Rockville, Md, 1984, Aspen Systems Corp.

Digest of Educational Statistics, NCES86-643, Washington, DC, 1989, US Department of Education Office of Educational Research and Improvement.

Dock LL: School-nurse experiment in New York, *Am J Nurs* 3:108-110, 1902.

Family health in an era of stress: General Mills American Family Report, 1979, General Mills, Inc.

Flinn Foundation special report: The health of Arizona's school children: key findings of two surveys by Louis Harris and Associates and the UCLA School of Medicine, Phoenix, Ariz 1989, Flinn Foundation.

Goodwin L: The effectiveness of school nurse practitioners: a review of the literature, *J Sch Health* 51:623-624, 1981.

Goodwin L: *Immunizations in schools: pros and cons,* Unpublished report, 1978.

Green LW: Health education models. In Matarazzo JD, Weiss SM, Herd JA, Miller N, Weiss SM, editors: *Behavioral health: a handbook of health enhancement and disease prevention*, New York, 1984, John Wiley & Sons.

Green M, editor: *Bright futures: guidelines for health supervision on infants, children and adolescents*, Arlington, Va, 1994, National Center for Education in Maternal and Child Health.

Guide to Clinical Preventive Services: *Report of the US preventive services task force*, Baltimore, 1989, Williams and Wilkins, pp 305-313.

Guidelines for a model school nursing services program, Scarborough, Maine, 1990, National Association of School Nurses.

Guidelines for the delineation of roles and responsibilities for the safe delivery of specialized health care in the educational setting, Developed by the joint task force for the management of children with special health needs of the American Federation of Teachers (AFT), The Council for Exceptional Children (CEC), National Association of School Nurses (NASN), National Education Association (NEA), Scarborough, Maine, 1990, National Association of School Nurses.

Health: United States, 1993, USDHHS Pub No (PHS) 73-1232, Washington, DC, 1994, USDHHS.

Healthy People 2000: national health promotion and disease prevention objectives, Washington, DC, 1991, USDHHS, Public Health Service.

Igoe J: Healthy long-term attitudes on personal health can be developed in school-age children, *Pediatrician* 15:127-136, 1988.

Igoe J: *Empowering the health care consumer, pediatric nursing forum on the future: looking toward the 21st century*, New Jersey, 1989, Anthony Jannetti.

Igoe J: School nursing and school health. In Natapoff J and Wieczarek R, editors: *Maternal child health policy: a nursing perspective*, New York, 1990, Springer.

Igoe J: Is health a school issue? School-based health services. In Aiken L and Fagin C, editors: *Nursing and health policy: issues of the 1990's*, Philadelphia, 1991, JB Lippincott.

Igoe J, Campos EL: Report of a national survey of school nurse supervisors, *Sch Nurs* 6:8-20, 1991.

Iowa Department of Education: *Administering medications to students in Iowa schools: a training guide*, unpublished report, 1991.

Kaplan D: *School health care ONLINE!!!! School-based clinic management information system*, Denver, Colo, 1991, Medical and Educational Software, Inc.

Kids count data book: state profiles of child well-being, Washington, DC, 1991, The Center for the Study of Social Policy.

Klerman L: School absence—a health perspective, *Pediatr Clin North Am* 35:1253-1269, 1988.

Kolbe L, Iverson D: Comprehensive school health education programs. In Matarazzo J, Weiss S, Herd J, Miller N, Weiss S, editors: *Behavioral health: a handbook of health enhancement and disease prevention*, New York, 1984, John Wiley & Sons.

Kornguth M: School absences for illness: who's absent and why, *Pediat Nurs* 16:95-99, 1990.

Kovar M: The health status of preschool and school-age children. In Wallace H, Ryan G, Oglesby A, editors: *Maternal and child health practices*, Oakland, Calif, 1988, Third Party Publishing Company.

Lewis C, Lewis MA: Consequences of empowering children to care for themselves, *Pediatrician* 17:63-67, 1990.

Lovato C, editor: *School health in America*, Kent, Ohio, 1990, American School Health Association.

Mann K: Screening for scoliosis: a review of the evidence. In Goldbloom RB, Lawrence R, editors: *Preventing disease beyond the rhetoric*, New York, 1990, Springer-Verlag.

Meeker R, De Angelis C, Berman B, et al: A comprehensive school health initiative, *Image* 18:86-91, 1986.

Model school health programs, unpublished report, Center for Disease Control and Prevention, Washington, DC, 1991.

National Council on Patient Information and Education: *Guidelines for improving prescription medicine use among children and teenagers: a report of the national council on patient information and education*, Washington, DC, 1989, The Council.

Northern J, Downs M: *Hearing in children*, Baltimore, 1989, Williams & Wilkins.

Rogers L: The nurse in the public school, *Am J Nurs* 5:763-769, 1905.

Rogers L: Some phases of school nursing, *Am J Nurs* 8:966-974, 1908.

Schneider M, Friedman S, Fisher Mil: Stated and unstated reasons for visiting a high school nurse's office, *J Adolesc Health* 16:35-41, 1995.

School health in America, Kent, Ohio, 1989, American School Health Association.

School nurses working with handicapped children: a statement of the American Nurses Association Divisions on Nursing Practice, The American School Health Association and the National Association of School Nurses, Kansas City, Mo, 1980, American Nurses Association.

Schwab N, Hass M: Delegation and supervision in school settings: standards, issues and guidelines for practice (Part 1), *J Sch Nurs* 11(1), Feb, 1995, pp 26-34.

Starfield B: Family income, ill health and medical care of US children, *J Public Health Policy* 3:244-259, 1982.

Stember M: *Kids as consumers: effectiveness of HealthPACT, final report of "a study of school nurses' use of project HealthPACT,"* Division of Nursing, Bureau of Health Professions, Health Resources and Services Administration, US Public Health Service, R01NU0093, 1988.

Stoto M, Behrens R, Rosemont C, editors: *Healthy People 2000: citizens chart the course*, Institute of Medicine, Washington, DC, 1990, National Academy Press.

Struthers LR: *The school nurse*, New York, 1917, GP Putnam's Sons.

US Department of Education: *National Goals for Education*, Washington, DC, 1990.

Walker D, Butler J, Bender A: Children's health care and the schools. In Schlesinger M, Eisenberg L, editors: *Children in a changing health system: assessments and proposals for reform*, Baltimore, 1990, John Hopkins University Press.

Waters Y: *Visiting nursing in the United States*, New York, 1909, Charities Publications Committee.

Whetten D, Cameron K: *Developing management skills*, New York, 1991, Harper Collins.

Wold SJ: *School nursing: a framework for practice*, North Branch, Minn, 1981, Sunrise River Press.

Woodfill M, Beyrer M: *The role of the nurse in the school setting: an historical view as reflected in the literature*, Kent, Ohio, 1991, American School Health Association.

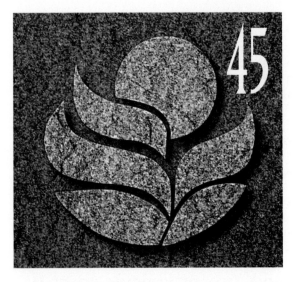

45

Community Health Nurse in Occupational Health

Charlene C. Ossler ◆ Marcia Stanhope ◆ Jeanette Lancaster

Objectives ▼

After reading this chapter, the student should be able to do the following:

◆ Describe the nursing role in occupational health.
◆ Describe at least three characteristics of the American work force.
◆ Describe the extent of work-related illnesses and injuries.
◆ Use the epidemiological model to explain work-health interactions.
◆ Cite at least three host factors associated with increased risk from an adverse response to hazardous workplace exposure.
◆ Define hypersusceptible workers.
◆ Explain one example each of biological, chemical, ergonomic, physical, and psychosocial workplace hazards.
◆ Differentiate between health promotion programs and employee assistance programs.
◆ Describe functions of OSHA and NIOSH.
◆ Describe an effective disaster plan.
◆ Complete an occupational health history.

Key Terms ▼

agents
biological agents
chemical agents
communication standards
cumulative trauma
employee assistance programs
environment
epidemiological triad
ergonomic agents
ergonomists
Hazard Communication Standard
host
hypersusceptible
National Institute for Occupational Safety and Health (NIOSH)
occupational health history
occupational health nursing
Occupational Safety and Health Act
Occupational Safety and Health Administration (OSHA)
physical agents
psychosocial agents
standards
workers' compensation act
work-health interactions
work site survey

Outline ▼

During the past two decades, there have been revolutionary changes in the nature of work and the workplace, the global economy, and the health care system. These complex changes are shaping future health priorities. An analysis of these trends suggests that **work-health interactions** will continue to grow in importance, especially as the demand for healthy workers exceeds the supply. As a result, impressive developments have occurred in occupational health and safety programs to control and prevent work-related illness and injury. Nurses, particularly occupational health nurses, have performed critical roles in planning and delivering work site health and safety services, which must continue to grow in comprehensiveness and cost effectiveness. The continuing escalation of the cost of health care and concern about the quality of care have prompted American businesses to add management of nonwork-related health problems to their health services programs.

The health impact of work is an important issue for most clients for whom the community health nurse provides care. At least one-third of the average adult's life is spent at work; therefore, the workplace has significant influence on individuals' health and is a primary site for the delivery of preventive health care. As a result of the influence of health care reform and the movement toward managed care, institutions, such as hospitals will lose some of their importance in the health care delivery system. The home, the clinic, the nursing home and other community-based sites such as the workplace will become the dominant areas where health and illness care will be sought.

The prevalence and significance of the interactions between health and work underscore the importance of incorporating principles of occupational health and safety into general nursing practice. The types of interactions and the frequent use of the general health care system for the identification, treatment, and prevention of occupational illnesses and injuries require nurses to use this knowledge in all practice settings.

This chapter describes the community health nurse's role with the working population and provides an introduction to work-related health and safety concerns and the principles for the prevention and control of adverse work-health interactions. The focus is on the knowledge and skills needed to promote the health and safety of workers through work site occupational health programs, as well as through offsite interventions from agencies other than the employing business organizations. The epidemiological triad is used as the model for understanding these interactions, as well as risk factors and effective nursing care for promoting health and safety among employed populations. The assessment, prevention, and management of occupational health problems are skills that can be applied in all types of nursing care settings.

The American Association of Occupational Health Nurses (AAOHN) defines **occupational health nursing** as "The application of nursing principles to conserve the health of workers in all organizations. It emphasizes prevention, recognition, and treatment of illness and injury, and requires special skills and knowledge in the fields of health education and counseling, environmental health, rehabilitation, and human relations" (AAOHN, 1988).

Occupational health nurses work in traditional manufacturing and industry settings, hospitals, construction sites, and university and government settings. Their scope of practice includes health history, assessment, surveilence, primary care, counseling, health promotion/protection, administration, management, quality assurance, research, and community collaboration. The nurse is guided in decision-making by the Code of Ethics of the AAOHN (Rogers, 1994).

THE EVOLUTION OF NURSING ROLES IN OCCUPATIONAL SETTINGS

Nursing care for workers began in 1888 and was called industrial nursing. A group of coal miners hired Betty Moulder, a graduate of the Blockley Hospital School of Nursing in Philadelphia, to take care of their ailing co-workers and their families (Rogers, 1994). Ada Mayo Stewart, hired in 1985 by the Vermont Marble Company in Rutland, Vermont, is considered the first industrial nurse. Riding a bicycle, Miss Stewart visited sick employees in their homes, provided emergency care, taught mothers how to care for their children, and taught healthy living habits (Felton, 1985). In the early days of occupational health nursing, the nurse's work was family-centered and holistic.

Employee health services grew rapidly during the early 1900s as companies recognized that the provision of work site health services led to a more productive workforce. At that time, workplace accidents were seen as an inevitable part of having a job. However, the public did not support this attitude, and a system for worker's compensation arose.

Industrial nursing grew rapidly during the first half of the twentieth century. Educational courses were established, as were professional societies. By World War II, there were approximately 4000 industrial nurses (Brown, 1981). The American Association of Industrial Nursing (AAIN), the precursor to the current American Association of Occupational Health Nurses, was established as the first national nursing organization in 1942. The aim of the AAIN was to improve industrial nursing education and practice and to promote interdisciplinary collaborative efforts (Rogers, 1994).

The enactment of several laws in the 1960s and 1970s to protect workers' safety and health led to an increased need for occupational health nurses. In particular, the passage in 1970 of the Occupational Health and Safety Act stimulated a large demand for nurses at the work site to meet the demands of the many newly-legislated occupational health services.

As American industry has shifted from agrarian to industrial to highly technological processes, the role of the occupational health nurse has continued to evolve. The focus on work-related health problems now includes the spectrum of human responses to multiple, complex interactions of biopsychosocial factors that occur in the community, home, and work environments. The customary role of the occupational health nurse has extended beyond emergency treatment and prevention of illness and injury to include the promotion and maintenance of health, overall risk management, and efforts to reduce health-related costs in businesses.

The occupational health nurse (OHN) offers direct care to employees and performs managerial functions such as program evaluation and analysis of work-related injuries and illnesses. The role changes with an organization's occupational health and safety program goals and is therefore diversified. The interdisciplinary nature of occupational health nursing has become more critical as occupational health and safety problems require more complex solutions. The OHN frequently collaborates closely with multiple disciplines and management, as well as representatives of labor.

OHNs constitute the largest group of occupational health professionals. The most recent national survey of registered nurses indicates that there are approximately 19,000 licensed occupational health nurses (U.S. Department of Health and Human Services, 1992). In the most recent survey conducted about OHNs, nearly 70% report that they are employed as staff nurses; the majority of these manage one-nurse units in a variety of businesses. Other OHNs hold positions as nurse practitioners, clinical nurse specialists, managers, supervisors, consultants, and edu-cators. The occupational health nursing role is unique in that the nurse adapts to an organization's needs as well as to the needs of specific groups of workers.

The professional organization for occupational nurses, the American Association of Occupational Health Nurses, Inc. (AAOHN), describes five job titles for OHNs: Solo practioner, administrator, educator,

---

Use of the Nursing Process in the Five Functional Roles of the Occupational Health Nurse

NURSE CLINICIAN/PRACTITIONER

◆ Assesses the work environment for actual or potential health hazards.

◆ Collects data about the health status of the worker through an occupational health history, physical assessment, and appropriate laboratory measurements.

◆ Develops a nursing diagnosis to formulate a plan of nursing care in collaboration with the employee and other health care professionals.

◆ Records health data and maintains accurate employee health records.

◆ Provides counseling for worker health problems, health promotion, and disease prevention interventions (e.g., immunization, respiratory protection, hypertension screening, hearing conservation programs).

◆ Develops liaison relationships with community health care providers and organizations for worker health enhancement (e.g., referral to private providers and non-profit and governmental agencies).

NURSE ADMINISTRATOR

◆ Assesses the health needs of the workforce to help plan and develop cost-effective health services.

◆ Defines goals and objectives for the occupational health nursing service.

◆ Determines resources, such as facilities, staff, and operating expenses necessary to accomplish unit goals and develops an appropriate, realistic budget, as well as develops policies and procedures aimed at fostering goal attainment and work performance.

◆ Provides nursing leadership in the management and evaluation of human and operational resources, such as opportunities for enhancement of professional growth and quality management.

NURSE EDUCATOR

◆ Assesses the needs of the workforce with respect to health information and educational interventions.

◆ Develops, implements, and evaluates health promotion and education programs and materials.

◆ Acts as a liaison to community agencies in establishing networks for health education and promotion resources.

◆ Provides current information to all workers regarding health issues, trends, and factors that influence health behaviors and impact on health outcomes.

NURSE RESEARCHER

◆ Identifies issues to be considered through an occupational health and safety research effort.

◆ Participates with others in the conduction of research.

◆ Disseminates research findings.

◆ Incorporates research findings into the delivery of occupational health nursing services.

NURSE CONSULTANT

◆ Provides advice about the scope and development of occupational health services and programs, considering regulatory and other trends in health care.

◆ Serves as a resource to management on occupational health nursing issues.

◆ Serves as a resource for information and professional networking.

From Rogers B: In McCunnery RM, Brandt-Rauf PW: *A practical approach to occupational and environmental medicine*, Boston, 1994, Little, Brown, and Company.

consultant, and researcher (AAOHN, 1988). The majority of OHNs work as solo practitioners, but an increasing number of positions have developed in other categories (see box on p. 909). New roles in case management and in environmental assessment and control have developed in larger firms. In many companies, management positions have been pared, and the OHN has assumed expanded responsibilities in job analysis, safety, and benefits management. Specialization in the field is often a requirement for the other positions. Graduate education in occupational health nursing is currently available through 15 universities (see box on p. 911).

With the current changes in health care delivery and the movement toward managed care, OHNs will need significant skills in primary care, including health promotion and disease prevention. The aim of the occupational health nurse will be to devote considerable attention to keeping the workers and, in some cases, their families, healthy and free from illness and work site injuries. There is a significant health education role within occupational health nursing.

Certification in occupational health nursing is provided by the American Board for Occupational Health Nurses, Inc. (ABOHN). OHNs must meet requirements for experience, continuing education, and professional activities before they are eligible to take the ABOHN certification examination. Approximately 25% of OHNs practicing in the specialty are certified occupational health nurses (COHN).

WORKERS AS A POPULATION AGGREGATE

There are more than 100 million workers over 16 years of age in the United States, employed in about 6.3 million different work sites (*Healthy People 2000*, 1991). More than 91% of those who are able to work outside of the home do so for some portion of their lives (Bureau of Labor Statistics, 1995). Neither of these statistics indicates the full number of individuals who have potentially been exposed to work-related health hazards. Although some individuals may currently be unemployed or retired, they continue to bear the health risks of past occupational hazards. The number of affected individuals may be even larger as work-related illnesses are found among spouses, children, and neighbors of exposed workers (Emergency Medicine, 1990).

Americans are employed in diverse industries that range in size from one to tens of thousands of employees. Types of industries include traditional manufacturing (e.g., automotive and appliances), service industries (e.g., banking, health care, and restaurants), agriculture, and the newer high-technology firms, such as computer chip manufacturers. Approximately 95% of business organizations are considered small; they employ fewer than 500 people (Bureau of Labor Statistics, 1995). Although some industries are noted

for the high degree of hazards associated with their work (e.g., manufacturing, mines, construction, and agriculture), no work site is free of occupational health and safety hazards. The larger the company, the more likely it is that there will be health and safety programs for employees. Smaller companies are more apt to rely on the external community to meet their needs for health and safety services.

Characteristics of the Workforce

The demographic trends in the American workforce describe a changing population aggregate that has implications for the preventive services targeted to that group. Major changes in the working population are reflected in the increasing numbers of women, older individuals, and those with chronic illnesses who are part of the workforce. Because of changes in the economy, extension of life span, legislative initiatives, and societal acceptance of working women, the proportion of the employed population that these three groups represent will probably continue to grow.

In an era in which the demand for workers is expected to outstrip the available supply, businesses must be concerned about strategies to enhance the health, employment longevity, and satisfaction of workers. For example, nearly 60% of women are employed, and it is predicted that women will account for 67% of the increase in the labor force over the next decade (Rix, 1990; US Department of Labor Statistics, 1995). These workers tend to be married, with children and aging parents for whom they are responsible. This aggregate of workers poses new issues for individual and family health promotion, such as child care and elder care), that can be addressed in the work environment. Other trends shaping the profile of the workforce include more education and mobility, as well as increasing mismatches in the 1990s between skills of workers and types of employment.

Characteristics of Work

There has been a dramatic shift in the types of jobs held by workers. Following the evolution from an agrarian economy to a manufacturing society and then to a highly technological workplace, the greatest proportion of paid employment is now in the occupations of service (e.g., health care, information processing, banking, and insurance), professional and technical positions (e.g., managers and computer specialists), and clerical work (e.g., word processors and secretaries). Of the new jobs created from 1984 to 1994, 73% were in the categories of professional administrative, sales and technical, and precision crafts (Bureau of Labor Statistics, 1995). In the traditional manufacturing setting, modernization with robots and other mechanization of work processes have altered job requirements. This change in the nature of work has

NIOSH Educational Resource Centers

The National Institute for Occupational Safety and Health (NIOSH) funds Educational Resource Centers (ERCs) that conduct research and administer graduate training programs in occupational medicine, occupational health nursing, industrial hygiene, and safety. It also provides continuing education programs for safety and health professionals and outreach programs for the community.

ALABAMA

Deep South Center for Occupational Health and Safety
University of Alabama at Birmingham
School of Public Health
Birmingham, AL 35294-2010
(205) 934-7178, FAX (205) 975-7179

CALIFORNIA

Northern California ERC
Center for Occupational and Environmental Health
University of California at Berkeley
Richmond Field Station
1301 South 46th St., Bldg., 102
Richmond, California 94804
(510) 231-5645, FAX (510) 231-5648

Southern California ERC
University of Southern California
Institute of Safety and Systems Management
Professional Programs
927 West 35th Place, Room 102
Los Angeles, CA 90089-0021
(213) 740-3995, FAX (213) 740-8789

ILLINOIS

Illinois ERC
Great Lakes Center for Occupational and Environmental Health
  & Safety
University of Illinois
School of Public Health
2121 West Taylor St., Room 216A
Chicago, Illinois 60612-7260
(312) 413-0459, FAX (312) 413-7369

MARYLAND

Johns Hopkins ERC
Johns Hopkins University
School of Hygiene and Public Health
615 North Wolfe St., Room 6001
Baltimore, MD 21205
(410) 955-3602, FAX (410) 955-9334

MASSACHUSETTS

Harvard ERC
Harvard Educational Resource Center
665 Huntington Avenue
Boston, MA 02115
(617) 432-3314, FAX (617) 432-0219

MICHIGAN

Michigan ERC
University of Michigan
Center for Occupational Health and Safety Engineering
1205 Beal, IOE Building
Ann Arbor, MI 48109-2117
(313) 936-0148, FAX (313) 764-3451

MINNESOTA

Midwest Center for Occupational Health and Safety
University of Minnesota
640 Jackson Street
St. Paul, MN 55101
(612) 221-3992, FAX (612) 292-4773

NEW YORK/NEW JERSEY

UMDNJ-Robert Wood
New York/New Jersey ERC
EOHSI Centers for Education and Training
45 Knightsbridge Road, Brookwood II
Piscataway, NL 08854-3923
(908) 235-5062, FAX (908) 235-5133

NIOSH

NIOSH-Division of Training and Manpower Development
4676 Columbia Parkway (C11)
Cincinnati, OH 45226
(513) 533-8225, FAX (513) 533-8560

NORTH CAROLINA

North Carolina ERC
Center for Occupational Safety and Health
University of North Carolina
109 Conner Drive, Suite 1101
Chapel Hill, NC 27514
(919) 962-2101, FAX (919) 966-7579

OHIO

University of Cincinnati ERC
University of Cincinnati
Department of Environmental Health
PO Box 670056
Cincinnati, OH 45267-0056
(513) 558-1729, FAX (513) 558-1756

TEXAS

Southwest Center of Occupational and Environmental Health
RASW-1026 P.O. Box 20186
Houston, TX 77225-0186
(713) 792-4648, FAX (713) 792-4407

UTAH

Rocky Mountain Center for Occupational and Environmental
  Health
University of Utah
Building 512
Salt Lake City, UT 84112
(801) 581-4055, FAX (801) 585-5275

WASHINGTON

Northwest Center for Occupational Health and Safety
Department of Environmental Health
School of Public Health and Community Medicine
University of Washington, SC-34
Seattle, WA 98195
(206) 543-1069, FAX (206) 685-3872

been accompanied by many new occupational hazards such as complex chemicals, non-ergonomic workstation design (the adaptation of the workplace or work equipment to meet the employee's health and safety needs), and job stress. In addition, the emergence of a global economy with free trade and multinational corporations presents new challenges for health and safety programs that are culturally relevant.

Work-Health Interactions

The influence of work on health is shown by statistics on illnesses, injuries, and deaths associated with employment. In 1993, 2.2 million reported work-related illnesses and injuries resulted in lost time from work. Of these, approximately 70,000 were severe enough to result in temporary or permanent disabilities that prevented the workers from returning to their usual jobs. Over the past few years, the incidence and severity of work-related injuries have increased (Bureau of Labor Statistics, 1995). During 1988, 3270 deaths were attributed to the work environment, in 1993 there were 6,271; another 100,000 deaths resulted from primary illnesses in which work was a contributing or exacerbating factor. More than 482,000 cases of occupationally induced illnesses were diagnosed in

1993 (Office of Technology Assessment, 1995). These figures are often described as the "tip of the iceberg" because many work-related health problems go unreported; but even the recorded statistics are significant in depicting the amount of human suffering, economic loss, and decreased productivity associated with workplace hazards.

NIOSH estimates that 17 American workers die everyday while trying to earn a living, and 137 additional workers die each day from workplace disease.

APPLICATION OF THE EPIDEMIOLOGICAL MODEL

The **epidemiological triad** can be used to understand the relationship between work and health (Figure 45-1). With a focus on the health and safety of the employed population, the **host** is described as any susceptible human being. Because of the ubiquitous nature of work-related hazards, nurses must assume that

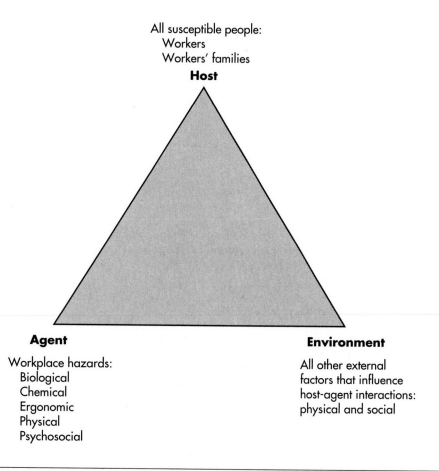

FIGURE 45-1

Elements of the epidemiological triad applied to occupational health.

all employed individuals and groups are at risk of being exposed to occupational hazards. The **agents,** factors associated with illness and injury, are occupational hazards that are classified as biological, chemical, ergonomic, physical, or psychosocial. The third element, the **environment,** includes all external conditions that influence the interaction of the host and agents. These may be workplace conditions such as temperature extremes, crowding, shift work, and inflexible management styles. The basic principle of epidemiology is that health status interventions for restoring and promoting health are the result of complex interactions among these three elements. To understand these interactions and to design effective nursing strategies for dealing with them in a proactive manner, nurses must look at how each element influences the others.

Host

Each worker represents a host within the worker population group. Certain host factors correlate with increased risk of adverse response to the hazards of the workplace. These include age, gender, chronic illness, work practices, immunological status, ethnicity, and lifestyle habits. For example, the population group at greatest risk for experiencing work-related accidents with subsequent injuries are males (18 to 30 years old) with less than 6 months experience on their current job. The host factors of age, gender, and work experience combine to increase this group's risk of injury because of characteristics such as risk-taking, lack of knowledge, and low dexterity on the new job. This population aggregate of workers is also more likely to be impaired by chronic use and abuse of drugs and alcohol.

Older workers may be at increased risk in the workplace because of diminished sensory abilities, the effects of chronic illnesses, and delayed reaction times. A third population group that may be very susceptible to workplace exposure is women in their childbearing years. The hormonal changes during these years, along with the increased stress of new roles and additional responsibilities, are host factors that may influence this group's response to potentially toxic exposures.

In addition to these host factors, there may be other, less well-understood individual differences in responses to occupational hazard exposures. Even if employers maintain exposure levels below the level recommended by occupational health and safety standards, 15% to 20% of the population may have health reactions to the "safe" low-level exposures. This group has been termed **hypersusceptible.** A number of host factors appear to be associated with this hypersusceptibility: light skin, malnutrition, compromised immune system, glucose 6-phosphate dehydrogenase deficiency, serum alpha 1-antitrypsin deficiency, chronic obstructive pulmonary disease, sickle cell trait, and hy-

pertension. Individuals who have known hypersusceptibility to chemicals that are respiratory irritants, hemolytic chemicals, organic isocyanates, and carbon disulfide may also be hypersusceptible to other agents in the work environment (Zenz, 1988, p. 109). Although this has prompted some industries to consider preplacement screening for such risk factors, the associations between these individual health markers and hypersusceptible response are speculative and require further research.

Agents

Work-related hazards, or agents, present potential and actual risks to the health and safety of workers in the millions of business establishments in the United States. These agents are classified in five categories: *biological, chemical, ergonomic, physical,* and *psychosocial.* Any worksite commonly presents multiple and interacting exposures from all five categories of agents. Table 45-1 lists some of the more common workplace exposures, their known health effects, and the types of jobs associated with these hazards.

Biological Agents

Biological agents are living organisms whose excretions or parts are capable of causing human disease, usually by an infectious process. Biological hazards are common in workplaces such as hospitals and clinical laboratories where employees are potentially exposed to a variety of infectious agents including viruses, fungi, and bacteria. Health services workers are at increased risk of contracting diseases from these exposures. For example, hepatitis B and tuberculosis rates are generally higher than expected among hospital personnel; a hospital employee is 41% more likely than the average worker to lose work time because of a serious occupational injury or illness (National Safety Council, 1989). Many workers in these settings are employed as maintenance workers, security guards, aides, or cleaning people, who tend not to be well-protected from inadvertent exposures which include contaminated bed linen in the laundry, soiled equipment, and trash containing contaminated dressings or specimens.

Other occupations with exposures to biological agents include agriculture (farmer's lung) and commercial baking (baker's asthma) (McCunney, 1988). In addition, new biological agents, such as AIDS, *Legionella* infection, and herpes, have developed.

Chemical Agents

Over 300 billion pounds of **chemical agents** are produced annually in the United States. Of the approximately 2 million known chemicals in existence, only several hundred have been adequately studied for their effects on humans. Of those chemicals that have been assayed for carcinogenicity, approximately one-half test positive as animal carcinogens. Most chemi-

Table 45-1   Selected Job Categories, Exposures, and Associated Work-Related Diseases and Conditions

Job categories	Exposures	Work-related diseases and conditions
Agricultural workers	Pesticides, infectious agents, gases, sunlight	Pesticide poisoning, "farmer's lung," skin cancer
Anesthetists	Anesthetic gases	Reproductive effects, cancer
Animal handlers	Infectious agents, allergens	Asthma
Automobile workers	Asbestos, plastics, lead, solvents	Asbestosis dermatitis
Bakers	Flour	Asthma
Battery makers	Lead, arsenic	Lead poisoning, cancer
Butchers	Vinyl plastic fumes	"Meat wrappers' asthma"
Caisson workers	Pressurized work environments	"Caisson disease," "the bends"
Carpenters	Wood dust, wood preservatives, adhesives	Nasopharyngeal cancer, dermatitis
Cement workers	Cement dust, metals	Dermatitis, bronchitis
Ceramic workers	Talc, clays	Pneumnoniosis
Demolition workers	Asbestos, wood dust	Asbestosis
Drug manufacturers	Hormones, nitroglycerin, etc.	Reproductive effects
Dry cleaners	Solvents	Liver disease, dermatitis
Dye workers	Dyestuffs, metals, solvents	Bladder cancer, dermatitis
Embalmers	Formaldehyde, infectious agents	Dermatitis
Felt makers	Mercury, polycyclic hydrocarbons	Mercuralism
Foundry workers	Silica, molten metals	Silicosis
Glass workers	Heat, solvents, metal powders	Cataracts
Hospital workers	Infectious agents, cleansers, radiation	Infections, accidents
Insulators	Asbestos, fibrous glass	Asbestosis, lung cancer, mesothelioma
Jack hammer operators	Vibration	Raynaud phenomenon
Lathe operators	Metal dusts, cutting oils	Lung disease, cancer

cals have not been studied epidemiologically to determine the effects of exposure on humans (Levy and Wegman, 1988, pp. 22-1223). As a consequence of general environmental contamination with chemicals from work, home, and community activities, a variety of chemicals are found in the body tissues of the general population. These tissue loads may result in part from the accidental release of chemicals into the environment, such as that which occurred in Love Canal when chemicals leached out from buried industrial wastes. In many workplaces, significant exposure to a daily, low-level dose of workplace chemicals may be below the exposure standards but still may constitute a potentially chronic and perhaps cumulative assault on workers' health. Predicting human responses to such exposures is further complicated because several chemicals are often combined to create a new chemical agent; human effects may be associated with the interaction of these agents rather than with a single chemical.

An evolving concern about occupational exposure to chemicals is reproductive health effects. Workplace reproductive hazards have become important legal and scientific issues. Toxicity to male and female reproductive systems has been demonstrated in common agents such as lead, mercury, cadmium, nickel, and zinc, as well as in antineoplastic drug administration. These concerns are addressed in a governmental report that calls for additional legislative intervention with occupational reproductive hazards (Office of Technology Assessment, 1986).

On March 20, 1991, the U.S. Supreme Court issued a decision, *Auto Workers vs. Johnson Controls, Inc.,* that will have far-reaching health effects. The Court ruled that women of childbearing age cannot be excluded from jobs that could result in reproductive hazards. Parents are to be informed about the potential work-related hazards, but they must make the decision about whether the women continue to work in a potentially dangerous environment. The Court based its decision, in part, on the aim of being non-discriminatory in allowing women to work in better-paying jobs even though these jobs may pose hazards to the fetus. In this case, the women working in a battery manufacturing plant were exposed to lead, which can cause anomalies in a developing fetus.

Since data for predicting human responses to many chemical agents are inadequate, workers should be assessed for all potential exposures and cautioned to work preventively with these agents. High-risk or vulnerable workers should be carefully screened and monitored for optimal health protection.

Ergonomic Agents

Ergonomic agents are those that involve the transfer of mechanical energy from the work processes or pose postural or other strains that can produce adverse health effects when certain tasks are performed repetitively. Examples are vibration, repetitive motion, poor workstation-worker fit, and lifting heavy loads. Vibration, which accompanies the use of power tools and vehicles such as trucks, affects internal organs, supportive ligaments, the upper torso, and the shoulder-girdle structure. Localized effects are seen with hand-held power tools; the most common is Raynaud's phenomenon. Carpal tunnel syndrome, tendonitis, and tendosynovitis are the most frequently seen occupational diseases observed in workers who are chronically exposed to repetitive motion (Putz-Anderson, 1988). The research on these hazards, related human responses, and prevention is evolving. Injuries and illnesses related to this category of agents have been termed **cumulative trauma,** which comprises the largest category of work-related illness and disability claims in the United States. The most productive strategy in preventing these exposures appears to be redesigning the workplace and the work machinery or processes.

Physical Agents

Physical agents are those that produce adverse health effects through the transfer of physical energy. Commonly encountered physical agents in the workplace include temperature extremes, noise, radiation, and lighting. The control of worker exposure to these agents frequently depends on the worker's compliance with preventive actions, such as practicing safe work habits and wearing personal protective equipment. Examples of safe work habits including taking appropriate breaks from environments with temperature extremes and not eating or smoking in radiation-contaminated areas. Personal protective equipment includes hearing protection, eye guards, protective clothing, and devices for monitoring exposures to agents such as radiation. This class of agents is considered one of the most easily controlled. Frost bite, heat stroke, hearing loss, radiation sickness, and headaches from improper lighting can be prevented through en-

Research Brief

Triolo P.: Occupational Health Hazards of Hospital Staff nurses: implications for practice and education. The University of Iowa, 1988, PhD (187p), Dissertation Abstract.

Researchers surveyed 197 registered nurses employed full-time in 11 Iowa hospitals with bed capacities of 250 or greater. The study investigated nurses' knowledge of occupational health, the incidence of physical, chemical, biological and psychosocial health stressors and outcomes, and the nurses' reporting practices and treatment patterns. The study explored the effect of length of shifts, shift patterns, length of employment in nursing, participation in a routine stress management program, age, smoking, alcohol intake, and role success on the incidence of occupational stress outcomes. Findings indicate that nurses experience a wide variety of occupational stress outcomes and inconsistently report and treat the injuries. Back pain was the most common injury experienced by 45% of the sample in the six-month period prior to the survey. Over 82% of the respondents rated their overall level of work-related stress as moderate or high. The five major causes of stress were intensity of patient care, lack of support from administration, physical demands of work, inadequate staffing, and responsibility for life and death decisions. Though nurses reported a high level of stress and the majority reported a poor attitude about work, only 51% engaged in exercise to reduce stress levels. Mediating variables which demonstrated statistically significant associations with occupational stress outcomes were length of shifts and perceived role success as a nurse. Nurses demonstrated the greatest need for knowledge related to transmission of disease, in particular hepatitis B, as well as other diseases transmitted via accidental needle sticks. The majority of nurses were interested in learning more about occupational health, and the preferred format of education was a one-hour inservice while on duty. Nurses demonstrated knowledge deficits in the reporting and treatment of injuries and knowledge related to occupational safety. Educational programs should focus on an improvement of participation of the nurse in occupational health.

gineering controls and appropriate education of workers in preventive work practices.

Psychosocial Agents

Psychosocial agents are conditions that pose a threat to the psychological and/or social well-being of individuals and groups. A psychosocial response to the work environment occurs as an employee acts selectively toward his environment in an attempt to achieve a harmonious relationship. When such a human attempt at adaptation to the environment fails, an adverse psychosocial response may occur. Work-related "burnout" is a response to excessive and continuous occupationally induced stress. Responses to negative interpersonal relationships, particularly those with authority figures in the workplace, are often the cause of vague health symptoms and increased absenteeism. Epidemiological work in mental health has pointed to environmental variables such as these in the incidence of mental illness and emotional disorder.

Environment

Environmental factors influence the occurrence of host-agent interactions and may mediate the course and outcome of those interactions. While there may be aspects of the physical environment (e.g., heat, odor, or ventilation) that influence the host-agent interaction, the psychological environment can be of equal importance. Consider an employee who is working with a potentially toxic liquid. Providing education about safe work practices and fitting the employee with protective clothing may not be adequate if the work must occur in a very hot and humid environment. As the worker becomes uncomfortable in the hot clothing, his or her protection may be compromised by rolling up a sleeve, taking off a glove, or wiping his face with a contaminated piece of clothing. If the psychosocial norms in the workplace condone such work practices (i.e., "Everyone does it when it's too hot."), the interventions that address only the host and agent will be ineffective.

The psychosocial environment includes characteristics of the work itself, as well as the interpersonal relationships required in the work setting. Job characteristics such as low autonomy, poor job satisfaction, and limited control over the pace of work have been associated with an increased risk of heart disease among clerical and blue collar workers (Haynes, 1980). Interpersonal relationships among employees and co-workers or bosses and managers are often sources of conflict and stress. Another environmental aspect is organizational culture. This refers to the norms and patterns of behavior that are sanctioned within a particular organization. Such norms and patterns set guidelines for the types of work behaviors that will enable employees to succeed within a particular firm. Examples include following organizational norms for working overtime, expressing dissatisfaction with management, and making work the first priority. These factors and the employee's response to them must be assessed if strategies for influencing the health and safety of workers are to be effective.

The epidemiological triad can be used as the basis for planning interventions to restore and promote the health of workers. These efforts are influenced by societal and organizational activities related to occupational health and safety.

ORGANIZATIONAL AND SOCIETAL EFFORTS TO PROMOTE WORKER HEALTH AND SAFETY

Promotion of worker health and safety is the goal of occupational health and safety programs. These programs are offered primarily by the employer at the workplace, but the range of services and the models for delivering them have been changing dramatically over the past few years. In addition to specific services, legislation at the federal and state levels has had a significant impact on efforts to provide a healthy and safe environment for all workers. Although the initial response to this legislation was an increased use of occupational health and safety professionals, the 1980s were a time of decreased enforcement of these laws. This effect, along with economic compression and cost cutting, resulted in *down-sizing:* Occupational health and safety services decreased in scope in some firms and were provided by paraprofessionals such as medical technicians, licensed practical nurses, or first aiders employed as production workers in the company. Under new administration of the Occupational Safety and Health Act and increased public concern about worker health and safety, there have recently been citations of companies that do not meet minimal occupational health and safety standards. Criminal charges have been filed against business owners when preventable work-related deaths occurred. These events have redirected an emphasis on preventive occupational health and safety programming.

Unless a company has OSHA-regulated exposures, business firms are not required to provide occupational health and safety services that meet any specified standards. With few exceptions, there is no legal mandate for specific services or level of personnel provided by employers to protect worker health and safety. Therefore, the range of services offered and the qualifications of the providers of occupational health and safety vary widely across industries. An important stimulus for health and safety programs is cost avoidance that can be attributed to the effectiveness of preventive services.

On-site Occupational Health and Safety Programs

Optimally, on-site occupational health and safety services are provided by a team of occupational health and safety professionals. The core members of this team are the occupational health nurse, occupational physician, industrial hygienist, and safety professional. The largest group of health care professionals in business settings is occupational health nurses; therefore, the most frequently seen model is that of the one nurse unit or solo-practicing occupational health nurse. This nurse collaborates with a community physician who provides consultation and accepts referrals for specific employee medical problems. The collaboration may occur primarily through telephone contact, or the physician may be under contract with the company to spend a certain amount of time on-site each week. As companies become larger, they are likely to hire additional nurses, part-time or full-time physicians, safety professionals, and industrial hygienists. An increasingly popular option is to contract some health, safety, and industrial hygiene work to external providers. The largest firms often have corporate occupational health and safety professionals who set policy and participate in company decision-making at the corporate level. These professionals work with the nurses employed at the individual sites within the company.

Depending on the needs of the company and the workers, additional professionals may be on the occupational health and safety team, including employee assistance counselors or social workers, health educators, physical fitness specialists, toxicologists, and human factors engineers **(ergonomists)**. The personnel and services in an organization's occupational health and safety program differ across companies and result from decisions made by management.

The services provided by on-site occupational health programs range from those focused only on work-related health and safety problems to a wide scope of services that includes primary health care (see box at right). In industries that have exposures regulated by law, certain programs are mandated. The ability of a company to offer additional programs depends on management's attitudes and understanding about health and safety, acceptance by the workers, and the economic status of the firm. A significant increase in the number of health promotion and **employee assistance programs** offered in industry has occurred over the past few years. Health promotion programs focus on life-style habits that pose risks to health (e.g., obesity, smoking, stress responses, or lack of exercise). Employee assistance programs are designed to address personal problems (e.g., marital discord, substance abuse, or financial difficulties) that affect the employee's productivity. Since such efforts are cost-effective for businesses, they should continue to increase (Healthy People 2000, 1991).

A similar array of occupational health and safety programs is available on a contractual basis from community-based providers. These may be offered by free-standing industrial clinics, health maintenance organizations, hospitals, emergency clinics, and other health care organizations. In addition, consultants in each discipline work in the private sector (self-employed, in group practice, or in insurance companies) and in the public sector (in local and state health departments or departments of labor and industry). These services may be brought on site, delivered elsewhere in the community, or offered through a mobile van that visits companies. These multiple resources have increased the options for companies that need occupational health and safety services and have also broadened the employment opportunities for health and safety professionals.

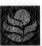 Scope of Services Provided Through an Occupational Health and Safety Program

Health assessments
  Preplacement
  Periodic: mandatory, voluntary
  Transfer
  Retirement/termination
  Executive
  Health risk appraisal
Preventive health screening with education
Employee assistance programs
Lifestyle classes: smoking cessation, weight control, stress management, physical fitness, and conditioning
Rehabilitation
Treatment of illness and injury
Primary health care for workers and dependents
Fitting of protective equipment
Worker safety and health education related to occupational hazards
Job analysis and design
Prenatal and postnatal care and support groups
Medical self-help and consumerism classes
Safety audits and accident investigation
Plant surveys and environmental monitoring
Workers' compensation and processing of OSHA claims and reports
Health-related cost-containment strategies, such as medical care utilization review, case management, and advice on benefit use
Risk management, loss control
Emergency preparedness
Preretirement counseling

Legislation

The occupational health and safety services provided by an employer are influenced by specific legislation at federal and state levels. Although the relationship between work and health has been known since the second century (Ramazzini, 1713), public policy that effectively controlled occupational hazards was not enacted until the 1960s. The Mine Safety and Health Act of 1968 was the first legislation that specifically mandated certain preventive programs for workers. This was followed by the **Occupational Safety and Health Act** of 1970, which established two agencies to carry out the act's purpose of ensuring "safe and healthful working conditions for working men and women" (PL 91-596, 1970). The functions of these agencies are described in the box on p. 918.

The **Occupational Safety and Health Administration (OSHA)** is a federal agency within the U.S. Department of Labor.

The **National Institute for Occupational Safety and Health (NIOSH)** was established by the Occupational Safety and Health Act of 1970 and is part of the Centers for Disease Control and Prevention (CDC). NIOSH is the federal institute responsible for conducting research and making recommendations about

Functions of Federal Agencies Involved in Occupational Health and Safety

OSHA

Determine and set standards for hazardous exposures in the workplace.

Enforce the occupational health standards (including the right of entry for inspection).

Educate employers about occupational health and safety.

Develop and maintain a database of work-related injuries, illnesses, and deaths.

Monitor compliance with occupational health and safety standards.

NIOSH

Conduct research and review of research findings to recommend permissible exposure levels for occupational hazards to OSHA.

Identify and research occupational health and safety hazards.

Educate occupational health and safety professionals.

Distribute research findings relevant to occupational health and safety.

---

ways to prevent work-related illness and injury. The Institute's responsibilities include: (1) Investigating potentially hazardous working conditions as requested by employers or employees. (2) Evaluating hazards in the workplace, ranging from chemicals to machinery. (3) Creating and disseminating methods for preventing disease, injury, and disability. (4) Conducting research and providing scientifically valid recommendations for protecting workers. (5) Providing education and training to individuals preparing for or actively working in the field of occupational safety and health (NIOSH, 1994).

Although NIOSH and OSHA were both created by the same act of Congress, they have different functions. Specifically, OSHA is located in the Department of Labor and has responsibility for creating and enforcing workplace safety and health regulations. In contrast, NIOSH is in the Department of Health and Human Services and is a research agency that identifies the causes of work-related illnesses and injuries and examines potential hazards of new work technologies and practices (NIOSH, 1994).

NIOSH publications, many of which are free, are available by writing or faxing a request to: NIOSH Publications, Mail stop C-13, 4676 Columbia Park-way, Cincinnati, OH 45226-1998, (513) 533-8573 (FAX), or E-Mail: Pubstaft@NIOSDT1.em.cdc.gov, 1-800-356-4674.

OSHA sets the **standards** that regulate workers' exposure to potentially toxic substances, enforcing these at the federal, regional, and state levels. Specific standards and information about compliance can be obtained from federal, regional, and state OSHA offices. NIOSH maintains a computerized database that can be accessed for the most recent international research and recommendations for occupational hazards.

One of the most far-reaching OSHA standards is the **Hazard Communication Standard.** Also known as the federal "right-to-know" law, this standard is based on the premise that working environments cannot eliminate *all* potentially toxic agents; therefore, an important line of defense is an educated workforce. The Hazard Communication Standard, which took effect in May 1986, required that all manufacturing firms inventory their toxic agents, label them, and develop information sheets, called *Material Safety Data Sheets* (MSDSs), for each agent. In addition, the employer must have in place a Hazard Communication Program that provides workers with education about these agents. This education must include identification, toxic effects, and protective measures. In 1988, this standard was extended to all employers covered by the Occupational Safety and Health Act. Noncompliance with the standard has been one of the most frequently cited OSHA violations. Similar right-to-know legislation exists at many state and local levels. The next legislative approach will focus on the right to act: standards and guidelines that protect workers' rights to use the information from right-to-know efforts to change unsafe or unhealthy working conditions.

In addition to standards, which are prescriptive laws, OSHA recently has been publishing non-binding *guidelines* that may be used by OSHA compliance officers to determine conformity with general health and safety recommendations. An example is the "Guidelines for Worker Protection Against Hepatitis, AIDS, and Other Bloodborne Diseases," which requires specific employer and employee actions to safeguard employees in human services jobs.

Workers' compensation acts are important state laws that govern financial compensation of employees who suffer work-related health problems. These acts vary by state; each sets rules for the reimbursement of employees with occupational health problems for medical expenses and lost work time associated with the illness or injury. Workers' Compensation also pays death benefits. The increased costs and frequency of workers' compensation claims and the experience-based insurance premiums paid by industry have been important motivations for increasing the health and safety of the workplace.

What Do You Think?
Small business of 50 employees or less should be required to offer occupational health and safety programs for their workers.

Healthy People 2000

In an attempt to meet the National Health goal of *increasing the span of healthy life for Americans*, health pro-

National Health Objectives Related to Occupational Safety and Health

Reduce deaths from work-related injuries to no more than 4 per 100,000 full-time workers.

Reduce work-related injuries resulting in medical treatment, lost time from work, or restricted work activity to no more than 6 cases per 100 full-time workers.

Reduce cumulative trauma disorders to an incidence of no more than 60 cases per 100,000 full-time workers.

Reduce occupational skin disorders or disease to an incidence of no more than 55 per 100,000 full-time workers.

Reduce hepatitis B infections among occupationally exposed workers to an incidence of no more than 125 cases and increase immunizations to 90 percent of exposed workers.

Increase the proportion of work sites that mandate employee use of occupant protection systems, such as seatbelts.

Reduce the proportion of workers exposed to high noise levels.

Eliminate lead exposures which result in workers having high blood level concentrates.

Implement occupational safety and health plans in 50 states.

Establish exposure standards in 50 states to prevent major occupational-related lung diseases.

Increase work site programs on health and safety.

Increase programs related to back injury prevention and rehabilitation.

Establish through public health or labor departments in 50 states, consultation and assistance to small businesses to implement health and safety programs.

Increase the proportion of primary care providers who routinely include occupational health histories and provide relevant counseling.

From *Healthy People 2000: national health promotion and disease prevention objectives,* Washington, DC, 1991, USDHHS, Public Health Service.

tection strategies are proposed to address the needs of large population groups. One such group is the American workforce. *Healthy Communities 2000: model standards 1991* identifies the national occupational safety and health strategy as the promotion of good health and well-being among workers, including the elimination of factors in occupational environments that cause death, injury, disease, or disability. In addition, this document promotes the minimizing of personal damage from existing occupationally related illness.

Establishing such priorities will assist the nation meet the occupational safety and health goals by the year 2000 (see box above). In order to improve the health of the workforce, more personnel need to be trained and more work sites need to provide on-site health care.

DISASTER PLANNING AND MANAGEMENT

Although disaster planning and management have been functions of occupational health and safety programs (Lee, 1978), this is an area of new legislation that affects businesses and health professionals. The legislation of the Superfund Amendment and Reauthorization Act (SARA) requires that written disaster plans be shared with key resources in the community, such as fire departments and emergency rooms (McCunney, 1988). Public concern about disasters, such as the methyl isocyanate leak in Bhopal, India, or the community exposure to chemicals at Times Beach, Missouri, has mandated more attention to disaster planning.

The goals of a disaster plan are to prevent or minimize injuries and deaths of workers and residents, minimize property damage, effectively triage, and facilitate the resumption of necessary business activities. A disaster plan requires the cooperation of different personnel within the company and community. The nurse is often a key person on the disaster planning team, along with safety professionals, physicians, industrial hygienists, the fire chief, and company management. The potential for disaster (e.g., explosions, fires, and leaks) must be identified, and this is best achieved by completing an exhaustive chemical and hazard inventory of the workplace. The material safety data sheets and plant blueprints are critical for correctly identifying substances and work areas that may be hazardous. Work site surveys are the first step to completing this inventory.

Effective disaster plans are designed by those with knowledge of the work processes and materials, the workers and workplace, and the resources in the community. Specific steps must be detailed for actions to be put in place by specific individuals in the event of a disaster. The written plan must be shared with all who will be involved in its execution. Employees should be prepared in first aid, CPR, and fire brigade procedures. Plans must be clear, specific, and comprehensive (i.e., covering all shifts and all work areas) and must include activities to be conducted within the work site and those that require community resources. Transportation plans, fire response, and emergency services response should be coordinated with the agencies that would be involved in an actual disaster. The disaster plan, emergency and safety equipment, and the first response team's capabilities should be tested annually with a drill. Practice results should be carefully evaluated with changes incorporated as needed.

Hospitals and other emergency services, such as fire departments, should be involved in developing the disaster plan and should receive a copy of the plan and a current hazard inventory. It is imperative that the plan and hazard inventory be periodically updated. The occupational health nurse or another company representative should provide emergency health care providers with updated clinical information on exposures and appropriate treatment. It should never be assumed that local services will have current information on substances used in industry. Representatives of these agencies should visit the work site and accompany the nurse on a work site walk-through so that they are familiar with the operations.

In disaster planning, the nurse is often assigned or assumes the responsibility for coordinating the planning and implementation efforts, working with appropriate key people within the company and in the community to develop a workable, comprehensive plan. Other tasks include providing ongoing communication to keep the plan current, planning the drills, educating the employees, management, and community providers, and assessing the equipment and services that may be used in a disaster.

In the event of a disaster, the nurse should play a key role in coordinating the response. Principles of triage may be employed as the response team determines the extent of the disaster and the ability of the company and community to respond. Postdisaster nursing interventions are also critical. Examples include identification of ongoing disaster-related health needs of workers and community residents, collection of epidemiological data, and assessment of the cause and the necessary steps to prevent a recurrence.

NURSING INTERVENTIONS WITH WORKING POPULATIONS

The nurse is often the first health care provider seen by an individual with a work-related health problem. Consequently, nurses are in key positions to intervene with working populations at all three levels of prevention.

Assessment of Individuals and Families

The initial step of assessment involves the traditional history and physical assessment, emphasizing exposure to occupational hazards and individual characteristics that may predispose the client to increased health risk at certain jobs.

The **occupational health history** is an indispensable component of the health assessment of individuals. Since work is a part of life for most people, incorporating an occupational health history into all routine nursing assessments is important. Many workers in the United States do not have access to health care services in their workplaces. Yet it is not unusual to encounter health care providers in the community who have little or no knowledge about workplaces or expertise in occupationally-related illnesses and injuries. Because of the large number of small businesses that do not have the resources for maintaining on-site health care, injured and ill workers are first seen in the public and private health care sector (i.e., in clinics, emergency rooms, physicians' offices, hospitals, HMOs, and ambulatory care centers). Nurses are often the first-line assessors of these individuals and perhaps the only contact for education about self-protection from workplace hazards. The identification of workplace exposures as sources of adverse health effects may influence the client's course of illness and rehabilitation and also prevent similar illnesses among others with potential for exposure.

Incorporating occupational health data into client assessments begins with recognizing the possible relationship between health and occupational factors. The next step is to integrate into the history-taking procedure some routine assessment questions that will provide the data necessary to confirm or rule out occupationally-induced symptoms. Symptoms of hazardous workplace exposures may be indicated by vague complaints involving any bodily system and often mimicking common medical problems. Three points that occupational health histories should include are a list of current and past jobs the client has held; questions about exposures to specific agents and relationships between the symptoms and activities at work, job titles, or history of exposures; and other factors that may enhance the client's susceptibility to occupational agents (e.g., smoking history, underlying illness, previous injury, or handicapping condition) (Emergency Medicine 1990).

Questions about the client's occupational history can be woven into existing assessment tools. The more complete the data collected, the more likely the nurse is to notice the influence of work-health interactions. All clients should be queried about their employment history. To describe only a current status of "retired" or "housewife" may lead to the omission of relevant data. The nurse should be aware that not all workers are well informed about the materials with which they work or about potential hazards. For this reason the nurse must develop basic knowledge about the types of jobs held by clients and the possible hazards associated with them. Since there is an increased likelihood of multiple exposures from other environments that may interact with workplace exposures, the nurse should extend the questioning to include this information.

Identification of work-related health problems does not require an extensive knowledge of occupational agents and their effects. A systematic approach for evaluating the potential for workplace exposures is the most effective intervention for detection and prevention of occupational health risks. Figure 45-2 shows one short assessment tool that can be incorporated into routine history-taking. Similar questions can be included in the assessment of workers' spouses and dependents, who may receive second-hand or indirect exposure to occupational hazards.

During these health assessments, the nurse has the opportunity to teach about workplace hazards and preventive measures the worker can use. At the same time, the nurse is obtaining information that will be valuable in optimizing worker-job fit. Such assessments may be done as preplacement exams before the client begins a job, on a periodic basis during employment, or with the onset of a work-related health problem or exposure. Work-related health assessments can also be conducted when an employee is being transferred to another job with different requirements and exposures, at termination, and at retirement. The goal of these assessments is to identify agent and host fac-

I. Present Job
   A. What do you do for a living? _____
   B. How long have you had this job? _____
   C. Describe the specific tasks this job involves: _____
_____

   D. What product or service is produced by the company where you work?

   E. Are you exposed to any of the following on your present job?

Chemicals	Vapors, gases	Radiation
Loud noise	Vibration	Extreme heat or cold
Infectious agent	Dusts	Stress
		Others:

   F. Do you feel you have any health problems related to your work?

     If yes, describe:

   G. How would you describe your satisfaction with your job?

Very satisfied	Satisfied	Somewhat satisfied
Dissatisfied	Very dissatisfied	

   H. Have there been any recent changes in your job or the hours you work?

     Comments:

   I. Do you use protective clothing and/or equipment on your job?

     If yes, describe:

   J. Have any of your co-workers been complaining of illnesses or injuries that they associate with their jobs?

     If yes, describe:

II. All Past Work
Starting with your first job, please provide the following information:

Job Title	Years Held from to	Description of work	Exposures	Injuries/Illnesses

III. Other Exposures
   A. Do you have any hobbies which involve exposure to chemicals, metals or any of the other agents mentioned before? If yes, describe:

   B. Are any other members of your household exposed to any of the substances listed above? If yes, describe:

   C. Do you live near any factories, dump sites, or other sources of pollution? If yes, describe:

FIGURE 45-2
Occupational health history.

Name of company _____ Date _____

  Address _____

_____

Parent company (if any) _____

  Location of corporate offices _____

SIC code _____ Major products _____

Major processes and operations:

Raw materials used/created:

Potential health hazards:

Organizational chart that includes the occupational health professionals:

Employees

  Total number: _____ Number in production: _____ Others: _____

  % Fulltime _____ % Men _____ % Women _____

  First shift _____ Second shift _____ Third shift _____

  Age distribution _____

  % Unionized _____ Names of unions _____

Health Data

  Work related illnesses, injuries, deaths per annum: _____

  OSHA recordable _____ Workers' Compensation _____

    Other _____ Most frequent complaints: _____

  Average number of monthly calls to the health unit: _____

  Absenteeism rate: _____

Description of health and safety services:

  Providers:

  Examinations offered:

  Employee assistance programs:

  Treatment if illness/injury:

  Health education: Preventive screening:

  Physical fitness, health promotion activities:

  Mandatory programs:

  Health and safety committee;

  Safety audits:

  Environmental monitoring:

Comments:

FIGURE 45-3

Guide for work site survey.

tors that could place the employee at risk and to determine preventive steps that can be taken to eliminate or minimize the exposure and potential health effect.

When the health data from such assessments are considered collectively, the nurse may determine some patterns in risk factors associated with the occurrence of work-related injuries and illnesses. For example, a nurse practitioner in a clinic noted a dramatic increase in the number of bladder cancer cases among her clients. When she looked at factors in common among these individuals, she determined that they all worked at a firm that used benzidine dyes, which are known bladder carcinogens. She worked with the union and the company to assess the environmental exposures to the employees. This nursing intervention led to a safer work environment and a subsequent decrease in bladder cancer among this population group.

Such an approach can be used at the company, industry, and community levels; the initial collection of data and the questioning about workplace exposures are vital steps for any intervention.

Assessment of the Workplace

The nurse may conduct a similar assessment of the workplace itself. The purpose of this assessment, known as a **work site survey** or *walk-through,* is to become knowledgeable about the work processes and materials, the requirements of various jobs, the presence of actual or potential hazards, and the work practices of employees (AAOHN, 1988). Figure 45-3 shows a brief outline that can be used to guide a walk-through. More complex surveys are performed by industrial hygienists and safety professionals when the purpose of the walk-through is environmental monitoring or a safety audit. Some occupational health nurses have developed expertise in these areas and include such tasks as part of their functions. For any health care provider who assesses workers, this information makes up an important data base. For the on-site health care provider, work site walk-throughs assist the professional in establishing rapport with and credibility among the employees.

A work site survey begins with an understanding of the type of work that occurs in the workplace. All business organizations are classified by the U.S. Department of Commerce with a numerical code, the Standard Industrial Classification (SIC) Code. This code, usually a two- to four-digit number, indicates a firm's product and, therefore, the possible types of occupational health hazards that may be associated with the processes and materials used by its employees. SIC codes are used to collect and report data on businesses. For example, illness and injury rates of one company are compared to the rates of other companies of similar size with the same SIC code to determine whether the company is experiencing an excess of illness or injury. All OSHA and workers' compensation data are reported by the SIC code. In addition, by knowing the SIC code of a company, a health care professional can access reference books that describe the usual processes, materials, and by-products of that kind of firm. A simple drawing of the work processes and work areas categorizes information by jobs or locations in the workplace. These preliminary data provide clues about what hazards may be present and an understanding of the types of jobs and health requirements that may be involved in a particular industry.

Characteristics of the employee group comprise the second area of important information. The nature, availability, and utilization of health and safety services are also assessed. The structure of the organization, the chain of command for occupational health professionals, and the incidence rates for work-related illnesses and injuries complete the survey data. The more information that can be collected before the walk-through, the more efficient will be the process of the survey. After the survey is conducted, the nurse can use the information with the aggregate health data to evaluate the effectiveness of the occupational health and safety program and to plan future programs.

Table 45-2 Areas to be Assessed in Applying the Epidemiological Model to the Use of VDTs in an Office Setting

Host: workers	Agent: VDTs	Work environment: office
Previous musculoskeletal injury	Height of work station	Pacing of work
Age	Adjustable keyboard	Worker control of work
Other use of VDT outside of employment	Lighting	Noise, other distractions
Underlying chronic illness	Wrist supports	Employee-supervisor relationships
Eyeglasses or other sign of visual impairment	Tiltable screen	Policies about rest breaks
Work habits	Chair with lumbar support and stability	Adequate space for rest breaks
	CRT shield	

Clinical Application

An example of how the epidemiological triad can be used to assess clients and plan nursing care illustrates the usefulness of approaching occupational health problems with an epidemiological perspective. An insurance company recently renovated its claims-processing office area. All typewriters were replaced with video display terminals (VDTs) and associated hardware for handling all future work by computer. The company's occupational health nurse noticed an increase in visits to the health unit for complaints of headaches, stiff neck muscles, and visual disturbances. These health problems have been associated with VDT operation. To conduct a complete investigation of this problem, the nurse assessed the workers, the new agent (the VDTs), previously existing potential agents, and the work environment. Table 45-2 depicts the factors that the nurse assessed for each of these areas. By collecting data for each of the three elements of the epidemiological triad, the nurse could respond most effectively to the aggregate health problem suggested by the increased use of the health unit.

This information led to the conclusion that certain workers may be at increased risk of adverse responses to this new agent; workstation design contributes to these unhealthy responses; and the work environment influences the host-agent interaction. Interventions should always focus on designing the health hazard out of the work process, if possible; for example, with hazardous chemicals the strategy may include substituting a safer chemical, isolating the chemical in the work process, or isolating the worker from the chemical. In the present example, the first level of intervention was design of the workstation, the component used by the VDT operators in doing their work. Minimizing the possible hazards of the agent involved recommendations for desks, chairs, and lighting designs that would accommodate the individual worker and allow shielding of the VDT. The nurse's recommendations about designing these components to minimize strain on the worker's comfort and health were based on principles of ergonomics—the study of adapting work and workplaces to fit humans.

The nursing interventions could include strengthening the resistance of the host by prescribing appropriate rest breaks, eye exercises, and relaxation strategies. Recognizing that previous cervical neck injury or impaired vision may increase the risk of adverse effects from VDT work, the nurse would include assessment for these factors in employees' preplacement and periodic health examinations.

For the environmental concerns, the nurse could educate the manager about the health risks of paced, externally controlled work expectations and recommend alternatives. Such an approach is likely to address most factors involved in this example of a work-related illness and to result in interventions that are effective in promoting worker health and safety while increasing the productivity and morale of the work group.

Key Concepts

♦ The health impact of work is an important aspect for most clients for whom the community health nurse provides care.

♦ Two major changes in the working population are the increasing number of women and older individuals in the workplace.

♦ Host factors known to be associated with increased risk of adverse response to exposures in the workplace are age, gender, underlying chronic illness, work practices, immunological status, ethnicity, and lifestyle.

♦ Work-related hazards, or agents, are classified as biological, chemical, ergonomic, physical, and psychosocial.

♦ Promotion of worker health and safety is the goal of occupational health and safety programs. Effective programs are proactive. The work should be redesigned to eliminate or minimize health hazards. Using personal protective equipment is an important strategy, but it should not substitute for redesigning.

♦ Services provided by on-site occupational health programs range from those focused only on work-related health and safety problems to a wide scope of services that may include primary care.

♦ The ability of a company to offer health and safety programs depends on the management's attitudes and understanding about health and safety, acceptance of the program by workers, and the economic status of the company.

Key Concepts—cont'd

♦ Although the relationship between work and health has been known since the second century, public policy that effectively controlled occupational health hazards was not enacted in the United States until the 1960s.

♦ Nurses are often the first health care providers seen by individuals with work-related health problems. Consequently, nurses are in key positions to intervene with working populations at all three levels of prevention.

♦ The occupational health history is an indispensable component of the health assessment of individuals, and it should include all prior potential occupational health exposures.

♦ A work site survey, or walk-through, is important in assessing the workplace for actual and potential hazards. It enables the nurse to gain knowledge of the requirements of various jobs, the presence of actual or potential hazards, and work practices of employees.

♦ The primary focus of occupational health nurses' practice is the health and safety of workers, with an emphasis on the prevention of illness and injury.

♦ As American industry has shifted from agrarian to industrial to highly technological processes, the occupational health nurse's role has evolved and expanded.

♦ Although nurses can specialize and become certified in occupational health, the principles of occupational health and safety are important to the practice of all nurses.

Critical Thinking Activities

1. Visit a work site and describe the workers. What are their ages? What percentage are women? What type of work are the employees doing? Can you detect anything about the workers' or management's attitudes about health and safety? Ask to see a Material Safety Data Sheet and the company's disaster plan.

2. After your work site visit, describe at least two real or potential occupational health hazards that you observed.

3. Describe at least one preventive strategy that could be used or that you observed being used for each hazard.

4. Select an individual with an injury or illness that could be work-related and ask to trace his or her work history. Look for risk factors that may have precipitated these symptoms or health problems.

5. Interview a worker to evaluate the psychosocial environment of the work setting. Identify hazards and possible interventions. Ask what the worker has done to minimize work stress.

6. Review your own work history and identify the potential hazards to which you have been exposed. What controls existed or could have been put in place?

7. Complete a thorough assessment of a workplace, and develop a model occupational health and safety plan. Include hazards, goals, resources, and deficits.

8. Identify at least one community resource for workers and employers that provides occupational health and safety-related services. What programs are available? How are they accessed? How can potential users contact them most effectively?

Bibliography

Adams J, et al: Primary Care at the worksite: the use of health risk appraisal in a nursing center, *AAOHN J* 43(1):17-22, 1995.

American Association of Occupational Health Nurses: *A comprehensive guide for establishing an occupational health service*, Atlanta, 1988, AAOHN.

American Nurses Association, Division of Governmental Affairs, *Capital Update* 9(6):1, March 29, 1991.

Barratt A, et al: Worksite-cholesterol screening and dietary intervention: the Staff Healthy Heart Project, Steering Committee, *Am J Public Health* 84(5):779-782, 1994.

Bellingham R, Cohen B, editors: *The corporate wellness sourcebook*, Amherst, Mass, 1987, Human Resource Development Press.

Bellows J, Rudolph L: The initial impact of a workplace lead-poisoning project, *Am J Public Health* 83(3):406-410, 1993.

Blouin A, Brent N: Legal concerns related to workers with HIV or AIDS, *J Nurs Adm* 25(1):17-18, 1995.

Brown, M: *Occupational health nursing*, New York, 1981, MacMillan.

Bureau of Labor Statistics: *Handbook of labor statistics*, Washington, DC, 1995, US Department of Labor.

Callahan E: Quality in occupational health care: management's view, *J Occup Med* 36(4):410-413, 1994.

Campos-Outcalt D: Occupational health epidemiology and objectives for the year 2000: primary care, *Clinics in Office Practice* 21(2):213-223, 1994.

Concerning occupational illness, *Emerg Med* Feb 15:22-44, 1990.

Controlling lead toxicity in bridge workers. Connecticut, 1991-1994, *MMWR Morb Mortal Wkly Rep* 44(4):76-79, 1995.

Cox AR: Profile of the occupational health nurse, *Occup Health Nurs* 33(12):591-593, 1988.

Ehlers JK, Connon C, Themann CL, et al: Health and safety hazards associated with farming, *AAOHN J* 41(9):414-421, 1993.

Felton J: The genesis of American occupational health nursing, Part 1, *Occup Health Nurs* 33:615, 1985.

Girgis A, et al: A workplace intervention for increasing outdoor workers' use of solar protection, *Am J Public Health* 84(1):77-81, 1994.

Grajny AE, Christie D, Tichy AM, et al: Chemotherapy: how safe for the caregiver? *Home Health Nurse* 11(5):51-58, 1993.

Haynes S, Feinleib M: Women, work, and coronary heart disease, *Am J Public Health* 70(2):133-141, 1980.

Healthy People 2000: national health promotion and disease prevention objectives, Washington, DC, 1991, USDHHS, Public Health Service.

Hodgson M, Storey E: Patients and the sick building syndrome, *J Allergy Clin Immunol* 94(2 Pt 2):335-343, 1994.

Hoffman C, Turner T: Strategies for using university health services for cholesterol screening, *J Am Coll Health* 43(2):86-89, 1994.

Jeffrey RW, Forster JL, French SA, et al: The Healthy Worker Project: a work-site intervention for weight control and smoking cessation, *Am J Public Health* 83(3):395-401, 1993.

Jenkins E, et al: Homicide in the workplace: the US experience, 1980-1988, *AAOHN J* 40(5):215-8, 1992.

Katz E, et al: Exposure assessment in epidemiologic studies of birth defects by industrial hygiene review of maternal interviews, *Am J Ind Med* 26(1):1-11, 1994.

Klinger C, Jones M: The OSHA standard setting process...role of the occupational health nurse, *AAOHN J* 42(8):374-8, 1994.

LaDou J, editor: *Occupational medicine*, Norwalk, Conn, 1990, Appleton & Lange.

Lee J: *New nurse in industry*, USDHEW, NIOSH, Pub No 78-143, US Government Printing Office, 1978.

Levin P, et al: Female workplace homicides: an integrative research review, *AAOHN J* 40:(229-236), 1992.

Levy BS, Wegman DH: *Occupational health: recognizing and preventing occupational disease*, Boston, 1988, Little, Brown & Co.

Marlenga B, Parker-Conrad J: Knowledge of occupational hazards in photography: a pilot study, *AAOHN Journal* 41(4):175-179, 1993.

McCunney R: *Handbook of occupational medicine*, Boston, 1988, Little, Brown, & Co.

Modesti PA, Pieri F, Cecioni I, et al: Comparison of ambulatory blood pressure monitoring and conventional office measurement in the workers of a chemical company, *Int J Cardiol* 46(2):151-157, 1994.

Morris S: Academic occupational safety and health training programs, *Occup Med* 9(2):189-200, 1994.

National Safety Council: *Accident facts*, Chicago, 1989.

NIOSH, US Dept of Health and Human Services, Public Health Service, Washington, DC, DHHS (NIOSH) Pub No 94-108.

Office of Technology Assessment, US Congress: *Preventing illness and injury in the workplace*, Pub No OTA-H-256, Washington, DC, 1986, US Government Printing Office.

Paskett ED, Case LD, Masten KB, et al: Breast cancer screening education in the workplace, *J Cancer Educ* 9(2):101-104, 1994.

Payling K: A hazard we can no longer ignore: effects of excessive noise on wellbeing, *Prof Nurse* 9(6):418, 420-421, 1994.

Platt J: Radon: its impact on the community and the role of the nurse, *AAOHN J* 41(11):547-550, 1993.

Porru S, Donato F, Apostoli P, et al: The utility of health education among lead workers: the experience of one program, *Am J Ind Med* 23(3):473-481, 1993.

Poster E, Ryan J: A multiregional study of nurses' beliefs and attitudes about work safety and patient assault, *H & CP* 45(11):1104-1108, 1994.

Postol T: Public health and working children in twentieth-century America: an historical overview, *J Public Health Policy* 14(3):348-354, 1993.

Prevalence of work disability, United States, 1990, *MMWR Morb Mortal Wkly Rep* 42(39):757-759, 1993.

Proctor NH, Hughes JP, Fischman ML: *Chemical hazards of the workplace*, ed 2, Philadelphia, 1988, JB Lippincott.

Putz-Anderson V: *Cumulative trauma disorders: a manual for musculoskeletal diseases of the upper limbs*, London, 1988, Taylor & Francis.

Rabinowitz S, Feinin M, Ribak J, et al: Teaching interpersonal skills to occupational and environmental health professionals, *Psycho Rep* 74(3 Pt 2): 1299-1306, 1994.

Ramazzini B: *De Morbis Artificum* [Diseases of Workers], 1713. Translated by WC Wright, Chicago, 1940, University of Chicago Press.

Rigotti N Stoto MA, Schelling TC, et al: Do businesses comply with a no-smoking law? Assessing the self-enforcement approach, *Prev Med* 23(2):223-229, 1994.

Rix S: *The American woman*, 1990-91, New York, 1990, WW Norton.

Rogers B: The role of the occupational health nurse. In McCunnery RM, Brandt-Rauf PW, editors: *A practical approach to occupational and environmental medicine*, Boston, 1994, Little, Brown & Co.

Rom WN: *Environmental and occupational medicine*, ed 2, Boston, 1992, Little, Brown & Co.

Rosenstock L, Cullen M: *Textbook of clinical occupational and environmental medicine*, Philadelphia, 1986, Saunders.

Sax NI: *Dangerous properties of industrial materials*, ed 5, New York, 1994, Saunders.

Sepkowitz K: Tuberculosis and the health care worker: a historical perspective, *Ann Intern Med* 120(1):71-79, 1994.

Silverstein M: Analysis of medical screening and surveillance in 21 Occupational Safety and Health Administration standards: support for a generic medical surveillance standard, *Am J Ind Med* 26(3):283-295, 1994.

Snyder M, Ruth V, Sattler B, et al: Environmental and occupational health education: a survey of community health nurses' need for educational programs, *AAOHN J* 42(7):325-328, 1994.

Stellman J: Where women work and the hazards they may face on the job, *J Occup Med* 36(8):814-825, 1994.

Triolo P: *Occupational health hazards of hospital staff nurses: implications for practice and education*, The University of Iowa, 1988, PhD (187p), Dissertation Abstract.

US Department of Health and Human Services: *Data from the national sample survey of registered nurses*, Rockville, Md, Bureau of Health Professions, 1992.

US Department of Labor, Bureau of Labor Statistics: *Handbook of labor statistics*, Washington, DC, 1989, US Government Printing Office.

US Department of Labor, Bureau of Labor Statistics: *Occupational injuries and illnesses in the United States by industry*, Washington, DC 1988, US Government Printing Office.

Wicher C: AIDS and HIV: the dilemma of the health care worker, *AAOHN J* 41(6):282-288, 1993.

Wollersheim J: Depression, women and the workplace, *J Occup Med* 8(4):787-795, 1993.

Workplace injury/illness rates for 1991 show a 10-year record drop in incidence, *Occup Health and Safety* 62(1):8, January 1993.

Zenz C: Occupational medicine: *Principles and practical applications*, ed 2, Chicago, 1988, Year Book Medical Publishers.

Zhou C, Roseman J: Agricultural injuries among a population-based sample of farm operators in Alabama, *Am J Ind Med* 25(3):385-402, 1994.

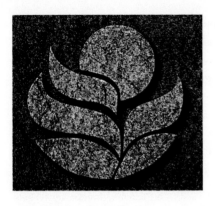

Appendixes

Continued.

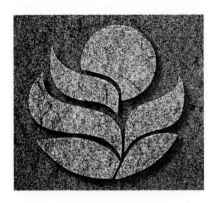

Appendix A
International/National Agendas for Health Care Delivery

A.1 YEAR 2000: NATIONAL HEALTH OBJECTIVES

1. Physical Activity and Fitness

Health Status Objectives

1.1 Reduce coronary heart disease deaths to no more than 100 per 100,000 people.

1.2 Reduce overweight to a prevalence of no more than 20% among people aged 20 and older and no more than 15% among adolescents 12 through 19.

Risk Reduction Objectives

1.3 Increase to at least 30% the proportion of people aged 6 and older who engage regularly, preferably daily, in light to moderate physical activity for at least 30 minutes per day.

1.4 Increase to at least 20% the proportion of people aged 18 and older and to at least 75% the proportion of children and adolescents aged 6 through 17 who engage in vigorous physical activity that promotes the development and maintenance of cardiorespiratory fitness 3 or more days per week for 20 or more minutes per occasion.

1.5 Reduce to no more than 15% the proportion of people aged 6 and older who engage in no leisure-time physical activity.

1.6 Increase to at least 40% the proportion of people aged 6 and older who regularly perform physical activities that enhance and maintain muscular strength, muscular endurance, and flexibility.

1.7 Increase to at least 50% the proportion of overweight people aged 12 and older who have adopted sound dietary practices combined with regular physical activity to attain appropriate body weight.

Services and Protection Objectives

1.8 Increase to at least 50% the proportion of children and adolescents in first through twelfth grade who participate in daily school physical education.

1.9 Increase to at least 50% the portion of school physical education class time that students spend being physically active, preferably in lifetime physical activities.

1.10 Increase the proportion of work sites offering employer-sponsored activity and fitness programs.

1.11 Increase community availability and accessibility of physical activity and fitness facilities.

1.12 Increase to at least 50% the proportion of primary care providers who routinely assess and counsel their patients regarding the frequency, duration, type, and intensity of each patient's physical activity practices.

2. Nutrition

Health Status Objectives

2.1 Reduce coronary heart disease deaths to no more than 100 per 100,000 people.

2.2 Reverse the rise in cancer deaths to achieve a rate of no more than 130 per 100,000 people.

2.3 Reduce overweight to a prevalence of no more than 20% among people aged 20 and older and no more than 15% among adolescents aged 12 through 19.

2.4 Reduce growth retardation among low-income children aged 5 and younger to less than 10%.

Risk Reduction Objectives

2.5 Reduce dietary fat intake to an average of 30% of calories or less and average saturated fat intake to less than 10% of calories among people aged 2 and older.

2.6 Increase complex carbohydrate and fiber-containing foods in the diets of adults to five or more daily servings for vegetables (including

From *Healthy People 2000: national health promotion and disease prevention objectives*, Washington, DC, 1991, USDHHS, Public Health Service.

legumes) and fruits, and to six or more daily servings for grain products.

2.7 Increase to at least 50% the proportion of overweight people aged 12 and older who have adopted sound dietary practices combined with regular physical activity to attain appropriate body weight.

2.8 Increase calcium intake so at least 50% of youth aged 12 through 24 and 50% of pregnant and lactating women consume 3 or more servings daily of foods rich in calcium, and at least 50% of people aged 25 and older consume two or more servings daily.

2.9 Decrease salt and sodium intake so at least 65% of home meal preparers prepare foods without adding salt, at least 80% of people avoid using salt at the table, and at least 40% of adults regularly purchase foods modified or lower in sodium.

2.10 Reduce iron deficiency to less than 3% among children aged 1 through 4 and among women of childbearing age.

2.11 Increase to at least 75% the proportion of mothers who breastfeed their babies in the early postpartum period and to at least 50% the proportion who continue breastfeeding until their babies are 5 to 6 months old.

2.12 Increase to at least 75% the proportion of parents and caregivers who use feeding practices that prevent baby tooth decay.

2.13 Increase to at least 85% the proportion of people aged 18 and older who use food labels to make nutritious food selections.

Services and Protection Objectives

2.14 Achieve useful and informative nutrition labeling for virtually all processed foods and at least 40% of fresh meats, poultry, fish, fruits, vegetables, baked goods, and ready-to-eat carry-away foods.

2.15 Increase to at least 5000 brand items the availability of processed food products that are reduced in fat and saturated fat.

2.16 Increase to at least 90% the proportion of restaurants and institutional food service operations that offer identifiable low-fat, low-calorie food choices, consistent with the *Dietary Guidelines for Americans.*

2.17 Increase to at least 90% the proportion of school lunch and breakfast services and child care food services with menus that are consistent with the nutrition principles in the *Dietary Guidelines for Americans.*

2.18 Increase to at least 80% the receipt of home food services by people aged 65 and older who have difficulty in preparing their own meals or are otherwise in need of home-delivered meals.

2.19 Increase to at least 75% the proportion of the nation's schools that provide nutrition education from preschool through twelfth grade, preferably as part of quality school health education.

2.20 Increase to at least 50% the proportion of work sites with 50% or more employees that offer nutrition education and/or weight management programs for employees.

2.21 Increase to at least 75% the proportion of primary care providers who provide nutrition assessment and counseling and/or referral to qualified nutritionists or dietitians.

3. Tobacco

Health Status Objectives

3.1 Reduce coronary heart disease deaths to no more than 100 per 100,000 people.

3.2 Slow the rise in lung cancer deaths to achieve a rate of no more than 42 per 100,000 people.

3.3 Slow the rise in deaths from chronic obstructive pulmonary disease to achieve a rate of no more than 25 per 100,000 people.

Risk Reduction Objectives

3.4 Reduce cigarette smoking to a prevalence of no more than 15% among people aged 20 and older.

3.5 Reduce the initiation of cigarette smoking by children and youth so that no more than 15% have become regular smokers by age 20.

3.6 Increase to at least 50% the proportion of cigarette smokers aged 18 and older who stopped smoking cigarettes for at least one day during the preceding year.

3.7 Increase smoking cessation during pregnancy so that at least 60% of women who are cigarette smokers at the time they become pregnant quit smoking early in pregnancy and maintain abstinence for the remainder of their pregnancy.

3.8 Reduce to no more than 20% the proportion of children aged 6 and younger who are regularly exposed to tobacco smoke at home.

3.9 Reduce smokeless tobacco use by males aged 12 through 24 to a prevalence of no more than 4%.

Services and Protection Objectives

3.10 Establish tobacco-free environments and include tobacco-use prevention in the curricula of all elementary, middle, and secondary schools, preferably as part of quality school health education.

3.11 Increase to at least 75% the proportion of worksites with a formal smoking policy that prohibits or severely restricts smoking in the workplace.

3.12 Enact in all 50 states comprehensive laws on clean indoor air that prohibit or strictly limit smoking in the workplace and enclosed public places (including health care facilities, schools, and public transportation).

3.13 Enact and enforce in all 50 states laws prohibiting the sale and distribution of tobacco products to youths under age 19.

3.14 Increase to 50 the number of states with plans to reduce tobacco use, especially among youth.

3.15 Eliminate or severely restrict all forms of tobacco product advertising and promotion to which youths under age 18 are likely to be exposed.

3.16 Increase to at least 75% the proportion of primary care and oral health care providers who routinely advise cessation and provide assistance and follow-up for all of their tobacco-using patients.

4. Alcohol and Other Drugs
Health Status Objectives

4.1 Reduce deaths caused by alcohol-related motor vehicle crashes to no more than 8.5 per 100,000 people.

4.2 Reduce cirrhosis deaths to no more than 6 per 100,000 people.

4.3 Reduce drug-related deaths to no more than 3 per 100,000 people.

4.4 Reduce hospital emergency department visits related to drug abuse by at least 20%.

Risk Reduction Objectives

4.5 Increase by at least 1 year the average age of first use of cigarettes, alcohol, and marijuana by adolescents ages 12 through 17.

4.6 Reduce the proportion of young people who have used alcohol, marijuana, and cocaine in the past month.

4.7 Reduce the proportion of high school seniors and college students engaging in recent occasions of heavy drinking of alcoholic beverages to no more than 28% of high school seniors and 32% of college students.

4.8 Reduce alcohol consumption by people aged 14 and older to an annual average of no more than 2 gallons of ethanol per person.

4.9 Increase the proportion of high school seniors who perceive social disapproval associated with heavy use of alcohol, occasional use of marijuana, and experimentation with cocaine.

4.10 Increase the proportion of high school seniors who associate risk of physical and psychological harm with the heavy use of alcohol, regular use of marijuana, and experimentation with cocaine.

4.11 Reduce to no more than 3% the proportion of male high school seniors who use anabolic steroids.

Services and Protection Objectives

4.12 Establish and monitor in all 50 states comprehensive plans to ensure access to alcohol and drug treatment programs for traditionally underserved people.

4.13 Provide to children in all school districts and private schools primary and secondary school educational programs on alcohol and other drugs, preferably as a part of quality school health education.

4.14 Extend adoption of alcohol and drug policies for the work environment to at least 60% of worksites with 50 or more employees.

4.15 Extend to all 50 states administrative driver's license suspension/revocation laws or programs of equal effectiveness for people determined to have been driving under the influence of intoxicants.

4.16 Increase to 50 the number of states that have enacted and enforce policies to reduce access to alcoholic beverages by minors.

4.17 Increase to at least 20 the number of states that have enacted statutes to restrict promotion of alcoholic beverages that is focused principally on young audiences.

4.18 Extend to all 50 states legal blood alcohol concentration tolerance levels of .04% for motor vehicle drivers aged 21 and older and .00% for those younger than age 21.

4.19 Increase to at least 75% the proportion of primary care providers who screen for alcohol and other drug use problems and provide counseling and referral as needed.

5. Family Planning
Health Status Objectives

5.1 Reduce pregnancies among girls aged 17 and younger to no more than 50 per 1000 adolescents.

5.2 Reduce to no more than 30% the proportion of all pregnancies that are unintended.

5.3 Reduce the prevalence of infertility to no more than 6.5%.

Risk Reduction Objectives

5.4 Reduce the proportion of adolescents who have engaged in sexual intercourse by age 15 to no more than 15% and by age 17 to no more than 40%.

5.5 Increase to at least 40% the proportion of adolescents aged 17 and younger who have ever been sexually active that have abstained from sexual activity for the previous 3 months.

5.6 Increase to at least 90% the proportion of sexually active unmarried people aged 19 and younger who use contraception, especially combined-method contraception that both effectively prevents pregnancy and provides barrier protection against disease.

5.7   Increase the effectiveness with which family planning methods are used, as measured by a decrease to no more than 5% in the proportion of couples experiencing pregnancy despite use of a contraceptive method.

Services and Protection Objectives

5.8   Increase to at least 85% the proportion of people aged 10 through 18 who have discussed human sexuality, including values surrounding sexuality, with their parents and/or have received information through other parentally endorsed sources, such as school, religious, or youth programs.

5.9   Increase to at least 90% the proportion of pregnancy counselors who offer positive, accurate information about adoption to their unmarried patients with unintended pregnancies.

5.10   Increase to at least 60% the proportion of primary care providers who provide age-appropriate preconception care and counseling.

5.11   Increase to at least 50% the proportion of the following kinds of clinics that screen, diagnose, treat, counsel, and provide (or refer for) partner notification services for HIV infection and bacterial sexually transmitted diseases (gonorrhea, syphilis, and chlamydia): family planning clinics, maternal and child health clinics, sexually transmitted disease clinics, tuberculosis clinics, drug treatment centers, and primary care clinics.

6. Mental Health and Mental Disorders
Health Status Objectives

6.1   Reduce suicides to no more than 10.5 per 100,000 people.

6.2   Reduce by 15% the incidence of injurious suicide attempts among adolescents aged 14 through 19.

6.3   Reduce to less than 10% the prevalence of mental disorders among children and adolescents.

6.4   Reduce the prevalence of mental disorders (exclusive of substance abuse) among adults living in the community to less than 10.7%.

6.5   Reduce to less than 35% the proportion of people aged 18 and older who within the past year have experienced adverse health effects from stress.

Risk Reduction Objectives

6.6   Increase to at least 30% the proportion of people aged 18 and older with severe, persistent mental disorders who use community support programs.

6.7   Increase to at least 45% the proportion of people with major depressive disorders who obtain treatment.

6.8   Increase to at least 20% the proportion of people aged 18 and older who seek help in coping with personal and emotional problems.

6.9   Decrease to no more than 5% the proportion of people aged 18 and older who report experiencing significant levels of stress who do not take steps to reduce or control their stress.

Services and Protection Objectives

6.10   In order to facilitate identification and appropriate intervention to prevent suicide by jail inmates, increase to 50 the number of states with officially established protocols that engage mental health, alcohol, drug, and public health authorities with corrections authorities.

6.11   Increase to at least 40% the proportion of work sites employing 50 or more people that provide programs to reduce employee stress.

6.12   Establish mutual-help clearinghouses in at least 25 states.

6.13   Increase to at least 50% the proportion of primary care providers who routinely review with patients their patients' cognitive, emotional, and behavioral functioning and the resources available to deal with any problems that are identified.

6.14   Increase to at least 75% the proportion of providers of primary care for children who include assessment of cognitive, emotional, and parent-child functioning, with appropriate counseling, referral, and follow-up, in their clinical practices.

7. Violent and Abusive Behavior
Health Status Objectives

7.1   Reduce homicides to no more than 7.2 per 100,000 people.

7.2   Reduce suicides to no more than 10.5 per 100,000 people.

7.3   Reduce weapon-related violent deaths to no more than 12.6 per 100,000 people.

7.4   Reverse to less than 25.2 per 1000 children the rising incidence of maltreatment of children younger than age 18.

7.5   Reduce physical abuse directed at women by male partners to no more than 27 per 1000 couples.

7.6   Reduce assault injuries among people aged 12 and older to no more than 10 per 1,000 people.

7.7   Reduce rape and attempted rape of women aged 12 and older to no more than 107 per 100,000 women.

7.8   Reduce by 15% the incidence of injurious suicide attempts among adolescents aged 14 to 19.

Risk Reduction Objectives

7.9   Reduce by 20% the incidence of physical fighting among adolescents aged 14 through 17.

7.10 Reduce by 20% the incidence of weapon-carrying by adolescents aged 14 through 17.

7.11 Reduce by 20% the proportion of weapons that are inappropriately stored and therefore available and dangerous.

Services and Protection Objectives

7.12 Extend protocols to at least 90% of hospital emergency departments for routinely identifying, treating, and properly referring victims of sexual assault, victims of spouse, elder, and child abuse, and those who have attempted suicide.

7.13 Extend to at least 45 states implementation of unexplained child death review systems.

7.14 Increase to at least 30 the number of states in which at least 50% of children identified as physically or sexually abused receive physical and mental evaluation with appropriate follow-up as a means of breaking the intergenerational cycle of abuse.

7.15 Reduce to less than 10% the proportion of battered women and their children turned away from emergency housing because of lack of space.

7.16 Increase to at least 50% the proportion of elementary and secondary schools that teach nonviolent conflict resolution skills, preferably part of quality school health education.

7.17 Extend coordinated, comprehensive violence prevention programs to at least 80% of local jurisdictions with populations over 100,000.

7.18 In order to facilitate identification and appropriate intervention to prevent suicide by jail inmates, increase to 50 the number of states with officially established protocols that engage mental health, alcohol, drug, and public health authorities with corrections authorities.

8. Educational and Community-Based Programs

Health Status Objective

8.1 Increase years of healthy life to at least 65 years.

Risk Reduction Objective

8.2 Increase the high school graduation rate to at least 90%, thereby reducing risks for multiple problem behaviors and poor mental and physical health.

Services and Protection Objectives

8.3 Achieve for all disadvantaged children and children with disabilities access to high quality and developmentally appropriate preschool programs that help prepare children for school, thereby improving their prospects with regard to school performance, behavior, and mental and physical health.

8.4 Increase to at least 75% the proportion of the nation's elementary and secondary schools that provide planned and sequential quality school health education from kindergarten through twelfth grade.

8.5 Increase to at least 50% the proportion of postsecondary institutions with institution-wide health promotion programs for students, faculty, and staff.

8.6 Increase to at least 85% the proportion of workplaces with 50 or more employees that offer health promotion activities for their employees, preferably as part of a comprehensive employee health promotion program.

8.7 Increase to at least 20% the proportion of hourly workers who participate regularly in employer-sponsored health promotion activities.

8.8 Increase to at least 90% the proportion of people aged 65 and older who during the preceding year had the opportunity to participate in at least one organized health promotion program through a senior center, lifecare facility, or other community-based setting serving older adults.

8.9 Increase to at least 75% the proportion of people aged 10 and older who have discussed issues related to nutrition, physical activity, sexual behavior, tobacco, alcohol, other drugs, or safety with family members on at least one occasion during the preceding month.

8.10 Establish community health promotion programs that separately or together address at least three of the *Healthy People 2000* priorities and reach at least 40% of each state's population.

8.11 Increase to at least 50% the proportion of counties that have established culturally and linguistically appropriate community health promotion programs for racial and ethnic minority populations.

8.12 Increase to at least 90% the proportion of hospitals, health maintenance organizations, and large group practices that provide patient education programs, and to at least 90% the proportion of community hospitals that offer community health programs addressing the priority health needs of their communities.

8.13 Increase to at least 75% the proportion of local television network affiliates in the top 20 television markets that have been become partners with one or more community organizations in working toward one of the health problems addressed by the *Healthy People 2000* objectives.

8.14 Increase to at least 90% the proportion of people who are served by a local health department that is effectively carrying out the core functions of public health.

9. Unintentional Injuries
Health Status Objectives

9.1   Reduce deaths caused by unintentional injuries to no more than 29.3 per 100,000 people.

9.2   Reduce nonfatal unintentional injuries so that hospitalizations for this condition are no more than 754 per 100,000 people.

9.3   Reduce deaths caused by motor vehicle crashes to no more than 1.9 per 100 million vehicle miles traveled and 17 per 100,000 people.

9.4   Reduce deaths from falls and from fall-related injuries to no more than 2.3 per 100,000.

9.5   Reduce deaths by drowning to no more than 1.3 per 100,000 people.

9.6   Reduce deaths resulting from residential fire to no more than 1.2 per 100,000 people.

9.7   Reduce hip fractures among people aged 65 and older so that hospitalizations for this condition are no more than 620 per 100,000 people.

9.8   Reduce nonfatal poisoning to no more than 88 emergency department treatments per 100,000 people.

9.9   Reduce nonfatal head injuries so that hospitalizations for this condition are no more than 106 per 100,000 people.

9.10   Reduce nonfatal spinal cord injuries so that hospitalizations for this condition are no more than 4.5 per 100,000 people.

9.11   Reduce the incidence of secondary disabilities associated with head injuries to no more than 16 per 100,000 people, and the incidence of secondary disabilities, associated with spinal cord injuries to no more than 2.6 per 100,000 people.

Risk Reduction Objectives

9.12   Increase use of occupant protection systems, such as safety belts, inflatable safety restraints, and child safety seats, to at least 85% of motor vehicle occupants.

9.13   Increase use of helmets to at least 80% of motorcyclists and at least 50% of bicyclists.

Services and Protection Objectives

9.14   Extend to all 50 states laws requiring safety belt and motorcycle helmet use for all ages.

9.15   Enact in all 50 states laws requiring that new handguns be designed to minimize the likelihood of discharge by children.

9.16   Extend to 2000 the number of jurisdictions whose codes address the installation of fire suppression sprinkler systems in those residences at highest risk for fires.

9.17   Increase the presence of functional smoke detectors to at least one on each habitable floor of all inhabited residential dwellings.

9.18   Provide academic instruction on injury prevention and control, preferably as part of quality school health education, in at least 50% of public school systems (grades K through 12).

9.19   Extend requirement of the use of effective head, face, eye, and mouth protection to all organizations, agencies, and institutions sponsoring sporting and recreation events that pose risks of injury.

9.20   Increase to at least 30 the number of states that have design standards for signs, signals, markings, lighting, and other characteristics of the roadway environment to improve the visual stimuli and protect the safety of older drivers and pedestrians.

9.21   Increase to at least 50% the proportion of primary care providers who routinely provide age-appropriate counseling on safety precautions to prevent unintentional injury.

9.22   Increase to 50 the number of states having emergency medical services and trauma systems that link prehospital, hospital, and rehabilitation services in order to prevent trauma deaths and long-term disability.

10. Occupational Safety and Health
Health Status Objectives

10.1   Reduce deaths from work-related injuries to no more than 4 per 100,000 full-time workers.

10.2   Reduce work-related injuries resulting in medical treatment, lost time from work, or restricted work activity to no more than 6 cases per 100 full-time workers.

10.3   Reduce cumulative trauma disorders to an incidence of no more than 60 cases per 100,000 full-time workers.

10.4   Reduce occupational skin disorders or diseases to an incidence of no more than 55 per 100,000 full-time workers.

10.5   Reduce hepatitis B infections among occupationally exposed workers to an incidence of no more than 1250 cases.

Risk Reduction Objectives

10.6   Increase to at least 75% the proportion of work sites with 50 or more employees that mandate employee use of occupant protection systems, such as seat belts, during all work-related motor vehicle travel.

10.7   Reduce to no more than 15% the proportion of workers exposed to average daily noise levels that exceed 85 decibels.

10.8   Eliminate exposures that result in workers having blood lead concentrations greater than 25 μg/dl of whole blood.

10.9   Increase hepatitis B immunization levels to 90% among occupationally exposed workers.

Services and Protection Objectives

10.10 Implement occupational safety and health plans in all 50 states for the identification, management, and prevention of leading work-related diseases and injuries within each state.

10.11 Establish in all 50 states exposure standards adequate to prevent the major occupational lung diseases to which their worker populations are exposed (byssinosis, asbestosis, coal workers' pneumoconiosis, and silicosis).

10.12 Increase to at least 70% the proportion of work sites with 50 or more employees that have implemented programs on worker health and safety.

10.13 Increase to at least 50% the proportion of work sites with 50 or more employees that offer back injury prevention and rehabilitation programs.

10.14 Establish in all 50 states either public health or labor department programs that provide consultation and assistance to small businesses to implement safety and health programs for their employees.

10.15 Increase to 75% the proportion of primary care providers who routinely elicit occupational health exposures as part of patient history and provide relevant counseling.

11. Environmental Health
Health Status Objectives

11.1 Reduce asthma morbidity, as measured by a reduction in asthma hospitalizations to no more than 160 per 100,000 people.

11.2 Reduce the prevalence of serious mental retardation among school-aged children to no more than 2 per 1000 children.

11.3 Reduce outbreaks of waterborne disease from infectious agents and chemical poisoning to no more than 11 per year.

11.4 Reduce among children aged 6 months through 5 years the prevalence of blood lead levels exceeding 15 μg/dl and 25 μg/dl to no more than 500,000 and zero, respectively.

Risk Reduction Objectives

11.5 Reduce human exposure to criteria air pollutants, as measured by an increase to at least 85% in the proportion of people who live in counties that have not exceeded any Environmental Protection Agency standard for air quality in the previous 12 months.

11.6 Increase to at least 40% the proportion of homes in which homeowners/occupants have tested for radon concentrations and that have either been found to pose minimal risk or have been modified to reduce risk to health.

11.7 Reduce human exposure to toxic agents by confining total pounds of toxic agents released into the air, water, and soil each year to no more than:

- ◆ 0.24 billion pounds of those toxic agents included on the Department of Health and Human Services list of carcinogens.
- ◆ 2.6 billion pounds of those toxic agents included on the Agency for Toxic Substances and Disease Registry list of the most toxic chemicals.

11.8 Reduce human exposure to solid waste-related water, air, and soil contamination, as measured by a reduction in the average amount of municipal solid waste produced per person each day to no more than 3.6 pounds.

11.9 Increase to at least 85% the proportion of people who receive a supply of drinking water that meets the safe drinking water standards established by the Environmental Protection Agency.

11.10 Reduce potential risks to human health from surface water, as measured by a decrease to no more than 15% in the proportion of assessed rivers, lakes, and estuaries that do not support beneficial uses, such as fishing and swimming.

Services and Protection Objectives

11.11 Perform testing for lead-based paint in at least 50% of homes built before 1950.

11.12 Expand to at least 35 the number of states in which at least 75% of local jurisdictions have adopted construction standards and techniques that minimize elevated indoor radon levels in those new building areas locally determined to have elevated radon levels.

11.13 Increase to at least 30 the number of states requiring that prospective buyers be informed of the presence of lead-based paint and radon concentrations in all buildings offered for sale.

11.14 Eliminate significant health risks from National Priority List hazardous waste sites, as measured by performance of clean-up at these sites sufficient to eliminate immediate and significant health threats as specified in health assessments completed at all sites.

11.15 Establish programs for recyclable materials and household hazardous waste in at least 75% of counties.

11.16 Establish and monitor in at least 35 states plans to define and track sentinel environmental diseases.

12. Food and Drug Safety
Health Status Objectives

12.1 Reduce infections caused by key foodborne pathogens (e.g., *Salmonella, Campylobacter jejuni, Escherichia coli 0157:H7,* and *Listeria monocytogenes*).

12.2 Reduce outbreaks of infections due to *Salmonella enteritidis* to fewer than 25 outbreaks yearly.

Risk Reduction Objective

12.3   Increase to at least 75% the proportion of households in which principal food preparers routinely refrain from leaving perishable food out of the refrigerator for over 2 hours and wash cutting boards and utensils with soap after contact with raw meat and poultry.

Services and Protection Objectives

12.4   Extend to at least 70% the proportion of states and territories that have implemented model food codes for institutional food operations and to at least 70% the proportion that have adopted the new uniform food protection code ("Unicode") that sets recommended standards for regulation of all food operations.

12.5   Increase to at least 75% the proportion of pharmacies and other dispensers of prescription medications that use linked systems to provide alerts to potential adverse drug reactions among medications dispensed by different sources to individual patients.

12.6   Increase to at least 75% the proportion of primary care providers who routinely review with their patients aged 65 and older all prescribed and over-the-counter medicines taken by their patients each time a new medication is prescribed.

13. Oral Health
Health Status Objectives

13.1   Reduce dental caries (cavities) so that the proportion of children with one or more caries in permanent or primary teeth is no more than 35% among children aged 6 through 8 and no more than 60% among adolescents aged 15.

13.2   Reduce untreated dental caries so that the proportion of children with untreated caries in permanent or primary teeth is no more than 20% among children aged 6 through 8 and no more than 15% among adolescents aged 15.

13.3   Increase to at least 45% the proportion of people aged 35 through 44 who have never lost a permanent tooth due to dental caries or periodontal disease.

13.4   Reduce to no more than 20% the proportion of people aged 65 and older who have lost all of their natural teeth.

13.5   Reduce the prevalence of gingivitis among people aged 35 through 44 to no more than 30%.

13.6   Reduce destructive periodontal diseases to a prevalence of no more than 15% among people aged 35 through 44.

13.7   Reduce deaths due to cancer of the oral cavity and pharynx to no more than 10.5 per 100,000 men aged 45 through 74 and to 4.1 per 100,000 women aged 45 through 74.

Risk Reduction Objectives

13.8   Increase to at least 50% the proportion of children who have received protective sealants on the occlusal (chewing) surfaces of permanent molar teeth.

13.9   Increase to at least 75% the proportion of people served by community water systems providing optimal levels of fluoride.

13.10   Increase use of professionally or self-administered topical or systemic (dietary) fluorides to at least 85% of people not receiving optimally fluoridated public water.

13.11   Increase to at least 75% the proportion of parents and caregivers who use feeding practices that prevent baby bottle tooth decay.

Services and Protection Objectives

13.12   Increase to at least 90% the proportion of all children entering school programs for the first time who have received an oral health screening, referral, and follow-up for necessary diagnostic, preventive, and treatment services.

13.13   Extend to all long-term institutional facilities the requirement that oral examinations and services be provided no later than 90 days after entry into these facilities.

13.14   Increase to at least 70% the proportion of people aged 35 and older using the oral health care system during each year.

13.15   Increase to at least 40 the number of states that have an effective system for recording and referring infants with cleft lips and/or palates to craniofacial anomaly teams.

13.16   Extend requirement of the use of effective head, face, eye, and mouth protection to all organizations, agencies, and institutions sponsoring sporting and recreation events that pose risks of injury.

14. Maternal and Infant Health
Health Status Objectives

14.1   Reduce the infant mortality rate to no more than 7 per 1000 live births.

14.2   Reduce the fetal death rate (20 or more weeks of gestation) to no more than 5 per 1000 cases of live births and fetal deaths combined.

14.3   Reduce the maternal mortality rate to no more than 3.3 per 100,000 live births.

14.4   Reduce the incidence of fetal alcohol syndrome to no more than 0.12 per 1000 live births.

Risk Reduction Objectives

14.5   Reduce low birth weight to an incidence of no more than 5% of live births and very low birth weight to no more than 1% of live births.

14.6   Increase to at least 85% the proportion of mothers who achieve the minimum recommended weight gain during their pregnancies.

14.7 Reduce severe complications of pregnancy to no more than 15 per 100 deliveries.

14.8 Reduce the Caesarean delivery rate to no more than 15 per 100 deliveries.

14.9 Increase to at least 75% the proportion of mothers who breastfeed their babies in the early postpartum period and to at least 50% the proportion who continue breastfeeding until their babies are 5 to 6 months old.

14.10 Increase abstinence from tobacco use by pregnant women to at least 90% and increase abstinence from alcohol, cocaine, and marijuana by pregnant women by at least 20%.

Services and Protection Objectives

14.11 Increase to at least 90% the proportion of all pregnant women who receive prenatal care in the first trimester of pregnancy.

14.12 Increase to at least 60% the proportion of primary care providers who provide age-appropriate preconception care and counseling.

14.13 Increase to at least 90% the proportion of women enrolled in prenatal care who are offered screening and counseling on prenatal detection of fetal abnormalities.

14.14 Increase to at least 90% the proportion of pregnant women and infants who receive risk-appropriate care.

14.15 Increase to at least 95% the proportion of newborns screened by state-sponsored programs for genetic disorders and other disabling conditions and to 90% the proportion of newborns testing positive for disease who receive appropriate treatment.

14.16 Increase to at least 90% the proportion of babies aged 18 months and younger who receive recommended primary care services at the appropriate intervals.

15. Heart Disease and Stroke
Health Status Objectives

15.1 Reduce coronary heart disease deaths to no more than 100 per 100,000 people.

15.2 Reduce stroke deaths to no more than 20 per 100,000 people.

15.3 Reverse the increase in end-stage renal disease (requiring maintenance dialysis or transplantation) to attain an incidence of no more than 13 per 100,000.

Risk Reduction Objectives

15.4 Increase to at least 50% the proportion of people with high blood pressure whose blood pressure is under control.

15.5 Increase to at least 90% the proportion of people with high blood pressure who are taking action to help control their blood pressure.

15.6 Reduce the mean serum cholesterol level among adults to no more than 200 mg/dl.

15.7 Reduce the prevalence of blood cholesterol levels of 240 mg/dl or greater to no more than 20% of the adult population.

15.8 Increase to at least 60% the proportion of adults with high blood cholesterol who are aware of their condition and are taking action to reduce their blood cholesterol to recommended levels.

15.9 Reduce dietary fat intake to an average of 30% of calories or less and average saturated fat intake to less than 10% of calories among people aged 2 and older.

15.10 Reduce overweight to a prevalence of no more than 20% among people aged 20 and older and no more than 15% among adolescents aged 12 through 19.

15.11 Increase to at least 30% the proportion of people aged 6 and older who engage regularly, preferably daily, in light to moderate physical activity for at least 30 minutes per day.

15.12 Reduce cigarette smoking to a prevalence of no more than 15% among people aged 20 and older.

Services and Protection Objectives

15.13 Increase to at least 90% the proportion of adults who have had their blood pressure measured within the preceding 2 years and can state whether their blood pressure was normal, high, or low.

15.14 Increase to at least 75% the proportion of adults who have had their blood cholesterol checked within the preceding 5 years.

15.15 Increase to at least 75% the proportion of primary care providers who initiate diet for patients with high blood cholesterol and, if necessary, drug therapy at levels of blood cholesterol consistent with current management guidelines.

15.16 Increase to at least 50% the proportion of work sites with 50 or more employees that offer high blood pressure and/or cholesterol education and control activities to their employees.

15.17 Increase to at least 90% the proportion of clinical laboratories that meet the recommended accuracy standard for cholesterol measurement.

15. Cancer
Health Status Objectives

16.1 Reverse the rise in cancer deaths to achieve a rate of no more than 130 per 100,000 people.

16.2 Slow the rise in lung cancer deaths to achieve a rate of no more than 42 per 100,000 people.

16.3 Reduce breast cancer deaths to no more than 20.6 per 100,000 women.

16.4 Reduce deaths from cancer of the uterine cervix to no more than 1.3 per 100,000 women.

16.5 Reduce colorectal cancer deaths to no more than 13.2 per 100,000 people.

Risk Reduction Objectives

16.6   Reduce cigarette smoking to a prevalence of no more than 15% among people aged 20 and older.

16.7   Reduce dietary fat intake to an average of 30% of calories or less and average saturated fat intake to less than 10% of calories among people aged 2 and older.

16.8   Increase complex carbohydrate and fiber-containing foods in the diets of adults to five or more daily servings for vegetables (including legumes) and fruits, and to six or more daily servings for grain products.

16.9   Increase to at least 60% the proportion of people of all ages who limit sun exposure, use sunscreens and protective clothing when exposed to sunlight, and avoid artificial sources of ultraviolet light (e.g., sun lamps, tanning booths).

Services and Protection Objectives

16.10   Increase to at least 75% the proportion of primary care providers who routinely counsel patients about tobacco use cessation, diet modification, and cancer screening recommendations.

16.11   Increase to at least 80% the proportion of women aged 40 and older who have ever received a clinical breast examination and a mammogram, and to at least 60% those aged 50 and older who have received them within the preceding 1 to 2 years.

16.12   Increase to at least 95% the proportion of women aged 18 and older with uterine cervix who have ever received a Pap test, and to at least 85% those who received a Pap test within the preceding 1 to 3 years.

16.13   Increase to at least 50% the proportion of people aged 50 and older who have received fecal occult blood testing within the preceding 1 to 2 years, and to at least 40% those who have ever received proctosigmoidoscopy.

16.14   Increase to at least 40% the proportion of people aged 50 and older visiting a primary care provider who have received oral, skin, and digital rectal examinations during a visit within the preceding year.

16.15   Ensure that Pap tests meet quality standards by monitoring and certifying all cytology laboratories.

16.16   Ensure that mammograms meet quality standards by monitoring and certifying at least 80% of mammography facilities.

17. Diabetes and Chronic Disabling Conditions
Health Status Objectives (Chronic Disabling Conditions)

17.1   Increase years of healthy life to at least 65 years.

17.2   Reduce to no more than 8% the proportion of people who experience a limitation in major activity due to chronic conditions.

17.3   Reduce to no more than 90 per 1000 people the proportion of all people aged 65 and older who have difficulty in performing two or more personal activities, thereby preserving independence.

17.4   Reduce to no more than 10% the proportion of people with asthma who experience activity limitation.

17.5   Reduce activity limitation due to chronic back conditions to a prevalence of no more than 19 per 1000 people.

17.6   Reduce significant hearing impairment to a prevalence of no more than 82 per 1000 people.

17.7   Reduce significant visual impairment to a prevalence of no more than 30 per 1000 people.

17.8   Reduce the prevalence of serious mental retardation in school-aged children to no more than 2 per 1000 children.

Diabetes

17.9   Reduce diabetes-related deaths to no more than 34 per 100,000.

17.10   Reduce the most severe complications of diabetes (i.e., end-stage renal disease, blindness, lower extremity amputation, perinatal mortality, and major congenital malformations).

17.11   Reduce diabetes to an incidence of no more than 2.5 per 1000 people and a prevalence of no more than 25 per 1000 people.

Risk Reduction Objectives

17.12   Reduce overweight to a prevalence of no more than 20% among people aged 20 and older and no more than 15% among adolescents aged 12 through 19.

17.13   Increase to at least 30% the proportion of people aged 6 and older who engage regularly, preferably daily, in light to moderate physical activity for at least 30 minutes per day.

Services and Protection Objectives

17.14   Increase to at least 40% the proportion of people with chronic and disabling conditions who receive formal patient education including information about community and self-help resources as an integral part of the management of their conditions.

17.15   Increase to at least 80% the proportion of providers of primary care for children who routinely refer or screen infants and children for impairments of vision, hearing, speech, and language, and assess other developmental milestones as part of well-child care.

17.16   Reduce the average age at which children with significant hearing impairment are identified to no more than 12 months.

17.17 Increase to at least 60% the proportion of providers of primary care for older adults who routinely evaluate people aged 65 and older for urinary incontinence and impairments of vision, hearing, cognition, and functional status.

17.18 Increase to at least 90% the proportion of perimenopausal women who have been counseled about the benefits and risks of estrogen replacement therapy (combined with progestin, when appropriate) for prevention of osteoporosis.

17.19 Increase to at least 75% the proportion of work sites with 50 or more employees that have a voluntary established policy or program for hiring people with disabilities.

17.20 Increase to 50 the number of states that have service systems for children at risk of or having chronic and disabling conditions, as required by Public Law 101-239.

18. HIV Infection

Health Status Objectives

18.1 Confine annual incidence of diagnosed AIDS cases to no more than 98,000 cases.

18.2 Confine the prevalence of HIV infection to no more than 800 per 100,000.

Risk Reduction Objectives

18.3 Reduce the proportion of adolescents who have engaged in sexual intercourse by age 15 to no more than 15% and by age 17 to no more than 40%.

18.4 Increase to at least 50% the proportion of sexually active unmarried people who used a condom during last sexual intercourse.

18.5 Increase to at least 50% the estimated proportion of all intravenous drug users who are in drug abuse treatment programs.

18.6 Increase to at least 50% the estimated proportion of intravenous drug users not in treatment who use only uncontaminated drug paraphernalia ("works").

18.7 Reduce to no more than 1 per 250,000 units of blood and blood components the risk of transfusion-transmitted HIV infection.

Services and Protection Objectives

18.8 Increase to at least 80% the proportion of HIV-infected people who have been tested for HIV infection.

18.9 Increase to at least 75% the proportion of primary care and mental health care providers who provide age-appropriate counseling on the prevention of HIV and other sexually transmitted diseases.

18.10 Increase to at least 95% the proportion of schools that have age-appropriate HIV education curricula for students in fourth through twelfth grade, preferably as part of quality school health education.

18.11 Provide HIV education for students and staff in at least 90% of colleges and universities.

18.12 Increase to at least 90% the proportion of cities with populations over 100,000 that have outreach programs to contact drug users (particularly intravenous drug users) to deliver HIV risk reduction messages.

18.13 Increase to at least 50% the proportion of the following kinds of clinics that screen, diagnose, treat, counsel, and provide (or refer for) partner notification services for HIV infection and bacterial sexually transmitted diseases (gonorrhea, syphilis, and chlamydia): family planning clinics, maternal and child health clinics, sexually transmitted disease clinics, tuberculosis clinics, drug treatment centers, and primary care clinics.

18.14 Extend to all facilities where workers are at risk for occupational transmission of HIV regulations to protect workers from exposure to blood-borne infections, including HIV infection.

19. Sexually Transmitted Diseases

Health Status Objectives

19.1 Reduce gonorrhea to an incidence of no more than 225 cases per 100,000 people.

19.2 Reduce *Chlamydia trachomatis* infections, as measured by a decrease in the incidence of nongonococcal urethritis, to no more than 170 cases per 100,000 people.

19.3 Reduce primary and secondary syphilis to an incidence of no more than 10 cases per 100,000 people.

19.4 Reduce congenital syphilis to an incidence of no more than 50 cases per 100,000 live births.

19.5 Reduce genital herpes and genital warts, as measured by reductions to 142,000 and 385,000, respectively, in the annual number of first-time consultations with a physician for the conditions.

19.6 Reduce the incidence of pelvic inflammatory disease, as measured by a reduction in hospitalizations for the condition to no more than 250 per 100,000 women aged 15 through 44.

19.7 Reduce sexually transmitted hepatitis B infection to no more than 30,500 cases.

19.8 Reduce the rate of repeat gonorrhea infection to no more than 15% within the previous year.

Risk Reduction Objectives

19.9 Reduce the proportion of adolescents who have engaged in sexual intercourse by age 15 to no more than 15% and by age 17 to no more than 40%.

19.10   Increase to at least 50% the proportion of sexually active unmarried people who used a condom during last sexual intercourse.

Services and Protection Objectives

19.11   Increase to at least 50% the proportion of the following kinds of clinics that screen, diagnose, treat, counsel, and provide (or refer for) partner notification services for HIV infection and bacterial sexually transmitted disease (gonorrhea, syphilis, and *Chlamydia*): family planning clinics, maternal and child health clinics, sexually transmitted disease clinics, tuberculosis clinics, drug treatment centers, and primary care clinics.

19.12   Include instruction in preventing transmission of sexually transmitted diseases in the curricula of all middle and secondary schools, preferably as part of quality school health education.

19.13   Increase to at least 90% the proportion of primary care providers treating patients with sexually transmitted diseases who correctly manage cases, as measured by their use of appropriate types and amounts of therapy.

19.14   Increase to at least 75% the proportion of primary care and mental health care providers who provide age-appropriate counseling on the prevention of HIV and other sexually transmitted diseases.

19.15   Increase to at least 50% the proportion of all patients with bacterial sexually transmitted diseases (gonorrhea, syphilis, and chlamydia) who are offered provider referral services.

20. Immunization and Infectious Diseases

Health Status Objectives

20.1   Reduce indigenous cases of vaccine-preventable diseases (i.e., diphtheria, tetanus, polio [wild-type virus], measles, rubella, congenital rubella syndrome, mumps, and pertussis).

20.2   Reduce epidemic-related pneumonia and influenza deaths among people aged 65 and older to no more than 7.3 per 100,000 people.

20.3   Reduce viral hepatitis.

20.4   Reduce tuberculosis to an incidence of no more than 3.5 cases per 100,000 people.

20.5   Reduce by at least 10% the incidence of surgical wound infections and nosocomial infections in intensive care patients.

20.6   Reduce incidence among international travelers of typhoid fever, hepatitis A, and malaria.

20.7   Reduce bacterial meningitis to no more than 4.7 cases per 100,000 people.

20.8   Reduce infectious diarrhea by at least 25% among children in licensed child care centers and children in programs that provide an Individualized Education Program (IEP) or Individualized Health Plan (IHP).

20.9   Reduce acute middle ear infections among children aged 4 and younger, as measured by days of restricted activity or school absenteeism, to no more than 105 days per 100 children.

20.10   Reduce pneumonia-related days of restricted activity.

Risk Reduction Objectives

20.11   Increase immunization levels as follows:
- Basic immunization series among children under age 2: at least 90%.
- Basic immunization series among children in licensed child care facilities and kindergarten through postsecondary education institutions: at least 95%.
- Pneumococcal pneumonia and influenza immunization among institutionalized chronically ill or older people: at least 80%.
- Pneumococcal pneumonia and influenza immunization among noninstitutionalized, high-risk populations, as defined by the Immunization Practices Advisory Committee: at least 60%.
- Hepatitis B immunization among high-risk populations, including infants of surface antigen-positive mothers to at least 90%; occupationally exposed workers to at least 90%; IV-drug users in drug treatment programs to at least 50%; and homosexual men to at least 50%.

20.12   Reduce postexposure rabies treatments to no more than 9000 per year.

Services and Protection Objectives

20.13   Expand immunization laws for schools, preschools, and day care settings to all states for all antigens.

20.14   Increase to at least 90% the proportion of primary care providers who provide information and counseling about immunizations and offer immunizations as appropriate for their patients.

20.15   Improve the financing and delivery of immunizations for children and adults so that virtually no American has a financial barrier to receiving recommended immunizations.

20.16   Increase to at least 90% the proportion of public health departments that provide adult immunization for influenza, pneumococcal disease, hepatitis B, tetanus, and diphtheria.

20.17   Increase to at least 90% the proportion of local health departments that have ongoing programs for actively identifying cases of tuberculosis and latent infection in populations at high risk for tuberculosis.

20.18   Increase to at least 85% the proportion of people found to have tuberculosis infection who completed courses of preventive therapy.

20.19   Increase to at least 85% the proportion of tertiary care hospital laboratories and to at least

50% the proportion of secondary care hospital and health maintenance organization laboratories possessing technologies for rapid viral diagnosis of influenza.

21. Clinical Preventive Services

Health Status Objective

21.1   Increase years of healthy life to at least 65 years.

Risk Reduction Objective

21.2   Increase to at least 50% the proportion of people who have received, as a minimum within the appropriate interval, all of the screening and immunization services and at least one of the counseling services appropriate for their age and sex as recommended by the U.S. Preventive Services Task Force.

Services and Protection Objectives

21.3   Increase to at least 95% the proportion of people who have a specific source of ongoing primary care for coordination of their preventive and episodic health care.

21.4   Improve financing and delivery of clinical preventive services so that virtually no American has a financial barrier to receiving, at a minimum, the screening, counseling, and immunization services recommended by the U.S. Preventive Services Task Force.

21.5   Assure that at least 90% of people for whom primary care services are provided directly by publicly funded programs are offered, at a minimum, the screening, counseling, and immunization services recommended by the U.S. Preventive Services Task Force.

21.6   Increase to at least 50% the proportion of primary care providers who provide their patients with the screening, counseling, and immunization services recommended by the U.S. Preventive Services Task Force.

21.7   Increase to at least 90% the proportion of people who are served by a local health de-partment that assesses and assures access to essential clinical preventive services.

21.8   Increase the proportion of all degrees in the health professions and allied/associated health profession fields awarded to members of underrepresented racial/ethnic minority groups.

22. Surveillance and Data Systems

Objectives

22.1   Develop a set of health status indicators appropriate for federal, state, and local health agencies and establish use of the set in at least 40 states.

22.2   Identify, and create where necessary, national data sources to measure progress toward each of the Year 2000: National Health Objectives.

22.3   Develop and disseminate among federal, state, and local agencies procedures for collecting comparable data for each of the Year 2000: National Health Objectives and incorporate these into Public Health Service data collection systems.

22.4   Develop and implement a national process to identify significant gaps in the nation's disease prevention and health promotion data, including data for racial and ethnic minorities, people with low incomes, and people with disabilities, and establish mechanisms to meet these needs.

22.5   Implement in all states periodic analysis and publication of data needed to measure progress toward objectives for at least 10 of the priority areas of the National Health Objectives.

22.6   Expand in all states systems for the transfer of health information related to the National Health Objectives among federal, state, and local agencies.

22.7   Achieve timely release of national surveillance and survey data needed by health professionals and agencies to measure progress toward the National Health Objectives.

A.2   SCHEDULE OF CLINICAL PREVENTIVE SERVICES

Table A.2-1   Birth to 18 Months—Schedule: 2, 4, 6, 15, 18 Months[1]

Leading Causes of Death:

Conditions originating in
  perinatal period
Congenital anomalies
Heart disease
Injuries (non–motor vehicle)
Pneumonia influenza

Remain Alert for:

Ocular misalignment
Tooth decay
Signs of child abuse or neglect

SCREENING

Height and weight
Hemoglobin and hematocrit[2]
High-risk groups
Heanng[3] (HR1)
Erythrocyte protoporphyrin (HR2)

PARENT COUNSELING

Diet

Breastfeeding
Nutrient intake, especially iron-rich foods

Injury Prevention

Child safety seats
Smoke detector
Hot water heater temperature
Stairway gates, window guards, pool fence
Storage of drugs and toxic chemicals
Syrup of ipecac, poison control telephone number

Dental Health

Baby bottle tooth decay

**Other Primary
Preventive Measures**

Effects of passive smoking

IMMUNIZATIONS AND CHEMOPROPHYLAXIS

Diphtheria-tetanus-pertussis (DTP)
  vaccine[4]
Oral poliovirus vaccine (OPV)[5]
Measles-mumps-rubella (MMR)
  vaccine[6]
Haemophilus influenzae type b (Hib)
  conjugate vaccine[7]
High-risk groups
Fluoride supplements (HR3)

FIRST WEEK

Ophthalmic antibiotics[8]
Hemoglobin electrophoresis (HR4)[8]
T4 TSH[7]
Phenylalanine[9]
Hearing (HR1)

HIGH RISK CATEGORIES

HR1   Infants with a family history of childhood hearing impairment or a personal history of congenital, perinatal infection with herpes, syphilis, rubella, cytomegalovirus, or toxoplasmosis; malformations involving the head or neck (e.g., dysmorphic and syndromal abnormalities, cleft palate, abnormal pinna); birthweight below 1500 g; bacteria, meningitis; hyperbilirubinemia requiring exchange transfusion; or severe perinatal asphyxia (Apgar scores of 0-3, absence of spontaneous respirations for 10 minutes, or hypotonia at 2 hours of age).

HR2   Infants who live in or frequently visit housing built before 1950 that is dilapidated or undergoing renovations who come in contact with other children with known lead toxicity; who live near lead processing plants or whose parents or household members work in a lead-related occupation; or who live near busy highways or hazardous waste sites.

HR3   Infants living in areas with inadequate water fluoridation (less than 0.7 parts per million).

HR4   Newborns of Caribbean, Latin American, Asian, Mediterranean, or African descent.

From Fisher M, editor: *Guide to clinical preventive services: report of the* US *Preventive Services Task Force*, Baltimore, 1989, Williams & Wilkins.
NOTE: **This list of preventive services is not exhaustive.** It reflects only those topics reviewed by the U.S. Preventive Services Task Force. Clinicians may wish to add other preventive services on a routine basis, and after considering the patient's medical history and other individual circumstances. Examples of target conditions not specifically examined by the Task Force include developmental disorders, musculoskeletal malformations, cardiac anomalies, genitourinary disorders, metabolic disorders, speech problems, behavioral disorders, and parent-family dysfunction.
[1]Five visits are required for immunizations. Because of lack of data and differing patient risk profiles, the scheduling of additional visits and the frequency of the individual preventive services listed in this table are left to clinical discretion (except as indicated in other footnotes). [2]Once during infancy. [3]At age 18-month visit, if not tested earlier. [4]At ages 2, 4, 6, and 15 months. [5]At ages 2, 4, and 15 months. [6]At age 15 months. [7]At age 18 months. [8]At birth. [9]Days 3 to 6 preferred for testing.

Table A.2-2 Ages 2-6—Schedule: See Footnote[1]

Leading Causes of Death:

Injuries (nonmotor vehicle)
Motor vehicle crashes
Congenital anomalies
Homicide
Heart disease

SCREENING

Height and weight
Blood pressure
Eye exam for amblyopia and strabismus[2]
Urinalysis for bacteriuria
High-risk groups
Erythrocyte protoporphyrin[3] (HR1)
Tuberculin skin test (PPD) (HR2)
Hearing[4] (HR3)

Remain Alert for:

Vision disorders
Dental decay, malalignment, premature loss of
    teeth, mouth breathing
Signs of child abuse or neglect
Abnormal bereavement

PATIENT AND PARENT COUNSELING
Diet and Exercise

Sweets and between-meal snacks, iron-
    enriched foods, sodium
Caloric balance
Selection of exercise program

Injury Prevention

Safety belts
Smoke detector
Hot water heater temperature
Window guards and pool fence
Bicycle safety helmets
Storage of drugs, toxic chemicals, matches, and
    firearms
Syrup of ipecac, poison control telephone
    number

Dental Health

Tooth brushing and dental visits

Other Primary
Preventive Measures

Effects of passive smoking
High-risk groups
Skin protection from ultraviolet light (HR4)

IMMUNIZATIONS AND
CHEMOPROPHYLAXIS

Diphtheria-tetanus-pertussis
    (DTP) vaccine[5]
Oral poliovirus vaccine (OPV)[5]
High Risk groups
Fluoride supplements (HR5)

HIGH RISK CATEGORIES

HR1   Children who live in or frequently visit housing built before 1950 that is dilapidated or undergoing renovation; who come in contact with other children with known lead toxicity; who live near lead processing plants or whose parents or household members work in a lead-related occupation; or who live near busy highways or hazardous waste sites.

HR2   Household members of persons with tuberculosis or others at risk for close contact with the disease; recent immigrants or refugees from countries in which tuberculosis is common (e.g., countries in Asia, Africa, Central and South America, and the Pacific Islands); family members of migrant workers: residents of homeless shelters; or persons with certain underlying medical disorders.

HR3   Children with a family history of childhood hearing impairment or a personal history of congenital perinatal infection with herpes, syphilis, rubella, cytomegalovirus, or toxoplasmosis malformations involving the head or neck (e.g., dysmorphic and syndroma abnormalities cleft palate, abnormal pinna), birthweight below 1500 g, bacterial meningitis; hyperbilirubinemia requiring exchange transfusion or severe perinatal asphyxia (Apgar scores of 0-3 absence of spontaneous respirations for 10 minutes, or hypotonia at 2 hours of age).

HR4   Children with increased exposure to sunlight.

HR5   Children living in areas with inadequate water fluoridation (less than 0.7 parts per million).

NOTE: **This list of preventive services is not exhaustive.** It reflects only those topics reviewed by the U.S. Preventive Services Task Force. Clinicians may wish to add other preventive services on a routine basis, and after considering the patient's medical history and other individual circumstances. Examples of target conditions not specifically examined by the Task Force include developmental disorders, speech problems, behavioral and learning disorders, and parent-family dysfunction.
[1]One visit is required for immunizations. Because of lack of data and differing patient risk profiles, the scheduling of additional visits and the frequency of the individual preventive services listed in this table are left to clinical discretion (except as indicated in other footnotes). [2]Ages 3-4.
[3]Annually. [4]Before age 3, if not tested earlier. [5]Once between ages 4 and 6.

Table A.2-3   Ages 7-12—Schedule: See Footnote[1]

Leading Causes of Death:

Motor vehicle crashes
Injuries (non–motor vehicle)
Congenital anomalies
Leukemia
Homicide
Heart disease

Remain Alert for:

Vision disorders
Diminished hearing
Dental decay, malalignment, mouth breathing
Signs of child abuse or neglect
Abnormal bereavement

SCREENING

Height and weight
Blood pressure
High-risk groups
Tuberculin skin test (PPD) (HR1)

PATIENT AND PARENT COUNSELING
Diet and Exercise

Fat (especially saturated fat), cholesterol, sweets
    and between-meal snacks, sodium
Caloric balance
Selection of exercise program

Injury Prevention

Safety belts
Smoke detector
Storage of firearms, drugs, toxic chemicals, matches
Bicycle safety helmets

Dental Health

Regular tooth brushing and dental visits

Other Primary
Preventive Measures
High-risk groups
Skin protection from ultraviolet light (HR2)

CHEMOPROPHYLAXIS

High-risk groups
Fluoride supplements (HR3)

HIGH RISK CATEGORIES

HR1   Household members of persons with tuberculosis or others at risk for close contact with the disease; recent immigrants or refugees from countries in which tuberculosis is common (e.g., countries in Asia, Africa, Central and South America, and the Pacific Islands); family members of migrant workers, residents of homeless shelters; or persons with certain underlying medical disorders.

HR2   Children with increased exposure to sunlight.

HR3   Children living in areas with inadequate water fluoridation (less than 0.7 parts per million).

NOTE: **This list of preventive services is not exhaustive.** It reflects only those topics reviewed by the U.S. Preventive Services Task Force. Clinicians may wish to add other preventive services on a routine basis, and after considering the patient's medical history and other individual circumstances. Examples of target conditions not specifically examined by the Task Force include developmental disorders, scoliosis, behavioral and learning disorders, parent-family dysfunction.

[1]Because of lack of data and differing patient risk profiles, the scheduling of visits and the frequency of the individual preventive services listed in this table are left to clinical discretion.

Table A.2-4   Ages 13-18—Schedule: See Footnote[1]

Leading Causes of Death:

Motor vehicle crashes
Homicide
Suicide
Injuries (non–motor vehicle)
Heart disease

Remain Alert for:

Depressive symptoms
Suicide risk factors (HR11)
Abnormal bereavement
Tooth decay, malalignment, gingivitis
Signs of child abuse and neglect.

SCREENING
History

Dietary intake
Physical activity
Tobacco alcohol drug use
Sexual practices

Physical Exam

Height and weight
Blood pressure
High-risk groups
Complete skin exam (HR1)
Clinical testicular exam (HR2)

Laboratory/Diagnostic Procedures
High-risk groups
Rubella antibodies (HR3)
VDRL RPR (HR4)
Chlamydial testing (HR5)
Gonorrhea culture (HR6)
Counseling and testing for HIV (HR7)
Tuberculin skin test (PPD) (HR8)
Hearing (HR9)
Papanicolaou smear (HR10)[2]

COUNSELING
Diet and Exercise

Fat (especialy salturated fat). cholesterol, sodium, iron,[3] calcium[3]
Caloric balance
Selection of exercise program

Substance Use

Tobacco: cessation primary prevention
Alcohol and other drugs: cessation primary prevention
Driving other dangerous activities while under the influence
Treatment for abuse
High-risk groups
Sharing using unsterilized needles and syringes (HR12)

Sexual Practices

Sexual development and behavior[4]
Sexually transmitted diseases, partner selection, condoms
Unintended pregnancy and contraceptive options

Injury Prevention

Safety belts
Safety helmets
Violent behavior[5]
Firearms[5]
Smoke detector

Dental Health

Regular tooth brushing, flossing, dental visits

Other Primary Preventive Measures
High-risk groups
Discussion of hemoglobin testing (HR13)
Skin protection from ultraviolet light (HR14)

IMMUNIZATIONS AND CHEMOPROPHYLAXIS

Tetanus-diphtheria (Td) booster[6]
High-risk groups
Fluoride supplements (HR15)

HIGH RISK CATEGORIES

HR1   Persons with increased recreational or occupational exposure to sunlight, a family or personal history of skin cancer, or clinical evidence of precursor lesions (e.g., dysplastic nevi, certain congenital nevi).

HR2   Males with a history of cryptorchidism, orchiopexy, or testicular atrophy.

NOTE: **This list of preventive services is not exhaustive.** It reflects only those topics reviewed by the U.S. Preventive Services Task Force. Clinicians may wish to add other preventive services on a routine basis, and after considering the patient's medical history and other individual circumstances. Examples of target conditions not specifically examined by the Task Force include developmental disorders, scoliosis, behavioral and learning, disorders, and parent-family dysfunction. [1]One visit is required for immunizations. Because of lack of data and differing patient risk profiles, the scheduling of additional visits and the frequency of the individual preventive services listed in this table are left to clinical discretion (except as indicated in other footnotes). [2]Every 1-3 years. [3]For females. [4]Often best performed early in adolescence and with the involvement of parents. [5]Especially for males. [6]Once between ages 14 and 16.

Continued.

Table A.2-4   Ages 13-18—Schedule: See Footnote[1]—cont'd

HIGH RISK CATEGORIES—cont'd

HR3   Females of childbearing age lacking evidence of immunity.

HR4   Persons who engage in sex with multiple partners in areas in which syphilis is prevalent, prostitutes, or contacts of persons with active syphilis.

HR5   Persons who attend clinics for sexually transmitted diseases; attend other high-risk health care facilities (e.g., adolescent and family planning clinics); or have other risk factors for chlamydial infection (e.g., multiple sexual partners or a sexual partner with multiple sexual contacts).

HR6   Persons with multiple sexual partners or a sexual partner with multiple contacts, sexual contacts of persons with culture-proven gonorrhea, or persons with a history of repeated episodes of gonorrhea.

HR7   Persons seeking treatment for sexually transmitted diseases; homosexual and bisexual men; past or present intravenous (IV) drug users; persons with a history of prostitution or multiple sexual partners; women whose past or present sexual partners were HIV-infected bisexual or IV drug users; persons with long-term residence or birth in an area with high prevalence of HIV infection; or persons with a history of transfusion between 1978 and 1985.

HR8   Household members of persons with tuberculosis or others at risk for close contact with the disease; recent immigrants or refugees from countries in which tuberculosis is common (e.g., countries in Asia, Africa, Central and South America, and the Pacific Islands); migrant workers; residents of correctional institutions or homeless shelters; or persons with certain underlying medical disorders.

HR9   Persons exposed regularly to excessive noise in recreational or other settings.

HR10   Females who are sexually active of (if the sexual history is thought to be unreliable) age 18 or older.

HR11   Recent divorce, separation, unemployment, depression, alcohol, or other drug abuse; serious medical illnesses; living alone or recent bereavement.

HR12   Intravenous drug users.

HR13   Persons of Caribbean, Latin American, Asian, Mediterranean, or African descent.

HR14   Persons with increased exposure to sunlight.

HR15   Persons living in areas with inadequate water fluoridation (less than 0.7 parts per million).

Table A.2-5 Ages 19-39—Schedule: Every 1-3 Years[1]

Leading Causes of Death:

Motor vehicle crashes
Homicide
Suicide
Injuries (non–motor vehicle)
Heart disease

Remain Alert for:

Depressive symptoms
Suicide risk factors (HR17)
Abnormal bereavement
Malignant skin lesions
Tooth decay, gingivitis
Signs of physical abuse

SCREENING

History

Dietary intake
Physical activity
Tobacco/alcohol/drug use
Sexual practices

Physical Exam

Height and weight
Blood pressure
Papanicolaou smear[2]
High-risk groups
Complete oral cavity exam (HR1)
Palpation for thyroid nodules (HR2)
Clinical breast exam (HR3)
Clinical testicular exam (HR4)
Complete skin exam (HR5)

Laboratory/Diagnostic Procedures

Nonfasting total blood cholesterol
High-risk groups
Fasting plasma glucose (HR6)
Rubella antibodies (HR7)
VDRL/RPR (HR8)
Urinalysis for bacteriuria (HR9)
Chlamydial testing (HR10)
Gonorrhea culture (HR11)
Counseling and testing for HIV (HR12)
Hearing (HR13)
Tuberculin skin test (PPD) (HR14)
Electrocardiogram (HR15)
Mammogram (HR3)
Colonoscopy (HR16)

COUNSELING

Diet and Exercise

Fat (especially saturated fat), cholesterol, complex carbohydrates, fiber, sodium, iron,[3] calcium[3]
Caloric balance
Selection of exercise program

Substance Use

Tobacco: cessation/primary prevention
Alcohol and other drugs:
    Limiting alcohol consumption
    Driving/other dangerous activities while under the influence
    Treatment for abuse
High-risk groups
Sharing/using unsterilized needles and syringes (HR18)

Sexual Practices

Sexually transmitted diseases: partner selection, condoms, anal intercourse
Unintended pregnancy and contraceptive options

Injury Prevention

Safety belts
Safety helmets
Violent behavior[4]
Firearms[4]
Smoke detector
Smoking near bedding or upholstery
High-risk groups
Back-conditioning exercises (HR19)
Prevention of childhood injuries (HR20)
Falls in the elderly (HR21)

Dental Health

Regular tooth brushing, flossing, dental visits

Other Primary Preventive Measures
High-risk groups
Discussion of hemoglobin testing (HR22)
Skin protection from ultraviolet light (HR23)

IMMUNIZATIONS

Tetanus-diphtheria (Td) booster[5]
High-risk groups
Hepatitis B vaccine (HR24)
Pneumococcal vaccine (HR25)
Influenza vaccine[6] (HR26)
Measles-mumps-rubella vaccine (HR27)

NOTE: **This list of preventive services is not exhaustive.** It reflects only those topics reviewed by the U.S. Preventive Services Task Force. Clinicians may wish to add other preventive services on a routine basis, and after considering the patient's medical history and other individual circumstances. Examples of target conditions not specifically examined by the Task Force include chronic obstructive pulmonary disease, hepatobiliary disease, bladder cancer, endometrial disease, travel-related illness, prescription drug abuse, and occupational illness and injuries.
[1]The recommended schedule applies only to the periodic visit itself. The frequency of the individual preventive services listed in this table is left to clinical discretion, except as indicated in other footnotes. [2]Every 1-3 years. [3]For women. [4]Especially for young males. [5]Every 10 years. [6]Annually.

Continued.

HIGH RISK CATEGORIES

HR1   Persons with exposure to tobacco or excessive amounts of alcohol, or those with suspicious symptoms or lesions detected through self-examination.

HR2   Persons with a history of upper-body irradiation.

HR3   Women aged 35 and older with a family history of premenopausally diagnosed breast cancer in a first-degree relative.

HR4   Men with a history of cryptorchidism, orchiopexy, or testicular atrophy.

HR5   Persons with family or personal history of skin cancer, increased occupational or recreational exposure to sunlight, or clinical evidence of precursor lesions (e.g., dysplastic nevi, certain congenital nevi).

HR6   The markedly obese, persons with a family history of diabetes, or women with a history of gestational diabetes.

HR7   Women lacking evidence of immunity.

HR8   Prostitutes, persons who engage in sex with multiple partners in areas in which syphilis is prevalent or contacts of persons with active syphilis.

HR9   Persons with diabetes.

HR10   Persons who attend clinics for sexually transmitted diseases; attend other high-risk health care facilities (e.g., adolescent and family planning clinics); or have other risk factors for chlamydial infection (e.g., multiple sexual partners or a sexual partner with multiple sexual contacts, age less than 20).

HR11   Prostitutes, persons with multiple sexual partners or a sexual partner with multiple contacts, sexual contacts of persons with culture-proven gonorrhea, or persons with a history of repeated episodes of gonorrhea.

HR12   Persons seeking treatment for sexually transmitted diseases; homosexual and bisexual men; past or present intravenous (IV) drug users; persons with a history of prostitution or multiple sexual partners; women whose past or present sexual partners were HIV-infected, bisexual, or IV drug users; persons with long-term residence or birth in an area with high prevalence of HIV infection; or persons with a history of transfusion between 1978 and 1985.

HR13   Persons exposed regularly to excessive noise.

HR14   Household members of persons with tuberculosis or others at risk for close contact with the disease (e.g., staff of tuberculosis clinics, shelters for the homeless, nursing homes, substance abuse treatment facilities, dialysis units, correctional institutions); recent immigrants or refugees from countries in which tuberculosis is common; migrant workers; residents of nursing homes, correctional institutions, or homeless shelters; or persons with certain underlying medical disorders (e.g., HIV infection).

HR15   Men who would endanger public safety were they to experience sudden cardiac events (e.g., commercial airline pilots).

HR16   Persons with a family history of familiar polyposis coli or cancer family syndrome.

HR17   Recent divorce, separation, unemployment, depression, alcohol or other drug abuse, serious medical illnesses, living alone, or recent bereavement.

HR18   Intravenous drug users.

HR19   Persons at increased risk for low back injury because of past history, body configuration or type of activities.

HR20   Persons with children in the home or automobile.

HR21   Persons with older adults in the home.

HR22   Young adults of Caribbean, Latin American, Asian, Mediterranean, or African descent.

HR23   Persons with increased exposure to sunlight.

HR24   Homosexually active men, intravenous drug users, recipients of some blood products, or persons in health-related jobs with frequent exposure to blood or blood products.

HR25   Persons with medical conditions that increase the risk of pnenumococcal infection (e.g., chronic cardiac or pulmonary disease, sickle cell disease, nephrotic syndrome, Hodgkin's disease, asplenia, diabetes mellitus, alcoholism, cirrhosis, multiple myeloma, renal disease, or conditions associated with immunosuppression).

HR26   Residents of chronic care facilities or persons suffering from chronic cardiopulmonary disorders, metabolic diseases (including diabetes mellitus), hemoglobinopathies, immunosuppression, or renal dysfunction.

HR27   Persons born after 1956 who lack evidence of immunity to measles (receipt of live vaccine on or after first birthday, laboratory evidence of immunity, or a history of physician-diagnosed measles).

Table A.2-6   Ages 40-64—Schedule: Every 1-3 Years[1]

Leading Causes of Death:	**Remain Alert for:**
Heart disease	Depressive symptoms
Lung cancer	Suicide risk factors (HR17)
Cerebrovascular disease	Abnormal bereavement
Breast cancer	Signs of physical abuse or neglect
Colorectal cancer	Malignant skin lesions
Obstructive lung disease	Peripheral arterial disease (HR18)
	Tooth decay, gingivitis, loose teeth

SCREENING

History

Dietary intake
Physical activity
Tobacco/alcohol/drug use
Sexual practices

Physical Exam

Height and weight
Blood pressure
Clinical breast exam[2]
High-risk groups
Complete skin exam (HR1)
Complete oral cavity exam (HR2)
Palpation for thyroid nodules
   (HR3)
Auscultation for carotid bruits
   (HR4)

Laboratory/Diagnostic Procedures

Nonfasting total blood cholesterol
Papanicolaou smear[3]
Mammogram[4]
High-risk groups
Fasting plasma glucose (HR5)
VDRL/RPR (HR6)
Urinalysis for bacteriuria (HR7)
Chlamydial testing (HR8)
Gonorrhea culture (HR9)
Counseling and testing for HIV
   (HR10)
Tuberculin skin test (PPD) (HR11)
Hearing (HR12)
Electrocardiogram (HR13)
Fecal occult blood
   sigmoidoscopy (HR14)
Fecal occult blood/colonoscopy
   (HR15)
Bone mineral content (HR16)

COUNSELING

Diet and Exercise

Fat (especially saturated fat), cholesterol, complex carbo-
   hydrates, fiber, sodium, calcium[5]
Caloric balance
Selection of exercise program

Substance Use

Tobacco cessation
Alcohol and other drugs:
   Limiting alcohol consumption
   Driving other dangerous activities while under the influence
   Treatment for abuse
High-risk groups
Sharing/using unsterilized needles and syringes (HR19)

Sexual Practices

Sexually transmitted diseases; partner selection, condoms,
   anal intercourse
Unintended pregnancy and contraceptive options

Injury Prevention

Safety belts
Safety helmets
Smoke detector
Smoking near bedding or upholstery
High-risk groups
Back-conditioning exercises (HR20)
Prevention of childhood injuries (HR21)
Falls in the elderly (HR22)

Dental Health

Regular tooth brushing, flossing, and dental visits

Other Primary Preventive Measures
High-risk groups
Skin protection from ultraviolet light (HR23)
Discussion of aspirin therapy (HR24)
Discussion of estrogen replacement therapy (HR25)

IMMUNIZATIONS

Tetanus-diphtheria (Td)
   booster[6]
High-risk groups
Hepatitis B vaccine (HR26)
Pneumococcal vaccine
   (HR27)
Influenza vaccine (HR28)[7]

NOTE: **This list of preventive services is not exhaustive.** It reflects only those topics reviewed by the U.S. Preventive Services Task Force. Clinicians may wish to add other preventive services on a routine basis, and after considering the patient's medical history and other individual circumstances. Examples of target conditions not specifically examined by the Task Force include chronic obstructive pulmonary disease, hepatobiliary disease, bladder cancer, endometrial disease, travel-related illness, prescription drug abuse, and occupational illness and injuries.
[1]The recommended schedule applies only to the periodic visit itself. The frequency of the individual preventive services listed in this table is
left to clinical discretion, except as indicated in other footnotes.[2]Annually for women. [3]Every 1-3 years for women. [4]Every 1-2 years for women beginning at age 50 (age 35 for those at increased risk). [5]For women. [6]Every 10 years. [7]Annually.

Continued.

Table A.2-6   Ages 40-64—Schedule: Every 1-3 Years[1]—cont'd

HIGH RISK CATEGORIES

HR1   Persons with family or personal history of skin cancer, increased occupational or recreational exposure to sunlight, or clinical evidence of precursor lesions (e.g., dysplastic nevi, certain congenital nevi).

HR2   Persons with exposure to tobacco or excessive amounts of alcohol, or those with suspicious symptoms or lesions detected through self-examination.

HR3   Persons with a history of upper-body irradiation.

HR4   Persons with risk factors for cerebrovascular or cardiovascular disease (e.g., hypertension, smoking, CAD, atrial fibrillation, diabetes); or those with neurologic symptoms (e.g., transient ischemic attacks); or a history of cerebrovascular disease.

HR5   The markedly obese, persons with a family history of diabetes, or women with a history of gestational diabetes.

HR6   Prostitutes, persons who engage in sex with multiple partners in areas in which syphilis is prevalent, or contacts of persons with active syphilis.

HR7   Persons with diabetes.

HR8   Persons who attend clinics for sexually transmitted diseases; attend other high-risk health care facilities (e.g., adolescent and family planning clinics); or have other risk factors for chlamydial infection (e.g., multiple sexual partners or a sexual partner with multiple sexual contacts).

HR9   Prostitutes, persons with multiple sexual partners or a sexual partner with multiple contacts, sexual contacts of persons with culture-proven gonorrhea, or persons with a history of repeated episodes of gonorrhea.

HR10   Persons seeking treatment for sexually transmitted diseases; homosexual and bisexual men; past or present intravenous (IV) drug users; persons with a history of prostitution or multiple sexual partners; women whose past or present sexual partners were HIV-infected, bisexual, or IV drug users; persons with long-term residence or birth in an area with high prevalence of HIV infection; or persons with a history of transfusion between 1978 and 1985.

HR11   Household members of persons with tuberculosis or others at risk for close contact with the disease (e.g., staff of tuberculosis clinics, shelters for the homeless, nursing homes, substance abuse treatment facilities, dialysis units, correctional institutions); recent immigrants or refugees from countries in which tuberculosis is common (e.g., countries in Asia, Africa, Central and South America, and the Pacific Islands); migrant workers; residents of nursing homes, correctional institutions, or homeless shelters; or persons with certain underlying medical disorders (e.g., HIV infection).

HR12   Persons exposed regularly to excessive noise.

HR13   Men with two or more cardiac risk factors (high blood cholesterol, hypertension, cigarette smoking, diabetes mellitus, family history of CAD); men who would endanger public safety were they to experience sudden cardiac events (e.g., commercial airline pilots); or sedentary or high-risk males planning to begin a vigorous exercise program.

HR14   Persons aged 50 and older who have first-degree relatives with colorectal cancer, a personal history of endometrial, ovarian, or breast cancer, or a previous diagnosis of inflammatory bowel disease, adenomatous polyps or colorectal cancer.

HR15   Persons with a family history of familial polyposis coli or cancer family syndrome.

HR16   Perimenopausal women at increased risk for osteoporosis (e.g., Caucasian race, bilateral oopherectomy before menopause, slender build) and for whom estrogen replacement therapy would otherwise not be recommended.

HR17   Recent divorce, separation, unemployment, depression, alcohol or other drug abuse, serious medical illnesses, living alone, or recent bereavement.

HR18   Persons over age 50, smokers, or persons with diabetes mellitus.

HR19   Intravenous drug users.

HR20   Persons at increased risk for low back injury because of past history, body configuration, or type of activities.

HR21   Persons with children in the home or automobile.

HR22   Persons with older adults in the home.

HR23   Persons with increased exposure to sunlight.

HR24   Men who have risk factors for myocardial infarction (e.g., blood cholesterol, smoking, diabetes mellitus, family history of early-onset CAD) and who lack a history of gastrointestinal or other bleeding problems, and other risk factors for bleeding or cerebral hemorrhage.

Table A.2-6 Ages 40-64—Schedule: Every 1-3 Years[1]—cont'd

HIGH RISK CATEGORIES—cont'd

HR25 Perimenopausal women at increased risk for osteoporosis (e.g., Caucasian, low bone mineral content, bilateral oopherectomy before menopause or early menopause, slender build) and who are without known contraindications (e.g., history of undiagnosed vaginal bleeding, active liver disease, thromboembolic disorders, hormone-dependent cancer).

HR26 Homosexually active men, intravenous drug users, recipients of some blood products, or persons in health-related jobs with frequent exposure to blood or blood products.

HR27 Persons with medical conditions that increase the risk of pneumococcal infection (e.g., chronic cardiac or pulmonary disease, sickle cell disease, nephrotic syndrome, Hodgkin's disease, asplenia, diabetes mellitus, alcoholism, cirrhosis, multiple myeloma, renal disease, or conditions associated with immunosuppression).

HR28 Residents of chronic care facilities and persons suffering from chronic cardiopulmonary disorders, metabolic diseases (including diabetes mellitus), hemoglobinopathies, immunosuppression, or renal dysfunction.

Table A.2-7 Ages 65 and Over—Schedule: Every Year[1]

Leading Causes of Death:

Heart disease
Cerebrovascular disease
Obstructive lung disease
Pneumonia/influenza
Lung cancer
Colorectal cancer

Remain Alert for:

Depression symptoms
Suicide risk factors (HR11)
Abnormal bereavement
Changes in cognitive function
Medications that increase risk of falls
Signs of physical abuse or neglect
Malignant skin lesions
Peripheral arterial disease
Tooth decay, gingivitis, loose teeth

SCREENING

History

Prior symptoms of transient ischemic
  attack
Dietary intake
Physical activity
Tobacco/alcohol/drug use
Functional status at home

Physical Exam

Height and weight
Blood pressure
Visual acuity
Hearing and hearing aids
Clinical breast exam[2]

High-risk groups

Auscultation for carotid bruits (HR1)
Complete skin exam (HR2)
Complete oral cavity exam (HR3)
Palpation of thyroid nodules (HR4)

COUNSELING

Diet and Exercise

Fat (especially saturated fat), cholesterol, complex
  carbohydrates, fiber, sodium, calcium[4]
Caloric balance
Selection of exercise program

Substance Use

Tobacco cessation
Alcohol and other drugs:
  Limiting alcohol consumption
  Driving other dangerous activities while under
    the influence
  Treatment for abuse

Injury Prevention

Prevention of falls
Safety belts
Smoke detector
Smoking near beeding or upholstery

IMMUNIZATIONS

Tetanus-diphtheria (Td)
  booster[6]
Influenza vaccine[2]
Pneumococcal vaccine
High-risk groups
Hepatitis B vaccine (HR16)

NOTE: **This list of preventive services is not exhaustive.** It reflects only those topics reviewed by the U.S. Preventive Services Task Force. Clinicians may wish to add other preventive services on a routine basis, and after considering the patient's medical history and other individual circumstances. Examples of target conditions not specifically examined by the Task Force include chronic obstructive pulmonary disease, hepatobiliary disease, bladder cancer, endometrial disease, travel-related illness, prescription drug abuse, and occupational illness and injuries.
[1]The recommended schedule applies only to the periodic visit itself. The frequency of the individual preventive services listed in this table is left to clinical discretion, except as indicated in other footnotes. [2]Annually. [3]Every 1-2 years for women until age 75, unless pathology detected. [4]For women. [5]Every 1-3 years. [6]Every 10 years.

Continued.

Table A.2-7 Ages 65 and Over—Schedule: Every Year[1]—cont'd

SCREENING—cont'd
Laboratory/Diagnostic Procedures

Nonfasting total blood cholesterol
Dipstick urinalysis
Mammogram[3]
Thyroid function tests[4]
High-risk groups
Fasting plasma glucose (HR5)
Tuberculin skin test (PPD) (HR6)
Electrocardiogram (HR7)
Papanicolaou smear[5] (HR8)
Fecal occult blood Sigmoidoscopy
  (HR9)
Fecal occult blood Colonoscopy
  (HR10)

COUNSELING—cont'd
Injury Prevention

Hot water heater temperature
Safety helmets
High-risk groups
Prevention of childhood injuries (HR12)

Dental Health

Regular dental visits, tooth brushing, flossing

Other Primary
Preventive Measures

Glaucoma testing by eye specialist
High-risk groups
Discussion of estrogen replacement therapy
  (HR13)
Discussion of aspirin therapy (HR14)
Skin protection from ultraviolet light (HR15)

HIGH RISK CATEGORIES

HR1 Persons with risk factors for cerebrovascular or cardiovascular disease (e.g., hypertension, smoking, CAD, atrial fibrillation, diabetes) or those with neurologic symptoms (e.g., transient ischemic attacks) or a history of cerebrovascular disease.

HR2 Persons with a family or personal history of skin cancer or clinical evidence of precursor lesions (e.g., dysplastic nevi, certain congenital nevi) or those with increased occupational or recreational exposure to sunlight.

HR3 Persons with exposure to tobacco or excessive amounts of alcohol, or those with suspicious symptoms or lesions detected through self-examination.

HR4 Persons with a history of upper-body irradiation.

HR5 The markedly obese persons with a family history of diabetes, or women with a history of gestational diabetes.

HR6 Household members of persons with tuberculosis or others at risk for close contact with the disease (e.g., staff of tuberculosis clinics, shelters for the homeless, nursing homes, substance abuse treatment facilities, dialysis units, correctional institutions); recent immigrants or refugees from countries in which tuberculosis is common (e.g., countries in Asia, Africa, Central and South America, and the Pacific Islands); migrant workers, residents of nursing homes, correctional institutions, or homeless shelters; or persons with certain underlying medical disorders (e.g., HIV infection).

HR7 Men with two or more cardiac risk factors (high blood cholesterol, hypertension, cigarette smoking, diabetes mellitus, family history of CAD); men who would endanger public safety were they to experience sudden cardiac events (e.g., commercial airline pilots); or sedentary or high-risk males planning to begin a vigorous exercise program.

HR8 Women who have not had previous documented screening in which smears have been consistently negative.

HR9 Persons who have first-degree relatives with colorectal cancer; a personal history of endometrial, ovarian, or breast cancer; or a previous diagnosis of inflammatory bowel disease, adenomatous polyps, or colorectal cancer.

HR10 Persons with a family history of familial polyposis coli or cancer family syndrome.

HR11 Recent divorce, separation, unemployment, depression, alcohol or other drug abuse, serious medical illnesses, living alone, or recent bereavement.

HR12 Persons with children in the home or automobile.

HR13 Women at increased risk for osteoporosis (e.g., Caucasian, low bone mineral content, bilateral oopherectomy before menopause or early menopause, slender build) and who are without known contraindications (e.g., history of undiagnosed vaginal bleeding, active liver disease, thromboembolic disorders, hormone-dependent cancer).

HR14 Men who have risk factors for myocardial infarction (e.g., high blood cholesterol, smoking, diabetes mellitus, family history of early-onset CAD) and who lack a history of gastrointestinal or other bleeding problems, or other risk factors for bleeding or cerebral hemorrhage.

Table A.2-7 Ages 65 and Over—Schedule: Every Year[1]—cont'd

HIGH RISK CATEGORIES—cont'd

HR15 Persons with increased exposure to sunlight.

HR16 Homosexually, active men, intravenous drug users, recipients of some blood products, or persons in health-related jobs with frequent exposure to blood or blood products.

Table A.2-8 Pregnant Women[1]

First prenatal visit		Follow-up visits	
Remain Alert for:		**Remain Alert for:**	
Signs of physical abuse		Signs of physical abuse Schedule: See Footnote[2]	
SCREENING History	**COUNSELING** Nutrition	**SCREENING** Blood pressure	**COUNSELING** Nutrition
Genetic and obstetric history	Tobacco use	Urinarlysis for bacteriuria	Safety belts
Dietary intake	Alcohol and other drug use		Discuss meaning
Tobacco alcohol drug use	Safety belts	**Screening Tests at Specific**	of upcoming
Risk factors for intrauterine growth	*High-risk groups*	**Gestational Ages**	tests
retardation and low birthweight	Discuss amniocentesis	**14-16 Weeks:**	*High-risk groups*
Prior genital herpetic lesions	(HR5)	Maternal serum alpha-fetoprotein	Tobacco use (HR6)
	Discuss risks of HIV infec-	(MSAFP)	Alcohol and other
Laboratory/Diagnostic	tion (HR4)	Ultrasound cephalometry (HR8)	drug use (HR7)
Procedures		**24-28 Weeks:**	
Blood pressure		50 g oral glucose tolerance test	
Hemoglobin and hematocrit		Rh(D) antibody (HR9)	
ABO Rh typing		Gonorrhea culture (HR10)	
Rh(D) and other antibody screen		VDRL/RPR (HR11)	
VDRL RPR		Hepatitis B surface antigen	
Hepatitis B surface antigen (HBsAg)		(HBsAg) (HR12)	
Urinalysis for bacteriuria		Counseling and testing for HIV	
Gonorrhea culture		(HR13)	
High-risk groups		**36 Weeks:**	
Hemoglobin electrophoresis (HR1)		Ultrasound exam (HR14)	
Rubella antibodies (HR2)			
Chlamydial testing (HR3)			
Counseling and testing for HIV (HR4)			

HIGH RISK CATEGORIES

HR1 Black women.

HR2 Women lacking evidence of immunity (proof of vaccination after the first birthday or laboratory evidence of immunity).

NOTE: **This list of preventive services is not exhaustive.** It reflects only those topics reviewed by the U.S. Preventive Services Task Force. Clinicians may wish to add other preventive services on a routine basis, and after considering the patient's medical history and other individual circumstances. Examples of target conditions not specifically examined by the Task Force include counseling on warning signs and symptoms, physical findings of abdominal and cervical examination, Tay-Sachs disease, childbirth education, and teratogenic and fetotoxic exposures. Women with access to counseling and follow-up services, skilled high-resolution ultrasound and amniocentesis capabilities, and reliable standardized laboratories.

[1]See also Tables 4–6 for other preventive services for women. [2]Because of lack of data and differing patient risk profiles, the scheduling of visits and the frequency of the individual preventive services listed in this table are left to clinical discretion, except for those indicated at specific gestational ages.

Continued.

Table A.2-8 Pregnant Women[1]—cont'd

HIGH RISK CATEGORIES—cont'd

HR3   Women who attend clinics for sexually transmitted diseases, attend other high-risk health care facilities (e.g., adolescent and family planning clinics) or have other risk factors for chlamydial infection (e.g., multiple sexual partners or a sexual partner with multiple sexual contacts)

HR4   Women seeking treatment for sexually transmitted diseases, past or present intravenous (IV) drug users; women with a history of prostitution or multiple sexual partners; women whose past or present sexual partners were HIV-infected, bisexual, or IV drug users; women with long-term residence or birth in an area with high prevalence of HIV infection in women; or women with a history of transfusion between 1978 and 1985.

HR5   Women aged 35 and older.

HR6   Women who continue to smoke during pregnancy.

HR7   Women with excessive alcohol consumption during pregnancy.

HR8   Women with uncertain menstrual histories or risk factors for intrauterine growth retardation (e.g., hypertension, renal disease, short maternal stature, low prepregnancy weight, failure to gain weight during pregnancy, smoking, alcohol and other drug abuse, and history of a previous fetal death or growth-retarded baby).

HR9   Unsensitized Rh-negative women.

HR10   Women with multiple sexual partners or a sexual partner with multiple contacts, or sexual contacts of persons with culture-proven gonorrhea.

HR11   Women who engage in sex with multiple partners in areas in which syphilis is prevalent or contacts of persons with active syphilis.

HR12   Women who engage in high-risk behavior (e.g., intravenous drug use) or in whom exposure to hepatitis B during pregnancy is suspected.

HR13   Women at high risk (see HR4) who have a nonreactive HIV test at the first prenatal visit.

HR14   Women with risk factors for intrauterine growth retardation (see HR8).

A.3   SELECT MAJOR HISTORICAL EVENTS DEPICTING FINANCIAL INVOLVEMENT OF FEDERAL GOVERNMENT IN HEALTH CARE DELIVERY*

1798   Marine Hospital Service Act was passed to provide medical care to Merchant Marines.

1878   Port Quarantine Act was passed to prevent epidemic diseases from entering the country through seaports.

1879   National Health Department was established by Congress with a budget of $500,000.

*Sources for this listing were Hanlon J, Pickett G: *Public health administration and practice,* ed 2, St Louis, 1984, Mosby; Congressional Research Service: *Summary of health legislation, 1959-1981.* Library of Congress, Pub No 82-127 EPW, Washington, DC, May 7, 1981, US Government Printing Office; Congressional Research Service: *Major legislation of the 97th Congress,* Library of Congress, Pub No 9, Washington, DC, Oct 6, 1982 US Government Printing Office; Congressional Research Service: *Major Legislation of the 98th Congress,* Library of Congress, Pub No 9, Washington, DC, Oct, 1986 US Government Printing Office; Congressional Information Service Index, 1990, 1992, and 1993 editions of the Legislative Histories of US Public Laws.

1887   Laboratory of Hygiene at Staten Island Marine Hospital marked the beginning of Public Health Service research activities. This bacteriologic research laboratory later evolved into the National Institute of Health.

1890   Marine Hospital Service was given authority to inspect all immigrants to bar "lunatics and others unable to care for self" from entering the country.

1902   National Health Department was renamed the Public Health and Marine Hospital Service.

1912   National Institute of Health functions were expanded to study and investigate diseases of persons and the conditions influencing the origin and spread of disease.

1912   The Public Health and Marine Hospital Service was renamed the United States Public Health Service.

1912   The Child Health Bureau was established within the USPHS.

1917   National leprosarium was established at Carville, Louisiana under the aegis of the USPHS.

1917   USPHS became responsible for the physical and mental examination of all aliens.

1917 Congress appropriated $25,000 to USPHS to study and provide demonstration projects sharing state and federal cooperative rural health services.

1918 Because of increased veneral disease incidence during World War I, the Division of Venereal Disease was established in USPHS providing for cooperative federal and state control and prevention programs.

1921 Shepherd-Towner Maternity Infancy Act was passed to provide for the establishment of state maternal and infant programs. The Act provided for mother-child health conferences, home delivery supplies, improved prenatal care, improved infant and child care, more public health nurses, and health education.

1929 USPHS Narcotics Division was developed to provide facilities for the confinement and treatment of drug addicts (renamed Division of Mental Hygiene in 1939).

1935 Congress passed the Social Security Act. Title VI of the Act was written for the purpose of assisting states, counties, health districts, and other political subdivisions in establishing and maintaining adequate public health service, including the training of personnel for state and local health work.

1935 The Social Security Act provided for grants-in-aid to states to finance the public's health. *Grants-in-aid* resulted in increased numbers of new health departments and the strengthening and expansion of existing health departments.

1937 National Cancer Act called for the establishment of the National Cancer Institute for research into the causes, diagnosis, and treatment of cancer; for assistance to public and private agencies; and for the promotion of the most effective prevention and treatment.

1938 The second Federal Veneral Disease Control Act was passed to promote investigation and control and to provide funds for the development and maintenance of state and local programs.

1939 The Federal Security Agency was established to bring health, welfare, and education services of the federal government together.

1940 Communicable Disease Center (National Center for Disease Control) was established in Atlanta for the purpose of conducting epidemiological studies, providing health personnel training, and establishing methods of communication and education.

1940 National Office of Vital Statistics (National Center for Health Statistics) was authorized to provide data about health, illness, injuries, and death.

1941 Nurse training appropriations provided monies to nursing programs to increase enrollment and improve programs.

1943 Nurse Training Act established the U.S. Nurse Cadet Corps in USPHS to support nurse training.

1946 National Mental Health Act was passed for constructing and equipping hospitals and laboratories to stimulate research and training in mental health.

1946 Hill-Burton Act provided for hospital services and construction.

1947 National Institute of Health Division of Research Grants were established to administer and award grants for research projects and training.

1947 A permanent Nursing Corps in the Army and Navy was established.

1948 National Heart Institute was established (renamed Heart, Lung, and Blood Institute in 1976).

1948 Microbiological, Experimental Biology, and Medicine Institutes were established (renamed National Institute of Allergy and Infectious Diseases in 1955).

1948 National Institute of Dental Research was authorized.

1948 National Institute of Health became National Institutes of Health (NIH).

1949 National Institute of Mental Health was established (renamed Alcoholism, Drug Abuse, and Mental Health Administration in 1974).

1950 National Institute of Neurological Diseases and Blindness was established (renamed National Eye Institute in 1968 and the National Institute of Neurological and Communicative Disorders and Strokes in 1975).

1950 Health Manpower Training Acts evolved to provide for training of Health Personnel.

1953 National Clinical Center was founded to accelerate research and to confirm and apply research findings. A 600-bed research hospital evolved.

1954 Congress extended Hill-Burton Act to allow monies for construction of other types of health facilities, such as general, mental, tuberculosis, and chronic disease hospitals; public health centers; diagnostic and treatment centers; rehabilitation facilities; nursing homes; state health laboratories; and nurse training facilities.

1954 Taft Sanitary Engineering Center was founded in Cincinnati for research and training in environmental health.

1955 National Institutes of Health Division of Biological Standards was established to oversee the growth of the pharmaceutical industry and market.

1955 Polio Vaccination Assistance Act was passed to aid state vaccination programs.

1956 U.S. Army Medical Library was transferred to USPHS, which became the Library of Medicine at the National Institutes of Health. The library provides MEDLARS, the Medical Literature Analysis and Retrieval System.

1956   CHAMPUS program was established for dependents of military personnel.

1956   National Health Survey was established for continuous monitoring of sickness and disability in the United States.

1959   National Institute of Arthritis and Metabolic Diseases was established (renamed National Institute of Arthritis, Metabolic, and Digestive Diseases in 1981).

1960   Social Security Amendments provided grants to states for medical assistance to the aged.

1962   National Institute of Child Health and Human Development was founded.

1962   Program for state assistance in preschool vaccination programs was authorized.

1963   Aid program was established for the construction of mental retardation and community mental health facilities and the development of programs to combat health problems (e.g., maternal health, crippled children, and the mentally retarded).

1965   Heart disease, cancer, and stroke legislation was provided for the establishment of Regional Medical Programs to coordinate existing services for these three health problems.

1965   Appalachian Regional Development Act was passed to provide for construction of health services facilities in economically depressed area.

1965   Social Security Act was amended to provide for Medicare and Medicaid programs.

1966   Division of Environmental Health Services was established in Public Health Service.

1966   Partnership for health legislation consolidated preexisting projects and *formula grants* to states through a new system of grants for comprehensive health planning. The legislation allowed health planning but did not give authority to control program development, spending, or construction of health facilities.

1968   Fogarty International Center for Advanced Study in Health Sciences was founded at NIH for international collaboration, study, and research by world scholars.

1970   Occupational Health and Safety Act was passed to assure safe and healthy working conditions.

1971   Environmental Protection Agency was founded to establish an umbrella agency for all environmental programs.

1971   National Center for Toxicological Research was established at Pine Bluff, Arkansas under the aegis of the Food and Drug Administration of USPHS.

1972·   National programs were established for research, screening, counseling, and treatment of sickle cell anemia and Cooley's anemia.

1972   Social Security Act amended to encourage Professional Standards Review Organizations (PSRO). PSROs were designed to review hospital services ordered by physicians to determine overuse and underuse of services for patient care.

1972   National commission was established to study and investigate causes, cures, and treatment of multiple sclerosis.

1973   Social Security Act was amended to provide for the development of health maintenance organizations (HMOs)—prepaid comprehensive health care delivery systems designed to introduce competition into the health care arena.

1973   Program of grants (contracts for establishing and operating emergency medical services systems) was authorized.

1974   National Health Planning and Resources Development Act was passed to provide a triad health planning system. The system was designed as a comprehensive planning structure to review health services and facilities and to control and limit the expenditure of federal monies by discouraging the development and continuation of unnecessary new and existing programs.

1974   National Diabetes Mellitus Research and Education Act was passed to authorize NIH to establish a National Commission on Diabetes to formulate long-range plans to combat the disease.

1974   Sudden Infant Death Syndrome Act was passed to provide a program of dissemination of research and information to the public.

1976   National Swine Flu Immunization Program was established and implemented.

1976   Toxic Substances Control Act was passed to require testing of certain chemical substances to protect human health and environment.

1977   Rural Health Clinics Services Act was passed to provide for the establishment of health clinics in rural underserved communities. The clinics were to be staffed by nurse practitioners or physician assistants. The bill marked the first national legislation passed for reimbursement of nurse practitioner and physician assistant services under Medicare and Medicaid.

1980   Civil Rights of Institutionalized Persons Act was passed to protect mentally ill, disabled, retarded, chronically ill, or handicapped persons from flagrant conditions in state-affiliated institutions.

1980   Infant Formula Act was passed to require that such formulas meet certain standards of nutrition, quality, and safety in manufacturing.

1980   Department of Health, Education, and Welfare reorganized. Department of Health and Human Services oversees the regulation of health programs.

1981   Omnibus Budget Reconciliation Act (OBRA) provided for maternal and child health block grants to states under Title V of the Social Security Act to assist the states in advancing the health of mothers and children. Legislation allows states to make decisions on how to spend monies for nine maternal-child health programs.

1981 Omnibus Budget Reconciliation Act provided preventive health services block grants to allow states to make decisions about monies spent for 10 preventive health programs like hypertensive screening, rape crisis centers, etc.

1981 Omnibus Budget Reconciliation Act provided alcohol, drug abuse, and mental health block grants for states to provide direct service through community health centers and alcohol and drug abuse programs.

1981 Omnibus Budget Reconciliation Act provided primary care block grants to states for community health center funding.

1982 Defense appropriations amendments allowed for direct, independent nurse practitioner reimbursement under CHAMPUS.

1982 The Tax Equity and Fiscal Responsibility Act established reductions in Medicare and Medicaid spending, called for the development of a prospective reimbursement system, authorized Medicare payments for hospice service, and replaced PSRO with a new utilization and quality control peer review program.

1983 Public Health Emergency Act provided for a permanent revolving fund for use by the Secretary of DHHS in responding to public health emergencies.

1983 Social Security Amendments of 1983 contained provisions providing for the establishment of a prospective payment system under Medicare.

1983 Amendments to the Public Health Act authorized grants, contracts, and loans for the development of home health agencies and training of home health personnel.

1985 Health Research Extension Act establishes a new National Center for Nursing Research.

1986 Supplemental appropriations bill passed to allow hospitals to include capital building costs in payment requests under PPS beginning in 1987.

1987 Omnibus Budget Reconciliation Act provided increased quality control measures for the nursing home industry, and required nurse aid training for nursing home and home health.

1989 Medicare/Medicaid regulations established a PPS for ambulatory surgery; provided Medicaid coverage for children 6 years of age and under and pregnant women with incomes of 133% of poverty level; provided reimbursement of certified pediatric nurse practitioners and family nurse practitioners for Medicaid services; and provided for nurse practitioners and clinical nurse specialists to certify patients needs for nursing home care.

1990 Americans with Disabilities Act prohibits discrimination against disabled individuals in employment, public transportation, accommodations, and services.

1992 The Older Americans Act Amendments were established to revise and extend assistance programs for the elderly. Authorizes grants to States and localities for services to the elderly, including food assistance and nutrition services, in-home services for the frail elderly, disease prevention, and health promotion programs.

1992 The Preventive Health Amendments to the Public Health Service Act to revise and extend the program of block grants for preventive health and health services.

1993 Family and Medical Leave Act grants eligible employees of up to 12 weeks unpaid medical leave for a serious health condition, childbirth, adoption, care of infants or seriously ill children, spouses or parents.

1993 National Institute of Health Revitalization Act amends the Public Health Service Act to revise and extend the programs of the National Institute of Health, including the formation of the National Institute of Nursing Research.

A.4 DECLARATION OF ALMA ATA

The International conference on primary health care, meeting in Alma-Ata this twelfth day of September in the year nineteen hundred and seventy-eight, expressing the need for urgent action of all governments, all health and development workers, and the world community to protect and promote the health of all the people of the world, hereby makes the following Declaration:

I

The Conference strongly reaffirms that health, which is a state of complete physical, mental, and social well-being, and not merely the absence of disease or infirmity, is a fundamental human right and that the attainment of the highest possible level of health is a most important worldwide social goal, whose realization requires the action of many other social and economic sectors in addition to the health sector.

II

The existing gross inequality in the health status of the people, particularly between developed and developing countries and within countries, is politically, socially, and economically unacceptable and is therefore of common concern to all countries.

III

Economic and social development, based on a new international economic order, is of basic importance to the fullest attainment of health for all and to the reduction of the gap between the health status of developing and developed countries. The promotion and protection of the health of the people are essential to sustained economic and social development and contribute to a better quality of life and to world peace.

IV

The people have the right and duty to participate individually and collectively in the planning and implementation of their health care.

V

Governments have a responsibility for the health of their people, which can be fulfilled only by the provision of adequate health and social measures. In the coming decades a main social target of governments, international organizations, and the whole world community should be the attainment by all peoples of the world by the year 2000 of a level of health that will permit them to lead a socially and economically productive life. Primary health care is the key to attaining this target as part of development in the spirit of social justice.

VI

Primary health care is essential health care based on practical, scientifically sound, and socially acceptable methods and technology made universally accessible to individuals and families in the community through their full participation and at a cost that the community and country can afford to maintain at every stage of their development in the spirit of self-reliance and self-determination. It forms an integral part both of the country's health system, of which primary health care is the central function and main focus, and of the overall social and economic development of the community. It is the first level of contact for individuals, the family, and the community with the national health system bringing health care as close as possible to where people live and work, and it constitutes the first element of a continuing health care process.

VII

Primary health care
1. reflects and evolves from the economic conditions and sociocultural and political characteristics of the country and its communities and is based on the application of the relevant results of social, biomedical, and health services research and public health experience;
2. addresses the main health problems in the community, providing promotive, preventive, curative, and rehabilitative services accordingly;
3. includes at least education concerning prevailing health problems and the methods of preventing and controlling them; promotion of food supply and proper nutrition; an adequate supply of safe water and basic sanitation; maternal and child health care, including family planning; immunization against the major infectious diseases; prevention and control of locally endemic diseases; appro-

priate treatment of common diseases and injuries; and provision of essential drugs;
4. involves, in addition to health sector, all related sectors and aspects of national and community development, in particular agriculture, animal husbandry, food industry, education, housing, public works, communication, and other sectors; and demands the coordinated efforts of all those sectors;
5. requires and promotes maximum community and individual self-reliance and participation in the planning, organization, operation, and control of primary health care making fullest use of local, national and other available resources; and to this end, develops through appropriate education the ability of communities to participate;
6. should be sustained by integrated, functional, and mutually supportive referral levels, on health workers, including physicians, nurses, midwives, auxiliaries, and community workers, as applicable, as well as on traditional practitioners as needed, suitably trained socially and technically to work as a health team and to respond to the expressed health needs of the community; and
7. relies, at local and referral levels, on health workers, including physicians, nurses, midwives, auxiliaries, and community workers, as applicable, as well as on traditional practitioners as needed, suitably trained socially and technically to work as a health team and to respond to the expressed health needs of the community.

VIII

All governments should formulate national policies, strategies, and plans of action to launch and sustain primary health care as part of a comprehensive national health system and in coordination with other sectors. To this end, it will be necessary to exercise political will, to mobilize the country's resources, and to use available external resources rationally.

IX

All countries should cooperate in a spirit of partnership and service to ensure primary health care for all people because the attainment of health by people in any one country directly concerns and benefits every other country. In this context the joint WHO-UNICEF report* on primary health care constitutes a solid basis for the further development and operation of Primary Health Care through the world.

X

An acceptable level of health for all the people of the world by the year 2000 can be attained through a fuller and better use of the world's resources, a considerable part of which is now spent on armaments

---

*World Health Organization: *Primary health care: report of the International Conference on Primary Health Care,* Alma-Ata, USSR, Sept 6-12, 1978, Geneva, 1978, WHO.

and military conflicts. A genuine policy of independence, peace, détente, and disarmament could and should release additional resources that could well be devoted to peaceful aims and in particular to the acceleration of social and economic development of which primary health care, as an essential part, should be allotted its proper share.

A.5 NURSING'S AGENDA FOR HEALTH CARE REFORM

Executive Summary

America's nurses have long supported our nation's efforts to create a health care system that assures access, quality, and services at affordable costs. This document presents nursing's agenda for immediate health care reform. We call for a basic "core" of essential health care services to be available to everyone. We call for a restructured health care system that will focus on the consumers and their health, with services to be delivered in familiar, convenient sites, such as schools, workplaces, and homes. We call for a shift from the predominant focus on illness and cure to an orientation toward wellness and care. The basic components of nursing's "core of care" include:

- A restructured health care system that:
  - enhances consumer access to services by delivering primary health care in community-based settings;
  - fosters consumer responsibility for personal health, self-care, and informed decision making in selecting health care services; and
  - facilitates utilization of the most cost-effective providers and therapeutic options in the most appropriate settings.
- A federally-defined standard package of essential health care services available to all citizens and residents of the United States, provided and financed through an integration of public and private plans and sources:
  - A public plan, based on federal guidelines and eligibility requirements, will provide coverage for the poor and create the opportunity for small businesses and individuals, particularly those at risk because of preexisting conditions and those potentially medically indigent, to buy into the plan.
  - A private plan will offer, at a minimum, the nationally standardized package of essential services. This standard package could be enriched as a benefit of employment or individuals could purchase additional services if they so choose. If employers do not offer private coverage, they must pay into the public plan for their employees.
- A phase-in of essential services, in order to be fiscally responsible:
  - Coverage of pregnant women and children is critical. This first step represents a cost-effective investment in the future health and prosperity of the nation.
  - One early step will be to design services specifically to assist vulnerable populations who have had limited access to our nation's health care system. A "Healthstart Plan" is proposed to improve the health status of these individuals.
- Planned change to anticipate health service needs that correlate with changing national demographics.
- Steps to reduce health care costs include:
  - required usage of managed care in the public plan and encouraged in private plans;
  - incentives for consumers and providers to utilize managed care arrangements;
  - controlled growth of the health care system through planning and prudent resource allocation;
  - incentives for consumers and providers to be more cost efficient in exercising health care options;
  - development of health care policies based on effectiveness and outcomes research;
  - assurance of direct access to full range of qualified providers; and
  - elimination of unnecessary bureaucratic controls and administrative procedures.
- Case management will be required for those with continuing health care needs. Case management will reduce the fragmentation of the present system, promote consumers' active participation in decisions about their health, and create an advocate on their behalf.
- Provisions for long-term care, which include:
  - public and private funding for services of short duration to prevent personal impoverishment;
  - public funding for extended care if consumer resources are exhausted; and
  - emphasis on the consumers' responsibility to financially plan for their long-term care needs, including new personal financial alternatives and strengthened private insurance arrangements.
- Insurance reforms to assure improved access to coverage, including affordable premiums, reinsurance pools for catastrophic coverage, and other steps to protect both insurers and individuals against excessive costs.
- Access to services assured by no payment at the point of service and elimination of balance billing in both public and private plans.
- Establishment of public/private sector review—operating under federal guidelines and including payers, providers, and consumers—to determine resource allocation, cost-reduction approaches, allowable insurance premiums, and fair and consistent reimbursement levels for providers. This review would progress in a climate sensitive to ethical issues.

Additional resources will be required to accomplish this plan. Although significant dollars can be obtained through restructuring and other strategies, responsibility for any new funds must be shared by individuals, employers, and government, phased in over several years to minimize the impact.

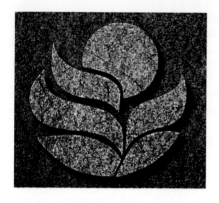

Appendix B
Community Resources

B.1 PARTIAL LIST OF HEALTH-RELATED ORGANIZATIONS

Agency for Toxic Substances and Disease Registry (ATSDR)

1600 Clifton Road, NE, Mail Stop E-28, Atlanta, GA 30333 (404) 639-0501

Created by Superfund legislation in 1980 as a part of the U.S. Department of Health and Human Services, ATSDR's mission is to prevent or interrupt adverse human health effects and diminished quality of life that results from exposure to hazardous substances in the environment. Agency activities include public health assessments, health investigations, exposure and disease registry, emergency response, toxicological profiles, health education, and applied research.

AL-ANON Family Group Headquarters, Inc.

1372 Broadway, New York, NY 10018

Founded in 1951, Al-Anon, including Alateen for teenagers, offers a self-help recovery program for relatives and friends who have been adversely affected by someone else's drinking problem. Members share experiences, strength, and hope in an effort to make their own lives manageable. Membership: 15,600 groups worldwide.

Alcoholics Anonymous World Services

PO Box 459, Grand Central Station, New York, NY 10163

Founded in 1935, AA is a program of recovery from alcoholism.

Alcohol and Drug Problems Association of North America, Inc.

444 North Capitol Street, NW, Suite 181, Washington, DC 20001

Founded in 1949, the association serves as a focal point for action and a medium of exchange for professionals in the alcohol and drug problems field at the national, state, and local governmental levels and in the private sector.

Alexander Graham Bell Association for the Deaf

3417 Volta Place, NW, Washington, DC 20007-2778

Alzheimer's Disease and Related Disorders Association

919 N. Michigan Avenue, Suite 1000, Chicago, IL 60611

American Association of Homes for the Aging

901 East Street, NW, Suite 500, Washington, DC 20004-2037

American Association of Retired Persons (AARP)

601 East Street NW, Washington, DC, 20049

American Burn Association

c/o Shriners Burns Institute, 202 Goodman Street, Cincinnati, OH 45219

Founded in 1967.

American Cancer Society's Cancer Response System

1599 Clifton Road, NE, Atlanta, GA 30329

American Dental Association

211 East Chicago Avenue, Chicago, IL 60611

Founded in 1859, the ADA is the national voluntary organization for the U.S. dental profession and is the second largest health profession in the country.

American Dental Hygienists' Association

1-800-847-6718

American Diabetes Association National Service Center

PO Box 25757, 1660 Duke Street, Alexandria, VA 22313

Founded in 1940, ADA funds research and conducts education programs in the field of diabetes. Publishes patient magazine and two medical journals.

American Epilepsy Society

c/o Priscilla S. Bourgeois, 179 Allyn Street, #304, Hartford, CT 06103

Founded in 1946, AES works to foster research and treatment of epilepsy in all of its phases—biological, clinical, and social—and the promotion of better care and treatment of persons subject to seizures.

American Fertility Society

2140 11th Avenue, S, Suite 200, Birmingham, AL 35205

Founded in 1944, the primary objective of the Society is to disseminate that body of knowledge that encompasses all aspects of infertility, related endocrinology, conception control, and reproductive biology. The greater emphasis is on those matters that are clinical in nature.

American Foundation for the Blind

15 West 16th Street, New York, NY 10011

Founded in 1921, the objective of the foundation is to stimulate, facilitate, and coordinate a national effort for improving services to blind and psychological, technological/social research, gathering, preparation, and publishing information to professional and general public, sponsoring workshops, seminars, and conferences.

American Foundation for Maternal and Child Health (AFMC)

439 East 51st Street, New York, NY 10022

Founded in 1972, AFMC serves as a clearinghouse for interdisciplinary research on maternal and child health and focuses on the perinatal or birth period and its effect on infant development. It sponsors medical research designed to improve application of technology in maternal and child health, conducts educational programs, compiles statistics, and operates extensive reference library.

American Geriatrics Society

770 Lexington Avenue, Suite 400, New York, NY 10021

Founded in 1942, AGS provides dissemination of information relating to the etiology, prevention, diagnosis, and treatment of diseases of the aging and aged, rehabilitation of patients and problems relating to the health care of the older patient.

American Health Care Association (AHCA)

1200 15th Street, NW, Washington, DC 20005

Founded in 1949. Members: 9000. The AHCA is a federation of state associations of long-term health care facilities. It promotes standards for professionals in long-term health care delivery and quality care for patients and residents in a safe environment; focuses on issues of availability, quality, affordability, and fair payment; conducts seminars and conferences that provide continuing education for nursing home personnel; maintains liaison with governmental agencies, Congress, and professional associations; presents awards; and compiles statistics. Publications: (1) Notes, biweekly; (2) Provider, monthly; also publishes Health Career Opportunities; Thinking About a Nursing Home; Welcome to Our Nursing Home; and training manuals and audiovisual aids.

American Health Foundation

320 East 43rd Street, New York, NY 10018

Founded in 1969, AHF is a unique, nonprofit insitution, totally committed to disease prevention and health promotion. Today, on national and community levels, AHF is achieving its goals through laboratory and clinical research, preventive health care services and public education.

American Heart Association

7272 Greenville Avenue, Dallas, TX 75231-4596

Founded in 1948, the AHA mission is to reduce death and disability from cardiovascular diseases.

American Hepatitis Association (AHA)

30 East 40th Street, Room 305, New York, NY 10016

Founded in 1983, AHA members are persons having hepatitis in any form, persons who have a high risk of contracting hepatitis, and interested individuals. The AHA conducts educational and prevention programs concerning hepatitis; provides low-cost blood screening and vaccines; offers support groups for individuals with hepatitis; sponsors talks for high risk groups, including health care workers, medical personnel, homosexual men, IV drug abusers, and those who work with infants with hepatitis; facilitates research on the treatment and prevention of hepatitis; sponsors Hepatitis Awareness Week; offers blood screenings and vaccinations; maintains speakers' bureau; and operates children's services. Publications: AHA Newsletter, periodic; also publishes dietary guidelines, pamphlets, and brochures.

American Liver Foundation

998 Pomptom Avenue, Cedar Grove, NJ 07009

Founded in 1976, the ALF seeks to improve the understanding, prevention, and cure of liver diseases through professional and public education and by supporting vitally needed research training of young scientific investigators.

American Lung Association

1740 Broadway, New York, NY 10019

Founded in 1904. ALA is primarily an educational organization to fight lung disease and work for lung health. It also works against cigarette smoking and air pollution.

American Lupus Society Information

260 Maple Court, Suite 123, Ventura, CA 93003

American Mental Health Foundation

2 East 86th Street, New York, NY 10028

Founded in 1924, the AMHF is dedicated to extensive and intensive research in the theories of psychotherapy and to the implementation of needed reforms.

American Parkinson Disease Association

116 John Street, Suite 417, New York, NY 10038

American Physical Fitness Research Institute

654 N Sepulveda Boulevard, Los Angeles, CA 90049

Founded in 1958, APFRI provides research and development of motivational and educational information on all aspects of health, fitness, and well-being directed toward personal responsibility for one's health.

American Red Cross

17th and D Streets, NW, Washington, DC 20006

Founded in 1881, the aims of the Red Cross are to improve the quality of human life and enhance individual self-reliance and concern for others. It works toward these aims through national and chapter services governed and directed by volunteers.

American School Health Association

PO Box 708, Kent, OH 44240

Founded in 1927. The ASHA's members include school physicians, dentists, nurses, nutritionists, health educators, dental hygienists, and public health workers. Its purposes are to promote comprehensive and constructive school health programs including the teaching of health, health services, and promotion of a healthful school environment. It offers a professional referral service, classroom teaching aids, and professional reference materials. It also conducts research programs, maintains a placement service and compiles statistics.

American Society on Aging

833 Market Street, Suite 4511, San Francisco, CA 94103

Arthritis Foundation

1314 Spring Street, NW, Atlanta, GA 30309

Founded in 1948.

Arthritis Society

920 Yonge Street, Suite 420, Toronto, Ontario, M4W 3J7, Canada

Founded in 1948, the AS is organized for the development of rheumatological manpower through associateships and fellowships, the support of research projects deemed relevant to the rheumatic disease, and the communication about arthritis with general public and medical profession.

Association for the Care of Children's Health

3615 Wisconsin Avenue, NW, Washington, DC 20016.

Founded in 1965, ACCH seeks to foster and promote the health and well-being of children and families in health care settings by education, interdisciplinary interaction and planning, and research.

Association for Children and Adults with Learning Disabilities

4156 Library Road, Pittsburgh, PA 15234

Founded in 1963.

Association for Children with Retarded Mental Development

162 Fifth Avenue, 11th Fl, New York, NY 10010

Founded in 1951, ACRMD is a nonprofit membership corporation offering services to mentally retarded adults throughout New York City. Services include rehabilitation and sheltered workshops, day training and activities centers, day treatment centers, job placement, evening and weekend social centers, and various community services.

Association for Education and Rehabilitation of the Blind and Visually Impaired

206 N. Washington Street, Suite 320, Alexandria, VA 22314

Founded in 1984, the association works to expand the opportunities for the visually handicapped in society.

Association of Occupational and Environmental Clinics (AOEC)

1010 Vermont Avenue, Suite 513, Washington, DC 20005

The AOEC is a network of clinics affiliated with medical schools throughout the United States. Member clinics provide professional training, community education about toxic substances, exposure and risk assessment, clinical evaluations, and consultation. A lending library of training materials is maintained for use by members. Membership is open to any person who shares the goals of the Association. Clinicians can contact the AOEC office for referrals.

Association for Retarded Citizens

500 East Border Street, Suite 300, Arlington, TX 76010

Founded in 1950.

Association for Vital Records and Health Statistics

c/o George van Amburg, Michigan Department of Public Health, 3423 Logan Street, North, PO Box 30195, Lansing, MI 48909

Founded in 1933, the AVRHS provides the only national forum for the study, discussion, and solution of the problems related to programs of vital and health statistics by state and local representatives without undue influence of Federal government officials.

Asthma and Allergy Foundation of America

1717 Massachusetts Avenue, Suite 305, Washington, DC 20036

Founded in 1953, the AAFA provides public education booklets and newletters, answers inquiries on asthma and allergy, arranges for professional speakers and audio-visual materials, and encourages community activities through its local chapters.

Autism Society for America

1234 Massachusetts Avenue, NW, Suite C-1017, Washington, DC 20005

Founded in 1965, the ASA is a nonprofit organization of parents, professionals and other concerned citizens working for better education, research, treatment, and legislation on behalf of autistic persons.

Braille Institute

741 North Vermont Avenue, Los Angeles, CA 90029

Founded in 1919. The institute provides training, education, and special services for the blind of all ages.

Centers for Disease Control and Prevention (CDC)

1600 Clifton Road, NE, Atlanta, GA 30333

The CDC is charged to protect the public's health by providing leadership and direction in the prevention and control of diseases and other preventable conditions and responding to public health emergencies.

Child Abuse Listening Mediation

PO Box 718, Santa Barbara, CA 93102

Founded in 1971, CALM is organized for the prevention of child abuse and neglect, and provides a hotline listener, child care to reduce stress, a speakers bureau, and parent support groups.

Children's Foundation

815 15th Street, NW, Suite 928, Washington, DC 20005

The foundation was established in 1969 as a national, nonprofit advocacy organization focusing upon the quality and availability of the federal food assistance programs for children and their families.

Consumer Product Safety Commission

East West Towers 4340 East West Highway, Bethesda MD 20814

This agency provides information on health and safety effects related to consumer products and has direct jurisdiction over chronic and chemical hazards in consumer products, assists consumers to evaluate product safety, develops uniform safety standards, and promotes research and legislation regarding the causes and prevention of product-related deaths, illnesses, and injuries.

Environmental Protection Agency (EPA)

401 M Street, SW, Washington, DC, 20460

The EPA was established in 1970 to abate and control pollution systematically through research, monitoring, standard setting, and enforcement. This agency is designed to serve as the public's advocate for producing a livable environment.

Gray Panthers

2025 Pennsylvania Avenue, NW Suite 831 Washington, DC 20006

Founded in 1970, the Gray Panthers are people of all ages, working for social change. It tries to develop creative alternatives to the injustices in society that confront people at every phase of life.

Health Care Financing Administration

6325 Security Boulevard, Baltimore, MD 21207

Healthy America

315 West 105th Street, #1F, New York, NY 10025

Founded in 1977, the coalition is a national, nonprofit organization emphasizing health advocacy, disease prevention and promotion of good health habits as means to attain lasting good health. It encourages health promotion policies and programs at all levels of government and within private sectors, sponsors seminars, conferences, etc, and serves as congressional liaison for membership.

Hospice Education Institute

190 Westbrook Road Essex, CT 06426

Huntington's Disease Society of America

140 West 22nd Street, 6th Floor, New York, NY 10011-2420

Founded in 1986, this agency is comprised of individuals and groups of volunteers concerned with Huntington's disease, an inherited and terminal neurological disease causing progressive brain and nerve deterioration. Goals are to identify HR families; educate the public and professionals, with emphasis on increasing consumer awareness of HR; promote and support basic and clinical research into the causes and cure of HR; maintain patient services program, coordinated with various community services, to assist families in meeting the social, economic, and emotional problems resulting from HR.

International Association of Cancer Victims and Friends

7740 W. Manchester Avenue, Suite 110, Playa del Rey, CA 90293

Founded in 1963, IACVF is a nonprofit (tax exempt) corporation organized under the laws of state of California. Its purpose is the dissemination of educational materials concerning the prevention and control of cancer through the use of nontoxic therapies. Chapters have symposiums and seminars in their respective areas throughout the year.

International Childbirth Education Association

PO Box 20048, Minneapolis, MN 55420

Founded in 1960, the ICEA promotes family-centered maternity care and helps groups and individuals promote same through classes in prepared childbirth, teacher training, publications, conferences, and conventions.

Job Accommodation Network

West Virginia University, PO Box 6080 Morgantown, WV 26506-6080

Juvenile Diabetes Foundation International

432 Park Avenue, South, New York, NY 10016

Founded in 1970, JDFI is a nonprofit voluntary agency whose prime objective is to support and fund research aimed at preventing the complications of and curing the disease itself. JDF chapters provide educational and counseling services in addition to fund raising.

La Leche League International

9616 Minneapolis Avenue, PO Box 1209, Franklin Park, IL 60131

Founded in 1956, the league is a nonprofit organization that provides help for breastfeeding mothers in a series of four meetings, annual seminar for physicians, biennial international conferences for parents and professionals, and a 24-hour telephone hotline.

Leukemia Society of America

733 Third Avenue, New York, NY 10017

Founded in 1949, the LSA promotes and provides support into the causes, treatment, and cure or control of the leukemias and related lymphomas. Allied programs are patient service, public and professional education, and community services.

Living Bank

PO Box 6725, Houston, TX 77625

Founded in 1968, the LB is an organ and body donor registry, educating the public about the importance of organ and body donations, registration, and referral of donations, at the time of death, to the appropriate medical facility closest to the point of death.

Lupus Foundation of America

1717 Massachusetts Ave, NW, Suite 203, Washington, DC 20036

Founded in 1977, the corporation is organized exclusively for charitable, educational, and scientific purposes to encourage development of research programs designed to discover the causes of, and to improve the methods of treating, diagnosing, curing and preventing lupus erythematosus.

March of Dimes Birth Defects Foundation

1275 Mamaroneck Avenue, White Plains, NY 10605

Founded in 1938. The goal of the foundation is the prevention of birth defects, our most serious child health problem, through support of research, medical services, and education.

Mended Hearts

c/o American Heart Association, 7320 Greenville Ave, Dallas, TX 75231

Founded in 1951.

MotherRisk Program

Hospital for Sick Children

555 University Avenue, Toronto, Ontario M5G1X8

The MotherRisk Program counsels callers about the safety of an exposure to drugs, chemicals, or radiation during pregnancy or breastfeeding. The team of physicians and information specialists gives advice on whether medications, x-rays, or chemicals in the work environment will harm the developing fetus or breast-fed baby. Genetic counseling is available from the Genetic Department of the Hospital for Sick Children.

Multiple Sclerosis Association of America

601 White Horse Pike, Oaklyn, NJ 08107

Muscular Dystrophy Association

810 Seventh Avenue, New York, NY 10019

The MDA is a voluntary national health agency—a dedicated partnership between scientists and concerned citizens aimed at conquering neuromuscular diseases that affect thousands of Americans.

Myasthenia Gravis Foundation

53 W Jackson Blvd, Suite 909, Chicago, IL 60604

Founded in 1952, the foundation fosters, coordinates, and supports research into the cause, prevention, alleviation, and cure of myasthenia gravis; gives research grants to MG clinics, hospitals, medical schools throughout the United States; and awards at least 10 medical student fellowships each year and a $20,000 postdoctoral fellowship.

National Association for Down's Syndrome

PO Box 4542, Oak Park, IL 60522

Founded in 1960, NADS is a not-for-profit organization comprised of parents and professionals involved with the individual with Down's Syndrome.

National Association of the Physically Handicapped

76 Elm Street, London, OH 43140

Founded in 1958, the NAPH advances the social, economic, and physical welfare of the physically handicapped. It is not a resource center for information. It neither provides services, nor gives financial aid. It supports legislation to benefit the handicapped, trying to make public aware of needs of handicapped.

National Association of School Nurses

PO Box 1300, Scarborough, ME 04074

Founded in 1969, Members include school nurses who conduct comprehensive school health programs in public and private schools. Objectives are to provide national leadership in the promotion of health services for school children, to promote school health interests to the nursing and health community and the public, and to monitor legislation pertaining to school nursing. It provides continuing education programs at the national level and assistance to states for program implementation and offers certification for school nurses.

National Association for Visually Handicapped

22 West 21st Street, New York, NY 10010

Founded in 1954, the NAVH offers guidance and counsel for all partially-seeing people and professionals and paraprofessionals working with them, as well as informational literature. It publishes and distributes large print books, textbooks, and testing material and serves as referral agency for all services for partially seeing. It is the only national health agency serving only the partially-seeing (not the totally blind).

National Cancer Institute

NIOH, 900 Rockville Pike, Bethesda, MD 20892

National Center for Health Promotion and Aging

c/o National Council on Aging

409 Third Street, SW, 2nd Floor, Washington, DC 20024

National Center for Learning Disabilities

99 Park Avenue, 6th Floor, New York, NY 10016

National Center for Nutrition and Dietetics Consumer Hotline

1-800-366-1655

National Committee for the Prevention of Alcoholism and Drug Dependency

RR 1, Box 635, Appomattox, VA 24522

Founded in 1950, the committee periodically holds institutes and seminar-workshops throughout the United States. It gathers and distributes information and materials concerning the effects of alcohol and other drugs on the physical, mental, and moral powers of the individual citizen and promotes an educational program for prevention with visual and teaching aids throughout the country. It is willing to cooperate with other organizations in holding seminar-workshops in their area.

National Council on Alcoholism
12 West 21st Street, New York, NY 10010
Founded in 1944, the council is the only national voluntary agency founded to combat the disease of alcoholism.

National Council of Senior Citizens
1331 F Street NW, Washington, DC 20004

National Council on Stuttering
PO Box 8171, Grand Rapids, MI 49518
Founded in 1965, this agency promotes and encourages programs and studies on the problems of stuttering.

National Genetics Foundation
PO Box 1374, New York, NY 10101
Founded in 1903.

National Health Council
622 Third Avenue, 34th Floor, New York, NY 10017
Founded in 1920, NHC is a membership organization of national voluntary, professional, and related organizations interested in improving the health of all Americans in the areas of planning, coordination, and delivery of health services.

National Hemophilia Foundation
110 Green Street, Rm 406, New York, NY 10012
Founded in 1948, the foundation provides information for those interested in the field, and promotes research.

National Information Center for Children and Youth with Disabilities
PO Box 1492, Washington, DC 20013-1492

National Institute of Neuro Disorders and Stroke
Bldg. 31, Room 8AOy, 31 Center Drive, MSC 2540
Bethesda, MD 20892-2540

National Institute for Occupational Safety and Health (NIOSH)
Robert A. Taft Laboratories, 4676 Columbia Parkway, Cincinnati, OH 45226-1998
NIOSH was established by the Occupational Safety and Health Act of 1970 to conduct research on occupational diseases and injuries, respond to requests for assistance by investigating health and safety problems in the workplace, recommend standards to the Occupational Safety and Health Administration (OSHA) and the Mine Safety and Health Administration (MSHA), and train professionals in occupational safety and health.

National Kidney Foundation
2 Park Avenue, New York, NY 10003
Founded in 1958, NKF is a national voluntary health organization supporting research and public information on the diagnosis and treatment of diseases of the kidney.

National Lupus Erythematosus Foundation
5430 Van Nuys Boulevard, Suite 206, Van Nuys, CA 91401
Founded in 1950, NLEF is a nonprofit organization for the distribution of Lupus literature. It compiles information gathered from Lupus patients, funds Lupus research, and establishes Lupus City of Hope Chapters throughout the country.

National Mental Health Association
1021 Prince Street, Alexandria, VA 22314
Founded in 1909, the MHA is a lay, volunteer organization that provides social action and public education in the area of mental health.

National Nurses' Society on Addictions (NNSA)
4101 Lake Boone Trail, Suite 201, Raleigh, NC 27607-6518

National Organization on Disability
910 16th Street, NW, Room 600, Washington, DC 20006

National Organization for Rare Disorders
PO Box 8923 New Fairfield, CT 06812-8923

National Parent Network on Disabilities
1600 Prince Street, #115, Alexandria, VA 22314

National Sudden Infant Death Syndrome Foundation
8200 Professional Plaza, Suite 104, Landover, MD 20785
Founded in 1962, NSIDSF provides support for SIDS research, services to families of victims of SIDS and SIDS-related disorders, and educational programs for health and emergency personnel. It also fulfills a consumer advocacy role for SIDS families.

National Support Center for Families of Aging
PO Box 245, Swarthmore, PA 19081

National Tay-Sachs and Allied Diseases Association
385 Elliot Street, Newton, MA 02164
Founded in 1957, the association conducts programs in support of research, family counseling, and public and professional education into the genetic disease Tay-Sachs and many other diseases caused by inborn errors of metabolism.

Planned Parenthood Federation of America
810 Seventh Avenue, New York, NY 10019
PPF works to make effective means of birth control available for all.

Society for the Advancement of Travel for the Handicapped
327 5th Avenue, Suite 610, New York, NY 10016

Synanon Foundation, Inc.
6055 Marshall Petalvma Road, Marshall, CA 84840
Founded in 1958, Synanon was the first community designed for the reeducation of drug addicts and other character disorders, and it continues to do that work. Since 1974 Synanon has been providing reeducation for children as young as 10. Facilities in Marshall, San Francisco, Los Angeles,

and Badger, CA; Kerhonkson and New York, NY; Chicago, IL; and Detroit, MI.

Toys "R" Us
(with National Parent Network on Disabilities)
(Toy) Guide for Differently-Abled Kids (free)
PO Box 8501 Nevada, IA 50201-9968

United Cerebral Palsy Association
66 East 34th Street, New York, NY 10016
Founded in 1948, UCP is the only nationwide voluntary organization targeting its services on the specific and multiple needs of persons with cerebral palsy and their families. UCP's more than 240 affiliates provide a variety of community services, support research and conduct programs of public education pertaining to cerebral palsy.

Winners on Wheels
2842 Business Park Avenue, Fresno, CA 93727
Nonprofit organization, modeled on Boy and Girl Scouts, for social and educational needs of children in wheelchairs.

W.K. Kellogg Foundation
400 North Avenue, Battle Creek, MI 49017
Founded in 1930, the foundation is committed to the application of existing knowledge to problems of people in the areas of health, education, and agriculture. It currently assists programs of four continents, including the United States and Canada, Latin America, Europe, and Australia. A grant-making organization, the foundation does not operate programs.

B.2   AAPCC—CERTIFIED REGIONAL POISON CONTROL CENTERS*

Poison Control Centers were established in 1953 to help physicians deal with poisonings of adults and children in the United States. In 1983 the American Association of Poison Control Centers (AAPCC) was established as the professional organization for Poison Control Centers. The Regional Poison Control Centers can act as valuable resources in providing information about the toxicity and health effects of hazardous exposures involved in poisonings.

ALABAMA
Birmingham

Children's Hospital of Alabama Poison Control Center
(205) 939-9201
(800) 292-6678 (in state)
(205) 933-4050

---

*From *Case studies in environmental medicine: taking an exposure history,* Atlanta, Ga, 1994, USDHHS, PHS, ATSDR, in conjunction with CDC, NIOSH.

ARIZONA
Phoenix

Samaritan Regional Poison Center
(602) 253-3334

Tucson

Arizona Poison and Drug Information Center
(800) 362-0101 (in state)
(602) 626-6016

CALIFORNIA
Fresno

Fresno Regional Poison Control Center
(800) 346-5922 (central CA only)
(209) 445-1222

Los Angeles

Los Angeles Regional Drug and Poison Control Center
(800) 825-2722 (physicians)
(800) 777-6476
(213) 222-8086
(213) 222-3212
(714) 634-5988

Sacramento

University of California, Davis Medical Center Regional Poison Control Center
(800) 342-9293 (Northern CA only)
(916) 734-3692 (in state)

San Diego

San Diego Regional Poison Control Center
(619) 543-6000
(800) 876-4766 (619 area only)

San Francisco

SF Bay Area Regional Poison Control Center
(800) 523-2222 (415 and 707 area codes only)

San Jose

Santa Clara Valley Medical Center Regional Poison Center
(408) 299-5112
(800) 662-9886 (CA only)

COLORADO
Denver

Rocky Mountain Poison and Drug Center
(303) 629-1123
(800) 332-3073 (in state)

DISTRICT OF COLUMBIA
Washington

National Capitol Poison Control Center
(202) 625-3333
(202) 362-8563 (TTY)

FLORIDA
Tampa

Florida Poison Information Center and Toxicology
Resource Center
(800) 282-3171 (in state)
(813) 253-4444

GEORGIA
Atlanta

Georgia Regional Poison Control Center
(800) 282-5846 (in state)
(404) 616-9000
(404) 616-9287 (TTY)

INDIANA
Indianapolis

Indiana Poison Center
(800) 382-9097 (in state)
(317) 929-2323

KENTUCKY
Louisville

Kentucky Regional Poison Center of Kosair Children's Hospital
(800) 722-5725 (in state)
(502) 589-8222

MARYLAND
Baltimore

Maryland Poison Center
(800) 492-2414 (in state)
(410) 528-7701

MASSACHUSETTS
Boston

Massachusetts Poison Control System
(800) 682-9211 (in state)
(617) 232-2120

MICHIGAN
Detroit

Poison Control Center
(313) 745-5711

Grand Rapids

Blodgett Regional Poison Center
(800) 632-2727 (in state)

MINNESOTA
Minneapolis

Hennepin Regional Poison Center
(612) 347-3141

St. Paul

Minnesota Regional Poison Center
(800) 222-1222 (in state)
(612) 221-2113

MISSOURI
St. Louis

Cardinal Glennon Children's Hospital
(800) 366-8888
(800) 392-9111
(314) 772-5200
(314) 577-5336 (TTY)

MONTANA
Denver (Colorado)

Rocky Mountain Poison and Drug Center
(303) 629-1123

NEBRASKA
Omaha

Omaha Poison Center
(402) 390-5555 (Omaha only)
(800) 955-9119 (NE & WY)

NEW JERSEY
Newark

New Jersey Poison Information and Education
System
(800) 962-1253
(201) 923-0764

NEW MEXICO
Albuquerque

New Mexico Poison and Drug Information Center
(800) 432-6866 (NM only)
(505) 843-2551

NEW YORK
Mineola

Long Island Regional Poison Control Center
(516) 542-2323, 2324, 2325, 3813

New York

New York City Poison Center
(212) 340-4494
(212) 764-7667
(212) 689-9014 (TDD)

Nyack

Hudson Valley Poison Center
(800) 336-6997
(914) 353-1000

OHIO
Cincinnati

Regional Poison Control System and Cincinnati Drug and Poison Information Center
(513) 558-5111
(800) 872-5111 (in state)

Columbus

Central Ohio Poison Center
(800) 682-7625
(614) 228-1323
(614) 461-2012
(614) 228-2272 (TTY)

OREGON
Portland

Oregon Poison Centr
(503) 494-8968
(800) 452-7165 (in state)

PENNSYLVANIA
Hershey

Central Pennsylvania Poison Center
(800) 521-6110

Philadelphia

The Poison Control Center serving the greater Philadelphia metropolitan area
(215) 386-2100

Pittsburgh

Pittsburgh Poison Center
(412) 681-6669

RHODE ISLAND
Providence

Rhode Island Poison Center
(401) 277-5727
(401) 277-8062 (TDD)

TEXAS
Dallas

North Texas Poison Center
(800) 441-0040 (in state)
(214) 590-5000

Galveston

Texas State Poison Center
(800) 392-8548 (in state)
(409) 765-1420 (Galveston)
(713) 654-1701 (Houston)

UTAH
Salt Lake City

Utah Poison Control Center
(801) 581-2151
(800) 456-7707 (in state)

VIRGINIA
Charlottesville

Blue Ridge Poison Center
(804) 924-5543
(800) 451-1428

Richmond

Virginia Poison Center
(800) 552-6337 (in state)

WEST VIRGINIA
Charleston

West Virginia Poison Center
(800) 642-3625 (in state)
(304) 348-4211

WYOMING
Omaha (Nebraska)

The Poison Center
(401) 390-5555 (Omaha)
(800) 955-9119 (NE & WY)

B.3 COMPUTERIZED INFORMATION SYSTEMS FOR ENVIRONMENTAL AND OCCUPATIONAL HEALTH*†

The development of electronic data bases has revolutionized the retrieval of up-to-date, accurate, and com-

---

*From *Case studies in environmental medicine: taking an exposure history,* Atlanta, Ga, 1994, USDHHS, PHS, ATSDR, in conjunction with CDC, NIOSH.
†The use of trade names is for identification only and does not imply endorsement by the Public Health Service or the U.S. Department of Health and Human Services.

prehensive information on hazardous exposures. Data bases are commonly accessed through (1) on-line retrieval of information, (2) floppy disk, or (3) CD-ROM (Compact Disk—Read Only Memory). The advantage of on-line systems is that they provide the greatest versatility and are the most comprehensive in obtaining different kinds of information because several databases can be cross-searched. CD-ROMs may be easier to search and may be cost effective depending on use.

Toxicology Data Network

The Toxicology Data Network (TOXNET), developed by the National Library of Medicine (NLM), is a computerized system of files oriented to toxicology and related areas. Three options are available for searching NLM files. The user may purchase a software package, GRATEFUL MED, to formulate searches off line and then dial into the files. Users also may be direct or menu searching when connected directly to TOXNET files. The following files are currently included in TOXNET.

Hazardous Substance Data Bank

Hazardous Substance Data Bank (HSDB) is a toxicology data base developed by NLM and ATSDR. It is a factual, peer-reviewed data base of more than 4200 chemicals. Records are in 12 different information categories: substance identification, manufacturing/use, chemical/physical properties, safety and handling, toxicity, biomedical effects, pharmacology, environmental fate/exposure summary, exposure standards and regulations, monitoring and analysis methods, additional references, and express data. HSDB includes annotated medical treatment information derived from the Poisindex data base. This data base is partially funded by ATSDR.

Registry of Toxic Effects of Chemical Substances

The Registry of Toxic Effects of Chemical Substances (RTECS) data base provides information on more than 100,000 potentially toxic chemicals and includes toxicity data, chemical identifiers, NTP test status, and exposure standards. RTECS is built and maintained by NIOSH.

Chemical Carcinogenesis Research Information System

The Chemical Carcinogenesis Research Information System (CCRIS) resource provides scientifically evaluated data from carcinogenicity, mutagenicity, and tumor-promotion and tumor-inhibition tests on 2100 substances that have been evaluated according to criteria and protocols widely accepted by experts in carcinogenesis.

Toxic Release Inventory

Toxic Release Inventory (TRI) was created by NLM and the Environmental Protection Agency (EPA). It is a record of estimated releases to the environment, reported by industries, of more than 300 toxic chemicals based on information collected by EPA.

Toxic Chemical Release Inventory Facts

Toxic Chemical Release Inventory Facts (TRIFACTS) supplements the environmental release data on chemicals in the TRI with information related to the health and ecological effects and safety and handling of these chemicals. The data may be especially useful to workers, employers, community residents, and health professionals.

The Integrated Risk Information System

The Integrated Risk Information System (IRIS) is an EPA data base that contains chemical-specific information on more than 370 chemicals. It contains information on reference doses, carcinogenicity, drinking water health advisories, risk management, and supplementary data.

Environmental Teratology Information Center Backfile

The Environmental Teratology Information Center Backfile (ETICBACK) is a bibliographic data base containing more than 49,000 citations to publications concerning teratology and developmental toxicology. It contains publications dating from pre-1950 through 1988. This data base was produced by Oak Ridge National Laboratory in Oak Ridge, Tennessee. ETICBACK is continued in the Developmental and Reproductive Toxicology Database (DART) data base.

Developmental and Reproductive Toxicology Data Base

The Developmental and Reproductive Toxicology Data Base (DART) is a bibliographic data base containing citations to literature published on birth defects and other aspects of reproductive and developmental toxicology since 1989. The file currently contains more than 1500 records. Plans call for the addition of approximately 3600 records each year. DART is a continuation of the ETICBACK file. DART is funded by the National Institute of Environmental Health Sciences (NIEHS) and EPA.

Environmental Mutagen Information Center

The Environmental Mutagen Information Center (EMIC) is a bibliographic data base on chemical, biologic, and physical agents that have been tested for genotoxic activity. It contains citations from literature after 1988. The data base is produced by the Oak Ridge National Laboratory in Oak Ridge, Tennessee, and is funded by the federal government.

Environmental Mutagen Information Center Backfile

The Environmental Mutagen Information Center Backfile (EMICBACK) is the backfile for the Environmental Mutagen Information Center (EMIC) data base. EMICBACK is a bibliographic data base on chemical, biologic, and physical agents that have been tested for genotoxic activity. It contains approximately 71,000 citations from literature published from 1950 through 1988. The data base is produced by the Oak Ridge National Laboratory in Oak Ridge, Tennessee, and is funded by the federal government.

Directory of Biotechnology Information Resources

The Directory of Biotechnology Information Resources (DBIR) is a multicomponent data bank containing information on a wide range of resources related to biotechnology. The resources include on-line data bases and networks, bulletin boards, organizations, collections, and publications such as books and compendiums. The DBIR file currently contains 1400 records.

Other Data Bases

NLM also offers the following data bases:

- **Toxicology Information On-Line (TOXLINE/ TOXLIT)** is designed specifically to offer comprehensive bibliographic coverage of toxicology information. It includes the pharmacologic, biochemical, physiologic, environmental, and toxicologic effects of chemicals and drugs. Sixteen subfiles containing approximately 2.5 million references can be searched. Subfiles are from Chemical Abstracts, Biological Abstracts, International Pharmaceutical Abstracts, and others. TOXLINE is available through the NLM MEDLARS System.
- **MEDLINE** is the data base used by most health care practitioners. It is the on-line version of *Index Medicus*. It is a bibliographic data base that indexes more than 3200 journals published in the United States and abroad. It can be accessed easily through the menu-driven Grateful Med software.

Other on-line systems include the following data bases:

- **Chemical Abstracts** data base provides worldwide information about chemical sciences, patents, books, conference proceedings, government research reports, and literature from more than 12,000 journals.
- **NIOSH Technical Information Center (NIOSHTIC)** is a compilation in abstract form of information about toxicology, epidemiology, industrial hygiene, and other areas of occupational safety and health. It is produced by the National Institute for Occupational Safety and Health.
- **Hazardline** provides emergency response, safety, regulatory, and health information on more than 4000 chemicals. Produced by Occupational Health Services, Hazardline contains an extensive companion file on Material Safety Data Sheets.
- **Online Library System (OLS)** is a free data base from the EPA and is available through Internet or a commercial phone number. OLS provides information on EPA publications and documents.
- **Reproductive Toxicology (REPROTOX)** includes information on reproductive toxicology. It is an inexpensive data base, easy to search, providing a beginning for more extensive evaluation of toxic exposures.
- **National Pesticide Information Retrieval System (NPIRS)** contains registration information on 45,000 pesticides registered by the EPA and the states. It includes specific information about the chemicals, studies, and related documents submitted to the EPA by companies seeking registration.

Compact Disk—Read Only Memory Systems

The Compact Disk—Read Only Memory (CD-ROM) systems use a compact disk reader and a computer software package to read the information on a compact disk. Because the CD-ROM data bases are generally updated quarterly, the information is not as current as that obtained from on-line searches. Two of the better known CD-ROM producers are Micromedex and SilverPlatter. Micromedex products include Poisindex and TOMES. SilverPlatter products include CHEM-BANK, OSH-ROM, and PEST-BANK. (For a complete listing of environmental health data bases and vendors see *Environmental On-Line . . . the Greening of Databases* published by On-Line, Inc., Wilton, CT, ISBN 0-910965-05-6.)

Micromedex developed the Poisindex CD-ROM System used in poison control centers. Poisindex contains toxicology information on drugs and consumer products.

The **TOMES-PLUS System (Toxicology, Occupational Medicine and Environmental Series Information System)** provides toxicology information about acute and chronic exposure to occupational and environmental chemicals. The **TOMES-Plus** System includes the following data bases: Meditext: detailed information on the evaluation and treatment of persons exposed to industrial chemicals. OSHA Permissible Exposure Limits (PEL) information is also supplied; Hazardtext: information on spills, leaks, and fires that may occur in hazardous materials incidents; protocols for first accident/injury/illness response; Department of Transportation Emergency Response Guides; the Hazardous Substances Data Bank (HSDB); the U.S. Coast Guard's Chemical Hazard Response Information System (CHRIS); the Oil and Hazardous Materials/Technical Assistance Data System (OHM/TADS); the Registry of Toxic Effects of Chemical Substances (RTECS); the New Jersey Department of Health's Fact Sheets; the EPA's Integrated Risk Information System (IRIS); and Reproductive Toxicology (REPROTOX).

SilverPlatter has various CD-ROM disks of toxicology information. Compact disks available include the following: **CHEM-BANK,** which includes the Registry of Toxic Effects of Chemical Substances (RTECS), the Oil and Hazardous Materials/Technical Assistance Data System (OHMTADS), the Chemical Hazard Response Information System (CHRIS), and the Hazardous Substance Data Bank (HSDB).

OSH-ROM includes the NIOSH Technical Information Center (NIOSHTIC), the HSALINE data base of the Health and Safety Executive (U.K.), and CISDOC from the International Labor Organization. The Major Hazard Incident Data Service (MHIDS) provides information on more than 3000 major accidents involving chemicals.

PEST-BANK contains information on the U.S. Registered pesticides used in agriculture, industry, and general commerce. The information comes from the National Pesticide Information Retrieval System (NPIRS). It contains information on synonyms, registration dates and registering companies, composition and formulation, sites, and pests affected by the pesticide.

TOXLINE contains toxicologic information from NLM that includes references to published materials on topics such as drugs, food, chemicals, occupational hazards, pesticides, and toxicologic analysis.

MEDLINE contains bibliographic citations and abstracts of biomedical literature.

B.4   ENVIRONMENTAL AND OCCUPATIONAL HEALTH HOTLINES*

Chemical Emergencies

Chemical Spills Emergency Hotline
(800) 535-0202
EPA Hazardous Waste Hotline
(800) 535-0202

Hazardous Waste

Emergency Planning and Community Right-To-Know Hotline (EPA)
Developing chemical contingency plans, gathering site-specific information, list of more than 400 acutely toxic chemicals
(800) 535-0202
Superfund Records of Decision
Hazardous waste, sites to be cleaned up, actions being taken
(703) 412-9810 or
(800) 535-0202
Integrated Risk Information System (IRIS)
Hazardous chemicals information, including health effects
(301) 496-6531
IRIS User Support
(513) 569-7254

Lung Disease

Lungline/National Jewish Hospital
Information on lung disease from chemical exposure
(800) 222-5864

Lead

National Center for Environmental Health (CDC)
Lead poisoning prevention
(404) 488-7330

National Maternal and Child Health Clearinghouse publications on lead poisoning
(703) 821-8955
National Lead Information Center
(800) LEAD-FYI

Occupational Health

NIOSH (CDC)
Information and publications on health effects of occupational exposures
(800) 356-4674
Medical Section
(513) 841-4386
Industrial Hygiene
(513) 841-4374
OSHA (Occupational Safety and Health Administration)
Regulations for toxic and hazardous substances in the workplace
(202) 219-8036

Pesticides

Pesticide Docket
(703) 305-5805
National Pesticide Telecommunications Network Pesticides
(800) 858-7378 or
(806) 743-3095
National Pesticides Information Retrieval System (NPIRS) (funded by EPA/USDA, managed by Purdue University) Help number for searching NPIRS data base to get fact sheets on pesticides, insecticides, fungicides, state and federally registered chemicals
(317) 494-6614

Radon

Radon Hotline
(800) SOS-RADON
EPA Office of Radon Programs
(202) 233-9370

Toxic Substances

Toxicology Information Response Center (Oak Ridge)
General toxicology information, searches on chemicals
(615) 576-1746
Agency for Toxic Substances and Disease Registry (ATSDR)
Toxicological profiles in draft (Final profiles available from National Technical Information Service)
(404) 639-6000
Toxic Substances Control Act (TSCA)
Hotline/Public Information Office (EPA)
Answers questions and gives general technical as-

---

*From *Case studies in environmental medicine: taking an exposure history,* Atlanta, Ga, 1994, USDHHS, PHS, ATSDR, in conjunction with CDC, NIOSH.

sistance on TSCA. Guidance on TSCA regulations
(202) 554-1404

Toxic Chemical Release Inventory System (EPA)
Information about which chemicals are used, stored, released by companies
(800) 535-0202

Chemical Referral Center (American Chemical Society)
Nonemergency health and safety information on chemicals

Outside continental United States
(800) 262-8200

Water

Environmental Protection Agency Safe Drinking Water-Hotline
(800) 426-4791

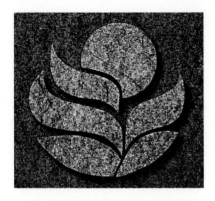

Appendix C
Contracts and Forms

C.1 COMMUNITY-ORIENTED HEALTH RECORD (COHR)

Community Health Assessment Model

Definition of community: A locality-based entity—composed of systems of formal organizations reflecting societal institutions, informal groups, and aggregates, which are interdependent—whose function (expressed intent) is to meet a wide range of collective needs.

Definition of community health: The meeting of collective needs, through identifying problems and managing interactions within the community and between the community and the larger society. This requires commitment; self-other awareness and clarity of situational definitions; articulateness; effective communication; conflict containment and accommodation; participation; management of relations with the larger society; and machinery for facilitating participant interaction and decision making.

Community Health Assessment Guide Categories

A. Community
   1. Place
      a. Geopolitical boundaries of community
      b. Local or folk name for community
      c. Size in square miles/areas/blocks/census tracts
      d. Transportation avenues
      e. Physical environment
   2. People
      a. Number and density of population
      b. Demographic structure of populations
      c. Informal groups
      d. Formal groups
      e. Linking structures
   3. Function
      a. Production—distribution—consumption of goods and services
      b. Socialization of new members
      c. Maintenance of social control
      d. Adapting to ongoing and unexpected change
      e. Provision of mutual aid
B. Community health
   1. Status
      a. Vital statistics
      b. Disease incidence and prevalence for leading causes of mortality and morbidity
      c. Health risk profiles
      d. Functional ability levels
   2. Structure
      a. Health facilities
      b. Health-related planning groups
      c. Health manpower
      d. Health resource utilization patterns
   3. Process
      a. Commitment
      b. Self-other awareness and clarity of situational definitions
      c. Articulateness
      d. Effective communication
      e. Conflict containment and accommodation
      f. Participation
      g. Management of relations with larger society
      h. Machinery for facilitating participant interaction and decision making

Data Base

This form provides a structured method for recording data. The name of the community and the assessment category and/or subcategory are noted at the top of the page. These categories correspond to those of the assessment guide. The data are collected and the source of the information and the data are recorded. Data are often entered using the SOAP format. An example of the COHR Data base form is depicted on the next page.

Community Health Nursing Diagnosis of the Problem

Headings of columns for the Community Health Diagnosis List are Date, Number, Diagnosis/Concern, and Supportive Data (title of appropriate section of Data base and capsule summary of relevant data).

Community Capability List

Heading of columns for this list are Date, Number, Capability, Supportive Data (title of appropriate section of Data base and capsule summary of relevant data).

Problem Analysis

Problems come from the Community Health Nursing Diagnosis. A line labeled Problem/Statement is included at the top of the form below Name of Community. Heading of columns are Problem Correlates, Relationship of Correlates of Problem and Data Supportive to Relationships (refer to appropriate sections of Data base and relevant research findings in current literature). An example of a completed Problem Analysis is depicted on page 302.

Problem Prioritization

Headings of columns are Criteria, Criteria Weights (1-10). Problem, Problem Rating (1-10), Rationale for Rating, Problem Significant/(Weight × Rate).

Data Base

Name of community _____

Assessment category _____ Subcategory _____

Date	Data source	Data*

*Note: With an asterisk the themes identified and meanings given.

Goals and Objectives

This form includes a line labeled Problem/Concern as well as lines for Goal Statement at the top under Name of Community. Column headings are Date, Objectives (number and statement) depicted on p. 303.

Plan

A line labeled Objective Number and Statement is included under Name of Community. Column headings are Date, Intervener Activities/Means, Value (1-10), and Activity/Means Selected for Implementation. Sample plan sheets from the interventions to infant malnutrition are presented on pp. 304-305.

Progress Notes

A line labeled Goal is included under Name of Community. Column headings are Date, Narrative, Assessment. Plan (NAP), and Budget and Time. A footnote to the second column explains the NAP procedure: Record both objective and subjective data. Interpret these data in terms of (1) whether the objectives were achieved and (2) whether the intervener activities utilized were effective. The plan is dependent on the assessment and may include both new (or revised) objectives and activities. Progress Notes reflecting evaluation of interventions aimed at the Nursing Diagnosis: Risk of infant malnutrition are presented on p. 307.

Windshield Survey Components

Element	Description
Housing and zoning	What is the age of the houses, their architecture, of what materials are they constructed? Are all the neighborhood houses similar in age, architecture? How would you characterize the differences? Are they detached from or connected to others? Do they have space in front and behind? What is their general condition? Are there signs of disrepair—broken doors, windows, leaks, locks missing? Is there central heating, modern plumbing, air conditioning?
Open space	How much open space is there? What is the quality of the space—green parks or rubble-filled lots? What is the lot size of the houses? Lawns? Flower boxes? Do you see trees on the pavements, a green island in the center of the streets? Is the open space public or private? Used by whom?
Boundaries	What signs are there of where this neighborhood begins and ends? Are the boundaries natural—a river, a different terrain? Physical—a highway, railroad? Economic—difference, in real estate or presence of industrial, commercial units along with residential? The neighborhood has an identity, a name? Do you see it displayed? Are there unofficial names?
"Commons"	What are the neighborhood hangouts? For what groups, at what hours? (e.g., schoolyard, candy store, bar, restaurant, park, 24-hour drugstore?) Does the "commons" have a sense of "territoriality" or is it open to the stranger?
Transportation	How do people get in and out of the neighborhood? Car, bus, bike, walk, etc.? Are the streets and roads conducive to good transportation and also to community life? Is there a major highway near the neighborhood? Whom does it serve? How frequent is public transportation available?
Service centers	Do you see social agencies, clients, recreation centers, signs of activity at the schools? Are there offices of doctors, dentists? Palmists, spiritualists, etc.? Parks? Are they in use?
Stores	Where do residents shop? Shopping centers, neighborhood stores? How do they travel to shop?
Street people	If you are traveling during the day, who do you see on the street? An occasional housewife, a mother with a baby? Do you see anyone you would not expect? Teenagers, unemployed males? Can you spot a welfare worker, an insurance collector, a door-to-door salesman? Is the dress of those you see representative or unexpected? Along with people, what animals do you see? Stray cats, dogs, pedigreed pets, "watchdogs"?
Signs of decay	Is this neighborhood on the way up or down? Is it "alive"? How would you decide? Trash, abandoned cars, political posters, neighborhood meeting posters, real estate signs, abandoned houses, mixed zoning usage?
Race	Are the residents white, black, or is the area integrated?
Ethnicity	Are there indices of ethnicity—food stores, churches, private schools, information in a language other than English?
Religion	Of what religion are the residents? Do you see evidence of heterogeneity or homogeneity? What denomination are the churches? Do you see evidence of their use other than on Sunday mornings?
Health and morbidity	Do you see evidence of acute or of chronic diseases or conditions? Of accidents, communicable diseases, alcoholism, drug addiction, mental illness, etc.? How far is it to the nearest hospital? Clinic?
Politics	Do you see any political campaign posters? Is there a headquarters present? Do you see any evidence of a predominant party affiliation?
Media	Do you see outdoor TV antennas? What magazines, newspapers do residents read? Do you see *Forward Times, Hampton Post, Enquirer, Readers' Digest* in the stores? What media seem most important to the residents? Radio, TV?

This example of a windshield survey is reprinted here with permission from Anderson ET, McFarlane J: *Community as client: application of the nursing process,* Philadelphia, 1988, Lippincott.

For students interested in a more thorough discussion of community as client with detailed step-by-step information and examples of the process, Anderson and McFarLane's book is an excellent resource and an updated edition is in press and due out in 1995. Their approach to community is congruent with the approach presented by the authors here. Anderson and McFarlanes' model emphasizes working with people (who are the community) and provides an in-depth approach showing how to analyze the eight subsystems (such as housing and government) that contribute to the makeup of the community. The model incorporates Neuman's theory within the community context.

C.2 THE LIVING WILL DIRECTIVE

The Living Will Directive

My wishes regarding life-prolonging treatment and artificially provided nutrition and hydration to be provided to me if I no longer have decisional capacity, have a terminal condition, or become permanently unconscious have been indicated by checking and initialing the appropriate lines below. By checking and initialing the appropriate lines, I specifically:

_____ Designate _____ as my health care surrogate(s) to make health care decisions for me in accordance with this directive when I no longer have decisional capacity. If

_____ refuses or is not able to act for me, I designate

_____ as my health care surrogate(s).
Any prior designation is revoked.

If I do not designate a surrogate, the following are my directions to my attending physician. If I have designated a surrogate, my surrogate shall comply with my wishes as indicated below:

_____ Direct that treatment be withheld or withdrawn, and that I be permitted to die naturally with only the administration of medication of the performance or any medical treatment deemed necessary to alleviate pain.
_____ DO NOT authorize that life-prolonging treatment be withheld or withdrawn.

_____ Authorize the withholding or withdrawal of artificially provided food, water, or other artificially provided nourishment or fluids.
_____ DO NOT authorize the withholding or withdrawal of artificially provided food, water, or other artificially provided nourishment or fluids.

_____ Authorize my surrogate, designated above, to withhold or withdraw artificially provided nourishment or fluids, or other treatment if the surrogate determines that withholding or withdrawing is in my best interest; but I no not mandate the withholding or withdrawing.

In the absence of my ability to give directions regarding the use of life-prolonging treatment and artificially provided nutrition and hydration, it is my intention that this directive shall be honored by my attending physician, my family, and any surrogate designated pursuant to this directive as the final expression of my legal right to refuse medical or surgical treatment and I accept the consequences of the refusal.

If I have been diagnosed as pregnant and that diagnosis is known to my attending physician, this directive shall have no force or effect during the course of my pregnancy.

I understand the full import of this directive and I am emotionally and mentally competent to make this directive.

Signed this _____ day of _____ 19 _____ .

_____
Signature and Address of the Grantor

In our joint presence, the grantor, who is of sound mind and eighteen years of age, or older, voluntarily dated and signed this writing or directed it to be dated and signed for the grantor.

_____   _____
Signature and Address of Witness   Signature and Address of Witness

or

STATE OF _____)
COUNTY OF _____)

Before me, the undersigned authority, came the grantor who is of sound mind and eighteeen (18) years of age, or older, and acknowledged that he voluntarily date and signed this writing or directed it to be signed and dated as above.

Done this _____ day of _____ 19 _____ .

_____
Signature or Notary Public or Other Officer

Date Commission Expires _____

Execution of this document restricts withholding of some medical procedures. Consult Revised Statutes or your attorney.

C.3 AUDIT FORM (SIMP-H)

Schmele Instrument to Measure the Process of Nursing Practice in Home Health

INSTRUCTIONS: On the scale provided for each item, please *circle the number* that best describes the nursing care observed during the home visit. If not observed or not applicable, indicate the reason under the item.

NOTE: Whenever "family" occurs in an item, consider it to mean "family or significant other." Whenever "nursing diagnoses" occurs in an item, consider it to mean "nursing diagnosis or nursing problem."

	Best care		Average care		Worst care	Not appli- cable	Not ob- served
	5	4	3	2	1	0	0

I. Assessing

Objective: To measure the quality of nursing care observed for the *intervention* component of the nursing process.

	5	4	3	2	1	0	0
1. The nurse collects data about the client's response to his/her medical illness.	5	4	3	2	1	0	0
2. The nurse collects data about the client's ability to care for self in the home.	5	4	3	2	1	0	0
3. The nurse collects data about client and/or family strengths that maintain or promote health.	5	4	3	2	1	0	0
4. During the visit, the nurse obtains pertinent data by questioning the client and/or family.	5	4	3	2	1	0	0
5. During the visit, the nurse's objective examination (auditory visual, palpable) of the client if either indicated* and made or *not* indicated and *not* made.	5	4	3	2	1	0	0
6. During the visit, the client is given an opportunity (time and encouragement) to initiate discussion or questions.	5	4	3	2	1	0	0
7. The nurse inquires about financial conditions of the client that affect his/her health.	5	4	3	2	1	0	0
8. Environmental data is collected (home, neighborhood, community).	5	4	3	2	1	0	0
9. The nurse collects data about cultural beliefs that affect his/ her health.	5	4	3	2	1	0	0
10. The nursing diagnoses are validated with the client and/or family during the visit.	5	4	3	2	1	0	0
11. The nurse collects data about client use and/or ability to use community health care resources.	5	4	3	2	1	0	0
12. The nurse asks questions about health history.	5	4	3	2	1	0	0
13. The data gathered supports the nursing diagnosis, which is noted in the record.	5	4	3	2	1	0	0
14. Nursing diagnoses are prioritized with the client during the visit.	5	4	3	2	1	0	0
15. The nursing diagnosis can be treated by nursing interventions.	5	4	3	2	1	0	0

II. Planning

Objective: To measure the quality of nursing care observed for the *planning* component of the nursing process.

	5	4	3	2	1	0	0
16. The client and family participate in goal setting.	5	4	3	2	1	0	0
17. A long-term goal (hoped for outcome) is established.	5	4	3	2	1	0	0
18. Short-term goals (steps to meet long-term goal) are established.	5	4	3	2	1	0	0
19. Action plans (steps to achieve goals) are established.	5	4	3	2	1	0	0
20. The client participates in action planning.	5	4	3	2	1	0	0
21. The nurse and client discuss the resources (community, agency, family, personal, etc.) needed to fulfill the plan.	5	4	3	2	1	0	0
22. The nurse and client mutually decide upon an expected date of goal accomplishment.	5	4	3	2	1	0	0
23. The nurse discusses costs and benefits of the nursing plan.	5	4	3	2	1	0	0
24. The plan includes community resources.	5	4	3	2	1	0	0
25. The plan is revised as goals are achieved or changed.	5	4	3	2	1	0	0
26. Goals are measurable.	5	4	3	2	1	0	0
27. Goals are achievable.	5	4	3	2	1	0	0
28. Goals are based on the nursing diagnosis.	5	4	3	2	1	0	0
29. The nursing plan indicates what the nurse will do.	5	4	3	2	1	0	0
30. The nursing plan indicates what the client will do.	5	4	3	2	1	0	0

Continued.

Schmele Instrument to Measure the Process of Nursing Practice in Home Health—cont'd

	Best care		Average care		Worst care	Not applicable	Not observed
	5	4	3	2	1	0	0

III. Intervention

Objective: To measure the quality of nursing care observed for the *intervention* component of the nursing process.

	5	4	3	2	1	0	0
31. The nurse periodically reinforces client and family strengths.	5	4	3	2	1	0	0
32. Nursing actions provide for client participation in health promotion, maintenance, or restoration.	5	4	3	2	1	0	0
33. During the visit, one of the following takes place regarding a referral to another agency or discipline: referral indicated* and made or referral *not* indicated and *not* made.	5	4	3	2	1	0	0
34. The communication pattern that illustrates the decision-making process during this visit is:							

Nurse ⟵ Client (⟶ / ⟵ / ⟶ / ⟵)

	5	4	3	2	1	0	0
35. Teaching regarding the client's problems or need is done during the visit.	5	4	3	2	1	0	0
36. The client participates in the intervention(s) if capable.	5	4	3	2	1	0	0
37. The intervention is performed to reach the nursing care goal.	5	4	3	2	1	0	0
38. The nurse explains the rationale for the intervention.	5	4	3	2	1	0	0
39. The nursing action reflects currently accepted standards of practice.	5	4	3	2	1	0	0
40. The nurse coordinates health care services when more than one discipline is involved.	5	4	3	2	1	0	0
41. The nurse advocates for the client.	5	4	3	2	1	0	0
42. The nurse informs the client about nursing interventions being carried out.	5	4	3	2	1	0	0
43. The nurse assists the client to modify the environment according to need.	5	4	3	2	1	0	0
44. The nurse explores the use of health care resources with the client and/or family.	5	4	3	2	1	0	0
45. The nurse adapts or uses alternative interventions based on the client's response.	5	4	3	2	1	0	0

IV. Evaluating

Objective: To measure the quality of nursing care observed for the *evaluation* component of the nursing process.

	5	4	3	2	1	0	0
46. The nurse refers to the nursing care goal set at the previous visit.	5	4	3	2	1	0	0
47. The communication pattern used to illustrate the evaluation of the client's progress to goal achievement is:							

Nurse ⟵ Client (⟶ / ⟵ / ⟶ / ⟵)

	5	4	3	2	1	0	0
48. The family and nurse discuss the accomplishment of the nursing care goal(s).	5	4	3	2	1	0	0
49. The nurse informs the client about his/her health status.	5	4	3	2	1	0	0
50. There is mutual consideration of the short-term goals.	5	4	3	2	1	0	0
51. There is mutual consideration of the long-term goals.	5	4	3	2	1	0	0
52. New data is validated with the client and family.	5	4	3	2	1	0	0
53. The nurse and the client discuss how actions will be evaluated.	5	4	3	2	1	0	0
54. Changes in the care plan are discussed with the client and family.	5	4	3	2	1	0	0
55. During the visit, there is evidence of ongoing assessment.	5	4	3	2	1	0	0
56. During the visit, there is consideration of priorities.	5	4	3	2	1	0	0
57. Revision of the nursing care plan is based on progress toward the goal.	5	4	3	2	1	0	0
58. The nurse and the client and/or family discuss progress toward goal achievement.	5	4	3	2	1	0	0
59. The client's ongoing response to the medical illness is discussed.	5	4	3	2	1	0	0
60. The client and/or family demonstrates the ability to follow the nursing care plan.	5	4	3	2	1	0	0

"Indicated" means that there was evidence of a problem requiring assistance of someone other than the nurse.

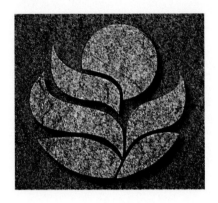

Appendix D
Drug and Immunization Information

D.1 RECOMMENDATIONS FOR PROPHYLAXIS OF HEPATITIS A

1. *Close personal contact.* Immune globulin (IG) is recommended for all household and sexual contacts of persons with hepatitis A.
2. *Day-care centers.* Day-care facilities with children in diapers can be important settings for HAV transmission. IG should be administered to all staff and attendees of day-care centers or homes if (1) one or more hepatitis A cases are recognized among children or employees, or (2) cases are recognized in two or more households of center attendees. When an outbreak (hepatitis cases in three or more families) occurs, IG should also be considered for members of households whose diapered children attend. In centers not enrolling children in diapers, IG need only be given to classroom contacts of an index case.
3. *Schools.* Contact at elementary and secondary schools is usually not an important means of transmitting hepatitis A. Routine administration of IG is not indicated for pupils and teachers in contact with a patient. However, when epidemiological study clearly shows the existence of a school- or classroom-centered outbreak, IG may be given to those who have close personal contact with patients.
4. *Institutions for custodial care.* Living conditions in some institutions, such as prisons and facilities for the developmentally disabled, favor transmission of hepatitis A. When outbreaks occur, giving IG to residents and staff who have close contact with patients with hepatitis A may reduce spread of disease. Depending on the epidemiologic circumstances, prophylaxis can be limited or can involve the entire institution.
5. *Hospitals.* Routine IG administration is not indicated. Rather, sound hygienic practices should be emphasized. Staff education should point out the risk of exposure to hepatitis A and emphasize precautions regarding direct contact with potentially infective materials. Outbreaks of hepatitis A among hospital staff occur occasionally, usually in association with an unsuspected index patient who is fecally incontinent. Large outbreaks have occurred among staff and family contacts of infected infants in neonatal intensive care units. In outbreaks, prophylaxis of persons exposed to feces of infected patients may be indicated.
6. *Offices and factories.* Routine IG administration is not indicated under the usual office or factory conditions for persons exposed to a fellow worker with hepatitis A. Experience shows that casual contact in the work setting does not result in virus transmission.
7. *Common-source exposure.* IG might be effective in preventing food-borne or waterborne hepatitis A if exposure is recognized in time. However, IG is not recommended for persons exposed to a common source of hepatitis infection after cases have begun to occur in those exposed, because the 2-week period during which IG is effective will have been exceeded.

If a food handler is diagnosed as having hepatitis A, common-source transmission is possible but uncommon. IG should be administered to other food handlers but is usually not recommended for patrons. However, IG administration to patrons may be considered if (1) the infected person is directly involved in handling, without gloves, foods that will not be cooked before they are eaten; (2) the hygienic practices of the food handler are deficient; and (3) patrons can be identified and treated within 2 weeks of exposure. Situations in which repeated exposures may have occurred, such as in institutional cafeterias, may warrant stronger consideration of IG use.

For postexposure IG prophylaxis, a single intramuscular dose of 0.02 ml/kg is recommended.

D.2   SUMMARY DESCRIPTION HEPATITIS A-E*

Type	Definition	Risk	Symptoms	Precautions	Prevention of spreading
A	Liver disease caused by picornavirus, commonly called "infectious hepatitis"	◆ Live in house with infected person ◆ Inject drugs ◆ Travel internationally to areas with high prevalence of hepatitis A ◆ Eat infected shell fish ◆ Consume contaminated food and water	◆ Skin, eye yellowing ◆ Loss of appetite ◆ Nausea ◆ Vomiting ◆ Fever ◆ Fatigue ◆ Diarrhea ◆ Stomach/joint pain ◆ Unable to work for extended periods	◆ Stricter handwashing by foodhandler ◆ Improved sanitary conditions ◆ Improved personal hygiene	◆ Immune gamma globulin injections ◆ Hepatitis A vaccine
B	A major cause of acute and chronic liver disease that can lead to cirrhosis and hepatocellular cancer; "serum hepatitis"	◆ Exposure to human blood ◆ Live with someone who is a carrier ◆ Inject drugs ◆ Have a sex partner infected with "B" ◆ Have sex with more than one partner ◆ A child born in Asia, Africa, Amazon, South America, Pacific Islands, or the Middle East	◆ Skin, eye yellowing ◆ Loss of appetite ◆ Nausea ◆ Vomiting ◆ Diarrhea ◆ Stomach/joint pain ◆ No symptoms—carrier ◆ Itching ◆ Skin erruptions	Vaccinate: ◆ Babies at birth ◆ Adolescents and others who have sex or inject drugs ◆ Persons whose job places them at risk	Hepatitis B vaccine
C	Virus causing chronic liver disease, found in blood caused by non-A and non-B hepatitis virus. May develop cirrhosis and liver failure	◆ Drug injection ◆ Exposure to human blood ◆ Hemodialysis patients ◆ Receipt of blood transfusion ◆ Multiple sex partners ◆ Live with person with "C"	Same as hepatitis "B"	◆ Do not take blood, organs, tissue, or sperm from "C" person ◆ Do not share toothbrushes, razors, or other items possibly contaminated with blood (including needles) ◆ Cover open sores or other skin breaks	◆ Practice safe sex ◆ Have only one sex partner ◆ Routine screening of blood/other donors
D	An incomplete virus requiring hepatitis B to be present to cause infection. This results in a more severe acute liver disease, leading to chronic liver disease with cirrhosis	◆ Injection drug users ◆ Hemophilia patients ◆ Developmentally disabled persons who are hospitalized	Same as hepatitis "B"	◆ Avoid sexual contact with injection drug users ◆ Do not use needle used by others ◆ Proper sterilization technique in institutions	◆ Individual screening for hepatitis B ◆ Blood screening for "B" and "D" ◆ Early vaccination for hepatitis B
E	Enterically transmitted non-A and non-B Hepatitis virus. Usually acute and does not usually cause chronic disease	◆ Ingestion of fecally contaminated water ◆ Pregnant women ◆ International travelers ◆ Persons in Asia and Indian countries	Same as hepatitis "B'	◆ Avoid contaminated waters	None at this time

*Data compiled from multiple sources provided by the Centers for Disease Control, Atlanta, 1995.

D.3   IMMUNIZATION INFORMATION

Routine Immunizing Agents

Agent	Age to administer	Administration	Reaction/treatment
DTP diphtheria toxoid, tetanus toxoid, and pertussis vaccine	2, 4, 6 months of age; 12-18 months of age; 4-6 years of age (may be given through the 6th year)	0.5 cc IM a. Primary series: 3 doses at 8-week intervals, followed by a fourth dose 6 to 12 months later b. Booster: First booster at 4-6 years. Td every 10 years thereafter. May begin 10-year cycles at 11 to 16 years of age. *Contraindications:* 1. Anaphylactic reaction to vaccine or vaccine components 2. Moderate to severe illness with or without fever 3. Fever of $\geq$40.5° C within 48 hours after prior DTP dose 4. Collapse or shocklike state within 48 hours of receiving prior DTP dose *Precautions:* (risks/benefits should be considered) 1. Seizures within 3 days of receiving a prior dose of DTP 2. Persistent inconsolable crying lasting $\geq$3 hours within 48 hours of receiving a prior dose of DTP 3. Neurologic disorder or history of seizures	a. Local: Induration, redness, or nodule at the injection site Treatment: Cool compress b. Systemic: Fever and irritability lasting 24 to 72 hours Treatment: Acetaminophen c. Moderate to severe reactions: Fever $\geq$40.5° C, seizure or shock, prolonged inconsolable crying $\geq$3 hours Refer to MD immediately and report to National Vaccine Injury Compensation Program
DTaP diphtheria toxoid, tetanus toxoid, and acellular pertussis vaccine	Not licensed for <15 months Not recommended for primary immunization at any age May be used for fourth and fifth doses	0.5 cc dose IM *Contraindications and Precautions:* See DTP	See DTP, however may be less likely to cause reactions
DT Pediatric diphtheria toxoid and tetanus toxoid	May be given through the sixth year	0.5 cc dose IM *Contraindications and Precautions:* See DTP. Indicated for use in infants and young children <7 years of age when the pertussis vaccine is contraindicated	See DPT
Td Adult tetanus toxoid and diphtheria toxoid	Used for $\geq$7 years 11-16 and every 10 years thereafter	0.5 cc dose IM Primary course: 2 doses at 8-week intervals, third dose 6 to 12 months after second	See DPT except less likely to produce reactions
Combination DTP/HIB products	May be used when DTP and HIB vaccines are administered simultaneously	0.5 cc dose IM *Contraindications and Precautions:* See DTP	See DTP

Modified from CDC, 1995; MMWR 43 (51, 52):960; and AAP: Report of the Committee on Infectious Diseases, ed 23, Elk Grove Village, IL, 1994, The Academy.

Continued.

Routine Immunizing Agents—cont'd

Agent	Age to administer	Administration	Reaction/treatment
Haemophilus influenzae Type b conjugate		0.5 cc dose IM	a. Local: Induration, redness, or nodule at the injection site
1. Oligosaccharide (HbOC) conjugated to diphtheria (HIBtiter)	1. 2,4,6 months of age and 12 to 15 months	1. Primary course: 3 doses at 8-week intervals; booster at 12 to 15 months	Treatment: Cool compress
2. Polyribosylribitol phosphate (PRP-T) conjugated to tetanus (Act HIB, Omni HIB)	2. 2,4,6 months of age and 12 to 15 months	2. Primary course: 3 doses at 8-week intervals; booster at 12 to 15 months	b. Systemic: Fever and irritability lasting 24 to 72 hours
3. H influenzae b (PRP-OMP) conjugated to meningococcal protein (Pedvax HIB)	3. 2-4 months of age and 12 to 15 months	3. Primary course: 2 doses at 8-week intervals; booster at 12 to 15 months	Treatment: Acetaminophen
		When feasible the same vaccine should be used for subsequent doses for children younger than 12 months. If not feasible, more than 3 doses for the primary series are not necessary	
		Any conjugate vaccine may be used for booster doses	
		Contraindications:	
		1. Anaphylactic reaction to vaccine or vaccine components	
		2. Moderate to severe illness with or without fever	
Hepatitis B live vaccine (for routine childhood immunizations) Two recombinant vaccines are available: Recombivax HB Energix B	1. Birth to 2 months of age	(For children <11 yrs old of HBsAg-neg mothers) 0.5 cc IM	a. Local: Induration, redness, or nodule at the injection site
	2. 2 to 4 months of age and 6 to 18 months of age	Total of 3 doses with 1 to 2 months between doses 1 and 2 and at least 2 months between doses 2 and 3. Highest titers are obtained if dose 2 and 3 are at least 4 months apart	Treatment: Cool compress b. Systemic: Fever and irritability lasting 24 to 72 hours
		When feasible the same vaccine should be used for all doses. If not feasible, the immune response of combined vaccines is appropriate	Treatment: Acetaminophen
		Contraindications:	
		1. Anaphylactic reaction to vaccine or vaccine components	
		2. Moderate to severe illness with or without fever	
OPV oral poliovirus vaccine-live	1. 2,4,6-12 months of age	Oral drops	Risks: Associated with paralysis in vaccines and their contacts—
	2. 4-6 years of age	Primary course: 2 doses at 2-month intervals, with a third dose 2-14 months later	1 per 6.8 million doses for recipient
	3. Do not give to persons over 18 years	Booster: 1 dose at 4-6 years	1 per 6.4 million doses for contacts
		Contraindications:	
		1. Anaphylactic reaction to vaccine or vaccine components	
		2. Moderate to severe illness with or without fever	
		3. Known altered immunodeficiency: hematologic and solid tumors, congenital immunodeficiency, long term immunosuppressive therapy, or HIV	
		4. Immunodeficient household contact	
		Precautions: (risks/benefits should be considered) Pregnancy	

Routine Immunizing Agents—cont'd

Agent	Age to administer	Administration	Reaction/treatment
MMR measles-mumps-rubella live attenuated virus vaccine	1. 12-15 months of age; 2. 4-6 or 11-12 years of age	1 subcutaneous injection of total volume of reconstituted vaccine Primary dose at 12-15 months Booster dose at 4-6 or 11-12 yrs *Contraindications:* 1. Anaphylactic reaction to vaccine or vaccine components including eggs and neomycin 2. Moderate to severe illness with or without fever 3. Known altered immunodeficiency: hematologic and solid tumors, congenital immunodeficiency, long term immunosuppressive therapy, or HIV 4. Pregnancy *Precautions:* IG administration within 3 mos	a. Local: Induration, redness, or nodule at the injection site Treatment-cool compress b. Systemic: Rash, fever, swollen lymph nodes 1-2 weeks after dose (very rarely a seizure may accompany fever) Treatment: Acetaminophen Pain, stiffness, or swelling in one or more joints 1-3 weeks after dose lasting for 3 days to 1 or more months

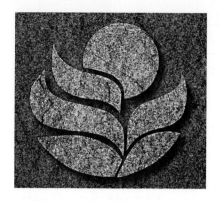

Appendix E
Guidelines for Practice

E.1 INFECTION CONTROL GUIDELINES FOR HOME CARE

The practice of universal precautions means that all blood and body fluids are treated as potentially infectious. Universal precautions is implemented to prevent exposure and infection of caregivers. It is an important practice because many infections are subclinical.

Use extreme care when handling needles, scalpels, and razors to prevent injuries. Do not recap, bend, break, or remove the needle from a syringe before disposal. Discard needles and syringes in puncture-resistant containers made of plastic or metal and dispose of them in a local landfill.

Barrier precautions, such as gloves, masks, eye covering, and gowns, should be worn when contact with blood and body fluids is expected. Gloves must be worn when in contact with body fluids, mucous membranes, nonintact skin, and when drawing blood. Masks and eye cover are recommended when droplets or splashes of blood or other body fluids is expected. Wear gowns, aprons, or smocks to protect regular clothing from splashes of blood or body fluids.

Handwashing is the single most important practice in preventing infections. Handwashing should be done before and after providing client care and before and after preparing food, eating, feeding, or using the bathroom.

Soiled dressings and perineal pads should be placed inside polyethylene garbage bags by using two bags and double lining them.

HIV is easily decontaminated by common disinfectants such as lysol and is rapidly killed by household bleach. Surfaces can be disinfected with a solution of 1 part bleach to 10 parts water. This solution must be mixed daily to retain its disinfectant properties. Bathrooms and kitchens can be safely shared with persons infected with HIV, but towels, razors, and toothbrushes should not be shared. Household cleaning can be done in a regular manner unless there are spills of blood or body fluids. If a spill occurs, wear gloves and decontaminate the area by flooding the spill with a disinfectant, then use paper towels to remove visible debris, and reapply disinfectant.

Kitchen counters, dishes, and laundry should be cleaned in warm water and detergent after use. Bathrooms may be cleaned with a household disinfectant.

E.2 SAFER SEX GUIDELINES

The following information is intended to be given to clients during risk reduction counseling.

Discuss injectable drug use, sexual history, and safer sex practices with potential partners before sexual activity. If you are infected with any sexually transmitted disease, such as genital herpes, HIV, or genital warts, let sexual partners know. Drugs and alcohol may impair judgment and reduce your ability to make wise decisions.

Recommendations for Use of Condoms

Use latex condoms to prevent exchange of body fluids because they offer greater protection against STD than natural membrane condoms. The use of condoms that contain spermicides, such as nonoxynol-9, can be effective in rendering HIV inactive. Nonoxynal-9 can also be put in the condom before putting it on. Oil-based lubricants, such as petroleum jelly (Vaseline), are unsafe because they weaken condoms and diminish protection. Only water-based lubricants, such as K-Y jelly, should be used. Condoms should be put on before any genital contact. Hold the tip of the condom and unroll it onto the erect penis. Leave a space at the tip for collection of semen but make sure that no air is trapped in the tip of the condom. Withdrawal should occur before loss of erection. The base of the condom should be held throughout withdrawal and the condom should be removed slowly to avoid tearing the condom or spilling body fluids. If the penis relaxes before withdrawal, the condom may fall off and body fluids may spill, thus causing potential exposure. Avoid mouth contact with the penis, vagina, or anus. Wear condoms during oral sex. Condoms should never be reused and should be stored in a cool, dry place.

E.3 GUIDE FOR EVALUATION OF GROUP EFFECTIVENESS

The following questions focus evaluation on group task accomplishment, member satisfaction, conflict management, and group purpose. Answer each question for the group, then write a descriptive summary of group effectiveness.

1. Describe the group's task goal. List the steps proposed or acted on by members relative to the goal. How well do members achieve these steps?
2. Describe leadership behavior for the group. How well do members carry out other group roles?
3. Describe comfort level for group members. Do members support each other? Is the level of tension conducive to productive behavior?
4. Is disagreement expressed clearly and openly? How do members manage and resolve conflict?
5. By what bonds are members attracted to each other and to the group?
6. Are there implicit goals for the group, and do these goals interfere with the group's work toward the explicit goal?

E.4 NORMAL VARIATIONS AND MINOR ABNORMALITIES IN NEWBORN PHYSICAL CHARACTERISTICS

Variant	Cause	Course	Nursing anticipatory guidance
HEAD			
Cephalhematoma	Usually caused by trauma of birth.	Soft, fluctuant, well-outlined mass of blood trapped beneath the pericranium and confined to one bone. This is a subperiosteal hematoma with no extension across suture lines.	Observe for any changes in the size or shape of the hematoma. Reassure parents. May not resolve for weeks to months.
Caput succedaneum	Caused by head pressing on the pelvic outlet in the last period of labor.	Clear fluid trapped between the scalp and bone. It is ill-defined, pits on pressure, not fluctuant. Fluid usually disappears in 1 to 2 weeks.	Explain the cause to parents and reassure them it will disappear.
Facial asymmetry	Overriding of the cranial sutures at birth caused by intrauterine molding or molding from delivery. Bones are soft and pliable.	Flattening of part of head or face. Generally disappears a few days after birth.	If the occipital area is flat because of labor and delivery, reassure parents about its disappearance in a few days. If it is caused by the "same" positioning of the child in the crib, instruct the parents to alternate the positioning of the child in the crib daily.
Asymmetry of the scalp	Usually occurs from molding during delivery or the use of forceps during delivery. Also can be caused by positioning the infant repeatedly on the same side without rotating.	Flattening of part of head.	Same as facial assymetry.
Craniotabes	Unknown.	Softening of localized areas in the cranial bone. Sometimes found in the parietal bones at the vertex near the sagittal suture. The areas are spongelike and can be indented by the pressure of a fingertip. They resume their shape when the pressure is removed.	Usually inconsequential, but if they persist, could be indicative of a pathological cause. There is no specific treatment. It is normal for these craniotabes to persist for months. They should eventually disappear.

Compiled by Nancy Dickenson-Hazard, RN, CPNP, MSN, for the 3rd edition of this text.

Continued.

E.4   Normal Variations and Minor Abnormalities in Newborn Physical Characteristics—cont'd

Variant	Cause	Course	Nursing anticipatory guidance
HEAD—cont'd			
Fontanelle	An irregular-shaped area enclosed by a membrane that occurs where the sutures of the bone of the skull meet. These areas are called anterior fontanelle, posterior fontanelle, and temporal fontanelles.	The anterior fontanelle should be open; the posterior fontanelle may be closed.	Explain to the parents that the open fontanelle helped to protect the baby's head during the birth process. The fontanelle allows the brain to grow and will continue to do so for the next 18 months. Reassure parents that fontanelle can be touched and scalp scrubbed without ill effect.
MOUTH			
Bednar's aphthae (ulcers)	Unknown. May be caused by vigorous sucking.	Usually located on hard palate posteriorly; generally bilateral.	Reassure and support parents. Explain to the parents that there is no specific treatment, and condition will disappear without any treatment.
Epstein's epithelial pearls	Small epithelial cysts.	Located along both sides of the middle of the hard palate or along the alveolar ridge.	Reassure parents that cysts will disappear. There is no specific treatment.
Bohn's pearls (nodules)	Small white papules.	Located on each side of the midline of the hard palate. They disappear spontaneously in several weeks.	Reassure and support parents. Parents sometimes think that these lesions look like thrush. Reassure that these lesions are not thrush and will go away without treatment.
High palatal arch		Of no significance if there are no other findings present.	Reassure, support, and explain the lack of significance.
EYES			
Chemical conjunctivitis	Irritation from silver nitrate solution instilled after birth.	Eyes red with purulent exudate. Lids swollen. Onset occurs within first 24 hours and lasts about 2 to 4 days.	Cleanse eyelids with cotton balls soaked in warm saline solution. Wipe the eyes from the inner canthus out toward the outer canthus. Reassure parents that the infant's eyesight will not be affected.
Subconjunctival hemorrhage	Caused from pressure in the birth process.	Occurs at the limbus. It may be crescent shaped or may form a red halo around the iris. The hemorrhage resolves itself without any specific treatment in a few days.	Reassure parents that no residual defects occur from the hemorrhage. The blood will reabsorb itself in a few days.
Pseudostrabismus	Poor muscle coordination of the eye.	Movements of the newborn's eyes are poorly coordinated. The eyes do not necessarily move together. Very common and usually disappears spontaneously.	Reassure parents that this generally disappears spontaneously as the eye muscles strengthen and the infant's eyes continue to develop and grow.

E.4   Normal Variations and Minor Abnormalities in Newborn Physical Characteristics—cont'd

Variant	Cause	Course	Nursing anticipatory guidance
SKIN			
Vernix caseosa	Cheeselike material that sticks to the skin. Protective covering for infant in utero.	Skin of newborn covered with varying amounts of this substance.	Will dry and disappear within a few days. Discourage mother from trying to vigorously rub it off. Encourage good skin care.
Lanugo	Fine downy type of hair.	Usually found on the back, shoulders, and ear lobes.	Usually disappears in time as a result of the friction of the skin rubbing on the bassinet linens. Reassure parents.
Desquamation	Skin in the newborn is very tender and soft. Following birth, the skin reacts to the changed environment by becoming very red. When the redness subsides, desquamation of the skin tends to occur.	Shedding, flaking, or peeling of the skin. Usually occurs during the first week of life. Can vary from extensive to so slight it almost goes unnoticed.	Reassure, support, and explain the cause to parents. Encourage good skin care, which avoids use of lotions, oils, and powders.
Ecchymosis	Blood under the skin caused by superficial trauma to the skin.	Bruise—disappears as the blood is reabsorbed.	Provide reassurance.
Acrocyanosis	Venous stasis.	Blue hands and feet.	No specific treatment. Make sure the baby is warm and that the cause of the acrocyanosis is not from being cold.
Erythema toxicum	Unknown.	A rash consisting of small red, flat, or raised lesions. Looks splotchy and sometimes resembles chicken pox or flea bites. Usually occurs during the first 2 weeks.	No specific treatment. Reassure, support, and explain.
Nevi, pigmented	Increased pigmentation.	Range from smooth, flat, hairless pigmented areas to those with hair; some can look like warts.	No treatment unless for cosmetic reasons. Provide reassurance.
Nevus flammeus (telangiectatic) or (storkbite)	Widening of surface capillaries.	Small red areas attributable to widening of surface capillaries; disappear momentarily with blanching of skin, but usually do not disappear completely.	Provide reassurance.
		Dull pink spots at the nape of the neck, eyelids, globella, or nasolabial folds. Gradually fade; usually disappear by 2 years (nape of the neck patches may persist).	Reassurance and support. No specific treatment.
Mongolian spots	Large aggregations of melanin—rich dark cells, which give the affected area a purple or blue/black color. Occur most frequently in black children but may occur in white children.	Generally found over the sacrum and coccygeal area of a large percentage of infants of black, Chicano, Mediterranean and Asiatic Indian origin. They do not have any significance and most disappear with time.	Explain cause and reassure parents. The spots usually disappear within the first year of life.

Continued.

E.4   Normal Variations and Minor Abnormalities in Newborn Physical Characteristics—cont'd

Variant	Cause	Course	Nursing anticipatory guidance
SKIN—cont'd			
Mottling (Cutis marmorata)	Vasoconstriction—general circulatory instability.	Overall red and white coloration of the skin. Generally occurs in fair children who become chilled. Disappears when child becomes warm.	Explain causes and reassure parents; use a blanket to warm the infant.
Milja	Retained sebum in the skin.	Yellow-white, pinpoint-size lesions located on the bridge of the nose, the chin, or the cheeks. Disappear after first few weeks of life.	No specific treatment necessary. Explain to parents that lesions will disappear.
Café au lait	Variations in pigment.	Light to dark brown pigmented spots. One or two patches considered normal. If infant has several patches, may indicate fibromas or neurofibromatosis.	Assess nature of spots. If number of spots exceeds five to six, refer to physician or neurologist. Reassurance and support.
Accessory nipples (supernumerary nipples)	Not adequately explained (sometimes referred to as developmental cutaneous defect).	Occurs in a unilateral or bilateral distribution along the "mammary lines" from midaxilla to the inguinal area.	Reassure parents that the nipples may be excised for cosmetic reasons.
Harlequin coloring	Thought to be caused by poorly developed vasomotor reflexes.	Half of the infant's body appears red/white, the other half is pale. Transitory condition, which usually occurs when the infant cries forcefully.	Explain to parents that this is not significant. It is apparently harmless and the cause is not adequately explained.
Cyanosis (localized)	Inadequate oxygenation of tissues; localized cyanosis because of immature peripheral circulation and venous stasis.	Usually involves lips, hands and feet, or cyanosis of the presenting parts. Usually present at birth and for variable number or days afterwards.	Keep child warm; cyanosis will decrease as peripheral circulation improves. Reassure and support parents. Explain cause.
Cyanosis (general)	Numerous causes of general cyanosis (e.g., atelectasis, congenital heart disease, central nervous system damage, obstructed airway).	Depends on the cause.	Reassurance and support. Try to determine the relationship of cyanosis to crying, (i.e., if cyanosis is relieved or improved when the child cries, then the cause may be atelectasis). Crying tends to make infants with cardiac malformations worse. Refer to physician.
ABDOMEN			
Umbilical cord variations	Natural process for sloughing tissues.	Blue/white at birth. Dull and yellow/brown within 24 hours, then black/brown and dry. Usually drops off at the end of the second week.	Keep cord area clean and dry. Reassure parents. Instruct parents in cord care.
Umbilical hernia	Occurs at the defect in the musculature of the abdominal wall near the umbilicus.	Skin-covered protuberance at the umbilicus. Very common in black infants and some Italian infants. Usually disappears spontaneously at the end of 1 to 3 years.	Reassure parents that it will probably disappear spontaneously. If it does not, it can be treated surgically when the child is older. Discourage home remedies (e.g., coin taped to hernia, binding, etc.)

E.4   Normal Variations and Minor Abnormalities in Newborn Physical Characteristics—cont'd

Variant	Cause	Course	Nursing anticipatory guidance
OTHER			
Vaginal discharge	Physiological manifestation of increased maternal hormonal influences.	Milky white discharge, sometimes blood-tinged or whole blood. Usually disappears in 2 weeks.	Reassure mother that this is nothing to worry about. It occurs quite frequently and is considered normal. Explain that it will disappear in a few weeks.
Brachial palsy	Sometimes caused when lateral traction is exerted on the head and neck during delivery of the shoulder in a vertex presentation, or in a breech presentation when the arms are extended over the head, or when there is excessive traction on the shoulders.	Should be suspected when there is asymmetric response of the upper extremities during a Moro response. The asymmetric response occurs because there is paralysis of the muscles of the upper arm or paralysis of the entire arm. Prognosis depends on the extent of damage to the nerves.	Treatment usually consists of partial immobilization, range of motion, and appropriate positioning. Problem needs to be evaluated and the appropriate treatment initiated. Depending on the severity of damage, there could be complete return of function within a few months or there may be permanent damage. Teach parents the importance of carrying out the immobilization-positioning treatment on a daily basis. Reassure and support parents. Observe for any changes in the movement of the upper extremities.

E.5   COMMON CONCERNS AND PROBLEMS OF FIRST YEAR (NEONATE AND INFANT)

Problem or concern	Assessment	Nursing intervention
Burping	Swallowed air bubbles trapped in stomach; occurs more frequently in bottle-fed infants who cry during feeding.	Burp frequently during feeding (i.e., before, during, and after, or after every 1 ounce of formula or after every 4-5 minutes at breast). Use upright position to burp (gently rub infant's back while baby sits on parent's knee and rests forward against parent's arm). Sit upright in infant seat for 30-45 minutes after feeding if awake or position with head elevated and on right side if sleeping.
Colic	Unexplained bouts of crying frequently occurring at same time of day (usually busiest) and often accompanied by abdominal distention, spasms, drawing up legs to stomach and/or passing gas. May be caused by feeding problems, maternal anxiety, allergy, and is aggravated by tension in household. Can last 3 months. Also see Crying.	Review basic infant needs with parents (i.e., is infant hungry, wet, have air bubble, in uncomfortable position)? Review feeding method, technique and burping; review maternal diet for offending foods if breastfed. Record time when colic episodes occur. Soothe and comfort before "attack." Walk, rock, and hold infant over shoulder. Try a monotonous soothing noise (music, ticking clock) or activity (ride in a car). Change infant position from stomach to side to back to sitting position.

Compiled by Nancy Dickenson-Hazard, RN, CPNP, MSN, for the 3rd edition of this text.

Continued.

E.5   Common Concerns and Problems of First Year (Neonate and Infant)—cont'd

Problem or concern	Assessment	Nursing intervention
		Rest infant on abdomen on warm hard surface (i.e., parent knee, warmed crib surface).
		Change household routine if indicated, create a quiet environment.
		Try pacifier or sugar water; if bottle fed, try soy formula.
		Reassure parents that infant is not ill, that they are providing good care, and that colic will definitely go away.
		Provide support to parents, giving opportunity to discuss feelings.
		Explain theories about origin and cycle of colic.
Crying	Periodic crying for unexplained reason; ascertain if a pattern exists for crying spells; may be related to colic; obtain a detailed history of time and length of spell; feeding frequency, method, technique and burping; stool patterns; meeting contact and sucking needs; parental handling of crying and feelings about crying; other household factors (i.e., siblings, relative advice, parental support of each other, presence of other symptoms and/or allergies).	See previous section on colic. Reinforce that babies cry for a reason. Best to respond to crying versus letting baby cry it out. Try to identify different types of cry (hungry, wet, sleepy, pain, boredom). Crying is a release and/or exercise for infant. One or two periods a day of 5-10 minutes is normal for most infants. Assist parents to develop positive, relaxed approach. Reassure and support parents in this time of stress. Suggest parents alternate infant care and alternate meeting infant demands.
Constipation	Consistency of stool which is hard, pebbly, rocklike. Not related to frequency, straining, grunting or number of days between stools. Ascertain color, consistency and frequency as well as presence of blood or mucus. Review infant diet and verify parent perception of constipation and expectation of normal stool patterns.	Discuss normal elimination/stool patterns for type of feeding method (i.e., breast-fed stools versus bottle-fed stools). Reassure that straining, grunting, infrequent number are normal. Reinforce that each infant has individual stool pattern and educate parents about *what* constipation actually is (i.e., consistency). Discuss parents' attitude regarding toilet habits and expectations about stool patterns. If constipated, increase liquids in diet; may offer water between meals. If introduced to solids too early or in too large a quantity, discontinue use until constipation clears, then begin again with smaller amounts. If appropriate for feeding stage, add prunes (up to 3 tb.) or prune juice to diet.
Flatus	Air in stomach or intestines causing abdominal distress, distension, and discomfort, frequently expelled through anus. May be caused by excess swallowing of air, overfeeding, underfeeding, or allergy. Ascertain details about feeding (i.e., frequency and size of nipple, type bottle used, breast-feeding technique, maternal diet, use of pacifier, propping of bottle, burping, etc.).	Burp frequently during and after feedings. See first section. Calm infant when crying and burp after crying. Place on left side to ease expelling of gas. If suspect allergies, try soy formula or elimination diet. Reassure parents. May offer water between feedings—5-10 cc may increase gastric mobility.
Hiccoughs	Sudden sharp involuntary spasms of diaphragm, usually occur following a meal.	Reassure patient that infant will cry if truly distressed. Offer infant something to suck (pacifier, breast, bottle with warm water).
Pacifier	Infants demonstrate a need for nonnutritional sucking.	Assist parents to understand aspects of positive and negative use of pacifier. Positive use: indicated immediately after birth before newborn can manipulate thumb into mouth; assists

E.5   Common Concerns and Problems of First Year (Neonate and Infant)—cont'd

Problem or concern	Assessment	Nursing intervention
		in developing sucking function; contributes to establishment of breast-feeding; good means of satisfying sucking need, especially for bottle-fed infants who need extra sucking time; does not usually become a habit unless child sucks beyond infancy; most infants substitute thumb for pacifier around 3 to 4 months. Parents should look for clues to eliminate pacifier use at this time and provide stimulation suitable for the age.
		Negative use: pacifiers do not replace holding; stimulation, or needs satisfaction; pacifiers should not be used constantly, especially before tending to infant's needs; parents should be encouraged to discontinue use by 5 months since continued use may become a hard habit to overcome.
		If thumb is substituted, generally it is used less frequently than pacifier.
Spoiling	Ascertain parent definition of spoiling. Generally it is the result of basic needs not being met in early infancy leading to a demanding, undisciplined child because need for gratification continues beyond normal time. Overgratification usually occurs then. Generally it is believed that infants cannot be spoiled under 6 months of age.	Parents require counseling and education that reinforces the following: Early infant needs must be gratified. A child cannot handle frustrations well until 8-9 months and is unable to delay gratification of needs until this age. A gradual and gentle approach to limits and delaying gratification is best. A relaxed, positive approach is helpful. Parents often find support groups helpful in dealing with this problem.
Biting	In first year, frequently related to teething. Particularly a problem for breast-feeding mothers. In toddlerhood related to normal aggressive impulses.	If related to teething, see later section on teething for alleviation of discomfort. Breast-feeding mothers should remove infant from breast at every occurrence and may accompany with a "no"; should also allow time to lapse before finishing feeding. If related to impulsivity of toddlerhood, see first section of table on p. 995.
Separation anxiety	Occurs at 9-10 months as infant is learning to differentiate self from mother. Can occur again in toddlerhood as child is learning to distance and separate self from mother in attempt to establish autonomy.	Reassure mother that this is normal developmental process. Advise parents, especially mother, to do the following: Play "peek-a-boo" games. Allow sufficient time (30-45 minutes for child to acquaint him/herself with new person (i.e., visitor, babysitter). Avoid "sneaking out." Tell child firmly that "mommy leaves, mommy comes back." Reinforce this with "peek-a-boo" or "hide and seek" games. Avoid making major changes in child's or household routines during this period (i.e., mother returning to work; changing child's room; changing regular babysitter or day care situation, etc.).
Stranger anxiety	Begins at 6-8 months, gradually diminishing by 18 months. Process of child development.	See preceding section on separation anxiety. Advise parents, particularly mother, to hold infant in presence of strangers. If infant is to be left, mother should spend a short time with stranger.

Continued.

E.5   Common Concerns and Problems of First Year (Neonate and Infant)—cont'd

Problem or concern	Assessment	Nursing intervention
Infant sleep patterns	Some infants have difficulty releasing into sleep or awaken easily. Separation anxiety, teething, illness are among the common causes. Ascertain history of problem to include how long infant sleeps, what feeding schedule is, bedtime and household routines, presence of illness or teething, and how problem is handled.	Counseling should be directed toward education of parents; infants need gratification and normal sleep patterns, emphasizing the following: Differences in temperament and incidence of sleep problems can be related. Infants generally sleep through the night by 6 months. Infant may need help transitioning to sleep by rocking, holding, pacifier, walking, etc., but should be put to bed drowsy, but awake Environment and atmosphere conducive to sleep, (e.g., quiet, dim) should be provided. If sleep problem is related to a physical problem, measures to remedy should be implemented.
Teething	Eruption of primary or deciduous teeth starting at about 6 months usually with lower incisors. Will continue every 2 months for first 2 years. Signs may include, but are not always present: red, swollen gums; irritable; crying and rubbing gums. Since other events in infant development are occurring simultaneously, nursing must assist parents to distinguish between these and teething as follows: Drooling, which normally occurs at 3-4 months and has little to do with teething, although it may persist throughout teething. Fevers do not usually accompany teething. Must be assessed separately because maternal antibody protection is diminishing and presence of fever is suspect for infectious process. Separation anxiety, sleep disturbances, or fussiness from other causes are all common developmental symptoms associated with infant age group, as is reaching for and mouthing objects.	Recommend to parents hard, clean objects for baby to chew on, such as rubber teething rings, or beads, hard rubber toys, cool spoon, teething biscuits or pretzels, etc. Parents should avoid use of teething toys or rings filled with liquid because plastic covers are easily broken and liquid can be ingested.
Diaper rashes	Rashes of varying types occurring in diaper area. Persistent rashes that do not respond to home management or continue to occur in spite of preventive measures should be referred for medical evaluation. Home management of diaper rash:	Preventive measures to keep area clean, dry, and aerated: Frequent diaper changing. Cleansing with water (and mild cleaner after bowel movement) at each changing, dry area well. Thick diapers and/or absorbent pads are recommended; plastic or rubber pants are not suggested. A *thin* film of protection may be used, such as A and D ointment, petroleum jelly, zinc oxide. Remove diapers for short periods every day. Wash diapers well as follows: 1. Soak soiled diapers in Borateen or borax solution (½ cup to 1 gallon of water). 2. Prerinse before washing. 3. Wash in full cycle with mild soap such as Ivory, Dreft, or Lux. 4. Avoid softeners and strong detergents. 5. Rinse diapers 2-3 times, and may be added ¼ to ½ cup vinegar to final rinse. 6. Dry in sun if possible. Follow preventive measures with emphasis on leaving diaper off more frequently, changing when wet, and cleaning area thoroughly during changes.

E.5   Common Concerns and Problems of First Year (Neonate and Infant)—cont'd

Problem or concern	Assessment	Nursing intervention
		Zinc oxide ointment often is helpful in checking early nonfungal rashes. Cornstarch is never recommended for rashes or their prevention. Seek medical help if rash worsens or does not improve.
Cradle cap	Form of seborrheic dermatitis in neonate characterized by scalping, flaking of scalp skin, especially over anterior fontanelle. May persist beyond neonate into infancy period.	Preventive measures: Teach parents how to shampoo infant head and recommend shampooing every other day. Reassure that vigorous scrubbing will not injure fontanelle or skull. Home management for mild cases: Shampoo head daily with warm water and soap, using firm pressure on scalp. Loosen cap by applying mineral or baby oil to scalp 15-20 minutes before shampooing. Remove with shampoo. Comb scalp with fine comb to loosen and dislodge scaly cap. Severe cases will require medical attention and are generally managed with nonsalicylate antiseborrheic shampoos.

PROBLEMS RELATED TO FEEDING

Problem or concern	Assessment	Nursing intervention
Parental concerns about overfeeding or underfeeding	Some parents find it difficult to determine appropriate amount of milk and/or solid food to give infant. Ascertain parent understanding, knowledge, and perceptions through the following: Diet history Height and weight measurement and charting on growth curve. Elimination habits and description.	Assist parents to construct a workable feeding schedule. Discuss normal feeding patterns for breast- and bottle-fed infants (see discussion in this chapter). Discuss infant need for nonnutrient sucking. Convey that infants will eat more than they need or require if food is offered at each cry. Offer water between feedings to postpone next feeding to reasonable time. Suggest schedule of solid food introduction (Appendix E.9, p. 1012). Reassure parents that if infant is gaining weight he is not underfed. Explain growth and appetite spurts.
Refusal of solids	Infant may refuse new foods for a number of reasons, e.g., temperature, texture, manner presented by person feeding, or too early introduction. Ascertain through diet history which foods accepted, and likes and dislikes, and parental feelings and perception regarding solid foods.	Discuss normal feeding patterns for age. Review indications for starting or not starting solid foods; No need before 4-6 months. Digestion begins with salivation around 4 months. Feeding of solid foods is not necessarily related to sleeping through the night. Tongue thrusting of solid food is normal and not a refusal. Discuss ways to encourage solid food acceptance: Allow infant to feed self. Avoid forcing infant to eat since this will only increase resistance. Solids may be stopped for a while, offering only ones that infant likes. Offer solid foods before milk when infant is hungriest. Offer food in calm positive manner.

Continued.

Problem or concern	Assessment	Nursing intervention

PROBLEMS RELATED TO FEEDING—cont'd

Problem or concern	Assessment	Nursing intervention
Refusal of food and variations in appetite	Once solid foods have been introduced and established, infants and especially toddlers will go through periods of refusal, pickiness, and preference. Obtain diet history as reviewed in preceding section (Refusal of solids).	See preceding section (Refusal of solids). Discuss following with parents: Refusal may be due to loss of interest in food when more active or due to form of negativism and means to control. Avoid use of food as substitute for attention or stimulation. Some degree of refusal and variation in appetite is normal for age. Try following approaches: Offer small amounts food frequently. Emphasize favorite foods as much as possible. Use as few nonnutritive foods as possible. Allow child to feed self if child desires to, and provide finger foods. Be patient as child tries to master use of utensils. Eating should be an enjoyable and sociable time. If hunger does not permit infant to wait until family dinner time, feed before and offer nibbles during family meal. Give older infant and toddler place, chair, utensils, plate at the table.
Spitting up	Regurgitation commonly following a feeding. Usually related to air swallowed with food, inability to relax esophageal sphincter, possible overfeeding, allergy to milk, gastroesophageal reflux. Ascertain nature of regurgitation (frequency, amount, color, consistency, etc.) as well as diet history and data regarding weight gain. Frequently outgrown by time infant is sitting well in upright position.	Reinforce the following with parents: Correct preparation of formula. Use of appropriate size nipple and nipple hole. Regular and frequent burping is needed. Place infant in an upright position for 30 minutes after feeding. Correct position of infant during feeding. Determine need to change method of feeding or formula.
Weaning	A transition of feeding methods. May be from bottle to cup or from breast to bottle and/or cup. Weaning from breast is difficult if parents (especially mother) have ambivalent feelings or if infant refuses alternative methods. Ascertain who wants baby weaned and why, as well as schedule of feedings. Weaning from bottle should be attempted gradually, when child is ready, usually around 1 year. Ascertain who wants child weaned, what has been tried, feeding schedule and number of bottles, and ability to use cup. Babies often begin to lose interest in one or two bottles between 9-12 months. Offering a cup at that time may ease weaning.	Assist parents to make decision to wean: Should be discussed and decided by both parents. Positive attitude toward weaning is essential, especially for breast-feeding mothers. Weaning at times of separation anxiety is not advised, especially in breast-fed infants. If possible, an infant should be weaned from breast to cup. This avoids having to wean from bottle later on. Active weaning for breast-feeding mothers: Start by substituting bottle or cup for breast at one feeding and allow 5-6 days before substituting second breast feeding. If resistance is encountered, try giving water or juice in bottle or cup before weaning starts, using nipple similar to breast or pacifier if one is used, heating milk before offering, and having someone other than mother offer bottle or cup. Keep to a schedule and be firm, positive, and patient. Active weaning to cup: continue preceding steps with following additions: Reinforce idea of accomplishment in using a cup to child. May give one bottle a day but should contain only water to avoid incidence of dental caries. Avoid forcing child to wean; forcing use of cup may increase need to suck. Calm, relaxed, positive approach is essential.

E.6 COMMON CONCERNS AND PROBLEMS OF TODDLER AND PRESCHOOL YEARS

Problem and assessment	Nursing intervention

AGGRESSIVE AND NEGATIVE BEHAVIORS
Biting and Hitting

Temporary behaviors occurring as a result of normal aggressive impulses and most frequently happening in new or difficult situations, when tired or hungry or frustrated or when expectations are too high in terms of social behaviors (ability to play with peers); used as a means of asserting control or power.

Reassure parents that behaviors are normal; discuss development and tasks child is trying to accomplish.
Advise parents to:
Avoid retaliation by hitting or biting back.
Cup chin or hold hand giving reminder that biting and/or hitting is unacceptable.
Anticipate circumstances in which behaviors occur and circumvent them.
Use limits, such as isolation, if helpful.
Limit playmates and playtime to what is reasonable for child and his age.
Allow child and playmate to work out difficulties as much as possible, redirecting their play when necessary.

Verbal Negativism

Use of the word "no" as means of control in striving for independence; often used indiscriminately and inappropriately.

Advise parents to:
Offer child a choice when possible, making alternatives simple.
Avoid bargaining and arguments.
If no choice is available, do not offer one—approach with a matter-of-fact attitude.
Develop strategy for times when child will choose and then change his mind.

Temper Tantrums

Developmental behavior directed at gaining control; Frequently triggered by unmet needs (tired, hungry), frustration and/or overgratification and need for limits; ascertain when tantrums occur and how they are handled.

Management by parents should be directed at finding cause and prevention; counseling is directed toward approaches to discipline and limit setting (see section on discipline) and the following:
Discussion of child's needs for limits at this age.
Diary can be kept to identify pattern when tantrums occur.
Intervention is made before tantrum begins.
Should tantrum occur, possible approaches include the following:
Calm, matter-of-fact approach by parents.
Isolation of child by removal to neutral place until control is achieved (time-out).
Hold child until control is achieved, possibly offering substitute for desired object or activity that triggered tantrum.
Discourage use of corporal punishment (spanking) to achieve control.

DISCIPLINE

Discipline is guidance offered by parents to assist child in demonstrating correct, acceptable safe behaviors; discipline is based on the parent's concepts, feelings, and attitudes regarding desirable behaviors and rules of conduct for them; mechanisms of discipline will set limits and control undesirable behaviors.

Advise parents regarding different approaches to discipline:
Permissiveness
Overpermissiveness
Authoritarianism.
Advise parents that setting limits should permit self-respect and protection of parent and child integrity; parents should be aware that discipline is essential to healthy growth.
Parent techniques include the following:
Set examples of desirable behaviors (honesty, unselfishness, good manners).
Be fair, clear, and consistent.
Agree on methods of discipline.
Give simple clear directions; bend a little by giving warnings.

Compiled by Nancy Dickenson-Hazard, RN, CPNP, MSN, for the 3rd edition of this text.

Continued.

E.6   Common Concerns and Problems of Toddler and Preschool Years—cont'd

Problem and assessment	Nursing intervention
DISCIPLINE—cont'd	Allow child to express feelings. Respect your child; be sure to praise, show approval, and encourage. Be realistic in behaviors expected. Avoid arguing, threatening, promising, sermonizing, over-permissiveness, and an overauthoritarian manner. Discipline (punishing the act).

PUNISHMENT
A method of controlling behaviors when limits are exceeded and based on child being made to feel responsible for misdeed; child will eventually learn to inhibit impulse to commit act; punishment may be verbal, restrictive, or physical and should always be appropriate to the act; punishment should not be the result of parent loss of temper.
	Advise parents to:
	   Allow a cooling-off period.
	   Direct anger at situation or act, not child.
	   Avoid retaliation by hitting, belittling, sarcasm, ridicule, humiliation, or shame.
	   Avoid sending to bed or going without food.
	   Avoid depriving child of love.
	Review points discussed in discipline section.

BREATHHOLDING Characterized by child holding breath and turning blue. May occur with episode of anger or crying. It has a high familial incidence. Ascertain circumstances that trigger episodes and how handled by parents.	Counseling directed toward guidance and education regarding parent-child relationship; parents will need reassurance and support as they attempt to ignore breathholding in an attempt to prevent child satisfaction in gaining control. See section on discipline.

ROCKING, HEAD BANGING, BED SHAKING
Forms of self-stimulation frequently occurs at bedtime; ascertain how child's needs are met.
	Counseling directed toward advising parents regarding:
	   Gratification of needs.
	   Provision of comfort and extra stimulation time.
	   Provision of relaxed, calm atmosphere through holding, singing, music.

MASTURBATION A normal reaction, which is an exploration of body that results in stimulation of pleasurable sexual feelings; generally occurs at bedtime and starts accidentally becoming more purposeful and frequent around 4 years. Ascertain frequency, how parents handle, and their attitude and feelings.	Advise parents that masturbation is normal and that censoring of open masturbation is appropriate; otherwise parents should convey to child that they are aware of and understand the behavior. Avoidance of placing excessive importance on masturbation, which may only encourage it; it is best to ignore it and/or set limits as appropriate to situation. A punitive attitude should be avoided.
PERSISTENT THUMB SUCKING A form of self-comfort occurring in times of stress or as a habit and persisting beyond 3-4 years; generally sporadic sucking is harmless and regular sucking until 2 or 3 is considered normal.	Assist parents to identify source of stress and ways to alleviate it. Reassure and support parents when thumb sucking is within normal range. Suggest parents remove fingers or thumb from mouth after asleep. Suggest parents avoid constant nagging and reminding; pulling thumb from mouth; and use of restraints. Contracting with child, rewarding alternate behaviors, and bad-tasting nail treatments may be useful to diminish thumb sucking.
FEEDING-RELATED PROBLEMS **Loss of Variations of Appetite; Refusal of Food** Common problems related to: "too busy to eat," development of food preferences; a normal decrease in amount of food required and/or an attempt to control and assert independence.	See Chapter 27 for anticipatory guidance.

E.6   Common Concerns and Problems of Toddler and Preschool Years—cont'd

Problem and assessment	Nursing intervention

SLEEP-RELATED PROBLEMS

Nightmares

Problems may follow a tiring, busy day, be associated with illness, or be the result of working things out in dreams.

Nightmares are frightening dreams that awaken child who feels fear and helplessness; they generally occur as a result of increased aggressive urges.

Review normal sleep patterns with parents (see Chapter 27).

Reassure parents that dreams and terrors are normal and tend to disappear spontaneously.

Parents should comfort child when awakened by dream—may attempt to explain why they are not "real."

Parents should avoid making a fuss over these sleep problems.

Night Terrors

These are dreams, generally frightening in nature, from which a child does not awaken; after acting out dream and/or a period of disorientation, child returns to sleep.

TOILET TRAINING

Achievement of control over bodily elimination; development of habits that make child self-sufficient in toileting; parents need to understand child's development and readiness before instituting a toilet training regime (see following); parent must ascertain attitude and expectations regarding toilet training as well as measures previously used.

Direct counseling toward parental understanding of realistic expectations, readiness of child, types of toilet training, and frequent problems encountered

Types of toilet training:

A. Early training from ages 10-15 months; points to emphasize:
   1. Child is not physiologically able to use toilet at this age.
   2. Parents may be ready to train child, but they will be the ones who will have to pick up signals, put child on toilet, undress and dress, etc.; therefore, they should be highly motivated.
   3. Bowel training may be accomplished but accidents will happen and will be due to trainer (parent), not trainee (child).
   4. Training should not be stressful for parent or child.
B. Training at 18-30 months; points to emphasize:
   1. Review readiness signs and check off which ones child has accomplished. If the majority has been achieved, probably appropriate to start training
   2. Select a good time, such as:
      When there are no major changes in household and child has shown some interest after observing others.
      When nursery school friends are trained.
      When child is aware of wet and dirty versus dry and clean.
   3. Select a method and stick to it.
   4. Training should not be stressful; if child resists it is best to forget for awhile then try again.
   5. Accomplishment of training is variable; it may be a few days or several weeks or months.
   6. Parents need to develop a relaxed, positive attitude.
   7. Alternative methods include:
      Placing child on own potty chair at given intervals during the day.
      Placing child on potty before elimination is expected.
      Placing child on potty when parent goes.
      Always positively reinforce a successful attempt.
C. "Natural" toilet training (children training themselves), points to emphasize:
   1. Toileting is brought to child's attention when readiness is indicated.
   2. Child handles situation by himself.
   3. Child needs to know parents are willing to help.
   4. Although enjoying a sense of independence and accomplishment, child also needs limits set at this age.

Indicators of readiness to toilet train	Approximate age (yr)
1. Manipulates sphincter muscles	1½-2
2. Manual dexterity needed to manipulate clothing	2-2½
3. Can hold urine for up to 4 to 5 hours	2-2½
4. Can understand simple directions	1½-2
5. Can communicate needs using words or gestures	1½-2
6. Developed a sense of self	1-2
7. Demonstrates trust in mother and desire to please	1½-2
8. Demonstrates sense of independence and a desire to do for self	2-2½
9. Is proud of own accomplishments	2-2½
10. Demonstrates behavioral control	2-2½

Continued.

E.6   Common Concerns and Problems of Toddler and Preschool Years—cont'd

Problem and assessment	Nursing intervention
TOILET TRAINING—cont'd	Problems are frequently encountered; reassure parents about naturalness, normalcy, and transient nature of these problems: 1. Problem with sitting or standing for boys; suggest starting training with sitting progressing to standing. 2. Problem using large toilet; suggest potty chair with portable seat, which can be taken on excursions. 3. Regression; suggest reinforcing as little as possible; depending on severity may require going back to diapers for a while. 4. Need help with wiping; suggest allowing child to try if wants to clean self. 5. Being able to communicate toilet needs to others; suggest parents make sure other caretakers are aware of child's progress in training, how he communicates need, what words and what degree of independence have been achieved. 6. Child does not wish to flush bowel movements; suggest this point not be emphasized; flush toilet later. 7. Playing with feces; suggest play with clay or fingerpaints; parent should matter-of-factly state displeasure when this occurs.

E.7   COMMON BEHAVIORS OF SCHOOL-AGE CHILD AND ADOLESCENT

Behavior	Development	Guidance
SCHOOL-AGE		
Cheating	Testing right and wrong; generally follow parents' rules and authority but may succumb to peer pressure to "break rules"; becoming more aware of their parents' "cheating" in different ways.	Assist parents to: Reinforce positive "good" behaviors. Maintain limits and discipline standards. Recognize that most children confess or are caught and that disciplinary action must be immediate. Identify what prompted cheating.
Lying	Differentiating between fantasies and realities; use of untruth to avoid the unpleasant; becoming more aware of parents not always telling the truth.	Confront and assess problem with assistance from teacher and involvement of child Reassure child that a real world of absolute truthfulness does not exist. Point out to child untruths that are fantasies, emphasizing the real component. Use discipline for act and discuss meaning of untruths. Reinforce honest behaviors positively.
Stealing	Curiosity about other possessions; continue to learn and internalize concept of "mine" versus "yours"; not easy to resist temptations; limited idea of property.	Act as role model; respect child's property and spouse's property; ask before use. Reinforce concept of property and ownership verbally as well as behaviorally. Discipline for petty acts, (e.g., have child return or pay back item; use verbal disapproval). Assess, help, and seek referral if problem is persistent.

Compiled by Nancy Dickenson-Hazard, RN, CPNP, MSN, for the 3rd edition of this text.

E.7 Common Behaviors of School-Age Child and Adolescent—cont'd

Behavior	Development	Guidance
SCHOOL-AGE—cont'd		
Fighting	More boys than girls fight; siblings usually fight; an attempt to establish position for self; may be result of frustration.	Act as role model; parents who verbally and physically fight indicate behavior is acceptable. Establish behaviors that are acceptable vents for frustration and anger. Emphasize the need to share, exchange, and interact in positive manner. Separate siblings when fighting; then allow them to work out differences once composure is regained. Avoid condoning physical assault as a means of retaliation with peers; assist child to find other solutions. Discover reason for fighting if it is continual.
Scatology	Uses dirty words as means of attention and testing parents; frequently has no understanding of meaning.	Set an example; do not use dirty words in front of child. Indicate unacceptability of dirty words; remind when child uses. Avoid a struggle, argument, or excessive discipline unless profound problem exists. Seek help if persistent.
Fears	Often learned from parents; indicative of struggle to cope with unknown or unpleasant experience; may be result of learning right from wrong.	Deal with each fear separately. Avoid overemphasis of own fear. Identify what specifically about situation evokes fear. Reassure child; reinforce that some fears are healthy and protective in nature. Seek help if fears interfere with daily life.
ADOLESCENT		

Moodiness/noncommunicative	Result of emotional conflicts of establishing an identity, developing sexually, and worries over body image and social relationships.	Assist adolescent and parents to:
		    Feel reassured about normalcy of wanting to be alone, mood swings, and fears.
		    Recognize and discuss family conflicts and possible solutions.
		    Recognize and discuss importance of communication and need to validate feelings.

Preoccupation with body image and sexuality	Physical changes are dramatic; need to be the same as peers; sexual fantasies and erotic urges and behaviors are heightened with physiological changes.	Recognize normalcy of feelings and preoccupation. Understand normal physical growth, physiological changes, and individual patterns. Accept self; develop constructive coping behaviors (e.g., sublimate into activity; need to verbalize feelings). Identify other resources of information: courses at school, books, etc. Encourage physical activity as tension release.
Rebellion	Need to establish own value and belief system.	Alleviate conflicts through open communication and validation of feelings. Role-play and offer reflective feedback to each other. Focus on individual needs and place value and pressure from others in perspective.

Continued.

E.7   Common Behaviors of School-Age Child and Adolescent—cont'd

Behavior	Development	Guidance
ADOLESCENT—cont'd		
Conformity	Need for allegiance and belonging; assists in challenge of authority and developing of self; serves as validation mechanism.	Reinforce positive aspects of peer group and what is taught by them. Recognize normalcy of need. Find solutions when conformity interferes with adolescent's and family's goals.
Inferiority feelings	Result of feelings of loneliness and being different when unable to conform to peer group.	Relate importance of social involvement to individual goals. Explore interest and participation in after-school activities. Recognize feelings about self (what he or she likes and dislikes and what are desired changes). Identify solutions to problem behaviors identified.
Poor study habits	May result from disinterest, preoccupation, excessive parent expectations.	Identify cause of poor habits; may need remedial help or assistance in developing constructive habits. Avoid nagging or conflict over issue. Identify constructive solutions. Identify feelings and attitudes. Discuss individual goals, methods of meeting goals as related to ability and consequences.
Ambivalence	An attempt to identify dependent versus independent needs; reflects conflict between parental rules and own wishes.	Identify conflict and possible solutions. Maintain a system of accountability for behavior and compliance with rules of system. Deal with feelings constructively (e.g., verbally, physical exercise). Recognize importance and normalcy of behavior.

E.8   HEALTH PROBLEMS OF SCHOOL-AGE CHILD AND ADOLESCENT

Health problem	Etiology	Incidence	Assessment	Management	Prevention
Acne	Sebaceous glands over produce sebum, which occludes skin pores.	70% of adolescents experience acne.	Noninflamed comedones or inflammed papules, pustules and nodulocystic lesions on face, neck, upper chest, back, and shoulders; hair and skin are often oily.	Use of benzoyl peroxide agent; more severe cases may require retinoic acid and/or antibiotics; thorough cleansing of the skin two or three times a day using warm water and a mild soap; drying and peeling lotions may be used overnight; avoid exposure to sun and wind; frequent shampooing of the scalp; proper diet with added liquids; no diet restrictions are indicated, but	No known prevention but severity of symptoms can be reduced with appropriate management.

Compiled by Nancy Dickenson-Hazard, RN, CPNP, MSN, for the 3rd edition of this text.

E.8   Health Problems of School-Age Child and Adolescent—cont'd

Health problem	Etiology	Incidence	Assessment	Management	Prevention
				should the adolescent feel a certain food aggravates the acne, it should be avoided; avoid greasy make-up, powder is better.	
Impetigo	Superficial skin lesion invaded by staphylococci or streptococci, spread by direct contact with incubation of 2-10 days.		Appearance of discolored spots that form vesicles or bullae; these vesicles break and form yellow, honey-colored seropurulent lesions. Most frequently on hands, face, or perineum and accompanied by regional lymphadenopathy. Culture fluid from lesion or at base of lesion.	Topical treatment with Bacitracin or neomycin ointment after soaking with warm compresses. Systemic antibiotic if numerous lesions are present. Follow-up if not improved within 3 days.	Teach child not to pick or scratch insect bites, healing lesions, etc. Keep nails short and clean. Frequent handwashing. Isolate child's washing and bed linen, drinking glass, and clothes. Inspect other family members. Adequate rest and nutrition.
Cellulitis	Bacterial invasion of skin (both dermis and subcutaneous tissue) caused by *Staphylococcus aureus*, group A *betahemolytic streptococcus*, or *Hemophilus influenza*. Less communicable than impetigo but suspect throughout infection; more apt to lead to septicemia.	Frequently a secondary infection to impetigo or other skin lesions.	Warm tender, erythematous, swollen, and indurated area on skin. Lymphangitis seen on extremities. Fever, malaise, lymphadenopathy often present.	Warm compresses. Immobilization of affected part. Rest and symptomatic measures. Systemic antibiotic therapy.	Prevention as for impetigo. All family members should be cultured and those with positive cultures treated.
Reye Syndrome	Acute encephalopathy may be sequelae of influenzae or varicella and is linked to aspirin use with viral illnesses.	Typical age of onset is 6-8 years of age. Incidence has declined in the past 10-15 years.	Characterized by encephalopathy, severe brain edema, increased intracranial pressure, hypoglycemia, and fatty infiltration of liver.	Immediate hospitalization and medical treatment of neurologic symptoms.	Educate parents and particularly school-age and adolescent children to eliminate use of aspirin for self-treatment of viral illnesses; develop school and/or community program about Reye syndrome, its

E.8   Health Problems of School-Age Child and Adolescent—cont'd

Health problem	Etiology	Incidence	Assessment	Management	Prevention
					prevention and early recognition.
Streptococcal pharyngitis	*Group A-beta hemolytic streptococcus.*	Increased incidence in winter and spring. 30%-50% of cases appear in school-age children. At risk for complications of cervical adenitis, otitis media, peritonsillar abscess, sinusitis, acute glomerulonephritis, acute rheumatic fever.	Must differentiate from viral pharyngitis. Obtain throat culture.	10-day course of appropriate antibiotic when strep confirmed by culture. Symptomatic treatment for fever reduction; normal saline gargles, hard sour candy for sore throat; hot or cold compresses for tender cervical nodes.	Culture all symptomatic exposed family contacts. Avoid contact with infected child and his eating/drinking utensils. Education regarding illness and necessity of full treatment course of medication.
Toxic shock syndrome	*Staphylococcus aureus* is causative agent, with use of super absorbant tampons a significant contributing factor.	42% of cases are adolescents.	Sudden onset of fever, headache, sore throat, nausea, vomiting, and diarrhea, abdominal pain, hypotension, rash, arthralgia and desquamation of soles and palms.	Immediate hospitalization, antibiotics, and monitoring and treatment of shock.	Counseling to avoid use of tampons; if must use tampons, use regular not superabsorbant and change every 3-4 hours; use sanitary pads at night; Employ general genitourinary hygiene measures.
Tuberculosis	Communicated through sputum and cough spray of infected person. Causative organism are *Mycobacterium tuberculosis* and M. *bovis.* Incubation range is 2-10 weeks.	Most at risk in first 3 years and the second year preceding puberty. For children of all ages, an average of 4000 new cases are reported annually. Predisposing factors include state of health and nutrition; age; environmental and socioeconomic circumstances (crowding, poor sanitation); virulence and number of bacilli.	Development of overt symptoms occurs in small percentage. Demonstrated systemic hypersensitivity as evidenced by positive skin test. Chest x-ray to determine presence and extent of active lesions. Sputum smears.	Rest, adequate diet, and gradual return to normal activity; prevention of other infection. Drug therapy. Counseling and support.	Screening tests, particularly for at-risk population. Identify, screen, and treat contacts. Hygiene and sputum precautions/measures.

E.8   Health Problems of School-Age Child and Adolescent—cont'd

Health problem	Etiology	Incidence	Assessment	Management	Prevention
Urinary tract infections	Bacteria enter urinary tract through urethra.	5%-10% of girls and 1% of boys experience a UTI before 18 years.	History of signs and symptoms: urgency, frequency, burning, dribbling, foul-smelling urine, fever, irritability, GI symptoms; *may be asymptomatic.*	Medication course based on causative organism, age, weight of child, sensitivity of organism to drug and previous occurrences.	
	Predisposing factors include: Short female urethra. Obstruction. Foreign body. Poor hygiene and/or fecal contamination. Incomplete bladder emptying resulting in urine stasis. Chemical irritants. Pinworms. Indwelling catheter or catheterization. Sexual intercourse. Pregnancy.	More frequent in girls than boys.	Laboratory signs: bacteria on clean-catch urine culture of greater than 100,000 colonies of a single bacteria per ml of urine confirms infection in symptomatic child.	Medications frequently used: Sulfisoxazole (Gantrisin). Ampicillin Nitrofurantoin (Furadantin). Cephalexin (Keflex).	Hygiene education: Wipe front to back. Frequent voiding (3-4 hours) with complete bladder emptying. Avoid bubble baths and harsh detergents. Use cotton versus nylon panties. Avoid tight clothing. Adequate fluid intake.
	Causative organisms: *Escherichia coli* accounts for 80% to 85% of cases. Gram-positive organisms (*Staphylococcus aureus*). *Klebsiella, enterobacteria, Pseudomonas,* and *Proteus* species.			Increased fluid and rest.	Prompt attention for recurrent symptoms.
				Symptomatic measures for generalized signs. Follow-up is essential: Urine culture 48-72 hours after medication is instituted.	

Continued.

E.8   Health Problems of School-Age Child and Adolescent—cont'd

Health problem	Etiology	Incidence	Assessment	Management	Prevention
				Urine culture on completion of medication. Further follow-up includes radiographic studies and regular urine cultures.	
Osteomyelitis	Causative organisms are *Staphylococcus aureus* in older children and *Haemophilus* in younger children; organisms may enter directly to bone or through a preexisting infection.	Occurs most frequently between the ages of 5 and 14 years and more commonly in boys than girls.	Frequently a history of trauma usually localized tenderness, warmth and redness with pain on movement. Laboratory signs: marked leukocytes, elevated erythrocyte sedimentation rate, and positive blood culture.	Antibiotic therapy for 3-4 weeks; complete bedrest and immobilization.	Prompt attention to penetrating injuries or suspect skin lesions. Proper treatment and hygiene of injuries and skin lesions.

PARASITIC INFECTIONS

Health problem	Etiology	Incidence	Assessment	Management	Prevention
Scabies	Caused by parasite, female mite that burrows into stratum corneum of skin and lays eggs in the tunnel. Transmitted by direct contact with infected person; can be contracted from infected bedding and clothing.	Pandemic in United States since 1974.	Vesicular or papulo-vesicular rash occurring typically on genitals, buttocks, between fingers and in folds of wrist, elbows, armpits, and at beltline. Appear as fine wavy line; gray to pink in color. Pruritus. Skin scrapings from over lesion reveal mite presence under microscope.	Scabicide applied to affected areas; one application is generally sufficient. Clothing and bedding should be washed.	Avoid contact with infected person's bedding and clothing. Family members should do self-skin inspection.
Tinea capitis (scalp), corporis (body), pedis (foot)	Fungal infection easily transmitted among children. Most frequently caused by Trichophyton tonsurans.	Permanent baldness may occur with severe capitis.	Capitis: bald patches with erythema, gray scaling, and crusting. Corporis: macule that enlarges peripherally, healing in center to present as scaly, circular lesions found on face, upper extremities, and trunk; may have mild pruritus.	Capitis: griseofulvin—follow-up cultures should be done. Corporis: tolnaftate (Tinactin) 1% solution or cream. Pedis: tolnaftate (Tinactin) solution or cream and Desenex or Tinactin powder prophylactically.	Capitis: avoid exchange of head gear; avoid/treat infected animal; wash scalp after haircuts; avoid use of infected person's personal care articles. Corporis: preceding plus avoiding exchange of clothing and community

Health problem	Etiology	Incidence	Assessment	Management	Prevention
PARASITIC INFECTIONS—cont'd					
			Pedis: vesicular eruptions with skin maceration between toes. Laboratory procedures: (1) microscopic exam with KOH; (2) ultraviolet light fluoresces Microsporum infections; (3) microscopic culture.		showers or bathing places. Pedis: preceding plus thoroughly dry between toes; use cotton socks and change frequently; wear well ventilated shoes; air feet; wear rubber sandals in community showers.
Pinworms	Ova are swallowed after scratching anal area and transfers fingers to mouth or inhaled from contaminated clothing or linens.	Most common of helminthic parasites in humans.	Nocturnal perianal or vaginal pruritus without systemic symptoms. Worm is seen as a whitish-yellow thread 8-13 mm long. Scotch tape test to confirm diagnosis.	Antihelmintic such as Piperzine citrate, Mebendazole, or Pyrantel pamoate. Clothing and linen should be washed.	Personal hygiene: Handwashing and trimming nails Education regarding transmission.
Pediculosis Capitis (head lice)	Causative agent is parasite, and lice infestations are communicable.	Very common among school children.	Itching of occipital area, behind ears and nape of neck; Diagnosis made by observation of eggs attached to hair shafts, which fluoresce white under wood light.	Application of pediculocidal shampoo, with manual removal of nits.	Wash clothing and bed linen of infected person in hot water; vacuum furniture; wash hair care items with louse shampoo; advise child against sharing hair care items or head coverings.
Insect bites	A variety of stinging and biting insects.	Very common in children of all ages.	Localized erythema, itching and a local wheal are common.	Cool compresses, antipruritic agents, and antihistamines are recommended; removal of stinger.	Wear shoes outside, avoid wooded, overgrown areas; use insect repellants; avoid scratching to prevent secondary infections.
Lyme disease	Causative agents is a spirochete, *Borrelia burdorferi.* Transmitted by tick bite.	High in Northeastern, coastal, Great Lakes, and western states.	Maculopapular rash at tick bite site progressing to an expanded area of erythema; progresses to neurologic and cardiac symptoms if not treated.	Careful removal of tick, pulling out with tweezers close to its mouth. Antibiotic therapy. Monitoring of progressive symptoms.	Avoid wooded, grassy areas; wear light colored clothing for easier visualization of ticks; wear hats, long sleeve shirts tucked inside

Continued.

E.8   Health Problems of School-Age Child and Adolescent—cont'd

Health problem	Etiology	Incidence	Assessment	Management	Prevention
PARASITIC INFECTIONS—cont'd					
					pants and white socks; check thoroughly for ticks if in woods; inspect children everyday if playing outside especially checking head, neck, ears, axilla, naval, buttocks and groin; and use DEET-containing insect repellants approved for children.
DENTAL					
Caries	Progressive lesions of calcified dental tissue characterized by tooth structure loss. Bacteria, carbohydrates, and plaque are definite factors producing tooth decay.	50%-97% of children have 1 or more cavities by 6 years of age. Greatest incidence occurs between 4 to 8 years and 12 to 18 years.	Characterized as discolored areas or actual lesion in fissures of chewing surfaces of teeth. May be visible on inspection. Dental equipment and x-rays most reliable in detecting caries.	Dental referral. Prevention.	Preventive measures: Early institution of dental care and visits. Brushing and flossing after every meal. Water fluoridation; oral supplemental fluoride if indicated; fluoride rinses. Topical fluoride application and use of toothpaste containing fluoride. Limit carbohydrate content of diet.
Malocclusion	Irregularities of tooth alignment and improper fitting of teeth. Causative factors: abnormal jaw alignment; abnormal muscle function; incompatibility of tooth and jaw size creating abnormal spacing, crowding, or teeth irregularities; delayed	Most frequently recognized in early school-age years. Not common in deciduous teeth.	Variation of normal occlusion of top molars meeting firmly on opposing bottom posterior teeth with upper incisors barely overlapping and touching bottom anterior incisors.	Dental referral. Prevention.	Preventive measures: Meeting early sucking needs. Avoidance of prolonged use of bottle over 2 years. Weaning to cup at 1 year to promote jaw and mouth development after sucking.

E.8   Health Problems of School-Age Child and Adolescent—cont'd

Health problem	Etiology	Incidence	Assessment	Management	Prevention
DENTAL—cont'd					
	permanent teeth eruption; prolonged retention of primary teeth; neglected teeth; prolonged occurrence of lip biting, mouth breathing, tongue twisting, teeth grinding, thumb sucking.				Gentle reminder about finger/thumb sucking, lip biting, etc. Remove finger, thumb from mouth when child is sleeping.
Enuresis	Exact cause is not known but potential factors include: delayed development of neuromuscular control, organic causes, deep sleep, and high threshold for nocturnal arousal; psychologic/emotional factors.	Up to 15% of 6- to 7-year olds and 3% of 13- to 14-year olds. Males affected more than females.	Primary: In children who have never achieved bladder control. Secondary: In children who have achieved bladder control for 3-6 months then lose it. Complete history to include: Amount and times of fluid intake. Number of enuretic episodes per week/month. Sleeping patterns. Voiding patterns. Any recent stressful events. Occurrence at home and/or away from home or both. Child's response to enuresis. Emotional atmosphere of home. Details of toilet training. Family history of enuresis. Past medical history. Laboratory tests. Routine urinalysis.	**INITIAL MEASURES** Fluids are restricted after supper. Child voids before bedtime. Before retiring for night, parents should wake child to void. A night light is provided. **CONDITIONING** Enuretone, a moisture-sensitive device that rings an alarm bell upon initiation of wetting, can be used. Imipramine (Tofranil), which exerts an anticholinergic effect on bladder muscle and/or an antidepressant effect on central nervous system, can be used.	Preventive measures: Avoid too early toilet training. Avoid negative reinforcement if accidents happen. Empty bladder before bedtime. Get up at night to void. Decrease fluid intake from dinner time on. Be supportive if accidents happen. Identify stresses child may have and help resolve.

Continued.

E.8   Health Problems of School-Age Child and Adolescent—cont'd

Health problem	Etiology	Incidence	Assessment	Management	Prevention

DENTAL—cont'd

BLADDER TRAINING (A BEHAVIOR MODIFICATION PROCEDURE)

Child drinks large fluid amount during day and retains urine as long as possible.

When child must void, urine is measured and recorded in a daily log.

Dry nights are recorded.

Wall charts are maintained.

Positive reinforcers, such as stars or points, are maintained for advances (e.g., two dry nights, dry all day, breaking record of previous voiding volume).

COUNSELING

Family and child should be encouraged to express feelings about enuresis.

Parents and child should be informed that enuresis is not intentional and is no one's fault.

Punitive or shaming techniques should be avoided.

Explanation of the many variables involved in enuresis is essential for parents and child.

Nurse should assist parents and child to accept problem.

Nurse should help provide support for child.

E.8   Health Problems of School-Age Child and Adolescent—cont'd

E.8   Health Problems of School-Age Child and Adolescent—cont'd

Health problem	Etiology	Incidence	Assessment	Management	Prevention
DENTAL—cont'd					
				Nurse should maintain a positive attitude and assist parents and child to do the same.	
Encopresis	Commonly caused by chronic constipation or psychogenic problems. Fecal incontinence with constipated movements; frequently impactions occur.	Occurs in children over 5 years. Boys affected more frequently than girls.	*Primary*: children have never been toilet trained. *Secondary*: children had established bowel control. Children state they are unaware of having bowel movement. Complete history focusing on patterns of occurrence, bowel habits, and toilet training. Explore psychosocial development for significant factors (i.e., illness, loss, stress).	Removal of fecal impactions by use of enemas. Use of stool softeners. High-residue diet. Counseling and support to child and parents. Establishment of regular bowel routine. Assist parents to help child deal with anxiety. Identify practical solutions (i.e., wear extra underwear) Skin care measures.	Preventive measures: Avoid too early toilet training. Avoid punitive techniques in toilet training. Avoid negative feedback when incontinent. Increase fluid intake. High-residue diet.
EATING DISORDERS					
Anorexia	Psychosomatic disorder that frequently begins with weight reduction diet even though weight is within normal range.	Primarily affects adolescent girls.	Weight loss and refusal of food accompanied by denial of hunger. Definitive diagnostic criteria include (1) loss of at least 25% of original body weight; (2) delay or cessation of menstruation for at least 3 months; and (3) distorted body image.	Frequently requires hospitalization for both anorexic and/or bulimic adolescent.	Promote healthy eating habits and attitudes; early recognition of behavioral indicators, such as: obsessive-compulsive traits; setting of perfectionistic standards for self; neat, clean, well-behaved manner; a general immaturity; and difficulty with peer and social relationships. Other nursing activities include (1) liaison contracts with the client, family, and teritary care management team; (2) provision of

E.8   Health Problems of School-Age Child and Adolescent—cont'd

Health problem	Etiology	Incidence	Assessment	Management	Prevention
EATING DISORDERS—cont'd					
					support and reassurance; and (3) faciliation of home management and follow-up care by assisting the discharged client and family to maintain normal eating patterns through use of a food journal and education about balancing caloric intake requirements and exercise.
Bulimia	Psychosomatic disorder of recurrent episodes of binge eating followed by self-induced vomiting.	Primarily affects adolescent girls.	Rapid consumption of large amounts of high-calorie, easily digested food in a short time period, sudden weight loss or dramatic weight fluctuations are common, dental erosion, electrolyte imbalance, and menstrual irregularities.		See measures under anorexia.
Obesity	Causes are related to organic problem and imbalance between caloric intake and energy expenditure. Influencing factors: Genetic. Activity patterns. Metabolic rate. Number and size of fat cells. Nutritional habits. Attitude about feeding. Quantity of food ingested.	Approximately 10% to 30% of American children are considered obese.	Clinically children with weight 20% above the mean for their age and height are obese with those 10% to 20% over mean defined as overweight. Organic problems must be ruled out. Nutritional status and diet history.	Referral, if organic problem indicated. Weight control or reduction plan that modifies eating habits, reduces caloric intake, increases energy expenditure, and promotes sense of well-being and self-esteem. Early prevention.	Preventive measures: Encourage breast feeding. Avoid overfeeding in infancy/early childhood, including milk. Teach nutritional needs to parents. Encourage healthful eating habits. Avoid extra-caloric foods (sweetened water, candy as reward). Delay early introduction of solids.

E.8   Health Problems of School-Age Child and Adolescent—cont'd

Health problem	Etiology	Incidence	Assessment	Management	Prevention
EATING DISORDERS—cont'd					
					Encourage home-prepared baby foods and meals for older children. Avoid commercially prepared baby dinners and meals for older children. Encourage physical activity.
DEVELOPMENTAL					
Stuttering	Child's advancing mental ability and level of comprehension exceeds vocabulary ability.	Common until 6 years, reversal difficult after 7 years.	Hesitancy or dysfluency in speech pattern.	Avoid helping child to speak; speak clearly to child, avoid rushing child, look at child when speaking, praise fluent speech.	Understand normalcy of dysfluency to age 6, avoid situations where stuttering increases.
PSYCHOSOCIAL					
Latch-key children	Increased number of single-, working-parent families and inadequacy of child-care options.	As many as 10 million children lack adequate adult supervision after school.	Inadequacy of care leaves children vulnerable to injury, delinquent behavior, feeling lonely, isolated, and fearful.	Teach self-help skills to children; develop programs that focus on safety, how to handle telephone calls, answering door, calling parent when arrives at home; explore alternative after-school activities; discuss feelings of loneliness, isolation and fear with child and explore ways to reduce these feelings; promote employer-based day care and after school care; assist parent and child to plan time alone with activities.	

E.9   FEEDING AND NUTRITION GUIDELINES FOR INFANTS

Age	Type of feeding	Specific recommendations
Birth-6 months	Breast-feeding	Most desirable complete diet for first half of year. Requires supplement of iron by 6 months of age (may be accomplished with solid foods). Average number of feedings 6-8 in first 2 weeks, decreasing to 4-5 by 6 months.
	Formula	Iron-fortified commercial formula is a complete food for the first half of the year. Requires fluoride supplements (0.25 mg) when the concentration of fluoride in the drinking water is below 0.3 parts per million (ppm). Average total of 22 oz at 2 weeks; 28-30 oz at 2 months; 32-34-oz at 3 months; 32-38-oz at 6 months. Frequency and amount ranges from 2-3 oz 6-8 times a day at 2 weeks to 5 oz, 5-6 times a day at 2 months to 7-8-oz, 4-5 times a day at 5 months
6-12 months	Solid foods	May begin to add solids by 4-6 months of age; earlier introduction tends to contribute to over-feeding, choking, and allergies. Cereals are offered first. First foods are strained, pureed, or finely mashed. "Finger foods" such as teething crackers, raw fruit, or vegetables can be introduced by 6 to 7 months. Chopped table food or commercially prepared junior foods can be started by 9 to 12 months. With the exception of cereal, the order of introducing foods is variable; a recommended sequence is weekly introduction of other foods, beginning with fruit or vegetables and then meat. As the quantity of solids increases, the amount of formula may be limited to 28-30 oz daily. Solids should be given with a spoon, not in a bottle or "feeder."
	Cereal	Introduce commercially prepared iron-fortified infant cereals, and offer daily until 12-18 months of age. Rice cereal is usually introduced first because of its low allergenic potential.
	Fruits and vegetables	Applesauce, bananas, and pears are usually well-tolerated. Avoid fruits and vegetables marketed in cans that are not specifically designed for infants, because of variable and sometimes high lead content and addition of salt, sugar, or preservatives.
	Meat, fish, and poultry	Avoid fatty meats. Prepare by baking, broiling, steaming, or poaching. Include organ meats such as liver, which has a high content of iron, vitamin A, and vitamin B complex. If soup is given, be sure all ingredients are familiar in child's diet.
	Eggs and cheese	Serve egg yolk hard-boiled and mashed, soft cooked, or poached. Introduce egg white in small quantities (1 tsp) toward end of first year to detect any allergic manifestation. Use cheese as a substitute for meat and as "finger food."
	Suggested progression of starting solids	Start enriched baby cereal 2-2½ tb at breakfast and supper at 4-6 months; progress to 3 tb at breakfast and supper by 6-7 months. Continue to progress not to exceed ½ cup by 9 months. Add 1½ to 3 tb strained fruits for breakfast and supper at 6 months; progress to 3 tb at breakfast and supper. Continue to progress, not to exceed 2-3 tb 2 to 3 times a day at 8 months. Add 1-2 tb strained vegetables at lunch at 6-7 months; progress to 2-3 tb. Continue to progress, not to exceed 3 tb 2 to 3 times a day by 8-9 months. Add strained meats, 1-2 tb at lunch at 7-9 months; progress to 1-2 tb at lunch and supper. Continue to progress to 2 to 2½ tb 2 to 3 times a day at 9-10 months. Add egg yolk, 1 yolk or 2 tb at 7 months. Add bread and starch at 8-9 months. Progress to mashed table food at 8-9 months and finger foods at approximately same time.
	Food texture	Liquids, birth to 4 months. Baby-soft, 4-6 months. Thickened soft, 6-7 months. Mashed table food, 8-9 months. Finger foods, 9 months. Finely cut, 11-12 months.

Modified from Wong D: *Whaley and Wong's nursing care of infants and children*, ed 5, St Louis, 1995, Mosby.

E.10 INFANT STIMULATION

BIRTH TO 1 MONTH

Babies like to
  Suck
  Listen to repeated soft *sounds*
  Stare at movement and light
  Be *held* and *rocked*
Give your baby
  Your *talking* and *singing*
  Lamps throwing light patterns
  Your *arms*
  Rocking

1 MONTH

Babies like to
  Listen to your voice
  Look up and to the side
  Hold things placed in
    their hands
Give your baby
  A lullaby *record*
  A *mobile* overhead
  Pictures on the walls
  Your *face* near his or hers
  A *change in scenery* and
    position

2 MONTHS

Babies like to
  Listen to musical sounds
  Focus, especially on their hands
  Reach and *bat* nearby objects
  Smile
Give your baby
  A *music box* or a soft *musical toy*
  A soft security *cuddle toy*
    tied to crib
  Your *smile*
  Play time with you

3 MONTHS

Babies like to
  Reach and *feel* with open hands
  Grasp crudely with two hands
  Wave their fists and *watch* them
Give your baby
  Musical records
  Rattles
  Dangling toys
  Textured toys

4 MONTHS

Babies like to
  Grasp things and *let go*
  Kick
  Laugh at unexpected sights and
    sounds
  Make *consonant sounds*
Give your baby
  Bells
  A *crib gym*
  More *dangling toys*
  Space to kick and move

5 MONTHS

Babies like to
  Shake, feel, and *bang* things
  Sit with support
  Play *peek-a-boo*
  Roll over
Give your baby
  A *high chair* with a rubber *suction toy*
  A *play pen*
  A *kicking toy*
  Toys that make noise

6 MONTHS

Babies like to
  Shake, bang and throw things down
  Gum objects
  Recognize familiar *faces*
Give your baby
  Many *household objects*
  Tin *cups, spoons,* and pot *lids*
  Wire *whisks*
  A *clutch ball* and *squeaky toys*
  A *teether* and *gumming toys*
  Bouncing, swinging seat

7 MONTHS

Babies like to
  Sit alone
  Use their *fingers* and *thumb*
  Notice *cause* and *effect*
  Bite on their *first tooth*
Give your baby
  Bath tub toys
  More 'things'
  String
  More *squeaky toys*
  Finger foods

8 MONTHS

Babies like to
  Pivot on their stomachs
  Throw, wave, and *bang* toys together
  Look for toys they have
  Make *vowel sounds*
Give your baby
  Space to pivot and creep
  2 *toys* at once to *bang* together
  Big *soft blocks*
  A *jack-in-the-box*
  Nested plastic *cups*
  Your *conversation*

9 MONTHS

Babies like to
  Pull themselves up
  Creep
  Place things generally where they're
    wanted
  Say "da-da"
  Play *pat-a-cake*
Give your baby
  A *safe corner* of the room to *explore*
  Toys tied to the *high chair*
  A metal *mirror*
  Jack-in-the-box

10 MONTHS

Babies like to
  Poke and *prod* with their forefingers
  Put things in other things
  Imitate sounds
Give your baby
  A big *pegboard* (small pegs could be dan-
    gerous at this age)
  Some *cloth books*
  Motion toys
  Textured toys

11 MONTHS TO 1 YEAR

Babies like to
  Use their fingers
  Lower themselves from standing
  Drink from a cup
  Mark on paper
Give your baby
  Pyramid disks
  A large *crayon*
  A baking *tin* with *clothespins*
  Personal *drinking cup*
  More *picture books*

E.11   ACCIDENT PREVENTION IN CHILDREN

Age	Development	Major accidents	Anticipatory guidance
Neonate to 1 month	Is unable to protect self; when on abdomen can lift and turn head; dependent, requires protection; little control over body and movements.	Motor vehicles	Use approved car seat. Do not hold infant in lap. Never leave infant in car unattended.
		Strangulation	Spacing between crib bars should be no more than $2\frac{3}{8}$ inches apart. Avoid tying anything, including pacifiers, around neck. Fasten mobiles securely.
		Suffocation and injuries	Crib mattress should fit firmly to sides. Do not use pillows; use bumper pads. Support infant's head when lifting, holding, or bathing.
		Burns, including sunburn	Avoid bathing near hot water faucets. Test water temperature before bath. Set home water temperature less than 120-130° F. Avoid handling hot liquids, and do not smoke while handling infant. Keep out of direct sunlight and use sun screen. Use flame-resistant clothing and furniture. Have smoke detectors and fire extinguishers in the home. Develop a fire plan for the home.
2-3 months	Begins gross motor movements of wiggling, squirming, thrashing, rolling.	Falls	Never leave infant unattended (at any age) for any reason. Keep one hand on infant while giving care. Keep crib sides up. Use infant seat on floor or playpen.
4-5 months	Mouths objects; brings hands to mouth.	Aspiration and choking	Do not prop bottles (at any age). Burp well before putting infant in crib. Toys should be too large for infant to swallow, nonbreakable, and free of sharp edges, strings, and detachable parts. Keep diaper pins closed during changing. Keep small objects (e.g., buttons, coins) out of reach. Use only one piece pacifiers with a large shield.
		Suffocation	Keep all plastic bags out of reach. Keep stuffed animals out of crib.
		Lead poisoning	Check toys and other objects for lead-free paint.
6-7 months	Sits without support; has a firm grasp; rolls and creeps.	Falls and falling objects	Use safety strap in stroller or high chair. Use sturdy high chair or feeding table. Keep doors to stairs and outside locked; use safety gates. Avoid use of hanging table cloths. Remove knickknacks and breakables.
		Ingestion	Keep small objects, medicine, and plants out of reach. Keep ipecac on hand and understand use. Have poison control number posted. Lock up medicine, cleaning agents, insecticides, etc. Keep trashcans out of reach or use locklids.

Compiled by Nancy Dickenson-Hazard, RN, CPNP, MSN, for the 3rd edition of this text.

E.11 Accident Prevention in Children—cont'd

Age	Development	Major accidents	Anticipatory guidance
		Injuries and electric shock	Cover wall outlets. Place furniture so cords are inaccessible. Check furniture for sharp corners—pad or remove. Inspect toys for breakage. Keep sharp objects out of reach.
8-12 months	Pulls to stand; crawls, grabs; beginning to walk; enjoys exploring.	Burns	Crawl around on floor and investigate what child could reach or get into. Keep all hot food and drinks away from table edge; turn pot handles inward on stove. Keep matches and lighters out of reach. Keep kitchen closed up or gated. Never leave child unattended near fireplace or stove. Place guards around open hearths, registers, stoves, and fans. Do not iron when child is crawling nearby.
		Choking	Do not give child small hard foods, such as peanuts, raw vegetables, popcorn. Inspect toys for broken parts. Keep floors, counters, tables free of small objects.
		Motor vehicle accidents	Continue use of car seat. Keep doors locked.
		Poisoning	See previous discussion.
1-2 years	Walks up and down stairs; stoops and recovers; climbs; likes to take things apart.	Falls and injuries	Supervise children in most activities, especially up and down stairs, out of doors, and at playgrounds. Lock all windows; when opening, do so from top only. Remove any objects or furniture in front of window that child could use as a ladder. Permit climbing within child's capabilities. Remove bumper pads or toys in crib which child could use to climb on. Check toys, especially riding ones, for damage. Keep small, pointed, or sharp objects out of reach. Keep out of way of swings.
		Burns	Teach child meaning of *hot*. Avoid use of flowing clothing.
		Drowning	Continue to supervise bath/toilet use. Supervise all water sport activity (e.g., wading pools, swimming, boating); use floats and/or life jackets. Teach child to respect water and seek swimming lessons.
		Automobile-related accidents	Continue to use appropriate car seat. Keep doors and windows locked. Do not permit child to hang out of windows. Hold onto child when crossing street or in parking lots. Do not permit child to ride toys near street.
		Poisoning and ingestion	Have ipecac in any household child frequents (babysitter, grandparents). Use childproof caps on medications. Do not regard medicine as candy. Do not give one child another's prescription.

Continued.

E.11   Accident Prevention in Children—cont'd

Age	Development	Major accidents	Anticipatory guidance
2-4 years	More adventuresome and curious; explores body orifices; more independent, with limited cognition, imitates.	Falls and injuries	Teach child to be cautious around strange animals. Supervise play at playground. Keep out of reach small objects and foods (peanuts, beans) that can be inserted into orifices; check buttons on clothes and toys. Discontinue use of crib when height of crib rail is ¾ of toddler's height. Keep stairs well lighted and free of clutter. Give toys a safety check. Discourage running in house and limit outdoor running to safe places. Teach child to respect street and cars. Teach child to stay away from and out of old appliances.
		Drowning	Continue to teach water safety. Supervise all water activities. Continue with swimming lessons.
		Automobile-related accidents	See previous discussion.
	Play increases to include rougher games and bike riding. Cognition improving and can identify good and bad.	Burns	Teach child what to do if fire breaks out; hold household drills. Teach child to roll and smother clothes if they catch on fire.
		Drowning	Continue swimming lessons. Use floats or lifejacket if child cannot swim. Swim only where supervision is available (parent or lifeguard).
		Automobile-related accidents	Teach pedestrian safety, providing example for child. Do not permit playing in street. Use adult seat belt, if child is over 40 pounds. If over 55 inches tall, use shoulder restraints. If under 55 inches tall, only lap belt is used.
		Falls, injuries	Make periodic checks on playground or play area used frequently. Check on child when out playing. Instruct child in safe use of toys; keep in good condition. Keep away from driveways and streets. If possible, provide fenced-in play area. Set a good example by using seat belt, looking before crossing street, etc.
		Burns	Teach child about danger of matches, lighters, stove. Recheck radiators, space heaters, fireplaces, and protective guards.
		Poisoning and ingestions	Do not become lax about keeping medication, etc., locked up. Teach child to respect harmful objects and use a symbol to indicate "danger or harmful" to child. Routinely check house, basement, and garage for harmful substances within reach.

E.11   Accident Prevention in Children—cont'd

Age	Development	Major accidents	Anticipatory guidance
4-6 years	Continues to be curious, daring, and imitative; frequently plays out of sight.		Involve child in safety discussions. Continue previously described activities when using household tools and equipment.
School age	Increased motor coordination and cognitive ability; increased peer and group activity and involvement in sports; assumes more responsibility for self and well-being.	Motor vehicle and bicycle accidents	Involve child in safety discussion and planning. Assign safety responsibilities, such as checking bike. Teach child not to ride with strangers. Teach child how to contact police and fire department and physician. Be certain child knows address and phone number. Discuss bicycle and pedestrian safety. Discuss bicycle riding rules: Always wear an approved bike helmet. Do not hitch ride on moving vehicles. Do not ride on dark street. Use headlight or reflector light at night; wear bright clothes. Do not dart from behind parked cars. Do not carry passengers on bicycle. Keep bike in good repair. Do not use street as a playground. Use seat belts.
		Injuries	Teach child to participate in sports safely using appropriate gear. Permit only supervised sport activities. Teach child proper use of household gadgets and equipment; supervise as necessary.
		Drowning	Teach the following swimming rules: Swim only where a lifeguard is present. Use buddy system. Know water depth before diving. Wear life jacket while boating or skiing or if non-swimmer. No horseplay or call for help jokingly.
		Falls	See bicycle rules. Discuss climbing trees: Avoid slippery shoes. Avoid weak or dead branches. Keep a secure handhold.
		Burns	Continue household drills. Camp with supervision. Teach proper campfire and barbecue care. Use safe camping gear, including flame-retardant clothes.

Continued.

E.11   Accident Prevention in Children—cont'd

Age	Development	Major accidents	Anticipatory guidance
Adolescence	Seeking identity and establishment of independence; subject to strong peer pressure; rejects unsought advice; has a need for physical activity; spends most of free time away from home.	Drowning	Most important to have cooperation of adolescent when discussing and implementing safety measures. See previous sections. Never too late to learn to swim. Enroll in lifesaving classes.
		Firearms accidents	Avoid having loaded guns in household. Learn safety handling if involved in sport hunting. Keep guns in locked closet and ammunition in separate locked area. Never assume gun is not loaded. Never point gun at another.
		Automobile-related accidents	Take drivers' education. Use seat belts for self and passengers. Practice pedestrian safety. Do not drive under influence of drugs or alcohol. Do not hitchhike or pick up hitchhikers.
		Alcohol, drugs, and tobacco	Discuss effects of substance use and abuse. Assist teen to identify other ways to achieve self-esteem, independence, and peer acceptance.

E.12   NURSING INTERVENTIONS FOR CHILD ABUSE PREVENTION

Observations of Parents-To-Be

1. Are the parents overconcerned with the baby's sex?
2. Are they overconcerned with the baby's performance? Do they worry that he will not meet the standard?
3. Is there an attempt to deny that there is a pregnancy (mother not willing to gain weight, no plans whatsoever, refusal to talk about the situation)?
4. Is this child going to be one child too many? Could he or she be the "last straw"?
5. Is there great depression over this pregnancy?
6. Is the mother alone and frightened, especially by the physical changes caused by the pregnancy? Do careful explanations fail to dissipate these fears?
7. Is support lacking from husband and/or family?
8. Where is the family living? Do they have a listed telephone number? Are there relatives and friends nearby?
9. Did the mother and/or father formerly want an abortion but not go through with it or waited until it was too late?
10. Have the parents considered relinquishing of their child? Why did they change their minds?

Modified from Kempe CH: Approaches to preventing child abuse, *Am J Dis Child* 130:941-947, 1976.

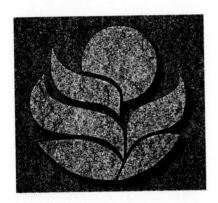

Appendix F
Screening Tools

F.1 GROWTH MEASUREMENTS: BIRTH TO 18 YEARS

Height and Weight Measurements for Boys

	Height by percentiles						Weight by percentiles					
	5		**50**		**95**		**5**		**50**		**95**	
Age*	cm	inches	cm	inches	cm	inches	kg	lb	kg	lb	kg	lb
Birth	46.4	18¼	50.5	20	54.4	21½	2.54	5½	3.27	7¼	4.15	9¼
3 months	56.7	22¼	61.1	24	65.4	25¾	4.43	9¾	5.98	13¼	7.37	16¼
6 months	63.4	25	67.8	26¾	72.3	28½	6.20	13¾	7.85	17¼	9.46	20¾
9 months	68.0	26¾	72.3	28½	77.1	30¼	7.52	16½	9.18	20¼	10.93	24
1	71.7	28¼	76.1	30	81.2	32	8.43	18½	10.15	22½	11.99	26½
1½	77.5	30½	82.4	32½	88.1	34¾	9.59	21¼	11.47	25¼	13.44	29½
2†	82.5	32½	86.8	34¼	94.4	37¼	10.49	23¼	12.34	27¼	15.50	34¼
2½†	85.4	33½	90.4	35½	97.8	38½	11.27	24¾	13.52	29¾	16.61	36½
3	89.0	35	94.9	37¼	102.0	40¼	12.05	26½	14.62	32¼	17.77	39¼
3½	92.5	36½	99.1	39	106.1	41¾	12.84	28¼	15.68	34½	18.98	41¾
4	95.8	37¾	102.9	40½	109.9	43¼	13.64	30	16.69	36¾	20.27	44¾
4½	98.9	39	106.6	42	113.5	44¾	14.45	31¾	17.69	39	21.63	47¾
5	102.0	40¼	109.9	43¼	117.0	46	15.27	33¾	18.67	41¼	23.09	51
6	107.7	42½	116.1	45¾	123.5	48½	16.93	37¼	20.69	45½	26.34	58
7	113.0	44½	121.7	48	129.7	51	18.64	41	22.85	50¼	30.12	66½
8	118.1	46½	127.0	50	135.7	53½	20.40	45	25.30	55¾	34.51	76
9	122.9	48½	132.2	52	141.8	55¾	22.25	49	28.13	62	39.58	87¼
10	127.7	50¼	137.5	54¼	148.1	58¼	24.33	53¾	31.44	69¼	45.27	99¾
11	132.6	52¼	143.3	56½	154.9	61	26.80	59	35.30	77¾	51.47	113½
12	137.6	54¼	149.7	59	162.3	64	29.85	65¾	39.78	87¾	58.09	128
13	142.9	56¼	156.5	61½	169.8	66¾	33.64	74¼	44.95	99	65.02	143¼
14	148.8	58½	163.1	64¼	176.7	69½	38.22	84¼	50.77	112	72.13	159
15	155.2	61	169.0	66½	181.9	71½	43.11	95	56.71	125	79.12	174½
16	161.1	63½	173.5	68¼	185.4	73	47.74	105¼	62.10	137	85.62	188¾
17	164.9	65	176.2	69¼	187.3	73¾	51.50	113½	66.31	146¼	91.31	201¼
18	165.7	65¼	176.8	69½	187.6	73¾	53.97	119	68.88	151¾	95.76	211

From Wong DL: *Whaley and Wong's nursing care of infants and children*, ed 5, St Louis, 1995, Mosby, pp 1919 and 1924 as adapted from National Center for Health Statistics, Health Resources Administration, Department of Health, Education and Welfare, Hyattsville, Md. Values correspond with NCHS percentile curves. Conversion of metric data to approximate inches and pounds by Ross Laboratories.

*Years unless otherwise indicated.

†Height data include some recumbent length measurements, which make values slightly higher than if all measurements had been of stature (standing height).

Height and Weight Measurements for Girls

Age*	Height by percentiles						Weight by percentiles					
	5		50		95		5		50		95	
	cm	inches	cm	inches	cm	inches	kg	lb	kg	lb	kg	lb
Birth	45.4	17¾	49.9	19¾	52.9	20¾	2.36	5¼	3.23	7	3.81	8½
3 months	55.4	21¾	59.5	23½	63.4	25	4.18	9¼	5.4	12	6.74	14¾
6 months	61.8	24¼	65.9	26	70.2	27¾	5.79	12¾	7.21	16	8.73	19¼
9 months	66.1	26	70.4	27¾	75.0	29½	7.0	15½	8.56	18¾	10.17	22½
1	69.8	27½	74.3	29¼	79.1	31¼	7.84	17¼	9.53	21	11.24	24¾
1½	76.0	30	80.9	31¾	86.1	34	8.92	19¾	10.82	23¾	12.76	28¼
2†	81.6	32¼	86.8	34¼	93.6	36¾	9.95	22	11.8	26	14.15	31¼
2½†	84.6	33¼	90.0	35½	96.6	38	10.8	23¾	13.03	28¾	15.76	34¾
3	88.3	34¾	94.1	37	100.6	39½	11.61	25½	14.1	31	17.22	38
3½	91.7	36	97.9	38½	104.5	41¼	12.37	27¼	15.07	33¼	18.59	41
4	95.0	37½	101.6	40	108.3	42¾	13.11	29	15.96	35¼	19.91	44
4½	98.1	38½	105.0	41¼	112.0	44	13.83	30½	16.81	37	21.24	46¾
5	101.1	39¾	108.4	42¾	115.6	45½	14.55	32	17.66	39	22.62	49¾
6	106.6	42	114.6	45	122.7	48¼	16.05	35½	19.52	43	25.75	56¾
7	111.8	44	120.6	47½	129.5	51	17.71	39	21.84	48¼	29.68	65½
8	116.9	46	126.4	49¾	136.2	53½	19.62	43¼	24.84	54¾	34.71	76½
9	122.1	48	132.2	52	142.9	56¼	21.82	48	28.46	62¾	40.64	89½
10	127.5	50¼	138.3	54½	149.5	58¾	24.36	53¾	32.55	71¾	47.17	104
11	133.5	52½	144.8	57	156.2	61½	27.24	60	36.95	81½	54.0	119
12	139.8	55	151.5	59¾	162.7	64	30.52	67¼	41.53	91½	60.81	134
13	145.2	57¼	157.1	61¾	168.1	66¼	34.14	75¼	46.1	101¾	67.3	148¼
14	148.7	58½	160.4	63¼	171.3	67½	37.76	83¼	50.28	110¾	73.08	161
15	150.5	59¼	161.8	63¾	172.8	68	40.99	90¼	53.68	118¼	77.78	171½
16	151.6	59¾	162.4	64	173.3	68¼	43.41	95¾	55.89	123¼	80.99	178½
17	152.7	60	163.1	64¼	173.5	68¼	44.74	98¾	56.69	125	82.46	181¾
18	153.6	60½	163.7	64½	173.6	68¼	45.26	99¾	56.62	124¾	82.47	181¾

From Wong DL: Whaley and Wong's nursing care of infants and children, ed 5, St Louis, 1995, Mosby, pp 1919 and 1924 as adapted from National Center for Health Statistics, Health Resources Administration, Department of Health, Education and Welfare, Hyattsville, Md. Values correspond with NCHS percentile curves. Conversion of metric data to approximate inches and pounds by Ross Laboratories.
*Years unless otherwise indicated.
†Height data include some recumbent length measurements, which make values slightly higher than if all measurements had been of stature (standing height).

F.2   INFANT REFLEXES

Reflex	How to elicit	Response of infant	Clinical implications
Acoustic blink	Produce a sharp loud noise (a clap of the hands) about 30 cm from the head.	By second or third day of life infant blinks both eyes. Disappearance of reflex is variable.	Absence may indicate decreased hearing.
Ankle clonus	Flex the leg at the hip and knee, sharply dorsiflex the foot, and maintain pressure.	Rhythmic flexions and extensions of the foot at the ankle.	Abnormal if more than 10 beats during the first 3 months or more than 3 beats after 3 months. Sustained clonus indicates upper motor neuron disease.
Babinski	Stroke lateral aspect of the plantar surface of foot from heel to toes. Use a blunt object.	Hyperextension or fanning of toes occurs. As myelinization is completed, the normal response becomes flexion (downward curling) of all toes; the positive (pathological) sign is hyperextension (dorsiflexion) of the great toe with or without fanning of the remaining toes.	After 2 years of age, a positive sign is the most significant clinical symptom of the presence of an upper motor neuron (pyramidal tract) lesion.

F.2   Infant Reflexes—cont'd

Reflex	How to elicit	Response of infant	Clinical implications
Blinking	Shine a light suddenly at the infant's open eyes.	Eyelids close in response to light. Disappears after first year.	Absence may indicate poor light perception or blindness.
Landau	Suspend infant carefully in prone position by supporting infant's abdomen with examiner's hand.	By 3 months of age the expected response consists of extension of head, trunk, and hips. Head is slightly above horizontal plane. Disappears by 2 years of age.	If newborn collapses into a limp concave position, it is abnormal.
Moro	With infant in supine position gently support head and lift it a few centimeters off the surface. As soon as neck relaxes, suddenly release the head and let it drop back to the surface. *or* Produce sudden loud noise, or jar the table or crib suddenly.	Normal response is present at birth and is one in which the arms extend outward, the hands open, and then are brought together in midline. The legs flex slightly. Usually disappears by 3 to 4 months. Infant may cry.	Asymmetry indicates possible paralysis. Absence suggests severe neurological problem. Persistence beyond 4 months may indicate neurological disease. If it lasts longer than 6 months, it is definitely abnormal.
Neck righting	With infant in supine position turn head to one side.	Infant's trunk rotates in direction in which head is turned. Appears at 4 to 6 months. Disappears at 24 months	Absent or decreased reflex may indicate spasticity.
Palmar grasp	With infant's head positioned in midline, place examiner's index fingers from ulnar side into infant's palm and press against palm.	Normal response is flexion of all fingers around examiner's fingers. Present at birth and disappears by 4 months when infant is ready to reach.	Note symmetry and strength. Persistence of grasp beyond 4 months suggests cerebral dysfunction.
Parachute	Infant is held in a prone position and is quickly lowered toward the surface of the examining table or floor.	Normal response is extension of arms, hands, and fingers, as if to break a fall. Appears by 9 months and persists.	Asymmetry or absence of response is abnormal.
Perez	Infant is held in a suspended prone position in one of the examiner's hands. The thumb of the other hand is moved firmly from sacrum along entire spine.	Normal response is extension of head and spine, flexion of knees on the chest, a cry, and emptying of the bladder. Present at birth and disappears by 3 months.	Absence indicates severe neurological disease.
Placing	Infant is held erect and the dorsum of one foot touches the undersurface of the examining table top.	Infant flexes hip and knee and places stimulated foot on top of the table. Present at birth and disappears at 6 weeks or variable.	Absent in paralysis or in infants born by breech delivery.
Plantar grasp	Examiner's finger is placed firmly across base of infant's toes.	Toes curl downward. Present at birth and disappears by 10 to 12 months.	Absent in defects of lower spinal column. Infant cannot walk until this reflex disappears.
Rooting	Infant is held in supine position with head in midline and hands against chest. Examiner strokes perioral skin at corner of mouth or cheek.	Infant opens mouth and turns head toward stimulated side. Present at birth and disappears by 3 to 4 months (awake); by 7 months (asleep).	Absence indicates severe central nervous system disease or depressed infant.
Rotation test	Infant is held upright facing examiner and rotated in one direction and then the other.	Infant's head turns in the direction in which the body is being turned. If head is restrained the eyes will turn in the direction in which the infant is turned.	If head and eyes do not move, it indicates a vestibular problem.

Continued.

F.2   Infant Reflexes—cont'd

Reflex	How to elicit	Response of infant	Clinical implications
Spontaneous crawling (Bauer's response)	Infant is lying prone and examiner presses soles of feet.	Infant makes crawling movements. Present at birth.	Crawling is absent in weak or depressed infants.
Stepping	Infant is held upright and soles of feet are put in touch with solid surface.	Infant "walks" along surface. Present at birth and disappears at 6 weeks.	Absence indicates depressed infant, breech delivery, or paralysis.
Sucking	With infant in supine position place nipple or finger 3 to 4 cm into mouth.	Vigorous sucking of finger or nipple. Present at birth and disappears by 3 to 4 months (awake) and 7 months (asleep). Tongue action should push finger up and back. Note rate of suck, amount of suction, and patterns or groupings of sucks.	Absence in term infants indicates central nervous system depression. Weak reflex may lead to feeding problems.
Tonic neck	With infant in supine position passively rotate head to one side.	Arm and leg on side to which head is turned extend, and opposite arm and leg flex (fencer's position). Present sometimes at birth but usually by 2 to 3 months. Disappears by 6 months.	Obligatory response is always abnormal. Persistence beyond 6 months is abnormal and indicates central motor lesions (e.g., cerebral palsy).
Trunk incurvation (Galant's)	Infant is held prone in examiner's hand. With the other hand the examiner moves a finger down the paravertebral portion of the spine, first on one side, then on the other.	Infant's trunk should curve to the side being stimulated. Present at birth and disappears by 2 months.	Presence of spinal cord lesions interrupts this reflex.
Vertical suspension positioning	Infant is held upright, head is maintained in midline.	Legs are flexed at the hips and knees. Present at birth and disappears after 4 months.	Scissoring or fixed extension indicates spasticity.

F.3   VISION AND HEARING SCREENING PROCEDURES

Method	Age	Procedure	Normal response
VISION			
Following	Infancy	Shine light or hold bright object directly in front of infant's line of vision; move slowly from side to side.	Follow light or bright object up to 180 degrees.
Turn to light response	Infancy	Hold back of head to bright light source.	Eyes turn toward source of light.
Optokinetic drum	Infancy	Twirl drum with stripes slowly in front of infant's eyes.	Nystagmus occurs.
Herschberg reflex (corneal light reflex)	Infancy through adolescence	Shine penlight into child's eyes; note where light reflex falls. For older children: have child focus and stare at point 14 inches and then 20 inches away before shining light into eyes.	Light reflex falls in same position in eye.
Cover test	Toddler through adolescence	Have child focus on specified spot first 14 inches, then 20 inches away. While child is focusing, one eye is completely covered for 5 to 10 seconds. Cover is then removed and	No wandering or sharp jerky movement of eyes noted, indicating ability to focus.

F.3   Vision and Hearing Screening Procedures—cont'd

Method	Age	Procedure	Normal response
		eye observed for movement. Procedure repeated for other eye.	
Snellen E	Preschool	Child is instructed to point finger in direction that the E or table legs are pointing from a distance of 20 feet. Test each eye separately, then together. Test as far down on chart as child can go.	Visual acuity of 20/30-20/40.
Snellen alphabet	School age through adolescence	Child stands 20 feet from chart and reads letters. Each eye is tested separately and then together. Testing usually started at 20/30 or 20/40 line and child allowed to test as far down chart as possible. Passing score consists of reading majority of letters (or Es) on each line.	Visual acuity of 20/20.
HEARING			
Startle reflex	Newborn	Loud noise or bang made near infant's ears.	Jumps at noise, blinks, cries or widens eyes.
Tracks sound	3-6 months	Make noise, call name, or sing.	Eyes shift toward sound; responds to mother's voice; coos to verbalization.
Recognizes sound	6-8 months	As preceding, from out of line of vision.	Turns head toward sound; responds to name, babbles to verbalization.
Localization of sound	8-12 months	Call name, or use tuning fork or say words.	Localizes source of sound; turns head (and body at times) toward sound, repeats words.
Pure tone screening— play	Toddler to preschool	Demonstrate to child by putting headphones on and making believe you hear sound. As you say "I hear it," put a block in box or ring on holder. Put headphones on child and give block or ring to use. Sound a 50 dB tone at 1000 Hz and guide child's hand with block to box. When child can do this alone, begin screening. Set at 25 dB at 1000 Hz. If child responds, go to 200, 4000, and 6000 Hz. Praise child and place new block in hand. Switch to other ear and test.	Should respond at 25 dB at any frequency.
Pure tone audiometry	School age through adolescence	Explain procedure to child. Place headphones on ears. Test one ear at a time in sequence as preceding (i.e., 25 dB at 1000, 2000, 4000 and 6000 Hz). Have child raise hand to indicate sound is heard.	Should respond at 25 dB at any frequency.
Tuning fork test	Some preschoolers; school age through adolescence		
A. Weber test		Strike tuning fork to make it vibrate and place the stem in midline of scalp. Ask child if sound is same in both ears or louder in either ear.	Sound heard equally well in both ears.
B. Rinne test		Strike tuning fork until it vibrates, place stem on child's mastoid until he no longer hears it. Then place vibrating fingers of fork 1 to 2 inches in front of concha. Ask child if he can still hear sound.	Sound from fingers of fork vibrating in air should be heard when child can no longer hear sound with stem against mastoid (i.e., air conduction is greater than bone conduction).

F.4   SCREENING FOR COMMON ORTHOPEDIC PROBLEMS

Deformity	Screening

CONGENITAL HIP DISLOCATION (CHD)

Complete or partial displacement of femoral head out of the acetabulum	Barlow's maneuver (for dislocation of femoral head): flex hip to 90 degrees; grasp symphysis in front and sacrum in back with one hand; with other hand, apply lateral pressure to medial thigh with thumb and longitudinal pressure to knee with palm; abduct flexed hip. A positive sign is sensation of abnormal movement. Reverse hands for examining other hip. See Figure F-1.
	Ortolani's maneuver (for reduction of femur): abduct hip to 80 degrees, lifting proximal femur anteriorly with fingers placed on lateral thigh. A positive sign is sensation of a jerk or snap with reduction into socket. See Figure F-2.
	Limited full abduction of hips: with child flat on back, abduct hips one at a time, then together. See Figure F-3 for degrees of hip abduction.
	Apparent shortening of femur:
	1. Allis sign: with child lying on back, pelvis flat, knees flexed and feet planted firmly, observe knees. If the knee projects further anteriorly, femus is longer; if one knee is higher, the tibia is longer.
	2. With child on back, both legs are extended out with pressure on knees. Heels are matched and observed for equal or unequal length.
	3. Trendelenburg sign: with child standing on one leg, observe pelvis. When child stands on abnormal leg, the pelvis drops on normal side. See Figure F-4.

METATARSUS ADDUCTUS (VARUS)

Adduction or turning in of forefoot with high longitudinal arch and wide space between first and second toes. Commonly associated with tibial torsion.	Test foot for flexibility and elicit tonic foot reflexes. Rigidity is indicated by eversion or inversion when foot does not move beyond neutral position or does not respond to toe grasping or by dorsiflexing. Signs of metatarsus adductus are illustrated in Figure F-5.

PES PLANUS (FLAT FEET)

When child is weight bearing, longitudinal arch of foot appears flat on floor	1. Observe feet in weighted and unweighted position
(1) Pseudo flat feet: very common until ages 2 to 3; created by plantar fat pad. Feet are flexible, exhibit hypermobility of joint, and have a low arch	2. Stand child on toes. Arch disappears with weight bearing in flexible flat foot and reappears when on toes. See Figure F-6.
	3. Elicit dorsal and plantar flexion to rule out tight heel cord.
	4. Elicit eversion and inversion flexion to rule out tarsal coalition.
(2) Rigid flat feet: Uncommon; created by tightness of heel cord or tarsal coalition (a cartilaginous fibrous or bony connection between bones)	Same as for preceding No. 1 (pseudo flat feet)

GENU VALGUM (KNOCK-KNEES)

A deviant axis of thighs and calves of more than 10 to 15 degrees; (normal from ages 2-6)	1. Observe axis of thighs and calves with child standing. Normally axes are parallel with 10 to 15 degrees deviance. See Figure F-7.
	2. Observe space between the knees from front to back. Normal spacing is $1\frac{1}{2}$ inches.
	3. Observe space between ankles from front and back. Normal spacing between medial malleoli at heel is 2 inches.

GENU VARUM (BOWLEGS)

Deviant axis of thighs and calves, which is	Same for genu valgum
(1) Physiological: normal until ages 2 to 3; occurs with internal tibial torsion and genu valgum	
(2) Pathological	

F.4   Screening for Common Orthopedic Problems—cont'd

Deformity	Screening
INTERNAL TIBIAL TORSION	
Twisting or torsion of tibia usually accompanied by metatarsus adductus	1. Examine legs for range of motion, flexibility of ankle and elicit tonic foot reflexes. 2. Holding knee firmly with foot in neutral position, observe medial and lateral malleoli. The normal angle between them is approximately 15 to 20 degrees. See Figure F-8. 3. Have child sit on examining table and draw a circle over patellar and external malleoli. With patella facing forward only anterior edge of malleolar circle should be seen. See Figure F-9.
SCOLIOSIS	

S-shaped lateral curvature of spine with rotation of vertical bodies.	Screening is implemented as follows:
	1. Ask the child to bend forward in a 50% flexing position with shoulders drooping forward, arms and head dangling. Observe the spine from above the head and inspect for any lateral curvature or prominent projection of the rib cage on one side (Figure F-10).
	2. While the child is standing erect with weight equal on both feet, observe for:
	    Difference in levels of shoulders, scapula, and hips;
	    Differences in the size of the spaces between the arms and the trunk;
	    Prominence of either scapula or hip;
	    A curve in the vertebral spinous process alignment.
	3. Ask the child to walk and make observations discussed in No. 2 and observe for the presence of a waddle, limp, or tilt.

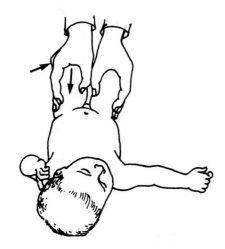

FIGURE F-1

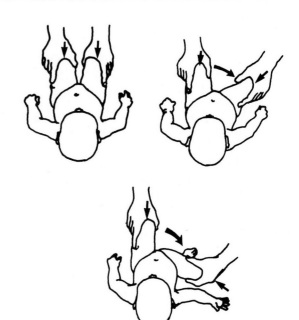

FIGURE F-2

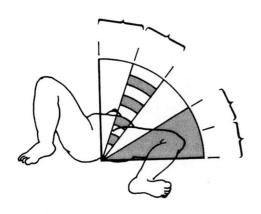

FIGURE F-3

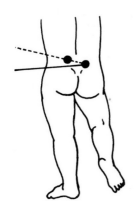

FIGURE F-4

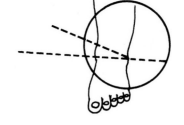

FIGURE F-8

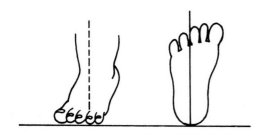

FIGURE F-5

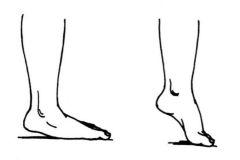

FIGURE F-6

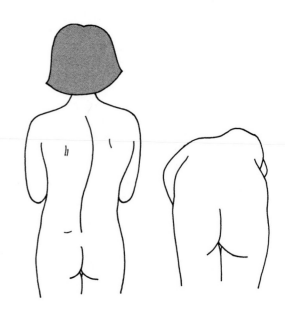

FIGURE F-9

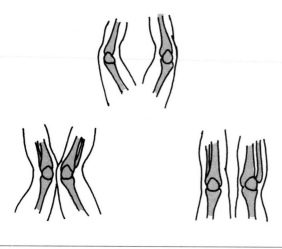

FIGURE F-7

FIGURE F-10

F.5 DEVELOPMENT CHARACTERISTICS: SUMMARY FOR CHILDREN
Waechter Developmental Guide: The First Year

Age	Physical and motor development	Intellectual development	Socialization and vocalization	Emotional development
1 month	Physiologically more stable than in newborn period. Waves hands as clenched fists. Objects placed in hands are dropped immediately. Momentary visual fixation on objects and human face. Tonic neck reflex position frequent and Moro reflex brisk. Able to turn head when prone, but unable to support head. Responds to sounds of bell, rattle, etc. Makes crawling motions when prone. Sucking and rooting reflex present. Coordinates sucking, swallowing, and breathing.	Reflexive. No attempt to interact with environment. External stimuli do not have meaning.	Cries, mews, and makes throaty noises. Responds in terms of internal need states. Interested in the human face.	Response limited generally to tension states. Panic reactions, with arching of back and extension and flexion of extremities. Derives satisfaction from the feeding situation when held and pleasure from rocking, cuddling, and tactile stimulation. Maximum need for sucking pleasures. Quiets when picked up.
2 months	Moro reflex still brisk. Posture still toward tonic neck reflex position. Has visual response to patterns. Eye coordination to light and objects. Follows objects vertically and horizontally. Responds to objects placed on face. Listens actively to sounds. Able to lift head momentarily from prone position. Turns from side to back. Able to swallow pureed foods.	Recognition of familiar face. Indicates inspection of the environment. Begins to show anticipation before feeding.	Begins to vocalize; coos. Beginning of social smile. Actively follows movement of familiar person or object with eyes. Crying becomes differentiated. Vocalizes to mother's voice. Visually searches to locate sounds of mother's voice.	Maximum need for sucking pleasures. Indicates more active satisfaction when fed, held, rocked.
3 months	Frequency of tonic neck reflex position and vigor of Moro response rapidly diminishing. Uses arms and legs simultaneously but not separately. Able to raise head from prone position; may get chest off bed. Holds head in fairly good control. Begins differentiation of motor responses. Hands are beginning to open, and objects placed in hands are retained for brief inspection; able to carry objects to mouth. Indicates preference for prone or supine position. "Stepping" reflex disappears. Landau reflex appears.	Shows active interest in environment. Can recognize familiar faces and objects such as bottle; however, objects do not have permanence. Recognition is indicative of recording of memory traces. Begins playing with parts of body. Follows objects visually. Begins to be able to coordinate stimuli from various sense organs. Shows awareness of a strange situation.	More ready and responsive smile. Facial and generalized body response to faces. Preferential response to adult voices. Has longer periods of wakefulness without crying. Begins to use prelanguage vocalizations, babbling and cooing. Laughs aloud and shows pleasure in vocalization. Shows anticipatory preparation to being lifted. Turns head to follow familiar person.	Maximum need for sucking pleasure. Wishes to avoid unpleasant situations. Not yet able to act independently to evoke response in others.

From Waechter EH, Blake FG: *Nursing care of children*, ed 9, Philadelphia, 1976, JB Lippincott.

Continued.

Age	Physical and motor development	Intellectual development	Socialization and vocalization	Emotional development
	Eyes converge as objects approach face. Has necessary muscular control to accept cereal and fruit.		Ceases crying when mother enters the room.	
4 months	Ability to carry objects to mouth. Inspects and plays with hands. Grasps objects with both hands. Turns head to sound of bell or bottle. Reaches for offered objects. Eyes focus on small objects. Begins to demonstrate eye-hand coordination. Ability to pick up objects. Rooting reflex disappears; tonic neck reflex disappearing. Sits with minimum support with stable head and back. Turns from back to side. Breathing and mouth activity coordination in relation to vocal cords. Holds head up when pulled to sitting position. Begins to drool.	Recognizes bottle on sight. Becomes bored when left alone for long periods of time. Actively interested in environment. Indicates beginnings of intentionality and interest in affecting the environment. Indicates beginning anticipation of consequences of action.	Vocalizes frequently and vocalizations change according to mood. Begins to respond to "no, no." Enjoys being propped in a sitting position. Turns head to familiar noise. Chuckles socially. Demands attention by fussing; enjoys attention.	Interest in mother heightens. Is affable and lovable. Shows signs of increasing trust and security.
5 months	Ability to recover near objects. Reaches persistently. Grasps with whole hand. Ability to lift objects. Begins to use thumb and finger in "pincer" movement. Able to sustain visual inspection. Able to sit for longer periods of time when well supported. Begins to show signs of tooth eruption. Ability to sleep through night without feeding. Moro reflex and tonic neck reflex finally disappear.	Able to discriminate strangers from family. Turns head after fallen object. Shows active interest in novelty. Attempts to regain interesting action in environment. Ability to coordinate visual impressions of an object. Begins differentiation of self from environment.	Enjoys play with people and objects. Smiles at mirror image. More exuberantly playful but also more touchy and discriminating.	Other members of the family become important as the baby's emotional world expands. Begins to be able to postpone gratification. Awaits anticipated routines with happy expectation. Begins to explore mother's body.
6 months	Ability to pick up small objects directly and deftly. Ability to lift cup by handle. Grasps, holds, and manipulates objects. Ability to pull self to sitting position. Begins to "hitch" in locomotion. Momentary sitting and hand support. When lying in prone position, supports weight with hands. Weight gain begins to decline. Ability to turn completely over.	Increasing awareness of self. Responds with attentiveness to novel stimuli. Begins to be able to recognize mother when she is dressed differently. Objects begin to acquire permanence; searches for lost object for brief period.	Very interested in sound production. Playful response to mirror. Laughs aloud when stimulated. Great interest in babbling, which is self-reinforcing. Begins to recognize strangers.	Begins to have sense of "self." Increased growth of ego.
7 months	Ability to transfer objects from one hand to another. Holds object in one hand.	Ability to secure objects by pulling on string.	Vocalizes four different syllables. Produces vowel sounds	Begins to show signs of fretfulness when

Age	Physical and motor development	Intellectual development	Socialization and vocalization	Emotional development
	Gums or mouths solid foods; exploratory behavior with food. Ability to bang objects together. Palmar grasp disappears. Bears weight when held in standing position. Sits alone for brief periods. Rolls over adeptly.	Repeats activities that are enjoyed. Discovers and plays with own feet. Drops and picks up objects in exploration. Searches for lost objects outside perceptual field. Has consciousness of desires. Growing differentiation of self from environment. Rudimentary sense of depth and space.	and chained syllables. Makes "talking sounds" in response to the talking of others. Crows and squeals.	mother leaves or in presence of strangers. Shows beginning fear of strangers. Orally aggressive in biting and mouthing.
8 months	Ability to ring bell purposively. Ability to feed self with finger foods. Begins to experience tooth eruption. Sits well alone. Ability to release objects at will.	Uncovers hidden toy. Increased interest in feeding self. Differentiation of means from end in intentionality. Has lively curiosity about the world.	Listens selectively to familiar words. Says "da da" or equivalent. Babbles to produce consonant sounds. Vocalizes to toys. Stretches out arms to be picked up.	Plays for sheer pleasure of the activity. Anxiety when confronted by strangers indicates recognition and need of mother; attachment behavior begins to be obvious and strong.
9 months	Rises to sitting position. Creeps and/or crawls; maybe backward at first. Tries out newly developing motor capacities. Ability to hold own bottle. Drinks from cup or glass with assistance. Begins to show regular patterns in bladder and bowel elimination. Good ability to use thumb and finger in pincer grasp. Pulls self to feet with help.	Ability to put objects in container. Examines object held in hand; explores objects by sucking, chewing, and biting.	Responds to simple verbal requests. Plays interactive games, such as peek-a-boo and patty cake.	Mother is increasingly important for her own sake; reacts violently to threat of her loss. Begins to show fears of going to bed and being left alone. Increasing interest in pleasing mother. Active search in play for solutions to separation anxiety.
10 months	Ability to unwrap objects. Pulls to standing position. Uses index finger to poke and finger and thumb to hold objects. Finger feeds self; controls lips around cup. Plantar reflex disappears. Neck-righting reflex disappears. Sits without support; recovers balance easily. Pulls self upright with use of furniture.	Begins to imitate. Looks at and follows pictures in book.	Extends toy to another person without releasing. Responds to own name. Inhibits behavior to "no, no" or own name. Begins to test reactions to parental responses during feeding and at bedtime. Imitates facial expressions and sounds.	Has powerful urge toward independence in locomotion, feeding; beginning to help in dressing. Experiences joy when achieving a goal and mastering fear.
11 months	Ability to hold crayon adaptively. Ability to push toys. Ability to put several objects in	Works to get toy out of reach. Growing interest in	Repeats performance laughed at by others. Imitates definite	Reacts to restrictions with frustration, but has abil-

Continued.

Age	Physical and motor development	Intellectual development	Socialization and vocalization	Emotional development
	container; releases objects at will. Stands with assistance; may be beginning attempts to walk with assistance. Begins to be able to hold spoon. "Cruises" around furniture.	novelty. Heightened curiosity and drive to explore environment.	speech sounds. Uses jargon. Communicates by pointing to objects wanted.	ity to master new situations with mother's help (weaning).
12 months	Turns pages in book; can make marks on paper. Babinski sign disappears. Begins standing alone and toddling. "Cruises" around furniture. Lumbar curve develops. Hand dominance becomes evident. Ability to use spoon in feeding.	Dogged determination to remove barriers to action. Further separation of means from ends. Experiments to reach goals not attained previously. Concepts of space, time, and causality begin to have more objectivity.	Jabbers expressively. Has words that are specific to parents. Few, simple words. Experimentation with "pseudo-words" of great interest and pleasure.	Ability to show emotions of fear, anger, affection, jealousy, anxiety. Is in love with the world.
15-18 months	Uses spoon and cup with little spilling; builds 2-cube tower; can undress; has refined pincer grasp.	Stoops and recovers; walks well; pushes furniture to climb; walks up stairs one at a time with assistance.	Rolls ball back and forth with one other person; imitates household chores; indicates desires without crying; drinks from a cup.	Vocabulary of 10 to 20 words; understands simple questions; forms 2-word phrases; beginning to name pictures.
2 years	Builds a 6-cube tower; turns pages of a book one at a time; begins to dress self; washes and dries hands.	Runs; walks up and down stairs alone; walks backwards; jumps in place; throws ball overhand.	Removes clothes; awareness of ownership; helps out; eats with family but cannot sit through entire meal.	Points to body parts; has 300-400 word vocabulary; uses "my" pronouns and prepositions; forms 3- to 4-word phrases.
3 years	Opens and closes doors using knob by self; uses fingers to hold pencil; builds 8- to 10-block tower; zips zippers; does simple buttoning.	Walks up and down stairs alternating feet; rides tricycle; broad jumps; dresses with assistance.	May have imaginary playmates; can put on simple garment; washes and dries hands; likes to have a choice.	Uses plurals; forms 3- to 4-word sentences, using correct grammatical structures.
4 years	Draws a 3-part man; buttons easily; can cut out pictures.	Catches ball with hands; broad jumps; climbs up and down stairs, alternating feet; balances on one foot momentarily.	Separates easily from mother; can button clothing; plays interactive and associative games, demonstrating some control; able to share.	Comprehends and uses opposites; has increased vocabulary and about 90% comprehensibility; speaks in full sentences, using prepositions, pronouns, adverbs, and adjectives.
5 years	Copies a square accurately; draws a 5-part man; begins to tie shoelaces.	Runs with speed and agility; dresses without supervision; skips crudely.	Developing attachment outside of family; engages in cooperative play; strives for independence.	Vocabulary expanding to 3-syllable words; composition increasing to spoken paragraphs.

F.6   DEVELOPMENTAL BEHAVIORS: SCHOOL-AGE CHILDREN

Age (years)	Physical competency	Intellectual competency	Emotional-social competency	Play	Safety
6-12 (General)	Gains an average of 2.5-3.2 kg/year (5½-7 lb/yr). Overall height gains of 5.5 cm (2 in) per year; growth occurs in spurts and is mainly in trunk and extremities. Loses deciduous teeth; most of permanent teeth erupt. Progressively more coordinated in both gross and fine motor skills. Caloric needs increase with growth spurts.	Masters concrete operations. Moves from egocentrism; learns he is not always right. Learns grammar and expression of emotions and thoughts. Vocabulary increases to 3000 words or more; handles complex sentences.	Central crisis: industry vs. inferiority; wants to do and make things. Progressive sex education needed. Wants to be like friends; competition important. Fears body mutilation, alterations in body image; earlier phobias may recur, nightmares; fears death. Nervous habits common.	Plays in groups, mostly of same sex; "gang" activities predominate. Books for all ages. Bicycles a must. Sports equipment. Cards, board, and table games. Most of play is active games requiring little or no equipment.	Enforce continued use of safety belts during car travel. Bicycle safety must be taught and enforced. Teach safety related to hobbies, handicrafts, mechanical equipment.
6-7	Depth perception developed. Vision reaches adult level of 20/20. Gross motor skill exceeds fine motor coordination. Balance and rhythm are good—runs, skips, jumps, climbs, gallops. Throws and catches ball. Dresses self with little or no help.	Vocabulary of 2500 words. Learning to read and print; beginning concrete concepts of numbers, general classification of items. Knows concepts of right and left; morning, afternoon, and evening; coinage. Intuitive thought process. Verbally aggressive, bossy, opinionated, argumentative. Likes simple games with basic rules.	Boisterous, outgoing, and know-it-all, whiney; parents should sidestep power struggles, offer choices. Becomes quiet and reflective during seventh year; very sensitive. Can use telephone. Likes to make things: starts many, finishes few. Give some responsibility for household duties.	Still enjoys dolls, cars, and trucks. Plays well alone but enjoys small groups of both sexes; begins to prefer same-sex peer during seventh year. Ready to learn how to ride a bicycle. Prefers imaginary, dramatic play with real costumes. Begins collecting for quantity, not quality. Enjoys active games such as hide-and-seek, tag, jump rope, roller skating, kickball. Ready for lessons in dancing, gymnastics, music. Restrict TV time to 1-2 hours/day.	Teach and reinforce traffic safety. Still needs adult supervision of play. Teach to avoid strangers, never take anything from strangers. Teach cold prevention and reinforce continued practice of other health habits. Restrict bicycle use to home ground; no traffic areas; teach bicycle safety. Teach and set examples regarding harmful use of drugs, alcohol, smoking.

Modified from Smith EC: Growth and development of school age child: maintaining wellness. In Foster R, Hunsberger M, Anderson I: *Family centered care of children and adolescents*, Philadelphia, ed 2, 1989, WB Saunders.

Continued.

F.6   Developmental Behaviors: School-Age Children—cont'd

Age (years)	Physical competency	Intellectual competency	Emotional-social competency	Play	Safety
8-10	Myopia may appear. Secondary sex characteristics begin in girls. Hand-eye coordination and fine motor skills well established. Movements are graceful, coordinated. Cares for own physical needs completely. Constantly on move; plays and works hard; enforce balance in rest and activity. Vision and hearing fully developed.	Learning correct grammar and to express feelings in words. Likes books he can read by himself; will read funny papers, scan newspaper. Enjoys making detailed drawings. Mastering classification, seriation, spatial and temporal, numerical concepts. Uses language as a tool; likes riddles, jokes, chants, word games. Rules guiding force in life now. Very interested in how things work, what and how weather, seasons, etc., are made.	Strong preference for same-sex peers; antagonizes opposite-sex peers. Self-assured and pragmatic at home; questions parental values and ideas. Has a strong sense of humor. Enjoys clubs, group projects, outings, large groups, camp. Modesty about own body increases over time; sex conscious. Works diligently to perfect skills he does best. Happy, cooperative, relaxed and casual in relationships. Increasingly courteous and well-mannered with adults. Gang stage at a peak; secret codes and rituals prevail. Responds better to suggestion than dictatorial approach.	Likes hiking, sports. Enjoys cooking, woodworking, crafts. Enjoys cards and table games. Likes radio and records. Begins qualitative collecting now. Continue restriction on TV time.	Stress safety with firearms. Keep them out of reach and allow use only with adult supervision. Know who the child's friends are; parents should still have some control over friend selection. Teach water safety; swimming should be supervised by an adult.
11-12	Vital signs approximate adult norms. Growth spurt for girls; inequalities between sexes increasingly noticeable; boys attain greater physical strength. Eruption of permanent teeth complete except for third molars. Secondary sex characteristics begin in boys. Menstruation may begin.	Able to think about social problems and prejudices; sees others' points of view. Enjoys reading mysteries, love stories. Begins playing with abstract ideas. Interested in whys of health measures and understands human reproduction. Very moralistic; religious commitment often made during this time.	Intense team loyalty; boys begin teasing girls and girls flirt with boys for attention; best-friend period. Wants unreasonable independence. Rebellious about routines; wide mood swings; needs some times daily for privacy. Very critical of own work. Hero worship prevails. "Facts of life" chats with friends prevail; masturbation increases. Appears under constant tension.	Enjoys projects and working with hands. Likes to do errands and jobs to earn money. Very involved in sports, dancing, talking on phone. Enjoys all aspects of acting and drama.	Continue monitoring friends; stress bicycle safety on streets and in traffic.

F.7 TANNER STAGES OF PUBERTY

BOTH SEXES	PUBIC HAIR
Stage 1	Prepubescent: no pubic hair.
Stage 2	Sparse growth along labia or at base of penis; long, slightly pigmented, downy.
Stage 3	Darker, coarser, curly hair spreading sparsely over junction of the pubes.
Stage 4	Dark, coarse, adult-like in texture but smaller area of distribution.
Stage 5	Adult-like in quantity and distribution; spread to medial surface of thighs.
Stage 6	Spread up linea alba.

BOYS	GENITALIA DEVELOPMENT
Stage 1	Prepubescent: no change from childhood.
Stage 2	Scrotum and testes enlarge; scrotal skin reddened and thicker in texture.
Stage 3	Penis enlongates; further enlargement of scrotum and testes.
Stage 4	Penis enlarges with increased size of glans; scrotal skin continues to darken.
Stage 5	Genitalia adult-like in size, shape, and pigmentation.

GIRLS	BREAST DEVELOPMENT
Stage 1	Prepubescent: elevation of papilla only.
Stage 2	Development of breast bud; diameter of areola increases; papilla and breast form small mound.
Stage 3	Enlargement of breast and areola with no separation of contours.
Stage 4	Areola and papilla form secondary mound above the level of the breast
Stage 5	Mature stage: Projection of papilla only, caused by recession of the areola to the general contour of the breast.

Developed From Tanner JM: *Growth at adolescence*, Oxford, 1962, Blackwell Scientific Publications.

F.8 SOURCES OF SCREENING AND ASSESSMENT TOOLS

Denver Articulation Screening Examination (Dase) by AF Drumwright
Source: LADOCA Project and Publishing Foundation
East 51st Avenue and Lincoln Street
Denver, CO 80216

Denver Developmental Screening Test (Denver II) by WK Frankenberg, JB Dodds, A Fandal, E Kazuk, and M Cohrs
Source: LADOCA Project and Publishing Foundation
East 51st Avenue and Lincoln Street
Denver, CO 80216

Development Profile II by GD Alpern. TJ Boll, and MS Shearer
Source: Western Psychological Services
12031 Wilshire Blvd
Los Angeles, CA 90025

Early Language Milestone Scale
Source: Modern Educational Corp
PO Box 721
Tulsa, OK 74101

Neonatal Behavioral Assessment Scale by TB Brazelton
Source: Spastic International Medical Publications
Lippincott Publications
Philadelphia, PA

Temperament Scales
Source: William Carey MD
Division of General Pediatrics
Childrens Hospital of Philadelphia
Philadelphia, PA 19104

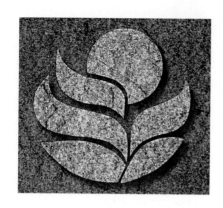

Appendix G

Health Risk Appraisal

G.1 LIFESTYLE ASSESSMENT QUESTIONNAIRE

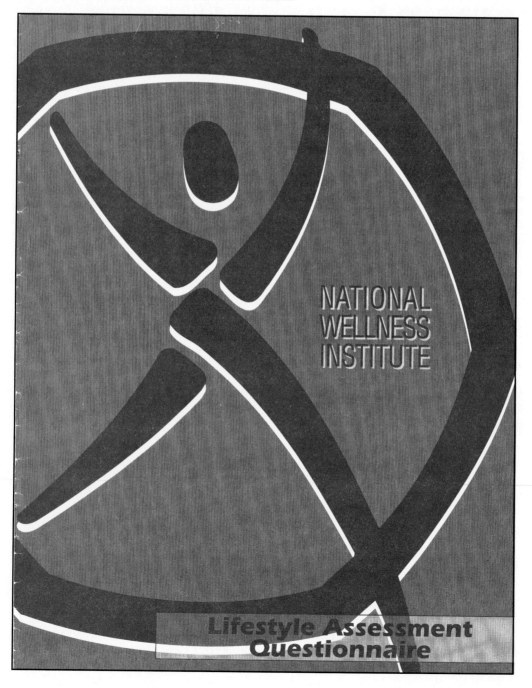

NATIONAL WELLNESS INSTITUTE

Lifestyle Assessment Questionnaire

Purpose

This assessment tool and the analysis it provides are designed to help you discover how the choices you make each day affect your overall health.

By participating in this assessment process, you will also learn how you can make positive changes in your lifestyle, enabling you to reach a higher level of wellness.

Some of the questions are personal. While you may leave them blank, the more information you provide about your current lifestyle, the more accurately the LAQ can assess your current level of wellness and risk areas.

Confidentiality

The National Wellness Institute, Inc. subscribes to the guidelines established by the Society of Prospective Medicine concerning confidentiality in the use of health risk appraisals and risk reduction systems. These guidelines specifically state that only the participant and health professionals authorized by the participant should receive copies of his/her own health risk appraisal results.

The National Wellness Institute, Inc. strongly encourages all users of the LAQ to strictly follow these guidelines and maintain the confidentiality of all answers.

What is Wellness?

Wellness is an active process of becoming aware of and making choices toward a higher level of well-being. **Remember,** leading a wellness lifestyle requires your **active involvement.** As you gain more knowledge about what enhances your well-being, you are encouraged to use this information to make informed choices which lead to a healthier life.

General Instructions

The enclosed answer sheet is for you to record your answers to the Lifestyle Assessment Questionnaire. Please make certain that you complete all of the information at the top of the answer sheet including your zip code, group code, and social security number. If a group code has not been provided for you, leave this item blank.

Your questionnaire will be scored by an optical mark reading instrument; therefore, please use only a No. 2 (soft) pencil for marking your responses. To assure the most accurate results, follow the instructions shown on the answer sheet. Only your answer sheet needs to be returned for scoring. You may keep this questionnaire.

The Lifestyle Assessment Questionnaire was written by the National Wellness Institute, Inc.'s Cofounders; Dennis Elsenrath, Ed.D., Bill Hettler, M.D., and Fred Leafgren, Ph.D.

LIFESTYLE ASSESSMENT QUESTIONNAIRE ANSWER SHEET

Please Do Not Mark In This Box

095290

NAME		INSTRUCTIONS	ZIP CODE	GROUP CODE	SOCIAL SECURITY #

LAST   FIRST

RETURN ADDRESS

INSTRUCTIONS
- USE #2 PENCIL ONLY
- MARK BUBBLE COMPLETELY
- DO NOT MAKE ANY STRAY MARKS
- ERASE ONLY MARKS YOU WISH TO CHANGE

Printed in U.S.A.   NCS Trans-Optic® MP30-78818-87   A2202

SECTION 1-PERSONAL DATA

1 Ⓐ Ⓑ

2 Ⓐ Ⓑ Ⓒ Ⓓ Ⓔ Ⓕ

3 ⓪①②③④⑤⑥⑦⑧⑨
  ⓪①②③④⑤⑥⑦⑧⑨

4 ⓪①②③④⑤⑥⑦⑧⑨
  ⓪①②③④⑤⑥⑦⑧⑨⑩⑪

5 ⓪①②③④⑤⑥⑦⑧⑨
  ⓪①②③④⑤⑥⑦⑧⑨
  ⓪①②③④⑤⑥⑦⑧⑨

6 Ⓐ Ⓑ Ⓒ

7 Ⓐ Ⓑ Ⓒ Ⓓ Ⓔ Ⓕ

8 Ⓐ Ⓑ Ⓒ Ⓓ Ⓔ Ⓕ Ⓖ

9 Ⓐ Ⓑ Ⓒ Ⓓ Ⓔ Ⓕ

10 Ⓐ Ⓑ Ⓒ Ⓓ

11 Ⓐ Ⓑ Ⓒ Ⓓ

12 Ⓐ Ⓑ Ⓒ Ⓓ Ⓔ

SECTION 2-LIFESTYLE

A. Physical Exercise

1 Ⓐ Ⓑ Ⓒ Ⓓ Ⓔ
2 Ⓐ Ⓑ Ⓒ Ⓓ Ⓔ
3 Ⓐ Ⓑ Ⓒ Ⓓ Ⓔ
4 Ⓐ Ⓑ Ⓒ Ⓓ Ⓔ
5 Ⓐ Ⓑ Ⓒ Ⓓ Ⓔ
6 Ⓐ Ⓑ Ⓒ Ⓓ Ⓔ
7 Ⓐ Ⓑ Ⓒ Ⓓ Ⓔ
8 Ⓐ Ⓑ Ⓒ Ⓓ Ⓔ
9 Ⓐ Ⓑ Ⓒ Ⓓ Ⓔ
10 Ⓐ Ⓑ Ⓒ Ⓓ Ⓔ

B. Nutrition

11 Ⓐ Ⓑ Ⓒ Ⓓ Ⓔ
12 Ⓐ Ⓑ Ⓒ Ⓓ Ⓔ
13 Ⓐ Ⓑ Ⓒ Ⓓ Ⓔ

14 Ⓐ Ⓑ Ⓒ Ⓓ Ⓔ
15 Ⓐ Ⓑ Ⓒ Ⓓ Ⓔ
16 Ⓐ Ⓑ Ⓒ Ⓓ Ⓔ
17 Ⓐ Ⓑ Ⓒ Ⓓ Ⓔ
18 Ⓐ Ⓑ Ⓒ Ⓓ Ⓔ
19 Ⓐ Ⓑ Ⓒ Ⓓ Ⓔ
20 Ⓐ Ⓑ Ⓒ Ⓓ Ⓔ
21 Ⓐ Ⓑ Ⓒ Ⓓ Ⓔ
22 Ⓐ Ⓑ Ⓒ Ⓓ Ⓔ
23 Ⓐ Ⓑ Ⓒ Ⓓ Ⓔ

C. Self-Care

24 Ⓐ Ⓑ Ⓒ Ⓓ Ⓔ
25 Ⓐ Ⓑ Ⓒ Ⓓ Ⓔ
26 Ⓐ Ⓑ Ⓒ Ⓓ Ⓔ
27 Ⓐ Ⓑ Ⓒ Ⓓ Ⓔ
28 Ⓐ Ⓑ Ⓒ Ⓓ Ⓔ
29 Ⓐ Ⓑ Ⓒ Ⓓ Ⓔ
30 Ⓐ Ⓑ Ⓒ Ⓓ Ⓔ
31 Ⓐ Ⓑ Ⓒ Ⓓ Ⓔ
32 Ⓐ Ⓑ Ⓒ Ⓓ Ⓔ
33 Ⓐ Ⓑ Ⓒ Ⓓ Ⓔ
34 Ⓐ Ⓑ Ⓒ Ⓓ Ⓔ
35 Ⓐ Ⓑ Ⓒ Ⓓ Ⓔ
36 Ⓐ Ⓑ Ⓒ Ⓓ Ⓔ
37 Ⓐ Ⓑ Ⓒ Ⓓ Ⓔ

D. Vehicle Safety

38 Ⓐ Ⓑ Ⓒ Ⓓ Ⓔ
39 Ⓐ Ⓑ Ⓒ Ⓓ Ⓔ
40 Ⓐ Ⓑ Ⓒ Ⓓ Ⓔ
41 Ⓐ Ⓑ Ⓒ Ⓓ Ⓔ
42 Ⓐ Ⓑ Ⓒ Ⓓ Ⓔ

43 Ⓐ Ⓑ Ⓒ Ⓓ Ⓔ
44 Ⓐ Ⓑ Ⓒ Ⓓ Ⓔ
45 Ⓐ Ⓑ Ⓒ Ⓓ Ⓔ
46 Ⓐ Ⓑ Ⓒ Ⓓ Ⓔ
47 Ⓐ Ⓑ Ⓒ Ⓓ Ⓔ
48 Ⓐ Ⓑ Ⓒ Ⓓ Ⓔ

E. Drug Usage Awareness

49 Ⓐ Ⓑ Ⓒ Ⓓ Ⓔ
50 Ⓐ Ⓑ Ⓒ Ⓓ Ⓔ
51 Ⓐ Ⓑ Ⓒ Ⓓ Ⓔ
52 Ⓐ Ⓑ Ⓒ Ⓓ Ⓔ
53 Ⓐ Ⓑ Ⓒ Ⓓ Ⓔ
54 Ⓐ Ⓑ Ⓒ Ⓓ Ⓔ
55 Ⓐ Ⓑ Ⓒ Ⓓ Ⓔ
56 Ⓐ Ⓑ Ⓒ Ⓓ Ⓔ
57 Ⓐ Ⓑ Ⓒ Ⓓ Ⓔ
58 Ⓐ Ⓑ Ⓒ Ⓓ Ⓔ
59 Ⓐ Ⓑ Ⓒ Ⓓ Ⓔ
60 Ⓐ Ⓑ Ⓒ Ⓓ Ⓔ
61 Ⓐ Ⓑ Ⓒ Ⓓ Ⓔ
62 Ⓐ Ⓑ Ⓒ Ⓓ Ⓔ
63 Ⓐ Ⓑ Ⓒ Ⓓ Ⓔ

F. Social/Environmental

64 Ⓐ Ⓑ Ⓒ Ⓓ Ⓔ
65 Ⓐ Ⓑ Ⓒ Ⓓ Ⓔ
66 Ⓐ Ⓑ Ⓒ Ⓓ Ⓔ
67 Ⓐ Ⓑ Ⓒ Ⓓ Ⓔ
68 Ⓐ Ⓑ Ⓒ Ⓓ Ⓔ
69 Ⓐ Ⓑ Ⓒ Ⓓ Ⓔ
70 Ⓐ Ⓑ Ⓒ Ⓓ Ⓔ
71 Ⓐ Ⓑ Ⓒ Ⓓ Ⓔ

72 Ⓐ Ⓑ Ⓒ Ⓓ Ⓔ
73 Ⓐ Ⓑ Ⓒ Ⓓ Ⓔ
74 Ⓐ Ⓑ Ⓒ Ⓓ Ⓔ
75 Ⓐ Ⓑ Ⓒ Ⓓ Ⓔ
76 Ⓐ Ⓑ Ⓒ Ⓓ Ⓔ
77 Ⓐ Ⓑ Ⓒ Ⓓ Ⓔ
78 Ⓐ Ⓑ Ⓒ Ⓓ Ⓔ
79 Ⓐ Ⓑ Ⓒ Ⓓ Ⓔ
80 Ⓐ Ⓑ Ⓒ Ⓓ Ⓔ
81 Ⓐ Ⓑ Ⓒ Ⓓ Ⓔ
82 Ⓐ Ⓑ Ⓒ Ⓓ Ⓔ
83 Ⓐ Ⓑ Ⓒ Ⓓ Ⓔ
84 Ⓐ Ⓑ Ⓒ Ⓓ Ⓔ

G. Emotional Awareness & Acceptance

85 Ⓐ Ⓑ Ⓒ Ⓓ Ⓔ
86 Ⓐ Ⓑ Ⓒ Ⓓ Ⓔ
87 Ⓐ Ⓑ Ⓒ Ⓓ Ⓔ
88 Ⓐ Ⓑ Ⓒ Ⓓ Ⓔ
89 Ⓐ Ⓑ Ⓒ Ⓓ Ⓔ
90 Ⓐ Ⓑ Ⓒ Ⓓ Ⓔ
91 Ⓐ Ⓑ Ⓒ Ⓓ Ⓔ
92 Ⓐ Ⓑ Ⓒ Ⓓ Ⓔ
93 Ⓐ Ⓑ Ⓒ Ⓓ Ⓔ
94 Ⓐ Ⓑ Ⓒ Ⓓ Ⓔ
95 Ⓐ Ⓑ Ⓒ Ⓓ Ⓔ
96 Ⓐ Ⓑ Ⓒ Ⓓ Ⓔ
97 Ⓐ Ⓑ Ⓒ Ⓓ Ⓔ
98 Ⓐ Ⓑ Ⓒ Ⓓ Ⓔ
99 Ⓐ Ⓑ Ⓒ Ⓓ Ⓔ
100 Ⓐ Ⓑ Ⓒ Ⓓ Ⓔ
101 Ⓐ Ⓑ Ⓒ Ⓓ Ⓔ

102 Ⓐ Ⓑ Ⓒ Ⓓ Ⓔ
103 Ⓐ Ⓑ Ⓒ Ⓓ Ⓔ
104 Ⓐ Ⓑ Ⓒ Ⓓ Ⓔ
105 Ⓐ Ⓑ Ⓒ Ⓓ Ⓔ
106 Ⓐ Ⓑ Ⓒ Ⓓ Ⓔ
107 Ⓐ Ⓑ Ⓒ Ⓓ Ⓔ
108 Ⓐ Ⓑ Ⓒ Ⓓ Ⓔ
109 Ⓐ Ⓑ Ⓒ Ⓓ Ⓔ
110 Ⓐ Ⓑ Ⓒ Ⓓ Ⓔ
111 Ⓐ Ⓑ Ⓒ Ⓓ Ⓔ
112 Ⓐ Ⓑ Ⓒ Ⓓ Ⓔ
113 Ⓐ Ⓑ Ⓒ Ⓓ Ⓔ
114 Ⓐ Ⓑ Ⓒ Ⓓ Ⓔ

H. Emotional Management

115 Ⓐ Ⓑ Ⓒ Ⓓ Ⓔ
116 Ⓐ Ⓑ Ⓒ Ⓓ Ⓔ
117 Ⓐ Ⓑ Ⓒ Ⓓ Ⓔ
118 Ⓐ Ⓑ Ⓒ Ⓓ Ⓔ
119 Ⓐ Ⓑ Ⓒ Ⓓ Ⓔ
120 Ⓐ Ⓑ Ⓒ Ⓓ Ⓔ
121 Ⓐ Ⓑ Ⓒ Ⓓ Ⓔ
122 Ⓐ Ⓑ Ⓒ Ⓓ Ⓔ
123 Ⓐ Ⓑ Ⓒ Ⓓ Ⓔ
124 Ⓐ Ⓑ Ⓒ Ⓓ Ⓔ
125 Ⓐ Ⓑ Ⓒ Ⓓ Ⓔ
126 Ⓐ Ⓑ Ⓒ Ⓓ Ⓔ
127 Ⓐ Ⓑ Ⓒ Ⓓ Ⓔ
128 Ⓐ Ⓑ Ⓒ Ⓓ Ⓔ
129 Ⓐ Ⓑ Ⓒ Ⓓ Ⓔ
130 Ⓐ Ⓑ Ⓒ Ⓓ Ⓔ
131 Ⓐ Ⓑ Ⓒ Ⓓ Ⓔ

132 Ⓐ Ⓑ Ⓒ Ⓓ Ⓔ
133 Ⓐ Ⓑ Ⓒ Ⓓ Ⓔ
134 Ⓐ Ⓑ Ⓒ Ⓓ Ⓔ
135 Ⓐ Ⓑ Ⓒ Ⓓ Ⓔ
136 Ⓐ Ⓑ Ⓒ Ⓓ Ⓔ
137 Ⓐ Ⓑ Ⓒ Ⓓ Ⓔ
138 Ⓐ Ⓑ Ⓒ Ⓓ Ⓔ
139 Ⓐ Ⓑ Ⓒ Ⓓ Ⓔ
140 Ⓐ Ⓑ Ⓒ Ⓓ Ⓔ

I. Intellectual

141 Ⓐ Ⓑ Ⓒ Ⓓ Ⓔ
142 Ⓐ Ⓑ Ⓒ Ⓓ Ⓔ
143 Ⓐ Ⓑ Ⓒ Ⓓ Ⓔ
144 Ⓐ Ⓑ Ⓒ Ⓓ Ⓔ
145 Ⓐ Ⓑ Ⓒ Ⓓ Ⓔ
146 Ⓐ Ⓑ Ⓒ Ⓓ Ⓔ
147 Ⓐ Ⓑ Ⓒ Ⓓ Ⓔ
148 Ⓐ Ⓑ Ⓒ Ⓓ Ⓔ
149 Ⓐ Ⓑ Ⓒ Ⓓ Ⓔ
150 Ⓐ Ⓑ Ⓒ Ⓓ Ⓔ
151 Ⓐ Ⓑ Ⓒ Ⓓ Ⓔ
152 Ⓐ Ⓑ Ⓒ Ⓓ Ⓔ
153 Ⓐ Ⓑ Ⓒ Ⓓ Ⓔ
154 Ⓐ Ⓑ Ⓒ Ⓓ Ⓔ
155 Ⓐ Ⓑ Ⓒ Ⓓ Ⓔ

J. Occupational

156 Ⓐ Ⓑ Ⓒ Ⓓ Ⓔ
157 Ⓐ Ⓑ Ⓒ Ⓓ Ⓔ
158 Ⓐ Ⓑ Ⓒ Ⓓ Ⓔ
159 Ⓐ Ⓑ Ⓒ Ⓓ Ⓔ
160 Ⓐ Ⓑ Ⓒ Ⓓ Ⓔ

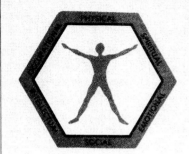

Lifestyle Assessment Questionnaire™

Answer Sheet

SIDE 2

J. Occupational (Cont.)

SECTION 3-HEALTH RISK APPRAISAL

161 Ⓐ Ⓑ Ⓒ Ⓓ Ⓔ
162 Ⓐ Ⓑ Ⓒ Ⓓ Ⓔ
163 Ⓐ Ⓑ Ⓒ Ⓓ Ⓔ
164 Ⓐ Ⓑ Ⓒ Ⓓ Ⓔ
165 Ⓐ Ⓑ Ⓒ Ⓓ Ⓔ
166 Ⓐ Ⓑ Ⓒ Ⓓ Ⓔ
167 Ⓐ Ⓑ Ⓒ Ⓓ Ⓔ
168 Ⓐ Ⓑ Ⓒ Ⓓ Ⓔ
169 Ⓐ Ⓑ Ⓒ Ⓓ Ⓔ
170 Ⓐ Ⓑ Ⓒ Ⓓ Ⓔ
171 Ⓐ Ⓑ Ⓒ Ⓓ Ⓔ

K. Spiritual

172 Ⓐ Ⓑ Ⓒ Ⓓ Ⓔ
173 Ⓐ Ⓑ Ⓒ Ⓓ Ⓔ
174 Ⓐ Ⓑ Ⓒ Ⓓ Ⓔ
175 Ⓐ Ⓑ Ⓒ Ⓓ Ⓔ
176 Ⓐ Ⓑ Ⓒ Ⓓ Ⓔ
177 Ⓐ Ⓑ Ⓒ Ⓓ Ⓔ
178 Ⓐ Ⓑ Ⓒ Ⓓ Ⓔ
179 Ⓐ Ⓑ Ⓒ Ⓓ Ⓔ
180 Ⓐ Ⓑ Ⓒ Ⓓ Ⓔ
181 Ⓐ Ⓑ Ⓒ Ⓓ Ⓔ
182 Ⓐ Ⓑ Ⓒ Ⓓ Ⓔ
183 Ⓐ Ⓑ Ⓒ Ⓓ Ⓔ
184 Ⓐ Ⓑ Ⓒ Ⓓ Ⓔ
185 Ⓐ Ⓑ Ⓒ Ⓓ Ⓔ

1 Ⓐ Ⓑ
2 Ⓐ Ⓑ Ⓒ
3 Ⓐ Ⓑ Ⓒ Ⓓ
4 Ⓐ Ⓑ
5a ⓪①②③④⑤⑥⑦⑧⑨ / ⓪①②③④⑤⑥⑦⑧⑨ / ⓪①②③④⑤⑥⑦⑧⑨
5b ⓪①②③④⑤⑥⑦⑧⑨ / ⓪①②③④⑤⑥⑦⑧⑨ / ⓪①②③④⑤⑥⑦⑧⑨
6 Ⓐ Ⓑ Ⓒ
7 ⓪①②③④⑤⑥⑦⑧⑨ / ⓪①②③④⑤⑥⑦⑧⑨
8 ⓪①②③④⑤⑥⑦⑧⑨ / ⓪①②③④⑤⑥⑦⑧⑨
9 ⓪①②③④⑤⑥⑦⑧⑨ / ⓪①②③④⑤⑥⑦⑧⑨
10 ⓪①②③④⑤⑥⑦⑧⑨ / ⓪①②③④⑤⑥⑦⑧⑨
11 ⓪①②③④⑤⑥⑦⑧⑨ / ⓪①②③④⑤⑥⑦⑧⑨
12 Ⓐ Ⓑ Ⓒ
13 ⓪①②③④⑤⑥⑦⑧⑨ / ⓪①②③④⑤⑥⑦⑧⑨
14a ⓪①②③④⑤⑥⑦⑧⑨ / ⓪①②③④⑤⑥⑦⑧⑨
14b ⓪①②③④⑤⑥⑦⑧⑨ / ⓪①②③④⑤⑥⑦⑧⑨

15a ⓪①②③④⑤⑥⑦⑧⑨ / ⓪①②③④⑤⑥⑦⑧⑨ / ⓪①②③④⑤⑥⑦⑧⑨
15b ⓪①②③④⑤⑥⑦⑧⑨ / ⓪①②③④⑤⑥⑦⑧⑨ / ⓪①②③④⑤⑥⑦⑧⑨
16 Ⓐ Ⓑ Ⓒ Ⓓ Ⓔ Ⓕ Ⓖ Ⓗ
17 ⓪①②③④⑤⑥⑦⑧⑨ / ⓪①②③④⑤⑥⑦⑧⑨ / ⓪①②③④⑤⑥⑦⑧⑨
18 Ⓐ Ⓑ Ⓒ Ⓓ
19 ⓪①②③④⑤⑥⑦⑧⑨ / ⓪①②③④⑤⑥⑦⑧⑨
20 ⓪①②③④⑤⑥⑦⑧⑨ / ⓪①②③④⑤⑥⑦⑧⑨
21 ⓪①②③④⑤⑥⑦
22 ⓪①②③④⑤⑥⑦⑧⑨ / ⓪①②③④⑤⑥⑦⑧⑨
23 ⓪①②③④⑤⑥⑦⑧⑨ / ⓪①②③④⑤⑥⑦⑧⑨
24 Ⓐ Ⓑ Ⓒ Ⓓ
25 ⓪①②③④⑤⑥⑦⑧⑨ / ⓪①②③④⑤⑥⑦⑧⑨
26 Ⓐ Ⓑ Ⓒ
27 Ⓐ Ⓑ Ⓒ Ⓓ Ⓔ
28 Ⓐ Ⓑ Ⓒ
29 Ⓐ Ⓑ Ⓒ Ⓓ Ⓔ
30 Ⓐ Ⓑ Ⓒ Ⓓ Ⓔ
31 Ⓐ Ⓑ Ⓒ Ⓓ Ⓔ
32 Ⓐ Ⓑ Ⓒ

33 Ⓐ Ⓑ Ⓒ
34 Ⓐ Ⓑ Ⓒ Ⓓ Ⓔ
35 Ⓐ Ⓑ Ⓒ Ⓓ
36 Ⓐ Ⓑ Ⓒ Ⓓ
37 Ⓐ Ⓑ Ⓒ
38 Ⓐ Ⓑ Ⓒ Ⓓ

39 Ⓐ Ⓑ
40 Ⓐ Ⓑ
41 Ⓐ Ⓑ Ⓒ
42 Ⓐ Ⓑ Ⓒ

SECTION 4-TOPICS FOR PERSONAL GROWTH

1 ◯   23 ◯
2 ◯   24 ◯
3 ◯   25 ◯
4 ◯   26 ◯
5 ◯   27 ◯
6 ◯   28 ◯
7 ◯   29 ◯
8 ◯   30 ◯
9 ◯   31 ◯
10 ◯ 32 ◯
11 ◯ 33 ◯
12 ◯ 34 ◯
13 ◯ 35 ◯
14 ◯ 36 ◯
15 ◯ 37 ◯
16 ◯ 38 ◯
17 ◯ 39 ◯
18 ◯ 40 ◯
19 ◯ 41 ◯
20 ◯ 42 ◯
21 ◯ 43 ◯
22 ◯

Section 1: *PERSONAL DATA*

INSTRUCTIONS:

Please complete the following general information about yourself by marking your answers in the appropriate places on the LAQ answer sheet. Please take your time and read each question carefully.

1. Sex
    a) male
    b) female
2. Race
    a) White
    b) Black
    c) Hispanic
    d) Asian
    e) American Indian
    f) other
3. Age
4. Height (feet and inches)
5. Weight (pounds)
6. Body frame size
    a) small
    b) medium
    c) large
7. Marital Status
    a) married
    b) widowed
    c) separated
    d) divorced
    e) single
    f) cohabiting
8. What was the total gross income of your household last year?
    a) under $12,000
    b) $12,000-$20,000
    c) $20,001-$30,000
    d) $30,001-$40,000
    e) $40,001-$50,000
    f) $50,001-$60,000
    g) over $60,000
9. What is the highest level of education you have completed?
    a) grade school or less
    b) some high school
    c) high school graduate
    d) some college or technical school
    e) college graduate
    f) postgraduate or professional degree
10. On the average day, how many hours do you watch television?
    a) 0 hours
    b) 1-3 hours
    c) 4-7 hours
    d) more than 8 hours
11. Where do you live?
    a) in the country
    b) in a city
    c) suburb
    d) small town
12. If you live in a city, suburb, or small town, what is the population?
    a) under 20,000
    b) 20,000-50,000
    c) 50,001-100,000
    d) 100,001-500,000
    e) over 500,000

Section 2: *LIFESTYLE*

INSTRUCTIONS:

This section will help determine your level of wellness. It will also give you ideas for areas in which you might improve. Some questions touch on very personal subjects. Therefore, if you prefer to skip certain questions, you may. However, the more questions you answer, the more you will learn about your health and how to improve it.

Please respond to these statements using the following responses. If an item does not apply to you, do not mark it.

A *Almost always (90% or more of the time)*
B *Very often (approximately 75% of the time)*
C *Often (approximately 50% of the time)*
D *Occasionally (approximately 25% of the time)*
E *Almost never (less than 10% of the time)*

PHYSICAL EXERCISE

Measures one's commitment to maintaining physical fitness.

1. I exercise vigorously for at least 20 minutes three or more times per week.
2. I determine my activity level by monitoring my heart rate.
3. I stop exercising before I feel exhausted.
4. I exercise in a relaxed, calm, and joyful manner.
5. I stretch before exercising.
6. I stretch after exercising.
7. I walk or bike whenever possible.
8. I participate in a strenuous activity (tennis, running, brisk walking, water exercise, swimming, handball, basketball, etc.)
9. If I am not in shape, I avoid sporadic (once a week or less often), strenuous exercise.
10. After vigorous exercise, I "cool down" (very light exercise such as walking) for at least five minutes before sitting or lying down.

NUTRITION

Measures the degree to which one chooses foods that are consistent with the dietary goals of the United States as published by the Senate Select Committee on Nutrition and Human Needs.

11. When choosing non-vegetable protein, I select lean cuts of meat, poultry, fish, and low-fat dairy products.
12. I maintain an appropriate weight for my height and frame.
13. I minimize salt intake.
14. I eat fruits and vegetables, fresh and uncooked.
15. I eat breakfast.
16. I intentionally include fiber in my diet on a daily basis.
17. I drink enough fluid to keep my urine light yellow.
18. I plan my diet to insure an adequate amount of vitamins and minerals.
19. I minimize foods in my diet that contain large amounts of refined flour (bleached white flour, typical store bread, cakes, etc.).
20. I minimize my intake of fats and oils including margarine and animal fats.

1

21. I include items from all four basic food groups in my diet each day (fruits and vegetables; milk group; breads and cereals; meat, fowl, fish or vegetable proteins).
22. To avoid unnecessary calories, I choose water as one of the beverages I drink.
23. I avoid adding sugar to my foods. I minimize my intake of pre-sweetened foods (sugarcoated cereals, syrups, chocolate milk, and most processed and fast foods).

SELF-CARE

Measures the behaviors which help one prevent or detect early illnesses.

24. I use footgear of good quality designed for the activity or the job in which I participate.
25. I record immunizations to maintain up-to-date immunization records.
26. I examine my breasts or testes on a monthly basis.
27. I have my breasts or testes examined yearly by a physician.
28. I balance the type and amount of food I eat with exercise to maintain a healthy percent body fat.
29. I take action to minimize my exposure to tobacco smoke.
30. When I experience illness or injury, I take necessary steps to correct the problem.
31. I engage in activities which keep my blood pressure in a range which minimizes my chances of disease (e.g., stroke, heart attack, and kidney disease).
32. I brush my teeth after eating.
33. I floss my teeth after eating.
34. My resting pulse is 60 or less.
35. I get an adequate amount of sleep.
36. If I were to have sex, I would take action to prevent unplanned pregnancy.
37. If I were to have sex, I would take action to prevent giving and/or getting sexually transmitted disease.

VEHICLE SAFETY

Measures one's ability to minimize chances of injury or death in a vehicle accident.

38. I do not operate vehicles while I am under the influence of alcohol or other drugs.
39. I do not ride with drivers who are under the influence of alcohol or other drugs.
40. I stay within the speed limit.
41. I practice defensive driving techniques.
42. When traffic lights change from green to yellow, I prepare to stop.
43. I maintain a safe driving distance between cars based on speed and road conditions.
44. Vehicles which I drive are maintained to assure safety.
45. Because they are safer, I use radial tires on cars that I drive.
46. When I ride a bicycle or motorcycle, I wear a helmet and have adequate lights/reflectors.
47. Children riding in my car are secured in an approved car seat or seat belt.
48. I use my seat belt while driving or riding in a vehicle.

DRUG USAGE AND AWARENESS

Measures the degree to which one functions without the unnecessary use of chemicals.

49. I use prescription drugs and over-the-counter medications only when necessary.
50. If I consume alcohol, I limit my consumption to not more than one drink per hour and no more than two drinks per day.
51. I avoid the use of tobacco.
52. Because of the potentially harmful effects of caffeine (e.g., coffee, tea, cola, etc.), I limit my consumption.
53. I avoid the use of marijuana.
54. I avoid the use of hallucinogens (LSD, PCP, MDA, etc.).
55. I avoid the use of stimulants ("uppers"—e.g., cocaine, amphetamines, "pep pills," etc.).
56. I avoid the use of nonmedically prescribed depressants ("downers"—e.g., barbituates, quaaludes, minor tranquilizers, etc.).
57. I avoid using a combination of drugs unless under medical supervision.
58. I follow the instructions provided with any drug I take.
59. I avoid using drugs obtained from illegal sources.
60. I understand the expected effect of drugs I take.
61. I consider alternatives to drugs.
62. If I experience discomfort from stress or tension, I use relaxation techniques, exercise, and meditation instead of taking drugs.
63. I get clear directions for taking my medicine from my doctor or pharmacist.

SOCIAL/ENVIRONMENTAL

Measures the degree to which one contributes to the common welfare of the community. This emphasizes interdependence with others and nature.

64. I conserve energy at home.
65. I consider energy conservation when choosing a mode of transportation.
66. My social ties with family are strong.
67. I contribute to the feeling of acceptance within my family.
68. I develop and maintain strong friendships.
69. I do my part to promote a clean environment (i.e., air, water, noise, etc.).
70. When I see a safety hazard, I take action (warn others or correct the problem).
71. I avoid unnecessary radiation.
72. I report criminal acts I observe.
73. I contribute time and/or money to community projects.
74. I actively seek to become acquainted with individuals in my community.
75. I use my creativity in constructive ways.
76. My behavior reflects fairness and justice.
77. When possible, I choose an environment which is free of **noise** pollution.
78. When possible, I choose an environment which is free of **air** pollution.
79. I participate in volunteer activities benefiting others.
80. I help others in need.
81. I beautify those parts of my environment under my control.

2

82. Because of limited resources, I do my part to conserve.
83. I recycle aluminum, glass, and paper products.
84. I involve myself with people who support a positive lifestyle.

EMOTIONAL AWARENESS AND ACCEPTANCE

Measures the degree to which one has an awareness and acceptance of one's feelings. This includes the degree to which one feels positive and enthusiastic about oneself and life.

85. I have a good sense of humor.
86. I feel positive about myself.
87. I feel there is a satisfying amount of excitement in my life.
88. My emotional life is stable.
89. I am aware of my needs.
90. I trust and value my own judgment.
91. When I make mistakes, I learn from them.
92. I feel comfortable when complimented for jobs well done.
93. It is okay for me to cry.
94. I have feelings of sensitivity for others.
95. I feel enthusiastic about life.
96. I find it easy to laugh.
97. I am able to give love.
98. I am able to receive love.
99. I enjoy my life.
100. I have plenty of energy.
101. My sleep is restful.
102. I trust others.
103. I feel others trust me.
104. I accept my sexual desires.
105. I understand how I create my feelings.
106. At times, I can be both strong and sensitive.
107. I am aware when I feel angry.
108. I accept my anger.
109. I am aware when I feel sad.
110. I accept my sadness.
111. I am aware when I feel happy.
112. I accept my happiness.
113. I am aware when I feel frightened.
114. I accept my feelings of fear.
115. I am aware of my feelings about death.
116. I accept my feelings about death.

EMOTIONAL MANAGEMENT

Measures the degree to which one controls and expresses feelings, and engages in effective, related behaviors.

117. I share my feelings with those with whom I am close.
118. I express my feelings of anger in appropriate ways.
119. I express my feelings of sadness in healthy ways.
120. I express my feelings of happiness in desirable ways.
121. I express my feelings of fear in appropriate ways.
122. I compliment myself for a job well done.
123. I accept constructive criticism without reacting defensively.
124. I set appropriate limits for myself.

125. I stay within the limits that I have set.
126. I recognize that I can have wide variations of feelings about the same person (such as loving someone even though you are angry with her/him at the moment).
127. I am able to develop close, intimate relationships.
128. I say "no" without feeling guilty.
129. I would feel comfortable seeking professional help to better understand and cope with my feelings.
130. I reduce feelings of failure by setting achievable goals.
131. I relax my body and mind without using drugs.
132. I can be alone without feeling lonely.
133. I am able to be spontaneous in expressing my feelings.
134. I accept responsibility for my actions.
135. I am willing to take the risks that come with making change.
136. I manage my feelings to avoid unnecessary suffering.
137. I make decisions with a minimum of stress and worry.
138. I accept the responsibility for creating my own feelings.
139. I can express my feelings about death.
140. I recognize grieving as a healthy response to loss.

INTELLECTUAL

Measures the degree to which one engages her/his mind in creative, stimulating mental activities, expanding knowledge, and improving skills.

141. I read a newspaper daily.
142. I read twelve or more books yearly.
143. On the average, I read one or more national magazines per week.
144. When I watch TV, I choose programs with informational/educational value.
145. I visit a museum or art show at least three times yearly.
146. I attend lectures, workshops, and demonstrations at least three times yearly.
147. I regularly use some of my time participating in hobbies such as photography, gardening, woodworking, sewing, painting, baking, art, music, writing, pottery, etc.
148. I read about local, state, national, and international political/public issues.
149. I learn the meaning of new words.
150. I engage in some type of writing activity such as a regular journal, letter writing, preparation of papers or manuscripts, etc.
151. I am interested in understanding the views of others.
152. I share ideas, concepts, thoughts, or procedures with others.
153. I gather information to enable me to make decisions.
154. I listen to radio and/or TV news.
155. I think about ideas different than my own.

OCCUPATIONAL

Measures the satisfaction gained from one's work and the degree to which one is enriched by that work. Please answer these items from your primary frame of reference, (e.g., your job, student, homemaker, etc.).

156. I enjoy my work.

3

157. My work contributes to my personal needs.
158. I feel that my job in some way contributes to my well-being.
159. I cooperate with others in my work.
160. I take advantage of opportunities to learn new work-related skills.
161. My work is challenging.
162. I feel my job responsibilities are consistent with my values.
163. I find satisfaction from the work I do.
164. I find healthy ways of reducing excessive job-related stress.
165. I use recommended health and safety precautions.
166. I make recommendations for improving worksite health and safety.
167. I am satisfied with the degree of freedom I have in my job to exercise independent judgments.
168. I am satisfied with the amount of variety in my work.
169. I believe I am competent in my job.
170. My co-workers and supervisors respect me as a competent individual.
171. My communication with others in my work place is enriching for me.

SPIRITUAL

Measures one's ongoing involvement in seeking meaning and purpose in human existence. It includes an appreciation for the depth and expanse of life and natural forces that exist in the universe.

172. I feel good about my spiritual life.
173. Prayer, meditation, and/or quiet personal reflection is/are important part(s) of my life.
174. I contemplate my purpose in life.
175. I reflect on the meaning of events in my life.
176. My values guide my daily life.
177. My values and beliefs help me to meet daily challenges.
178. I recognize that my spiritual growth is a lifelong process.
179. I am concerned about humanitarian issues.
180. I enjoy participating in discussions about spiritual values.
181. I feel a sense of compassion for others in need.
182. I seek spiritual knowledge.
183. My spiritual awareness occurs other than at times of crisis.
184. I believe in something greater or that I am part of something greater than myself.
185. I share my spiritual values.

Section 3: HEALTH RISK APPRAISAL

INSTRUCTIONS:

This section is intended to help you identify the problems most likely to interfere with the quality of your life. It will also show you choices you can make to stay healthy and avoid the most common causes of death for a person your age and sex.

This Health Risk Appraisal is not a substitute for a checkup or physical exam that you get from a doctor or nurse. It only gives you some ideas for lowering your risk of getting sick or injured in the future. It is NOT designed for people who already have HEART DISEASE, CANCER, KIDNEY DISEASE, OR OTHER SERIOUS CONDITIONS. If you have any of these problems and you want a Health Risk Appraisal anyway, ask your doctor or nurse to read this section of the printout with you.

If you don't know or are unsure of an answer, please leave that item blank.

1. Have you ever been told that you have diabetes (or sugar diabetes)?
   a. yes
   b. no
2. Does your natural mother, father, sister or brother have diabetes?
   a. yes
   b. no
   c. not sure
3. Did either of your natural parents die of a heart attack before age 60? (If your parents are younger than 60, mark no).
   a. yes, one of them
   b. yes, both of them
   c. no
   d. not sure
4. Are you now taking medicine for high blood pressure?
   a. yes
   b. no
5. What is your blood pressure now?
   a. _____ systolic (high number)
   b. _____ diastolic (low number)
6. If you *do not* know the number, select the answer that describes your blood pressure.
   a. high
   b. normal or low
   c. don't know
7. What is your TOTAL cholesterol level (based on a blood test)?
   _____ (mg/dl)
8. What is your High Density Lipoprotein (HDL) cholesterol level (based on a blood test)?
   _____ (mg/dl)
9. How many cigars do you usually smoke per day?
   _____
10. How many pipes of tobacco do you usually smoke per day? _____
11. How many times per day do you usually use smokeless tobacco (chewing tobacco, snuff, pouches, etc.)? _____
12. How would you describe your cigarette smoking habits?
    a. never smoked **Go to 15**
    b. used to smoke **Go to 14**
    c. still smoke **Go to 13**

4

13. How many cigarettes a day do you smoke?
    _____ cigarettes per day **Go to 15**

14. a. How many years has it been since you smoked cigarettes regularly?
       _____ years
    b. What was the average number of cigarettes per day that you smoked in the 2 years before you quit?
       _____ cigarettes per day

15. In the next 12 months, how many thousands of miles will you probably travel by each of the following? (NOTE: U.S. average = 10,000 miles)
    a. car, truck, or van: _____,000 miles
    b. motorcycle: _____,000 miles

16. On a typical day how do you USUALLY travel? (Check one only)
    a. walk
    b. bicycle
    c. motorcycle
    d. sub-compact or compact car
    e. mid-size or full-size car
    f. truck or van
    g. bus, subway, or train
    h. mostly stay home

17. What percent of the time do you usually buckle your safety belt when driving or riding?
    _____%

18. On the average, how close to the speed limit do you usually drive?
    a. within 5 mph of limit
    b. 6-10 mph over limit
    c. 11-15 mph over limit
    d. more than 15 mph over limit

19. How many times in the last month did you drive or ride when the driver had perhaps too much alcohol to drink?
    _____ times last month

20. When you drink alcoholic beverages, how many drinks do you consume in an average day? (If you *never* drink alcoholic beverages, write 0.)
    _____ alcoholic beverages/average day

21. On the average, how many days per week do you consume alcohol?
    _____ days/week

(MEN GO TO QUESTION 31)

WOMEN ONLY (QUESTIONS 22-30)

22. At what age did you have your first menstrual period?
    _____ years old

23. How old were you when your first child was born (if no children, write 0)?
    _____ years old

24. How long has it been since your last breast x-ray (mammogram)?
    a. less than 1 year ago
    b. 1 year ago
    c. 2 years ago
    d. 3 or more years ago
    e. never

25. How many women in your natural family (mother and sisters only) have had breast cancer?
    _____ women

26. Have you had a hysterectomy?
    a. yes
    b. no
    c. not sure

27. How long has it been since you had a pap smear test?
    a. less than 1 year ago
    b. 1 year ago
    c. 2 years ago
    d. 3 or more years ago
    e. never

28. How often do you examine your breasts for lumps?
    a. monthly
    b. once every few months
    c. rarely or never

29. About how long has it been since you had your breasts examined by a physician or nurse?
    a. less than 1 year ago
    b. 1 year ago
    c. 2 years ago
    d. 3 or more years ago
    e. never

30. About how long has it been since you had a rectal exam?
    a. less than 1 year ago
    b. 1 year ago
    c. 2 years ago
    d. 3 or more years ago
    e. never

WOMEN GO TO QUESTION 35

MEN ONLY (QUESTIONS 31-34)

31. About how long has it been since you had a rectal or prostate exam?
    a. less than 1 year ago
    b. 1 year ago
    c. 2 years ago
    d. 3 or more years ago
    e. never

32. Do you know how to properly examine your testes for lumps?
    a. yes
    b. no
    c. not sure

33. How often do you examine your testes for lumps?
    a. monthly
    b. once every few months
    c. rarely or never

34. About how long has it been since you had your testes examined by a physician or nurse?
    a. less than one year ago
    b. 1 year ago
    c. 2 years ago
    d. 3 or more years ago
    e. never

35. How many times in the last year did you witness or become involved in a violent fight or attack where there was a good chance of a serious injury to someone?
    a. 4 or more times
    b. 2 or 3 times
    c. 1 time or never
    d. not sure

5

36. Considering your age, how would you describe your overall physical health?
   a. excellent
   b. good
   c. fair
   d. poor

37. In an average week, how many times do you engage in physical activity (exercise or work which lasts at least 20 minutes without stopping and which is hard enough to make you breathe heavier and your heart beat faster)?
   a. less than 1 time per week
   b. 1 or 2 times per week
   c. at least 3 times per week

38. If you ride a motorcycle or all-terrain vehicle (ATV), what percent of the time do you wear a helmet?
   a. 75% to 100%
   b. 25% to 74%
   c. less than 25%
   d. does not apply to me

39. Do you eat some food every day that is high in fiber, such as whole grain bread, cereal, fresh fruits, or vegetables?
   a. yes
   b. no

40. Do you eat foods every day that are high in cholesterol or fat, such as fatty meat, cheese, fried foods, or eggs?
   a. yes
   b. no

41. In general, how satisfied are you with your life?
   a. mostly satisfied
   b. partly satisfied
   c. not satisfied

42. Have you suffered a personal loss or misfortune in the past year that had a serious impact on your life? (For example, a job loss, disability, separation, jail term, or the death of someone close to you.)
   a. yes, 1 serious loss or misfortune
   b. yes, 2 or more
   c. no

Section 4: TOPICS FOR PERSONAL GROWTH

This section will help you identify areas in which you would like more information. In response to your selection from the following topics, we will provide you with resources or services to meet your requests.

Select topics on which you would like information. (Maximum of 4 topics.)

1. Responsible alcohol use
2. Stop-smoking programs
3. Sexuality
4. Gay issues
5. Depression
6. Loneliness
7. Exercise programs
8. Weight reduction
9. Self-breast exam
10. Medical emergencies
11. Nutrition
12. Relaxation
13. Stress reduction
14. Parenting skills
15. Marital or couples problems
16. Assertiveness training (how to say "no" without feeling guilty)
17. Biofeedback for tension headache and pain
18. Overcoming fears (i.e., high places, crowded rooms, etc.)
19. Educational career goal setting/planning
20. Spiritual or philosophical values
21. Communication skills
22. Automobile safety
23. Suicide thoughts or attempts
24. Substance abuse
25. Anxiety associated with public speaking, tests, writing, etc.
26. Enhancing relationships
27. Time-management skills
28. Death and dying
29. Learning skills (i.e., speed-reading, comprehension, etc.)
30. Financial management
31. Divorce
32. Alcoholism
33. Men's issues
34. Women's issues
35. Medical self-care
36. Dental self-care
37. Self-testes exam
38. Aging
39. Self-esteem
40. Premenstrual syndrome (PMS)
41. Osteoporosis
42. Recreation and leisure
43. Environmental issues

IMPORTANT— If you have finished completing all sections of the LAQ, please make sure you have answered the questions in Section 1 requesting your sex, race, age, height and weight. Results cannot be generated for the Health Risk Appraisal section without this information.

6

You and Your Lifestyle Are the Major Determinants for Joyful Living

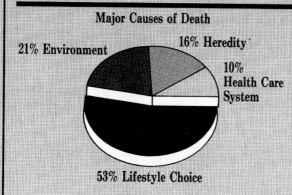

Major Causes of Death

21% Environment

16% Heredity

10% Health Care System

53% Lifestyle Choice

The circle graph to the left indicates the factors which contribute to your enjoyment and quality of life. While medical professionals contribute to the quality of your life, this graph clearly shows that the majority of those factors which contribute to your well-being are controlled by you. As you make responsible, informed choices, your chances of improving your health and well-being increase.

The LAQ's Role . . .

We believe this instrument is useful in helping individuals identify the most likely causes of death and disability. More importantly, it identifies those areas of self-improvement which will lead to higher levels of health and well-being.

The areas assessed in the LAQ emphasize the importance of creating a balance among the many different aspects of your lifestyle. Each of these areas affects one another and determines your overall wellness status. Also, each provides an opportunity for learning, making responsible decisions, and personal growth.

We invite you to use the information provided by the LAQ to your best advantage to increase your level of wellness.

Words from the Past

Wellness is a term that has enjoyed growing popularity during the past several decades. Although the term was introduced relatively recently, the concept of prevention has been present for centuries. The following passages provide a brief glimpse of the wellness philosophy through the years. Wellness is a movement which has become a major part of modern culture and is the most important weapon available to combat lifestyle illnesses.

"For many years, while engaged in the practice of medicine, the author of this volume has been more and more impressed with the idea that the causes of suffering, diseases, and premature deaths, which we witness around us on every hand, lie near our own doors . . . and that the men and women of today, are, at least, equally as responsible for existing suffering, as those who have gone before them, and often much more so. In fact, he feels satisfied that by far the greatest portion of all the suffering, disease, deformity, and premature deaths which occur are the direct result of either the violation of, or the want of compliance with the laws of our being; calamities, which, were the requisite knowledge possessed by the community, can and should be avoided."

—JOHN ELLIS, M.D., 1859

"It is universally admitted at the present time that preventive medicine is of far greater importance than curative medication, and many of the most eminent members of the profession are devoting themselves exclusively to this branch."

—J. H. KELLOGG, M.D., 1902

"To ward off disease or recover health, men as a rule find it easier to depend on the healers than to attempt the more difficult task of living wisely."

—RENE DUBOS, Ph.D., 1959

"It's what you do hour by hour, day by day, that largely determines the state of your health; whether you get sick, what you get sick with, and perhaps when you die."

—LESTER BRESLOW, M.D., 1969

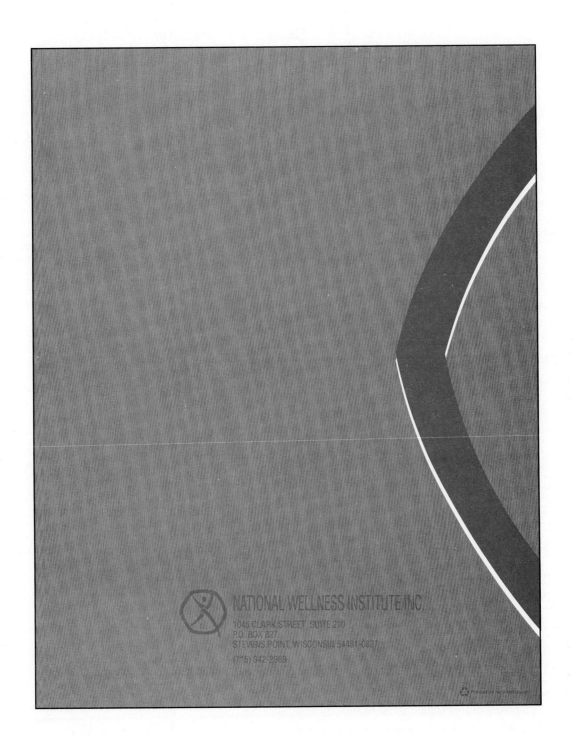

NATIONAL WELLNESS INSTITUTE INC.

1045 CLARK STREET, SUITE 210
P.O. BOX 827
STEVENS POINT, WISCONSIN 54481-0827

(715) 342-2969

Printed on recycled paper

G.2   HEALTHIER PEOPLE HEALTH RISK APPRAISAL

THE
CARTER CENTER
OF EMORY UNIVERSITY

Healthier People
Health Risk Appraisal

No. _____

Detach this coupon and put it in a safe place.
You will need it to claim your appraisal results.

✂ ─

Healthier People
Health Risk Appraisal
The Carter Center of Emory University

No. _____

_____

Health Risk Appraisal is an educational tool. It shows you choices you can make to keep good health and avoid the most common causes of death for a person your age and sex. This Health Risk Appraisal is not a substitute for a check-up or physical exam that you get from a doctor or nurse. It only gives you some ideas for lowering your risk of getting sick or injured in the future. It is NOT designed for people who already have HEART DISEASE, CANCER, KIDNEY DISEASE, OR OTHER SERIOUS CONDITIONS. If you have any of these problems and you want a Health Risk Appraisal anyway, ask your doctor or nurse to read the report with you.

DIRECTIONS: To keep your answers confidential DO NOT write your name or any identification on this form. Please keep the coupon with your participant number on it. You will need it to claim your computer report. To get the most accurate results answer as many questions as you can and as best you can. If you do not know the answer leave it blank. Questions with a ★ (star symbol) are important to your health, but are not used by the computer to calculate your risks. However, your answers may be helpful in planning your health and fitness program.

Please put your answers in the empty boxes. (Examples: ☒ or 125)

1. SEX	1 ☐ Male 2 ☐ Female
2. AGE	☐ Years
3. HEIGHT (Without shoes) (No fractions)	☐ Feet ☐ Inches
4. WEIGHT (Without shoes) (No fractions)	☐ Pounds
5. Body frame size	1 ☐ Small 2 ☐ Medium 3 ☐ Large
6. Have you ever been told that you have diabetes (or sugar diabetes)?	1 ☐ Yes 2 ☐ No
7. Are you now taking medicine for high blood pressure?	1 ☐ Yes 2 ☐ No
8. What is your blood pressure now?	☐ / ☐ Systolic (High number) / Diastolic (Low number)
9. If you *do not* know the numbers, check the box that describes your blood pressure.	1 ☐ High 2 ☐ Normal or Low 3 ☐ Don't Know
10. What is your TOTAL cholesterol level (based on a blood test)?	☐ mg/dl
11. What is your HDL cholesterol (based on a blood test)?	☐ mg/dl
12. How many cigars do you usually smoke per day?	☐ cigars per day
13. How many pipes of tobacco do you usually smoke per day?	☐ pipes per day
14. How many times per day do you usually use smokeless tobacco? (Chewing tobacco, snuff, pouches, etc.)	☐ times per day

From The Carter Center of Emory University, Decatur, Ga.

Health Risk Appraisal is an educational tool. It shows you choices you can make to keep good health and avoid the most common causes of death for a person your age and sex. This Health Risk Appraisal is not a substitute for a check-up or physical exam that you get from a doctor or nurse. It only gives you some ideas for lowering your risk of getting sick or injured in the future. It is NOT designed for people who already have HEART DISEASE, CANCER, KIDNEY DISEASE, OR OTHER SERIOUS CONDITIONS. If you have any of these problems and you want a Health Risk Appraisal anyway, ask your doctor or nurse to read the report with you.

Your report may be picked up at _____ on _____.

15. CIGARETTE SMOKING
How would you describe your cigarette smoking habits?

1 ☐ Never smoked ☛ Go to 18
2 ☐ Used to smoke ☛ Go to 17
3 ☐ Still smoke ☛ Go to 16

16. STILL SMOKE
How many cigarettes a day do you smoke?
☛ GO TO QUESTION 18

[____] cigarettes per day ☛ Go to 18

17. USED TO SMOKE
a. How many years has it been since you smoked cigarettes fairly regularly?

[____] years

b. What was the average number of cigarettes per day that you smoked in the 2 years before you quit?

[____] cigarettes per day

18. In the next 12 months how many thousands of miles will you probably travel by each of the following? (NOTE: U.S. average = 10,000 miles)
a. Car, truck, or van:
b. Motorcycle:

[____],000 miles
[____],000 miles

19. On a typical day how do you USUALLY travel?

(Check one only)

1 ☐ Walk
2 ☐ Bicycle
3 ☐ Motorcycle
4 ☐ Sub-compact or compact car
5 ☐ Mid-size or full-size car
6 ☐ Truck or van
7 ☐ Bus, subway, or train
8 ☐ Mostly stay home

20. What percent of the time do you usually buckle your safety belt when driving or riding?

[____] %

21. On the average, how close to the speed limit do you usually drive?

1 ☐ Within 5 mph of limit
2 ☐ 6-10 mph over limit
3 ☐ 11-15 mph over limit
4 ☐ More than 15 mph over limit

22. How many times in the last month did you drive or ride when the driver had perhaps too much alcohol to drink?

[____] times last month

23. How many drinks of alcoholic beverages do you have in a typical week?

☛ *(MEN GO TO QUESTION 33)*

(Write the number of each type of drink)
[____] Bottles or cans of beer
[____] Glasses of wine
[____] Wine coolers
[____] Mixed drinks or shots of liquor

WOMEN
24. At what age did you have your first menstrual period?

[____] years old

25. How old were you when your first child was born?

[____] years old
(If no children write 0)

26. How long has it been since your last breast x-ray (mammogram)?	1 ☐ Less than 1 year ago 2 ☐ 1 year ago 3 ☐ 2 years ago 4 ☐ 3 or more years ago 5 ☐ Never
27. How many women in your natural family (mother and sisters only) have had breast cancer?	☐ women
28. Have you had a hysterectomy operation?	1 ☐ Yes 2 ☐ No 3 ☐ Not sure
29. How long has it been since you had a pap smear test?	1 ☐ Less than 1 year ago 2 ☐ 1 year ago 3 ☐ 2 years ago 4 ☐ 3 or more years ago 5 ☐ Never
★ 30. How often do you examine your breasts for lumps?	1 ☐ Monthly 2 ☐ Once every few months 3 ☐ Rarely or never
★ 31. About how long has it been since you had your breasts examined by a physician or nurse?	1 ☐ Less than 1 year ago 2 ☐ 1 year ago 3 ☐ 2 years ago 4 ☐ 3 or more years ago 5 ☐ Never
★ 32. About how long has it been since you had a rectal exam?	1 ☐ Less than 1 year ago 2 ☐ 1 year ago 3 ☐ 2 years ago 4 ☐ 3 or more years ago 5 ☐ Never
☞ (WOMEN GO TO QUESTION 34)	
MEN ★ 33. About how long has it been since you had a rectal or prostate exam?	1 ☐ Less than 1 year ago 2 ☐ 1 year ago 3 ☐ 2 years ago 4 ☐ 3 or more years ago 5 ☐ Never
★ 34. How many times in the last year did you witness or become involved in a violent fight or attack where there was a good chance of a serious injury to someone?	1 ☐ 4 or more times 2 ☐ 2 or 3 times 3 ☐ 1 time or never 4 ☐ Not sure
★ 35. Considering your age, how would you describe your overall physical health?	1 ☐ Excellent 2 ☐ Good 3 ☐ Fair 4 ☐ Poor
★ 36. In an average week, how many times do you engage in physical activity (exercise or work which lasts at least 20 minutes without stopping and which is hard enough to make you breathe heavier and your heart beat faster)?	1 ☐ Less than 1 time per week 2 ☐ 1 or 2 times per week 3 ☐ At least 3 times per week
★ 37. If you ride a motorcycle or all-terrain vehicle (ATV) what percent of the time do you wear a helmet?	1 ☐ 75% to 100% 2 ☐ 25% to 74% 3 ☐ Less than 25% 4 ☐ Does not apply to me

★ 38. Do you eat some food every day that is high in fiber, such as whole grain bread, cereal, fresh fruits or vegetables?	1 ☐ Yes	2 ☐ No
★ 39. Do you eat foods every day that are high in cholesterol or fat, such as fatty meat, cheese, fried foods, or eggs?	1 ☐ Yes	2 ☐ No

★ 40. In general, how satisfied are you with your life?

1 ☐ Mostly satisfied
2 ☐ Partly satisfied
3 ☐ Not satisfied

★ 41. Have you suffered a personal loss or misfortune in the past year that had a serious impact on your life? (For example, a job loss, disability, separation, jail term, or the death of someone close to you.)

1 ☐ Yes, 1 serious loss or misfortune
2 ☐ Yes, 2 or more
3 ☐ No

★ 42a. Race

1 ☐ Aleutian, Alaska native, Eskimo or American Indian
2 ☐ Asian
3 ☐ Black
4 ☐ Pacific Islander
5 ☐ White
6 ☐ Other
7 ☐ Don't know

★ 42b. Are you of Hispanic origin such as Mexican-American, Puerto Rican, or Cuban?

1 ☐ Yes   2 ☐ No

★ 43. What is the highest grade you completed in school?

1 ☐ Grade school or less
2 ☐ Some high school
3 ☐ High school graduate
4 ☐ Some college
5 ☐ College graduate
6 ☐ Post graduate or professional degree

★ 44. What is your job or occupation?

(Check only one)

1 ☐ Health professional
2 ☐ Manager, educator, professional
3 ☐ Technical, sales or administrative support
4 ☐ Operator, fabricator, laborer
5 ☐ Student
6 ☐ Retired
7 ☐ Homemaker
8 ☐ Service
9 ☐ Skilled crafts
10 ☐ Unemployed
11 ☐ Other

★ 45. In what industry do you work (or did you last work)?

(Check only one)

1 ☐ Electric, gas, sanitation
2 ☐ Transportation, communication
3 ☐ Agriculture, forestry, fishing
4 ☐ Wholesale or retail trade
5 ☐ Financial and service industries
6 ☐ Mining
7 ☐ Government
8 ☐ Manufacturing
9 ☐ Construction
10 ☐ Other

V.3.0

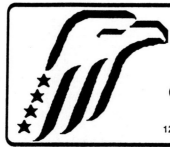

THE
CARTER CENTER
OF EMORY UNIVERSITY

1276 McConnell Drive, Suite D. Decatur, Ga. 30033

User's Guide to Interpreting the
HEALTH RISK APPRAISAL REPORT FORM

Unhealthy habits lead to early death or chronic illness. Every year 1.3 million people die prematurely in the United States from conditions which could be prevented or delayed. This Health Risk Appraisal (HRA) may help you avoid becoming one of these statistics by giving you a prediction of your health risks related to your particular characteristics and habits.

WHAT IS A HEALTH RISK APPRAISAL ?
The health risk appraisal is an estimation of your risk of dying in the next ten years from each of forty-two causes of death. The twelve most important of these are printed individually on your Report Form; the others are grouped together and printed as "All Other" on the form. These risks are calculated by a computer which compares your characteristics to national mortality statistics using equations developed by epidemiologists. The Health Risk Appraisal does not tell you how long you will live, nor does it diagnose or treat disease; it gives you a way to compare yourself to large groups of people on which medical data have been collected.

RISK FACTORS
Most chronic diseases develop slowly in the presence of certain risk factors. Risk factors are either controllable or uncontrollable. Uncontrollable risk factors include factors such as your age, sex, and the health history of your family. Controllable risk factors include lifestyle habits that you can change such as blood pressure, exercise, smoking, weight, cholesterol, and stress.

The Health Risk Appraisal uses both uncontrollable and controllable risk factors in calculating health risks, however, you should focus on controllable risk factors. To help you decide which controllable risk factors you should concentrate on, the Health Risk Appraisal identifies the controllable factors for each cause of death. The report gives you an idea of their relative importance by indicating the number of risk years you could gain by controling each factor.

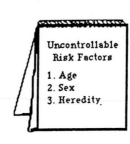

Uncontrollable
Risk Factors

1. Age
2. Sex
3. Heredity

Controllable
Risk factors
1. Blood Pressure
2. Exercise
3. Smoking
4. Weight
5. Cholesterol
6. Stress

To see what the numbers on your Report Form mean, where to find your relative risks, and which risk factors you need to control, turn the page.

User's Guide to Interpreting the Health Risk Appraisal Report Form

An example using a 48 year old woman: 57", 175 lbs, 250mg/dl cholesterol, 160/95 B.P., 30 cigarettes/day, 7 drinks/week, seat belt use 15%, drives 4,000 mi/yr, menarche 13 yrs, 1st child at 32.

Your actual age is here

Your **RISK AGE** compares your total risk from 42 causes of death to the total risk of those who are your age and sex. It merely gives you an idea of your risks compared with the population average in terms of an age. Your **TARGET** risk age indicates how much you could improve.

If your **TARGET** risk age seems too high, and you have medical factors you can not change, such as diabetes and a family history of breast cancer, it may be helpful for you to see how you compare with others who are more like you than just the same sex and age.

12345
Female Age 48

	YOUR NOW	TARGET
RISK AGE	55.57	47.68

THIS REPORT CONTAINS ESTIMATES DUE TO MISSING ITEMS, INCLUDING THE FOLLOWING

HDL Cholesterol

If you did not answer items on the questionnaire which are used for calculations, these missing items will be listed here. The computer substitutes national average values for the items you left blank and calculates your risks with these numbers.

Many serious injuries and health problems can be prevented. Your Health Risk Appraisal lists factors you can change to lower your risk. For causes of death that are not directly computable, the report uses the average risk for persons of your age and sex. More technical detail about the report is on page 2.

Beside each cause of death are listed the modifiable risk factors which your questionnaire responses indicate you need to work on. The list is specific for you unless you have none of the risk factors or if there are no known risk factors for a cause of death. In this case, a short statement of general advice related to risk reduction is printed.

MOST COMMON CAUSES OF DEATH	NUMBER OF DEATHS IN NEXT 10 YEARS FOR 1000 WOMEN AGE 48			MODIFIABLE RISK FACTORS
	YOUR GROUP	TARGET	POPULATION AVERAGE	
Heart attack	33	7	7	Avoid Tobacco Use, Blood Pressure, Cholesterol Level, HDL Level, Weight
Lung cancer	11	6	4	Avoid Tobacco Use
Stroke	7	2	3	Avoid Tobacco Use, Blood Pressure
Breast cancer	7	7	6	A Low-Fat Diet and Regular Exams Might Reduce Risk
Colon Cancer	2*	2*	2	A High-Fiber and Low-Fat Diet Might Reduce Risk
Cirrhosis of Liver	2*	2*	<2	Continue to Avoid Heavy Drinking
Ovary Cancer	2*	2*	2	Get Regular Exams
Emphysema/Bronchitis	1	1	1	Avoid Tobacco Use
Esophagus Cancer	1	<1	1	Avoid Tobacco Use
Diabetes mellitus	1	<1	1	Control Your Weight and Follow Your Doctor's Advice
Pancreas Cancer	1	<1	<1	Avoid Tobacco Use
All Other	22	21	22	* = Average Value Used
TOTAL:	91	49	51	Deaths in Next 10 Years Per 1,000 WOMEN, Age 48

The numbers in the YOUR GROUP column refer to the number of predicted deaths for each cause of death in the next 10 years from among 1,000 people who have habits and characteristics just like you.

The numbers in the TARGET column refer to those predicted to die in the next 10 years from among 1,000 people who have characteristics just like you, but who have adopted the habits recommended below in the **TO IMPROVE YOUR RISK PROFILE** box.

The numbers in the POPULATION AVERAGE column refer to the national average of deaths in 10 years for people of your same sex and age.

For Height 5'7" and Large Frame, 175 pounds is about 20% Overweight.   Desirable Weight Range: 139-153

Your **DESIRABLE WEIGHT RANGE** is based on your height and frame size.

TO IMPROVE YOUR RISK PROFILE:	RISK YEARS GAINED
- Quit smoking	4.07
- Lower your blood pressure	1.58
- Lower your cholesterol	1.27
- Improve your HDL Level	.76
- Bring your weight to desirable range	.11
- Always wear your safety belt.	.10

In this box is our prescription to lengthen your life and a prediction of how much life you may be expected to gain by adopting these health habits. The **TOTAL RISK YEARS** you could gain by making these habit changes are printed here. This is also the difference between your present Risk Age and your Target Age. Also important are the recommendations on page 2.

Total Risk Years you could gain = 7.89

HERE'S THE IMPORTANT PART!

GOOD HABITS
+ Regular pap tests
+ Safe driving speed
+ You don't use smokeless tobacco

This box GOOD HABITS lists your **GOOD HABITS**. Congratulations!

Page two of your Report Form lists some **ROUTINE PREVENTATIVE SERVICES**. These services are specific for people of your age and sex. The Report Form also lists some **GENERAL RECOMMENDATIONS FOR EVERYONE**. For the particular woman used in this example, the Report Form printed the following messages:

ROUTINE PREVENTIVE SERVICES FOR WOMEN YOUR AGE
Blood Pressure and Cholesterol test
Pap Smear test
Breast cancer screening (check with your doctor or clinic)
Rectal exam (or Sigmoidoscopy)
Eye exam for glaucoma
Dental Exam
Tetanus-Diptheria booster shot (every 10 years)

GENERAL RECOMMENDATIONS FOR EVERYONE
* Exercise briskly for 15-30 minutes at least three times a week
* Use good eating habits by choosing a variety of foods that are low in fat and cholesterol and high in fiber
* Learn to recognize and handle stress - get help if you need it.

The Standard Report Form also prints a message about AIDS and some additional information about the Report.

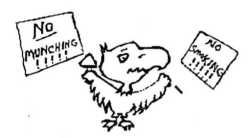

CHOOSING A HABIT TO WORK ON

Your Health Risk Appraisal is intended to encourage you to work on the habits you can change - to be the best that you can be. You don't have to change your entire lifestyle overnight - in fact, trying to change too many habits at once is probably the quickest way to discouragement and failure. The Health Risk Appraisal, therefore, may help you by showing you which behaviors should have priority. If you can not change the behavior that is top on the list (the one that would give the greatest amount of **RISK YEARS GAINED**), try to concentrate on changing the next highest on the list.

HRA LIMITS

Your Health Risk Appraisal does have limits. It is not a predictor, but rather an educational tool. It does not take into consideration whether or not you already have a medical condition and it does not consider more rare diseases and other health problems which are not fatal but can limit your enjoyment of life (such as arthritis).

What it does consider are the lifestyle factors over which you have a great degree of control and which account for a large number of premature deaths. Now that you are familiar with your particular health risks, it's time to do something about them!

MAKE A PLAN

Make a plan of how to change the habit you chose to work on. Write the plan down and keep it in sight. Be prepared for temptation! Observe the time, situation, or place that most often triggers your unhealthy habit and be ready to combat the urge when it appears. Let family and friends know of your goals, and ask for their encouragement.

REWARD YOURSELF

Rewards are an important part of changing behavior. Give yourself a reasonable reward when you accomplish your goal. Don't eat half a gallon of ice cream after losing 10 pounds! Choose a healthy and enjoyable reward. You've worked hard and are on the road to good health!

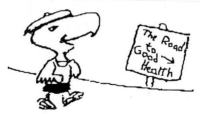

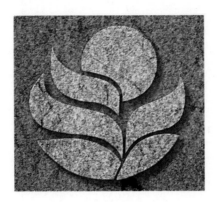

Appendix H
Community Assessment Tools

H.1 COMMUNITY-AS-PARTNER MODEL

The community-as-partner model was developed to illustrate public health nursing as a synthesis of public health and nursing. The model, originally titled community-as-client, has evolved to incorporate the philosophy that nurses work *with* communities as partners. This is congruent with what was learned about how communities (and people, for that matter) change and grow best, that is, by full involvement and self-empowerment, not by imposed programs and structures.

The model's "heart" is the assessment wheel (see Figure H-1), which depicts that the *people* actually *are* the community—the *core* elements. Without people there is no community, and it is the people (their demographics, values, beliefs, history) that is of interest to the public health nurse. Surrounding the people, and integral with them, are the identified eight subsystems of a community. These subsystems (housing, education, fire and safety, politics and government, health, communication, economics, and recreation) both affect and are affected by the people. In order to understand this interaction, one must understand each subsystem; therefore, incorporate its assessment into assessment of the people.

The "wheel" (actually the entire community, including the people and subsystems) is shown with broken lines between each subsystem to show that these are

Elizabeth T. Anderson, RN, FAAN, DrPH
Professor and Chair, Department of Community Health and Gerontology
University of Texas School of Nursing at Galveston
University of Texas Medical Branch
Galveston, TX 77555-1029
(409) 772-5029 (ETANDERS@BEACH.UTMB.EDU)

not discrete, but that all subsystems affect each other. Within the community are *lines of resistance*, those "strengths" that defend against stressors (e.g., a school-based program to prevent teen violence); identifying strengths in the community is as important as identifying "problems." Surrounding the community are lines of defense, depicted in the model as "flexible" and "normal" to indicate that there are two types of defense: one is the usual (normal) "health" of a community and the other is more dynamic (flexible) and changes more rapidly. Two illustrations may assist in clarifying these lines. The *flexible line of defense* may be a temporary response to a stressor. For instance, an environmental stressor like flash flooding or a major fire may call into play resources from within the community and from surrounding areas; these resources are considered the flexible lines of defense. The *normal line of defense* is the usual level of health a community has reached over time. Examples of normal lines of defense include the immunization rate, adequate housing, or access to Meals On Wheels for shut-ins; all of these contribute to the health of the community.

Stressors affect the community and may be *of* the community or from outside the community. Either way, the community's response to stressors is mitigated by its overall health state, that is, by the strength of its lines of resistance and defense. Knowing these strengths is one purpose of the community assessment. In the analysis phase of the nursing process, the nurse will weigh the stressor and the degree of reaction it causes in order to describe a community nursing diagnosis which, in turn, will give direction to goals and interventions. One method for stating the community nursing diagnosis is to state the "problem" as the *degree of reaction* (from which the goal is derived) and the "as related to" as *stressors* ("causes" that help define needed interventions). Using this method, an example of a community nursing diagnosis might be as follows: *High rate of tuberculosis* (the problem, the degree of reaction) *related to* poor hygiene and sanitation, crowded living conditions, poverty, and consumption of raw milk (stressors) *as manifested by* open garbage, and poor ventilation; an average of 5.6 persons per household, and sale of raw milk for income (the "data" collected in your assessment).

Think for a moment how each subsystem contributes to the health of the community. The nurse can see how an inadequate infrastructure, such as modern sewage treatment or unemployment, can affect the health of all of the citizens.

Many models exist to provide a framework for assessing a community. This systems model gives one other way to describe a community. Working *with* the community is a vital and challenging task for nurses. Using a model wherein the community is viewed as a partner will help formulate community-focused interventions and promote the health of the entire community.

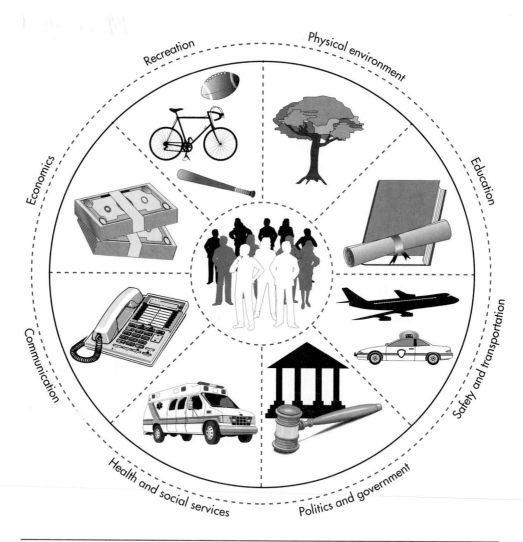

FIGURE H-1

The community assessment wheel, the assessment segment of the community-as-partner model. (From Anderson ET, McFarlane J. *Community-as-partner: theory and practice in nursing*, Philadelphia, 1995, JB Lippincott.)

H.2   COMMUNITIES WITH PHYSICALLY COMPROMISED MEMBERS: ASSESSMENT TOOLS

Use with Community/Population

Assessment tool	Purpose	Reference
Adequacy of Prenatal Care Utilization Index	Assesses the adequacy of prenatal care utilization and its association with low birthweight in the United States	In *Am J Public Health* 84:9: a) Kotelchuck, M: An evaluation of the Kessner-Adequacy of Prenatal Care Index and a Proposed Adequacy of Prenatal Care Utilization Index, 1414-1420. b) Kotelchuck M: The Adequacy of Prenatal Care Utilization Index: its U.S. distribution and association with low birthweight, 1486-1489.
Attitude towards Disabled People (ATDP)	Measures attitudes of people in community towards those who are disabled	Yuker HE, Block JR, Campbell WJ: *A scale to measure attitudes towards disabled persons*, Albertson, NY, 1960, Human Resources Foundation.
Health Related Quality of Life	Evaluates efforts in the prevention of disabling chronic diseases	Hennessey CH, Moriarty DG, Zack MM, Scherr PA, Brackbill R: Measuring health-related quality of life for public health surveillance, *Public Health Rep* 109(5):665-672, 1994.
Readily Available Checklist	Determines the frequency of architectural barriers to persons with disabilities	Ahn HC, McGovern EE, Walk EE, Edlich RF: Architectural barriers to persons with disabilities in businesses in an urban community, J *Burn Care Rehab* 15(2):176-179, 1994.
Revised Screening Survey	Measures the extent that populations are served by local health departments carrying out core functions of public health	Miller CA, Moore KS, Richards TB, McKaig C: A screening survey to assess local public health performance, *Public Health Rep* 109(5):659-664, 1994.
Wheelchair Accessibility Checklist	Assesses the accessibility of buildings to those who use wheelchairs	1) McClain L, et al: Restaurant wheelchair accessibility, *Am J Occup Ther* 47(7):619-623, 1993. 2) McLain L, Todd D: Food store accessibility, *Am J Occup Ther* 44(6):487-491, 1990.

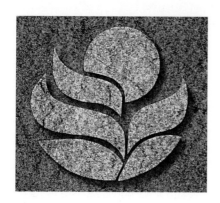

Appendix I

Family Assessment Tools

I.1 FAMILY ASSESSMENT TOOLS: COMPARISON

Assessment tool	Reference	Purpose
Calgary Family Assessment Model (CFAM)	Wright, LM, Leahey, M: *Nurses and families—a guide to family assessment and intervention*, Philadelphia, 1984, Davis.	Assessment based on strengths critical to healthy family functioning. Addresses family structure, development, and function.
Chronicity Impact and Coping Instrument: Parent Questionnaire (CICI:PQ)	Hymovich D: The chronicity impact and coping instrument: parent questionnaire, *Nurs Res* 32, 1983.	Assessment of parent perception of the effect of chronic childhood disorder on family and how families cope with the problems associated with the problems associated with the child's condition.
Family Assessment for School Nurses and Other Professionals (FAT)	Holt S, Robinson T: The school nurses's family assessment tool, *Am J Nurs* 79(5), 1979.	Assessment of home and environment; family interaction styles; child's growth, development, and health history; and family health and social history.
Family Health Protective Behavior Assessment Tool	Dandzari JH, Howard JR: *The well family: a developmental approach to assessment*, Boston, 1981, Little, Brown, & Co.	Assessment of specific health behaviors for each family developmental stage.
Feetham Family Functioning Survey (FFFS)	Feetham S, Humenick S: The Feetham family functioning survey. In Humenick S, editor: *Analysis of current assessment strategies in the health care of young children and childbearing families*, New York, 1982, Appleton-Century-Crofts.	Assessment of accomplishment of family tasks and functioning of families with normal or impaired child. Identifies specific areas of dysfunction during a period of stress.
Friedman's Guidelines for Function Assessment of the Family	Friedman M: *Family nursing—theory and assessment*, ed 2, New York, 1986, Appleton-Century-Crofts.	Assessment of variables (communication, role, power, values, and coping) and their effect on affective, socialization, and health care functions.
Home Observation for Measurement of the Environment (HOME)	Caldwell BM: *Home observation for measurement of the environment*, Little Rock, 1979, University of Arkansas.	Assessment of family influence through the child's environment. Assesses animate and inanimate aspects of the environment that support development. Identifies family strengths and weaknesses.

I.2 FAMILY PROBLEM-SOLVING GUIDE*

I. Types of family problems
  A. Problems that can be resolved by the family without the community health nurse
  B. Problems that can be resolved by the family with the community health nurse's assistance
  C. Problems that should be referred to another health care professional or other human services worker

II. Problem-solving process (family and community health nurse)
  A. Assessment of the problem
    1. Who identified problem—family, community health nurse, others?
    2. Extent of problem—is the problem a threat to the health and well-being of the family? An individual family member? Others? The community?
    3. Family's assessment of the problem—seriousness? Implications of the problem for the family? If family did not identify the problem, does the family view the situation as a problem?
    4. Community health nurse's assessment of the problem (using criteria regarding extent of problem)—if the problem is of a threatening nature but not recognized as a problem by the family, the nurse will need to assist the family to recognize and understand the implications of the problem.
  B. Problem solving
    1. What is the history of the problem—when started, who started, why existing, effect on family?
    2. If family attempting to resolve or handle problem?
      If yes
      How? How successful is approach? If approach is succeeding, support should be given to the family to continue its efforts.
      If approach is not successful, assist family to explore possible reasons for limited or lack of resolution.
      What other possible approaches has family considered?
      Have any of these approaches been tried with the present situation or similar situations in the past? If so, how effective was the approach? If approach was successful, why? If approach was unsuccessful, why?
      Would an approach used in the past be appropriate for the present situation? Would it meet with some degree of success? Explore possibilities regarding implementation and outcomes.

If family has considered alternate approaches but has not tried them, family should be assisted to (1) think how approach could be implemented and (2) consider effectiveness of outcomes.

If family perceives that implementation and outcomes will be successful, explore why—is the reasoning realistic? If not, explore other possibilities regarding implementation and outcomes that might be more realistic and workable.

If family perceives that implementation and/or outcomes will be unsuccessful, use same exploratory process as preceding example.

The family should be assisted to explore the implications for each possible approach to decide on the one most effective for the problem situation and the family.

If it becomes necessary for the community health nurse to supplement the family's ideas with other suggested approaches, the same exploratory approach as in the previous example should be used by the family—and the final decision regarding a problem-solving approach resides with the family.

If no (family not attempting to resolve problem)

Must the family do something because of the nature of the problem?

What are the family's reasons for not working on the problem? For example, is there some other family situation that must be resolved first? The problem-solving process may need to refocus unless both problems can be approached simultaneously.

The family is provided with information about the resolution of the problem and the risks associated with neglecting the problem to make an informed decision about a course of action.

The family is assisted in its problem solving in the same manner as discussed previously.

  C. Evaluation (jointly by family and community health nurse)
    1. Evaluation of problem-solving process and experience.
    2. Evaluation of the implementation and outcomes of the family's selected approach to the problem.

---

*Developed by Johnson R for Stanhope M, Lancaster J: *Community Health Nursing,* ed 1.

I.3 FAMILY SYSTEMS STRESSOR-STRENGTH INVENTORY (FS³I)*

Karen B. Mischke, RN, OGNP/WHCNP, PhD, CFLE

Hillsboro Womens Clinic
620 SE Oak Street
Hillsboro, OR 97123

Shirley M. H. Hanson, RN, PMHNP, PhD, FAAN, CFLE, LMFT†

Professor, School of Nursing
Department of Family Nursing
Oregon Health Sciences University
Portland, OR 97201
Telephone: (503) 494-3869
Fax: (503) 494-3878
E-Mail: hanson@ohsu.edu

Instructions for Administration

The Family Systems Stressor-Strength Inventory (FS³I) is an assessment/measurement instrument intended for use with families. It focuses on identifying stressful situations occurring in families and the strengths families use to maintain healthy family functioning. Each family member is asked to complete the instrument on an individual form prior to an interview with the clinician. Questions can be read to members unable to read.

Following completion of the instrument the clinician evaluates the family on each of the stressful situations (general and specific) and the available strengths they possess. This evaluation is recorded on the family member form.

The clinician records the individual family member's score and the clinician perception score on the Quantitative Summary. A different color code is used for each family member. The clinician also completes the Qualitative Summary synthesizing the information gleaned from all participants. Clinicians can use the Family Care Plan to prioritize diagnoses, set goals, develop prevention/intervention activities, and evaluate outcomes.

*From Mischke-Berkey K, Hanson SMH: *Pocket guide to family assessment and intervention,* St Louis, 1991, Mosby.
†Respondent to inquires

FAMILY SYSTEMS STRESSOR-STRENGTH INVENTORY (FS³I)

Family Name _____   Date _____

Family Member(s) Completing Assessment _____

Ethnic Background(s) _____

Religious Background(s) _____

Referral Source _____

Interviewer _____

Family members	Relationship in family	Age	Marital status	Education (highest degree)	Occupation
1. _____	_____	_____	_____	_____	_____
2. _____	_____	_____	_____	_____	_____
3. _____	_____	_____	_____	_____	_____
4. _____	_____	_____	_____	_____	_____
5. _____	_____	_____	_____	_____	_____
6. _____	_____	_____	_____	_____	_____

Families current reasons for seeking assistance?

_____

_____

_____

Part I: Family Systems Stressors (General)

DIRECTIONS: Each of the 25 situations/stressors listed here deals with some aspect of normal family life. They have the potential for creating stress within families or between families and the world in which they live. We are interested in your overall impression of how these situations affect your family life. Please circle a number (0 through 5) that best describes the amount of stress or tension they create for you.

Stressors:	Not applicable	Family perception score					Clinician perception
		Little stress		Medium stress		High stress	Score
1. Family member(s) feel unappreciated 0		1	2	3	4	5	_____
2. Guilt for not accomplishing more 0		1	2	3	4	5	_____
3. Insufficient "me" time 0		1	2	3	4	5	_____
4. Self-image/self-esteem/feelings of unattractiveness 0		1	2	3	4	5	_____
5. Perfectionism 0		1	2	3	4	5	_____
6. Dieting 0		1	2	3	4	5	_____
7. Health/Illness 0		1	2	3	4	5	_____
8. Communication with children 0		1	2	3	4	5	_____
9. Housekeeping standards 0		1	2	3	4	5	_____
10. Insufficient couple time 0		1	2	3	4	5	_____
11. Insufficient family playtime 0		1	2	3	4	5	_____
12. Children's behavior/discipline/sibling fighting 0		1	2	3	4	5	_____
13. Television 0		1	2	3	4	5	_____
14. Over-scheduled family calendar 0		1	2	3	4	5	_____
15. Lack of shared responsibility in the family 0		1	2	3	4	5	_____
16. Moving 0		1	2	3	4	5	_____
17. Spousal relationship (communication, friendship, sex) 0		1	2	3	4	5	_____
18. Holidays 0		1	2	3	4	5	_____
19. In-laws 0		1	2	3	4	5	_____
20. Teen behaviors (communication, music, friends, school) 0		1	2	3	4	5	_____
21. New baby 0		1	2	3	4	5	_____
22. Economics/finances/budgets 0		1	2	3	4	5	_____
23. Unhappiness with work situation 0		1	2	3	4	5	_____
24. Overvolunteerism 0		1	2	3	4	5	_____
25. Neighbors 0		1	2	3	4	5	_____

Additional stressors: _____

Family remarks: _____

Clinician: Clarification of stressful situations/concerns with family members.
Prioritize in order of importance to family members: _____

Part II: Family Systems Stressors (Specific)

DIRECTIONS: The following 12 questions are designed to provide information about your specific stress producing situation, problem, or area of concern influencing your family's health. Please circle a number (1 through 5) that best describes the influence this situation has on your family's life and how well you perceive your family's overall functioning.

The specific stress producing situation/problem or area of concern at this time is _____

_____
_____

Stressors:	Family perception score					Clinician perception
	Little		Medium		High	Score
1. To what extent is your family bothered by this problem or stressful situation? . . . . 1 (e.g., effects on family interactions, communication among members, emotional, and social relationships)		2	3	4	5	____

Family remarks: _____

Clinician remarks: _____

2. How much of an effect does this stressful situation have on your family's usual pattern of living? . . . . 1 (e.g., effects on life-style patterns and family developmental tasks)		2	3	4	5	____

Family remarks: _____

Clinician remarks: _____

3. How much has this situation affected your family's ability to work together as a family unit? . . . . 1 (e.g., alteration in family roles, completion of family tasks, following through with responsibilities)		2	3	4	5	____

Family remarks: _____

Clinician remarks: _____

Has your family ever experienced a similar concern in the past?
    1. YES   If YES, complete question 4.
    2. NO   If NO, complete question 5.

4. How successful was your family in dealing with this situation/problem/concern in the past? . . . . 1 (e.g., workable coping strategies developed, adaptive measures useful, situation improved)		2	3	4	5	____

Family remarks: _____

Clinician remarks: _____

5. How strongly do you feel this current situation/problem/concern will affect your family's future? . . . . 1 (e.g., anticipated consequences)		2	3	4	5	____

Family remarks: _____

Clinician remarks: _____

6. To what extent are family members able to help themselves in this present situation/ problem/concern? . . . . 1 (e.g., self-assistive efforts, family expectations, spiritual influence, and family resources)		2	3	4	5	____

Family remarks: _____

Clinician remarks: _____

Stressors:	Family perception score					Clinician perception
	Little		**Medium**		**High**	**Score**
7. To what extent do you expect others to help your family with this situation/problem/concern? . . . . 1 (e.g., What roles would helpers play? How available are extra-family resources?) Family remarks: _____ _____ Clinician remarks: _____ _____		2	3	4	5	___

Stressors:	Family perception score					Clinician perception
	Poor		**Satisfactory**		**Excellent**	**Score**
8. How would you rate the way your family functions overall? . . . . 1 (e.g., how your family members relate to each other and to larger family and community) Family remarks: _____ _____ Clinician remarks: _____ _____		2	3	4	5	___
9. How would you rate the overall physical health status of each family member by name? (Include yourself as a family member; record additional names on back.)						
a. _____ 1		2	3	4	5	___
b. _____ 1		2	3	4	5	___
c. _____ 1		2	3	4	5	___
d. _____ 1		2	3	4	5	___
e. _____ 1		2	3	4	5	___
10. How would you rate the overall physical health status of your family as a whole? . . . . 1 Family remarks: _____ _____ Clinician perceptions: _____		2	3	4	5	___
11. How would you rate the overall mental health status of each family member by name? (Include yourself as a family member; record additional names on back.)						
a. _____ 1		2	3	4	5	___
b. _____ 1		2	3	4	5	___
c. _____ 1		2	3	4	5	___
d. _____ 1		2	3	4	5	___
e. _____ 1		2	3	4	5	___
12. How would you rate the overall mental health status of your family as a whole? . . . . 1 Family remarks: _____ _____ Clinician perceptions: _____		2	3	4	5	___

Part III: Family Systems Strengths

Directions: Each of the 16 traits/attributes listed below deals with some aspect of family life and its overall functioning. Each one contributes to the health and well-being of family members as individuals and to the family as a whole. Please circle a number (0 through 5) that best describes the extent that the trait applies to your family.

My family:	Not applicable	Family perception score					Clinician perception
		Seldom		Usually		Always	Score
1. Communicates and listens to one another 0		1	2	3	4	5	____
Family remarks: _____							
Clinician remarks: _____							
2. Affirms and supports one another 0		1	2	3	4	5	____
Family remarks: _____							
Clinician remarks: _____							
3. Teaches respect for others 0		1	2	3	4	5	____
Family remarks: _____							
Clinician remarks: _____							
4. Develops a sense of trust in members 0		1	2	3	4	5	____
Family remarks: _____							
Clinician remarks: _____							
5. Displays a sense of play and humor 0		1	2	3	4	5	____
Family remarks: _____							
Clinician remarks: _____							
6. Exhibits a sense of shared responsibility 0		1	2	3	4	5	____
Family remarks: _____							
Clinician remarks: _____							
7. Teaches a sense of right and wrong 0		1	2	3	4	5	____
Family remarks: _____							
Clinician remarks: _____							
8. Has a strong sense of family in which rituals and traditions abound 0		1	2	3	4	5	____
Family remarks: _____							
Clinician remarks: _____							
9. Has a balance of interaction among members 0		1	2	3	4	5	____
Family remarks: _____							
Clinician remarks: _____							
10. Has a shared religious core 0		1	2	3	4	5	____
Family remarks: _____							
Clinician remarks: _____							

My family:	Not applicable	Seldom		Usually		Always	Clinician perception Score
11. Respects the privacy of one another 0		1	2	3	4	5	____
Family remarks: _____							
Clinician remarks: _____							
12. Values service to others 0		1	2	3	4	5	____
Family remarks: _____							
Clinician remarks: _____							
13. Fosters family table time and conversation 0		1	2	3	4	5	____
Family remarks: _____							
Clinician remarks: _____							
14. Shares leisure time 0		1	2	3	4	5	____
Family remarks: _____							
Clinician remarks: _____							
15. Admits to and seeks help with problems 0		1	2	3	4	5	____
Family remarks: _____							
Clinician remarks: _____							
16a. How would you rate the overall strengths that exist in your family? 0		1	2	3	4	5	____
Family remarks: _____							
Clinician remarks: _____							

16b. Additional Family Strengths: _____
_____
_____

16c. Clinician: Clarification of family strengths with individual members: _____
_____
_____
_____
_____

SCORING SUMMARY

The Family Systems Stressor-Strength Inventory (FS³I) Scoring Summary is divided into two sections: Section 1, Family Perception Scores and Section 2, Clinician Perception Scores. These two sections are further divided into three parts: Part I, Family Systems Stressors: General; Part II, Family Systems Stressors: Specific; and Part III, Family Systems Strengths. Each part contains a Quantitative Summary and a Qualitative Summary.

Quantifiable family and clinician perception scores are both graphed on the Quantitative Summary. Each family member has a designated color code. Family and clinician remarks are both recorded on the Qualitative Summary. Quantitative summary scores, when graphed, suggest a level for initiation of prevention/intervention modes: primary, secondary and tertiary. Qualitative summary information, when synthesized, contributes to the development and channeling of the Family Care Plan.

Section 1: Family Perception Scores

Part I   Family Systems Stressors (General)

Add scores from questions 1 to 25 and calculate an overall numerical score for Family System Stressors (General). Ratings are from 1 (most positive) to 5 (most negative). The Not Applicable (0) responses are omitted from the calculations. Total scores range from 25 to 125.

Family Systems Stressor Score: General

$$\frac{(\quad)}{25} \times 1 = \underline{\hspace{2cm}}$$

Graph score on Quantitative Summary, Family Systems Stressors: General, Family Member Perception. Color code to differentiate family members.

Record additional stressors and family remarks in Part I, Qualitative Summary: Family and Clinician Remarks.

Part II   Family Systems Stressors: Specific

Add scores from questions 1-8, 10, and 12 and calculate a numerical score for Family Systems Stressors: Specific. Ratings are from 1 (most positive) to 5 (most negative). Questions 4, 6, 7, 8, 10, and 12 are reverse scored.* Total scores range from 10-50.

Family Systems Stressor Score: Specific

$$\frac{(\quad)}{10} \times 1 = \underline{\hspace{2cm}}$$

Graph score on Quantitative Summary: Family Systems Stressor: Specific. (Family Member Perceptions). Color code to differentiate family members.

Summarize data from questions 9 and 11 (reverse scored) and record family remarks in Part II, Qualitative Summary: Family and Clinician Remarks

Part III   Family Systems Strengths

Add scores from questions 1 to 16 and calculate a numerical score for Family Systems Strengths. Ratings are from 1 (seldom) to 5 (always). The Not Applicable (0) responses are omitted from the calculations. Total scores range from 16 to 80.

Family Systems Strength Score

$$\frac{(\quad)}{16} \times 1 = \underline{\hspace{2cm}}$$

Graph score on Quantitative Summary: Family Systems Strengths (Family Member Perception).

Record additional family strengths and family remarks in Part III, Qualitative Summary: Family and Clinician Remarks.

*Reverse Scoring:
  Question answered as (1) is scored 5 points
  Question answered as (2) is scored 4 points
  Question answered as (3) is scored 3 points
  Question answered as (4) is scored 2 points
  Question answered as (5) is scored 1 point

Section 2: Clinician Perception Scores

Part I   Family Systems Stressors (General)

Add scores from questions 1 to 25 and calculate an overall numerical score for Family System Stressors (General). Ratings are from 1 (most positive) to 5 (most negative). The Not Applicable (0) responses are omitted from the calculations. Total scores range from 25 to 125.

Family Systems Stressor Score: General

$$\frac{(\quad)}{25} \times 1 = \underline{\hspace{2cm}}$$

Graph score on Quantitative Summary, Family Systems Stressors: General (Clinician Perception).

Record Clinicians' clarification of general stressors in Part I, Qualitative Summary: Family and Clinician Remarks

Part II   **Family Systems Stressors: Specific**

Add scores from questions 1-8, 10 and 12 and calculate a numerical score for Family Systems Stressors: Specific. Ratings are from 1 (most positive) to 5 (most negative). Questions 4, 6, 7, 8, 10, and 12 are reverse scored.* Total scores range from 10-50.

Family Systems Stressor Score: Specific

$$\frac{(\quad)}{10} \times 1 = \underline{\qquad}$$

Graph score on Quantitative Summary: Family Systems Stressor: Specific. (Clinician Perception).

Summarize data from questions 9 and 11 (reverse order) and record clinician remarks in Part II, Qualitative Summary: Family and Clinician Remarks

Part III   **Family Systems Strengths**

Add scores from questions 1 to 16 and calculate a numerical score for Family Systems Strengths. Ratings are from 1 (seldom) to 5 (always). The Not Applicable (0) responses are omitted from the calculations. Total scores range from 16 to 80.

Family Systems Strength Score

$$\frac{(\quad)}{16} \times 1 = \underline{\qquad}$$

Graph score on Quantitative Summary: Family Systems Strengths (Clinician Perception).

Record clinicians' clarification of family strengths in Part III, Qualitative Summary: Family and Clinician Remarks.

---

*Reverse Scoring:
   Question answered as (1) is scored 5 points
   Question answered as (2) is scored 4 points
   Question answered as (3) is scored 3 points
   Question answered as (4) is scored 2 points
   Question answered as (5) is scored 1 point

Quantitative Summary Family Systems Stressors: General and Specific Family and Clinician Perception Scores

DIRECTIONS: Graph the scores from each family member inventory by placing an "X" at the appropriate location. (Use first name initial for each different entry and different color code for each family member.)

Scores for Wellness and Stability	Family Systems Stressors: General		Scores for Wellness and Stability	Family Systems Stressors: Specific	
	Family Member Perception Score	Clinician Perception Score		Family Member Perception Score	Clinician Perception Score
5.0			5.0		
4.8			4.8		
4.6			4.6		
4.4			4.4		
4.2			4.2		
4.0			4.0		
3.8			3.8		
3.6			3.6		
3.4			3.4		
3.2			3.2		
3.0			3.0		
2.8			2.8		
2.6			2.6		
2.4			2.4		
2.2			2.2		
2.0			2.0		
1.8			1.8		
1.6			1.6		
1.4			1.4		
1.2			1.2		

PRIMARY Prevention/Intervention Mode: Flexible Line   1.0-2.3
SECONDARY Prevention/Intervention Mode: Normal Line   2.4-3.6
TERTIARY Prevention/Intervention Mode: Resistance Lines   3.7-5.0

*Breakdown of numerical scores for stressor penetration are suggested values.

Family Systems Strengths Family & Clinician Perception Scores

DIRECTIONS: Graph the scores from the inventory by placing an "X" at the appropriate location and connect with a line. (Use first name initial for each different entry and different color code for each family member.)

Sum of strengths available for prevention/ intervention mode	Family Systems Strengths	
	Family Member Perception Score	Clinician Perception Score
5.0		
4.8		
4.6		
4.4		
4.2		
4.0		
3.8		
3.6		
3.4		
3.2		
3.0		
2.8		
2.6		
2.4		
2.2		
2.0		
1.8		
1.6		
1.4		
1.2		
1.0		

PRIMARY Prevention/Intervention Mode: Flexible Line   1.0-2.3
SECONDARY Prevention/Intervention Mode: Normal Line   2.4-3.6
TERTIARY Prevention/Intervention Mode: Resistance Lines   3.7-5.0

*Breakdown of numerical scores for stressor penetration are suggested values.

Qualitative Summary Family and Clinician Remarks

Part I: Family Systems Stressors: General

Summarize general stressors and remarks of family and clinician. Prioritize stressors according to importance to family members.

_____

_____

_____

Part II: Family Systems Stressors: Specific

A. Summarize specific stressor and remarks of family and clinician.

_____

_____

_____

B. Summarize differences (if discrepancies exist) between how family members and clinician view effects of stressful situation on family.

_____

_____

_____

C. Summarize overall family functioning.

_____

_____

_____

D. Summarize overall significant physical health status for family members.

_____

_____

_____

E. Summarize overall significant mental health status for family members.

_____

_____

_____

Part III: Family Systems Strengths

Summarize family systems strengths and family and clinician remarks that facilitate family health and stability.

_____

_____

_____

Family Care Plan*					
Diagnosis general and specific family system stressors	Family systems strengths supporting family care plan	Goals family and clinician	Prevention/Intervention mode		Outcomes evaluation and replanning
			Primary, secondary or tertiary	Prevention/intervention activities	

*Prioritize the three most significant diagnoses.

I.4 THE FRIEDMAN FAMILY ASSESSMENT MODEL—SHORT FORM

Two words of caution are called for before using the following guidelines in completing family assessments. First, not all areas included below will be germane for each of the families visited. The guidelines are comprehensive and allow depth when probing is necessary. The student should not feel that every sub-area needs to be covered when the broad area of inquiry poses no problems to the family or concern to the health worker. Second, by virtue of the interdependence of the family system, one will find unavoidable redundancy. For the sake of efficiency, the assessor should try not to repeat data, but to refer the reader back to sections where this information has aleady been described.

Identifying Data

1. Family Name
2. Address and Phone
3. Family Composition (genogram)
4. Type of Family Form
5. Cultural (Ethnic) Background
6. Religious Identification
7. Social Class Status
8. Family's Recreational or Leisure-time Activities

Developmental Stage and History of Family

9. Family's Present Developmental Stage
10. Extent of Developmental Stage Fulfillment
11. Nuclear Family History
12. History of Family of Origin of Both Parents

Environmental Data

13. Home Characteristics
14. Characteristics of Neighborhood and Larger Community
15. Family's Geographic Mobility
16. Family's Associations and Transactions With Community
17. Family's Social Support Netowrk (ecomap)

Family Structure

18. Communication Patterns
    Extent of Functional and Dysfunctional Communication (types of recurring patterns)
    Extent of Affective Messages and How Expressed
    Characteristics of Communication within Family Subsystems
    Types of Dysfunctional Communication Processes Seen in Family
    Areas of Closed Communication
    Familial and External Variables Affecting Communication
19. Power Structure
    Power Outcomes
    Decision-making Process
    Power Bases
    Variables Affecting Power
    Overall Family Power
20. Role Structure
    Formal Role Structure
    Informal Role Structure
    Analysis of Role Models (optional)
    Variables Affecting Role Structure
21. Family Values
    Compare the family to American or family's reference group values and/or identify important family values and their importance (priority) in family.
    Congruence Between Family's Values and Values of Family's Subsystems, as well as Family's Reference Group and/or Wider Community
    Variables Influencing Family Values
    Are these values consciously or unconsciously held by the family?
    Presence of value conflicts in family.
    Effect of the above values and value conflicts on health status of family.

Family Functions

22. Affective Function
    Family's Need-Response Patterns
    Mutual Nurturance, Closeness, and Identification
    Separateness and Connectedness
23. Socialization Function
    Family Child-rearing Practices
    Adaptability of Child-rearing Practices for Family Form and Family's Situation
    Who Is (Are) Socializing Agent(s) for Child(ren)?
    Value of Children in Family
    Cultural Beliefs That Influence Family's Child-rearing Patterns
    Social Class Influence on Child-Rearing Patterns
    Estimation About Whether Family Is at Risk for Child-rearing Problems and if so, Indication of High-Risk Factors
    Adequacy of Home Environment for Children's Needs to Play
24. Health Care Function
    Family's Health Beliefs, Values, and Behavior
    Family's Definitions of Health-Illness and Their Level of Knowledge
    Family's Perceived Health Status and Illness Susceptibility
    Family's Dietary Practices
    Adequacy of family diet (recommended 24-hour food history record).
    Function of mealtimes and attitudes toward food and mealtimes.

From Friedman, M.M. (1992). Family nursing: theory and practice, ed 3, Norwalk, Conn, 1992.

Table I-I   Family Composition Form

Name (Last, First)	Gender	Relationship	Date/place of birth	Occupation	Education
1. (Father)					
2. (Mother)					
3. (Oldest child)					
4.					
5.					
6.					
7.					
8.					

Shopping (and its planning) practices.
Person(s) responsible for planning, shopping, and preparation of meals.
Sleeping and Resting Habits
Exercise and Recreation Practices
Family's Drug Habits
Family's Role in Self-care Practices
Family's Environmental Practices
Medically Based Preventive Measures (physicals, eye and hearing tests, and immunizations)
Dental Health Practices
Family Health History (both general and specific diseases—environmentally and genetically related)
Health Care Services Received
Feelings and Perceptions Regarding Health Services
Emergency Health Care Services
Dental Health Services

Source of Medical and Dental Payments
Logistics of Receiving Care

Family Coping

25. Short- and Long-term Familial Stressors
26. Family's Ability to Respond, Based on Objective Appraisal of Stress-producing Situations
27. Coping Strategies Utilized (present/past)
    Differences in family members' ways of coping
    Family's inner coping strategies
    Family's external coping strategies
28. Areas/Situations Where Family Has Achieved Mastery
29. Dysfunctional Adaptive Strategies Utilized (present/past)

I.5   FAMILIES WITH PHYSICALLY COMPROMISED MEMBERS: ASSESSMENT TOOLS

Use with Families

Assessment tool	Purpose	Reference
The Caregiver Reaction Assessment (CRA)	Assesses the reaction of family members caring for elderly persons with physical impairments.	Given CW, Given B, Stommel M, Collins C, King S, Franklin S: The Caregiver Reaction Assessment (CRA) for caregivers to persons with chronic physical and mental impairments, *Res Nurs Health*, 15(4):271-283, 1992.
Demands-of-Illness Scale	Can be used with individuals or families to assess impact of disease on entire family's health, coping, and functioning.	Haberman MR, Woods NF, Packard NJ: Demands of chronic illness: reliability and validity assessment of a Demands-of-Illness Inventory, *Holistic Nurs Practice* 5(1):25-35, 1990.
Family Needs Assessment Tool	Assesses needs of families of chronically ill children.	Rawlins PS, Rawlins TD, Horner M: Development of the Family Needs Assessment Tool, *Western J Nurs Res* 12(2):201-214, 1990.
Impact-on-Family Scale	Measures stressors related to childhood illness.	Stein R, Riessman C: The development of an Impact-on-Family Scale: preliminary findings, *Med Care* 18(2):324-330, 1980.

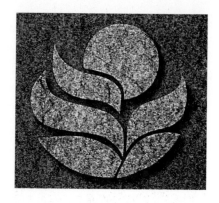

Appendix J
Individual Assessment Tools

J.1 DISCHARGE PATIENT QUESTIONNAIRE

VNA of Eastern Montgomery County/Department of Abington Memorial Hospital Discharge Patient Questionnaire

---

DISCHARGE PATIENT QUESTIONNAIRE # _____

1. What services were provided?

   Nursing —   Occupational Therapy —

   Home Health Aide (personal care) —   Speech Therapy —

   Social Worker —   Physical Therapy —

2. Was the service what you expected it to be? _____
   _____

3. VNA personnel considered my family's special needs.

Poor	Fair	Satisfactory	Very Good	Excellent
1	2	3	4	5

4. I was satisfied with ther personnel.

Poor	Fair	Satisfactory	Very Good	Excellent
1	2	3	4	5

5. Were there other services you would have liked us to provide? _____
   _____

6. Instructions provided by VNA personnel related to my health care needs were clear.

Poor	Fair	Satisfactory	Very Good	Excellent
1	2	3	4	5

7. Questions were answered adequately.

Poor	Fair	Satisfactory	Very Good	Excellent
1	2	3	4	5

8. This service helped me achieve my health care goals.

Poor	Fair	Satisfactory	Very Good	Excellent
1	2	3	4	5

9. Would you use this service again? _____
   _____

10. Would you recommend this service to others? _____
   _____

11. What suggestions would you make to improve the services? _____
   _____

VNA of Eastern Montgomery County/Department of Abington Memorial Hospital Discharge Patient Questionnaire—cont'd

12. Additional Comments: _____

_____

_____

Signature: _____   Date: _____

Please complete for those services received:

1. The nurse understood what my main health problem was.

Poor	Fair	Satisfactory	Very Good	Excellent
1		3	4	5

2. The nurse appeared skillful in carrying out procedures.

Poor	Fair	Satisfactory	Very Good	Excellent
1		3	4	5

3. The home health aide considered my individual needs.

Poor	Fair	Satisfactory	Very Good	Excellent
1		3	4	5

4. The home health aide provided personal care to my satisfaction.

Poor	Fair	Satisfactory	Very Good	Excellent
1		3	4	5

5. The physical therapist explained things in language that I could understand.

Poor	Fair	Satisfactory	Very Good	Excellent
1		3	4	5

6. The exercise program that the physical therapist gave me helped me achieve my goals.

Poor	Fair	Satisfactory	Very Good	Excellent
1		3	4	5

7. The social worker acted in a supportive manner.

Poor	Fair	Satisfactory	Very Good	Excellent
1		3	4	5

8. The social worker gave me information about available resources.

Poor	Fair	Satisfactory	Very Good	Excellent
1		3	4	5

9. The speech therapist visited according to the plan.

Poor	Fair	Satisfactory	Very Good	Excellent
1		3	4	5

10. The speech therapist helped me communicate.

Poor	Fair	Satisfactory	Very Good	Excellent
1		3	4	5

11. The occupational therapist enabled me to improve in my activities of daily living.

Poor	Fair	Satisfactory	Very Good	Excellent
1		3	4	5

12. The occupational therapy visit schedule met my needs.

Poor	Fair	Satisfactory	Very Good	Excellent
1		3	4	5

J.2　INSTRUMENTAL ACTIVITIES OF DAILY LIVING (IADL) SCALE

Name _____　Rated by _____　Date _____

1. **Can you use the telephone**
   without help,　　3
   with some help, or　　2
   are you completely unable to use the telephone?　　1

2. **Can you get to places beyond walking distance**
   without help,　　3
   with some help, or　　2
   are you completely unable to travel unless special arrangements are made?　　1

3. **Can you go shopping for groceries**
   without help,　　3
   with some help, or　　2
   are you completely unable to do any shopping?　　1

4. **Can you prepare your own meals**
   without help,　　3
   with some help, or　　2
   are you completely unable to prepare any meals?　　1

5. **Can you do your own housework**
   without help,　　3
   with some help, or　　2
   are you completely unable to do any housework?　　1

6. **Can you do your own handyman work**
   without help,　　3
   with some help, or　　2
   are you completely unable to do any handyman work?　　1

7. **Can you do your own laundry**
   without help,　　3
   with some help, or　　2
   are you completely unable to do any laundry at all?　　1

8a. **Do you take medicines or use any medications?**
   Yes (If yes, answer Question 8b.)　　1
   No (If no, answer Question 8c.)　　2

8b. **Do you take your own medicine**
   without help (in the right doses at the right time),　　3
   with some help (if someone prepares it for you and/or reminds you to take it), or　　2
   are you completely unable to take your own medicine?　　1

8c. **If you had to take medicine, could you do it**
   without help (in the right doses at the right time),　　3
   with some help (if someone prepared it for you and/or reminded you to take it), or　　2
   would you be completely unable to take your own medicine?　　1

9. **Can you manage your own money**
   without help,　　3
   with some help, or　　2
   are you completely unable to manage money?　　1

From Philadelphia Geriatric Center, Philadelphia, PA. Used with permission.

J.3　COMPREHENSIVE OLDER PERSONS' EVALUATION

Name (print): _____　Date of Visit: _____

Chief complaint: _____

Today, I will ask you about your overall health and function and will be using a questionnaire to help me obtain this information. The first few questions are to check your memory.

Preliminary Cognition Questionnaire: Record if answer is correct with (+); if answer is incorrect with (−).

1. What is the date today?　_____
2. What day of the week is it?　_____
3. What is the name of this place?　_____
4. What is your telephone number or room number?
   record answer: _____
   If subject does not have phone, ask:
   What is your street address?　_____
5. How old are you? record answer: _____　_____
6. When were you born? Record answer from records if patient cannot answer: _____　_____
7. Who is the president of the United States now?　_____

8. Who was the president just before him?　_____
9. What was your mother's maiden name?　_____
10. Subtract 3 from 20 and keep subtracting from each new number until you get all the way down　_____
    Total errors: _____

If more than 4 errors, ask 11. If more than 6 errors, complete questionnaire for informant.

11. Do you think you would benefit from a legal guardian, someone who would be responsible for your legal and financial matters? Do you have a living will? Would you like one?
    a. no
    b. has functioning legal guardian for sole purpose of managing money-describe:
    c. has legal guardian
    d. yes

From Pearlman R: Development of a functional assessment questionnaire for geriatric patients: the comprehensive older persons evaluation, J *Chronic Disease* 40(56): 85S-94S, 1987.

J.3   Comprehensive Older Persons' Evaluation—cont'd

Demographic Section:

1. Patient's race or ethnic background—record: _____
2. Patient's gender (circle)   male   female
3. How far did you go in school?
   a. post-graduate education
   b. four-year degree
   c. college or technical school
   d. high school complete
   e. high school incomplete
   f. 0-8 years

Social Support Section: Now there are a few questions about your family and friends.

4. Are you married, widowed, separated, divorced, or have you never been married?
   a. now married
   b. widowed
   c. separated
   d. divorced
   e. never married
5. Who lives with you? (circle all responses)
   a. spouse
   b. other relative or friend—specify: _____
   c. group living situation (non-health)
   d. lives alone
   e. nursing home, number of years: _____
6. Have you talked to any friends or relatives by phone during the last week?
   a. yes
   b. no
7. Are you satisfied by seeing your relatives and friends as often as you want to, or are you somewhat dissatisfied about how little you see them?
   a. satisfied—skip to #8
   b. dissatisfied—ask A
   A. Do you feel you would like to be involved in a Senior Citizens Center for social events, or perhaps meals?
      1. no
      2. is involved—describe: _____
      3. yes
8. Is there someone who would take care of you for as long as you needed if you were sick or disabled?
   a. yes—skip to C
   b. no—ask A
   A. Is there someone who would take care of you for a short time?
      1. yes—skip to C
      2. no—ask B
   B. Is there someone who could help you now and then?
      1. yes—ask C
      2. no—ask C
   C. Who would we call in case of an emergency? Record name and telephone: _____

Financial Section: The next few questions are about your finances and any problems you might have.

9. Do you own, or are you buying, your own home?
   a. yes—skip to #10
   b. no—ask A
   A. Do you feel you need assistance with housing?
      1. no
      2. has subsidized or other housing assistance
      3. yes—describe: _____
   B. What type of housing did you have prior to coming here?
10. Are you covered by private medical insurance, Medicare, Medicaid, or some disability plan? (Circle all that apply)
    a. private insurance—specify and skip to #11:
       _____
    b. medicare
    c. medicaid
    d. disability—specify and ask A:
       _____
    e. none
    f. other—specify: _____
    A. Do you feel you need additional assistance with your medical bills?
       1. no
       2. yes
11. Which of these statements best describes your financial situation?
    a. my bills are no problem to me—skip to #12
    b. my expenses make it difficult to meet my bills—ask A
    c. my expenses are so heavy that I cannot meet my bills—ask A
    A. Do you feel you need financial assistance such as: (circle all that apply)
       1. food stamps
       2. social security or disability payments
       3. assistance in paying your heating or electrical bills
       4. other financial assistance? describe: _____

Psychological Health Section: The next few questions are about how you feel about your life in general. There are no right or wrong answers, only what best applies to you. Please answer yes or no to each question.

12. Is your daily life full of things that keep you interested?   _____
13. Have you, at times, very much wanted to leave home?   _____
14. Does it seem that no one understands you?   _____
15. Are you happy most of the time?   _____
16. Do you feel weak all over much of the time?   _____
17. Is your sleep fitful and disturbed?   _____

Continued.

J.3 Comprehensive Older Persons' Evaluation—cont'd

18. Taking everything into consideration, how would you describe your satisfaction with your life in general at the present time?
    a. good
    b. fair
    c. poor
19. Do you feel you now need help with your mental health; for example, a counselor or psychiatrist?
    a. no
    b. has—specify: _____
    c. yes

Physical Health Section: The next few questions are about your health.

20. During the past month (30 days), how many days were you so sick that you couldn't do your usual activities, such as working around the house or visiting with friends? _____
21. Relative to other people your age, how would you rate your overall health at the present time?
    a. excellent—skip to #22
    b. very good—skip to #22
    c. good—ask A
    d. fair—ask A
    e. poor—ask A
        A. Do you feel you need additional medical services such as a doctor, nurse, visiting nurse or physical therapy?
            1. doctor
            2. nurse
            3. visiting nurse
            4. physical therapy
            5. none
22. Do you use an aid for walking, such as a wheelchair, walker, cane or anything else? (circle aid usually used)
    a. wheelchair
    b. other—specify _____
    c. visiting nurse
    d. walker
    e. none
23. How much do your health troubles stand in the way of your doing things you want to do?
    a. not at all—skip to #24
    b. a little—ask A
    c. a great deal—ask A
        A. Do you think you need assistance to do your daily activities; for example, do you need a live-in aide or choreworker?
            1. live-in aide
            2. choreworker
            3. has aide, choreworker or other assistance describe _____
            4. none needed

24. Have you had, or do you currently have, any of the following health problems? (if yes, place an "X" in appropriate box and describe; medical record information may be used to help complete this section.)

	HX	Current	Describe
a. Arthritis or rheumatism?			
b. Lung or breathing problem?			
c. Hypertension?			
d. Heart trouble?			
e. Phlebitis or poor circulation problems in arms or legs?			
f. Diabetes or low blood sugar?			
g. Digestive ulcers?			
h. Other digestive problem?			
i. Cancer?			
j. Anemia?			
k. Effects of stroke?			
l. Other neurological problem? specify: _____			
m. Thyroid or other glandular problem? specify: _____			
n. Skin disorders such as pressure sores, leg ulcers, burns?			
o. Speech problem?			
p. Hearing problem?			
q. Vision or eye problem?			
r. Kidney or bladder problems, or incontinence?			
s. A problem of falls?			
t. Problem with eating or your weight? specify: _____			
u. Problem with depression? specify: _____			
v. Problem with your behavior? specify: _____			
w. Problem with your sexual activity?			
x. Problem with alcohol?			
y. Problem with pain?			
z. Other health problems? specify: _____			

J.3   Comprehensive Older Persons' Evaluation—cont'd

Immunizations: _____
_____
_____

25. What medications are you currently taking, or have been taking, in the last month? (May I see your medication bottles?) (If patient cannot list, ask categories a-r and note dosage and schedule, or obtain information from medical or pharmacy records and verify accuracy with the patient.)

Allergies: _____

		Rx (dosage and Schedule)
a.	Arthritis medication	_____
b.	Pain medication	_____
c.	Blood pressure medication?	_____
d.	Water pills or pills for fluid?	_____
e.	Medication for your heat	_____
f.	Medication for your lungs	_____
g.	Blood thinners	_____
h.	Medication for your circulation	_____
i.	Insulin or diabetes medication	_____
j.	Seizure medication	_____
k.	Thyroid pills	_____
l.	Steroids	_____
m.	Hormones	_____
n.	Antibiotics	_____
o.	Medicine for nerves or depression	_____
p.	Prescription sleeping pills	_____
q.	Other prescription drugs	_____
r.	Other nonprescription drugs	_____

26. Many people have problems remembering to take their medications, especially ones they need to take on a regular basis. How often do you forget to take your medications? Would you say you forget often, sometimes, rarely or never?
   a. never
   b. rarely
   c. sometimes
   d. often

Activities of Daily Living: The next set of questions asks whether you need help with any of the following activities of daily living.

27. I would like to know whether you can do these activities without any help at all, or if you need assistance to do them. Do you need help to: (If yes, describe, including patient needs.)

		Yes	No	Describe (include needs)
a.	Use the telephone?			
b.	Get to places out of walking distance? (using transportation)			
c.	Shop for clothes and food?			
d.	Do your housework?			
e.	Handle your money?			
f.	Feed yourself?			
g.	Dress and undress yourself?			
h.	Take care of your appearance?			
i.	Get in and out of bed?			
j.	Take a bath or shower?			
k.	Prepare your meals?			
l.	Do you have any problem getting to the bathroom on time?			

28. During the past six months, have you had any help with such things as shopping, housework, bathing, dressing and getting around?
   a. yes—specify: _____
   b. no

Signature of person completing the form:

_____

J.4   THE GERIATRIC DEPRESSION SCALE

Choose the best answer for how you felt the past week.

1. Are you basically satisfied with your life?	YES	NO*
2. Have you dropped many of your activities and interests?	YES*	NO
3. Do you feel that your life is empty?	YES*	NO
4. Do you often get bored?	YES*	NO
5. Are you hopeful about the future?	YES	NO*
6. Are you bothered by thoughts you can't get out of your head?	YES*	NO
7. Are you in good spirits most of the time?	YES	NO*
8. Are you afraid that something bad is going to happen to you?	YES*	NO
9. Do you feel happy most of the time?	YES	NO*
10. Do you often feel helpless?	YES*	NO
11. Do you often get restless and fidgety?	YES*	NO
12. Do you prefer to stay at home, rather than going out and doing new things?	YES*	NO
13. Do you frequently worry about the future?	YES*	NO
14. Do you feel you have more problems with memory than most?	YES*	NO
15. Do you think it is wonderful to be alive now?	YES	NO*
16. Do you often feel downhearted and blue?	YES*	NO
17. Do you feel pretty worthless the way you are now?	YES*	NO
18. Do you worry a lot about the past?	YES*	NO
19. Do you find life very exciting?	YES	NO*
20. Is it hard for you to get started on new projects?	YES*	NO
21. Do you feel full of energy?	YES	NO*
22. Do you feel that your situation is hopeless?	YES*	NO
23. Do you think that most people are better off then you are?	YES*	NO
24. Do you frequently get upset over little things?	YES*	NO
25. Do you frequently feel like crying?	YES*	NO
26. Do you have trouble concentrating?	YES*	NO
27. Do you enjoy getting up in the morning?	YES	NO*
28. Do you prefer to avoid social gatherings?	YES*	NO
29. Is it easy for you to make decisions?	YES	NO*
30. Is your mind as clear as it used to be?	YES	NO*

From Yesavage HA, Brink TL, Rose TL, et al: Development and validation of a geriatric depression scale: a preliminary report, J *Psychiatric Res* 17:37-49, 1983. Elsevier Science Ltd, Pergamon Imprint, Oxford, England. Reprinted with permission.

*Each answer indicated by an asterisk counts 1 point. Scores between 15 and 22 suggest mild depression; scores above 22 suggest severe depression. Fifteen-item short form includes questions 1-4, 7-10, 12, 14, 17, 21-23. On the short form, scores between 5 and 9 suggest depression, scores above 9 generally indicate depression.

J.5   MINI-MENTAL STATE EXAMINATION

<table>
<tr><td></td><td align="right">**Points**</td></tr>
</table>

I.   **Orientation** (Maximum score: 10)
Ask "What is today's date?" Then ask specifically for parts omitted, such as "Can you also tell me what season it is?"

Ask "Can you tell me the name of this hospital?"
"What floor are we on?"
"What town (or city) are we in?"
"What county are we in?"
"What state are we in?"

	Points	
Date (e.g., January 21)	...1	___
Year	2	___
Month	3	___
Day (e.g., Monday)	4	___
Season	5	___
Hospital	6	___
Floor	7	___
Town/City	8	___
County	9	___
State	...10	___

II.   **Registration** (Maximum score: 3)
Ask the patient if you may test his memory. Then say "ball", "flag", "tree" clearly and slowly, allowing about one second for each. After you have said all three words, ask the patient to repeat them. This first repetition determines the score (0-3), but continue to say them (up to six trials) until the patient can repeat all three words. If he does not eventually learn all three, recall cannot be meaningfully tested.

"ball"	...11	___
"flag"	...12	___
"tree"	...13	___

Number of trials: _____

III.   **Attention and calculation** (Maximum score: 5)
Ask the patient to begin at 100 and count backward by 7. Stop after five subtractions (93, 86, 79, 72, 65). Score one point for each correct number.

If the subject cannot or will not perform this task, ask him to spell the word "world" backward (D, L, R, O, W). Score one point for each correctly placed letter, e.g., DLROW=5, DLORW=3.
Record how the patient spelled "world" backward: _____

"93"	...14	___
"86"	...15	___
"79"	...16	___
"72"	...17	___
"65"	...18	___
or		
Number of correctly placed letters	19	___

IV.   **Recall** (Maximum score: 3)
Ask the patient to recall the three words you previously asked him to remember (learned in Registration).

"ball"	...20	___
"flag"	...21	___
"tree"	...22	___

V.   **Language** (Maximum score: 9)
Naming: Show the patient a wristwatch and ask "What is this?"
Repeat for a pencil. Score one point for each item named correctly.

Watch	...23	___
Pencil	...24	___

Repetition: Ask the patient to repeat "No if's, and's or but's." Score one point for correct repetition.

Repetition	...25	___

Three-stage command: Give the patient a piece of blank paper and say "Take the paper in your right hand, fold it in half and put it on the floor." Score one point for each action performed correctly.

Takes in right hand	26	___
Folds in half	27	___
Puts on the floor	28	___

Reading: On a blank piece of paper, print the sentence "Close your eyes" in letters large enough for the patient to see clearly. Ask the patient to read it and do what it says. Score correct only if he actually closes his eyes.

Closes eyes	...29	___

Writing: Give the patient a blank piece of paper and ask him to write a sentence. It is to be written spontaneously. It must contain a subject and verb and make sense. Correct grammar and punctuation are not necessary.

Writes sentence	30	___

Copying: On a clean piece of paper, draw intersecting pentagons as illustrated, each side measuring about 1 inch, and ask the patient to copy it exactly as it is. All 10 angles must be present and two must intersect to score 1 point. Tremor and rotation are ignored.

Draws pentagons	31	___

Score: Add number of correct responses. In Section III, include items 14 through 18 or item 19, not both. (Maximum total score: 30).

Level of consciousness: ___ coma ___ stupor ___ drowsy ___ alert

Total Score: _____

From Folstein MS, Folstein SE, McHugh PR: Mini-mental state examination, J *Psychiatric Res* 12:189-198, 1995. Elsevier Science Ltd, Pergamon Imprint, Oxford, England. Reprinted with permission.

J.6   ASSESSMENT TOOLS FOR PHYSICALLY COMPROMISED INDIVIDUALS

Assessment tool	Purpose	Reference
Alcohol Consumption Questionnaire	Administered after the Semi-Quantitative Food Frequency Questionnaire as a way to enhance self-report of alcohol use.	King AC: Enhancing the self-report of alcohol consumption in the community: two questionnaire formats, *Am J Public Health* 84(2):294-296, 1994.
Assessment of older drivers: History and initial tests	Assesses older drivers' capacity to operate a motor vehicle safely.	Reuben DB: Assessment of older drivers, *Clin Geriatr Med* 9(2):449-459, 1993.
Barriers to Health-Promoting Activities for Disabled Persons Scale	Measures perceived barriers to health promotion behaviors of adults with disabilities.	Stuifbergen AK, Becker H, Sands D: Barriers to health promotion for individuals with disabilities, *Fam Community Health* 13(1):11-22, 1990.
Coping Health Inventory for Children (CHIC)	Designed to provide systematic assessment of coping behaviors of chronically ill school-aged children.	Austin JK, Patterson JM, Huberty TJ: Development of the Coping Health Inventory for Children, *J Pediatr Nurs* 6(3):166-174, 1991.
Denver II	Screen for developmental problems in children 1 month-6 years of age.	Frankenburg WK: Preventing developmental delays: is developmental screening sufficient? *Pediatrics* 93(4):586-593, 1994.
Dietary Behavior Questionnaire	Measures dietary practices related to fat intake.	Beerman KA, Dittus K: Assessment of a Dietary Behavior Questionnaire, *Health Values* 18(2);3-6, 1994.
Epilepsy Self-Efficacy Scale (ESES)	Assesses a person's confidence in managing epilepsy; explores epilepsy self-management.	Dilorio C, Faherty B, Manteuffel B: The development and testing of an instrument to measure self-efficacy in individuals with epilepsy, *J Neuroscience Nurs* 24(1):9-13, 1992.
Functional Disability Inventory	Measures functional limitations of children.	Walker LS, Greene JW: The Functional Disability Inventory: measuring a neglected dimension of child health status, *J Pediatr Psychol* 16(1):39-58, 1991.
Groningen Activity Restriction Scale (GARS)	Measures disability severity of several chronic conditions and changes over time in adults.	Suurmeijer TP, et al: The Groningen Activity Restriction Scale for measuring disability: its utility in international comparisons, *Am J Public Health* 84(8):1270-1273, 1994.
Health Assessment Questionnaire	Self-administered questionnaire. Disability score is specifically for function with arthritis.	Goeppinger T, Doyle AT, Charlton SL, Lorig K: A nursing perspective on the assessment of function in persons with arthritis, *Res Nurs Health* 11(5):321-331, 1988.
The Hearing Handicap Inventory for Adults	Questionnaire for adults <64 years of age to help describe a person's reaction to his hearing loss.	Newman CW, Weinstein BE, Jacobson GP, Huy GA: The Hearing Handicap Inventory for Adults Psychometric adequacy and audiometric correlates, *Ear and Hearing* 11(6):430-433, 1990.
Metro-Manila Developmental Screening Test (MMDST)	A Philippine version of the Denver Developmental Screening Test.	Williams PD: The Metro-Manila Developmental Screening Test: a normative study, *Nurs Res* 33:204-212, 1984.
Pediatric Evaluation of Disability (PEDI)	Assessment of children with physical disabilities.	Reid DT, Boschen K, Wright V: Critique of the Pediatric Evaluation of Disability Inventory (PEDI), *Phys Occup Ther Pediatr* 13(4):57-93, 1993.
Tinnitus Handicap Questionnaire	Compares a person's tinnitus handicap with the norm, identifies specific areas of handicaps, and monitors progress with particular treatment programs.	Kuk FK, Tyler RS, Russell D, Jordan H: The psychometric properties of a TInnitus Handicap Questionnaire, *Ear and Hearing* 11(6):434-445, 1990.
Torabi Cancer Prevention Behavior Scale	Measures behavior of college students with regard to cancer prevention.	Torabi MR: A cancer prevention behavior scale, *Health Values* 15(3):12-21, 1991.

Assessment Tools for Physically Compromised Individuals—cont'd

Type	Client	References
Development	Children	1. Fewell RR: Trends in the assessment of infants and children with disabilities, *Exceptional Children* 58(2):166-173, 1991. 2. Glascoe FP, Martin ED, Humphrey S: A comparative review of developmental screening tests, *Pediatrics* 86(4):547-554, 1990.
Disability	Adults	1. Kinney WB, Coyle CP: Predicting life satisfaction among adults with physical disabilities, *Arch Phys Med Rehab* 73(9):863-869, 1992. 2. Delitto A: Are measures of function and disability important in low-back care? *Phys Ther* 74(5):452-462, 1994. 3. Duncan PW: Stroke disability, *Phys Ther* 74(5):399-407, 1994. 4. Haley SM, Coster WJ, Binda-Simdberg K: Measuring physical disablement: the contextual challenge, *Phys Ther* 74(5):443-451, 1994.

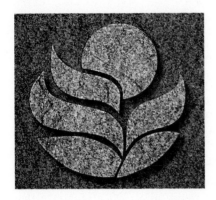

Glossary

A

abandonment Forsaking a client in need of service; determined through the judicial system.

absolute standard Standard used by the federal government to define a basic set of resources necessary for adequate (not poverty level) existence.

acceptant intervention mode Consultative mode of client intervention that is a process of catharsis intended to clear emotional blocks in order to engage in objective problem solving.

accommodation Ways in which children modify their view of the world as they have new experiences that influence their responses.

accountability Being answerable legally, morally, ethically or socially, to someone for something one has done.

accreditation A credentialing process used to recognize health care agencies or educational programs for provision of quality services and programs.

acid rain The precipitation of moisture as rain with high acidity caused by release of pollutants into the atmosphere.

acquired immunodeficiency syndrome (AIDS) The final stages of HIV infection, which follows a protracted and debilitating course, characterized by specific opportunistic diseases that have a poor prognosis.

active immunization Administration of all or part of a microorganism to stimulate active response by the host's immunological system, resulting in complete protection against a specific disease.

activities of daily living (ADLs) Basic personal care activities that include eating, toileting, dressing, bathing, transferring, walking, and getting outside.

activity theory A theory of aging that states that older persons need to and want to become involved with a variety of activities.

addiction Compulsive, uncontrolled psychological or physical dependence on a substance or a habit.

administrative law Branch of law dealing with organs of government power; prescribes the manner of their activity (e.g., state board of nurse examiners).

administrator One who manipulates the resources within an organization to meet the organizational goals.

adult day care center Congregate facility for activities, such as socialization, eating, and supervised care of older adults during specified day hours, with the person returning home for the evening hours.

adult nurse practitioner Registered nurse with additional education through a master's degree program in nursing or through a nondegree or certificate continuing education program preparing the nurse to deliver primary health care to adults.

advance directives Written or oral statements by which a competent person makes known treatment preferences and/or designates a surrogate decision maker.

advocacy Activities for the purpose of protecting the rights of others while supporting the client's responsibility for self-determination; involves informing, supporting, and affirming a client's self-determination in health care decisions.

affective domain The learning domain that deals with feelings, attitudes, values, and interests.

affirming Ratifying, asserting, or giving strength to the declarations of self or others.

ageism A term for prejudice about older people that is similar to racism or sexism.

Agency for Toxic Substances and Disease Registry (ATSDR) Federal agency mandated to prevent exposure and adverse health effects associated with exposure to hazardous substances from waste sites, unplanned releases, and other sources of environmental pollution.

agent Causative factor invading a susceptible host through an environment favorable to produce disease, such as a biologic or chemical agent.

agent factors Agent's characteristics that allow it to enter a host and cause disease.

aggregates Populations or defined groups.

Aid to Families with Dependent Children A federal and state program to provide financial assistance to needy children deprived of parental support because of death, disability, absence from the home, or in some states, unemployment.

air pollution The presence of foreign materials in the air, either natural or manmade.

Al-Anon Organization of relatives of alcoholic individuals, operated in many communities within the structure of Alcoholics Anonymous.

Alcoholics Anonymous Lay, self-help group that practices a 12-step approach to recovery.

alcoholism Addiction to alcohol.

alliance A formal relationship between two agencies in which they agree to cooperate in some way.

Alzheimer's type of dementia   The most frequent form of dementia, also called primary degenerative dementia. It is characterized by short-term memory loss, gradual loss of expressive and comprehensive language, visual perceptual defects, decreased olfactory sense, and problem-solving difficulties.

ambulatory care centers   Hospital or community-based facilities that offer a wide range of outpatient services to treat mental and physical health problems.

Amercians with Disabilities Act (ADA)   An act passed in 1990 to promote the mainstreaming of people with mental and physical disabilities.

amplification   Expanding a statement or idea; an objective of communication.

analytic epidemiology   An epidemiologic study designed to investigate associations between exposures or characteristics and health or disease outcomes, often with a goal of understanding the etiology (or origins and casual factors) of disease.

anhedonia   Lack of joy.

Antabuse   Drug used as a deterrent to alcohol consumption. When alcohol and Antabuse are mixed, the person experiences a variety of unpleasant physiological reactions.

anthrax   Illness with varying symptoms caused by a spore-forming organism; may be endemic to many agricultural areas.

antibody   An organism formed in the body that identifies and destroys initial and subsequent invasions of an identified disease-producing organism.

anticipatory guidance   Providing advice to clients before an event and discussing potential problems or risks so clients will be aware and may be able to prevent the occurrence of the problem.

antitoxin   Solution of antibodies derived from the serum of animals immunized with specific antigens (e.g., diphtheria, tetanus); used to achieve passive immunity.

appropriate technology   Social, biomedical, and health services that are relevant to people's health, needs and concerns and are affordable and acceptable to them.

artificial acquired immunity   Immune state that results from immunization or vaccination for a specific disease.

ascariasis (roundworm infection)   Infection caused by a parasitic worm, *Ascario lumbriacoides*, that migrates through the lungs in its larval stage; symptoms are coughing, wheezing, and fever.

assessment   Systematic use of data to assist in identifying needs, questions to be addressed, or abilities and available resources.

assessment of community resources   Procedure similar to the process used on behalf of individual clients. The scope of the investigation is more detailed and includes examination of data from health planning groups, including the number of public health facilities, availability of health personnel, availability of funds, and a multitude of other statistics, such as those on mortality and morbidity.

assessment of need   Verifying and mapping out the extent and location of a problem and the target population.

assimilation   Process of a minority group becoming absorbed into the dominant or majority culture by adopting its behaviors. Also the process of a child's responding to the environment in accordance with his cognitive structures so that elements in the environment are incorporated into his or her cognitive structures.

assisted living   Living arrangements, primarily for elders, that provide services in an environment that resembles a home. Assisted-living facilities have common areas (dining room, game room) that are available but also provide privacy and independence to the residents, fostering an increased sense of self.

attack rates   A type of incidence rate defined as the proportion of persons exposed to an agent who develop the disease, usually for a limited time in a specific population.

attention deficit disorder   Inappropiate degree of inattention, impulsiveness, and hyperactivity for age and development.

attributable risk   Statistical measure that estimates the reduction in the occurrence of a particular disease that could be affected by elimination of a specific causal agent.

audit process   A six-step process used concurrently or retrospectively for nursing peer review.

authorization   The process of placing a ceiling on money to be requested for a program.

autism   Autism is a developmental disability that significantly affects the way in which a person learns to communicate and develop social relationships.

autoimmunity   Abnormal condition in which the body reacts against parts of its own tissues.

autonomy   Freedom of action as chosen by an individual.

B

barriers to access   Financial or nonfinancial impediments to obtaining health care. May include lack of funds to pay for health care or inadequate insurance coverage. Also may include cultural obstacles and practical problems, such as lack of transportation or inconvenient clinic hours.

battered child syndrome   Term coined by Kempe to describe the pattern of abuse against children.

battered women   Women who are physically and/or emotionally abused by their spouses or partners.

BCG vaccines   Several vaccines that vary in their ability to induce active immunity and therefore prevent tuberculosis.

behavioral theory   Has as its goal changing behavior and uses target behavior, reinforcers, withdrawal of a reinforcer, and punishment.

beneficence   Ethical principle stating that one should do good and prevent or avoid doing harm.

benefit schedule   A list of services with monetary values specifying the amounts an insurer will pay for the services.

Bernhard and Walsh's decision-making model   A structured method for analyzing alternative choices in which the goals, risks, feasibility, and other unique desired characteristics of the optimal choice are weighted and compared.

bias   A systematic deviation of observed values from the true value.

biological agents   Disease-producing hazards primarily consisting of bacteria, viruses, and other microorganisms and parasites.

biosphere   The world of living things, consisting of numerous ecosystems.

black lung   Disease common among coal miners, characterized by a large, solid black lung mass; caused by deposits of black mining dust in the lungs.

blackouts Intervals of temporary memory loss during which a person remains conscious and active and may even appear sober, but after which there is no memory of what was said or done.

block nursing A contemporary term for district nursing.

botulism Often fatal form of blood poisoning caused by an endotoxin produced by the bacillus *Clostridium botulinum*.

boundary In systems theory, the line or border that defines the elements comprising the system.

breast self-examination A technique that enables a woman to detect changes in her breast.

brokering health services Coordinating services provided by multiple agencies. Case managers often coordinate services to provide comprehensive care for clients.

bromarker The substance or its metabolite that can be detected in body tissue without any apparent health effect.

brucellosis Infectious disease of nonhuman mammals, which is contagious to humans.

budget A plan stated in financial terms that identifies the costs associated with implementing a program.

byssinosis Type of lung disease common among cotton mill workers: similar to nonoccupational bronchitis.

C

capitation A payment system whereby one fee is charged the client to pay for all services received or needed.

carbon monoxide Colorless, odorless, poisonous gas produced by the combustion of carbon or organic fuels in a limited oxygen supply.

carcinogenic agent Single, cancer-inducing substance that triggers the change in behavior of cells resulting in uncontrolled growth.

care coordination Linking clients with services.

caregiver burden The physical, psychological or emotional, social, and financial problems that can be experienced by those who provide care for impaired others.

caregivers Those persons, professional and nonprofessional, who provide for the social and health needs of others.

case-control study An epidemiologic study design in which subjects with a specified disease or condition (cases) and a comparable group without the condition (controls) are enrolled and assessed for the presence or history of an exposure or characteristic.

case finding Careful, systematic observations of people to identify present or potential problems.

case law Decisions by the courts; judicial opinions.

case management Interchangeable term with care management. Used to describe a service given to clients that contains the following activities: screening, assessment, care planning, arranging for service delivery, monitoring, reassessment, evaluation, and discharge. Case management is a process that enhances continuity and appropriateness of care. Most often used with clients whose health problems are actually or potentially chronic and complex.

case register Systematic registration of acute, chronic, and contagious diseases.

case study A written analysis of program development and implementation throughout the life of the program; an historical depiction of the program.

catalytic intervention mode A situation whereby a consultant assists a client to broaden his or her view of an existing situation by gaining additional information or by unifying existing data.

causality The relationship of one factor to another such that the presumed causal factor produces or contributes to the occurrence of some outcome.

cellular interaction theory This theory suggests that an organism's individual cells are influenced by other cells and unless they are functioning in harmony, the feedback mechanism will fail and the cells will degenerate.

census data Composite data, provided by the federal government on the population of states, local and political jurisdictions, and defined geographic tracts in organized areas.

Centers for Disease Control Branch of the U.S. Public Health Service whose primary responsibility is to propose, coordinate, and evaluate changes in the surveillance of disease in the United States.

cerebral palsy Umbrella term for a group of disabling conditions resulting from central nervous system damage. Do not assume that a person with cerebral palsy also has mental retardation; the two disabilities do not necessarily or typically occur together.

certificate of need Determination in any given community of the need for new health care facilities on the basis of currently available resources and anticipated demands for use.

certification A mechanism, usually by means of written examination, that provides an indication of professional competence in a specialized area of practice.

chancroid A sexually transmitted disease caused by a bacteria, *Hemophilus ducreyi*, that results in a highly infectious ulcer located on the penis, urethra, vulva, or anus.

charter A mechanism by which a state government agency under state laws grants corporate status to institutions with or without rights to award degrees.

chemical agents Home, workplace, and community man-made hazards found in the environment that can produce disease.

chemical contamination Contamination of food, either deliberately or accidentally, by chemical additives.

chemical dependency Addiction to alcohol or other drugs.

child abuse Active forms of maltreatment of children.

child neglect Physical or emotional neglect. Physical neglect refers to failure to provide adequate food, clothing, shelter, hygiene, or necessary medical care; emotional neglect refers to the omission of basic nurturing, acceptance, and caring essential for healthy development.

chlamydia A sexually transmitted disease caused by the organism *Chlamydia trachomatis*, that causes infection of the urethra and cervix. Infections may be asymptomatic and, if untreated, result in severe morbidity.

chlorofluorocarbons A family of chemicals containing chlorine and fluorine that damages the ozone layer in the air; found in furniture and bedding foam, carpet padding, foam egg cartons and coffee cups, and insulation.

chronic homelessness Long-term homelessness.

cirrhosis Chronic degenerative liver disease, often caused by chronic alcohol abuse, but can also result from nutritional deprivation, hepatitis, or other infections.

CITYNET process A nine-step community problem-solving process for health promotion that emphasizes leadership development.

civil law Area of law concerned with the legal rights and duties of individuals.

clarification The process of attempting to make communication or expression clear or easier to understand.

Clean Water Act Legislation passed in 1963 to protect air quality. The goal of the 1990 Act is to reduce acid rain, urban smog, and toxic chemical emissions from industry.

client population Individuals, groups, families, organizations, or communities that are the targets of the consultant's interventions.

client problem A current, historic, or potential matter of difficulty or concern that adversely affects any aspect of a client's well-being.

client responsibilities Those tasks or areas for which the client is accountable. In the case of an individual health care client, responsibilities might be related to self-care or actively participating in a referral. In a consulting relationship, the client may be expected to provide information and engage in active problem solving.

clients' rights Those services, programs, goods, and provider behaviors to which consumers are entitled in order to maintain or achieve health or to exist.

clinical breast examination A periodic physical examination of the breast by a health care provider for both asymptomatic and symptomatic patients.

clinical nurse specialist An advanced practice nurse who provides direct care to clients and participates in consultative, health education, and program management.

clinician A nurse prepared at any level who provides direct care.

coaching Encouraging another in the acquisition of certain skills, including making suggestions, giving feedback at incremental intervals, and praising as goals are met.

coalition A relationship between individuals or people in which the group is working toward some shared goal. A coalition is similar to an alliance, except that individuals may be involved and the relationship may be informal.

Code for Nurses The American Nurses Association professional statement prescribing moral behavior and actions of nurses based on moral principles.

code of ethics Set of statements encompassing rules that apply to people in professional roles.

codependency A companion illness in drug or alcohol addiction in which the codependent is addicted to the addict. Strict rules typically develop in the family to maintain their relationship.

Codes of Regulation Federal and State legal documents in which finalized regulations are published.

coercive health measures Health care treatment and services required regardless of the client's wishes, choices, or life plans. Such care is usually regulated by law and is instituted to protect the public's health.

coercive sex Sexual relations that occur with force, intimidation, or authority.

cognitive development The progressive process of acquisition of skills for thinking, reasoning, and language use.

cognitive domain Learning domain that deals with the recall or recognition of knowledge and the development of intellectual skills.

cognitive theory Purports that by changing thought patterns and providing information, learner's behavior will change.

cognitive theories of motivation Theories that explain human motivation in terms of the beliefs, expectations, and goals held by individuals.

cohesion Attraction of group members to one another and to the group.

cohort Group of people born during the same era who are influenced by some of the same biological, psychological, and social factors.

cohort study An epidemiologic study design in which subjects without an outcome of interest are classified according to past or present (or future) exposures or characteristics and followed over time to observe and compare the rates of some health outcome in the various exposure groups.

collaboration Mutual sharing and working together to achieve common goals in such a way that all persons or groups are recognized and growth is enhanced.

collaborative practice Professionals working together in a collegial relationship to provide primary health care to a given population.

collectivism The culture tendency to include family and friends in one's own experiences.

combination agency A health care agency that provides home health and hospice services.

common law Law based on the opinion of the courts; comes from past court decisions or opinions based on fairness, respect for individuals, autonomy, and self-determination.

communicable disease A disease of human or animal origin caused by an infectious agent and resulting from transmission of that agent from an infected person, animal, or inanimate source to a susceptible host. Infectious disease may be communicable or noncommunicable, (i.e., tetanus is infectious but not communicable).

communicable period The time or times when an infectious agent may be transferred from an infected source directly or indirectly to a new host.

communication structure Descriptive framework that identifies message pathways and member participation in sending and receiving messages utilized for a group or groups.

community People and the relationships that emerge among them as they develop and use in common some agencies and institutions and a physical environment.

community client Target of service (i.e., the population group for whom healthful change is sought).

community forum An open meeting for members of a particular community or group to address an issue of interest.

community health Meeting collective needs by identifying problems and managing interactions within the community and larger society. The goal of community-oriented practice.

community health nurse consultant A community health nurse who assists another individual or organization with problem solving regarding provision of community health nursing services.

community health nursing Synthesis of nursing and public health practice applied to promoting and preserving the health of populations. The practice is general and comprehensive, with the dominant responsibility being to the population as a whole.

community health nursing leadership Refers to the influence that community health nurses exert to improve client health, whether clients are individuals, families, groups, or entire communities.

community health nursing management Refers to the ways that community health nurses manage resources in the provision of clinical services. Resources include people, time, supplies and equipment, and financial resources.

community health problem Actual or potential difficulties within a target population with identifiable causes and consequences in the environment.

community health services Services directed to meet the needs of groups; tend to reflect a public health orientation of health promotion and maintenance of capabilities.

community health strength Resources available to meet a community health need.

community mental health Orientation toward health care that seeks to provide a program of continuing and comprehensive mental health care to a specific population.

community-oriented practice A clinical approach in which the nurse and community join in partnership and work together for healthful change.

community participation Involvement of community members for whom programs are being developed in the early stages of program planning, implementation, and evaluation.

community preparedness A process whereby communities prepare and update a disaster plan and participate in regular mock disaster drills.

community resident survey A direct assessment of the population of a community to identify the need for a service, the acceptability of the service to the population, and the willingness of the people to use and pay for the service.

comorbidity Presence of multiple illnesses simultaneously in a person.

competitive medical plans Organization of services within a community for the purpose of bidding on delivery of health care to groups of individuals.

comprehensive assessment The process of identifying medical, physiological, functional, environmental, social, and other problems that elders may encounter.

Comprehensive Health Planning and Public Health Services Amendments of 1966 (CHP) Landmark legislation that emphasized regional planning; the first time each person's "right to health care" was acknowledged.

comprehensive services Services that completely meet an individual's or family's needs.

compromise An agreement between two or more people or groups with goals that cannot be met without modification of the positions of each person or group; implies "give and take" in the negotiating process.

concept Category or class of objects or phenomena that represents either an abstract version of the real world (e.g., an ideal) or a concrete idea (e.g., a chair or bench).

conceptual framework A group of concepts and a set of propositions that spells out the relationships between them.

conceptual model A set of concepts and the assumptions that integrate them into a meaningful configuration.

concurrent audit A method of evaluating quality of ongoing care through appraisal of the nursing process.

confidentiality Information kept private, such as between health care provider and client.

conflict Difference in perception, opinion, or priorities between people; can be spoken or unspoken.

conflict resolution Methods of handling conflict between individuals or groups. Some methods may lead to desirable outcomes for all parties, or for only some parties, or for none of the parties involved.

confounding A bias that results from the relation of both the outcome and study factor (exposure or characteristic) with some third factor not accounted.

confrontation intervention mode Consultant intervention mode that provides for presentation of ideas and facts to the client and reveals the client's values and assumptions that cannot be disputed.

confusion An imprecise term commonly used to describe a mental state in which inappropriate reactions are observed.

congenital disability A disability that has existed since birth. Do not use the term birth defect; the word "defect" is not a synonym of "disability."

constituents Clients, individuals, families, peers, groups, or communities represented by another person(s).

constitutional law Branch of law dealing with organization and function of government.

constructs Conceptual components that are not directly observable; deliberately created ideas of references that cannot be seen but allow for explanation and analysis.

consultant One who provides professional advice, services, or information.

consultation Interactional or communication process between two or more persons; one is a consultant, and the other is the consultee. The consultant seeks to help the consultee solve a problem or improve or broaden skills.

consultative contract A working agreement between the consultant and consultee for services provided by the consultant. The contract stipulates the responsibilities held by both the consultant and the consultee.

consultee Person seeking the help of an outside, usually impartial, person in problem resolution.

consumer The recipient of health care. Primary clients are the current or former recipients of care; secondary consumers are the client's family or significant others.

consumerism Organized movement and commitment to the belief that people have both a right and a responsibility to be knowledgeable about the choices they make for health and illness care.

contingency leadership theory A theory that predicts a single leadership style is not always the most effective in every situation. Instead, the best leadership style is determined by evaluating the characteristics of the situation. Fiedler, Blake and Mouton, and Hersey and Blanchard are considered to be contingency leadership theorists.

continuity of care A desirable goal in the delivery of health care services as a client utilizes multiple providers and services.

continuity theory This theory states that each person copes with the later years of life in much the same way as he or she coped with earlier periods of life.

continuous quality improvement An approach to managing quality that emphasizes continual improvement in real time, empowering employees to manage quality themselves, including client and family perceptions of quality, and making changes in organizational systems to better enable workers to provide high quality services.

contraceptive options Methods of birth control available for a client to use.

contract A promissory agreement between two or more persons that creates, modifies, or destroys a legal relation. It is a legally enforceable promise between two or more persons to do or not to do something.

contracting Any working agreement, continuously renegotiable and agreed upon by nurse and client.

coordination Conscious activity of assembling and directing the work efforts of a group of health providers so that they can function harmoniously in the attainment of the objective of client care.

core metropolitan Densely populated counties with more than 1 million inhabitants.

cost-accounting studies Studies finding the actual budgetary cost of a program, procedure, or technique.

cost-benefit studies Studies assessing the desirability of a program, procedure, or technique by placing a specific quantifiable value—a dollar amount—on all costs and benefits of the variable to be evaluated.

cost-effectiveness studies Studies analyzing the actual costs of performing a number of services at different volumes when the same standards are applied.

cost-efficiency studies Studies analyzing the actual costs of performing a number of services at different volumes when the same standards are applied.

cost-plus reimbursement Method of payment whereby an agency receives actual costs of services delivered plus added allowable expenses, such as depreciation of facilities and equipment and administrative costs.

credentialing A mechanism that seeks to produce performance of acceptable quality by individuals and programs of education and service. The four fundamental features of credentialing are quality, identify, protection, and control.

critical path method (CPM) A planning technique that focuses on activities, best use of time and resources, and estimated time to complete activities. The technique can be used for planning programs or individual client care as it is related to a specific diagnosis.

critical theory Approaches learning as an "ongoing dialogue" where the educator attempts to change the learner's belief by questioning the learner.

cross-sectional study An epidemiologic study in which health outcomes and exposures or characteristics of interest are simultaneously ascertained and examined for association in a population or sample, providing a picture of existing levels of all factors.

crude rates Statistical rates in which the events in the numerator and the denominator refer to the entire population.

cultural awareness An appreciation of and sensitivity to a client's values, beliefs, practices, life-style and problem-solving strategies.

cultural blindness Differences between cultures are ignored and persons act as though these differences do not exist.

cultural brokering Advocating, mediating, negotiating, and intervening on behalf of the client between the health care culture and the client's culture.

cultural competence An interplay of factors that motivate persons to develop knowledge, skill, and ability to care for others.

cultural conflict A perceived threat that may arise from a misunderstanding of expectations between clients and nurses when neither is aware of their cultural differences.

cultural encounter Interactions with clients related to all aspects of their lives.

cultural imposition The process of imposing one's values on others.

cultural knowledge The information necessary to provide nurses with an understanding of the organizational elements of cultures and to provide effective nursing care.

cultural relativism The value of the culture as defined by its meaning to its members.

cultural sensitivity Appreciation for and receptiveness to another's cultural heritage and values.

cultural skill The effective integration of cultural knowledge and awareness to meet client needs.

cultural values The prevailing and persistent guides influencing thinking and actions of people within a culture.

culturally sensitive communication Communication that recognizes the cultural meanings and values of multiple ways of communicating. Community health nurses that practice culturally sensitive communication are sensitive to diverse interpretations at a minimum, and ideally, develop ways of communicating that the receiver of the communication understands and is comfortable with.

culture Standards for decisions on what is, what can be, how to feel about it, and how to do it.

culture-bound illnesses Illnesses specific to a particular culture (e.g., *mal ojo* [evil eye] in the Mexican-American culture).

culture change The constant process of adding or deleting elements within a culture, such as language, customs, beliefs, attitudes, values, goals, laws, traditions, and moral codes.

culture of poverty A status not merely of economic deprivation but also entailing personality traits passed from one generation to another.

culture shock Feelings of helplessness, discomfort, and disorientation experienced by a person attempting to understand or effectively adapt to a different cultural group because of dissimilarities in practices, values, and beliefs.

cumulative risks The additive effects of multiple risk factors.

cumulative trauma *See* cumulative risks.

curandera Folk healers in Hispanic cultures.

cycle of vulnerability The feedback effect of factors that predispose one to vulnerability and lead to negative health outcomes, which then increase the predisposing factors and so on.

D

data collection The process of acquiring existing information or developing new information.

data generation The development of data, frequently qualitative rather than numerical, by the data collector.

data interpretation The process of analyzing and synthesizing data, which culminates in the identification of community health problems and strengths.

data management A method of collecting, organizing, and prioritizing information to use in resolving client problems.

death rates A statistical indicator comparing the number of deaths to the total population.

decentralization Services, authority, responsibility, etc., shared from the top of the organization throughout all levels.

deductive approach The reasoning process of developing specific predictions or ideas from general principles.

deinstitutionalization Effort to move long-term psychiatric patients out of the hospital and back into their own community.

delayed stress reaction Stress that occurs postdisaster that is related to a disaster; workers' feelings of exhaustion; frustration and guilt over not having been able to do more; disappointment from family and friends who don't seem as interested in what the worker has been through;

and a general inability to adjust to the slower pace of work and home.

delegation Sharing responsibility for a task with another who is competent to perform the task. The person who delegates the task retains responsibility and ultimate accountability for the effective completion of the task.

delirium A cause of confusion that is characterized by acute onset, disordered attention, and changes in cognition, psychomotor behavior, and the sleep-wake cycle.

delirium tremens Severe reaction to alcohol withdrawal; characterized by disorientation, paranoia, and outbursts of irrational behavior; symptoms also may include tachycardia, fever, rapid breathing, sweating, vomiting, and diarrhea.

dementia Progressive, organic mental disorder characterized by chronic personality disintegration, confusion, and deterioration of mental functioning.

demographic trends Population trends related to age at first marriage; fertility patterns; birth rates; numbers of individuals engaging in singlehood, divorce, and remarriage; number of dependent children experiencing divorce, life with a never-married parent; and the number of persons in specific age categories.

denial A primary symptom of addiction. The person may lie about use, play down use, and blame; also may use anger or humor to avoid acknowledging the problem to self and others.

deontology Doctrine that moral duty or obligation is binding; *also*: what makes acts right are nonconsequential characteristics such as fidelity, veracity, justice, and honesty.

Department of Health and Human Services (DHHS) A regulatory agency of the executive branch of government charged with overseeing health and welfare needs of U.S. citizens.

depression Mental state characterized by dejection, lack of hope, and absence of cheerfulness.

descriptive epidemiology An epidemiologic study designed to describe the distribution of health outcomes according to person, place, and time.

determinants Factors that influence the risk for or distribution of health outcomes.

detoxification Gradual withdrawal from an abused substance; best achieved in a controlled hospital setting.

developed countries Those countries with a stable economy and a wide range of industrial and technological capability.

development Increase in complexity of the function and progression of physical, social, and mental skills throughout life.

developmental disability Any mental or physical disability manifested before the age of 22 that may continue indefinitely and result in substantial limitation in three or more of the following life activities: self-care, receptive and expressive language, learning mobility, self-direction, independent living, economic sufficiency.

developmental tasks Age-appropriate physical, social, and mental skills to be accomplished by individuals throughout the lifespan.

developmental theory A way of thinking about how changes occur in human development; includes characteristics such as stages, phases, levels, direction, and forces.

diabetes Disorder of carbohydrate metabolism caused by the destruction and reduction of pancreatic insulin-producing cells.

diagnosis-related groups (DRGs) A patient classification scheme that defines 468 illness categories and the corresponding health care services that are reimbursable under Medicare.

digital rectal exam A procedure used to assess the condition of the prostate and rectum; generally used for early detection of cancer.

direct care Health care services that require face-to-face interaction between the nurse and client.

disability adjusted life years A measure of the numbers of years of life lost worldwide as a result of premature deaths.

disabled An individual who has a physical or mental impairment that substantially limits that person in some major life activity, such as walking, talking, breathing, or working; has a record of such an impairment; and/or is regarded as being "disabled."

disaster Any man-made or natural event that causes destruction and devastation that cannot be alleviated without assistance.

disaster action team A group of specially trained persons who can assist communities in implementing their disaster plans.

disaster medical assistance teams (DMAT) A team consisting of approximately 30 volunteers including physicians, nurses, and other allied health personnel who train as a group to perform specific emergency functions during a disaster. Upon activation of the National Disaster Medical System, each member becomes an automatic and temporary employee of the U.S. Public Health Service.

disaster planning The process of developing organized actions to prevent or minimize injuries or deaths of workers or residents, and property damage. To effectively triage and facilitate the resumption of normal activities.

discharge planning The process of activities facilitating the client's movement from one setting to another. Discharge planning is a process that enhances continuity of care.

disease/illness prevention Behavior directed toward reducing the threat of illness, disease, or complications.

disenfranchisement A sense of social isolation; a feeling of separation from mainstream society.

disengagement theory A theory of aging that views society and the older person in a process of mutual withdrawal.

distribution The pattern of a health outcome in a population, the frequencies of the outcome according to various personal characteristics, geographic regions, and time.

distribution effects The effects that a policy may have on people other than those for which it was intended.

distributive care Health care services that emphasize health promotion, maintenance, and disease prevention.

district nursing Early public health nursing whereby a nurse was assigned to each district in a town to provide home health care to needy people.

diversity Differences among and between individuals and groups of people. In the work setting, diversity refers to heterogeneity in cultural, ethnic, and racial heritage.

Division of Nursing A component of the Public Health Service, part of the Health Resources and Services Administration, which oversees nursing education and special nursing demonstration projects in the United States.

doctor-patient model of consultation A consulting mode in which the consultant is employed to diagnose a problem and suggest a remedy.

documentation   The process of recording data in client records.

dysfunctional family   A family unit that inhibits clear communication within family relationships and does not provide psychological support for individual members.

E

early adopters   Individuals and/or groups with cosmopolitan rather than local orientations, with abilities to adopt new ideas from mass media rather than face-to-face information sources and with specialized rather than global interests.

ecological fallacy   A bias that may occur in ecological studies because associations observed at the group level may not hold true for the individuals that comprise the groups, or associations that actually exist may be masked.

ecological studies   An epidemiologic study in which only aggregate or group data, such as population rates, are used rather than data on individuals.

ecology   The science of the relationship between living and nonliving things; concerned with both structure and function.

economics   Social science concerned with the problems of using or administering scarce resources in the most efficient way to attain maximum fulfillment of society's unlimited wants.

ecosystem   All living things and nonliving parts that support a chain of life within a selected area.

ectopic pregnancy   A pregnancy that develops outside of the uterus; usually refers to a pregnancy in the fallopian tubes.

effectiveness   A measure of an organization's performance as compared to its philosophy, goals, and objectives.

efficiency   The process of meeting goals in a way that minimizes costs and maximizes benefits.

elder abuse   A form of family violence against older members. May include neglect and failure to provide adequate food, clothing, shelter, and physical and safety needs; can also include roughness in care and actual violent behavior toward the elderly.

emancipated   Free from parental care and control.

emergency nurse practitioner   Registered nurse with additional education through a master's degree program in nursing or through a nondegree or certificate continuing education program preparing the nurse to deliver primary care within an emergency room setting.

emergency support functions   Activities that must be carried out as part of the Federal Response Plan by each of 26 federal agencies and the American Red Cross.

emotional abuse   Extreme debasement of a person's feelings so that he or she feels inept, uncared for, and worthless.

employee assistance programs   The range of services offered in the workplace to assist employees to cope with personal and work-related problems.

empowerment   Helping people acquire the skills and information necessary for informed decision making and ensuring that they have the authority to make decisions that affect them.

enabling   The act of shielding or preventing the addict from experiencing the consequences of the addiction. Also applies to shielding individuals from the consequences of their actions more generally.

enabling legislation   A bill or law passed by Congress to support the development of a specific program or service.

enculturation   The process of acquiring knowledge and internalizing values or learning about a culture.

endemic   Indigenous to an area or group; the constant presence of an infectious disease within a specific geographic area.

enterobiasis   Pinworm infestation.

entitlement theory   Theory that people have rights to resources as determined by the natural lottery and may increase their possessions in any way possible (by purchase, gift, or legitimate exchange), as long as they do not cheat others or acquire the possessions in an unjust manner.

entropy   A concept stating that elements in a closed environment will proceed toward greater randomness or less order.

environment   All those factors internal and external to the client that constitute the context in which the client lives and that influence and are influenced by the host and agent-host interactions.

environmental health   Aspect of community health concerned with those forms of life, substances, forces, and conditions in the surroundings of people that may exert an influence on their health and well-being.

Environmental Protection Agency (EPA)   Established in 1970 to be responsible for air, water, and land pollution control; never achieved its full goal.

epidemic   A rate of disease clearly in excess of the usual or expected frequency in that population.

epidemiologic triad   The host, agent, and environment relationship necessary for a disease to occur.

epidemiology   The study of the distribution of states of health and of the causes of deviations from health in populations and the application of this study to control the health problems.

epididymitis   Inflammation of the epididymis that may be a complication of gonorrhea or chlamydia, resulting in fever and chills, pain in the inguinal region, and a swollen epididymis.

epilepsy   Umbrella term for various disorders marked by disturbed electrical rhythms of the central nervous system and typically manifested by seizures—involuntary muscular contractions.

episodic care   Curative and restorative aspect of nursing practice.

episodic homelessness   Frequently being without permanent shelter.

equalitarian theory   Doctrine that takes the needs of all people into account equally.

equifinality   The end state of an open system is independent from the beginning state.

equity   Providing accessible services to promote the health of populations most at risk to health problems.

ERG theory   A motivation theory developed by Clayton Alderfer based on Maslow's earlier work. This theory says that people are motivated by existence, relatedness, or growth needs.

ergonomic agent   Agents that cause mechanical strain on the body resulting in illness (i.e., vibrations).

ergonomics   The study of people at work in order to understand the complex relationships associated with work.

error catastrophe theory   Errors occur in DNA, RNA, and protein synthesis. Each error augments the other and culminates in an error catastrophe.

erythema Reddened raised area on the skin produced by a tissue response to small doses of antigenic substances.

established group An existing group of persons linked by membership and group purpose.

estimation of risk Assessing the nature of a problem, size of the problem, and need for a program within a community to prevent occurrence of the problem.

ethical principles Abstract guides that serve as foundations for moral rules.

ethical theories Collection of principles and rules providing theoretical foundations for deciding what to do when moral principles or rules conflict.

ethics Science or study of moral values; *also*: a code of principles and ideals that guide action.

ethnicity Shared feeling or peoplehood among a group of individuals.

ethnocentrism Belief that one's own group or culture is superior to others.

eudaimonistic model of health A model in which health is viewed as maximizing individual and family well-being and potential.

eutrophication Process in which nutrients in lakes promote the growth of algae, which causes cloudy, odorous water.

evaluation Provision of information through formal means, such as criteria, measurement, and statistics, for making rational judgments necessary about outcomes of care.

evaluative research A method of collecting information according to the rigors of scientific inquiry for the purpose of evaluating the long-term effect of a program.

evaluative studies Systematic method for collecting information to assess the relevance, progress, effectiveness, efficiency, and impact of a program.

exchange theory A theory of aging in which elders are viewed with great esteem as a result of their experience and greater knowledge of lore and history. The elder "exchanges" his or her knowledge for a position of deferment and respect from younger individuals.

experimental epidemiology Third stage of epidemiological investigation that uses experimental design for studies to confirm the causal nature of relationships identified through observational studies.

exposure pathway The process by which an individual is exposed to contaminants that originate from some source of contamination.

extended care facility An agency that provides long-term care for chronic conditions.

F

facilitator One who provides an environment in which the client is assisted in meeting health care needs and is a participant in decision making.

familialism A culture belief that family needs take priority over individual needs.

family Two or more individuals coming from the same or different kinship groups who are involved in a continuous living arrangement, usually residing in the same household, experiencing common emotional bonds, and sharing certain obligations toward each other and toward others.

family assessment Systematic collection, classification, and analysis of family data for the purpose of identifying the family's health-related strengths and problems.

family-centered care A care arrangement enabling families to assume the role of advocates, decision makers, and caregivers.

family crisis A situation whereby the demands of the situation exceed the resources and coping capacity of the family.

family demography The study of the structure of families and households and the family-related events, such as marriage and divorce, that alter the structure through the number, timing, and sequence of the events.

family developmental framework A model that assumes that family development follows orderly, sequential changes throughout the family's lifespan.

family developmental task A growth responsibility that arises at a certain stage in the life of a family, the successful achievement of which leads to satisfaction, approval, and success with later tasks.

family dynamics Interactions and relationships within the family that influence the work of the family and its ability to complete its functions and tasks.

family functions Behaviors or activities performed to maintain the integrity of the family unit and to meet the family's needs, individual members' needs, and society's expectations.

family health A condition including the promotion and maintenance of physical, mental, spiritual, and social health for the family unit and for individual family members.

family health risks Those factors that predispose or increase the family's likelihood of ill health.

Family Life Cycle A developmental theory that divides family life into a series of stages or phases over time. The stages are qualitatively and quantitatively different from the preceding and succeeding stages.

family nurse practitioner/clinician Registered nurse with additional education through a master's degree program in nursing or a nondegree or certificate continuing education program preparing the nurse to deliver primary health care to individuals, groups, and communities of all ages.

family planning nurse practitioner (obstetric/gynecological nurse practitioner) Registered nurse with additional education through a master's degree program in nursing or a nondegree or certificate continuing education program preparing the nurse to deliver obstetrical and gynecological primary care to women.

family roles Behaviors assumed by family members to maintain the organizational structure of the family and to define the division of labor and the family processes.

family self-care A decision-making process that involves the family in self-observation, symptom perception and labeling, judgment of severity, and choice and assessment of treatment options.

family strengths Those factors or forces that contribute to family unity and solidarity and foster the development of the potentials inherent within the family.

family structure (configuration) Refers to the characteristics of the individual members (gender, age, number) who constitute the family unit.

farm residency Residence outside area zoned as "city limits"; usually infers involvement in agriculture industry.

Federal Emergency Management Agency (FEMA) The governmental agency responsible for directing the federal response to disasters.

Federal Poverty Guidelines A definition of poverty drafted by the Social Security Administration in 1964. The federal government defines poverty in terms of income, family size, the age of the head of household, and the number of children under 18 years of age. The guidelines change annually to be consistent with the consumer price index.

federal poverty level The income level for a certain family size that the federal government uses to define poverty.

Federal Register A legal document in which all U.S. government proposed new regulations are published.

federal response plan A federal emergency response system that may become activated when a disaster is assumed to overwhelm the capability of state and local governments to carry out the extensive emergency operations necessary to save lives and protect property. Twenty-six federal agencies and the American Red Cross are responsible for coordinating efforts in a particular area with all of its designated support agencies.

feedback Process in which the output of a system is returned as input to the same system.

fee-for-service benefit schedule List of health care services with monetary or unit values attached that specifies the amounts third parties must pay for specific services.

fee screen system The use of usual, customary, and reasonable charges (based on regional evaluations in all specialties) by physicians to set their own reimbursement levels for units of service.

feminization of poverty Refers to the growing number of women living in poverty and the growing number of female-headed households.

fetal alcohol syndrome A condition that may occur when a woman has consumed alcohol regularly during pregnancy (about six drinks per day). Infants tend to be of low birth weight, mentally retarded, and may have behavioral, facial, limb, genital, cardiac, or neurological impairments.

fiscal year Annual operating year of the government (October 1 to September 30 of the next calendar year).

flexible lines of defense In the Neuman System's Model, the outer concentric ring, which characterizes an open system that exchanges energy with the environment.

formal group Persons having a defined membership and specified purpose. The group may or may not have an official or public place in the community's organization.

formal operations Level of cognitive development in which thoughts are independent of physical experience and allow children to deal with hypothetical questions.

formal structure The established power and communication relationships within an organization.

formative evaluation An ongoing evaluation instituted for the purpose of assessing the degree to which objectives are met or activities are being conducted.

freebasing Homemade refining process that extracts a concentrated form of cocaine from its chemical base and then smokes it in a water pipe usually filled with liquor.

frontier Regions having fewer than six persons per square mile.

functional family A family unit that provides autonomy and is responsive to the particular interests and needs of individual family members.

G

gastrointestinal virus Viral infectious process causing inflammation of the stomach and intestines producing vomiting and diarrhea.

general systems theory As defined by von Bertalantfy, a complex of elements in mutual interaction. The elements are wholeness, organization, and order.

genital herpes A virus that attacks genitalia and sacral nerve. Infection is characterized by painful lesions that present as vesicles and progress to ulcerations on the male and female genitalia, buttocks, or upper thighs.

genital warts Lesions caused by the human papillomavirus.

geriatric day care facility Ambulatory health care facility for elderly people; uses a broad range of professional and community services to maximize functional independence for this age group in the home and community.

geriatric nurse practitioner Registered nurse with additional education through a master's degree program in nursing or a nondegree or certificate continuing education program preparing the nurse to deliver primary health care to older adults.

gerontology A field of study that explores the biopsychosocial issues of aging.

global burden of disease A world wide mortality indicator (death rate) that combines premature deaths and losses of healthy life that result from disability.

goal The end or terminal point toward which intervention efforts are directed.

goal attainment A process for assessing the efficacy of a program by examination or measurement of predetermined goals.

goals/objectives A consultative problem that involves the inability of a group or individual to accept new goals, change goals, or meet established goals.

goal setting theory A motivation theory developed by Edwin Locke and his associates that says that people are motivated to accomplish goals that they participate in setting, that are somewhat challenging, and for which they receive regular feedback about their progress.

gonorrhea A sexually transmitted disease caused by a bacteria, *Neisseria gonorrhoeae*, resulting in inflammation of the urethra and cervix and dysuria, or it may result in no symptoms.

greenhouse effect Global condition resulting from the burning of fossil fuel, which gives off carbon dioxide and is warming the earth's atmosphere, changing weather conditions throughout the world and decreasing water supplies in some parts of the world.

gross domestic product (GDP) A statistical measure used to compare health care spending between countries.

gross national product (GNP) The total value of all final goods and services produced in the United States in 1 year.

group A collection of interacting individuals who have a common purpose or purposes.

group cohesion Measurement of degree of attraction among members and toward the group.

group culture A composite of the group norms that come to dictate perceptions and behaviors.

group member Interaction member exchanges within a group setting; includes the processes that accomplish group tasks and maintenance.

group norms Unwritten and often unspoken standards for group members that guide their behavior and influence their attitudes and perceptions.

group purpose The reason two or more people come together; may be subtle or obvious and easily stated by members.

group structure The particular arrangement of group parts that comprise the whole.

growth Increase in size of the whole or parts of an organism.

growth charts Standardized tools that serve as norms to compare an individual's growth to a population.

gynecological age Number of years from menarche.

H

hallucinosis A condition that can result from alcohol withdrawal; the person remains oriented and rational but may be confused about time.

HBV *See* hepatitis B virus.

health Balanced state of well-being resulting from harmonious interaction of body, mind, and spirit.

health behavior Any health-related action undertaken by a person to prevent or detect disease, protect health, or promote a higher level of health.

health belief model A model that describes health, based on perceptions of susceptibility, seriousness, and advantages or disadvantages of action. Useful in promoting adherence to treatment regimen.

health care rationing *See* rationing.

health commodification The buying and selling of health and health care products.

health economics Branch of economics concerned with the problems of producing and distributing the health care resources of the nation in a way that provides maximum benefit to the most people.

health education Any combination of learning experiences designed to facilitate adaptations of behavior conducive to health.

health field concept A model of health which states that health results from the interactions between individual behavior, biology, the environment, and the health care system. Originally described by LaFramboise (1973) and expanded by Lalonde (1974) (both in Denver, 1988).

health hazards Biological, physical, chemical, or psychosocial threats to health that arise from the environment.

health index A summary of the health features of a community that enables us to determine health care delivery needs.

Health Maintenance Organization (HMO) Organized system of health care that provides a fixed fee for all needed health care services with an emphasis on primary care.

health personnel shortage areas (HPSAs) Geographical areas that have insufficient numbers of health professionals according to criteria established by the federal government.

health planning A continuous social process by which data about a client are collected and evaluated for the purpose of creating a plan to guide change in health care delivery.

health policy Public policy that affects health and health services. Delineates options from which individuals and organizations make their health-related choices. Made within a political context.

health promotion Strategies designed to increase the physical, social, and emotional health and well-being of individuals, families, and communities.

health promotion model A model organized like the health belief model and directed toward increasing the level of well-being in a person or group.

health risk appraisal Process of identifying and analyzing an individual's prognostic characteristics of health and comparing them with those of a standard age group, thereby providing a prediction of a person's likelihood of prematurely developing the health problems that have high morbidity and mortality in this country.

health risk/health risk factor Disease precursor whose presence is associated with higher-than-average morbidity and/or mortality. Disease precursors include demographic variables, certain individual behaviors, positive individual and/or family history, and some physiological changes.

health risk reduction Application of selected interventions to control or reduce risk factors and minimize the incidence of associated disease and premature mortality. Risk reduction is reflected in greater congruousness between appraised and achievable ages.

health status The state or level of health of an individual, family, or community at a given time.

health systems agency Federally funded agency that plans and approves the development of health care facilities in a community.

Healthy Cities An international movement of cities focused on mobilizing local resources and political, professional, and community members to improve the health of the community.

Healthy City A city whose priority is to improve its environment and expand its resources so that community members can support each other in achieving their highest potential.

Healthy People 2000 A government document that outlines the nation's health goals and objectives.

hearing impaired Or "hard of hearing" refers to partial hearing loss and a range of hearing disabilities from slight to severe. People with hearing impairments sometimes use American Sign Language (ASL), a visual gestural language.

hemiplegia Refers to full or partial paralysis of one side of the body caused by brain damage most often attributable to disease, trauma, or stroke.

hepatitis Inflammatory condition of the liver caused by viral or bacterial infection, parasites, alcohol, drugs, toxins, or transfusions of incompatible blood.

hepatitis B virus (HBV) A virus that is transmitted through exposure to body fluids. Infection results in a clinical picture that ranges from a self-limited acute infection to fulminant hepatitis or hepatic carcinoma, possibly leading to death.

herbicide Chemical agent used to destroy unwanted plants.

herpes Any one of five related viruses that attack skin, genitalia, or cranial, cervical, or spinal nerves; infection is characterized by severe pain and various acute symptoms.

heterosexism A belief in the superiority of heterosexuality.

HFA 2000 The 1977 goal of the World Health Assembly of WHO of the attainment of a level of health for all world citizens that will permit them to lead socially and economically productive lives.

hidden homeless Individuals who are not usually visible to members of a community because they may have shelter while they are in that community, but not on a permanent basis. Migrant workers are often among the hidden homeless.

Hill-Burton Act First U.S. legislation to focus on planning as a major area of concern. Its primary purpose was to provide for a more equal distribution of hospitals across the nation by matching federal funds for one-third to two-thirds of the total cost of a facility.

HIV *See* Human immunodeficiency virus.

HIV antibody test Enzyme linked immunosorbent assay (ELISA) is the test commonly used in screening blood for the antibody to HIV; the Western Blot is used as a confirmatory test.

HIV disease A disease involving a defect in cell-mediated immunity that is caused by HIV and has a spectrum of clinical expressions that includes AIDS and other symptoms not included in the clinical definition of AIDS.

HIV infection Infection with the human immunodeficiency virus. A phase of this infection is subclinical, but infected individuals remain capable of transmitting the virus through specific behaviors.

HIV seronegative/HIV seropositive Blood serum showing a positive or negative result to a specific test.

HIV seroprevalence The number of new and old cases of persons in the United States identified with human immunodeficiency virus in their blood.

HMO Act Legislation enacted in 1973 to provide a demonstration program for the development of health maintenance organizations.

home health agency An organization that provides skilled nursing and other related skills in the home.

home health care An arrangement of health-related services provided to people in their place of residence.

homeless child syndrome Combination of the effects of homelessness on children resulting in health problems, environmental dangers, and stress.

homelessness The federal government defines a homeless person as one who lacks a fixed, regular and adequate address or has a primary nighttime residence in a supervised publicly or privately operated shelter for temporary accommodations.

home visits Provision of community health nursing care where the individual resides.

homophobia An unfounded fear or hatred of lesbians and gays.

hospice Palliative system of health care for terminally ill people; takes place in the home with family involvement under the direction and supervision of health professionals, especially the visiting nurse. Hospice care takes place in the hospital when severe complications of terminal illness occur or when there is family exhaustion or loss of commitment.

hospital-based agencies Home health agencies that are extensions of hospitals.

host Human or animal that provides adequate living conditions for any given infectious agent.

household A single dwelling (apartment or house) occupied by an individual or a group of two or more individuals (related or untreated).

HPV Human pipillomavirus.

HSV Herpes simplex virus.

human capital The combined human potential of the people living in a community.

human immunodeficiency virus (HIV) The virus that causes AIDS and HIV disease.

human papillomavirus infection A sexually transmitted disease that results in genital warts (condyloma acuminata) that grow in the vulva, vagina, cervix, urinary meatus, scrotum, or perianal area. A link exists between HPV infections and cancer.

human subject review committees Members of various related disciplines brought together to review research proposals to protect research participants from physical or mental harm and the researcher from undue complaints.

humanistic theory Views individuals as unique, self-determined, worthy or respect, and guided by a variety of basic human needs.

hypersusceptible A condition in which individuals may have an illness related to safe, low-level exposure to an occupational hazard.

hypothesis A supposition or question that is raised to explain an event or guide investigation.

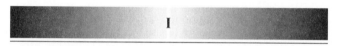

I

immune globulin (IG) Sterile solution containing antibodies from human blood. IG is primarily indicated for routine maintenance of certain immunodeficient individuals and for passive immunization.

immunity Natural or acquired ability to ward off disease.

immunization A process of protecting an individual from a disease through introduction of a live, killed, or partial component of the invading organism into the individual's system.

impairment A disturbance in structure or function resulting from anatomical, physiological, and/or psychological abnormalities.

implementation Carrying out a plan that is based on careful assessment of need.

incest Sexual abuse among family members, typically a parent and a child.

incidence rate The frequency or rate of new cases of an outcome in a population; provides an estimate of the risk of disease in that population over the period of observation.

incubation period Time interval beginning with invasion by an infectious agent and continuing until the organism multiplies to sufficient numbers to produce a host reaction and clinical symptoms.

independent practice Private practice of a professional who works independently from other professionals.

indirect care Nurse-provided services that support client care, (i.e., charting, referral, client case conferences).

inductive approach The reasoning process of developing general rules or ideas from specific observations.

infancy The age of a child between 1 month to 1 year.

infant stimulation Activities to encourage development of the infant, such as cognitive, emotional, and social development.

infection The state produced by the invasion of a host by an infectious agent. Such infection may or may not produce clinical signs.

infectious disease A disease of human or animal caused by the entry and development of an infectious agent (bacteria, rickettsia, virus, fungus, or parasite) in the body.

infectivity An organism's ability to spread rapidly from one host to another.

informal caregiver A voluntary caregiver who may or may not be related to the client. This caregiver usually does not receive payment for the caregiving services rendered but may actually give care more hours of the day than the formal (professional or ancillary) health care worker.

informal group A group whose membership and purposes are not articulated but are understood by members.

informant interviewing Directed conversation with selected members of a community about community members or groups and events; a direct method of assessment.

informed consent The client agrees to a treatment plan after receiving sufficient information concerning the proposal, its incumbent risks, and the acceptable alternatives.

informed group A social group such as those of friends and family. Membership and purposes usually are not articulated but are understood by members.

informing A communication process in which the nurse interprets facts and shares knowledge with clients.

injection drug use Includes intravenous and subcutaneous drug injection with the latter usually being over the abdominal area and called "popping." The sharing of paraphernalia to prepare or inject the drug can result in transmission of bloodborne pathogens, such as HIV.

injury Inflicted damage or harm, generally foreseeable, unlike accidents, and therefore preventable.

institutional licensure A mechanism for allowing employing agencies to be responsible for the competence of the people they hire.

institutional privileges Rights and responsibilities awarded to a nurse not employed by the agency to practice autonomously in the agency.

institutional theory An organizational theory that explains that much of what people do in organizations is based on values and norms. Institutional theory predicts that symbols, rituals, and habitual ways of working have a potentially stronger impact on behavior than formal policies and procedures.

instructive district nursing Nursing provision begun in Boston, which included health education provided by the family-centered health care.

instrumental activities of daily living Those activities of daily living that help individuals manage their lives, such as cooking, shopping, paying bills, cleaning house, and using the telephone.

interacting group A cluster of individuals who are linked by personal relationships. The links may be either primary, such as in a family, or secondary such as in a voluntary association.

Interagency Council on the Homeless A council comprised of the heads of 16 federal agencies that have programs or activities for the homeless; created by the Stewart B. McKinney Act to coordinate and direct federal homeless activities.

intercessor One who acts on behalf of the client when the client could act for self.

interdependent The involvement between different groups or organizations within the community that are mutually reliant upon each other.

interdisciplinary Activities involving the collaboration among personnel representing different disciplines (occupational therapists, nurses, physical therapists, physicians, environmental hygienists, etc.).

intergovernmental organizations Those agencies supported by more than one nation's government, e.g., WHO.

international cooperation Solving health problems that transcend national boundaries.

interpersonal theory A theory that involves the development of satisfactory interpersonal relationships as a sign of maturity. As relationships are lost, the individual may also experience the loss of interpersonal security.

intervention activities Means or strategies by which objectives are achieved and change is effected.

iterative assessment process Obtaining only as much assessment data as necessary at one time, then obtaining additional data as it is needed.

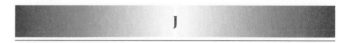

J

job enlargement Refers to adding task variety, task identity, and task significance to a job, but not increasing autonomy or feedback. Workers often believe that they have simply been given more to do, without any corresponding increase in autonomy or motivation.

job enrichment *See* job redesign theory.

job redesign theory Refers to ensuring that a job is designed to be high in task variety, task identity, task significance, autonomy, and feedback (i.e., job enrichment).

joint practice Practice in which professionals work together in a complementary and consultative manner.

judicial law Law based on court or jury decisions.

justice Ethical principle which claims that equals should be treated equally and those who are unequal should be treated differently according to their differences.

K

key informants Professional experts, community leaders, politicians, and entrepreneurs who are in touch with the needs of the community and who are in positions to support new community programs.

knowledge That which we know, our range of information.

L

law The sum total of man-made rules and regulations by which society is governed in a formal and legally binding manner.

lay advisors Individuals who are influential in approving or disapproving new ideas and who seek advice and information from others about these things.

leader An individual who is given informal power in an organization by followers.

leadership Influencing others to achieve a goal.

learning disability A disorder in one or more of the basic psychological processes involved in understanding or ill-using spoken or written language, which may affect one's ability to listen, think, speak, read, write, spell, or do mathematical calculations. The term includes such conditions as perceptual handicaps, brain injury, minimal brain dysfunction, dyslexia, and developmental aphasia.

learning organization Refers to organizations in which people not only learn to improve the way they work, but are encouraged to question even the basic assumptions and goals of work in an effort to constantly increase value.

least restrictive environment A response to institutionalization whereby mentally ill people remain in the community and are maintained with the least restrictions they can handle.

Legionnaires' disease (legionellosis) Pneumonia-like communicable disease caused by *Legionella pneumophilia*. Mode of transmission is presumed to be airborne.

legislation Bills introduced by Congress for the purpose of establishing laws that direct policy.

legislative process The process used within governments to make laws.

lesser developed countries Those countries that have not yet achieved economic and technologic stability.

level I disaster A disaster that requires activation by the local emergency medical system in cooperation with local community organizations.

level II disaster A disaster that requires activation of the local emergency medical system and local community organizations in cooperation with the regional response system.

level III disaster A disaster that requires activation of the federal emergency system to work in cooperation with local and regional emergency medical systems.

levels of prevention A three-level model of interventions based on the stages of disease, designed to halt or reverse the process of pathological change as early as possible, thereby preventing damage.

Lexis A computerized search tool of the legal literature.

liability An obligation one has incurred or might incur through any act or failure to act, or responsibility for conduct falling below a certain standard that is the cause of client injury.

licensure Legal sanction to practice a profession after attaining the minimum degree of competence to ensure protection of public health and safety.

life events Occurrences that are normative (generally expected to occur at a particular stage of life) and nonnormative (unanticipated) in a person or family's life.

life expectancy The average number of years that a man or woman can expect to live from the time of birth.

life review A universal process that can occur at any point in life where an individual is forced to confront his or her mortality.

life-style Behaviors associated with daily living, such as exercise, rest, sleep, nutrition, work, and play.

life-style risk Factors that predispose a family to ill health that are caused by the personal health behaviors of the members.

lines of resistance In the Neuman System's Model, refers to a series of circles between the normal lines of defense and the basic care that support the defense lines and protect the basic structure.

litigation Trial in court to determine legal issues and the rights and duties between the parties.

locus of control An individual's feeling of whether he or she controls his/her destiny (internal locus of control) or if his/her destiny is controlled by outside forces such as luck (external locus of control).

long-term care Care that is delivered to individuals who are dependent on others for assistance with basic tasks over a sustained period of time.

long-term care facility (nursing home) Where individuals receive minimum to maximum skilled nursing care, depending on the type of facility and the need of the client.

low-birth-weight Birth weight of less than 5.5 pounds.

M

machismo The male quality of dominance defined as courage, strength, honor, virility, pride, and dignity.

macro-level management theories Sociological theories that explain and predict the best ways to organize work, obtaining organizational resources, power dynamics, and organizational change.

mainstream smoke Smoke inhaled and exhaled by the smoker.

maintenance functions Behaviors that provide physical and psychological support and therefore hold the group together.

maintenance norms Norms that create group pressures to ensure affirming actions for members and are helpful in maintaining comfort.

malnutrition A condition in which a person has too much or too little to eat.

malpractice Professional misconduct, improper discharge of professional duties, or a failure to meet the standard of care by a professional that results in harm to another.

malpractice litigation A lawsuit resulting from client dissatisfaction with the provider and the content or quality of care received; a quality assurance measure.

mammography X-ray study of the breast; used in the diagnosis of cancer and other breast disease.

managed care Refers to integrating payment for services with delivery of services and emphasizing cost-effective service delivery along a continuum of care.

managed competition A creation of market conditions in which the more efficient providers will survive and the more costly will be put out of business.

mandatory credentialing Certification requiring statutory law (e.g., state nurse practice acts).

mandatory nurse licensure A law that requires all who practice nursing for compensation to be licensed.

man-made disaster An act of individuals that causes devastation and destruction, such as war, terrorist bombings, riots.

mass media Newspapers, TV, radio, or other modes of communication to large audiences.

mastery Attainment of task or skill.

maximum theory Economic theory of distribution of goods and resources to maximize the minimum position in society while at the same time allowing exercise of liberty on the span of all people.

Meals on Wheels Local programs in which one hot meal and sometimes a cold breakfast and sack lunch are delivered to elderly people in their homes.

mediating structures Institutions standing between the individual in private life and the larger institution of public life, such as one's neighborhood, family, church, or voluntary associations.

mediator A role in which the nurse acts to assist parties to understand each other's concerns and to determine their conclusion of the issues. The mediator has no authority to decide on behalf of another.

Medicaid A jointly sponsored state and federal program that pays for medical services for the aged, poor, blind, disabled, and families with dependent children.

medical technology A set of interventions, drugs, equipment, and services used to deliver health care.

medically indigent A portion of the population which is usually above the recognized poverty level and has money to buy the necessities of life but which cannot afford a catastrophic illness or an acute illness crisis.

medically underserved Not having an adequate number of health care providers and/or services.

Medicare A federally funded health insurance program for the elderly, disabled, and persons with end-stage renal disease.

menopause Permanent cessation of menstruation resulting from loss of ovarian, follicular activity.

men's health care practitioner A registered nurse who has advanced education and clinical training in the health care of men.

mental health problems Difficulties related to a person's ability to manage daily life events without experiencing undue social isolation, emotional distress, or behavioral incapacity.

mental illness/mental disorder Disturbances of thinking, feeling, and behaving that may be due to physical or psychological factors. Mental disorder is a more comprehensive term that describes any of the recognizable forms of mental illness or severe mental disorders. These specific forms include schizophrenia, psychosis, mania, or depression. Such terms have well-defined clinical meaning and should not be used casually. Also, people are not "schizophrenics," but should be described as persons with schizophrenia.

mental retardation A condition causing a person to have significant, below-average general intellectual functioning.

men-to-women death ratio A statistical comparison of death rates between men and women.

methadone A synthetic narcotic analgesic used for anesthesia or as a substitute for heroin.

micro-level management theories Psychological theories that help explain and predict individual behavior in organizations (e.g., work motivation) and interpersonal dynamics (e.g., leadership theories, group dynamics).

migrant farm worker A laborer whose principle employment involves moving from farm to farm, planting or harvesting agriculture, and attaining temporary housing.

minimental status exam A screening tool to check the level of cognitive functioning that has a maximum total score of 30.

minimum data set A minimum set of items of information concerning an aspect or dimension of the health care system. Nursing's minimum data set reveals the comparability of nursing data across clinical populations, settings, geographic areas, and time.

mobile clinics A method of providing ambulatory care in a variety of geographic locations via use of specially equipped vans.

model A representation of reality.

moral accountability A moral obligation that directs the professional nurse to act in a particular way according to moral norms and requires the nurse to be answerable for what has been done.

moral obligation Duty to act in a particular way in response to moral norms.

moral virtue Ideal standard of human behavior or thinking; excellence in response to moral norms, such as goodness.

morbidity Relative disease rate, usually expressed as incidence or prevalence of a disease.

mortality Relative death rate; the proportion of deaths at a particular time and place.

motivation theories Psychological theories that explain and predict those factors that help motivate work behavior.

multiattribute utility A planning method based on decision theory.

multiinfarct dementia Dementia that occurs as a result of either sustained or recurrent cortical or subcortical strokes.

multilevel intervention Intervention targeted to the individual, family, aggregate, and the community.

multiproblem family A family unit that faces a number of events within and without the family environment and does not have the ability to solve its own problems.

multisectoral cooperation Coordinated action by all sectors of a community from local government officials to grass-roots community members.

multiskilled workers Refers to people with a broad range of skills. Such individuals are considered to be more productive in day-to-day situations than more specialized workers because they are able to respond quickly and in a flexible way to needs in the work environment.

N

Narcotics Anonymous Support group for narcotics addicts.

national disaster Acts of nature that cause devastation and destruction, such as floods, tornados, earthquakes.

National Disaster Medical System (NDMS) A system comprised of approximately 75 local disaster medical assistance teams (DMAT) that can be activated (1) in a presidential declaration of a disaster (2) by request for major medical assistance from a state health official under provisions of the Public Health Service Act, or (3) in a foreign military conflict involving U.S. Armed Forces, where casualty levels are likely to exceed the capacity of the Department of Defense-Veterans' Administration Medical System.

national health objectives Indicate major health concerns for population aggregates and provide standards for researchers to evaluate program progress.

National Health Planning and Resources Development Act of 1974 (P.L. 93-641) Legislation set forth to coordinate and direct national health policy via state and regional regulatory agencies; its major goal was to establish a nationwide network of health system agencies.

National Health Service Corps Program established in 1970 by the Public Health Service to recruit health providers to areas experiencing shortages in health work forces.

National Institute for Nursing Research One of the National Institutes of health charged with promoting the growth and quality of research in nursing.

National Institute of Mental Health (NIMH) The federal agency charged with developing and supporting education and research programs for mental health.

National Institute of Occupational Safety and Health (NIOSH) The branch of the USPHS responsible for investigating workplace illnesses, accidents, and hazards.

National Joint Practice Commission Organization established by the American Nurses' Association and the American Medical Association to promote collaborative efforts between medicine and nursing; disbanded in 1981.

National Labor Relation Act Amendments of 1974 (P.L. 93-8360) Amended the Taft Hartley Act of 1947 and extended the right to organize collectively for matters concerning wages, hours, and working conditions to all employees of nonpublic health care facilities.

National Labor Relations Act Passed in 1935 and known as the Wagner Act; it protected employees' rights to organize and join unions and also provided for action against unfair labor practices of employers.

nationally notifiable conditions Certain communicable diseases defined by the Centers for Disease Control as requiring weekly, monthly, and annual reports of occurrence by all states.

natural history of disease The course of disease process from onset to resolution without intervention by humans.

natural radiation Radiation that comes from soil, certain rocks, body potassium, and ultraviolet sun rays.

near poor People who earn slightly more than the government defined poverty level, are unable to meet living expenses, and are not eligible for government assistance programs.

need theories of motivation Psychological theories that say that people are motivated to be productive workers when their needs are met. Two well-known examples are Maslow's theory and Aldefer's theory.

negentrophy Energy in a system that propels toward order or can be used for work.

negligence Failure to act as an ordinary, prudent person; conduct contrary to that of a reasonable person under a specific circumstance.

negotiation Working with others in a formal way to achieve agreement on areas of conflict, using principles of communication, conflict resolution, and assertiveness. Negotiation may be relatively informal, as when two staff members negotiate which vacation times they will have. It may also be formal, as when labor and management negotiate a contract in a unionized environment.

neighborhood poverty Refers to spatially defined areas of high poverty, characterized by dilapidated housing and high levels of unemployment.

neoclassical management A theoretical approach to management based on the idea that human needs, group dynamics, and cooperation are important to successful achievement of organizational goals.

neonate Age period from birth to 1 month.

Newton risk reduction The approach used to predict individual risks of dying, to provide recommendations for reducing the risks, and to promote healthful behavior changes. Also called health risk or health hazard appraisal.

Noise Control Act Legislation passed by Congress in 1972 to identify major sources of noise, establish noise emission standards, and provide a mechanism for people to take civil action on their own behalf when a person or agency violates the Act.

nonfarm residency Residence within area zoned as "city limits."

nongonococcal urethritis (NGU) Inflammation of the urethra from microorganisms other than *Neisseriae gonorrhea*; *Chlamydia trachomatis* has been implicated as the cause of 50% of cases.

non–metropolitan statistical area (non–MSA) Counties that do not meet SMSA criteria.

Nonoxynol-9 A spermicidal gel found in some contraceptive foams and jellies, in condoms, and in some sexual lubricants. Nonoxynol-9 has viricidal and bactericidal properties and can be used as a lubricant to protect against HIV.

nontraditional family Alternative family structures comprised of two or more individuals coming from the same or different kinship groups who are involved in a continuous living arrangement, usually residing in the same household, experiencing common emotional bonds, and sharing certain obligations toward each other and toward others.

normal lines of defense In the Neuman System's Model, is dynamic and defines the stability and integrity of the system.

norms Standards that guide, regulate, and control.

nuclear (traditional) family A unit comprised of mother, father, and young children.

nurse practitioner Nursing role that includes a primary care component that focuses on health maintenance and client counseling.

nursing centers Health care facilities in which the primary aim is to offer nursing services, including health assessment, promotion, screening, and health teaching.

nursing diagnosis A clinical judgment about individual, family, or community responses to actual or potential health problems/life processes.

nursing practice Nurse clinical activities and behaviors that are performed on behalf of clients.

nursing process A clinical decision-making method that involves assessing, planning, implementing, and evaluating client care. Assessment of client problems results in formulating a nursing diagnosis.

O

objective A precise behavioral statement of the achievement that will accomplish partial or total realization of a goal. The date by which the achievement is expected is specified.

occupational health The state in which a worker is able to function at an optimum level of well-being (see HEALTH) at the worksite; reflected by higher employee productivity, an increase in work attendance, a reduction in workers' compensation claims, and an increase in longevity in employment status.

Occupational Safety and Health Administration (OSHA) Federal agency charged with improving worker health and safety by establishing standards and regulations and by educating workers.

official agencies Agencies operated by state or local governments to provide home health care.

Older American's Act Legislation enacted in 1965 to mandate and provide funds for services, programs, and activities deemed essential to accomplish certain goals for older Americans meeting specified criteria.

Omaha Problem Classification Scheme A client-focused taxonomy of nursing diagnoses comprised of simple terms.

Omaha Problem Rating Scale for Outcomes A five-point Likert-type scale that provides a systematic, recurring way of measuring client progress throughout the time of service.

Omaha System A system of nursing diagnoses, interventions, and evaluations of outcomes of care developed by the Omaha Visiting Nurses Association.

ombudsman A role of a community health nurse in which the investigation of complaints about health care services and providers is the predominant activity.

operant behavior Behavior not elicited by a known stimulus but simply exhibited by the organism.

operating budget An agency's budget that includes all anticipated revenues and projected expenses that are related to the day-to-day costs of achieving the organization's goals.

Orem's self-care nursing theory Dorothea Orem's theory that explains that the goal of nursing is to assist people to meet their self-care needs when they are unable to do so themselves. Orem says that nurse managers should ensure that the nursing staff is adequate in number and skill mix to meet clients' self-care needs. Her theory can be applied to situations in which clients are individuals, families, groups, or communities.

organizational structure The formal and informal relationships that operationalize accomplishment of organizational goals.

osteoporosis Condition characterized by increased bone brittleness.

other metropolitan Fringe counties of core metropolitan areas; suburban areas.

Ottawa Charter for Health Promotion (1986) Provides a definition for health promotion and a framework for the Healthy Cities movement. Includes six elements: health promotion, building healthy public policy, creating supportive environments, strengthening community action, developing personal skills, and reorienting health services.

outcome A change in client health status as a result of care or program implementation.

outreach Making a special, focused effort to find people with a specific health problem for the purpose of increasing their access to health services.

ozone Unstable colorless gas with an oxidizing power surpassed only by fluorine.

P

pandemic A worldwide outbreak of an epidemic disease.

papanicolaou (PAP) test A technique of collecting vaginal and cervical cells to detect early abnormal changes of the cells of the cervix that may lead to cervical cancer.

paraplegia Refers to paralysis of the lower half of the body involving the partial or total loss of function of both legs.

parish nursing A nursing service provided by a church as a community outreach to its parishioners, usually focused on primary prevention.

participant observation Conscious and systematic sharing in the life activities and occasionally in the interests and activities of a group of persons; observational methods of assessment; a direct method of data collection.

partner notification Also known as contact tracing. Identifying and locating sexual and injectable drug-use partners of people who have been diagnosed with a sexually transmitted disease in order to notify them of exposure and encourage them to seek medical treatment.

partnership A relationship between individuals, groups, or organizations in which the parties are working together to achieve a joint goal. Often used synonymously with coalitions and alliances, although partnerships usually have focused goals, such as jointly providing a specific program. Partnerships generally involve shared power.

passive immunization Administration of a performed antibody to a susceptible host.

paternity fatherhood

path-goal leadership theory Robert House's leadership theory. He predicts that the most effective leaders remove obstacles to workers' goals achievement.

pathogenicity An agent's relative ability to produce disease.

Patients Bill of Rights A document prepared by the American Hospital Association that defines the provider-client relationship within an organization.

pediatric nurse practitioner Registered nurse with certificate or master's level advanced education in the areas of health assessment, diagnosis, and treatment of children. The program prepares the nurse to deliver primary health care to infants and children.

pelvic inflammatory disease (PID) Also known as salpingitis. Infection of the female reproductive organs, especially the fallopian tubes and endometrium resulting in infertility and/or ectopic pregnancy. Acute symptoms and signs include lower abdominal pain, increased vaginal discharge, urinary frequency, vomiting, and fever. PID results from untreated gonorrhea and chlamydia.

performance budget A financial plan that shows clearly and concisely the services to be provided in return for the funds available or income generated.

perimenopause The period immediately prior to menopause when endocrinological, biological, and clinical features of approaching menopause commence, continuing for at least the first year after permanent cessation of menstruation.

permissive nurse licensure A law that allows a person to practice nursing without a license as long as the term *registered nurse* is not used and the practitioner does not pretend to be licensed.

persistent poverty Refers to individuals and families that remain poor for long periods of time.

personalismo The cultural preference to see health care providers with backgrounds, culture, and language similar to one's own.

personal preparedness A process whereby the nurse keeps self healthy and plans for family and work responsibilities to continue in an organized manner if the nurse is called to participate in a disaster.

pesticides Chemical poisons used to eliminate pests and to increase annual crop production by generating healthy crops.

philanthropic organizations Those agencies who receive funds through private endowments and use those funds to support health-related projects.

physical abuse One or more episodes of extreme disciplining or displaced aggression or frustration, often resulting in serious physical damage to the internal organs, bones, central nervous system, or sense organs.

physical agent Extremes of temperature, noise, radiation and lighting that may cause illness.

physical dependency A state of neuroadaption in which continued use of a drug is necessary to prevent withdrawal symptoms.

physician assistant Health practitioner role created in the 1960s to free physician's time by completing tasks such as taking medical histories and conducting physical examinations.

planning Selecting a series of actions designed to achieve stated goals.

planning, programming, and budgeting An outcome-oriented accounting system, which helps to determine the most efficient use of resources to meet objectives.

point epidemic A concentration in space and time of a disease event, such that a graph of frequency of cases over time shows a sharp point, usually suggestive of a common exposure.

police power States' power to act to protect the health, safety, and welfare of their citizens.

political skills Bargaining and negotiation skills based on an understanding of others' wants and needs, and the effects of decisions on others' goals achievement.

pollution Addition of a substance (e.g., noise or toxic chemicals) to an environment that changes its natural qualities.

polysubstance abuse Use of drugs from different categories used together or at different times to regulate how the person feels.

population demography *See* demographic trends

positive predictive value The proportion of persons with a positive screening or diagnostic test who do have the disease (the proportion of "true positives" among all who test positive).

postmenopause A period dating form the menopause, although it cannot be determined until 12 months of spontaneous cessation of the menstrual period.

poverty Refers to having insufficient financial resources to meet basic living expenses. These expenses include cost of food, shelter, clothing, transportation, and medical care.

poverty guidelines A definition of poverty drafted by the Social Security Administration in 1964. The federal government defines poverty in terms of income, family size, the age of the head of household, and the number of children under 18 years of age. The guidelines change annually to be consistent with the consumer price index.

power The ability to influence others or the course of events.

Practice Acts State laws that govern the practice of health providers.

practice-based research Involves translating clinical hunches from community health nursing practice into questions that can be researched.

practice setting Context and/or environment within which nursing care is given.

PRECEDE model A health education model that is outcome oriented and asks "why" before it asks "how" and can be used with individuals, families, groups, or the community.

preconceptional counseling Education, assessment, diagnosis, and intervention to address risk of pregnancy and birth prior to conception.

Preferred Provider Organization (PPO) An organization of providers who contract on a fee-for-service basis with third-party payers to provide comprehensive medical services to subscribers.

prejudice The emotional manifestation of deeply held beliefs about other groups; involves negative attitudes.

prematurity Birth that occurs prior to 37 weeks' gestation.

preparedness The predisaster stage in which individuals and communities plan for and coordinate their response efforts.

prepathogenesis A stage in the natural history of a disease in which the disease has not yet developed, although the groundwork has been laid through the presence of factors that favor its occurrence.

preschooler A child between the ages of three to five.

prescriptive authority A legal right granted to nurses by states to write prescriptions for clients.

prescriptive intervention mode An intervention requiring less collaboration between consultant and client because the consultant explicitly tells the client how to solve the problem.

prevalence The proportion of existing cases of a health outcome in a population at a particular time.

prevention Behaviors designed to avoid disease.

price inflation Increases in costs of all goods and services in the United States.

primary care Typically the entry point into the health care system; emphasizes management of commonly occurring diseases or chronic disease.

primary health care A conceptual framework for providing public health and primary care services; it includes delivering essential, affordable, accessible, and acceptable health care to the community, with an emphasis on disease prevention and health promotion, community involvement, multisectoral cooperation, and appropriate technology.

primary prevention Actions that reduce the incidence of disease by promoting health and preventing disease processes from developing.

primary relationship Relationship consisting of at least two persons interacting together within both an immediate context and a larger environment.

principles The foundations for rules.

private/commercial organizations Those agencies who provide financial and technical support for investment, research, and employment.

private practice A clinical setting that is usually a single physician's office in which the nurse practitioner is employed.

private sector An individual or any part of society that is not part of the government.

probability Likelihood that an intervention activity can be implemented.

problem analysis Process of identifying problem correlates and interrelationships and substantiating them with relevant data.

problem prioritization Evaluation of problems and establishment of priorities according to predetermined criteria.

problem-solving A process of seeking to find solutions to situations that present difficulty or uncertainty.

process The ongoing activities and behaviors of health providers engaged in conducting client care.

process consultation A consultation model in which the consultant and client work in the partnership to identify and solve client problems. The consultant works more as a facilitator and coach, encouraging the client to identify the problem and helping the client develop a problem-solving strategy.

professional isolation The act of practicing in a setting where there are no colleagues.

professional negligence An unreasonable act or a failure to act when a duty is owed to another, leading to injuries that can be legally compensated.

professional preparedness A process whereby the nurse becomes aware and understands disaster plans in the workplace and the community.

Professional Standards Review Organizations/Professional Review Organizations Organizations established by law to monitor delivery of health care to clients of Medicaid, Medicare, and Maternal/Child health programs and to monitor implementation of prospective reimbursement.

program A health care service designed to meet identified health care needs of clients.

program budget A financial plan that shows expenses and income related to a specific service.

program evaluation Collection of methods, skills, and activities necessary to determine whether a service is needed, likely to be used, conducted as planned, and actually helps people.

Program Evaluation and Review Technique (PERT) A network programming method that focuses on key parts, objectives, and time needed to make decisions and evaluate objectives.

program planning method A program planning technique that uses normal groups to assess client problems and find ways to solve the problems.

promotor An advocacy role in which the nurse partners with the client and pushes the client's right to make their own decision.

proprietary agencies For-profit organizations.

prospective payment system The diagnosis-related group payment mechanism for reimbursing hospitals for inpatient health care services through Medicare.

prospective reimbursement Method of payment to an agency for services to be delivered based on predictions of what an agency's costs will be for the coming year.

protocols (algorithms) Written, standing orders that have been mutually agreed on by the nurse practitioner and the physician. The nurse practitioner uses them as a guide to manage certain illnesses or conditions.

provider service records A written summary of the provider's work activities on a daily, weekly, or monthly basis.

psychomotor domain The learning domain that includes performance of skills that require some degree of neuromuscular coordination.

psychosis Mental disorder often characterized by delusions and hallucinations.

psychosocial Development combination of emotional and social development.

psychosocial agents Workplace hazards that affect the emotional and social well-being of a worker.

psychotropic Drugs that affect psychic function, behavior, or experience.

public health Organized community efforts designed to prevent disease and promote health.

public health ethic Principle of providing health care services that will offer the greatest good for the greatest number.

public health nursing The field of nursing that synthesizes the public health sciences and the theory of nursing to improve the health of individuals, families, and communities.

public health service An arm of the Department of Health and Human Services that fulfills the function of overseeing health care services within the United States.

public sector A governmental entity.

purchase-of-expertise consultation A model of consultation in which the client hires an expert to provide information or suggest solutions to client-identified problems.

Q

quadriplegia Refers to paralysis of the body involving partial or total loss of function in both arms and both legs.

qualified person with a disability In order to be considered a qualified person with a disability for the purpose of employment, the individual must satisfy the requisite skills, experience, education, and other job-related requirements of the position. This determination must be based on the individual's current status, and not on speculation about his or her future ability to perform. Moreover, the job applicant must be able to perform the essential functions of the position with or without reasonable accommodations.

qualitative methods Characterized by inductive reasoning, subjectivity, discovery, description and the meaning of an experience to an individual.

quality Continuous striving for excellence and a conformance to specifications or guidelines.

quality assurance Monitoring of the activities of client care to determine the degree of excellence attained in the implementation of the activities.

quality improvement *See* total quality management/improvement.

quantitative methods Characterized by deductive reasoning, objectivity, quasiexperiments, statistical techniques and control.

quasivoluntary A form of accreditation that is linked to governmental regulations and encourages programs to participate in a voluntary accrediting process.

R

race A biological designation whereby group members share distinguishing features (e.g., skin color, bone structure, and genetic traits such as a blood grouping).

racism A form of prejudice and refers to beliefs that persons who are born into particular groups are inferior in intelligence, morals, beauty, and self-worth.

radiation Energy emitted by natural or synthetic radioactive sources. The natural forms come from the sun, soil, and some rocks; synthetic radiation comes from x-rays and radioisotopes in clinical facilities and industry.

radioactive Containing radiation.

radon A radioactive gas caused by the decaying or uranium that can enter homes through floors, cracks, and walls.

rape Natural or unnatural sexual intercourse forced on an unwilling person by threat of bodily injury or loss of life.

rate A measure of the frequency of a health event in a defined population during a specified period of time.

ratio Statistical measure in which the numerator is not included in the denominator.

rationing Limits placed on health care that may not be beneficial to a client's well-being.

recertification In home health care, the review and certification performed at least every 62 days by the health care team; it demonstrates that the client continues to need a specified plan of care.

reciprocity The recognition and acceptance of a professional's licensure between certain states.

recognition Process whereby one agency accepts the credentialing status of and the credentials conferred by another.

recovery The stage of a disaster when all involved agencies and individuals pull together to restore the economic and civic life of a community.

referral Guiding clients toward problem-resolution and assisting them in using available resources.

regulations Specific statements of law that relate to and clarify individual pieces of legislation.

relapse management Activities of a case manager designed to foster coping and competency and manage symptoms in order to prevent a relapse of illness.

relative risk ratio Statistical measure of how much the risk of acquiring a particular disease increases with exposure to a specific causal agent or risk factor.

relative standard Defines poverty in terms of the society's median standard of living.

reliability The consistency of a measure from person to person or over time.

report card An agency report card is a written listing of how the agency compares with others in the field on certain key indicators of quality, including morbidity and mortality measures, consumer satisfaction, and cost of care.

representative group Type of community group whose members are elected, appointed, or selected from various community sectors.

research process A comprehensive problem-solving process, including the stages of assessment, planning, implementation, evaluation and action.

resilience The ability to withstand stressors and multiple problems without developing health problems.

resource dependence theory An organizational theory that explains organizational power in terms of the extent of the organization's resources. According to this theory, an organization with a large budget would be more powerful in the community than one with a smaller budget.

respite Relief time provided by others to a caregiver from responsibilities for care of a family member.

response Responsibilities assumed and activities that occur as a result of a specific level of disaster. (*See* level I, II, and III disasters.)

retrospective audit A method of evaluating quality of care through appraisal of the nursing process after the client's discharge from the health care system.

retrospective cost reimbursement Method of payment to an agency based on units of service delivered.

return migration Geographical term for the return of elders, after retirement, to their hometown after having spent their working life elsewhere.

right That to which a person has a just claim; legal claim recognized as valid by a legal system; moral claim recognized as valid by moral principles that in turn may or may not be recognized by legal rules.

right to health Right to not have one's health affected by others (a negative right).

right to health care Right to goods, resources, and services to maintain and improve one's state of health (a positive right).

risk The probability of some event or outcome within a specified period of time.

risk appraisal A quantitative approach comparing data from epidemiologic studies and vital statistics with information supplied by individuals about their (1) health-related practices, (2) health habits, (3) demographic characteristics, and (4) personal and family medical history.

risk assessment Assessing the probability of developing a disease.

risk factor Disease precursor, the presence of which is associated with higher than average mortality. Disease precursors include demographic variables, certain everyday health practices, family history of disease, and some physiological changes.

risk management Intervention designed to induce and/or sustain changes in health-compromising behaviors, such as counseling, mass media campaigns, or increased production of low-fat dairy goods.

role Identifiable social position associated with a set of behavioral expectations.

role ambiguity Lack of clarity about what is expected.

role behavior What an actor in a position actually does in response to role expectations.

role conflict Presence of contradictory and often competing role expectations.

role negotiation Two or more persons deciding together which tasks, activities, or responsibilities each will accept in a defined situation.

role overload A situation that occurs when there is insufficient time to carry out all of the expected role functions.

role performance model of health A model in which health is viewed as the individual's ability to effectively perform roles and the family's ability to effectively meet their functions and developmental tasks.

role sequence Positions within the family and related behaviors that change over time.

role sharing Arrangement in which both partners have equal claims to the bread-winning role and equal responsibilities for the care of the home and children, including the obligations to contribute equally or equitably to family expenses.

role strain A situation resulting from conditions requiring complex role demands and the fulfillment of multiple roles.

role structure Arrangement of group-member positions according to the expected functions of members.

Roy's adaptation model of nursing administration Sr. Callista Roy's modification of her Adaptation Model to nursing administration. Roy explains that the role of nursing administrators is to help the organization adapt to changing circumstances in the best way.

rubeola (measles) Acute, highly contagious viral disease involving the respiratory tract and characterized by a rash.

rule of confidentiality Nondisclosure of personal information about others, such as clients, to those not authorized to have this information; also, a rule grounded in the principle of autonomy.

rule of utility Rule derived from the principle of beneficence. Includes the moral duty to weigh and balance benefits and reduce the occurrence of harms.

rules Guidelines, principles, or regulations that govern conduct.

rural areas Communities having less than 20,000 residents or fewer than 99 persons per square mile.

Rural Health Clinic Legislation enacted in 1978 to provide for the development of rural health clinics staffed by new health professionals in existing medically underserved areas of the United States.

S

salmonellosis A gastroenteritis caused by ingestion of food contaminated with a species of *Salmonella*; characterized by sudden, colicky, abdominal pain, fever, and bloody, watery diarrhea.

salpingitis Also referred to as pelvic inflammatory disease; inflammation of the fallopian tubes that may result from gonorrhea or chlamydia.

sampling Selecting a portion of the population to study; can use random or deliberate sampling techniques.

sanitary landfill Method of solid waste disposal whereby waste is taken to canyons, swamps, and ravines, compacted by heavy-machines, and covered with earth before rodent infestation occurs.

satellite clinic Health care facility generally operated under the auspices of a large institution but situated in a location away from the institution.

school-age adolescent Persons in the age range of 6 through 20 years.

school-based clinics Facilities that provide physical and/or mental health services to school-age children that are located within or near schools.

school nurse practitioner Registered nurse with certificate or master's level advanced education in the areas of health assessment, diagnosis, and treatment who is prepared to deliver primary health care to school-age children.

school phobia The persistent and abnormal fear of going to school.

scientific management The earliest theoretical approach to management; the best way to increase work productivity is to help people become expert at their jobs through repeating the same tasks over and over.

scope of practice The usual and customary practice of a profession taking into account how legislation defines the practice of a profession within a particular jurisdiction (Local, state, community, or nationally).

scorpio A service provided by the Library of Congress to assist in topic searches in the legal literature.

screening The application of a test to people who are as yet asymptomatic for the purpose of classifying them with respect to their likelihood of having a particular disease.

screening test sensitivity and specificity The extent to which screening tests identify all individuals with a particular health problem and do not inaccurately indicate that people have the problem when they actually do not.

seasonal farm worker Person who works during certain seasons in agriculture but does not relocate from one area or another to obtain work.

secondary analysis Method of assessment in which existing data are used.

secondary care Actions to treat disease in the early, acute phase.

second-hand smoke Smoke in environment inhaled by someone who is not currently smoking.

second-order change Changes that do not merely represent improvements over past ways of working, but are fundamental variations in the assumptions and goals of working.

secondary prevention Programs, such as screening, designed to detect disease in the early stages (early pathogenesis), before clinically evident signs and symptoms, in order to intervene with early diagnosis and treatment.

secular trend Long-term patterns of morbidity or mortality (i.e., over years or decades).

selected membership group A group of persons brought together for a specific purpose, such as health assessment or promotion. Some members may be linked to others through previous association, or members may be unacquainted before group formation.

self-care Activities that individuals initiate and perform on their own behalf to maintain life, health, and well-being.

self-determination The right and responsibility of one to decide and direct one's choices.

self-efficacy A sense of competence and capability.

self-regulation An essential characteristic of a profession involving activities that have as their goals the overseeing of the rights, obligations, responsibilities, and relationships of a provider to society, to the profession, and to the client. On the individual level, one's ability to exert self-control.

sensitivity The proportion of persons who actually have a disease who will have a positive screening or diagnostic test; or the probability that a person with disease will be correctly classified by the test.

sepsis Invasion of infecting organisms through the bloodstream to multiple organ systems.

seroconversion The appearance of antibodies in serum.

seroprevalence The overall occurrence of HIV antibodies within a specific population at any point in time.

service delivery network A group of organizations that provide health and human services. Generally, the services are complementary, although some overlap is often seen. Clients may receive comprehensive services from the agencies in the network.

service leadership A form of leadership that emphasizes the leader's role in providing service as a partner with others, as opposed to a more hierarchical approach to leadership.

settlement houses Early agencies for visiting nurses.

severe mental disorders Disorders that are persistent and disabling; they are determined by diagnosis and criteria that evaluate degree of functional disability.

sexual abuse Abuse ranging from fondling to rape; robs children of the feeling of being in control of themselves and emphasizes their vulnerability.

sexual behavior Behaviors or practices of a sexual nature.

sexual debut First intercourse.

sexual victimization Suffering from a destructive or injurious sexual action.

sexually transmitted diseases (STDs) Communicable diseases, such as gonorrhea, chlamydia, and HIV infection, that can be passed on during sexual activity.

short portable mental status questionnaire A screening tool to assess the level of cognitive functioning. As the score increases, so does the level of intellectual impairment.

sibling relationship The interaction among brothers and sisters.

sidestream smoke Smoke generated by a smoldering cigarette.

simpatia Some cultures have a goal of polite, respectful, nonconfrontational relationships with others; these tendencies may prevent clients from asking questions of health care providers.

social Darwinism A sense that only those people who are skillful and hardworking deserve to obtain social goods, such as a good income and comfortable life-style.

social learning theory A motivation theory developed by Albert Bandura that emphasizes the extent to which individuals are motivated by learning from others with whom they identify.

social network Individuals who may or may not include family members with whom others have contact because of proximity or reciprocity.

social reinforcement theories of motivation Motivation theories that emphasize the role of learning in motivation. Reinforcement theory focuses on the effects of learning from the consequences of past behavior. Social learning theory focuses on learning from other people. (*See* social learning theory.)

somatic mutagenesis theory As cells divide, they develop spontaneous mutations that eventually lead to death.

somatotropin Hormone responsible for growth released by the hypothalamus.

special population groups Groups identified as needing special consideration in *Healthy People 2000*. The special population groups include low income groups, minority groups, and people with disabilities.

specialist A nurse who provides services that are specific to an area of concentration of nursing (e.g., pediatric care).

specific immune globulin Special preparation obtained from human blood preselected for its high antibody count against a specific disease (e.g., varicella zoster immune globulin).

specific protection Measures aimed at protecting individuals against specific agents, such as immunization or attempts to remove agents from the environment.

specific rates Statistical rates in which the events in both the numerator and the denominator are restricted to a specified subgroup of the population.

specific screening test Laboratory examinations that correctly classify healthy persons as healthy.

specificity The proportion of persons who do not have a disease who will have a negative screening or diagnostic test, or the probability that a person without disease will be correctly classified by the test.

speech impairment Limited or difficult speech patterns. The presence of a speech impairment does not mean that there is a problem in hearing or in mental ability.

spouse abuse Physical or emotional mistreatment of one's partner.

staff review committees Committees whose function is to monitor client-specific aspects of care appropriate for certain levels of care.

Standard Metropolitan Statistical Area (SMSA) Region with a central city of at least 50,000 residents.

standard of care Those acts performed or omitted that an ordinarily prudent person in the defendant's position would or would not have done; a measure by which the defendant's conduct is compared to ascertain negligence.

standardized rates (adjusted rates) Artificial rates of disease that are calculated to allow comparison of rates in populations with differing distributions of characteristics, such as age or race.

standards Criteria for measuring conformity to established practice.

statistical indicators Measures of incidence, prevalence, mortality, and other data to estimate client problems, magnitudes of problems, and needs for programs to resolve the problems.

statutes Legislative enactments declaring, commanding, or prohibiting something.

statutory law Law enacted by a legislative body.

stereotypes Exaggerated beliefs and images that are generally false and serve to obscure important differences among members of a group and exaggerate the differences between groups.

Stewart B. McKinney Homelessness Act Public Law 100-77 passed in 1987 officially involved the federal government with meeting the needs of homeless persons. It was intended to respond to the range of emergency needs facing homeless Americans, such as food, shelter, and health care. The McKinney Act includes several demonstration projects that deal with issues such as mental health, education, job training, and substance abuse.

strategic planning A process in which client needs, specific provider strengths, and agency and community resources are successfully matched to offer a service to the community.

strategy Premeditated approach or method of dealing with a situation.

strength of the association Degree of a relationship between a causal factor and disease occurrence, usually measured by the relative risk ratio.

structural contingency theory An organizational theory that predicts that the optimal form of organizational structure is one that is matched to the characteristics of the situation, including the environment within which that organization is functioning, the nature of the work in that organization, and the skills of the workers.

structural-functional framework Framework that views the family as a social system with members who have specific roles and functions.

structure In groups, the particular arrangement of group parts that helps to describe the group as a whole. An organizational arrangement including mission, goals, services, and work force.

substance abuse Use of chemicals having actual or potential undesirable effects.

suburban Area adjacent to highly populated city.

sudden infant death syndrome (SIDS) Death that occurs during infancy for which there is no definite cause.

summative evaluation A method used to assess program outcomes or as a follow-up of the results of program activities.

supervision The process of directing, coaching, and monitoring the work of others to whom tasks have been delegated.

supplemental security income Money awarded to an individual with insufficient resources for the purpose of increasing the income level to a minimum standard.

supporter An advocacy role in which the nurse upholds the client's right to make a choice.

surveillance Systematic and ongoing observation and collection of data concerning disease occurrence in order to describe phenomena and detect changes in frequency or distribution.

survey Method of assessment in which data from a sample of persons are reported to the data collector.

susceptibility The stage prior to the development of disease at which a person is subject to or at risk of disease.

syphilis An infectious, chronic sexually transmitted disease caused by a bacteria, *Treponema Pallidum*; characterized by the appearance of lesions or chancres that may involve any tissue. Relapses are frequent, and after the initial chancre, syphilis may exist without symptoms for years.

system Complex of elements in interaction.

T

Taft-Hartley Act Passed in 1947, a revision of the Wagner Act of 1935. Included in the 1947 law was a provision that professional employees should not be organized in the same bargaining unit with nonprofessionals unless a majority of the professional employees voted for such an inclusion.

target of service Population group for whom healthful change is sought.

task Function with work or labor overtones assigned to or demanded of a person.

task functions Behaviors that focus or direct movement toward the main work of the group.

taxonomy A framework that provides order to a set of related terms or concepts.

temperament Basic behavioral style.

tertiary care Actions taken to limit the progression of disease or disability.

tertiary prevention Programs directed toward persons with clinically apparent disease, with the aim of ameliorating the course of disease, reducing disability, or rehabilitating.

testicular self-exam A procedure performed by one's self to assess the condition of the testicles and detect abnormalities.

theories of justice Doctrines that indicate how to distribute goods and resources among the population.

theory A clearly stated, operationally defined set of concepts, statements, and hypotheses. A collection of principles and rules.

theory principles intervention mode A consultation mode in which the client learns theories and their application to problem solving.

third-party payments Reimbursement made to health care providers by an agency other than the client for the care of the client (e.g., insurance companies, governments, or employers).

third-party payors Insurance companies, governments, and charitable organizations who pay a client's health care bill.

toddler A child between the ages of 1 to 3.

tolerance A state characterized by a need to continually increase the dosage of a drug to achieve the desired effects.

tort Legal or civil wrong committed by one person against the person or property of another.

total quality management/improvement An approach to managing quality that emphasizes continual improvement, employee empowerment, client input, and systems change as key principles.

toxic wastes Poisons, inflammables, infectious contaminants, explosives, and radionuclides.

toxicity Ability of a substance to cause injury to biological tissues.

tracer method A method of evaluating programs based on the premise that health status and care can be evaluated by observing the care and outcomes of specific health problems.

transformational leadership Leadership theory that explains that certain leaders are able to radically change organizations because they are able to communicate a new vision and to help others move toward achieving that vision.

trend An event that occurs over time and shows a series of fluctuations in its patterns.

triage Deciding which individuals need the most immediate attention and by whom.

triangulation Use of multiple assessment methods. In relationships, the involvement of a third party or object to avoid communication, closeness, or conflict between two individuals.

triggers Temptations that may lead to relapse in drug usage.

typology The study or classification of communities by types.

U

underclass poverty Poverty defined in terms of attitudes and behavior, especially behavior that indicates deviance from the norm.

unit of service An entity—individual, family, aggregate, organization, or community—to whom nursing care is given; the level at which service is delivered.

urban areas Geographic areas described as nonrural and having a higher population density; more than 99 persons per square mile; cities with a population of at least 20,000 but less than 50,000.

urban nonmetropolitan Urban areas having fewer than 50,000 persons.

urinary incontinence (UI) A condition in which involuntary loss of urine is a social or hygienic problem.

utilitarian theory Economic theory that holds that the best way to distribute resources among people is to decide how expenditures or the use of resources will bring about the greatest net total of good and serve the largest number of people.

utilization review   Review directed toward ensuring that care is actually needed and cost is appropriate for the level of care provided.

V

vaccine   Immunizing agent.

validity   The accuracy of a test or measurement; how closely it measures what it claims to measure. In a screening test validity is assessed in terms of the probability of correctly classifying an individual with regard to the disease or outcome of interest, usually in terms of sensitivity and specificity.

values   Ideas of life, customs and ways of behaving that members of a society regard as desirable.

variables   Key characteristics of the problem under study.

variance analysis   Analyzing variations from the expected goals or standards. It can be applied to analyzing variances from budgeted expenditures or to analyzing situations in which client goals on a critical pathway were not met.

vector   Agent that actively carries a germ to a susceptible host.

verification   A communication process used by a nurse advocate to establish accuracy and reality of facts.

violence   Nonaccidental acts, interpersonal or intrapersonal, that result in physical or psychological injury to one or more of the people involved.

virulence   Ability to produce severe disease.

vision impairment   Refers to partial vision, which may also be correctly called partial sight.

visiting nurses   A nurse who provides care wherever the client may be—residence, work, school.

voluntary agency   An agency that relies on staff and volunteers to provide a wide range of services; must seek operating funds from a variety of sources, including gifts, dues, and fees.

voluntary certification   Process of education, experience, or examination in which a professional elects to engage to be recognized as a specialist.

voluntary credentialing   The choice made by an agency or institution to participate in an accreditation process.

Vroom and Yetton's decision-making theory   Theory that predicts that the most effective approach to making decisions is based on the nature of the decision, the characteristics of the individuals who will be affected, and the urgency with which the decision must be made.

Vroom's expectancy theory   Victor Vroom's theory of motivation. Expectancy theory says that workers are motivated by their expectations of their abilities to achieve goals and the likely outcomes associated with goal achievement.

vulnerable population groups   A subgroup of the population that is more likely to develop health problems as a result of exposure to risk or to have worse outcomes from these problems than the population as a whole.

W

warts   Sexually transmitted, multiple, textured, cauliflower-like lesions that appear on the genitalia, anus, or mouth, caused by human papillomavirus.

wear and tear theory   A theory of aging that sees parts of the body wearing out with age, much as machines wear out with age.

web of causality   The complex interrelations of factors interacting with each other to influence the risk for or distribution of health outcomes.

wellness   Dynamic state of health in which individuals progress toward a higher level of functioning, thus maximizing their potential in the environment.

windshield survey   A community assessment, the motorized equivalent of a physical assessment for an individual; windshield refers to looking through the car windshield as the community health nurse drives through the community collecting data.

withdrawal   Physical and psychological symptoms that occur when a drug upon which a person is dependent is removed.

women, infants, and children (WIC)   A special supplemental food program administered by the Department of Agriculture through the State Health Departments. Provides nutritious foods that add to the diets of pregnant and nursing women, infants, and children under 5 years of age. Eligibility is based on income and nutritional risk as determined by a health professional.

Worker's Compensation Acts   Laws requiring employers to assume financial responsibility for wages lost by employees because of occupational injury or illness.

World Health Organization   An arm of the United Nations that provides worldwide services to promote health.

worthiness   A sense that some people are deserving of help from the community as a whole.

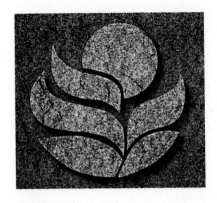

Index

Page numbers in *ital* include illustrations. Page numbers followed by a *t* indicates a table.

B

C

D

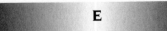

E

F

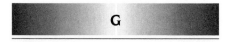

G

H

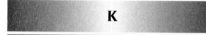

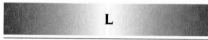

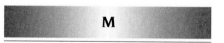

O

P

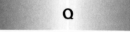

Q

R

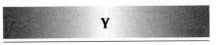

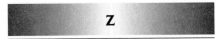